Antimicrobial Therapy in Infants and Children

Clinical Pediatrics

Series Editor: Fima Lifshitz
Cornell University Medical College, New York, New York
North Shore University Hospital, Manhasset, New York

Volume 1 Common Pediatric Disorders: Metabolism, Heart Disease, Allergies, Substance Abuse, and Trauma, *edited by Fima Lifshitz*

Volume 2 Congenital Metabolic Diseases: Diagnosis and Treatment, *edited by Raul A. Wapnir*

Volume 3 Pediatric Endocrinology: A Clinical Guide, *edited by Fima Lifshitz*

Volume 4 Antimicrobial Therapy in Infants and Children, *edited by Gideon Koren, Charles G. Prober, and Ronald Gold*

Other volumes in preparation

Antimicrobial Therapy in Infants and Children

edited by

Gideon Koren

The Hospital for Sick Children
Toronto, Ontario, Canada

Charles G. Prober

Stanford University School of Medicine
Stanford, California

Ronald Gold

The Hospital for Sick Children
Toronto, Ontario, Canada

MARCEL DEKKER, INC. New York and Basel

Library of Congress Cataloging-in-Publication Data

Antimicrobial therapy in infants and children.

(Clinical Pediatrics; v. 4)
Includes index.
1. Infection in children--Chemotherapy. 2. Anti-infective agents. I. Koren, Gideon.
II. Prober, Charles G. III. Gold, Ronald.
IV. Series. [DNLM: 1. Antibiotics--therapeutic use.
2. Bacterial Infections--in infancy & childhood.
W1 CL694I v.5 / QV 350 A6345]
RJ275.A58 1987 618.92'90461 87-20108
ISBN 0-8247-7745-X

MARCEL DEKKER, INC.
270 Madison Avenue, New York, New York 10016

Current printing (last digit):
10 9 8 7 6 5 4 3 2 1

PRINTED IN THE UNITED STATES OF AMERICA

This book is dedicated to
Andrew, Bath-Sheva, Gal, Helga, Laura,
Lee, Lonio, Meghan, and Tal

Series Introduction

Clinical Pediatrics is a continuing series of books designed to update the knowledge of the practicing physician in current and rapidly developing areas in pediatrics. Each of the topics discussed in these books presents the state of the art from the vantage point of recognized experts in the field.

The first book of the series, *Common Pediatric Disorders*, edited by Fima Lifshitz, deals with metabolic, cardiac, and allergic diseases. The second volume, *Congenital Metabolic Diseases*, edited by Raul A. Wapnir, deals with selective inborn errors of metabolism afflicting children. The third book, *Pediatric Endocrinology*, edited by Fima Lifshitz, is devoted in its entirety to this subject. The fourth book, and most recent addition to the series, *Antimicrobial Therapy in Infants and Children*, edited by Gideon Koren, Charles G. Prober, and Ronald Gold, includes the most recent developments in this field and provides explanations of the underlying pharmacokinetic principles of antibiotic therapy in the pediatric population.

This series constitutes an excellent data base for physicians who welcome authoritative, clearly written reviews to aid them in their clinical practice, and will serve as an invaluable reference source and complement any medical library.

Fima Lifshitz

Foreword

Older physicians will recall that in the early 1960s children were referred to as "therapeutic orphans." This sobriquet derived from the ubiquitous warnings in FDA-approved package inserts for newly marketed drugs that optimal dosages and the safety and efficacy of drugs X, Y, and Z in infants and children had not been established.

It was common practice in the "bad old days" to determine pharmacologic and pharmacokinetic properties of new drugs in healthy adult volunteers and to establish efficacy and pharmacodynamics in sick adults. Scant investigation was done in pediatric patients.

Physicians treating children floundered about and made guesses about "appropriate" dosages, usually scaled-down estimates based on body weight. We know now that this was a totally inappropriate approach. Drugs in infants and children have different dispositional characteristics than in adults, and pharmacology and toxicity are often significantly altered in metabolically immature infants.

The systematic, scientific evaluation of antibiotic and chemotherapeutic drugs in children began in the 1960s and flourished in the 1970s. The federal agencies did not support such studies, arguing that studies of commercial products should be supported by their manufacturers. That is probably a valid position to take in regard to new drugs under development; however, what about older antibiotics that had been used for many years in children without ever being critically evaluated from a pharmacokinetic and pharmacodynamic standpoint? It is a tribute to the pharmaceutical industry that several companies supported such studies when there was no potential financial gain. Even in the case of new drugs under development, the expected profits are minimal. Many children are treated with antibiotics, but the absolute amounts consumed are a small fraction of the total annual tonnage of antibiotic consumption.

These are happier times in terms of evaluation of antimicrobials in children. It is almost inconceivable that a new antibiotic gets to the marketplace without prior evaluation in infants and children, to the clear advantage of children and physicians alike.

There are many books about infectious diseases in children, and there is a plethora of handouts, handbooks, and therapeutic "cookbooks" about recommendations for treatment, but until now there has not been a comprehensive compilation of the mass of information about antimicrobial drugs in pediatric patients: antibacterial, antifungal, antiviral, and antiparasitic drugs.

Doctors Koren, Prober, and Gold have broad training and experience in clinical pharmacology and efficacy studies that qualify them as editors of this textbook, and they have assembled an able group of authors. The result is not suited to pleasurable bedtime reading: The concentrated amount of data and the outline format would be overwhelming in a short while. Rather, this book is intended as a resource for virtually everything known about antimicrobial drugs in infants and children. It is a treasure trove of facts, interpretations of those facts, recommendations for implementation and monitoring of drug therapy, and medical literature citations. We plan to keep our copies of this book close to our desks and anticipate reaching for them frequently when we come up short of a piece of needed information.

John D. Nelson, M.D.
George H. McCracken, Jr., M.D.
The University of Texas
Health Science Center at Dallas

Preface

In the last two decades we have witnessed the emergence of Pediatric Infectious Diseases and Pediatric Pharmacology as two independent disciplines.

It has become apparent that infants and children are not small adults. They suffer from a different array of infectious diseases. The disposition of antimicrobial drugs in their bodies is different and so is often their response to drug therapy. Moreover, there are substantial differences in these variables even within the pediatric age group, with preterm infants being very different from the healthy adolescent or the patient with cystic fibrosis. The intelligent use of antimicrobial agents in children requires more than simple extrapolation of observations made in adults.

Consequently, we now see a very intensive research effort into the pharmacokinetics and response to antimicrobial drugs in the pediatric age group. In several areas (e.g., aminoglycosides) the available data are relatively complete, whereas in others (e.g., antiparasitics) there are almost no pediatric data.

This book represents an attempt to summarize the current knowledge on antimicrobial drugs in children. A large international team of scientists was asked to review each antimicrobial agent in a standardized manner. In addition, we have chosen to include methodology chapters essential for the understanding of pharmacokinetics, laboratory procedures, and analytical tests.

We hope that this book will give clinicians and students access to the rapidly developing area of antimicrobial therapy in infants and children. We also hope that this book will highlight those areas in desperate need of expanded research.

We wish to thank the word processing team at the Research Institute, The Hospital for Sick Children, Toronto: Mrs. Eva McGrath, Supervisor; Beverly Li, Toni Smith, Leslie Pagana, Sophie Ku, Denise Agard, Eva East, and Kitty Yue. The secretarial help of Ms. Karen Foster is greatly appreciated. We thank Lee Koren and Dr. Neil H. Shear for their help in indexing this book.

Gideon Koren
Charles G. Prober
Ronald Gold

Contents

Contributors

Ann M. Arvin, M.D. Department of Pediatric Infectious Diseases, Stanford University School of Medicine, Stanford, California

James B. Besunder, D.O. Division of Pediatric Pharmacology and Critical Care, Rainbow Babies and Childrens Hospital, Department of Pediatrics, Case Western Reserve University School of Medicine, Cleveland, Ohio

Jeffrey L. Blumer, Ph.D., M.D. Division of Pediatric Pharmacology and Critical Care, Rainbow Babies and Childrens Hospital, Departments of Pediatrics and Pharmacology, Case Western Reserve University School of Medicine, Cleveland, Ohio

José Antonio Jesús Bodino, M.D., F.A.A.P. Department of Clinical Pediatrics, Children's Hospital of Buenos Aires, Buenos Aires, Argentina

John C. Christenson, M.D. Division of Pediatric Infectious Diseases, University of Oklahoma Health Sciences Center, Oklahoma City, Oklahoma

Pamela S. Diaz, M.D. Division of Pediatric Infectious Diseases, Department of Pediatrics, Stanford University School of Medicine, Stanford, California

L. Lee Dupuis, M.Sc.Phm. Department of Pharmacy, The Hospital for Sick Children, Toronto, Ontario, Canada

E. Lee Ford-Jones, M.D., F.R.C.P.(C) Department of Pediatrics, Division of Infectious Diseases, The Hospital for Sick Children, Toronto, Ontario, Canada

Charles M. Ginsburg, M.D. Department of Pediatrics, University of Texas Health Science Center at Dallas, Dallas, Texas

Ronald Gold, M.D. Department of Pediatrics, The Hospital for Sick Children, Toronto, Ontario, Canada

Daniel A. Goldstein, M.D., F.R.C.P.(C) Division of Clinical Pharmacology, The Hospital for Sick Children, Toronto, Ontario, Canada

Mark Greenwald, M.D. Department of Pediatrics, the University of Toronto, Toronto, Ontario, Canada

R. Brian Haynes, M.D., Ph.D., F.R.C.P.(C) Department of Clinical Epidemiology and Biostatistics, McMaster University, Hamilton, Ontario, Canada

Gideon Koren, M.D. Department of Pediatrics and Pharmacology, The Hospital for Sick Children, and the University of Toronto, Toronto, Ontario, Canada

Allan S. Lau, M.D., F.R.C.P.(C) Department of Pediatrics, Division of Infectious Diseases, The Hospital for Sick Children, Toronto, Ontario, Canada

J. Steven Leeder, Pharm.D. Department of Pediatrics and The Research Institute, Division of Clinical Pharmacology, The Hospital for Sick Children, Toronto, Ontario, Canada

Paul S. Lietman, M.D., Ph.D. Department of Medicine, The Johns Hopkins University School of Medicine, Baltimore, Maryland

Susan M. Lisby, Pharm.D. Section of Infectious Diseases, Children's Hospital, Columbus, Ohio

Eduardo L. López, M.D. Department of Clinical Pediatrics, Children's Hospital of Buenos Aires, Buenos Aires, Argentina

Donald E. Low, M.D. Department of Microbiology, Mount Sinai Hospital, and University of Toronto, Toronto, Ontario, Canada

Stuart M. MacLeod Faculty of Health Sciences, McMaster University, Hamilton, Ontario, Canada

*Melvin I. Marks, M.D.** Department of Pediatrics, Division of Infectious Diseases, University of Oklahoma Health Sciences Center, Oklahoma City, Oklahoma

John F. Milliken, Jr., M.D.† Division of Infectious Diseases, The Hospital for Sick Children, Toronto, Ontario, Canada

Michael J. Muszynski, M.D.‡ Division of Pediatric Infectious Diseases, University of Oklahoma Health Sciences Center, Oklahoma City, Oklahoma

Milap C. Nahata, Pharm.D. Colleges of Pharmacy and Medicine, The Ohio State University, and Children's Hospital, Columbus, Ohio

Charles G. Prober, M.D. Department of Pediatrics, Stanford University School of Medicine, Stanford, California

Edward D. Ralph, M.D., F.R.C.P.(C)§ Department of Medicine, The University of Western Ontario, London, Ontario, Canada

Michael D. Reed, Pharm.D. Division of Pediatric Pharmacology and Critical Care, Rainbow Babies and Childrens Hospital, Case Western Reserve University School of Medicine, Cleveland, Ohio

Michael J. Rieder, M.D. Department of Pediatrics and Research Institute, Division of Clinical Pharmacology, The Hospital for Sick Children, Toronto, Ontario, Canada

Ronald K. Scribner, M.S., M. (ASCP) Division of Pediatric Infectious Diseases, University of Oklahoma Health Sciences Center, Oklahoma City, Oklahoma

Itamar Shalit, M.D. Department of Pediatrics and Pediatric Infectious Disease Unit, Tel Aviv Medical Center, Sackler School of Medicine, Tel Aviv, Israel

Neil H. Shear, M.D., F.R.C.P.(C) The Hospital for Sick Children, Toronto, Ontario, Canada

Present affiliations:
*Miller Children's Hospital, Memorial Medical Center, Long Beach, California
†Blue Hill Memorial Hospital, Blue Hill, Maine
‡Orlando Regional Medical Center, Orlando, Florida
§University Hospital, London, Ontario, Canada

Susan Stansfield, B.Sc.Phm. Department of Pharmacy, The Hospital for Sick Children, Toronto, Ontario, Canada

H. Andrew Strong, Ph.D. Department of Pediatrics, Division of Clinical Pharmacology, The Hospital for Sick Children, Toronto, Ontario, Canada

E. Kanta Subbarao, M.B., B.S. Department of Pediatrics, Division of Infectious Diseases, University of Oklahoma Health Sciences Center, Oklahoma City, Oklahoma

Alan M. Sugar, M.D. Evans Memorial Department of Clinical Research, and Section of Infectious Diseases, Department of Medicine, University Hospital of the Boston University Medical Center, Boston, Massachusetts

Wayne M. Sullender, M.D. Division of Pediatric Infectious Disease, Department of Pediatrics, Stanford University School of Medicine, Stanford, California

*Elaine Wang, M.D.C.M., F.R.C.P.(C)** Department of Clinical Epidemiology and Biostatistics, McMaster University, Hamilton, Ontario, Canada

Richard J. Whitley, M.D. Department of Pediatrics and Microbiology, University of Alabama at Birmingham, Birmingham, Alabama

---

**Present affiliation*: The Hospital for Sick Children, Toronto, Ontario, Canada

Part I
General Principles

1

Laboratory Procedures and the Management of Antimicrobial Therapy

DONALD E. LOW
Mount Sinai Hospital, and the University of Toronto, Toronto, Ontario, Canada

The selection of appropriate antimicrobial therapy for the management of the infected patient usually requires knowledge of the results of in vitro antimicrobial susceptibility testing. A variety of susceptibility testing methods are available. Although they may not simulate the environment of the host, they do provide assessment of the in vitro activity of an antimicrobial agent against the organism being tested. Studies have demonstrated a good correlation between in vitro susceptibility testing and the outcome of clinical therapy. However, this correlation depends on accurate and reproducible susceptibility test results, which in turn depend on rigidly standardized techniques.

The need for standardization of antimicrobial susceptibility testing was recognized as early as 1961 by the Expert Committee on Antibiotics of the World Health Organization (WHO) (1). Bauer and his colleagues, 5 years later, published their paper describing a standard method for susceptibility testing by the disk diffusion method (2). In 1968, the National Committee for Clinical Laboratory Standards (NCCLS) was established as a primary standards-setting body for clinical laboratories in the United States.

Agar disk diffusion was the first accepted method of antimicrobial sensitivity testing used by the vast majority of microbiology laboratories. It was the first method to become standardized by the NCCLS.

The dilution test was the second method of antimicrobial susceptibility testing to become standardized. It determines the minimal inhibitory concentration (MIC), a concentration of antimicrobial that relates to achievable body fluid levels, as opposed to the qualitative category of susceptibility produced by the agar disk diffusion test. The dilution test has undergone many modifications that have allowed it to be more readily accessible for use in the routine laboratory. The commercial availability of the broth microdilution susceptibility test system has allowed even the smallest clinical laboratories to meet increasing requests for quantitative MIC.

There have been modifications in the antimicrobial susceptibility testing of anaerobes and in the determination of β-lactamase, which have made their results more reliable and the tests more assessible for use in the clinical laboratories. There have also been attempts to standardize tests used to determine the efficacy of antimicrobial combinations and the degree of serum bactericidal activity.

In order that the clinician may use the information now being provided by the microbiology laboratory, the limitations associated with each of these tests must first be understood.

I. DEFINITIONS

A. MIC

The degree of susceptibility of an organism has been defined as the lowest concentration of antimicrobial in micrograms per milliliter that prevents the in vitro growth of the organism (Figure 1). This is referred to as the minimal inhibitory concentration (3). The reference method for determining the MIC of an antimicrobial to an organism has been by the broth dilution susceptibility test as described by the NCCLS (4). The MIC is a reproducible parameter for a given antimicrobial agent against a specific pathogen if performed with standardized methodology. The MIC "break point" is the concentration of antimicrobial that defines resistant and susceptible categories for each antimicrobial agent. The MIC breakpoint for susceptibility must be lower than the level of antibiotic attainable in the blood or tissues with a clinically acceptable dosage and route of administration (5).

B. MBC

The minimal bactericidal concentration (MBC) is the lowest concentration of antimicrobial in micrograms per milliliter that results in a 99.9% kill of the bacteria being tested (6,7). This is determined by subculturing those tubes that show no visible growth in the broth dilution test. Unfortunately, there has been no universally accepted standard method for MBC determinations in clinical laboratories, and many technical factors influence the outcome of this test (7) (Table 1). In addition, there are considerable species differences and strain-to-strain variability in MBC results. Therefore, interpretation of the clinical relevance of much of the reported MBC data must be questioned. There is little evidence to support the clinical necessity for determination of MBC as a routine test in the clinical microbiology laboratory.

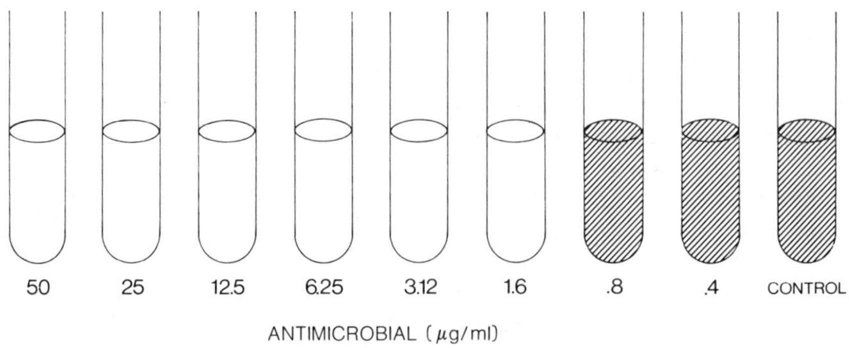

Figure 1 A broth dilution susceptibility test. The minimal inhibitory concentration is 1.6 μg/ml.

Table 1 Summary of Technical Factors that Influence the MBC Test

Variable factor	Effect
Phase of growth	Increased survivors in stationary phase
Type of tube	Adhesion varies with material and may falsely elevate counts of survivors if organisms adhere to tube walls above meniscus
Mode of inoculation	Small-volume inoculum and avoiding shaking eliminate adhesion above meniscus
Vortexing	Vigorous vortexing at 4 hr before tubes finally sampled and again at the time of sampling ensures that any organisms contaminating glassware above meniscus are exposed to antibiotic
Antibiotic carryover	Gives falsely low counts of survivors

Source: From Taylor et al. (7).

C. Tolerance

The term "tolerance" refers to the ability of some bacteria to survive the killing action of penicillins and other antimicrobials (3). This phenomenon differs from "persistence," which refers to those bacterial cells that have survived the lethal effect of the antimicrobial but remain susceptible to the drug when retested (3). The mechanism for tolerance may involve the absence or suppression of the cells' autolytic enzyme system, whereas persisters are thought to be metabolically inactive bacteria that were not growing and therefore were not susceptible to the antibiotic (8). Many authors define antimicrobial tolerance with the MBC is $\geqslant 32$ times the MIC (3,8–10). The technical difficulties associated with detecting tolerance are identical to those encountered in MBC determinations. Infections due to tolerant bacterial strains have been documented, but treatment failures are less frequently reported (8–10).

D. Susceptibility

The NCCLS has recently changed the categorization of susceptibility for both the disk and the dilution test (4,11). Previously, the disk test simply categorized isolates as susceptible or resistant with intermediate as a buffer zone. "Susceptible" implied that the infection due to the strain tested could be appropriately treated with a dosage of antimicrobial agent recommended for that type of infection. "Resistant" implied that the stain tested was not inhibited by a drug concentration achievable in blood or tissue within the normal dosage range. The "intermediate" category indicated strains that were not clearly resistant or fully susceptible and provided a buffer zone that minimized the significance of minor technical variables that can occur with routine testing. The additional interpretive category introduced by the NCCLS in the disk diffusion test standard M2-A3 was the "moderately" susceptible category (11). This has been recommended for use with some of the newer β-lactam antibiotics for strains that may be inhibited by the maximum safe dosage of the drug. The moderately susceptible category is not the same as the intermediate category.

The NCCLS has recommended major changes in the categorization of susceptibility based on MIC determined by dilution tests (4). The categories are now susceptible, moderately susceptible, resistant, and conditionally susceptible. "Susceptible" implies that the organism's MIC is lower than the levels of antibiotic attainable in the blood or tissues with clinically accepted dosage and route of administration. "Moderately susceptible" implies that the maximum safe dosage of the drug would be required. "Resistant" implies that the organism's MIC is greater than the levels of antimicrobial that are achievable in the blood or tissue. "Conditionally susceptible" is a new category proposed for those situations in which the drug is concentrated in an area of the body (e.g., urine) and the greater concentration is sufficient to inhibit the organism in question.

II. ANTIMICROBIAL SUSCEPTIBILITY TESTING FOR AEROBIC ORGANISMS

Susceptibility tests are indicated for organisms that are the causative agents of an infection and for which the susceptibility cannot be predicted from knowledge of their identity. Susceptibility testing is usually carried out by either the disk diffusion or dilution method.

A. Diffusion Tests

The disk diffusion test, using a single-potency disk, continues to be the most widely used antimicrobial susceptibility testing method. The test is essentially a qualitative test that allocates organisms to interpretive categories. Disk diffusion methods are designed particularly for testing the susceptibility of common rapidly growing bacterial pathogens, such as members of the Enterobacteriaceae family and the *Staphylococcus* spp. There are standardized methods for testing more fastidious organisms, such as *Streptococcus pneumoniae, Hemophilus influenzae*, and *Neisseria gonorrhoeae*. However, first the inoculum must be standardized and the agar medium supplemented with substances that permit a good growth rate and do not alter the diffusion and potency of the antibiotic (11). Strains whose growth requires enrichment or a special atmospheric environment and strains that are slow growing cannot be readily tested by this method.

The disk diffusion test is performed by inoculating a standardized suspension of organism onto specialized susceptibility agar (Mueller-Hinton agar). Paper disks impregnated with a specific amount of antibiotic are placed on the agar, and the plates are incubated in precisely controlled conditions. After overnight incubation, the zones of inhibited growth around the disks are measured and correlated with established interpretive categories (11).

The deficiences of the diffusion test are its nonquantiative interpretion, its inapplicability to many slow-growing organisms and anaerobes, and the failure of certain types of resistance to be fully expressed. Special modifications of routine testing procedure must be used in order to determine the susceptibility of *Neisseria meningitidis* to the sulfonamides (12); the *Staphylococcus* spp. to the penicillinase-resistant penicillins (3); β-lactamase-producing *Hemophilus* supp. and *N. gonorrhoeae* to the penicillins (3); and methicillin-resistant staphylococci to the cephalosporins (13). Overall, however, the disk diffusion test is an effective procedure for the most routine testing, but it should be supplemented with a dilution test when it is inapplicable or when more quantitive results are needed.

B. Dilution Tests

The primary purpose of the dilution test is to obtain quantitative results that are expressed as the MIC. Such results may be helpful in determining the degree of susceptibility of an organism and in defining quantitatively the intermediate category designated in the diffusion test. When a urinary tract infection is due to an organism that is qualitatively resistant, the precise degree of susceptibility may influence the choice for an antimicrobial agent that attains high concentrations in the urine.

Dilution tests are not influenced by the growth rate of the organism and avoid some of the complexities of diffusion properties of antimicrobial agents. Even though results are quantitative they may be reported qualitatively (4). The tests used to determine the MIC are the agar and broth dilution methods.

1. Agar Dilution

The agar dilution technique is best applied in large-volume laboratories processing large numbers of specimens because of the number of strains that can be tested simultaneously. Other advantages of the agar dilution method are low cost when large number of tests are performed; the ability to detect microbial heterogeneity or contamination; good reproducibility; and strict quality control of each plate by using three or more test organisms.

The procedure involves the use of a series of agar plates, each containing a different concentration of antimicrobial encompassing the attainable concentrations of the antimicrobial agent in serum. For example, if the therapeutic range for an antibiotic, such as gentimicin, is 2–8 μg/ml, a series of agar plates containing 1, 2, 4, 8, 16, and 32 μg/ml gentamicin are prepared. This system can be mechanized by use of an inoculum-replicating apparatus called the Steers replicator (14). This consists of an aluminum head of 32–36 equally spaced inoculating rods. The counterpart is an aluminum seed plate containing 32–36 wells. The head is lowered into the seed plate wells containing the test organisms, where a known volume of bacterial suspension is picked up on each inoculating pin. The head is then placed onto the agar surfaces containing the antibiotic. The procedure is repeated for all the antibiotic plates to be tested. The plates are then incubated at 35°C for 18 hr. The MIC represents the lowest concentration of antimicrobial agent that completely inhibits the growth of the organism.

2. Microdilution and Macrodilution Broth Procedures

The dilution antimicrobial susceptibility test in a broth medium are very similar in principle to the agar-based method. The macrodilution method with volumes $\geqslant$1.0 ml is cumbersome and is not applicable to the volume of tests performed in most clinical laboratories. It has been held in reserve to be used for determining MIC when only a few strains are to be tested. In addition, because technical variables have been more carefully defined for the macrotube procedure, it is a preferable reference procedure for determining MBC (3). The microdilution broth procedures are performed with plastic trays that may have a variable number of wells, each containing different concentrations of antibiotic solutions as explained in the agar dilution method. These wells are then inoculated with the test organisms and incubated at 35°C for 18 hr. After incubation, the microdilution trays are examined and the MIC then determined by taking the lowest concentration of drug at which the microorganism tested does not show visible growth. Both the broth macrodilution and microdilution have been standardized (4). Commercial microdilution products are increasing in popularity because of their accuracy, reproducibility, and convenience (15). The MIC by broth microdilution for gram-negative bacilli are often a twofold dilution lower than those obtained by broth macrodilution (16). In addition, the microdilution procedure may also fail to detect some β-lactamase-producing staphylococci (17). Caution is advised when attempting to determine MBC by the broth microdilution procedure because of the lack of standardization of the test and correlation with macrodilution method (18).

III. ANTIMICROBIAL SUSCEPTIBILITY TESTING FOR ANAEROBES

Antimicrobial susceptibility testing is generally not routinely indicated in patients with mixed infections due to both anaerobes and aerobes, as occurs in intra-abdominal sepsis. However, testing may prove beneficial when anaerobes are isolated in pure culture or from blood, bone, joint, or cerebrospinal fluid. Other reasons for performing anaerobic susceptibility tests are (1) in vitro activity may predict clinical outcome (19,20); (2) anaerobe susceptibilities are changing (21,22); and (3) the availability of standardized susceptibility testing procedures (23,24). In the rat, good correlation could be shown between the outcome of intra-abdominal sepsis and in vitro testing against isolates of *Bacteroides fragilis* (25). Antimicrobial activity against anaerobes was required for a favorable outcome when patients had bacteremias due to *Bacteroides* spp. and when infection due to anaerobes followed abdominal trauma (19,20).

The antimicrobial susceptibility of anaerobes is much less predictible than previously thought. Penicillin G had previously been recommended for most anaerobic infections of the head, neck, and respiratory tract, but reports have noted failures of penicillin used for these infections (26-29). Resistance is increasing both to members of the *Clostridium* genus and to *B. fragilis* (21,22,30,31). Many of the new cephalosporins are susceptible to hydrolysis by the β-lactamases produced by strains of *B. fragilis* and as a result have poor in vitro activity, which correlates with poor in vivo results (25,32-34).

The NCCLS subcommittee has provided a standard reference for performing anaerobic susceptibility testing (23), the agar dilution method. This standard can serve as a reference for comparing the accuracy of more practical methods, such as broth macrodilution, broth microdilution, and broth disk elution. Broth macrodilution and microdilution may be performed as described for testing aerobes, with modifications necessary for growth of anaerobic bacteria (35). Broth macrodilution is probably the least useful of the three methods because of its complexity. Broth microdilution tests are efficient and practical and provide a specific MIC value. Plates can be pre-prepared and, if kept frozen at −70°C, may be stored for as long as 3 weeks.

The broth disk elution test is a simple and an accurate method and is the most practical test for the average clinical laboratory. In this method, antimicrobials rapidly elute into broth from commercially available disks (35). By adding one or more disks of a particular antimicrobial to a specified volume of broth, it is possible to obtain a specific antimicrobial concentration. The isolate tested is considered resistant when turbidity in the broth containing antimicrobial is 50% or greater than that of the control. The results are reported as sensitive or resistant.

In addition to the above methods for performing antimicrobial susceptibility tests with anaerobes, the detection of β-lactamase activity can be used to predict the in vivo activity of penicillins and cephalosporins that are susceptible to inactivation by β-lactamases. The chromogenic cephalosporin, nitrocefin, is the most reliable method of detecting β-lactamases produced by anaerobes. At present, it is recommended that only the *Bacteroides* spp. be tested for β-lactamase (3).

The agar disk diffusion test and the MBC test are two tests that are not recommended for determining antimicrobial activity to anaerobes. The results of agar disk diffusion are unreliable, and there is no standardized test available for determining MBC for anaerobes (35).

IV. β-LACTAMASE DETECTION

Commercially available β-lactam antibiotics include penicillins, cephalosporins, and monobactams. Like many other antibiotics, these compounds are susceptible to enzyme modification and degradation. β-Lactamases are highly efficient enzymes that catalyze the hydrolysis of a variety of β-lactam antibiotics (36,37). β-Lactamases are produced by both gram-negative and gram-positive bacteria (37-40). The majority of β-lactamases produced by gram-positive organisms are inducible and extracellular (40); those produced by gram-negative organisms may be inducible or constitutive and are cell bound (38).

The primary mechanism by which staphylococci, *H. influenzae*, and *N. gonorrhoeae* are resistant to penicillins is by their elaboration of β-lactamases that hydrolyze the β-lactam ring to produce penicilloic acid. β-Lactamase production is only one of several factors accounting for resistance to β-lactam compounds (39).

Several reliable methods are available for the direct and rapid detection of β-lactamase produced by bacteria. The methods most commonly used are those in which penicilloic acid is detected by its ability to alter pH or reduce iodine and those in which an electron shift in a chromogenic cephalosporin gives rise to a color change (41-44). The acidometric methods detect penicilloic acid formed from the breakdown of the β-lactam ring of penicillin G when it is incubated with a test organism that produces β-lactamase (41). Phenol red is the acid-base indicator frequently used to detect the production of the penicilloic acid. Starch and iodine react to produce a purple color. When iodine reacts with penicilloic acid it becomes reduced and no longer available to react with the starch, resulting in a loss of color intensity (42).

Hydrolysis of the β-lactamase ring in a chromogenic cephalosporin results in the molecule undergoing a distinct color change (43,44). At present two chromogenic cephalosporins are available commercially: nitrocefin (Glaxo, Ltd.) and PADAC (Hoechst-Roussel Pharmaceuticals). PADAC is useful only with organisms that produce large quantities of β-lactamase. It frequently fails to detect the β-lactamase produced by the *Staphylococcus* spp. and the Enterobacteriaceae (3). Only the chromogenic cephalosporin methods should be used to test *Bacteroides* spp. β-Lactamase tests are not recommended for Enterobacteriaceae, nonfermentative gram-negative bacilli, or anaerobes other than *Bacteroides* spp.

V. ANTIBIOTIC COMBINATION TESTING

One of the rationales for the use of antimicrobial combinations is the concept of synergism, in which the net effect of an antimicrobial combination is greater than the sum of either antimicrobial alone. However, there is no uniformly accepted definition of synergism and only a few controlled trials showing agreement between the in vitro laboratory data and clinical experience (45-48). Despite this, most clinicians believe that infections in compromised hosts and in patients with infective endocarditis and osteomyelitis should be treated with antimicrobial combinations.

When choosing a drug combination, it is desirable that the drugs be synergistic or at least additive—not antagonistic. An additive or indifferent effect is produced when both drugs act independently without affecting each other. A synergistic effect is produced when a combined response gives a result significantly greater than that of either action alone at the same concentration. An antagonistic effect is produced when the activity of one drug is reduced by the presence of a second drug. There are two laboratory procedures commonly used for determining whether a two-drug combination is synergistic: the checkerboard titration method and the killing curve method.

The checkerboard technique is the method most frequently used by clinical laboratories to test drug combinations (49,50). The checkerboard consists of columns in which each well contains the same amount of the drug being diluted along the x axis and rows in which each well contains the same amount of the drug being diluted along the y axis (Figure 2). The first row contains only twofold dilutions of antibiotic A and the first column contains only twofold dilutions of antibiotic B. As a result, each well contains a unique combination of the drugs being tested. After the wells have been inoculated and incubated at 35°C for 18 hr, the checkerboard testing is read by examining for evidence of visible growth. The range of concentrations to be used must be close to that which is inhibitory for each drug acting alone. Most clinical laboratories usually perform the checkerboard technique using microtiter trays.

A method for evaluating the activity of the antimicrobial combination is the isobologram. The well of each column contains the minimum concentration of antibiotic to inhibit or kill the test organisms, which is determined and plotted on the appropriate axis for that antibiotic (Figure 3). A straight line joining the values obtained with each drug

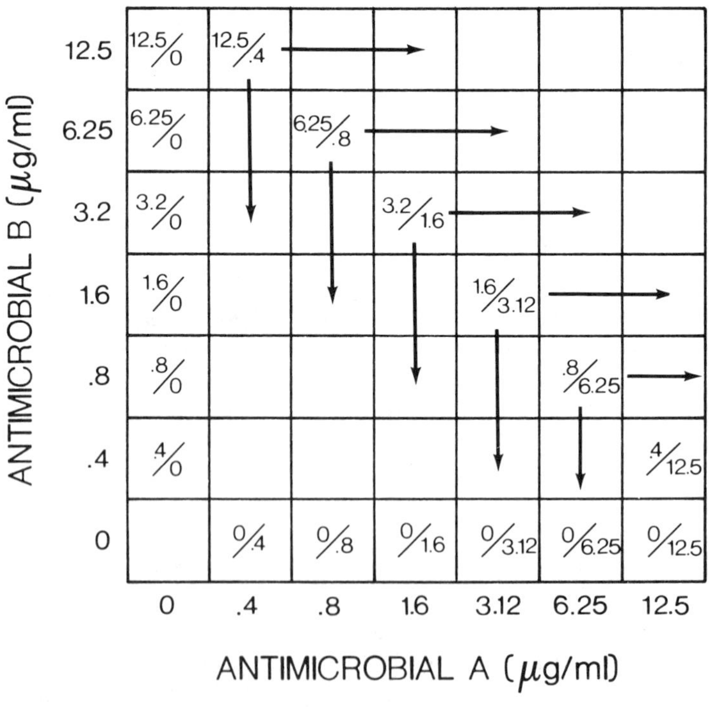

Figure 2 In the checkerboard technique, serial dilutions of two drugs being tested are performed so that each square, representing a tube or well, contains a unique combination of the two drugs being tested.

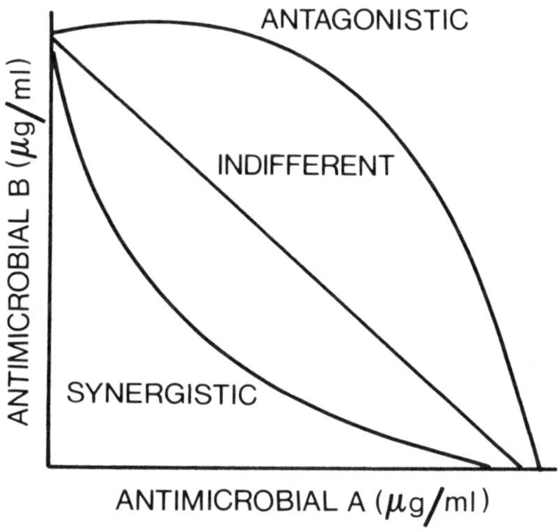

Figure 3 Isobologram portraying three possible results when two antimicrobial agents are tested singly and in various combinations. Indifference is indicated by a straight isobol. Antagonism is indicated by an isobol that bows upward. Synergism is indicated by an isobol that bows downward.

separately represents indifference. Antagonism is indicated by a convex bowing of the isobologram and synergy by concave bowing of the isobologram.

The checkerboard method using the microtiter tray has two major limitations: first, it provides only MIC, not MBC information, and second, the results are usually examined at only one point in time, therefore providing a static rather than a dynamic view of antimicrobial interactions.

The killing curve method measures bactericidal activity of the antimicrobials being tested at several points during the incubation period (51). In this method, appropriate dilutions of the antimicrobials to be tested, singly and in combination, are prepared in broth. At starting time 0 the inoculum of the test organism is added to each diluted antimicrobial broth suspension and the tubes are incubated at 35°C. At periodic intervals an accurate colony count is performed on each of the tubes and a time-killing curve is constructed (Figure 4). The definition of synergy requires that the combined effect be greater than the sum of the independent effects. The results are interpreted by the effect of the combination in comparison with the most active single drug alone. Synergism is defined as a ⩾100-fold increase in killing at 24 hr with the combination in comparison with the most active single drug. Antagonism is defined as ⩽100-fold decrease in killing at 24 hr, and additivity is defined as a less than 10-fold change at 24 hr with the combination in comparison with the most active single antimicrobial alone (51). This definition assumes that at least one of the drugs being tested produces no significant inhibition or killing alone. At present, there are no established criteria with which to evaluate the results obtained using two drugs, each of which has significant activity alone. The major limitation of the killing curve technique is the need for repetitive sampling and colony counts. As a result, the number of antibiotic concentrations that can be tested are limited.

In contrast to the numerous in vitro studies, there are only two clinical situations in which the results of antimicrobial drug combination testing have been shown to predict

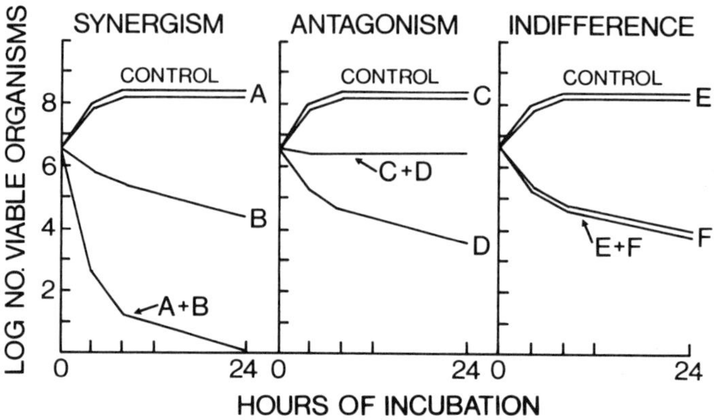

Figure 4 Rate of killing with antimicrobial agents singly and in combination: A + B = synergism, C + D = antagonism, E + F = indifference.

the outcome of clinical therapy: the neutropenic patient with gram-negative rod sepsis, and the patient with endocarditis due to *Pseudomonas aeruginosa* (52-54).

VI. SERUM BACTERICIDAL ACTIVITY TESTING

The serum bactericidal activity has been used for many years to monitor antibiotic therapy in the treatment of patients with infective endocarditis, osteomyelitis, bacteremia, and other serious bacterial infections. The test measures the ability of serial dilutions of serum to inhibit or kill the growth of a standard concentration of the organism causing the infection. The original test determined inhibitory activity rather than bactericidal activity of the serum (55). The test was later amended to determine bactericidal activity (56). There has been no accepted method of standardization of the test, and as a result it is difficult to evaluate the few good studies that correlates serum bactericidal activity with clinical outcome (57-59,62). No data exist pertaining to whether serum bactericidal activity is helpful in the management of infective endocarditis, the disease for which this test is most often performed.

Determination of the serum bactericidal activity is very similar to measurement of the broth MBC. A number of variables are known to affect its measurement (Table 2) (57,58,63-79). The optimal time to obtain a specimen remains uncertain; therefore,

Table 2 Factors That May Affect Measurement of Serum Bactericidal Activity

Time of collection of sample
Phase of growth and size of initial bacterial inoculum
Definition of bactericidal end point
Type of broth and diluent
Method of mixing samples
Presence or absence of serum complement
Antibiotic carryover onto antibiotic-free medium on subculture

Source: From Wolfson et al. (57).

recommendations vary (72-76). Measurement of serum bactericidal activity may be influenced by variation in size of the bacterial inoculum: a large inoculum may include spontaneously resistant bacterial cells, and a small inoculum makes it statistically difficult to detect 99.9% killing (77,78). The use of human serum rather than broth as a diluent influences the results (79). In addition, variables that affect determination of minimal bactericidal concentration affect the determination of serum bactericidal activity. Because of this lack of standardization, the results of the serum bactericidal activity test must be used with caution and should not be used as the sole guide in making major therapeutic decisions (78).

REFERENCES

1. World Health Organization Expert Committee on Antibiotics: WHO Technical Report Series No. 210. WHO, Geneva, 1961.
2. Bauer, A, Kirby, WMM, Sherris, JC, Turck, M: Antibiotic susceptibility testing by a standardized single disk methods. *Am. J. Clin. Pathol. 45*:493–496, 1966.
3. Schoenknecht, FD, Sabath, LD, Thornsberry, C: Susceptibility tests: Special tests. In: *Manual of Clinical Microbiology*, 4th ed. (EH Lennette, A. Balows, WJ Hausley, Jr., and HJ Shadomy, eds.), American Society of Microbiology, Washington, D.C., 1985, pp. 1000–1008.
4. National Committee for Clinical Laboratory Standards: *Tentative Standard. Methods for Dilution Antimicrobial Susceptibility Tests for Bacteria That Grow Aerobically*. Villanova, Pa., 1983.
5. Hewitt, WL, McHenry, MC: Blood level determinations of antimicrobial drugs. *Med. Clin. North Am. 62*:1119–1140, 1978.
6. Murray, PR, Jorgensen, J: Quantitative susceptibility test methods in major U.S. medical centers. *Antimicrob. Agents Chemother. 20*:66–70, 1981.
7. Taylor, PC, Shoenknecht, FD, Sherris, JC, Linner, EC: Determination of minimum bactericidal concentration of oxacillin for *Staphylococcus aureus*: Influence and significance of technical factors. *Antimicrob. Agents Chemother. 23*:142–150, 1983.
8. Sabath, LD, Wheeler, N, Laverdiere, M, Blazevic, D, Wilkinson, B: A new type of penicillin resistance of *Staphylococcus aureus. Lancet 1*:443–447, 1977.
9. Mayhall, CG, Medoff, G, Marr, JJ: Variation in susceptibility of strains of *Staphyloccus aureus* to oxacillin, cephalothin, and gentamicin. *Antimicrob. Agents Chemother. 10*:707–712, 1977.
10. Rajasherkaraiah, KR, Rice, T, Rao, VS, Marsh, D, Ramakrishna, B, Kallick, CA: Clinical significance of tolerent strains of *Staphylococcus aureus* in patients with endocarditis. *Ann. Intern. Med. 93*:796–801, 1980.
11. National Committee for Clinical Laboratory Standards: *Approved Standard. Performance Standards for Antimicrobial Disk Susceptibility Tests*, 3rd ed. Villanova, Pa., 1984.
12. Bennett, JV, Camp, HM, Eickhoff, TC: Rapid sulfonamide disc sensitivity test for meningococci. *Appl. Microbiol. 16*:1056–1060, 1968.
13. Archer, GL, Tenenbaum, MJ: Antibiotic resistant *Staphylococcus epidermidis* in patients undergoing cardiac surgery. *Antimicrob. Agents Chemother. 17*:269–272, 1980.
14. Steers, E, Foltz, EL, Graves, BS, Riden, J: An inocula replicating apparatus for routine testing of bacterial susceptibility to antibiotics. *Antibiot. Chemother. 9*: 307–311, 1959.
15. Jones, RN, Edson, DC: Antibiotic susceptibility testing accuracy. *Arch. Pathol. Lab. Med. 109*:595–601, 1985.

16. Barry, AL, Jones, RN, Gavan, TL: Evaluation of the Micro-Media System for quantitative antimicrobial drug susceptibility testing: A collaborative study. *Antimicrob. Agents Chemother. 13*:61–69, 1978.
17. Thornsberry, C, Gavan, TL, Gerlach, EH: New developments in antimicrobial agent susceptibility testing. In: *Cumitech 6* (JC Sherry, ed.), American Society for Microbiology, Washington, D.C., 1977.
18. Shanholtzer, CJ, Peterson, LR, Mohn, ML, Moody, JA, Gerding, DN: MBCs for *Staphylococcus aureus* as determined by macrodilution and microdilution techniques. *Antimicrob. Agents Chemother. 26*:214–219, 1984.
19. Thadepalli, H, Gorbach, SL, Broido, PW, Norsen, J, Nyhus, L: Abdominal trauma, anaerobes, and antibiotics. *Surg. Gynecol. Obstet. 137*:270–276, 1973.
20. Wilson, WR, Martin, WJ, Wilkowske, CJ, Washington, JA, II: Anaerobic bacteremia. *Mayo Clin. Proc. 47*:639–646, 1972.
21. Edson, RS, Rosenblatt, JE, Lee, DT, McVey, EA: Recent experience with antimicrobial susceptibility of anaerobic bacteria. Increasing resistance to penicillin. *Mayo Clin. Proc. 57*:737–741, 1982.
22. Tally, FP, Cuchural, GJ, Jacobus, NV, Gorbach, SL, Aldridge, KE, Clearly, TJ, Finegold, SM, Hill, GB, Iannini, PB, McCloskey, RV, O'Keefe, JP, Pierson, CL: Susceptibility of the *Bacteroids fragilis* group in the United States in 1981. *Antimicrob. Agents Chemother. 23*:536–540, 1983.
23. National Committee for Clinical Laboratory Standards: *Approved Standard. Reference Agar Dilution Procedure for Antimicrobial Susceptibility Testing of Anaerobic Bacteria*. Villanova, Pa., 1985.
24. Slutter, VL: Susceptibility testing of anaerobes. In: *Manual of Clinical Microbiology*, 4th ed. (EH Lennette, A Balows, WJ Hausler, Jr., and HJ Shadomy, eds.), American Society of Microbiology, Washington, D.C., 1985, pp. 988–990.
25. Bartlett, JG, Louie, TJ, Gorbach, SL, Onderdonk, AB: Therapeutic efficacy of 29 antimicrobial regimens in experimental intraabdominal sepsis. *Rev. Infect. Dis. 3*: 535–542, 1981.
26. Brook, I, Calhoun, L, Yocum, P: β-Lactamase-producing isolates of *Bacteroides* species from children. *Antimicrob. Agents Chemother. 18*:164–166, 1980.
27. Heimdahl, A, Von Konow, L, Nord, CE: Isolation of β-lactamase producing *Bacteroides* strains associated with clinical failures with penicillin treatment of orofacial infections. *Arch. Oral Biol. 25*:689–692, 1980.
28. Tuner, K, Nord, CE: β-Lactamase-producing anaerobic bacteria in recurrent tonsillitis. *J. Antimicrob. Chemother. 10* (Suppl. A):153–156, 1982.
29. Levison, ME, Mangura, CT, Lorber, B, Abrutyn, E, Pesanti, EL, Levy, RS, Macgregor, RR, Schwartz, AR: Clindamycin compared with penicillin for the treatment of anaerobic lung abscess. *Ann. Intern. Med. 98*:466–471, 1983.
30. Privitera, G, Dublanchet, A, Sebald, M: Transfer of multiple antibiotic resistance between subspecies of *Bacteroides fragilis. J. Infect. Dis. 139*:97–100, 1979.
31. Tally, FP, Snydman, DR, Gorbach, SL, Malamy, MH: Plasmid-mediated, transferable resistance to clindamycin and erythromycin in *Bacteroids fragilis. J. Infect. Dis. 139*:83–88, 1979.
32. Brown, JE, Del Bene, VE, Collins, CD: In vitro activity of *N*-formimidoyl-thienamycin, moxalactam and other new β-lactam agents against *Bacterioides fragilis*: Contribution of β-lactamase to resistance. *Antimicrob. Agents Chemother. 19*:248–252, 1981.
33. Ryan, RW, Kwasnik, I, Tilton, RC: Modified microdilution antimicrobial susceptibility test for anaerobic bacteria. *Curr. Microbiol. 3*:365–368, 1980.
34. Joiner, K, Lowe, B, Dzink, J, Bartlett, JG: Comparative efficacy of 10 antimicrobial agents in experimental infections with *Bacteroides fragilis. J. Infect. Dis. 145*: 561–568, 1982.

35. Rosenblatt, JE: Antimicrobial susceptibility testing of anaerobes. In: *Antibiotics in Laboratory Medicine*, 2nd ed. (V Lorian, ed.), Williams and Wilkins, Baltimore, 1985, pp. 159–179.
36. Neu, HC: What do β-lactamases mean for clinical efficacy. *Infection II*:S74–S80, 1983.
37. Neu, HC: Antibiotic inactivating enzymes and bacterial resistance. In: *Antibiotics in Laboratory Medicine*, 2nd ed. (V Lorian, ed.), Williams and Wilkins, Baltimore, 1985, pp. 757–789.
38. Richmond, MH, Sykes, RB: The β-lactamases of gram-negative bacteria and their possible physiological role. *Adv. Microb. Physiol. 9*:31–88, 1973.
39. Sykes, RB, Matthew, M: The β-lactamases of gram-negative bacteria and their role in resistance to β-lactam antibiotics. *J. Antimicrob. Chemother. 2*:115–157, 1976.
40. Citri, N, Pollock, MR: The biochemistry and functions of β-lactamase (penicillinase). *Adv. Enzymol. 28*:237–323, 1966.
41. Thornsberry, C, Kirven, LA: Ampicillin resistance in *Haemophilus influenza* as determined by a rapid test for β-lactamase production. *Antimicrob. Agents Chemother. 6*:653–654, 1974.
42. Catlin, BW: Iodometric detection of *Haemophilus* β-lactamase: Rapid presumptive test for ampicillin resistance. *Antimicrob. Agents Chemother. 7*:265–270, 1975.
43. Jorgensen, JH, Crawford, SA, Alexander, GA: Pyridinium-2-azo-*p*-dimethylanilne chromophore, a new chromogenic cephalosporin for rapid β-lactamase testing. *Antimicrob. Agents Chemother. 22*:162–164, 1982.
44. O'Callaghan, CH, Morris, A, Kirby, SM, Shingler, AH: Novel method for detection of β-lactamases by using a chromogenic cephalosporin substrate. *Antimicrob. Agents Chemother. 1*:283–288, 1972.
45. Lau, WK, Young, LS, Black, RE, Winston, DJ, Linne, SR, Weinstein, RJ, Hewitt, WL: Comparative efficacy and toxicity of amikacin/carbenicillin versus gentamicin/carbenicillin in leukopenic patients: A randomized prospective trial. *Am. J. Med. 62*:959–966, 1977.
46. Chang, HY, Rodriguez, V, Narboni, G, Bodey, GP, Luna, MA, Freireich, EJ: Causes of death in adults with acute leukemia. *Medicine (Baltimore) 55*:259–268, 1976.
47. Moellering, RC, Jr., Wennersten, CBG, Weinberg, AN: Studies on antibiotic synergism against enterococci. I. Bacteriologic studies. *J. Lab. Clin. Med. 77*:821–828, 1971.
48. Moellering, RC, Jr., Wennersten, CBG, Weinberg, AN: Synergy of penicillin and gentamicin against enterococci. *J. Infect. Dis. 124*:S207–S209, 1971.
49. Garrod, LP, Waterworth, PM: Methods of testing combined antibiotic bactericidal action and the significance of the results. *J. Clin. Pathol. 15*:328–338, 1962.
50. Sabath, LD: Synergy of antibacterial substances by apparently known mechanisms. *Antimicrob. Agents Chemother. 1967*:210–217, 1968.
51. Marymont, JH, Jr., Marymont, J: Laboratory evaluation of antibiotic combinations: A review of methods and problems. *Lab. Med. 12*:47–55, 1980.
52. Anderson, ET, Young, LS, Hewitt, WL: Antimicrobial synergism in the therapy of gram-negative rod bacteremia. *Chemotherapy 24*:45–54, 1978.
53. Klastersky, J: Empiric treatment of infections in neutropenic patients with cancer. *Rev. Infect. Dis. (Suppl. 1) 5*:521–531, 1983.
54. Reyes, MP, Raid El-Khatib, M, Brown, WJ, Smith, F, Lerner, AM: Synergy between carbenicillin and an aminoglycoside (gentamicin or tobramycin) against *Pseudomonas aeruginosa* isolated from patients with endocarditis and sensitivity of isolates to normal human serum. *J. Infect. Dis. 140*:192–202, 1979.
55. Schlichter, JG, Maclean, H: A method of determining the effective therapeutic level in the treatment of subacute bacterial endocarditis with penicillin: A preliminary report. *Am. Heart J. 34*:209–211, 1947.

56. Fisher, AM: A method for the determination of antibacterial potency of serum during therapy of acute infections: A preliminary report. *Bull. Johns Hopkins Hosp. 90*:313–320, 1952.
57. Wolfson, JS, Swartz, MN: Serum bactericidal activity as a monitor of antibiotic therapy. *N. Engl. J. Med. 312*:968–975, 1985.
58. Bryan, CS, Marney, SR, Alford, RH, Bryant, RE: Gram-negative bacillary endocarditis: Interpretation of serum bactericidal test. *Am. J. Med. 58*:209–215, 1975.
59. Sande, MA, Scheld, WM: Combination antibiotic therapy of bacterial endocarditis. *Ann. Intern. Med. 92*:390–395, 1980.
60. Bisno, AL, Dismukes, WE, Durack, DT: Treatment of infective endocarditis due to viridans streptococci. *Circulation 63*:730A–733A, 1981.
61. Prober, CG, Yeager, AS: Use of the serum bactericidal titer to assess the adequacy of oral antibiotic therapy in the treatment of acute hematogenous osteomyelitis. *J. Pediatr. 95*:131–135, 1979.
62. Weinstein, MP, Stratton, CW, Ackley, A, Hawley, HB, Robinson, PA, Fisher, BD, Alcid, D, Stephens, DS, Reller, LB: Multicenter collaborative evaluation of a standardized serum bactericidal test as a prognostic indicator in infective endocarditis. *Am. J. Med. 78*:262–269, 1985.
63. Pien, FD, Vosti, KL: Variation in performance of the serum bactericidal test. *Antimicrob. Agents Chemother. 6*:330–333, 1974.
64. Edberg, SC: The measurement of antibiotics in human body fluids: Techniques and significance. In: *Antibiotics in Laboratory Medicine*, 2nd ed. (V Lorian, ed.), Williams and Wilkins, Baltimore, 1985, pp. 381–476.
65. Anhalt, JP, Washington, JA, II: Bactericidal tests. In: *Laboratory Procedures in Clinical Microbiology*, 2nd ed. (JA Washington, ed.), Springer-Verlag, New York, 1985, pp. 731–743.
66. Levy, J, Klastersky, J: Serum bactericidal test: A review with emphasis on its role in the evaluation of antibiotic combination. In: *Combination Antibiotic Therapy in the Compromised Host* (J Klastersky, MJ Staquet, eds.), Raven Press, New York, 1982, pp. 43–58.
67. Rosenblatt, JE: Laboratory tests used to guide antimicrobial therapy. *Mayo Clin. Proc. 58*:14–20, 1983.
68. Coleman, DL, Horwitz, RI, Andriole, VT: Association between serum inhibitory and bactericidal concentrations and therapuetic outcome in bacterial endocarditis. *Am. J. Med. 73*:260–267, 1982.
69. Washington, JA, II: The role of the microbiology laboratory in the diagnosis and antimicrobial treatment of infective endocarditis. *Mayo Clin. Proc. 57*:27–32, 1982.
70. Stratton, CW, Weinstein, MP, Reller, LB: Correlation of serum bactericidal activity with antimicrobial agent level and minimal bactericidal concentration. *J. Infect. Dis. 145*:160–168, 1982.
71. Dunlop, SG: The serum-dilution bactericidal test for antibiotic effectiveness. *Am. J. Med. Technol. 31*:69–76, 1965.
72. Archer, GL, Fekety, FR: Experimental endocarditis due to *Pseudomonas aeruginosa*. II. Therapy with carbenicillin and gentamicin. *J. Infect. Dis. 136*:327–335, 1977.
73. Carrizosa, J, Kaye, D: Antibiotic concentrations in serum bactericidal activity, and results of therapy of streptococcal endocarditis in rabbits. *Antimicrob. Agents Chemother. 12*:479–483, 1977.
74. Tight, RR: Ampicillin therapy of experimental enterococcal endocarditis. *Antimicrob. Agents Chemother. 18*:307–310, 1980.
75. Hamburger, M, Garancis, JC, Sott, NJ, Carleton, J, Beasley, JS: Studies in experimental staphylococcal endocarditis in dogs. V. Treatment with oxacillin. *J. Lab. Clin. Med. 70*:786–799, 1967.

76. Scheld, WM, Van Ness, MM, Sande, MA: Therapy of experimental *Stapylococcus aureus* endocarditis: Relative importance of serum bactericidal activity. In: *Current Chemotherapy and Infectious Disease* (JD Nelson, C Grassi, eds.), American Society for Microbiology, Washington, D.C., 1980, pp. 909–911.
77. Gould, JC: The laboratory control of antibiotic therapy. *Br. Med. Bull. 16*:29–34, 1960.
78. Reller, LB, Stratton, CW: Serum dilution test for bactericidal activity. II. Standardization and correlation with antimicrobial assays and susceptibility tests. *J. Infect. Dis. 136*:196–204, 1977.
79. Kunin, CM: Clinical pharmacology of the new penicillins. I. The importance of serum protein binding in determining antimicrobial activity and concentration in serum. *Clin. Pharmacol. Ther.* 7:166–179, 1966.

2
Analytical Methods and Measurement of Antimicrobial Drugs

H. ANDREW STRONG
The Hospital for Sick Children, and the University of Toronto, Toronto, Ontario, Canada

Measurement of antimicrobial drugs in body fluids is required during drug development and to monitor concentrations during therapy. The principal requirements of the assays used in these two applications are often very different. During development, determination of the pharmacokinetics and metabolism of the drug demands assays of high sensitivity and specificity. In recent years, high-performance liquid chromatography (HPLC) has become the method of choice for such studies. In therapeutic drug monitoring, antibiotics are measured at higher concentrations over narrower ranges so sensitivity of the assays is less important. However, the assays must be rapid, simple, and reliable to allow clinicians to make effective dose adjustments before the next dose. Most antibiotics have a large therapeutic index, and for these therapeutic monitoring is usually not required as toxicity is not likely to occur. The rule of thumb is often to administer doses that result in serum concentrations of antibiotic many times the minimum inhibitory concentrations of the infecting organism. However, chloramphenicol, vancomycin, and the aminoglycosides have narrow therapeutic margins and reliance on the recommended dosage regimen is not sufficient to ensure therapeutic concentrations or to avoid potentially toxic concentrations. Thus therapeutic drug monitoring for these compounds is essential, especially when their pharmacokinetics may be subject to interindividual variation (i.e., in patients with hepatic or renal impairment, in neonates and young children, and in patients in whom there is a potential for drug interactions). The choice of assay depends on many factors, such as speed, reliability, specificity, cost, and technical ease, and these may be tempered by the specific requirements and/or the facilities of individual hospitals and research institutes.

The purpose of this chapter is to describe the basis of the different methods used for both pharmacological and therapeutic drug monitoring purposes and to discuss their relative advantages and disadvantages.

No attempt is made in this chapter to provide a review of the different methods available for the various families of antimicrobial drugs, let alone individual species. Such methods have been previously reviewed and are referenced in each chapter for the different drugs. In addition, the most recent reviews for each assay type are included in the References at the end of this chapter.

I. BASIS OF THE DIFFERENT ASSAY METHODS

A. Microbiologic Assays

These assays use the degree of effect of an antibiotic on a bacterial population as a measure of the antibiotic concentration. They are the oldest methods for antibiotic determination, first described over 40 years ago, and are based upon methods used for bacterial sensitivity testing. Four major types of microbiologic assays have been described: agar diffusion assays, turbidimetric assays, dilution assays, and the urease assay (1). Of these, only the agar diffusion assay is described here since it is by far the most commonly used (2) and it is a good example of the principle of these assay types.

In the assay, appropriate volumes of seeded agar (agar containing the indicator bacteria or its spores) are poured into sterilized plates or petri dishes. The number of bacteria added to the agar is carefully controlled since too large a number of bacteria lead to smaller zones of inhibition but small numbers can lead to difficulty in defining the edge of the zone of inhibition (see below).

The plates must be on a completely horizontal surface to obtain an agar layer of uniform thickness. Once set, the plates are dried at 37°C for 30 min and they are used either immediately or after storage at 4°C for up to a week. Wells are punched into the agar in a selected design, using, for example, a sterile 9-mm diameter cork borer and a paper template positioned below the plate. The agar plugs are removed using a sterile needle or a fine scalpel blade. The wells are filled with a constant volume (anything from 20 to 200 μl) of sample in duplicate or triplicate in a suitable random fashion (Figure 1). For a large 30 × 30 plate this arrangement can be used for the assay of up to 36 samples, which should include four to five standards over the concentration range of the specimens being assayed.

The plates are incubated, usually overnight at 37°C, although rapid assays (3-6 hr) are usually at 40°C. Movement of the antibiotic from the well into the agar occurs by

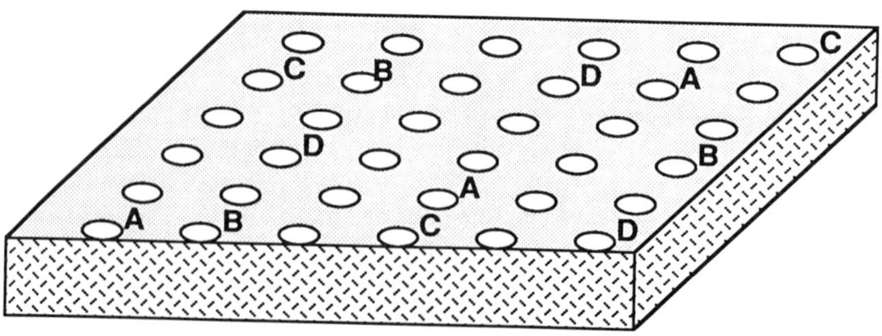

Figure 1 A typical arrangement of wells used in an agar diffusion assay. To limit errors that may be caused by variations in bacterial growth and/or agar thickness, each sample is applied to three wells spaced at random across the plate.

simple diffusion and forms a circular zone of inhibition, the perimeter of which is at the antibiotic concentration that is just able to inhibit bacterial growth. The rate of diffusion is constant under controlled conditions and is affected by the molecular weight of the antibiotic, the temperature of the incubation, and also the viscosity, ion content, and pH of the agar.

Normally, diffusion is complete by 6–8 hr, after which the zones of inhibition can be measured. Within the first hours of incubation the concentration gradient of antibiotic radiating from the wells is very steep. Therefore, early measurements of the zone of inhibition are liable to large errors owing to rapid changes in the antibiotic concentration. However, in many "same-day" assays, conditions have been designed to facilitate maximal diffusion rates, which enables accurate readings after as short as 3 hr incubation.

The zones of inhibition can be measured accurately using a commercially available zone reader, which projects a magnified image of the circular zone onto a screen.

There are numerous variables in the methodology, depending on the antibiotic being assayed:

Media. Differences in the composition of the media can affect not only the diffusion rate of the antibiotic but also its antibacterial activity and the growth rate of the indicator organism.

Indicator organisms. A large variety of indicator organisms are used. Bacilli, staphylococci, *Escherichia coli*, and other coliforms are the most common but they are not exclusive. The organisms are chosen for their sensitivity to the antibiotic being assayed, their specificity to the antibiotic being determined (important when patients are receiving multiple antibiotic therapy), and their ability to produce clearly defined inhibition zones and to grow rapidly. The latter is especially important when results are required for therapeutic drug monitoring.

Inoculation. The indicator organism is not always incorporated into the agar prior to plating. Sometimes a suspension of an indicator organism is flooded over the surface of sterile agar. The excess fluid is removed, and the plate is dried and can be stored as above before cutting the wells. This method is usually employed when the assay is not routine. Generally, greater reproducibility is found when the bacteria or their spores are incorporated into the agar before plating, because it is easier to control the numbers of bacteria applied to the plate and thereby achieve more confluent growth. Spores are often used because of their greater heat tolerance since the agar must be warmed to about 50°C for pouring.

Dosing. Agar wells are sometimes replaced with either sterile high-quality blotting paper disks, surface-mounted cups, or fish spines containing a small volume of the sample being assayed.

B. Immunoassays

As in classic immunologic reactions, antibiotic immunoassays depend on the reaction of a specific antibody with an antigen; in this case the antibiotic represents the antigen. The antibody or antiserum with specificity for an antibiotic is usually raised in sheep, goats, or rabbits by their immunization with the antibiotic covalently linked to a carrier protein, such as bovine serum albumin. The antibody-antigen reaction is reversible and obeys the law of mass action. Thus, if antigen (Ag) and antibody (Ab) are mixed and their reaction allowed to proceed, the amount of bound complex (Ag·Ab) formed and the amount of free Ag and Ab will eventually reach an equilibrium that is dependent on the two rate constants: k_1 (association) and k_2 (dissociation).

$$Ag + Ab \underset{k_2}{\overset{k_1}{\rightleftharpoons}} Ag{:}Ab$$

1. Radioimmunoassays

Of the immunoassay techniques, radioimmunoassays were the first to achieve widespread use. A small constant amount of isotopically labeled antigen (i.e., the antibiotic being assayed) is mixed with a constant amount of its antiserum; the quantity of antiserum is carefully selected so that not all the labeled antigen is bound at equilibrium. The sample or standard undergoing analysis is added to this mixture. With increasing concentrations of antibiotic in the analysate, increasing concentrations of labeled antibiotic are displaced from antibody (Figure 2). After equilibrium is reached, the bound and free fractions are separated by physical, chemical, or immunologic means and the radioactivity in one or both the fractions determined. Because the reaction between antibody and antigen is

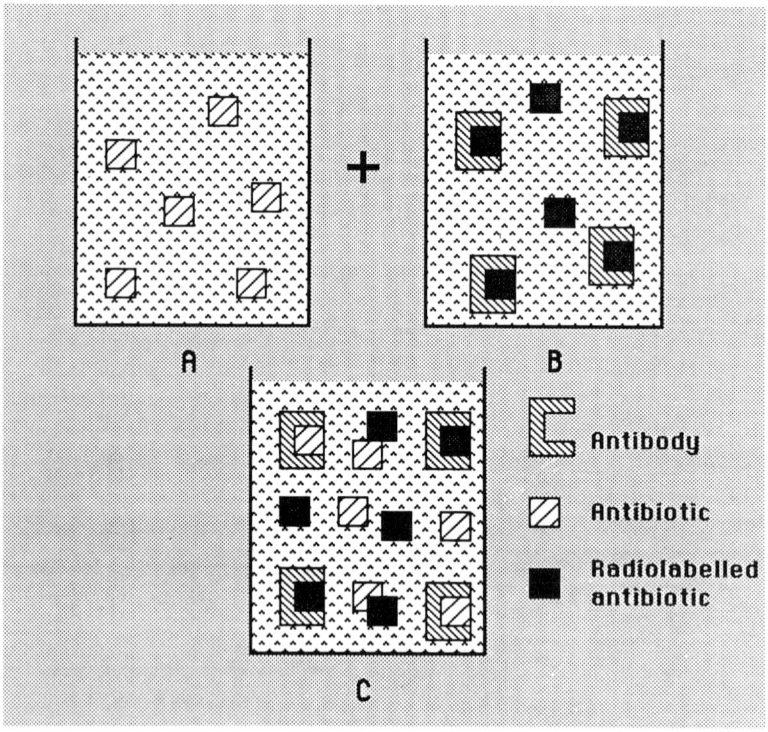

Figure 2 Radioimmunoassay. The sample (A) containing an unknown concentration of antibiotic (e.g., gentamicin) is added to a mixture of antiserum and radiolabeled gentamicin (sample B) to give sample C. After equilibration, the antibody-antigen complex and free antigen are separated and the radioactivity of one or both is determined. The amount of free radiolabeled gentamicin is proportional to the concentration of gentamicin in sample A (see Figure 3).

stoichiometric (i.e., one antibody can bind only to one antigen), the amount of bound or free label is directly proportional to the antibiotic concentration in the sample undergoing analysis. The concentration can be determined simply by comparing the radioactivity of samples with standard curves that have been prepared over the concentration range expected in the samples. A typical standard curve for a radioimmunoassay is shown in Figure 3.

Although the first immunoassays employed β emitters (usually tritium) as the radiolabel, these radionuclides have largely been replaced with low-energy γ emitters, such as Iodine 125. This was due mainly to the lower cost and ease of quantitation of the latter radionuclide. β Emitters require the use of expensive liquid scintillation counters, liquid scintillants, and low-background vials. Also, standardization is more complex owing to chemical or color quenching of the scintillations by the sample.

2. Nonisotopic Immunoassays

The γ-emitting radiolabels themselves have many disadvantages compared with nonisotopic immunoassays (Table 1) since they require the use of expensive γ counters, they are subject to specific regulations (transport, handling, and disposal), they have a relatively short shelf life, and they require a separation step. As a result, commercially available nonisotopic immunoassays for the aminoglycosides and vancomycin have become the methods of choice in therapeutic drug monitoring laboratories. Consequently, numerous nonisotopic immunoassays have been developed recently (3), and it is likely that they will replace radioimmunoassays for most routine antibiotic and drug determinations.

The basis of nonisotopic immunoassays is not significantly different from their isotopic counterparts except that the label and the method of measuring it are different. Also, some of the newer methods do not require the separation of bound and free label

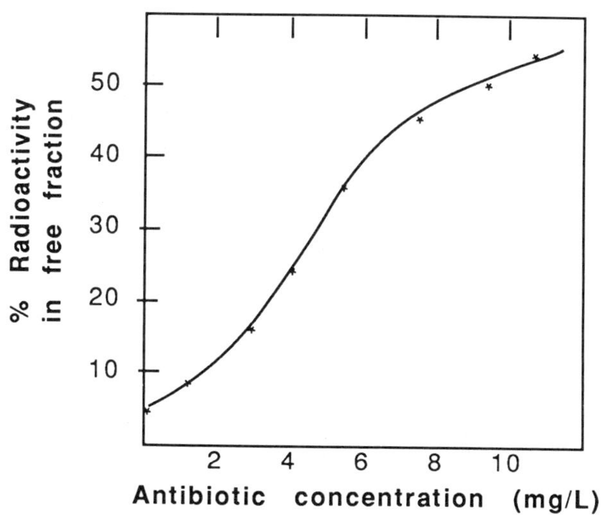

Figure 3 A typical standard curve obtained by radioimmunoassay. With increasing concentrations of the standard or sample, increased amounts of radioactive antibiotic are displaced from the antibody and are measured in the free fraction.

Table 1 Comparison of Different Assay Methods for Antibiotics

Method	Assay time	Assay sensitivity	Advantages	Disadvantages
Microbiologic	Min 4 hr Max 48 hr	0.1–2.0 μg/ml	Technical competence, versatile, low cost	Long assay time, interference by other antibiotics, day-to-day variation
Immunoassays				
Radioimmunoassay	1–2 hr	1–100 ng/ml	Sensitive, specific, accurate	Require costly equipment for radioactivity measurement, handling of isotopes, separation step needed
Nonisotopic immunoassays	<1 hr	1–100 ng/ml	Rapid, sensitive, specific, accurate, simple	Relatively high cost/sample, commercial kits available only for the aminoglycosides and vancomycin, more prone to interference than isotopic assays unless separation step is included
Chromatography				
HPLC	1 hr	1–100 ng/ml	Specific, sensitive, accurate, automation	Expertise required, costly equipment, extraction of samples
GLC	1 hr	0.1–10 ng/ml	Sensitive, specific, accurate	Expertise required, costly equipment, extraction of samples, derivitization of most antibiotics excludes GLC as method of choice

prior to determination. The nonisotopic immunoassays that are currently available can be subdivided according to the label used into (1) fluoroimmunoassays, which employ fluorophore-labeled antigen, (2) enzymimmunoassays, in which the antigen is labeled with an enzyme, and (3) those using particles as the label. Further subdivision can be made as to whether a separation step is required.

a. Nonseparation Nonisotopic Immunoassays. Polarization Fluorophore Immunoassays: In these assays, the reaction mixture consists of fluorescein-labeled antibiotic together with its antibody. Polarized light is passed through the reaction mixture. Excitation of the fluorescein is followed a few nanoseconds later by light emission. Free labeled drug undergoes considerable random movement so that the emitted light is no longer in the same plane as the excitatory light. A detector set to read light only in the plane of the excitatory light will therefore have a low signal. When drug-fluorophore is bound to antibody, the large size of the antibody-fluorophore complex leads to a decrease in random movement between excitation and emission and thereby an increase in the signal (Figure 4A). Addition of sample containing unlabeled antibiotic results in less fluorophore-labeled drug being bound with a corresponding decrease in the signal (Figure 4B). It has proved simple to synthesize fluorescein-labeled gentamicin and other aminoglycosides with excellent shelf lives. Suitable instrumentation, which includes a polarization fluori-

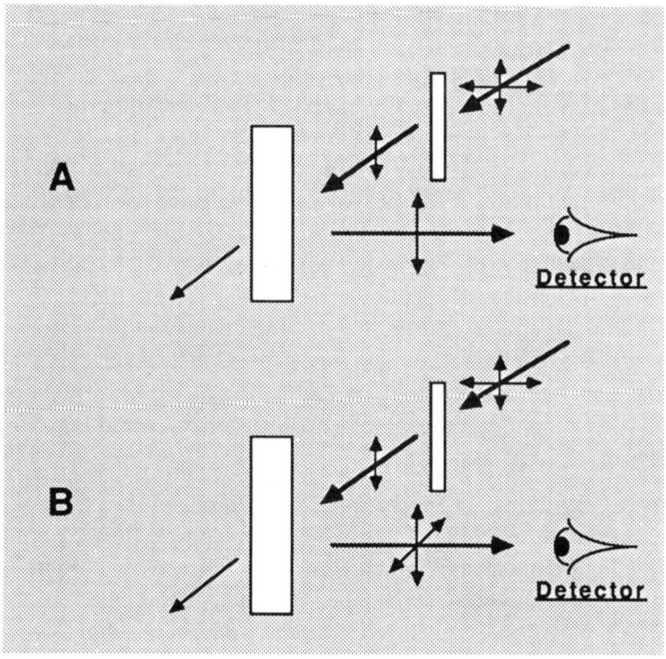

Figure 4 Polarization fluoroimmunoassay. In sample A, the majority of fluorophore-labeled antibiotic is bound to antibody. Between light excitation and emission of the bound fluorophore, there is relatively little random movement. Thus, a high signal is obtained on a photon counter set to detect emitted light in the same plane as the excitatory light. Addition of a sample containing antibiotic to A results in an increase in free fluorophore, which, because it has more rapid random movement than when in the bound state, results in a decrease in signal (B).

meter incorporating a photon counter, has been produced by Abbott. The assay is extremely rapid (2 min) and requires only very low volumes of serum (2-5 μl). These factors, together with the simplicity of the instrumentation, have resulted in this technique becoming very popular for the routine assay of aminoglycosides so that more than 50% of laboratories in North America use this method or one similar for the assay of gentamicin (4).

Direct Quenching Fluoroimmunoassay: In this assay, the antibody binding of the fluorophore results in quenching (i.e., the antibody binding to the fluorphore-labeled antibiotic prevents either the activation or the emission of the fluorophore). Thus, in direct contrast to the polarization fluoroimmunoassay, antibody binding results in a decrease in signal. However, this method is limited by the ability to raise antisera that,when bound to the labeled drug, causes such impairment in the excitation of or the emission from the fluorophore. The lack of need for a separation step enables the use of a simple fluorimeter. The assay for gentamicin has been automated using standard Technicon Auto-Analyzer equipment (5), which allows the reporting of results within 10 min of specimen receipt, also making the method suitable for therapeutic drug monitoring.

Substrate-labeled Fluoroimmunoassay: These assays were developed by Miles Laboratories for gentamicin, tobramicin, and amikacin. In this case, the antibiotic label is umbelliferyl-β-D-galactoside, which is nonfluorescent when it is conjugated to the galactoside. Upon addition of the enzyme β-galactosidase, fluorescent products are formed from the labeled antibiotic in the free fraction but not from that in the bound fraction, where the presence of antibody inhibits the enzyme from cleaving the fluorescent conjugate. The need for accurate timing between enzyme addition and fluorescence measurement may be a problem in busy laboratories, and so this assay has not been the method of choice for therapeutic drug monitoring.

Nonseparation Enzyme Immunoassay: In these assays, the label attached to the antibiotic is an enzyme. When antibody binds to the labeled antibiotic there is a reduction in enzyme activity. Thus in the presence of unlabeled antibiotic, less enzyme-labeled drug will be bound to the antibody, which results in increased enzyme activity in the reaction mixture. The Syva Company has marketed these type of assays as the EMIT system for the aminoglycosides netilmicin, amikacin, tobramycin, and gentamicin; a kit for vancomycin is in development and is expected to be marketed in 1987. These systems have rapidly achieved a dominant position in routine therapeutic drug monitoring of the aminoglycosides. [About 25% of North American centers were using enzyme immunoassay for gentamicin in 1986 (4).]

b. Nonisotopic Immunoassay Employing a Separation Step. Nonisotopic immunoassays can be prone to interference by nonspecific factors present in biologic fluids. For example, in nonseparation enzyme immunoassays, endogenous enzymes may be present with similar effects to those of the enzymes used as the label. Similarly, nonseparation fluoroimmunoassays can be affected by endogenous fluorophores, such as bilirubin, and by light scattering in turbid specimens. In practice, these kinds of problems are overcome by extensive predilution of the sample or by running appropriate controls and blanks. To avoid the need for these procedures, some investigators include separation steps in fluoroimmunoassays for the aminoglycoside antibiotics (3).

C. Chromatography

In all chromatographic methods, separation of molecules is obtained by virtue of their physicochemical properties. The sample undergoing analysis is applied to a stationary phase and eluted with a mobile phase. The stationary phase may either be packed into a column, as in gas chromatography (GC) and high-performance liquid chromatography (HPLC), or it may be spread in a layer on a glass or plastic sheet, as in thin-layer chromatography (TLC). The mobile phase in GC is a gas; in HPLC and TLC it is a liquid. Separation is dependent on the relative tendencies of different molecules in the sample to associate more strongly with one or the other of the phases.

Chromatographic methods available for the determination of antibiotics include all three of the techniques above, although GC and TLC are used much less often than HPLC. Gas-liquid chromatography (GLC) is used for only a very few antibiotics (chloramphenicol and aminoglycosides) because it requires a cumbersome derivatization of the antibiotic into a volatile compound and most antibiotics cannot be volatilized. TLC is used rarely in pharmacological studies and has little application in therapeutic drug monitoring. Large numbers of HPLC methods have been developed for virtually all antibiotics in common use (for major reviews, see References 6-10).

HPLC methods can be subdivided into a number of modes based on the nature of the stationary phase and the method of separation. The most commonly used modes are adsorption chromatography and partition chromatography. Additional modes, such as ion-exchange chromatography and size-exclusion chromatography, are rarely used for antibiotics and are not described here. The adsorption and partition modes are often defined as normal and reversed-phase chromatography, respectively. In the normal phase, the stationary phase is highly polar in nature (e.g., silica or alumina) and the mobile phase is nonpolar (e.g., hexane, chloroform, or isopropanol). Thus separation is based on repeated adsorption-desorption of molecules to the adsorbent, with polar compounds retained on the column longer than nonpolar compounds because their affinity to the stationary phase is higher (Figure 5A).

Reversed-phase chromatography is the exact opposite in that the surface hydroxyl groups of silica particles are bonded to a nonpolar material and the mobile phase is a polar liquid, such as water or an alcohol (Figure 5B). The bonded phases most commonly used are alkyl chains (usually octadecyl or octyl). These alkyl chains on the stationary phase can be thought of as a liquid into which partitioning of compounds occurs. Thus, nonpolar compounds partition strongly into the stationary nonpolar "liquid" and are retained longer on the column than polar compounds, which partition more strongly into the relatively polar mobile phase (Figure 5B). Polar bonded phases are also available (e.g., cyano or amino groups) but these are used in the normal mode.

Alkyl-bonded phases are used almost without exception for HPLC analyses of most antibiotic families. The carbon chain length is normally 18, although sometimes C8 and rarely C12 and C2 have been employed. A mixture of buffer and methanol or acetonitrile is used as the mobile phase. The pH of the buffer is chosen according to the pK_a of the antibiotic undergoing analysis to provide sufficient suppression of ionization in order to obtain a suitable retention relative to potentially interfering molecules in the sample. Similarly, the concentrations of methanol or acetonitrile, which are nonpolar relative to the buffer, depend on the polarity of the reversed-phase packing and the physicochemical nature of potentially interfering molecules.

The size of the silica particles vary from 3 to 30 μm, although in most analytic methods the size is 3-10 μm. Packing materials (of the same particle size) supplied by different manufacturers invariably differ in their characteristics so it is important, when a published method is followed, that the same column type be obtained.

The deproteinized or extracted sample is injected either manually or automatically onto the column through which the mobile phase is pumped at a constant flow rate of

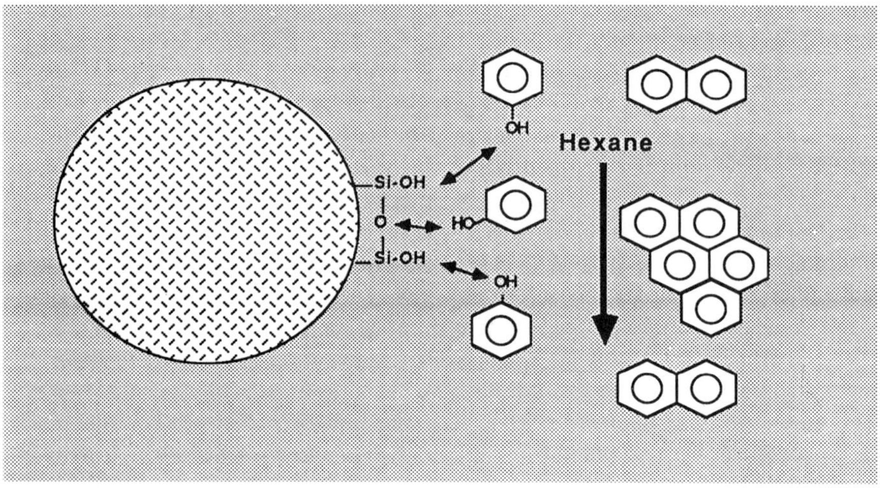

(A)

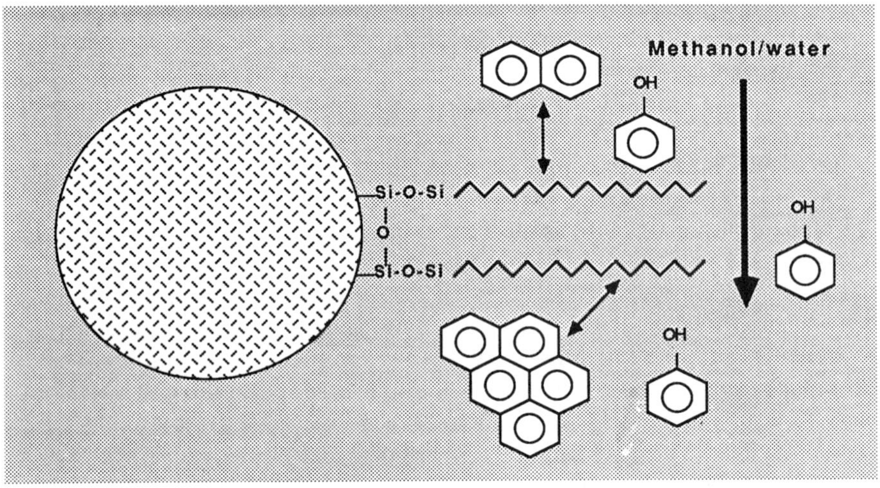

(B)

Figure 5 (A) Normal-phase (adsorption) and (B) reversed-phase (partition).

1-2 ml/min. A short guard column packed with a large (30-μm) alkyl-bonded phase is normally included before the main column to prevent insoluble particles from blocking and shortening the life of this expensive commodity. On the main column, the sample separates into its molecular components by virtue of their relative affinities for the mobile and stationary phases (as described above). The mobile phase containing the separated sample then passes through a detector whose signal is visualized on a recorder. Data storage and integration modules may also be coupled to the system.

Detection is usually by ultraviolet (UV) absorbance since most antibiotics have a high UV molar absorptivity and this mode of detection allows sensitive determinations. There are exceptions, such as the aminoglycosides and erythromycin, for which fluorometric or electrochemical detection has been used. Fluorescence detection requires that the antibiotic be derivatized with such agents as O-phthalaldehyde, fluorescamine, and dansyl chloride. Derivatization is performed on the extracted samples before injection onto the column or on line after the sample has been eluted from the column.

II. COLLECTION OF SAMPLES FOR ANALYSIS

Whole blood, plasma, serum, and urine are the biologic samples most commonly used in the assay of antibiotics and can be readily obtained. The sample volume required depends on the sensitivity of the method and the concentration of the antibiotic in samples. In chemical assays, such as HPLC, sample volumes of 200 μl to 2 ml are normally employed, and these must undergo extraction and/or deproteinization before analysis. Because large errors can arise owing either to intersample variation in extraction efficiency and/or to losses of sample during cleanup procedures a fixed amount of an internal standard is added to each sample prior to cleanup. The internal standard is a molecule that has similar physicochemical properties to the drug undergoing analysis. Thus loss or poor extraction of the sample will result in a corresponding loss in the amount of the internal standard and can be corrected.

Biologic assays (immunoassays and microbiologic assays) can be performed with sample volumes from 10 to 200 μl and often do not require any cleanup procedure. However, these assays do require carefully prepared controls to determine the effects of protein binding and/or interference with any endogenous materials.

It is important to be able to measure antibiotic concentrations achieved in tissues, especially during the development stages of the antibiotic, since it is in the tissues that most bacterial infections occur. Tissue concentrations of antibiotic can be measured in either tissue fluid or processed or intact samples of tissue itself. Although the antibiotic can be measured in these samples by all the methods described here, obtaining and preparation of samples pose special problems.

A number of techniques have been described to provide a sufficient volume of tissue fluid. These include inducing skin blisters by using local irritants or suction or by implantation of cotton threads and paper disks. Each technique has limitations when applied to the pharmacokinetics of antibiotics in actual compartments, and these are discussed in detail elsewhere (11,12).

Tissue samples are usually obtained by various biopsy techniques. Often the size of the sample is small and care must be taken to prevent evaporation, which can lead to overestimation of the antibiotic concentration. The samples are usually homogenized and extracted prior to analysis, although small samples of unmanipulated muscle tissue have been measured reliably using the agar diffusion technique. Problems associated with the interpretation of results are usually similar to those found in the assay of body fluids (i.e., binding to protein or other macromolecules) and can usually be overcome by careful preparation of standard curves (13).

III. COMPARISON OF THE AVAILABLE TECHNIQUES

A. Microbiologic Assays

These assays have the advantages of economy, simplicity, and easy applicability to all antibiotics (Table 1). Also, sample cleanup is not required. However, numerous factors may affect their accuracy and sensitivity and careful attention to detail and full use of controls are required. The controls should take into account the presence of substances in the sample that may effect either the growth of the indicator organism (e.g., blood and those tissues that contain lysozyme or spermatine) or the diffusion rate of the antibiotic through the media (e.g., protein and salt concentration) (2). Interference by metabolites and degradation products may arise, although it should be stated that these are exceptions rather than the rule since most antibiotics are relatively stable and do not normally have active metabolites. Interactions with coadministered antimicrobials can be limited by using indicator organisms that have a specific sensitivity to the antibiotic being assayed. For most methods the limits of sensitivity are 0.1-0.5 mg/liter which is adequate for therapeutic drug monitoring, but for this application they have the major disadvantage of a long turnaround time (4-24 hr). Also, microbiologic assays are not considered as reproducible as HPLC or immunology, and in terms of specificity and sensitivity they fall short of the requirements for pharmacokinetic studies or other developmental investigations and cannot be used to assess the metabolism of an antibiotic. However, their widespread use has resulted in a high level of technical competence; some authors have reported methods that claim to be as reliable and as sensitive as more modern and sophisticated techniques, such as HPLC.

B. Immunoassays

Immunoassays are sensitive, specific, and reliable, and they require only a few microliters of a sample that does not need to undergo a cleanup procedure (Table 1). Although commercially available radioimmunoassays employing γ emitters are still used for therapeutic drug monitoring of the aminoglycosides in some centers in North America, they have a number of disadvantages (outlined in Section I.B.2) and have largely been replaced with nonisotopic immunoassays. Of 340 centers, less than 5% now use radioimmunoassays compared with 64 and 25% using polarization fluorophore immunoassay and enzyme immunoassay, respectively (4). The relatively high costs of the commercial kits are compensated for by their simplicity and by the savings in time. In addition, the kits permit small laboratories to carry out determinations. The major disadvantage with immunoassays is that they are limited to only a small number of antibiotics. Few laboratories have the expertise to develop their own assays by preparing suitably labeled antibiotics and specific antisera to those antibiotics. The nonisotopic immunoassays are prone to interference by nonspecific factors, such as metabolites (although aminoglycosides are not metabolized significantly), similar drugs and endogenous fluorophores, and enzymes. However, most problems of interference can be overcome by running controls that correct for background positive reading or by using immunoassays with a separation step.

C. Chromatography

HPLC is the chromatographic procedure essentially used for antibiotic quantitation. The greatest advantage of HPLC is its almost unlimited potential. It is accurate, sensitive, specific, selective, and rapid and can be fully automated, allowing unattended operation round the clock (Table 1). It allows simultaneous assay of a drug and its metabolites, two different antibiotics from the same family and possibly different families, and even different isomers of the same drug. Almost every antibiotic in clinical use has at least one published HPLC method for its assay (6-10). Most of the methods use the reversed-phase mode, which affords great selectivity by the choice of mobile and stationary phases. The development of microbore columns permits smaller sample volumes to be used together with great reduction in the consumption of mobile phase. Also, new mass spectrometric and diode-array UV detectors have recently been marketed that may prove to be valuable, particularly in studies of metabolism when the structures of compounds are investigated.

The disadvantages of HPLC include the high cost of the equipment and the requirement for highly trained personnel to operate it. Although the development of assays can be time consuming, they can rapidly be applied to antibiotics of the same family with only minor modification. The requirement of cleanup from a biologic matrix makes HPLC time consuming; however, with large numbers of samples automation can make the process efficient. Analysis of aminoglycosides involves derivitization, another time-consuming operation that can also involve additional equipment if postcolumn derivitization is employed. Routine analysis of an antibiotic by HPLC becomes efficient if there are large numbers of analyses. Compared to commercially available immunoassays, a HPLC system can be at least 10 times cheaper per sample. However, for less routine analyses a laboratory can rarely afford to designate one HPLC system to a single assay, which makes the application inefficient economically and temporally owing to the constant changing from one method to another.

IV. CONCLUSIONS

Although antibiotic levels were originally measured by microbiologic methods, the lack of specificity, sensitivity, and speed of this method has resulted in the application of alternative techniques. Immunoassays are rapid and reliable, and they have achieved a dominant position in therapeutic drug monitoring of aminoglycosides and vancomycin. Pharmacological studies of most antibiotics and therapeutic monitoring of chloramphenicol is by HPLC, which although more complex and time consuming is a powerful technique for all antibiotics because of its unique selectivity.

REFERENCES

1. Reeves, DS, Phillips, I, Williams, JD, Wise, R (eds.): *Laboratory Methods in Antimicrobial Chemotherapy*, Churchill Livingstone, Edinburgh, 1978.
2. de Louvois, J: Factors influencing the assay of antimicrobial drugs in clinical samples by the agar plate diffusion method. *J. Antimicrob. Chemother. 9*:253–265, 1982.
3. Munro, AJ, Landon, J, Shaw, EJ: The basis of immunoassays for antibiotics. *J. Antimicrob. Chemother. 9*:423–342, 1982.
4. American Association of Clinical Chemistry: *Quality Control Report*, 1986.
5. Shaw, EW, Watson, RAA, Smith, DS: Continuous flow fluorimmunoassay of serum gentamicin, with automatic sample blank correction. *Clin. Chem. 25*:322–324, 1979.
6. Nilsson-Ehle, I: High-pressure liquid chromatography as a tool for the determination of antibiotics in body fluids. *Acta Pathol. Microbiol. Scand. 259 (Suppl.)*:61–66, 1977.
7. Nilsson-Ehle, I: High-pressure liquid chromatography for analysis of antibiotics in biological fluids. *J. Liq. Chromatogr. 6* (S2):251, 1983.

8. Yoshikawa, TT, Maitra, SK, Schotz, MC, Guze, LB: High-pressure liquid chromatography for quantitation of antimicrobial drugs. *Rev. Infect. Dis. 2*:169–181, 1980.
9. Rouan, MC: Antibiotic monitoring in body fluids. *J. Chromatogr. (Biomed. Appl.) 340*:361–400, 1985.
10. Schwarz, V: Drug level monitoring: Chromatography of some minor groups of drugs. *J. Chromatogr. (Biomed. Appl.) 340*:401–479, 1985.
11. Raeburn, JA: A review of experimental models for studying the tissue penetration of antibiotics in man. *Scand. J. Infect. Dis. Suppl. 14*:225–227, 1978.
12. Ryan, DM: Influence of surface area/volume ratio on the kinetics of different antibiotics in tissues and tissue fluids. *Scand. J. Infect. Dis. Suppl. 44*:24–33, 1985.
13. Cars, O, Ogren, S: Antibiotic tissue concentrations: Methodological aspects and interpretation of results. *Scand. J. Infect. Dis. Suppl. 44*:7–15, 1985.

3
Clinical Relevance of Pharmacokinetic Principles for Antimicrobial Therapy

GIDEON KOREN
The Hospital for Sick Children, and the University of Toronto, Toronto, Ontario, Canada

Various pharmacokinetic concepts are discussed in association with the antimicrobial agents reviewed in this book. These include serum or plasma concentrations, distribution, elimination, and half-life. This chapter will define various pharmacokinetic concepts relevant to antimicrobial therapy. This will enable the reader to better understand the advantages and limitations of a pharmacokinetically oriented approach.

I. BASIC ASSUMPTION

For decades, antimicrobial therapy was based on the dose-response approach. A correlation was assumed between the dose given and the effects on the microorganisms. It was appreciated that the key determining an effect was related to the concentration of the active drug at the site of infection. However, as appropriate methodology was lacking, it was impossible to readily measure concentrations of antimicrobial drugs in body fluids. Parallel to the development of analytic methods for the measurement of drug concentrations, mathematical models of drug movement in the body were constructed. These concentration-time concepts are the cornerstone of pharmacokinetics. By properly using pharmacokinetic principles, the physician should be able to design a dosing schedule for an antimicrobial agent that results in the desired serum concentration. Yet in most cases physicians still do not know the drug concentrations at the site of infection. It must be assumed that concentrations at the site of infection are proportional to measured concentrations in the blood. As will be shown in this chapter, this assumption is true in some cases but false in others.

Antimicrobial drugs are unique in that their target is an exogenous agent, a microorganism; whereas the target of most other drugs is one or more body tissues. Therefore, the characteristics of the offending microorganism must be considered in conjunction with the host's biology. The following discussion introduces pharmacokinetic principles that must be considered in association with any antimicrobial drug.

II. ADMINISTRATION

Antimicrobial drugs are mainly administered orally, intramuscularly, and intravenously. Topical use of antimicrobials (such as for the skin and eye) are common. In special cases they may be administered directly into the infected compartment (e.g., the cerebrospinal fluid or the peritoneum). Generally, it is assumed that the intravenous route of drug administration guarantees complete delivery of the dose. However, especially in small neonates, this may not be the case. This issue is discussed in detail in Chapter 8.

A. Absorption

Many factors may influence the absorption of antimicrobial agents after oral administration. In general, such influences may affect the rate of absorption which is measured in terms of time, and/or the extent of absorption, which is expressed as the fraction of the given dose that has eventually been absorbed.

1. Rate of Absorption

The rate of absorption may be an important determinant of antimicrobial drug efficacy. A drug that is absorbed slowly may not create a sufficient concentration gradient to result in high enough concentrations at the infected site, even if the entire dose is eventually absorbed. For example, when taken together with food, the rate of absorption of penicillin, ampicillin, oxacillin, dicloxacillin, lincomycin, and some erythromycins is reduced (1-5). Pharmacokinetically, the rate of absorption is characterized by K_a, the absorption rate constant, which expresses the fraction of the dose that has been absorbed in a unit of time. In the clinical setting, K_a is not often available, as its calculation may be quite complicated. In contrast, the value of T_{max}, which is defined as the time needed for a drug to achieve its peak concentration following administration, is often available. T_{max} is influenced by the rate of absorption K_a and the rate of elimination K according to the formula

$$T_{max} = \frac{2.3 \log (K_a/K)}{K_a - K}$$

2. Extent of Absorption

Many factors may influence the extent of absorption of antimicrobial agents. Administration with food will reduce the amount of isoniazid absorbed by 50%. This reduction probably results from a change in gastric emptying and gastrointestinal pH induced by food (6). Similarly, antacids exert an inhibitory effect on isoniazid absorption (7).

Other antimicrobial drugs that are absorbed to a lesser extent in the presence of food include rifampin, tetracyclines, penicillins, erythromycin, and lincomycin (1.3,8,9).

Food does not appear to affect the extent of absorption of amoxicillin, metronidazole, or esterified ampicillin (10-12), and it appears to improve the absorption of erythromycin stearate, nitrofurantoin, and griseofulvin (13-15).

It appears that the food-induced delay in gastric emptying improves the poor dissolution of nitrofurantoin, whereas a high fat content of food increases the dissolution of the lipophilic griseofulvin.

Many drugs, including antihistamines, phenothiazines, tricyclic antidepressants, narcotics, and sedative hypnotics, may decrease gastric motility (16) and are capable of modulating both the rate and the extent of absorption of antimicrobial drugs.

The extent of absorption is measured mathematically by comparing the amount absorbed after an oral dose to that absorbed after an equivalent amount given intravenously. Figure 1A demonstrates a patient receiving the same milligram dose of penicillin by the oral route and then intravenously. Although the initial concentration is higher after the intravenous injection, the total concentration over time, expressed as area under concentration-time curve (AUC), is equal. This indicates that the total dose was absorbed. In Figure 1B, the same patient took the oral dose with food, and it is apparent that the AUC after the oral dose is much smaller than after the intravenous dose. In this case, the ratio

$$\frac{\text{AUC oral}}{\text{AUC intravenous}} = 0.5$$

means that only 50% of the oral dose was absorbed. This ratio is often referred to as *oral bioavailability* and is denoted F. Many factors other than food or drugs may impair the absorption and reduce the bioavailability of antimicrobial drugs. Vomiting soon after an oral dose, malabsorption syndromes, and changes of gastric pH are but a few examples.

Low oral bioavailability may result from the *first-pass effect* in the presence of complete absorption. It is possible that after being completely absorbed, a drug is rapidly metabolized during the first passage through the liver and before entering the systemic circulation. In such a case, systemic concentration is low although absorption is complete. This phenomenon has been shown with the lidocaine, quinidine, 6-mercaptopurine, and others. However, antimicrobial agents have not yet been shown to undergo measurable first-pass metabolism.

Recently, the oral absorption of amoxicillin and bacampicillin has been shown to be dose dependent; with a higher dose the AUC is proportionally lower then with a lower dose (17). This phenomenon, which reflects saturation of intestinal absorption above a certain dose, has also been documented with chlorothiazide (18).

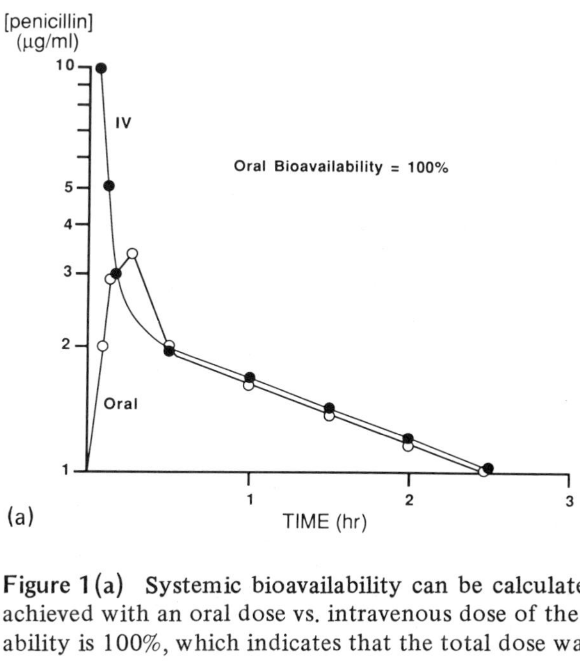

(a)

Figure 1(a) Systemic bioavailability can be calculated from the proportion of AUC achieved with an oral dose vs. intravenous dose of the same amount of the drug. Bioavailability is 100%, which indicates that the total dose was absorbed.

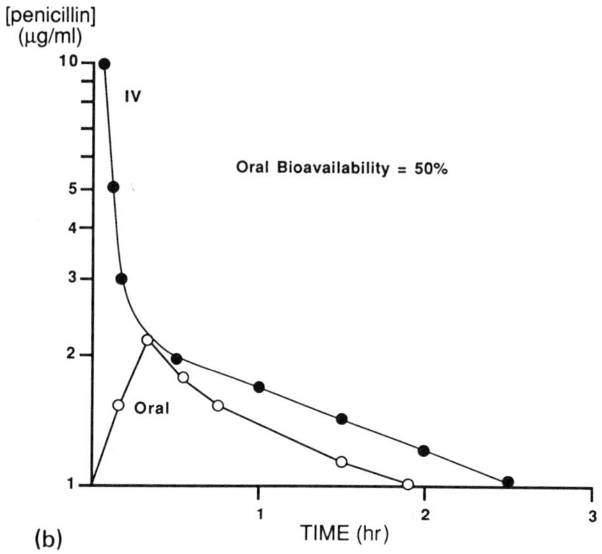

Figure 1 (b) When the drug was taken with food, the AUC is much smaller than after the intravenous dose.

B. Distribution

The distribution of antimicrobial drugs from the blood into various tissues is a complex process that will define the accessability of the agent to the site of infection. The degree of distribution of a drug is characterized by its volume of distribution V_d, which is the relationship between the concentration of the drug in the blood C_p and the total amount of the drug in the body A_b

$$V_d = \frac{A_b}{C_p} \tag{2}$$

As shown in this formula, the volume of distribution is calculated from the concentration of the drug in the blood, assuming it is homogeneously distributed throughout the body. This assumption is never true, as drugs tend to be concentrated in some tissues but not in others. Consequently, the distribution volume does not have a physiological identity and it will not indicate where or how the drug is distributed. It reflects only how much of the drug stays in the blood after distribution has been completed.

The practical use of V_d is in predicting the serum concentration of the drug after distribution, simply by changing formula (2) to

$$C_p = \frac{A_b}{V_d} \tag{3}$$

As therapeutic drug monitoring is based mainly on serum concentrations of antimicrobial drugs, knowing the value of V_d is essential for predicting serum concentration for a given dose.

From the above discussion it becomes apparent that the volume of distribution is too vague a concept to furnish the physician with information on whether an antimicrobial agent achieves high enough concentrations at the site of infection. As early as 1946, it became evident that penicillin can be recovered in wound exudates and lymph nodes long after it is undetectable in the blood (19). As the major goal of antimicrobial therapy is to achieve high enough levels at the site of infection to inhibit or kill the pathogen, accurate information on concentrations of antibiotics at these sites is very important.

Over the past few decades, several factors have been documented as important in determining the distribution of antimicrobial drugs into normal and infected tissues. They are summarized by Bergeron in a recent review (20) and are briefly mentioned here.

1. Chemical Characteristics of a Drug

Lipid-soluble antimicrobials, like rifampin and chloramphenicol, easily penetrate the cerebrospinal fluid (CSF) and other tissues, whereas penicillins, which are hydrophilic, penetrate to a much more limited extent. The pK_a of a drug may determine its movement along a pH gradient (see below), and the affinity of the drug molecules for a specific tissue may determine relative binding and hence the concentrations attained (e.g., aminoglycosides in renal tubular lysosomes).

2. Method of Administration of a Drug

For many drugs, including vasoactives, analgesics, antiepileptics, and antiasthmatics, it is considered desirable to maintain steady concentrations. This may be accomplished by establishing a continuous infusion during acute illness. The advantage of such a strategy is in avoiding potentially toxic "peaks" or subtherapeutic "troughs." This approach, however, may not be valid for antimicrobial agents. As shown in animal studies, single large boluses of certain antibiotics (aminoglycosides, penicillin, or aztreonam) may be far more effective than equivalent doses given as a continuous infusion or as an intermittent divided dose. Peak concentrations and AUC in serum, interstitial fluid, and fibrin clot are higher with the single bolus. Although most of this information is derived from animal models, it certainly illustrates the concept that the concentration ratio of tissue fluid over serum concentration is much lower following a continuous infusion than after a bolus. Consequently, a large bolus is more likely to result in the rapid achievement of higher antimicrobial concentrations at the site of infection (20).

3. Protein Binding

The distribution of antimicrobial agents is significantly influenced by their plasma protein binding. In general, the higher the protein binding of a drug, the lower are the concentrations attained in tissue fluids. Although most antimicrobials are bound reversibly to albumin, other proteins may also participate in this process [e.g., most of the plasma load of clindamycin is bound to α_1-glycoprotein (21)]. As a rule, acidic drugs are bound to plasma albumin whereas basic drugs are bound to α_1-glycoproteins or lipoproteins (22).

Although protein binding may be influenced by the relative concentrations of protein and drug, within the usual serum concentration ranges of most antimicrobial agents and physiologic concentrations of serum albumin, protein binding is quite constant. Once saturation of protein binding occurs, the free drug fraction will be increased. As only the free fraction of antimicrobial drugs is distributed into various tissue compartments, hypoproteinemia may be associated with higher tissue concentrations. Consequently, in cases of hypoproteinemia (e.g., uremia), the calculated distribution volume of cephalosporins, penicillins, and sulfamethoxasole is significantly larger (23). Various drugs have been shown to compete with protein binding of sulfonamides and penicillins (22). High concentrations of bilirubin may cause displacement of sulfonamides, tetracyclines, penicillins, and cephalosporins. Because the affinity of bilirubin to binding sites on the albumin molecule is higher than the affinity of drugs, it will probably displace antimicrobial agents, such as ampicillin and penicillin in neonates with hyperbilirubinemia, whereas it is unlikely that the drugs will displace bilirubin already bound to its primary binding sites. Conversely, previous binding of ampicillin or sulfonamides to albumin may significantly increase the available number of bilirubin molecules that can enter the brain to cause kernicterus. In spite of these pharmacokinetic considerations, the clinical importance of protein binding in antimicrobial therapy is still unknown. It is impossible to compare the efficacy of two different drugs merely according to their protein binding as there are numerous other factors influencing in vivo antimicrobial activity, including the intrinsic antimicrobial in vivo activity of the drug and various host factors. Yet is is evident that, for a given antimicrobial agent, an effect will be produced when the concentrations of free drug in the site of infection exceed the minimal inhibitory concentration following penetration from the blood compartment. The theoretical application is that for any given total serum concentration of an antimicrobial drug, the value of protein binding will permit the estimation of free drug concentration that may be achieved in various tissues.

4. Antimicrobial Transport Through Membranes

Being relatively small molecules, antimicrobials easily penetrate the porous capillary endothelium into the interstitial fluid. In several organs, including the brain, the prostate, and the eye, such pores are unavailable owing to the existence of tightly junctioned endothelium (18). During infections, there is apparent creation of pores in the blood-brain barrier, accounting for the significantly higher rate of penetration of antimicrobial agents into CSF and brain.

In two eliminating systems, the renal and the biliary, some antimicrobials have been shown to be actively secreted against their concentration gradient. Penicillins and cephalosporins share the organic acid channel of secretion at the renal tubular cell. Classically, coadministration of probenecid can block this pathway, causing accumulation of these drugs in the blood and increasing their efficacy. Similarly, cefoperazone may be actively secreted into the bile against its concentration gradients.

5. Tissue Binding

In comparison with protein binding, the binding of antimicrobial agents to tissues is more stable and may not readily equilibrate after depletion of the drug from the blood. Both amphotericin B and aminoglycosides have been shown to accumulate in certain tissues and then to be slowly released over several months, long after the drug has been eliminated from other tissues and the blood. The accumulation of aminoglycosides in the parenchyma of the kidney may explain both their renal toxicity and, possibly, their efficacy in infections involving the kidney (24).

6. Perfusion of Infected Areas

Whereas the concepts of protein binding and distribution volume may reflect the overall penetration of an antimicrobial agent, disease states may dramatically impair perfusion to the site of infection, thus reducing the ability of the drug to achieve therapeutic concentration there. Osteomyelitis and diabetic cellulitis are good examples of this state, when even very high serum concentrations of antibiotics may not guarantee therapeutic levels at the infected site.

C. Elimination

Several mechanisms are active in lowering the body load of antimicrobial agents. The kidneys are responsible for elimination of many drugs through filtration (penicillins, aminoglycosides, and vancomycin) and active tubular secretion (penicillins and nitrofurantoins). Impairment of renal function is expected to decrease the elimination of such drugs, and appropriate adjustment of dose schedules should take place (see Chapter 5).

The liver is capable of metabolizing various antimicrobial agents, including clindamycin, chloramphenicol, and isoniazid. As a rule, the metabolite is less lipophilic and more polar and appears to be better eliminated by glomerular filtration. In most cases, liver metabolism results in a molecule that is less active against pathogens. Metabolism involves either nonsynthetic reactions (oxidation, reduction, or hydrolysis) or conjugation in which new moieties (e.g., sulfate) are added to the drug molecule.

Several pharmacokinetic concepts are useful in characterizing the elimination pattern of drugs. The *elimination constant* K_e is the fraction of drug eliminated each unit of time. For example, if each hour one-sixth of the body load of gentamicin is excreted from the body, then

$$K_e = 0.166\ \text{hr}^{-1}$$

This term is practical, as all antimicrobial agents have *first-order elimination* kinetics; that is, in each unit of time the same fraction of remaining drug will be eliminated. This means that, in this example, if 100 mg gentamicin are in the body, during the first hour one-sixth (0.16) of this amount will be eliminated (16.6 mg), leaving 83.6 mg. During the next hour, one-sixth of the remaining dose will be eliminated, that is, 83.6 × 0.16 = 13.8 mg, and so on.

From this calculation it is apparent that the higher the amount of a drug in the body, the higher is the amount that is expected to be eliminated. For some drugs (although not antimicrobial agents), there is a *limit* to the ability of the liver to inactivate them through metabolism even at therapeutic concentrations. When the body load of ethanol or phenytoin, for instance, exceeds a certain level, saturation of the metabolic process will cause a *zero-order elimination*. This means that during each unit of time the same amount of drug will be metabolized, not the same fraction as in first-order kinetic elimination.

The elimination rate constant K_e is not a convenient parameter to work with in the clinical setting. Instead, it can be easily converted into elimination $T_{1/2}$ by

$$T_{1/2} = \frac{0.693}{K_e} \tag{4}$$

Using the example given before, if one-sixth of the body load of gentamicin is eliminated from the body each hour, then $K_e = 0.166\ \text{hr}^{-1}$; therefore, the elimination $T_{1/2}$ of gentamicin in this case is

$$T_{1/2} = \frac{0.693}{0.166\ \text{hr}^{-1}} = 4.2\ \text{hr}$$

This means that every 4.2 hr half of the body load of gentamicin is eliminated.

The first-order kinetic behavior of drugs is described mathematically as

$$C_t = C_0 \, e^{-Ke}$$

where C_t is the serum concentration at time t, C_0 is the concentration at time zero, and K_e is the elimination rate constant.

Elimination $T_{1/2}$ is a very useful parameter in planning dose schedules of antimicrobial agent. The shorter the $T_{1/2}$, the more rapid is the elimination of the drug from the body and the faster the levels of the drug would fall below the MIC for a pathogen.

The dosing interval T for a drug is given by the formula

$$T = 1.44 T_{1/2} \ln \frac{C_{max}}{C_{min}} \tag{5}$$

where C_{max} is the desired peak and C_{min} the desired trough of the drug. It is apparent from this formula that the longer the $T_{1/2}$, the longer is the optimal dosing interval for a given C_{max}/C_{min}.

The term "clearance" is used routinely in medicine to quantify the glomerular filtration rate (GFR) by measuring creatinine clearance. In pharmacokinetics, the same concept is used to determine the volume of blood that is completely cleared of a drug in a unit of time. Clearance of a drug depends upon the velocity with which the eliminating organ (liver, kidney, or other) clears the blood of the drug. Many clinicians erroneously identify clearance as a synonym of elimination $T_{1/2}$, whereas $T_{1/2}$ is dependent on *both* clearance Cl and distribution volume V_d according to the formula

$$T_{1/2} = \frac{0.693 \, V_d}{Cl} \tag{6}$$

In order to clarify the interrelations among the three, the following example may be helpful.

In a large stadium, the *clearance* of spectators is dependent on the number of gates. Let us assume that 2000 people are sitting very close to the gates; that is, their distribution V_d is small. Therefore, at the end of the show, they will quickly find their way out ($T_{1/2}$ will be short). If these 2000 people are scattered throughout the stadium (large V_d), then it will take them more time to leave the stadium (longer $T_{1/2}$). Similarly, if they are located near the gates (small V_d) but only two of five gates are open (lower clearance rate), then it will take them more time (prolonged $T_{1/2}$).

There are various ways to measure the clearance of drugs; however, unlike $T_{1/2}$, which can be readily calculated by plotting serum concentrations during the elimination phase on semilogarithmic paper, the calculation of clearance is more complicated.

Following a single dose of a drug, the clearance can be calculated as

$$Cl = \frac{\text{infusion rate}}{\text{serum concentration}} \tag{8}$$

As early as 1930, it was realized that even if a drug is given in a very high unchanged dose, it will not accumulate indefinitely, but rather reach a level at which the rate in (i.e., the given dose) will equal the rate out (elimination) (25). At this point, concentrations are expected to stay unchanged provided that the dose schedule is fixed. The time to achieve the steady state depends *only* on the elimination $T_{1/2}$ of the drug and is equal to approximately 5 half-lives of the drug. The dose itself will determine the *level* achieved during a steady state but not the time necessary to achieve it. With a dose of 25 mg/kg, the steady-state level is twice as high as that achieved with 12.5 mg/kg, because

$$\text{Concentration at steady state} = \frac{\text{dose (mg/kg hr}^{-1})}{\text{clearance}} \tag{9}$$

From this concept it is apparent that for any given dose schedule of an antimicrobial drug, the physician should allow the drug to achieve a steady-state level before assuming that the dose is too small or too large based on prematurely measured concentrations. However, in various cases, especially in the severely sick child, time is most valuable and it is often thought that the desired concentration should be achieved more quickly (26). In order to waver this lag time of 4–5 half-lives, a *loading dose* may be given. This initial dose will fill the distribution volume according to the formula

$$\text{Loading dose} = V_d\, C_{max} \tag{10}$$

It is important to realize that the concentration produced by a loading dose is determined by the distribution volume (V_d) whereas the steady-state concentration depends upon the clearance (Cl) [according to Eq. (9)].

III. THE CONCEPT OF COMPARTMENTS

Clinicians are often puzzled by the meaning and applicability of such terms as "one-compartment open model" or "two-compartment open model." These models represent attempts to describe mathematically the distribution and elimination of drugs. In most cases the researcher has a number of serum or plasma concentration values obtained at various time points after a dose. Figure 1(a) is the typical profile of a two-compartment open model following an intravenous bolus. Following the injection, concentrations are extremely high as all the drug is still in the blood. The rapid initial decrease in levels represents a distribution of the drug into a "peripheral" compartment. Simultaneously, elimination of the drug takes place (by the liver or kidney or any other eliminating organ from the blood). According to this model, there is equilibrium between the peripheral and central compartments; thus elimination of drug molecules from the blood prompts re-entry of molecules from the peripheral into the central compartment. It is important to stress that these mathematical compartments do not have an anatomic or physiological identity as is often believed. These models are, however, very useful for the calculation of pharmacokinetic parameters, such as bioavailability, V_d, clearance, and elimination $T_{1/2}$. Consequently, they are essential for the prediction of serum concentrations following the administration of an antimicrobial agent.

For the interested reader, several texts are recommended for a deeper insight into pharmacokinetic concepts (27-29).

REFERENCES

1. Hirsch, HH, Finland, M: Effect of food on the absorption of erythromycin propionate, erythromycin stearate and triacetyloleandomycin. *Am. J. Med. Sci. 237*: 693-699, 1959.
2. Pierpaeli, PG: Drug therapy and diet. *Drug. Intell. Clin. Pharm. 6*:89-99, 1972.
3. Klein, JO, Finland, M: Medical progress: The new penicillins. *N. Engl. J. Med. 269*: 1019-1024, 1963.
4. Doluisio, JT, La-Piana, JC, Vilkinson, GR, Ditter, LW: Pharmacokinetic interpretation of dicloxacillin levels in serum after extravascular administration. *Antimicrob. Agents Chemother. 9*:49-55, 1969.
5. Welling, PG: How food and fluid affect drug absorption. *Postgrad. Med. 62*:73-82, 1977.
6. Melander, A, Danielson, K, Hanson, A, Jansson, L, Renup, C, Schersten, B, Thulin, T, Whalin, E: Reduction of isoniazid bioavailability in normal men by concomitant intake of food. *Acta Med Scand. 20*:93-97, 1976.
7. Hurwitz, A, Schlozman, DL: Effects of antacids on gastrointestinal absorption of isoniazid in rat and man. *Am. Rev. Respir. Dis. 109*:41-44, 1974.
8. Acocella, G: Clinical pharmacokinetics of rifampicin. *Clin. Pharmacokinet. 3*:128-143, 1978.
9. Neuvonen, PJ: Interactions with the absorption of tetracyclines. *Drugs 11*:45-54, 1976.
10. Neu, HC: Antimicrobial activity and human pharmacology of amoxycillin. *J. Infect. Dis. 129 (Suppl)*:123, 1974.
11. Melander, A, Kahlmeter, G, Kamme, C, Ursing, B: Bioavailability of metronidazole in fasting and non-fasting healthy subjects and in patients with Crohn's disease. *Eur. J. Clin. Pharmacol. 12*:69-72, 1977.
12. Jordan, MC, de Moine, J, Kirby, W: Clinical pharmacology of pivampicillin as compared with ampicillin. *Antimicrob. Agents Chemother. 2*:438-441, 1970.
13. Bates, TR, Segueiras, Tembo, AV: Effect of food on nitrofurantoin absorption. *Clin. Pharmacol. Ther. 16*:63-68, 1974.
14. Crounse, RG: Effective use of griseofulvin. *Arch. Dermatol. 87*:176-180, 1963.
15. Malmborg, AS: Absorption of erythromycin stearate after oral administration. *Curr. Med. Res. Opin. 5 (Suppl. 2)*:15-18, 1978.
16. Goldfrank, LR: *Toxicologic Emergencies*, Appleton-Century-Crofts, New York, 1982.
17. Sjovall, J, Alvan, G, Westerlund, D: Dose-dependent absorption of amoxicillin and bacampicillin. *Clin. Pharmacol. Ther. 38*:241-250, 1985.
18. Dressman, JB, Fleister, D, Amidon, GL: Physicochemical model for dose-dependent drug absorption. *J. Pharm. Sci. 73*:1274-1279, 1984.
19. Florey, ME, Turton, EC, Duthie, ES: Penicillin in wound exudates. *Lancet 2*:405-409, 1946.
20. Bergeron, MG: Tissue penetration of antibiotics. *Clin. Chem.* 1986 (In Press).
21. Suh, B, Craig, WA, England, AC, Eliott, RL: Effect of free fatty acids on protein binding of antimicrobials. *J. Infect. Dis.* 1981.
22. Craig, WA, Welling, PG: Protein binding of antimicrobials. In: *Handbook of Clinical Pharmacokinetics* (M Gibaldi and L Prescott, eds.), ADIS Health Science Press, New York, 1983, pp. 55-74.
23. Craig, WA, Welling, PG, Wagnild, JP, Kunin, CM: Reduced protein binding of antimicrobial agents in serum of patients with impaired renal function. In: *Progress in*

Chemotherapy (Daikos, ed.), Hellenic Society of Chemotherapy, Athens, 1974, pp. 722–725.
24. Bergeron, MG, Bastille, A, Lessard, C, Gagnon, P: Significance of intrarenal concentrations of gentamicin for the outcome of experimental pyelonephritis in rats. *J. Infect. Dis. 146*:91–96, 1983.
25. Gold, H, De Graff, AC: Studies on digitalis in ambulatory cardiac patients: Newer principles of digitalis dosage. *JAMA 95*:1237–1243, 1930.
26. Rajgchot, P, Prober, CG, Soldins, Golas, C, Good, F, Harding, E, MacLeod, SM: Initiation chloramphenicol therapy in the newborn infant. *J. Pediatr. 101*:1018–1021, 1982.
27. Gibaldi, M, Perrier, D: *Pharmacokinetics*, Marcel Dekker, New York, 1982.
28. Gibaldi, M, Prescott, L (eds.): *Handbook of Clinical Pharmacokinetics*, ADIS Health Science Press, New York, 1983.
29. Benet, LZ, Massoud, N, Gambertoglio, JG: *Pharmacokinetic Basis of Drug Treatment*, Raven Press, New York.

Part II
Specific Aspects of Antimicrobial Therapy in the Pediatric Age Group

4

Clinical Pharmacology of Antimicrobial Drugs During Development: How Are Infants and Children Different?

GIDEON KOREN
The Hospital for Sick Children, and the University of Toronto, Toronto, Ontario, Canada

During the last few decades it has become apparent that infants and children are very different from adults in their disposition of and response to drugs. Yet information is almost always collected after the drug has been tried in adults. Moreover, the accumulation of these data in children is often slow and incomplete as ethical considerations hinder proper studies and in many cases the lack of micromethods for drug analysis in small volumes hampers detailed trials in infants and small children. Perinatal medicine now treats many high-risk, very low birth weight infants with combinations of antibiotics, and over the last decade this group has prompted very intensive research into the disposition of and response to antimicrobial drugs in preterm infants.

This chapter will review differences in disposition of antimicrobial drugs in infants and children. Developmental changes will be dealt here, but the effect of various disease states on the handling of antimicrobial drugs will be discussed in Chapter 5.

I. ABSORPTION

The two major determinants of gastrointestinal absorption, gastric acidity and gastric emptying time, are very different in the newborn infant compared with adults.

A. Gastric Acidity

At birth, gastric pH is in the neutral range (between 6 and 8) owing to the presence of alkaline amniotic fluids. It generally falls to a pH between 1 and 3 within 1 day. However, gastric acidity is poorly maintained in neonates. Only by 3 years of age does the production of acidity reach adult capacity (0.15 mEq per 10 kg per hr in neonates vs. 2 mEq per 10 kg per hr in adults following stimulation test) (1,2). These age-dependent changes closely correspond to the development of the gastric mucosa. The relatively alkaline milk consumed by the infant further decreases gastric acidity.

These differences in gastric pH have been shown to affect the absorption of several antimicrobial drugs. For example, oral penicillin, ampicillin, and nafcillins, which are all acid labile, achieve higher concentrations in neonates than in children or adults (3-6). Higher concentrations of these agents in neonates may also be due to lower elimination rates (see below). The relative contributions of these two mechanisms have yet to be defined.

On the other hand, the absorption of acidic drugs, such as nalidixic acid, is better in the nonionized form. In alkaline pH a larger fraction of the drug is ionized and therefore absorption is reduced in the small infant (7).

B. Gastric Emptying

In infants less than 6 months of age, gastric emptying is significantly slower than in older children and adults. In normal adults, gastric emptying is biphasic, with a rapid (10-20 min) phase followed by an exponentially slower phase. In the preterm infant, gastric emptying is slow and linear. The prolonged gastric emptying in the small infant (6-8 hr) may result in an unexpected rate and/or extent of absorption.

Theoretically, it may be expected that drugs that have relatively poor absorption in the adult may have an improved absorption rate owing to prolonged contact with the gastrointestinal mucosa secondary to slow gastric emptying. However, although data are limited, certain antibiotics, including amoxicillin, rifampin, chloramphenicol, and cephalosporins, demonstrate delayed and incomplete absorption in neonates and small infants (8-10). After birth, there is a gradual improvement of gastrointestinal absorption of drugs, and by 3 months of age absorption may be comparable to or even more complete than in adults (11).

C. Intramuscular Absorption

The bioavailability of antimicrobial drugs following intramuscular injection depends upon the perfusion in the area of injection, the rate of penetration of the drug through capillary endothelium, and the apparent volume into which the drug has been distributed. Several physiological factors distinguish neonates from older children and adults, including vasomotor instability, smaller muscular mass and subcutaneous fat, and a higher proportion of water. In addition, the pathologic states of hypovolemia, hypothermia, and hypoxemia may decrease perfusion and potentially decrease intramuscular bioavailability. Only sparse information exists comparing intramuscular administration of antimicrobial drugs in various age groups. It appears that the time needed to achieve peak concentration (T_{max}) is comparable for infants, children, and adults for aminoglycosides, ampicillin, and carbenicillin (11-14), whereas preterm infants have a delayed absorption of chloramphenicol, rifampicin, cephalexin, cephaloridine, and benzylpenicillin administered by the intramuscular route (10,11,15,16).

D. Percutaneous Absorption

Two major factors determine the rate and extent of percutaneous absorption and may cause excessive absorption of an agent applied to the skin in the neonate and small infants. The thickness of the epidermal stratum corneum is inversely related to absorption, whereas the state of skin hydration directly influences absorption. Several antiseptic agents have been implicated in cases of severe toxicity following percutaneous absorption in neonates. Hexachlorophene (PHisohex) was used routinely for many years for the "total body bath" against skin bacteria. It was first believed that absorption occurs only through wounds and burns; however, following cases of severe central nervous system (CNS) toxicity with generalized seizures in neonates with intact skin, it was found that in 3% of infants blood levels of hexachlorophene were comparable to those causing seizures in animals (17). Subsequently, the American Academy of Pediatrics recommended it not be used on extensive areas (18). Similarly, increased skin permeability was shown with boric acid when used as a skin antiseptic in infants. Owing to severe intoxications and the existence of safer and less penetrating antiseptic agents, it is now thought that boric acid should not be used at all.

II. DISTRIBUTION

Several determinants of antimicrobial distribution are markedly different in neonates and infants compared with adults. Some of these parameters, such as protein binding and compartmentalization of body water, change continuously during the first years of life, influencing the distribution of antimicrobial drugs.

A. Protein Binding

In general, protein binding of antimicrobials is lower in the newborn than in older children and adults. This is the result of lower albumin values, lower affinity of fetal albumin for drugs, and the existence of endogenous compounds, such as bilirubin, which compete for protein binding. Examples of antibiotics for which lower protein binding has been noted in neonates are ampicillin, benzylpenicillin, nafcillin, sulfaphenazole, sulfisoxazole and sulfamethoxyphrazine (3,19-21). Consequently, higher proportions of antimicrobial drugs are free to penetrate various tissue compartments, yielding higher distribution volumes.

B. Body Water

In the newborn infant, water makes up 70-75% of the body weight compared with 50-55% in adults, with a larger extracellular water component (40 vs. 20% of body weight in adults). There is less fat tissue, 15% compared with 20% of body weight in adults, and there is less muscle tissue (25%). These parameters affect the volume of distribution of drugs that are mainly distributed in body water and, to a lesser extent, the distribution of lipophilic drugs. Kanamycin, gentamicin, and amikacin have all been shown to have a larger distribution in neonates, and this tends to gradually decrease during childhood (11). These changes are explained mainly by changes in body water, as the aminoglycosides are minimally bound to plasma proteins.

Larger distribution volumes V_d in infants and small children mean that, following an equal dose (per body weight), a lower peak level will be produced in their blood compared with that of adults. However, during steady state, the *mean* serum concentration is independent of distribution according to the equation

$$\text{Mean concentration at steady state} = \frac{\text{dose (mg/kg}\cdot\text{hr)}}{\text{clearance}} \tag{1}$$

As will be discussed later, differences in drug clearance rates during infancy and childhood are likely to affect the mean steady-state concentration.

III. ELIMINATION

A. Hepatic Metabolism

Although almost all liver metabolic processes can be demonstrated even in the human fetus, their rates are by far slower in the newborn infant, especially if preterm, than in the older child and adult. The maturation of different phase 1 reactions (hydroxylation, deacetylation, oxidation, and so on) and phase 2 reaction (e.g., conjugation) may vary extensively. For almost all the antimicrobials studied that are metabolized by the liver, clearance rates are slower at birth. The deacetylation of rifampicin (9), glucuronidation of chloramphenicol (8), oxidation of nalidixic acid (7), and hydrolysis of clindamycin (22) appear to be much slower in newborn infants. Similarly, the clearance rate of tetracyclines appears to increase with age (23). The direct result of this immaturity of metabolic degradation of antimicrobial drugs is a prolonged $T_{1/2}$, as half-life is inversely correlated with clearance rate:

$$T_{1/2} = \frac{0.69\ V_d}{Cl} \tag{2}$$

Clinically this means that in the newborn and small infant antimicrobial drugs that are metabolically eliminated tend to stay for longer periods in the body. As a result, therapeutic levels and prevention of toxicity are achieved with lower unit doses and/or longer dose intervals. This issue is addressed as it relates to each agent and in the chapter dealing with therapeutic drug monitoring (Chapter 6).

B. Renal Elimination

Many antimicrobial drugs, including penicillins, cephalosporins, several sulfonamides, and the aminoglycosides, are eliminated unchanged by the kidney. All of them are filtrated in the glomerulus, whereas some of them are also reabsorbed and secreted by the tubular cell (e.g., penicillins, cephalosporins, and nitrofurantoins). At birth, both the glomerular filtration rate (GFR) and tubular secretion processes are reduced; however, filtration is relatively more developed. The preterm infant has fewer glomeruli than the full-term neonate, who in fact has the same number as an adult (24-27). The maturation process of kidney structure and function is associated with prolongation and maturation of the tubules, increase in renal blood flow, and improvement of the filtration coefficient. In addition, there is a shift in blood flow from the deeper to the more superficial nephrons. Improvement of the GFR depends on both gestational and postnatal age. Similarly, the rate of tubular secretion is impaired owing to poor perfusion and undeveloped energy supply. It generally takes 6-12 months for the various renal functions to reach adult values.

It is often assumed that drugs that are metabolically inactivated by the liver are not influenced by reduced renal function. However, in most cases the inactive metabolite is eliminated by filtration and/or tubular secretion in the kidney. With chloramphenicol, for example, the conjugated metabolite is mainly secreted by the renal tubules. Reduced tubular secretion in preterm infants may result in increased serum concentrations of the inactivated drug. Subsequently, due to intestinal β-glucuronidase hydrolysis of the inactive metabolite, increased enterohepatic recycling of the parent drug would result.

These dynamic principles are crucial in planning a rational dose schedule for antimicrobial drugs. In general, the preterm infant would need lower doses and/or longer dose intervals than the full-term infant to maintain similar steady-state concentrations.

The clinician must consider both the degree of maturation of renal function and possible disease or drug-induced impairment (e.g., aminoglycosides) of renal elimination of antimicrobial drugs. Methods for the estimation of renal functions are delineated in Chapter 6.

REFERENCES

1. MacLeod, SM, Radde, JC: Mechanisms of drug absorption and their development. In: *Textbook of Pediatric Clinical Pharmacology* (SM MacLeod and J Radde, eds.), PSG Publication Co., Littleton, Manitoba, 1985, pp. 17-31.
2. Yaffe, SJ, Jucham, MR: Perinatal pharmacology. *Annu. Rev. Pharmacol. 14*:219-238, 1974.
3. Marselli, PL: Clinical pharmacokinetics in neonates. *Clin. Pharmacokinet. 1*:82-98, 1976.
4. Huang, NN, High, RH: Comparison of serum levels following the administration of oral and parenteral preparation of penicillin to infants and children of various age groups. *J. Pediatr. 42*:657-668, 1953.
5. O'Connor, WJ, Warren, GH, Edrada, LS, Mandala, PS, Rosenman, SB: Serum concentrations of sodium nafaillin in infants during the perinatal period. *Antimicrob. Agents Chemother. 2*:220-222, 1965.
6. Silvers, J, Poole, JW: Serum concentrations of ampicillin in newborn infants after oral administration. *Pediatrics 51*:578-580, 1973.
7. R'Ohwedder, HJ, Simon, C, Kubler, W, Hohfnauer, M: Untesuchungen uber die pharmakokinetick von nalidixin sause bei kinder verschiedenen alten. *Z. Kinderchir. 109*:124-134, 1970.
8. Meissner, HC, Smith, AL: The current status of chloramphenical. *Pediatrics 64*:348-356, 1979.
9. Acocella, G: Clinical pharmacokinetics of rifampicin. *Clin. Pharmacokinet. 3*:108-127, 1978.
10. McCracken, GH, Ginsburg, CM, Clahsen, JC, Thomas, ML: Pharmacologic evaluation of orally administered antibiotics in infants and children: Effect of feeding on bioavailability. *Pediatrics 68*:738-743, 1978.
11. Morselli, PL, Morselli, RF, Bossi, L: Clinical pharmacokinetics in newborns and infants. In: *Handbook of Clinical Pharmacokinetics*, Section II, (M Gibaldi and L Prescott, eds.), 1983, pp. 98-141.
12. McCracken, GH, Chrane, DH, Thomas, ML: Pharmacologic evaluation of gentamicin in newborn infants. *J. Infect. Dis. 124 (Suppl.)*:S214-S223, 1971.
13. Paisley, JW, Smith, AL, Smith, DH: Gentamicin in newborn infants. Comparison of intramuscular and intravenous administration. *Am. J. Dis. Child. 126*:473-477, 1973.
14. Driessen, OMJ, Sorgedrager, N, Michel, MF, Kerrebijn, KF, Hermans, J: Pharmacokinetic aspects of therapy with ampicillin and kanamycin in newborn infants. *Eur. J. Clin. Pharmacol. 13*:449-457, 1978.
15. Tognoni, G: Antibiotics. In: *Drug Disposition During Development*, (PL Morselli, ed.), Spectrum, New York, 1977, pp. 123-217.
16. Rolewitcz, TF, Minkin, BL, Cooper, MJ, Anders, NW: Metabolic disposition of cephalotin and deacetylcepholatin in children and adults. *Clin. Pharmacol. Ther. 22*:928-935, 1977.

17. Arena, JM: *Poisoning*, Charles C Thomas, Springfield, Illinois, 1974, pp. 575–577.
18. Committee on Fetus and Newborn: *Standards and Recommendations for Hospital Care of Newborn Infants*, 5th ed., American Academy of Pediatrics, Evanston, Illinois, 1971.
19. Ehrnebo, M, Agurell, S, Jalling, B, Boreus, LO: Age differences in drug binding by plasma proteins: Studies on human foetuses, neonates and adults. *Eur. J. Clin. Pharmacol. 3*:189–193, 1971.
20. Krasner, J, Giacocia, GP, Yaffe, SJ: Drug-protein binding in the newborn infant. *Ann. N.Y. Acad. Sci. 226*:101–114, 1973.
21. Chignell, CF, Vesell, ES, Starkweather, DK, Berlin, CM: The binding of sulfaphenazole to feto-neonatal and adult human plasma albumin. *Clin. Pharmacol. Ther. 12*: 897–901, 1971.
22. Bell, MJ, Shackelford, P, Smith, R, Schroeder, K: Pharmacokinetics of clindamycin phosphate in the first year of life. *J. Pediatr. 105*:482–486, 1984.
23. Rane, A, Wilson, JT: Clinical pharmacokinetics in infants and children. In: *Handbook of Clinical Pharmacokinetics*, Section II (M Gibaldi and L Prescott, eds.), ADIS Health Sciences Press, New York, 1983, pp. 142–168.
24. Arant, BS: Developmental patterns of renal functional maturation compared in the human neonate. *J. Pediatr. 92*:705–712, 1978.
25. Barnett, HL, Hare, WK, McNamara, N, Hare, RS: Influence of postnatal age on kidney function of premature infants. *Proc. Soc. Exp. Biol. Med. 69*:55–67, 1948.
26. Leake, RD, Trygstad, CW: Glomerular filtration rate during the period of adaptation to extrauterine life. *Pediatr. Res. 11*:959–962, 1977.
27. Siegel, SR, Oh, W: Renal function as a marker of human fetal maturation. *Acta Paediatr. Scand. 65*:481–492, 1976.

5

Effect of Disease State and Organ Failure on Antimicrobial Disposition in Children*

JAMES B. BESUNDER, MICHAEL D. REED, AND JEFFREY L. BLUMER
Rainbow Babies and Childrens Hospital, and Case Western Reserve University School of Medicine, Cleveland, Ohio

Antibiotic selection is based initially on the organism(s) likely to be responsible for the illness and the antimicrobial activity of available agents. However, once an agent has been selected, determination of a dose and dosing interval must be based on knowledge of the biodisposition of the drug in the body. Drug biodisposition reflects a complex interplay between the physicochemical properties of the drug and a variety of host factors. For the pediatric patient, developmental changes in pharmacokinetic processes, as well as disease-induced physiologic perturbations, may profoundly influence these choices. Following previous chapters that have dealt with developmental aspects of drug disposition during infancy and childhood, the present chapter focuses on the effects of disease states and organ failure on the handling of antimicrobial agents in the pediatric age group.

I. DRUG ABSORPTION

Disease-associated alterations in drug absorption are among the derangements most often recognized (Table 1). Obviously, gastrointestinal diseases impact mostly on the absorption of orally administered agents. Malabsorption syndromes may impair both the rate and extent of drug absorption. The amount of drug absorbed influences the steady-state concentration; a reduced absorption rate will blunt the peak plasma concentration. Thus, therapeutic concentrations of antibiotics may not be achieved in patients with malabsorption syndromes when using standard dosing regimens.

Celiac disease and cystic fibrosis (CF) are the most common causes of chronic malabsorption in the pediatric age group (1). In the former, clinical symptoms are caused by gluten-induced mucosal damage in the small bowel. The effects of the disease on antibiotic absorption are variable (2). Sulfamethoxazole, trimethoprim, and cephalexin peak plasma concentrations have been reported to be increased, but the time to the peak con-

*With an Appendix (Adjustment of Antimicrobial Dosage Schedule in Renal Failure) by Gideon Koren.

Table 1 Disease States That Affect Gastrointestinal Absorption of Antibiotics

Celiac disease	Crohn's disease	Diarrhea
Short bowel syndrome	Pyloric stenosis	Thyroid dysfunction
Protein-calorie mulnutrition	Congestive heart failure	Cystic fibrosis

centration for amoxicillin is delayed. Parsons (3) also showed reduced absorption of the ampicillin ester pivampicillin, which may imply malabsorption of other penicillin esters. Abnormalities in celiac disease, such as increased mucosal permeability and increased intraluminal pH with a reduction in solubility of some drugs, as well as certain small bowel esterase deficiencies, may explain these variable effects on peak plasma concentrations.

CF is a relatively common cause of malabsorption in children. In a recently completed study at our institution by Dickenson et al. (4), the biodisposition of three forms of chloramphenicol, an oral capsule (CAP-base), the palmitate oral liquid (CAP-P), and the intravenous succinate ester (CAP-S) were evaluated in patients with CF. The CAP-P and CAP-S formulations require hydrolysis to liberate antimicrobially active chloramphenicol, the former by pancreatic lipase in the intestinal lumen, and the latter by hepatic esterases (5). The CAP-P peak concentration was significantly lower and the time to the peak concentration significantly delayed when compared with the other formulations. The biodisposition of the CAP-S and CAP-base forms were similar. These data suggest that pancreatic exocrine insufficiency may influence the bioavailability of antibiotics requiring hydrolysis by pancreatic enzymes.

Malabsorption in infants and children may also occur secondary to the short bowel syndrome. Massive resection of the bowel in a neonate may be required following necrotizing enterocolitis, malrotation with volvulus, or certain congenital anomalies of the gastrointestinal tract. In older infants and children, massive bowel resection may be required in some cases of intussusception or Crohn's disease. The magnitude of the absorptive defect depends upon the type of resection (1). Complications are unusual following extensive mid-small bowel resections, whereas significant malabsorption may follow the resection of smaller segments of the proximal or distal small bowel (1). Gastric hyperacidity is common after proximal small bowel resections (6), and therapy with antacids may interfere with the bioavailability of some oral antibiotics, such as isoniazid (2). This occurs with the aluminum hydroxide antacids and is due to a delay in gastric emptying.

Acute diarrhea may affect the rate and extent of antibiotic absorption by decreasing intestinal transit time, altering the mucosal absorptive surfaces, and/or by causing dehydration (2). This effect on antibiotic disposition has been demonstrated in pediatric patients with infectious diarrhea secondary to *Shigella* (7). Patients in this study received either ampicillin or nalidixic acid orally. Two distinct groups were identified, the "good absorbers" with normal absorption and the "poor absorbers," who had delayed and reduced peak plasma concentrations. The poor absorbers of ampicillin were statistically younger, had more severe diarrhea, and were less than the third percentile for weight.

Protein-calorie malnutrition (PCM), through a variety of pathophysiologic changes, may also result in perturbations in drug absorption (8). Some of these changes include delayed gastric emptying and increased intestinal transit time, pancreatic exocrine dysfunction with depressed enzyme activity, small intestinal malabsorption secondary to villous atrophy, and diarrhea secondary to infection or fat malabsorption (8). These effects are important since patients with PCM have a higher incidence of intercurrent infections and require frequent treatment with antibiotics (9).

Abnormalities seen in Crohn's disease have led to unpredictable effects on the disposition of oral antibiotics (2). These include a reduced surface area for drug absorption, thickened bowel wall, which may lead to reduced diffusion or malabsorption, and delayed intestinal transit time. Parsons and Paddock (10) showed disparate absorption rates of the components of the fixed drug combination trimethoprim-sulfamethoxazole in patients with Crohn's disease. These different absorption rates may affect the timing of the peak plasma concentrations and lead to a suboptimal plasma concentration ratio of the constituents, thus interfering with maximal antimicrobial activity.

Disorders of the stomach may also affect the absorptive process. Prolonged gastric emptying, as seen for example with pyloric stenosis (2), may delay or reduce the peak concentration of antibiotics. Achlorhydria, by affecting the antibiotic dissolution rate, may alter the bioavailability of phenoxymethylpenicillin and cephalexin, although the available data conflict (11,12).

There is little information available concerning the effect of liver disease on drug absorption. One can speculate, however, that drugs requiring micelle formation may have a low bioavailability in diseases associated with reduced bile flow.

II. EXTRAINTESTINAL DISEASES AFFECTING ANTIBIOTIC ABSORPTION

A. Cardiac

Congestive heart failure is a common complication of heart disease in children. Mucosal edema has been used to explain the impaired absorption in patients with heart failure although supportive evidence is lacking (13). Sympathetic tone is increased in patients with heart failure. This physiologic compensation may affect drug absorption by delaying gastric emptying time and by shunting blood flow away from visceral organs to the heart and brain.

B. Endocrine

Hypo- and hyperthyroidism may influence the rate and extent of drug absorption by prolonging or reducing intestinal transit time (14). However, there are no studies to date evaluating the effect of an altered thyroid state on antibiotic biodisposition. Predicting the overall effect of hypo- or hyperthyroidism on antibiotic disposition is further complicated by their secondary effects on metabolic activity and cardiac function.

C. Drug-Drug Interactions

Drug-drug interactions may also influence drug absorption. Cholestyramine, which is occasionally used in the management of diarrhea secondary to bile acid malabsorption, will reduce the absorption of cephalexin, trimethoprim, and clindamycin by binding these drugs in the intestinal lumen (2). The biocarbonate in antacids alters tetracycline solubility, and the Al^{3+}, Ca^{2+} and Mg^{2+} salts may chelate tetracycline (2).

III. CUTANEOUS DRUG ABSORPTION

Drug absorption may also occur through the skin. The amount absorbed through intact skin is generally insignificant; however, the absorption of topical antimicrobial agents is enhanced by damage to the integument. The review by Sawchuk and Rector (15) of the literature on the pharmacokinetics of topical and systemic drugs in burn patients shows variable absorption of such topical agents as mafenide acetate, povidone iodide, silver sulfadiazine, and gentamicin. The degree of absorption and hence the risk of toxicity probably depend upon the degree of the burn, the percentage of surface area involved, the amount of drug applied, and the hydration status of the patient (15). The risk of toxicity may also depend upon the underlying renal function of the patient.

The same principles should apply to most conditions in which the skin barrier has been violated. One must therefore exercise caution with the use of topical antimicrobial agents in other relatively common pediatric disease states, such as Stevens-Johnson syndrome, staphylococcal scalded skin syndrome, and toxic epidermal necrolysis.

IV. DRUG DISTRIBUTION

Drug distribution is influenced by the fraction of unbound drug in the circulation and tissues and by the size of the individual compartments into which a given drug distributes (Table 2). Albumin is the most important drug-binding protein in plasma. Although it binds both acidic and basic drugs, the former appear to be bound with greater affinity (16). Basic drugs may bind to albumin but will also bind to other plasma proteins, such as lipoprotein, α_1-acid glycoprotein, and gammaglobulin (17). A reduction in protein binding due to hypoproteinemia, qualitative changes in the binding protein, or displacement by endogenous ligands as seen in hyperbilirubinemic states or uremia (18) may increase the V_d of highly bound drugs. Since primary liver disease, cystic fibrosis, protein-losing enteropathies secondary to such conditions as celiac disease and the short bowel syndrome, and nephrotic syndrome can all lead to hypoproteinemia, these states may also be associated with altered antibiotic distribution.

Drugs that are extensively bound to hepatic ligands will have a smaller V_d in liver disease if tissue uptake is significantly affected (19). This may limit the increase in elimination half-life that would otherwise result from a decrease in hepatic clearance. Marshall et al. (20) reported findings consistent with this theory in a study on nafcillin disposition in patients with liver disease or extrahepatic biliary obstruction. The steady-state V_d was 27.1 liters in normal subjects compared with 19.93 liters in patients with cirrhosis and 15.85 liters in patients with extrahepatic biliary obstruction ($p < 0.05$). In contrast to the reduction in the V_d, there was a significant reduction in hepatic clearance in patients with biliary obstruction (435 ml/min in normal patients vs. 46 ml/min in cirrhotics vs.

Table 2 Disease States Affecting Drug Distribution

Decreased circulating plasma protein	Decreased protein affinity or displacement
Nephrotic syndrome	Uremia
Protein-calorie malnutrition	Hyperbilirubinemia
Short bowel syndrome	Drug-drug interactions
Celiac disease	Genetic alterations in albumin
Hepatic failure	Increased tissue water
Decreased intracellular binding	Congestive heart failure
Cirrhosis	Renal failure
Biliary obstruction	Liver failure with ascites

83 ml/min in patients with extrahepatic biliary obstruction). The overall effect on the elimination half-life was minimal even though there was a statistically significant difference between patients with extrahepatic biliary obstruction and controls (1.02 hr controls vs. 1.23 hr cirrhosis vs. 1.73 hr in extrahepatic obstruction).

Disease states that lead to expansion of the extracellular fluid space will increase the V_d of drugs that mainly distribute in this compartment. This may be of importance in edematous patients secondary to liver or renal disease or congestive heart failure (21). For example, aminoglycosides in the presence of ascites have an increased V_d (22).

V. EFFECT OF DISEASE ON HEPATIC DRUG METABOLISM AND ELIMINATION

The pharmacokinetics of antibiotics that undergo hepatic biotransformation and/or hepatobiliary elimination may be affected by diseases that affect hepatocyte function (Tables 3 and 4). Compromised function in the neonate may be secondary to viral infections, such as herpesvirus, echovirus, and andenovirus (1), overwhelming bacterial sepsis, inborn errors of metabolism, such as galactosemia, α_1-antitrypsin deficiency, tyrosinemia, and hereditary fructose intolerance, congenital heart disease associated with a low flow state, or fatty liver secondary to parenteral hyperalimentation (1). In older patients, non-A,non-B viral hepatitis is probably the most common cause of fulminant hepatic necrosis (1). Other causes of liver disease in the older patient include hepatitis B, cytomegalovirus, Epstein-Barr virus, graft-versus-host disease, and CF. Severe hepatic functional impairment may occur with overdoses of such drugs as acetaminophen and exposure to chemicals or naturally occurring plant toxins (*Amanita phalloides*) (1).

Since there are no tests that indicate the degree of hepatic impairment relative to drug absorption and disposition, it becomes difficult to predict empirically how a given hepatobiliary disease will affect the biodisposition of a specific drug. We will review several studies, mostly performed in adults, that evaluated antibiotic disposition in the face of compromised liver function.

Chloramphenicol is metabolized in the liver to inactive products. The primary metabolite is a glucuronide that is then eliminated by the kidney (23). Of an oral dose of chloramphenicol, 90% is recovered in the urine in 24 hrs with 5-10% of the dose excreted unchanged in the urine (23). Azzolini et al. (24) demonstrated a prolonged half-life in patients with cirrhosis. Koup et al. (23) demonstrated a lower total body clearance (TBC) in cirrhotic patients with total bilirubin concentrations >1.5 mg per 100 ml when compared with patients with normal liver function. They also showed a correlation between

Table 3 Disease States Affecting Drug Metabolism

Viral infections
Inborn errors in metabolism
Congestive heart failure
Bacterial sepsis
Cystic fibrosis
Protein-calorie malnutrition
Chemical intoxications

Table 4 Disease States Affecting Hepatobiliary Drug Excretion

Biliary tract obstruction
Hepatic cirrhosis
Cystic fibrosis
Protein-calorie malnutrition

the dose and serum concentration in patients with normal liver function. This relationship was not seen in patients with cirrhosis. The decreased clearance of chloramphenicol in liver disease may increase the plasma concentration and the risk of toxicity. Koup et al. (23) also reported a 23% reduction in protein binding, which increased the plasma free chloramphenicol concentration. However, since chloramphenicol clearance is capacity limited and binding insensitive, this probably is of little clinical significance except for the interpretation of plasma drug concentrations. Thus, in the presence of liver disease, there may exist antimicrobially significant free chloramphenicol concentrations in the plasma associated with "subtherapeutic" total plasma concentrations.

Slaughter et al. (25) did not find a correlation between total body or metabolic clearance of chloramphenicol and indices of hepatic function (SGOT, LDH, alkaline phosphatase, total bilirubin, and albumin), whereas Azzolini et al. (24) showed a significant correlation between chloramphenicol $t_{1/2\beta}$ and either serum albumin or total bilirubin. In summary, liver disease may impair chloramphenicol elimination so that reduced doses should be given and blood levels monitored carefully to avoid toxicity.

Clindamycin clearance is capacity limited and binding sensitive such that hepatic clearance is dependent both on the fraction of free drug delivered to the liver and the intrinsic rate of conversion to its major metabolites desmethylclindamycin and clindamycin sulfoxide (26). Hinthorn et al. (27) reported significantly higher clindamycin concentrations in patients with cirrhosis versus controls, but not in patients with acute or chronic hepatitis. The $t_{1/2\beta}$ was 2.5 hr in patients with cirrhosis versus 1.8 hr in normal patients. In addition, there was no significant accumulation of clindamycin noted after three doses given every 12 hr, and no patient suffered an exacerbation of underlying disease. In conclusion, clindamycin appears to be safe in acute and chronic hepatitis but should be used cautiously in patients with significant liver disease since hepatotoxicity from clindamycin is dose related.

Only a few β-lactam antibiotics are metabolized in the liver. Hepatic clearance of nafcillin is reduced with liver disease, although the $t_{1/2\beta}$ is not prolonged. This is most likely due to an increase in renal excretion of nafcillin. Marshall et al. (20) found an increase in urinary excretion of nafcillin from 30 to 50% in the patients with liver disease or extrahepatic biliary obstruction.

Of a dose of cefotaxime, 40–50% is metabolized to an active desacetyl form, which is then cleared by the kidneys along with its inactive metabolites (19). Wise et al. (28) demonstrated reduced formation of the desacetyl derivative with liver dysfunction, although significant drug accumulation and $t_{1/2\beta}$ prolongation occurred only with severe renal impairment (Cl_{Cr} <10 ml/min). These authors recommended reducing the dose and increasing the dosing interval to every 12 hr in patients with severe renal impairment owing to the extreme variability in $t_{1/2\beta}$.

The effect on other cephalosporins that are desacetylated, such as cephalothin, although not studied, is also likely to be small. In addition, desacetylating enzymes are found in the kidney and other tissues (19).

Studies have demonstrated longer half-lives for isoniazid (29) and rifampin (29,30) in patients with liver disease. Isoniazid is eliminated via acetylation in the liver and rifampin by desacetylation and subsequent excretion in the urine and bile. However, since the prolonged half-lives are still far shorter than the dosing intervals, changes need only be made in the face of severe liver impairment or when the drugs themselves are responsible for the liver disease.

Changes in the hepatic metabolism of antibiotics have also been documented in malnourished children. Mehta et al. (9) evaluated chloramphenicol disposition in 10 infants with PCM and 4 normal infants following an oral dose of 25 mg/kg of body weight. The normal children had a mean peak serum concentration of 17.8 μg/ml (range, 15.0-20.4) 2 hr postdose, compared with peak levels of 21.3 μg/ml (range 17-52 μg/ml) 4-6 hr postdose in patients with PCM. Repeat studies in 5 children with PCM following 4-8 weeks of nutritional rehabilitation showed improvement in peak serum levels and half-lives toward normal.

Of significance is the altered pattern of chloramphenicol metabolism seen in malnourished patients. In the patients with PCM, only 35-55% of the chloramphenicol recovered in the urine was conjugated compared with 75-80% in normal patients. Nutritional rehabilitation was again associated with a significant increase in the urinary recovery of the conjugated chloramphenicol metabolites. The implications of these data are twofold: (1) the longer time to achieve peak serum concentrations is probably due to a slower rate of absorption, and (2) the higher peak concentration reflects reduced hepatic metabolism of chloramphenicol. In fact, electron microscopic alterations in the endoplasmic reticulum in humans with PCM have been demonstrated (31). Cefoperazone is primarily eliminated in the bile and its $t_{1/2\beta}$ is prolonged in patients with severe liver disease (32,33), whereas its $t_{1/2\beta}$ in functionally anephric patients is similar to that of patients with normal renal function (34). Greenfield et al. (32) reviewed the pharmacokinetics of cefoperazone in normal patients and in patients with hepatic or renal dysfunction. They reported a two- to fourfold increase in the $t_{1/2\beta}$ of cefoperazone in patients with severe biliary tract obstruction or cirrhosis. This is similar to the results in the study by Boscia et al. (33) in which the mean half-life in patients with cirrhosis was 4.5 hr compared with 1.5 hr in normal controls. Boscia et al. (33) also reported significantly lower serum concentrations, a higher V_d, and a larger percentage of renal excretion (50 vs. 21%). The lower serum concentration was due to the larger V_d, which reflected the increased extracellular fluid space secondary to ascites, and to a reduction in protein binding. The longer half-life was a consequence of reduced biliary excretion. These pharamacokinetic alterations were all confirmed by Greenfield et al. (32). The prolongation of the half-life of cefoperazone was limited by the increased renal excretion of the drug. Since cefoperazone is highly protein bound, a reduction in binding will increase the fraction of free drug available for elimination by glomerular filtration. In fact, three patients studied by Greenfield et al. (32) had relatively complete biliary tract obstruction. Of the dose of cefoperazone, 90% was recovered in the urine within 24 hr in these patients. Also, urinary recovery of the drug was directly related to the extent of hyperbilirubinemia, which displaces ceforperazone from its albumin binding sites (5). It should also be noted that the biliary concentrations of cefoperazone were still potentially therapeutic in patients with severe biliary tract obstruction. Dosage modification is only necessary if there is concomitant renal dysfunction since the half-life of cefoperazone in patients with liver disease is still much less than the every 12-hr dosing interval.

Although similar studies have not been performed in children, we expect the pharmacokinetics to be altered similarly in pediatric diseases, such as extrahepatic biliary atresia, or diseases causing severe intrahepatic cholestasis, such as inborn errors of metabolism, or Allagille's syndrome. However, further studies to substantiate this claim are needed.

Ceftriaxone is a capacity-limited, binding-sensitive, third-generation cephalosporin that has been studied in patients with hepatic functional impairment (35,36). It is extensively protein bound and distributes throughout the extracellular fluid compartment. Of a dose, 30-60% is eliminated in the bile; renal elimination is solely by glomerular filtration. The $t_{1/2\beta}$ of 8 hr in adults and 4-5 hr in children is due to the extensive protein binding and absence of renal tubular secretion. Therefore, a reduction in biliary elimination or albumin synthesis may alter its biodisposition in liver disease. Stoeckel et al. (35) studied the pharmacokinetics in 8 normal subjects and 15 patients with liver disease; 5 with alcoholic fatty liver, 4 with cirrhosis, and 6 with cirrhosis and ascites. They demonstrated a decrease in protein binding with an increase in free drug concentration in the groups with liver disease. However, the V_d was only greater in the group with ascites. The half-lives in all three groups were similar. The steady-state concentration of free drug increased by only 50–100% in patients with liver disease but up to 600% with concomitant renal impairment. Therefore, the dose need only be adjusted in patients with both hepatic and renal dysfunction. Stoeckel and Koup (36) did not find significant changes in TBC, V_d, or $t_{1/2\beta}$ in patients with liver disease. The $t_{1/2\beta}$ was 9.7 hr in cirrhotics with ascites compared with 8 hr in normal subjects.

Hepatic elimination of other penicillins, such as ampicillin (37) and carbenicillin (38), is not markedly affected by liver disease alone, and no dosing adjustments are necessary.

Brown et al. (39) found a prolonged elimination $t_{1/2\beta}$ (2.6 vs. 37 hr) and a lower rate of TBC (162 vs. 48 ml/min) for vancomycin in patients with impaired liver function when compared with normal subjects. The $t_{1/2\beta}$ did not correlate with the severity of liver impairment, and these changes were not due to decreased protein binding since patients in both groups were hypoalbuminemic. Although this study examined renal function, it did not measure vancomycin concentration in the urine, so that altered renal excretion could not be assessed. In addition, all these patients had leukemia or cancer with sepsis, which may alter drug disposition (39). Therefore, more data on vancomycin disposition in liver disease are needed before recommending dosage adjustments.

Finally, tissue hypoxia and passive congestion secondary to congestive heart failure may compromise hepatic function and reduce the clearance of drugs dependent on the liver for metabolism.

VI. EFFECT OF RENAL DISEASE ON DRUG ELIMINATION

It is important to quantitate a patient's renal function so that predictions of antimicrobials that are renally eliminated can be made. A Cl_{Cr} determination is preferable to a serum creatinine as an indicator of renal function in children. Because of their reduced muscle mass, children have lower serum creatinine concentrations than adults. This may explain, for example, the higher ratio of gentamicin $t_{1/2\beta}$ to creatinine seen in children. However, a serum creatinine determination is more practical. A table listing antimicrobial dose adjustments in renal failure appears in the Appendix.

Vancomycin is eliminated by the kidneys and is excreted unchanged in the urine. Moellering et al. (40) constructed a dosing nomogram for nondialysis patients with renal impairment. The nomogram is based on their study, which showed an excellent correlation between Cl_{Cr} and clearance of vancomycin. Vancomycin is not cleared by dialysis.

Aminoglycosides are not metabolized and are eliminated in the urine solely by glomerular filtration. Dosage modifications are necessary in renal impairment, and because of their narrow therapeutic index, blood levels need to be monitored carefully. Sirinaven et al. (41) studied gentamicin pharmacokinetics in children with renal failure. They demonstrated a highly significant linear correlation between gentamicin half-life and serum creatinine. Linear regression analysis indicated the $t_{1/2\beta}$ was 3.8 times the serum creatinine concentration. These authors suggest using one-half the normal dose every half-life, or three-quarters the normal dose every 2 half-lives, or a full dose every 3 half-lives. A comibnation of dose reduction and/or interval extension is most practical clinically. This avoids low peak levels when using lower doses at normal intervals and avoids long periods of subtherapeutic concentrations that are possible when using normal doses at extended intervals. Since the aminoglycosides are less than 5% bound to plasma proteins, a significant percentage of a dose is removed by hemodialysis or peritoneal dialysis (42). Therefore, supplemental doses are necessary following dialysis. A similar correlation between renal function and half-life was demonstrated by Lanao et al. (43) for amikacin in children.

The calculated $t_{1/2\beta}$ of aminoglycosides depends upon the cumulative dose of drug received. Blaser et al. (44) showed that the half-life of amikacin with the first dose is a function of both renal elimination and tissue accumulation, mainly by the kidneys. These tissue sites are rapidly saturated, so that by the time steady state is reached (5 half-lives), the $t_{1/2\beta}$ is dependent only upon renal elimination. In patients with renal insufficiency, Blaser et al. (44) saw a rise in $t_{1/2\beta}$ between the first dose and last dose of amikacin from 11.2 to 21.5 hr compared with 2.27 and 2.33 hr in patients with normal renal function.

In functionally anephric patients, the $t_{1/2\beta}$ for clindamycin may be altered. Since this may lead to serum concentrations two times normal (45), serum concentrations should be monitored in these patients. The $t_{1/2\beta}$ of lincomycin (45) is prolonged to a greater extent in functionally anephric patients for 10-13 hr compared with 4-5 hr in normal renal function (45) so that dosage adjustment is necessary in anephric patients. Lincomycin is also not removed by dialysis.

Most tetracyclines accumulate in the body in renal failure, except minocycline, which is eliminated primarily by enterohepatic mechanisms (46,47). Macdonald et al. (46) found the highest concentration of minocycline following oral administration in the tissues of the intestinal tract, liver, gallbladder, and bile, with only 9% of the total dose excreted in the urine, thus suggesting a role for the hepatobiliary system in its excretion.

Heaney and Eknoyan (47) demonstrated an independent relationship between minocycline clearance and renal function. In the same study, they demonstrated a prolonged $t_{1/2\beta}$ for doxycycline in patients with Cl_{Cr} <5 ml/min. Of a dose of doxyclycline, 57% was excreted in the urine within 72 hr in normal patients compared with 2% in the patients with severe renal failure. Compensation by enterohepatic mechanisms limits the reduction in doxycycline clearance seen in renal failure. Whelton et al. (48) provide evidence for transmucosal diffusion of doxycycline from the bloodstream into the intestinal lumen and excretion into the feces. However, owing to a greatly prolonged $t_{1/2\beta}$ in patients with severe renal impairment, the dosing interval should be increased to 24 hr when the Cl_{Cr} is <10 ml/min. Neither minocycline nor doxycycline is removed by dialysis.

The urinary tract antiseptics, methenamine, mandelamine, nalidixic acid, and nitrofurantoin, should be avoided in patients with renal failure (42). These drugs are ineffective in renal failure and may exacerbate gastrointestinal symptoms or cause a metabolic acidosis (nalidixic acid) or peripheral sensory neuropathy (nitrofurantoin) due to accumulation of parent drug and metabolites (42).

Most penicillins are renally excreted, and therefore, dosage modifications are often suggested in the face of severe renal impairment (Cl_{Cr} <10 ml/min). However, only a few clinical studies have been performed in children. Arancibia et al. (49) evaluated the pharmacokinetics of penicillin in patients with renal failure. This study demonstrated the prolonged $t_{1/2\beta}$ and reduced TBC of parenteral and oral amoxicillin in patients with renal impairment. The $t_{1/2\beta}$ in normal patients was 1.1 hr. Patients with a mean Cl_{Cr} of 49 ml/min (range, 39-60) had a $t_{1/2\beta}$ of 1.5 hr. The $t_{1/2\beta}$ of patients with a mean Cl_{Cr} of 20 ml/min (range, 7-19) was 7.4 hr, and a $t_{1/2\beta}$ of 10.7 hr was observed in patients with a mean Cl_{Cr} of 5 ml/min (range, 1-8). Dialysis patients had a $t_{1/2\beta}$ of 2.3 hr. The dose modification necessary could be calculated from the following equation:

$$B = 0.516Cl_{Cr} + 0.0149 \qquad r = 0.97$$

where B is the elimination rate constant. Again, the $t_{1/2\beta}$ was not significantly affected until the Cl_{Cr} approached 20 ml/min. The results of this study also support the use of a supplemental dose of ampicillin following hemodialysis (42,49). Penicillin may also require supplemental dosing following hemodialysis (42,49); ticarcillin and carbenicillin require supplemental doses after both hemodialysis and peritoneal dialysis (42).

Several studies have examined the disposition of the acylureidopenicillins in patients with various degrees of renal impairment (50–57). Of a dose of azlocillin, a capacity-limited antibiotic that exhibits dose-dependent pharmacokinetics, 60–75% is excreted unchanged in the urine (51). The $t_{1/2\beta}$ in patients with normal renal function increases with the use of higher doses. This is due to reduced renal and nonrenal clearance. The relatively lower renal clearance with increased dose suggests that active renal tubular secretion of azlocillin is capacity limited. In patients with renal impairment, the renal clearance of azlocillin is appreciably reduced only at Cl_{Cr} <30 ml/min. The use of the drug in patients with renal failure is limited by the capacity of the nonrenal pathways to eliminate the drug. In end-stage renal disease, the $t_{1/2\beta}$ ranges from 2.5 to 6 hr. Because of the apparent dose-dependent clearance exhibited by the drug, dosage nomograms must deal separately with each dose size given to a patient.

Whelton et al. (52) studied azlocillin disposition in patients undergoing hemodialysis or peritoneal dialysis. With hemodialysis, 8.4% of the total drug dose was removed each hour compared with 5.4% of the total dose in 7.5 hr of peritoneal dialysis. Therefore, supplemental dosing may be required only following hemodialysis.

Mezlocillin (55) and piperacillin (56,57) exhibit pharmacokinetic properties similar to those of azlocillin in patients with renal impairment, including dose-dependent kinetics. Dosage adjustments in patients with renal failure and supplementation following hemodialysis should be undertaken as described for azlocillin (42). Despite the profound effects of renal failure on the elimination of these drugs, the acylureidopenicillins achieve sufficient urinary concentrations to treat most urinary tract pathogens (54) in patients with renal impairment. This is in contrast to amoxicillin and ampicillin, of which higher doses may be necessary in patients with end-stage renal disease (42).

Like the penicillins, most of the cephalosporins are eliminated via the kidney and may require dosage adjustments in the presence of renal impairment. Cefazolin, a first-generation cephalosporin, has been studied in children with renal failure. Hiner et al. (58) demonstrated a prolongation in $t_{1/2\beta}$ with decreasing Cl_{Cr}. The effect was most pronounced when the Cl_{cr} <50 ml/min. The $t_{1/2\beta}$ is variably prolonged in patients undergoing hemodialysis (58); however, a significant amount of drug is cleared during hemodialysis, and a supplemental dose following hemodialysis may be warranted (42,58).

The second-generation cephalosporins are also eliminated primarily by the kidneys. The TBC and renal clearance of cefuroxime parallel the Cl_{Cr} (59). The dose must be reduced in patients with Cl_{Cr} <20 ml/min (59). Supplemental doses are needed following both hemodialysis and peritoneal dialysis (42). Regardless of the severity of the renal disease, cefuroxime urinary concentrations are adequate to treat most urinary tract pathogens (59).

Cefoxitin is a cephamycin that is 75% protein bound, and up to 80% of the drug is eliminated by tubular secretion (60). Kampf et al. (60) demonstrated a significant prolongation of the $t_{1/2\beta}$ and reduction in TBC when the Cl_{Cr} was <40 ml/min. Although the clearance of para-aminohippurate (Cl_{PAH}) was the best indicator of cefoxitin clearance, Cl_{Cr} should guide changes in dosing since the latter is more readily available. The dosing interval should be increased from 6-8 hr with $Cl_{Cr} < 40$ ml/min to 12 hr with $Cl_{Cr} = 20–40$ ml/min, to 24 hr with $Cl_{Cr} = 10–20$ ml/min, and to 48 hr with $Cl_{Cr} = 5–10$ ml/min (60). Supplemental dosing is required after hemodialysis but not peritoneal dialysis (42).

The disposition of many third-generation cephalosporins in renal functional impairment has been studied in adults (34–36,61–66). Most of these agents, except cefoperazone and ceftriaxone, are mainly eliminated by the kidney and require dosage modification in patients with compromised renal function. Of a dose of ceftriaxone, 30–60% is cleared in the bile (34), and dose adjustments in most patients are unnecessary. The half-life is increased to 8–12 hr in anephric patients (35). There is great variability in clearance and $t_{1/2\beta}$ in patients with $Cl_{Cr} < 5$ ml/min, and plasma levels should be monitored. The V_d is unchanged, and ceftriaxone is not removed by dialysis (66).

There is excellent correlation between ceftazidime clearance and Cl_{Cr} (61–63), since ceftazidime is eliminated solely by glomerular filtration. Welage et al. (61) recommended a 12-hr dosing interval if the Cl_{Cr} is 30-50 ml/min, a 24-hr interval if the Cl_{Cr} is 15-30 ml/min, and 36–48 hr or one-half the dose every 24 hr if the $Cl_{Cr} < 15$ ml/min. A repeat dose may be needed following hemodialysis (62).

Cefotaxime, as described earlier, is desacetylated in the liver to an active metabolite that has 1/10 the activity of cefotaxime (64). Matzke et al. (65), in the most recent review of cefotaxime kinetics in renal impairment, recommended multiplying the normal dosing interval by 1.5, 2.0, and 3.0 for patients with Cl_{Cr} of 60, 30, and 10 ml/min, respectively.

Tissue hypoxia and hypotension secondary to congestive heart failure may also compromise renal function and reduce the clearance of drugs dependent upon the kidney for elimination. This should be considered when selecting a drug dose and dosing interval.

A. Renal Elimination During Protein-Calorie Malnutrition

The influence of PCM on renal function was demonstrated by Mehta et al. (9), who showed that malnourished children had slower rates of total chloramphenicol urinary excretion and that this improved with nutritional repletion. Buchanan et al. (67) found a similar prolongation of penicillin urinary excretion in malnourished children. However, renal function and free drug concentrations were not monitored.

B. Renal Elimination in Burn Trauma

Burn trauma may have variable effects on renal function (15). Renal impairment, with reduced Cl_{Cr}, may occur secondary to acute tubular necrosis (68). Several studies, however, have demonstrated increased creatinine clearances in burn patients (69–71). Loirat et al. (69) found elevated glomerular filtration rates in 13 of 20 burn patients. They also demonstrated a shortened $t_{1/2\beta}$ for tobramycin in burn patients (69), as did Zaske et al. in their studies on the pharmacokinetics of gentamicin (70) and amikacin (71) in burn patients.

Elimination of drugs via the skin may also occur in burn patients (72). Glew et al. (72) found 20% of a daily dose of gentamicin in wound dressings of an adolescent with 45% body surface area burns. They suggested that this route of elimination may be more significant in small infants and children owing to the higher ratio of surface area to volume.

VII. EFFECTS OF CYSTIC FIBROSIS ON ANTIMICROBIAL ELIMINATION

The pharmacokinetics of many antibiotics have been shown to be different in patients with CF compared with unaffected individuals. Studies consistently demonstrate lower serum concentrations, a larger V_d, and a more rapid TBC of antibiotics in patients with CF, including the aminoglycosides (73-76), ceftazidime (77), trimethoprim-sulfamethoxazole (78), and the penicillin derivatives cloxacillin, dicloxacillin (79,80), and methicillin (81). One of the first studies to examine antibiotic disposition in CF was in 1975 by Jusko et al. (79). Their 10 CF patients and 8 normal patients were given a single oral dose of 6.25 mg/kg of dicloxacillin. Peak serum concentrations were achieved in both groups at about 1 hr postdose. The urinary recovery of dicloxacillin in CF patients was equal to or greater than that in normal controls. Both these results suggest normal absorption of the drug in CF; however, the peak serum concentrations in the CF patients were 2 1/2 times lower than the controls. Dicloxacillin is highly protein bound, but the lower serum concentrations were not due to decreased binding since there was no statistically significant difference in the percentage of bound drug between the two groups. Jusko proposed the major reason for the lower peak levels was probably an increased renal clearance of dicloxacillin in the CF patients, which averaged three times the renal clearance seen in normal patients.

Spino et al. (80) also studied cloxacillin absorption and disposition in 16 patients with CF and 12 controls. All patients received one dose orally and then intravenously. The doses were separated by 2 days. Following the intravenous dose, the CF patients had a significantly lower mean concentration. This was due to a statistically significant increase in TBC and in V_d (78 and 38%, respectively). There was no difference in protein binding between the two groups. The CF patients also had lower mean serum levels following the oral administration of cloxacillin. Bioavailability was more variable in the CF patients, but there was no significant difference between the two groups. The greater TBC in CF patients was due to a 2 1/2-fold larger nonrenal clearance of cloxacillin. The authors conclude that an increase in the nonrenal clearance of cloxacillin is responsible for the lower serum levels and the increased clearance may be a result of increased biotransformation.

Yaffe et al. (81) compared intravenous methicillin disposition in patients with CF and young adult volunteers. The results demonstrated lower serum concentrations in CF patients in association with significantly higher TBC and renal clearance rates ($p < 0.05$ and $p < 0.01$, respectively). There was no difference in the V_d.

Levy et al. (74) prospectively compared the pharmacokinetics of tobramycin in patients with CF and in age-matched controls. Aminoglycosides are eliminated by the kidney by glomerular filtration, but tubular reabsorption does occur (74). Patients with CF had a significantly higher TBC of tobramycin than did controls (20%) without a corresponding difference in renal clearance between the two groups. There was also no significant change in TBC in either group following water overload, indicating the lower TBC in the control group was not due to a greater amount of tubular reabsorption. When these data were normalized to body surface area, there was not a significantly larger V_d in patients with CF. This study suggests that extrarenal clearance of tobramycin is significant in CF patients and that dosages of tobramycin should be increased by approximately 20% in patients with CF. In another study by Hsu et al. (75), the TBC of tobramycin in patients with CF increased with the age of the patient. Significant differences were demonstrated for $t_{1/2\beta}$, V_d, TBC, and K_d between infants less than 12 months of age and patients 5-27 years old. In addition to requiring higher doses of tobramycin, the data suggested that the majority of CF patients may also require shorter dosing intervals (every 4 hr) owing to a shortened mean $t_{1/2\beta}$ of 1.0-1.5 hr.

In summary, there is strong evidence to suggest increased TBC of many antibiotics in patients with cystic fibrosis. Some studies have concluded that this observation is the result of increased renal clearance, but the results are not consistent. On the other hand, an increase in nonrenal clearance in CF is supported by studies evaluating the biodisposition of theophylline (82), cimetidine (83), and trimethoprim-sulfamethoxazole (78) in patients with CF. Of note, all of these undergo primarily hepatic elimination.

VIII. SUMMARY

The rational dosing of drugs in pediatric patients has been hampered by both a lack of understanding of the impact of organ development on drug biodisposition and the paucity of information concerning the modification of these biodisposition parameters in the presence of diseases. During the last two decades, research has been concentrated on the newborn. As a result, there is now a significant data base that can be employed to describe the handling of a number of therapeutic agents by the normal and preterm newborn infant. However, outside the newborn period, the fundamental determinants of drug biodisposition have not been well defined.

Only limited attempts have been made to ascertain the impact of the combined effects of organ dysfunction and functional ontogeny on drug biodisposition. Thus, predictions regarding the effect of systemic illness on antimicrobial pharmacokinetics remain largely empirical. Although some of the problems may occur infrequently (e.g., inborn errors in metabolism), and therefore preclude a rigorous evaluation of their impact on antimicrobial therapeutics, others occur with an incidence that mandates thorough pharmacokinetic investigation.

REFERENCES

1. Silverman, A, Roy, C (eds.): Malabsorption syndrome. In: *Pediatric Clinical Gastroenterology*, 3rd ed., C. V. Mosby Co., St. Louis, 1983, pp. 265, 290, 655.
2. Parsons, RL: Drug absorption in gastrointestinal disease with particular reference to malabsorption syndromes. *Clin. Pharmacokinet. 2*:45–60, 1977.
3. Parsons, RL, Hossack, GA, Paddock, GM: The absorption of antibiotics in adult patients with coeliac disease. *J. Antimicrob. Chemother. 1*:39–50, 1975.
4. Dickenson, CJ, Reed, MD, Stern, RC, Aronoff, SC, Yamashita, TS, Blumer, JL: Chloramphenicol biodisposition in cystic fibrosis. *Pediatr. Res. 18*:151A, 1984.
5. Ambrose, PJ: Clinical pharmacokinetics of chloramphenicol and chloramphenicol succinate. *Clin. Pharmacokinet. 9*:222–238, 1984.
6. Hamilton, JR: Short small intestine. In: *Nelson's Textbook of Pediatrics*, 12th ed. (WE Nelson, RD Behrman, and VC Vaughan, eds.), W. B. Saunders Co., Philadelphia, 1983, p. 932.
7. Nelson, JD, Shelton, S, Kusmiesz, HT, Haltalin, KC: Absorption of ampicillin and nalidixic acid by infants and children with acute shigellosis. *Clin. Pharmacol. Ther. 13*:879–886, 1972.

8. Krishnaswamy, K: Drug metabolism and pharmacokinetics in malnutrition. *Clin. Pharmacokinet. 3*:216–240, 1978.
9. Mehta, S, Kalsi, HK, Jayaraman, S, Mathur, VS: Chloramphenicol metabolism in children with protein-calorie malnutrition. *Am. J. Clin. Nutr. 28*:977–981, 1975.
10. Parsons, RL, Paddock, GM: Absorption of two antibacterial drugs, cephalexin and co-trimoxazole, in malabsorption syndromes. *J. Antimicrob. Chemother. 1 (Suppl.)*: 59–67, 1975.
11. Davies, JA, Strangeways, JEM, Holt, JM: Absorption of cephalexin from the gastro-intestinal tract in diseased subjects. *Postgrad. Med. J. 46 (Suppl.)*:16–19, 1970.
12. Davies, JA: Absorption of cephalexin in diseased and aged subjects. *J. Antimicrob. Chemother. 1 (Suppl.)*:69–70, 1975.
13. Benowitz, NL, Meister, W: Pharmacokinetics in patients with cardiac failure. *Clin. Pharmacokinet. 1*:182–200, 1976.
14. Shenfield, GM: Influence of thyroid dysfunction on drug pharmacokinetics. *Clin. Pharmacokinet. 6*:275–297, 1981.
15. Sawchuck, RJ, Rector, TS: Drug kinetics in burn patients. *Clin. Pharmacokinet. 5*: 548–556, 1980.
16. MacLeod, SM, Radde, IC: Mechanisms of drug absorption and their development. In: *Textbook of Pediatric Clinical Pharmacology* (SM MacLeod and IC Radde, ed.), PSG Publishing Co., Littleton, Massachusetts, 1985, pp. 17–43, 56–71, 109.
17. Borga, O, Piafsky, KM, Nilsen, G: Plasma protein binding of basic drugs. *Clin. Pharmacol. Ther. 22*:539–544, 1977.
18. Boreus, LO: *Principles of Pediatric Pharmacology*, Monographs in Clinical Pharmacology (DL Azarnoff, ed.), Vol. 6, Churchill Livingstone, New York, 1982, pp. 48–49, 95, 117–118, 146.
19. Turnidge, JD, Craig, WA: β-Lactam pharmacology in liver disease. *J. Antimicrob. Chemother. 11*:499–501, 1983.
20. Marshall, JP, Salt, WB, Elam, RO, Wilkinson, GR, Schenker S: Disposition of nafcillin in patients with cirrhosis and extra hepatic biliary obstruction. *Gastroenterology 73*:1388–1392, 1977.
21. Williams, RL, Benet, LZ: Drug pharmacokinetics in cardiac and hepatic disease. *Annu. Rev. Pharmacol. Toxicol. 20*:389–413, 1980.
22. Lanao, JM, Dominguez-Gil, A, Macias, JG, Diez, JL, Nieto, MJ: The influence of ascites on the pharmacokinetics of amikacin. *Int. J. Clin. Pharmacol. Ther. Toxicol. 18*:57–61, 1980.
23. Koup, JR, Lou, AH, Brodsky, B, Slaughter, RL: Chloramphenicol pharmacokinetics in hospitalized patients. *Antimicrob. Agents Chemother. 15*:651–657, 1979.
24. Azzolini, F, Gozzaniga, A, Lodola, E, Natangelo, R: Elimination of chloramphenicol and thiamphenicol in subjects with cirrhosis of the liver. *Int. J. Clin. Pharmacol. 6*: 1059–1065, 1972.
25. Slaughter, RL, Pieper, JA, Cerra, RB, Brodsky, B, Koup, JR: Chloramphenicol sodium succinate kinetics in critically ill patients. *Clin. Pharmacol. Ther. 28*:69–77, 1980.
26. Lesar, TS, Zaske, DE: Antibiotics and hepatic disease. *Med. Clin. North Am. 66*: 257–266, 1982.
27. Hinthorn, DR, Baker, LH, Romig, DA, Hassanein, K, Liu, C: Use of clindamycin in patients with liver disease. *Antimicrob. Agents Chemother. 9*:498–501, 1976.
28. Wise, R, Wright, N, Willis, PJ: Pharmacology of cefotaxime and its desacetyl metabolite in renal and hepatic disease. *Antimicrob. Agents Chemother. 19*:526–531, 1981.
29. Acocella, G, Bonollo, L, Garimoldi, M, Mainardi, M, Tenconi, LT, Nicolis, FB: Kinetics of rifampin and isoniazid administered alone and in combination to normal subjects and patients with liver disease. *Gut 13*:47–53, 1972.

30. Pozzi, E, Menghini, P: Blood levels of rifampin in liver diseases. *Int. J. Clin. Pharmacol. 10*:44, 1974.
31. Theron, JJ, and Lienberg, N: Some observations on fine cytology of parenchymal liver cells in kwashiorkor. *J. Pathol. Bacteriol. 86*:109, 1963.
32. Greenfield, RA, Gerber, AU, Criag, WA: Pharmacokinetics of cefoperazone in patients with normal and impaired hepatic and renal function. *Rev. Infect. Dis. 5*: S127–S136, 1983.
33. Boscia, JA, Korzeniowski, OM, Snepar, R, Kobasa, WD, Levinson, ME' Koye, D: Cefoperazone pharmacokinetics in normal subjects and patients with cirrhosis. *Antimicrob. Agents Chemother. 23*:385–389, 1983.
34. Bolton, WK, Scheld, WM, Spyker, DA, Sande, MA: Pharmacokinetics of cefoperazone in normal volunteers and subjects with renal insufficiency. *Antimicrob. Agents Chemother. 19*:821–825, 1981.
35. Stoeckel, K, Tuerk, H, Trueb, V, McNamara, PJ: Single-dose ceftriaxone kinetics in liver insufficiency. *Clin. Pharmacol. Ther. 36*:500–509, 1984.
36. Stoeckel, K, Koup, JR: Pharmacokinetics of ceftriaxone in patients with renal and liver insufficiency and correlations with a physiologic nonlinear protein binding model. *Am. J. Med. 77*:26–32, 1984.
37. Lewis, GP, Jusko, WJ: Pharmacokinetics of ampicillin in cirrhosis. *Clin. Pharmacol. Ther. 18*:475–484, 1975.
38. Hoffman, TA, Cestero, R, Bullock, WE: Pharmacodynamics of carbenicillin in hepatic and renal failure. *Ann. Intern. Med. 73*:173–178, 1970.
39. Brown, N, Ho, DHW, Fong, KLL, Bogerd, L, Maksymiuk, A, Bolivar, R, Fainstein, V, Bodey, GP: Effects of hepatic function on vancomycin clinical pharmacology. *Antimicrob. Agents Chemother. 23*:603–609, 1983.
40. Moellering, RC, Krugstad, DJ, Greenblatt, DJ: Vancomycin therapy in patients with impaired renal function: A nomogram for dosage. *Ann. Intern. Med. 94*:343–346, 1981.
41. Sirinaven, S, McCracken, G, Nelson, JD: Determining gentamicin dosage in infants and children with renal failure. *J. Pediatr. 96*:331–334, 1980.
42. Bennett, WM, Aronoff, GR, Morrison, G, Golper, TA, Pulliam, J, Wolfson, M, Singer, I: Drug prescribing in renal failure: Dosing guidelines for adults. *Am. J. Kidney Dis. 3*:155–193, 1983.
43. Lanao, JM, Dominguez-Gil, AA, Dominguez-Gil, A, Malaga, S, Crespo, M, Santos, F: Pharmacokinetics of amikacin in children with normal and impaired renal function. *Kidney Int. 20*:115–121, 1981.
44. Blaser, J, Ruttiman, S, Bhend, H, Luthy, R: Increase of amikacin half-life during therapy in patients with renal insufficiency. *Antimicrob. Agents Chemother. 23*: 888–891, 1983.
45. Kucer, A, Mck Bennett, N: *Clindamycin in the Use of Antibiotics*, William Heinemann Medical Books, London, 1979, pp. 475–476.
46. Macdonald, H, Kelly, RG, Allen, ES, Noble, JF, Kanegis, LA: Pharmacokinetic studies on minocycline in man. *Clin. Pharmacol. Ther. 14*:852–861, 1973.
47. Heaney, D, Eknoyan, G: Minocycline and doxycycline kinetics in chronic renal failure. *Clin. Pharmacol. Ther. 24*:233–239, 1978.
48. Whelton, A, Von Wittenau, MS, Twomey, TM, Walker, WG, Bianchine, JR: Doxycycline pharmacokinetics in the absence of renal function. *Kidney Int. 5*:365–371, 1974.
49. Arancibia, A, Droguett, MT, Fuentes, G, Gonzalez, G, Gonzalez, C, Thambo, S, Palombo, G: Pharmacokinetics of amoxicillin in subjects with normal and impaired renal function. *Int. J. Clin. Pharmacol. Ther. Toxicol. 20*:447–453, 1982.

50. Barza, M, Weinstein, L: Pharmacokinetics of the penicillins in man. *Clin. Pharmacokinet. 1*:297–308, 1976.
51. Whelton, A, Stout, RL, Delgado, FA: An azlocillin dosing nomogram for renal insufficiency. *J. Antimicrob. Chemother. 11 (Suppl. B)*:97–99, 1983.
52. Whelton, A, Stout, RL, Delgado, FA: Azlocillin kinetics during extracorporeal haemodialysis and peritoneal dialysis. *J. Antimicrob. Chemother. 11 (Suppl. B)*: 89–95, 1983.
53. Bergan, T: Review of the pharmacokinetics and dose dependency of azlocillin in normal subjects and patients with renal insufficiency. *J. Antimicrob. Chemother. 11 (Suppl. B)*:101–114, 1983.
54. Leroy, A, Humbert, G, Godin, M, Fillastre, JP: Pharmacokinetics of azlocillin in subjects with normal and impaired renal function. *Antimicrob. Agents Chemother. 17*:344–349, 1980.
55. Mangione, A, Boudinot, D, Schultz, RM, Jusko, WJ: Dose-dependent pharmacokinetics of mezlocillin in relation to renal impairment. *Antimicrob. Agents Chemother. 21*:428–435, 1982.
56. Welling, PG, Craig, WA, Bundtzen, RW, Kwok, FW, Gerber, AU, Modsen, PO: Pharmacokinetics of piperacillin in subjects with various degrees of renal function. *Antimicrob. Agents Chemother. 23*:881–887, 1983.
57. Thompson, MIB, Russo, ME, Masten, JM, Atkin-Thor, E: Piperacillin pharmacokinetics in subjects with chronic renal failure. *Antimicrob. Agents Chemother. 19*: 450–453, 1981.
58. Hiner, LB, Baluarte, J, Polinsky, MS, Gruskin, AB: Cefazolin in children with renal insufficiency. *J. Pediatr. 96*:335–339, 1980.
59. Bundtzen, RW, Toothaker, RD, Nielson, OS, Maden, PO, Welling, PG, Craig, WA: Pharmacokinetics of cefuroxime in normal and impaired renal function: Comparison of high-pressure liquid chromatography and microbiological assays. *Antimicrob. Agents Chemother. 19*:443–449, 1981.
60. Kampf, D, Schurig, R, Korsukewitz, I, Bruckner, O: Cefoxitin pharmacokinetics: Relation to three different renal clearance studies in patients with various degrees of renal insufficiency. *Antimicrob. Agents Chemother. 20*:741–746, 1981.
61. Welage, LS, Schultz, RW, Schentag, JJ: Pharmacokinetics of ceftazidime in patients with renal insufficiency. *Antimicrob. Agents Chemother. 25*:210–204, 1984.
62. Leroy, A, Leguy, F, Borsa, F, Spencer, GR, Fillastre, JP, Humbert, G: Pharmacokinetics of ceftazidime in normal and uremic subjects. *Antimicrob. Agents Chemther. 25*:638–642, 1984.
63. Ackerman, BH, Ross, J, Tofte, RW, Rotschafer, JC: Effect of decreased renal function on the pharmacokinetics of ceftazidime. *Antimicrob. Agents Chemother. 25*: 785–786, 1984.
64. Ohkawa, M, Okasho, A, Motoi, I, Tokunaga, S, Shoda, R, Kawaguchi, S, Sawaki, M, Shimamura, M, Hirano, S, Kurock, K, Awazu, S: Elimination kinetics of cefotaxime and desacetyl cefotaxime in patients with renal insufficiency and during hemodialysis. *Chemotherapy 29*:4–12, 1983.
65. Matzke, GR, Abraham, PA, Halstenson, CE, Keane, WF: Cefotaxime and desacetyl cefotaxime kinetics in renal impairment. *Clin. Pharmacol. Ther. 38*:31–36, 1985.
66. Patel, IH, Sugihara, JG, Weinfeld, RE, Wong, EGC, Siemsen, AW, BErman, SJ: Ceftriaxone pharmacokinetics in patients with various degrees of renal impairment. *Antimicrob. Agents Chemother. 25*:438–442, 1984.
67. Buchanan, N, Hansen, JDL, Van der Walt, LA, Robinson, R, Koornhof, HJ: Chloramphenicol metabolism in children with PCM (letter). *Am. J. Clin. Nutr. 29*:327–330, 1976.

68. Graber, IG, Sevitt, S: Renal function in burned patients and its relationship to morphological changes. *J. Clin. Pathol. 12*:25–44, 1959.
69. Loirat, P, Rohan, J, Baillet, A, Beaufils, F, David, R, Chapman, A: Increased glomerular filtration rate in patients with major burns and its effect on the pharmacokinetics of tobramycin. *N. Engl. J. Med. 299*:915–919, 1978.
70. Zaske, DE, Sawchuck, RJ, Gerding, DN, Strate, RG: Increased dosage requirements of gentamicin in burn patients. *J. Trauma 16*:824–828, 1976.
71. Zaske, DE, Sawchuck, RJ, Strate, RG: The necessity of increased doses of amikacin burn patients. *Surgery 84*:603–698, 1978.
72. Glew, RH, Moellering, RJ, Jr., Burke, JF: Gentamicin dosage in children with extensive burns. *J. Trauma 16*:819–823, 1976.
73. Kelly, HB, Menendez, R, Fan, L, Murphy, S: Pharmacokinetics of tobramycin in cystic fibrosis. *J. Pediatr. 100*:318–321, 1982.
74. Levy, J, Smith, AL, Koup, JR, Williams-Warren, J, Ramsey, B: Disposition of tobramycin in patients with cystic fibrosis: A prospective controlled study. *J. Pediatr. 105*:177–124, 1984.
75. Hsu, MC, Aquila, HA, Schmidt, VL, Munzenberger, PJ, Kauffman, RE, Polgar, G: Individualization of tobramycin dosage in patients with cystic fibrosis. *Pediatr. Infect. Dis. 3*:526–529, 1984.
76. Kearns, GL, Hilman, BC, Wilson, JT: Dosing implications of altered gentamicin disposition in patients with cystic fibrosis. *J. Pediatr. 100*:312–317, 1982.
77. Leeder, JS, Spino, M, Isles, AF, Tesoro, AM, Gold, R, MacLeod, SM: Ceftazidime disposition in acute and stable cystic fibrosis. *Clin. Pharmacol. Ther. 36*:355–362, 1984.
78. Reed, MD, Stern, RC, Bertino, JS, Myers, CM, Yamashita, TS, Blumer, JL: Dosing implications of rapid elimination of trimethoprim-sulfamethoxazole in patients with cystic fibrosis. *J. Pediatr. 104*:303–307, 1984.
79. Jusko, WJ, Mosovich, LL, Gerbracht, LM, Mattar, ME, Yaffe, SJ: Enforced renal excretion of dicloxacillin in patients with cystic fibrosis. *Pediatrics 56*:1038–1044, 1975.
80. Spino, M, Chai, RP, Isles, AF, Thiessen, JJ, Tesoro, A, Gold, R, MacLeod, SM: Cloxacillin absorption and disposition in cystic fibrosis. *J. Pediatr. 105*:829–835, 1984.
81. Yaffe, SJ, Gerbracht, LM, Mosovich, LL, Mattar, ME, Danish, M, Jusko, WJ: Pharmacokinetics of methicillin in patients with cystic fibrosis. *J. Infect. Dis. 135*: 828–831, 1977.
82. Isles, A, Spino, M, Tabachni, KE, Levinson, H, Thiessen, J, MacLeod, S: Theophylline disposition in cystic fibrosis. *Am. Rev. Respir. Dis. 127*:417–421, 1983.
83. Ziemniak, JA, Assael, BM, Padoan, R, Schentag, JJ: The bioavailability and pharmacokinetics of cimetidine and its metabolites in juvenile cystic fibrosis patients: Age related differences as compared to adults. *Eur. J. Clin. Pharmacol. 26*:183–189, 1984.

APPENDIX

Adjustment of Antimicrobial Dosage Schedule in Renal Failure

GIDEON KOREN
The Hospital for Sick Children, and the University of Toronto, Toronto, Ontario, Canada

I. INTRODUCTION

Drugs excreted in their active form by the kidney depend upon renal function for their elimination from the body. Unlike adults, for whom adjustment of dose in renal failure is based upon the assumption of 70 kg body weight or 1.73 m^2 body surface area, in infants and children the $t_{1/2}$ and clearance of drugs, body weight, and surface area are changed continuously. The following table does not include the $t_{1/2}$ of each drug for each age group within the pediatric population. These can be found in each chapter. Rather, the changes in $t_{1/2}$ during renal failure are summarized and the necessary adjustment of dose indicated. A "change" is always in comparison to the normal values of *renal function* or *drug dose* in the specific age group. In the recommendation for adjustment in renal failure, it is commonly suggested to increase dose interval according to the ratio of

$$\frac{\text{Normal creatinine clearance (CrCl)}}{\text{Present creatinine clearance}}$$

In most cases during infancy and childhood, plasma creatinine has a good correlation with creatinine clearance. Only during the first weeks of life, when the infant has his mother's plasma creatinine concentration, this measurement may not accurately reflect creatinine clearance.

Specific references on the disposition of a certain drug in renal failure can be found in the relevant chapters.

Table 1 Adjustment of Antimicrobial Dosage in Renal Failure

	Route of elimination	$t_{1/2}$	Adjustment in renal failure	Supplement for dialysis	Comments
Aminoglycosides	R	A	B,C	Yes (H,P)	Tobramycin, gentamicin: peak < 8–10 μg/ml; trough < 2–3 μg/ml amikacin: peak < 30 μg/ml; trough < 10 μg/ml
Amphothericin B	Nonrenal	$t_{1/2}$ not increased in renal failure	Increase dose interval in 50% in end stage renal failure	No (H,P)	Careful monitoring of renal function as the drug is nephrotoxic to some degree in every patient. Decrease in dose of coadministered drugs eliminated by the kidney (e.g., flucytosine).
Acyclovir	R	A	B	Yes (H)	
Amantadine	R	A	B	Yes (H,P)	Check for signs of CNS toxicity in renal failure.
Amipicillin	R	A	B	Yes (H) No (P)	In renal failure, high doses may be needed to achieve therapeutic urinary concentrations.
Amoxicillin	R	A	B	Yes (H) No (P)	In renal failure, high doses may be needed to achieve therapeutic urinary concentrations.
Azlocillin	R	A	B	Yes (H) No (P)	
Cephalosporin					Nephrotoxic when coadministered with aminoglycosides and diuretics; cannot achieve urinary concentrations in advanced renal failure.
Cefaclor	R+(H)	A	C	Yes (H)	
Cefotaxime	R+(H)	A	B	Yes (H)	Active metabolite has prolonged $T_{1/2}$ in renal failure.
Cephalothine	R+(H)	$t_{1/2}$ increased in severe renal failure	B	Yes (H,P)	
Cephapirin	R+(H)	$t_{1/2}$ increased in severe renal failure	B		

Table 1 (Continued)

	Route of elimination	$t_{1/2}$	Adjustment in renal failure	Supplement for dialysis	Comments
Cefoperazone	NR (+R)	No change in $t_{1/2}$	No changes needed	Yes (H)	
Ceftriaxone	NR (+R)	$t_{1/2}$ increased in anephric patients	Dose interval should be increased only in end stage disease and anephric patients	No	
Cefadroxil, Ceftazidime, Cefoxitin, Cefuroxime, Cefamandole, Cephalexin, Cefazolin, Moxaloctam, Ceforanide	R	A	B	Yes (H)	
Cefroxadine, Cefsulodine, Ceftizoxime, Cephradine	R	A	C	Yes (H,P) for Cephradine Yes (H) for Cefsulodine Not known for Cefroxadine and Ceftizoxime	
Chloramphenicol	H(R)	$t_{1/2}$ may be pro-	No changes	Yes (H)	Therapeutic concentrations 10–25 μg/ml

		longed in end stage	needed	No (P)	$T_{1/2}$ may be markedly prolonged in combined hepatic and renal insufficiency.
Chloroquine	R(H)	$t_{1/2}$ not studied in end stage renal failure	Decrease dose to 50% in end stage renal failure	No (H)	
Clindamycin	H	$t_{1/2}$ may be prolonged in end stage renal failure	No change	No (H,P)	
Carbenecillin	R(H)	A	B	Yes (H,P)	In severe renal failure, inadequate urinary concentrations are achieved.
Cloxacillin	R(H)	A	No changes needed	No (H)	
Doxycycline	R+(H)	A	B	No (H,P)	In severe renal failure, appropriate concentrations for urinary infections cannot be achieved.
Erythromycin	H	$t_{1/2}$ increase in end stage renal failure	No change needed	No (H,P)	
Ethambutal	R	A	B		
Flucytosine	R	A	B	Yes (H,P)	Drug accumulation in renal failure may cause hepatic dysfunction and bone marrow suppression.
Isoniazid	H+(R)	$t_{1/2}$ increased in renal failure only in slow acetylators	Reduce dose to 66–75% in cases of end stage renal disease	Yes (H,P)	
Ketoconazole	H	No change in $t_{1/2}$ in renal failure	No change needed	No (H)	
Lincomycin	H+(R)	A	B	No (H,P)	
Miconazole	H	No change in $t_{1/2}$ in renal failure	No change needed	No (H,P)	

Table 1 (Continued)

	Route of elimination	$t_{1/2}$	Adjustment in renal failure	Supplement for dialysis	Comments
Methenamine	R	$t_{1/2}$ probably increase proportionally to degree of renal failure	Do not prescribe in renal failure		Inappropriate urinary concentrations are achieved in renal failure. Increases GiT symptoms during chronic renal failure.
Minocycline	H	$t_{1/2}$ prolonged in renal failure	No change needed		
Mezlocillin	R(+H)	A	B	Yes (H)	
Methicillin	R(+H)	A	B	No (H,P)	
Metronidazole	H+(R)	$t_{1/2}$ of drug is not changed but active metabolite is renally secreted and its $t_{1/2}$ prolonged	B	Yes (H) No (P)	
Nafcillin	H+(R)	$t_{1/2}$ increased in renal failure	No change needed	No (H)	Dose should be reduced in combined renal and hepatic failure.
Nalidixic acid	H+(R)	$t_{1/2}$ is increased in renal failure	Do not use in renal failure		Metabolites accumulate; not effective for urinary infection in renal failure.
Nitrofurantoin	H+(R)	$t_{1/2}$ in renal failure not known. Metabolites accumulate in renal failure	Do not use in renal failure	Yes (H)	Appropriate urinary concentrations cannot be achieved in renal failure.

Oxacillin	R(+H)	$t_{1/2}$ increased in renal failure	No change needed	Yes (H,P)	
Piperacillin	R(+H)	A	B	Yes (H)	
Penicillin G	R(+H)	A	B	Yes (H) No (P)	
Rifampin	H	No change in $t_{1/2}$ in renal failure	No change needed	No (H)	May induce acute renal failure.
Sulfamethoxazole	H+(R)	A	B	Yes (H) No (P)	Decreased protein binding in uremia may result in higher concentrations of free drug.
Sulfisoxazole	R+(H)	A	B	Yes (H,P)	Decreased protein binding in uremia may result in higher concentrations of free drug; large dose needed to achieve therapeutic urinary concentration in renal failure.
Ticarcillin	R	A	B	Yes (H,P)	Ineffective for UTI in renal insufficiency.
Trimethoprim	R+(H)	A	B	Yes (H) No (P)	May increase serum creatinine by competition on tubular secretion. Appropriate urinary concentrations achieved even in severe renal failure.
Vancomycin	R	A	B,C	No (H,P)	Peak $\leqslant$ 30–40; trough $\leqslant$ 5–10 μg/ml.
Vidarabine	R+(H)	$t_{1/2}$ increased in renal failure	Decrease dose to 75% in severe renal failure	Yes (H)	A total of 50% of active metabolite is excreted by the kidney.

A, $t_{1/2}$ increased proportionally to degree of renal failure; B, increase dose interval according to the ratio $\frac{\text{normal Cr clearance for age}}{\text{present Cr clearance}}$; C, decrease dose according to the ratio $\frac{\text{normal Cr clearance for age}}{\text{present Cr clearance}}$; H, hemodialysis; P, peritoneal dialysis; R, renal; H, hepatic.

REFERENCES

1. Bennett WM, Aronoff GB, Morrison G, Golper TA, Pulliam J, Wolfson M, Singer J: Drug prescribing in renal failure: dosing guidelines for adults. *Am. J. Kidney Dis 3*: 155–193, 1983.
2. Anderson RJ, Schrier RW, Gambertoglio JG: Clinical use of drugs in patients with kidney and liver disease. WB Saunders Co., Philadelphia, 1981.
3. Bennett WN: Drugs and the kidney. In *Contemporary Nephrology* (S Klahr, SG Massry, eds.), Plenum Medical, New York, pp. 657–694, 1981.
4. Chennavasin P, Brater DC: Normograms for drug use in renal disease. *Clin Pharmacokinet 6*:193–214, 1981.
5. Knepshield JH, Winchester JF: Hemodialysis and hemoperfusion for drugs and poisons. *Trans. Am. Soc. Artif. Intern. Organs 28*:666–669, 1982.
6. Reidenberg MM, Dryer DE: Drug therapy in renal failure. *Ann. Rev. Pharmacol. Toxicol. 20*:45–54, 1980.

6
Therapeutic Drug Monitoring of Antimicrobial Drugs in Children

GIDEON KOREN
The Hospital for Sick Children, and the University of Toronto, Toronto, Ontario, Canada

Therapeutic drug monitoring (TDM) is the area in which pharmacokinetic and pharmacodynamic principles are incorporated to ensure optimal antimicrobial effect with minimal toxicity. TDM has emerged as an important clinical tool during the last decade, parallel to the development of accurate micromethods for the measurement of antimicrobial concentration in the body fluids of infants and children.

Several basic conditions must be fulfilled before TDM of a specific drug can be utilized effectively. There should be a known correlation between the concentrations measured in the serum and those at the site of infection. A drug may be maintained at serum concentrations above the minimal inhibitory concentration (MIC) of a certain microorganism, but at the site of infection concentrations may be lower because of poor penetration (abcess, poor vascularization, and other factors). In such a case, the measurement of drug concentrations in the blood may not reflect the real picture of the drug's effectiveness. Penetration of antimicrobial drugs into the tissue compartment is a dynamic process, dependent upon various factors delineated in Chapter 3. During the acute phase of meningitis, the penetration of antibiotics through the blood-brain barrier is much better than during convalescence. Consequently, the same serum concentration may be adequate during the early phase of the disease, but not later. Conversely, drugs that are eliminated unchanged by the kidney may achieve very high concentrations in the urine in spite of serum concentrations below the MIC of the specific microorganism (e.g., aminoglycosides, cephalosporins, and penicillins).

In addition, host factors may modify the antimicrobial need. Equilibrium between the drug load in the blood and in the various tissue compartments, including the site of infection, must be assumed. As only the unbound fraction of the drug is free to penetrate various tissue compartments and arrive at the infection site, it is postulated that by measuring the *total concentration* of the drug one can extrapolate the active portion of the drug.

Even in the presence of a good correlation between drug concentrations in the blood and in the infection site, the measured blood level may not be easily correlated with the minimal inhibitory concentrations of the microorganism: the MIC is based on the total drug concentration surrounding the microorganism, whereas apparent activity may be modified by the degree of protein binding, as only the free drug reaches the infection site. In the case of the aminoglycosides, which are the antibiotics for which TDM is most often used, this is merely a theoretical question, as their protein binding is negligible. Most importantly, correlations between blood concentrations and clinical efficacy should be known. Unfortunately, in spite of the generation of large amounts of pharmacokinetic data, this most important correlation is the least known.

In addition, a known correlation between antimicrobial concentrations and toxic manifestations must be documented. Classic examples are the aminoglycosides, for which there is a relatively confined "therapeutic window" above which nephrotoxicity and autotoxicity may occur.

In many cases, measurement of serum concentration of drugs is unnecessary even though they have good correlation with effect, as the therapeutic effect can be accurately assessed clinically. Such drugs as diuretics, hypoglycemics, antipyretics, analgesics, antihypertensives, and anticoagulants have clear and measurable therapeutic effects. Consequently, the concentration of the drug in the blood will not provide more accurate information about the response of the target organ. This concept is also true with respect to most antimicrobial drugs. The clinical course in conjunction with laboratory tests (e.g., cultures) may yield more relevant information about the effectiveness of the drug than will determining serum concentrations.

I. INDICATIONS FOR THERAPEUTIC DRUG MONITORING

Bochner and Carruthers and their colleagues have summarized the different indications for TDM (1). Only those indications relevant to the use of antimicrobial drugs are included in this review.

A. Determining Effective Serum Concentrations

In general, antimicrobial therapy is thought optimal if concentrations of the drug in the blood or in other fluids are 4- to 10-fold in excess of the MIC of the specific microorganism. Most antimicrobials have a wide therapeutic range, with serum concentrations exceeding the infecting organism's MIC often by several hundredfold. Effective serum concentrations are thus assumed rather than determined. In a recent study, Moore and his associates could show that peak concentrations of gentamicin above 5 μg/ml of amikacin above 20 μg/ml were associated with reduced mortality in patients with gram-negative septicemia (2).

B. Narrow Therapeutic Index

Several antimicrobial agents have a narrow ratio between therapeutic and toxic serum concentrations. The best examples are chloramphenicol and the aminoglycosides. Because of large variability in the ability of patients to eliminate chloramphenicol, even recommended doses may result in toxic serum concentrations in some patients. This is particularly so in the newborn infant, in whom routine TDM is mandatory.

Both ototoxicity and nephrotoxicity caused by aminoglycosides are associated with high serum concentrations. Although an exact therapeutic window is difficult to predict, it is generally agreed that a peak concentration (30-60 min after intravenous dose) $>$ 8-10 μg/ml and a trough (before next dose) concentration $>$ 2-3 μg/ml are associated with a higher rate of toxicity (see Chapter 13) (3–11). It is relatively easy to exceed it with a slight variation of the daily dose. The frequency of excessive concentrations is reduced with maturation of renal function and increase in glomerular filtration rate (GFR) (Figure 1). However, in spite of the improvement in renal elimination of aminoglycosides, there is a wide overlapping in values. As shown in Figure 2, the large variability in measured creatinine clearance and gentamicin clearance in neonates can be related only in part

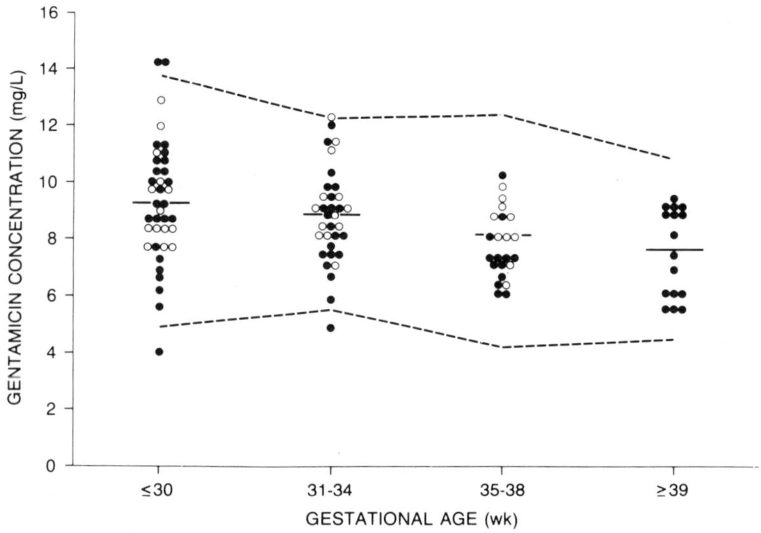

(a)

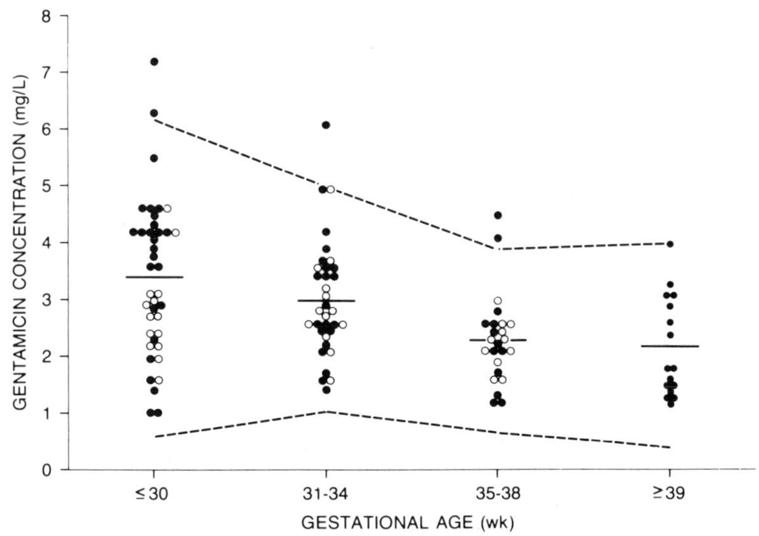

(b)

Figure 1 Age-dependent changes in peak (a) and trough (b) concentrations of gentamicin in newborn infants after receiving 2.5 mg/kg twice daily for 2 days.

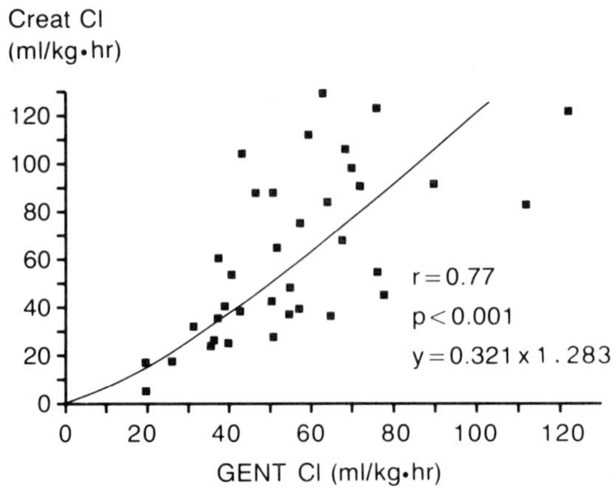

Figure 2 Variability in measured creatinine clearance and gentamicin clearance in neonates. (From Reference 18, with permission of Mosby Ltd., St. Louis.)

to age-related maturation. Although there is a tendency of renal clearance to improve, such a general trend would not suffice in the specific case. Often the neonate needing aminglycosides has other factors that may impair renal function, such as sepsis, shock, or asphyxia.

From a pharmacokinetic standpoint it is clear that, after administration of a dose of aminoglycoside, concentrations are not static but rather change constantly. The best estimation of the degree of exposure of a patient to the dose is the area under concentration time curve (AUC); however, in the clinical setting the AUC cannot be easily calculated. Instead, investigators base their estimation of efficacy and potential toxicity on peak (C_{max}) and trough (C_{min}) concentrations. Several studies in adult patients have correlated C_{max} and C_{min} with toxicity (3-11). In the pediatric age group, similar relations have not been described. It has been suggested that infants and small children are less sensitive to these toxic effects (12). Dean has reported two cases of definite aminoglycoside-induced nephrotoxicity in 345 courses (0.6%) of therapy in children. In both cases, adjustment of the dose to obtain a peak level of 5–8 μg/ml and trough level of <2 μg/ml resulted in a rapid decline of creatinine concentrations (13).

Chloramphenicol therapy in infants and children may be associated with several toxic manifestations. Both bone marrow suppression and the "gray baby" syndrome (see Chapter 16) are associated with serum concentrations above 25 μg/ml. However, this is only a statistical figure; there are many cases in whom concentrations in the potentially toxic range are harmless. In a group of 37 neonates with excessive serum concentrations of chloramphenicol (27 with concentrations above 25 μg/ml and 7 cases above 50 μg/ml), no toxicity was documented (14). It appears that the gray baby syndrome rarely occurs at concentrations below 80 μg/ml, and pancytopenia is rare below 40 μg/ml.

Similarly to the aminoglycosides, toxic concentrations of vancomycin may cause nephrotoxicity and ototoxicity. Although older studies coupled toxicity with serum concentration in excess of 20–30 μg/ml, some investigators currently believe that toxicity occurs at much higher concentrations (50--80 μg/ml) (15). However, such high concentrations are not needed because most bacteria for which vancomycin is indicated are inhibited or killed at concentrations of 12–15 μg/ml. Consequently, a peak of <50 μg/ml and a trough of 15 μ/ml appear reasonable to guarantee an optimal effect. In children, vancomycin-induced nephrotoxicity in 2 of 19 patients was reported by Dean in children not concurrently receiving aminoglycosides. When doses were adjusted to maintain peak concentrations of 20-40 μg/ml and trough concentrations of 5-10 μg/ml, serum creatinine concentrations returned to normal (13).

When aminoglycosides are given concurrently with vancomycin, the rate of nephrotoxicity appears to increase significantly [35% according to Farber and Moallering (16) and 27% in the report by Dean et al. (13)] above the incidence caused by each agent independently. It is therefore mandatory to carefully monitor both aminoglycoside and vancomycin peak and trough concentrations in patients receiving both together (16,17). According to retrospective studies, in most cases of nephrotoxicity induced by the aminoglycoside-vancomycin combination, concentrations of vancomycin were not excessive. Although more studies are needed in order to clarify this question, it is conceivable that because of the cumulative toxic effect of the two drugs, lower concentrations may result in nephrotoxicity.

C. Overlapping Signs of Drug Toxicity and Disease

TDM is indicated when toxicity is easily confused with the signs of the disease. This indication is best demonstrated with the aminoglycosides. Gentamicin may cause nephro-

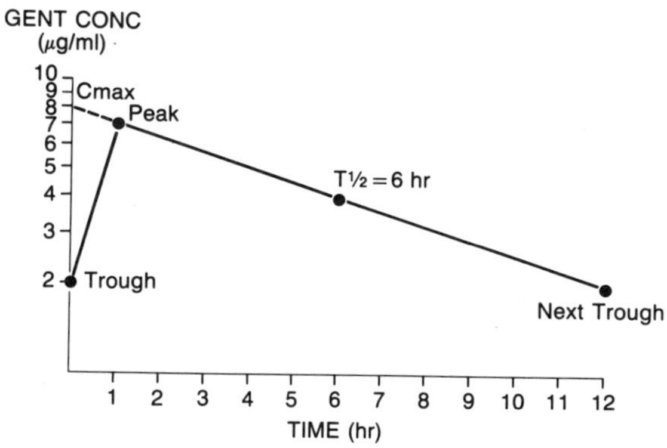

Figure 3 Graphic estimation of gentamicin $t_{1/2}$, volume of distribution, and clearance from trough, peak, and next trough serum concentrations. $T_{1/2}$ (the time taken for the concentration to decrease by one-half) is derived from the line connecting the measured peak and the next trough concentrations. When this line is back-extrapolated to time zero, the y intercept yields the C_{max}. Volume of distribution V_d can then be calculated as

$$V_d = \frac{\text{intravenous dose}}{C_{max} - \text{trough}}$$

Clearance Cl is calculated as

$$Cl = \frac{0.69\, V_d}{t_{1/2}}$$

(From Reference 18, with permission of Mosby Ltd., St. Louis.)

Table 1 Translation of Calculated Gentamicin Cl or $t_{1/2}$ into CR_{Cl} in Newborns[a]

Calculated gentamicin Cl range (ml/kg hr^{-1})	0–25	26–40	41–60	>60
Predicted Cl_{cr} (ml/kg hr^{-1})	16 ± 10	35.7 ± 14	58.4 ± 26	88.5 ± 30
Calculated gentamicin $t_{1/2}$ range (hr)	>10	6–10	4–6	<4
Predicted Cl_{cr} (ml/kg hr^{-1})	22.8 ± 10	69 ± 33	78.9 ± 29	106.3 ± 15

[a]Data are $\bar{X} \pm SD$.

(From Reference 18, with permission of Mosby Ltd., St. Louis.)

toxicity, with a potential decrease in GFR. If toxicity is not recognized and gentamicin dose is not reduced proportionally, its accumulation may further insult renal function in a positive feedback effect.

It is often difficult to define whether the initial reason for the gradually increasing serum creatinine in conjunction with a parallel elevation of gentamicin concentrations are due to an underlying kidney disease or are secondary to aminoglycoside therapy. The differentiation between these two mechanisms may be based on the fact that, typically, aminoglycoside nephrotoxicity is usually reversible following cessation of therapy.

Generally, a careful assessment of renal function by measuring plasma creatinine concentrations or creatinine clearance, in conjunction with monitoring aminoglycoside concentrations, may help the clinician to adjust the aminoglycoside dose. However, in the newborn infant, creatinine plasma concentrations may be more difficult to interpret as the neonate has at birth the mother's creatinine values, and it may take several days to several weeks to achieve that of infancy (0.2–0.4 mg/dl). During this period, the physiological fall in the creatinine level may hamper a gradual impairment of renal function. We have recently suggested the use of gentamicin disposition for the estimation of GFR (18). It appears that both gentamicin elimination $T_{1/2}$ and clearance rates correlate well with creatinine clearance. The employment of this simple technique is demonstrated in Figure 3, and a nomogram for translation of gentamicin $T_{1/2}$ and clearance to creatinine clearance is presented in Table 1.

II. PRACTICE OF TDM OF ANTIMICROBIAL DRUGS

In the next paragraphs, practical aspects of TDM will be discussed in order to familiarize the clinician with the employment of this clinical tool. In general, at the outset of antimicrobial therapy, the recommended dosage is given. This dose is based on age, weight, and disease state, including eliminating organ malfunction (kidney, liver, and so on; see Chapter 5). The dose is based upon the assumption that, in a steady state,

$$\text{Mean steady-state concentration} = \frac{\text{dose (mg/kg hr}^{-1}) \times F}{\text{clearance (ml/kg hr}^{-1})} \qquad (1)$$

where F is the bioavailability (the percentage of the administered drug that enters the systemic circulation; see Chapter 3). This formula incorporates all the possible reasons for concentrations that are lower or higher than expected from the dose in the specific age group and disease state.

A. Reasons for Suboptimal Concentrations

1. Steady State Not Achieved

It takes 4–5 elimination $T_{1/2}$ to reach steady-state concentrations. If assessment of concentrations is performed *before* steady state, concentrations will be lower than expected, leading to increased doses that will eventually result in potentially toxic concentrations. For example, if the $T_{1/2}$ of gentamicin in newborn infants is 6 hr, a steady state will be achieved after about 30 hr (or almost three doses given every 12 hr). A concentration obtained earlier is likely to be lower than steady-state concentrations. In the case of the ill patient, the clinician may not wish to wait 5 half-lives for a steady state. In this situation a loading dose may be indicated, as discussed in Chapter 3.

2. Impaired Bioavailability

In the case of oral administration, impaired bioavailability may be caused by poor dissolution of a product, the presence of food, gastrointestinal diseases, vomiting, and various other reasons delineated in Chapter 4.

Even if a drug is infused intravenously, it may be sequestered in the intravenous set or in a filter chamber, especially in the small infant in whom infusion rates are extremely slow (see Chapter 8). For the same reason, it is possible that the determination of an assumed peak concentration was performed before the total dose was infused, resulting in a *falsely* low concentration.

3. Erroneous Dose

Errors in the calculation of drug dose are probably much more common than reported in the literature (18,19). Therefore, this possibility must be considered and checked whenever steady-state concentrations are unexpectedly low. In addition, it is possible that the dose ordered is lower than needed for the child's size or that the error stems from transcription error or dilution error.

4. Increased Clearance Rate

Depending upon the eliminating organ, an improved clearance rate of a drug may cause a decrease in its serum concentrations. In a neonate, improved GFR due to maturation or secondary to successful treatment of shock or sepsis will probably result in lower serum concentrations of aminoglycosides or vancomycin with a parallel need to increase the dose (Figure 1). Drug-drug interaction may result in an increased clearance (e.g., rifampin increasing chloromphenicol clearance).

B. Reasons for Excessive Concentrations

1. Dose Higher Than Needed for Age Group

Dosing guidelines are often erroneously extrapolated from older age groups. This may result in excessive doses of certain agents. The best examples are the excessive doses of aminoglycosides and chloramphenicol that were formerly prescribed to newborn infants. In the case of the latter, a dose of 100 mg/kg day^{-1} given to older infants and children may be disastrous in the newborn infant, who would accumulate chloramphenicol to toxic concentrations, often with any dose above 25 mg/kg day^{-1}.

2. Medication Errors

Tenfold calculation errors of drug doses are common in infants owing to the small amounts needed (see Chapter 8). This possibility must be seriously considered in any case of excessive concentration. This is especially so if previous determinations were within the therapeutic range. Here, too, a transcription error or a dilutional error may result in acute toxicity.

3. Improved Bioavailability

Improvement of the bioavailability of a product (20) may cause inadvertent toxic concentrations if the physician is not aware of the need to decrease the dose. Simiarly, food may increase the bioavailability of various drugs, especially those with poor dissolution characteristics, such as nitrofurantoin and griseofulvin.

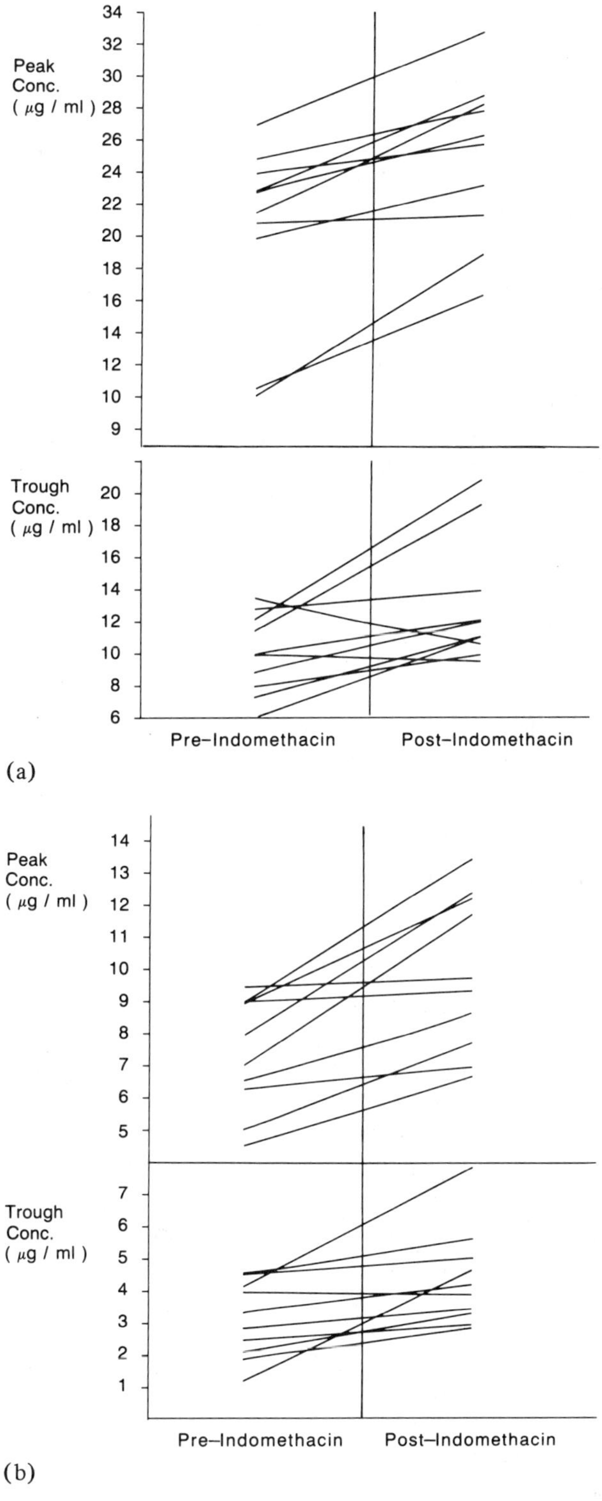

Figure 4 Indomethacin causes elevation in steady-state concentrations of amikacin (a) and gentamicin (b) due to impairment of renal function.

4. Decreased Clearance

Renal disease results in the decreased clearance of drugs that are eliminated unchanged by the kidney. Similarly, impairment or immaturity of hepatic metabolism is associated with the decreased clearance of agents eliminated by the liver (e.g., chloramphenicol and clindamycin). In a recent study, we could show accumulation of gentamicin and amikacin following the administration of indomethacin for the closure of patent ductus arteriosus (Figure 4) (21). This elevation was coupled with an increase in plasma creatinine and a decrease in urine output.

5. Slow Equilibration with a Deep Compartment

For practical purposes, aminoglycoside pharmacokinetics are described as a one-compartment open model with elimination $T_{1/2}$ between 2 hr (in adults) and 10–14 hr (in some very low birth weight infants). However, recent studies have documented the existence of an additional slow-equilibrating compartment with a half-life of about 40 hr to several days (7). This compartment is probably consistent with deep tissue accumulation. Consequently, a gradual increase in peak and trough concentrations may occur over weeks, as 5 half-lives are needed for a steady state to be achieved (five times several days).

In this case, the gradual elevation in peak and trough concentrations does not reflect changes in dose, bioavailability, or clearance rate but rather that a steady state has not yet been achieved after the first few days of treatment.

6. Error in Sampling Time

It often happens that a trough concentration is assumed; however a new dose has already been given or is still being given (22). This may lead to an erroneous assumption of toxicity. In addition, when steady-state concentrations are found to be high or low and the dose is readjusted, it will take another 4–5 half-lives of the drug to achieve the new steady state; if samples are drawn before permitting a new steady state to be achieved, concentrations may be interpreted erroneously as too high or too low.

C. Appropriate Collection of Samples

In order for a peak concentration to be accurate, one must guarantee the full delivery of the dose in an intravenous administration or the complete absorption of an intramuscular or an oral dose. In the case of a prodrug (e.g., chloramphenicol or clindamycin esters), the real peak may be achieved only after hydrolysis of the ester.

In order to interpret serum concentrations, it is essential to accurately document the time of sampling. Samples must be collected into tubes not containing any additives that might interfere with the assays. In some cases, antimicrobials are very stable even at room temperature (e.g., aminoglycoside), whereas for others stability cannot be assumed even at $-20°C$ (e.g., some penicillins and β-lactam antibiotics).

D. Assay Methods

A discussion of the various analytic methods for the measurement of drug concentrations is included in Chapter 2. In most cases, the technical aspects of these tests are beyond the interest or expertise of the clinician. However, several characteristics of each method should be evaluated by the physician.

Specificity: Does the assay measure only the drug in question or also its metabolites, endogenous substances, or other drugs from the same group?
Sensitivity: Even if the method is specific for the drug, it must be guaranteed that it is sensitive enough to measure the drug at the concentrations in question.
Accuracy: Is the reported concentration accurate? The degree of accuracy is routinely reported as the coefficient of variation. If the same sample is measured several times under the same conditions then the coefficient of variations (CV) is

$$CV = \frac{\text{standard deviation}}{\text{mean}}$$

A higher coefficient of variation indicates a less accurate test due to a larger variation. Generally, a test is least accurate at very low concentrations.

E. Effectiveness of TDM of Antimicrobials

It is conceivable that a rational therapeutic drug monitoring of antimicrobial drugs may result in improved efficacy and lower toxicity rates for aminoglycosides, chloramphenicol, and vancomycin. However, such improvement is difficult to prove scientifically. Zaske and his colleagues, who employed a TDM program to monitor aminoglycoside concentrations, found only 0.9% changes of serum creatinine in 1640 patients receiving gentamicin. They attributed these favorable results to their monitoring program. However, they lacked a control group in their own series (23). This factor may be crucial in evaluating the results as, in series with septicemia, there is a high rate of renal and cochlear insult in patients receiving aminoglycosides (6).

We have recently shown that by using a consultation service for therapeutic drug monitoring in a pediatric hospital, we could decrease by twofold the rate of potentially toxic concentrations (24,25). The vast majority of potentially toxic measurements occurred with aminoglycosides (59%). Although it is conceivable that by reducing potentially toxic concentrations we might have reduced the actual toxicity rate, this question is very difficult to answer, especially in newborn infants, who appear to be less sensitive to the toxic effects of aminoglycosides.

As mentioned above, several studies have documented that gentamicin and tobramycin concentrations above >5 μg/ml or higher than 20 μg/ml of amikacin were associated with lower mortality rates in septic patients. However, there is a delicate interplay between efficacious and toxic concentrations of aminoglycosides, and it is possible that by achieving better control of toxicity one may compromise efficacy, and vice versa. More controlled studies are still needed to prove the efficiency of present modalities in both guaranteeing efficacy and preventing toxicity in the same patients.

REFERENCES

1. Bochner, F, Carruthers, G, Kampmann, P, Steiner, J: *Handbook of Clinical Pharmacology*. Little, Brown, Boston, 1983.
2. Moore, RD, Smith, CR, Lietman, PS: The association of aminoglycoside plasma levels with mortality in patients with gram-negative bacteremia. *J. Infect. Dis. 149*:443–448, 1984.
3. Mawer, EE, Ahmed, R, Dobbs, SM, McGough, JG, Lucas, SB, Tooth, JA: Prescribing aids for gentamicin. *Br. J. Clin. Pharmacol. 1*:45–50, 1974.

4. Dahlgren, JG, Anderson, ET, Hewitt, WL: Gentamicin blood levels: A guide to nephrotoxicity. *Antimicrob. Agents Chemother. 8*:58–62, 1975.
5. Black, RE, Lau, WK, Weinstein, RJ, Young, LS, Hewitt, WL: Ototoxicity of amikacin. *Antimicrob. Agents Chemother. 9*:956–961, 1976.
6. Smith, CR, Banghan, KL, Edwards, CQ, Rogerst, F, Lietman, PS: Controlled comparison of amikacin and tobramycin. *N. Engl. J. Med. 296*:349–353, 1977.
7. Schentag, JJ, Jusko, WJ, Vance, JW, Cumbo, TJ, Abrulyn, E, DeLallre, M, Gerbracht, LM: Gentamicin disposition and tissue accumulation on multiple dosing. *J. Pharmacokinet. Biopharmacol. 5*:559–577, 1977.
8. Gailiunas, P, Dominguez-Mareno, M, Lazarus, JM, Lowrie, EG, Gaulieb, MN, Merill, JP: Vestibular toxicity of gentamicin: Incidence in patients receiving long-term hemodialysis therapy. *Arch. Intern. Med. 1387*:621–624, 1978.
9. Feld, R, Tuffnell, PG, Curtio, JE, Messner, HA, Hasselback, R: Empiric therapy for infections in granulocytopenic cancer patients: Continuous infusion of amikacin plus cephalothin. *Arch. Intern. Med. 139*:310–314, 1979.
10. Bock, BV, Edelstein, PH, Meyer, RD: Prospective comparative study of efficacy and toxicity of netilmicin and amikacin. *Antimicrob. Agents Chemother. 17*:217–225, 1980.
11. Rajchot, P, Prober, CG, Soldin, SJ, Perlman, M, Good, F, Harding, E, Klein, J, MacLeod, SM: Aminoglycoside-related nephrotoxicity in the premature newborn. *Clin. Pharmacol. Ther. 35*:394–401, 1984.
12. Assael, BM, Parini, R, Rusconi, F: Ototoxicity of aminoglycoside antibiotics in infants and children. *Pediatr Infect. Dis. 1*:357–365, 1982.
13. Dean, RP, Wagner, DJ, Tolpin, MD: Vancomycin/aminoglycoside nephrotoxicity. *J. Pediatr. 106*:861–862, 1985.
14. Mulhall, A, deLouvois, J, Hurley, R: Chloramphenicol toxicity in neonates: Its incidence and prevention. *Br. Med. J. 287*:1424–1427, 1983.
15. Moellering, RC, Krogstad, DJ, Greewslatt, DJ: Vanconycin therapy in patients with impaired renal function: A nomogram for dosage. *Ann. Intern. Med. 94*:343–346, 1981.
16. Farber, BF, Moallering, RC: Retrospective study of the toxicity of preparations of vancomycin from 1974 to 1981. *Antimicrob. Agents Chemother. 23*:138, 1983.
17. Odio, C, McCracken, GH, Nelson, JD: Nephrotoxicity associated with vancomycin-aminoglycoside therapy in four children. *J. Pediatr. 105*:491–493, 1984.
18. Koren, G, James, A, Perlman, M: A simple method for the estimation of GFR in neonates using routine monitoring of gentamicin. *Clin. Pharmacol. Ther. 38*:680–685, 1985.
19. Koren, G, Barzilay, Z, Greenwald, M: Ten-fold errors in drug dose administration; a neglected iatrogenic disease in pediatrics. *Pediatrics 77*:848–849, 1986.
20. Tyrer, JH, Eadie, MJ, Sutherland, JM, Hooper, WD: Outbreak of anticonvulsant intoxication in an Australian city. *Br. Med. J. 3*:271–273, 1970.
21. Zarfin, Y, Koren, G, Perlman, M, MacLeod, SM: Possible interaction of indomethacin with aminoglycosides. *J. Pediatr. 106*:511–513, 1985.
22. Koren, G, Parker, R: Interpretation of excessive serum concentrations of digoxin in children. *Am. J. Cardiol. 55*:1210–1214, 1985.
23. Zaske, DE, Cipalle, RJ, Rotschafer, JC, Solem, LD, Moiser, NR, Strate, RG: Gentamicin pharmacokinetics in 1640 patients: Method for control of serum concentrations. *Antimicrob. Agents Chemother. 21*:407–411, 1982.
24. Koren, G, Soldin, S, MacLeod, SM: A therapeutic drug monitoring consultation service in a pediatric hospital. *Ther. Drug Monit. 7*:295–298, 1985.
25. Soldin, SJ, Koren, G: Optimization of a therapeutic drug monitoring program. *Am. Assoc. Clin. Chem. 2*:8, 1984.

7

Exposure of the Embryo and Fetus to Antimicrobial Agents

GIDEON KOREN
The Hospital for Sick Children, and the University of Toronto, Toronto, Ontario, Canada

Antimicrobial drugs are indicated for various maternal diseases during pregnancy. In some of them (e.g., amnionitis and syphilis), treatment is also aimed at the fetus.

In many instances, antimicrobial therapy is planned knowing that the woman is pregnant. However, in other cases therapy is given during the first few weeks after conception, before pregnancy is evident to the woman. This chapter summarizes common uses of antimicrobial drugs during pregnancy, for both maternal and maternofetal diseases, the pharmacokinetics of their penetration into the fetus, and their disposition by the immature organism. Finally, current evidence for antimicrobial teratogenicity will be presented with special focus on methodological evaluation of these data from our Motherisk Program.

I. PHARMACOKINETICS OF THE MATERNAL-FETAL UNIT

Several pharmacokinetic models have been utilized to describe the movement of different drugs between the maternal and fetal circulations (1). In general, two principal groups of changes characterize pregnancy with respect to drug disposition.

A. Alterations in Drug Kinetics Due to Maternal Changes

There is a gradual increase in renal function in the pregnant woman. This will result in augmented elimination rate of antimicrobial agents that are eliminated by the kidney (e.g., ampicillin, gentamicin, and amikacin) (2-4). Distribution volume may be altered during pregnancy because of increases of 50% in blood (plasma) volume and 30% in cardiac output (5-7). A parallel 50% increment in renal flow and a substantial increase of uterine blood flow to 600-700 ml/min has been noted. During pregnancy there is a mean increase of 8 liters in body water, 60% of which is distributed to the placenta, fetus, and amniotic fluid and 40% distributed to maternal tissues (5,8-10). Consequently, a decrease in serum concentrations of such drugs as ampicillin and oxacillin has been documented. It is very likely that similar effects occur with other agents.

Changes in hepatic elimination patterns during pregnancy are less consistent. Hepatic blood flow appears to be unchanged during pregnancy (1). However, there is evidence that the elimination rate of clindamycin, which is metabolized by the liver, is increased during pregnancy (3), suggesting a possible increase in hepatic clearance. It is also possible that the faster elimination of trimethoprim-sulfamethoxazole observed during pregnancy is due to higher hepatic clearance, although increased renal clearance may be the major determinant of this change (11).

As shown in Table 1, the above-mentioned changes in the pharmacokinetics of many antibiotics administered during pregnancy result in a decrease in serum concentrations when compared with concentrations observed in nonpregnant women. Thus, the standard dose schedule may result in lower concentrations in the pregnant woman. This may have important implications in treating both maternal and fetal infections.

B. The Placental-Fetal Compartment

Almost all drugs, including most antimicrobial agents, have been shown to penetrate the placenta and to appear in measurable concentrations in the fetal blood. In general, the ratio between antibiotic concentration in the fetus vs. mother is different from (in most cases less than) unity (Table 2). Several mechanisms govern the movement of drugs across the placental barrier and determine the maternofetal ratio of drug concentrations.

1. Differences in Protein Binding

Fetal protein appears to bind less avidly various drugs, including ampicillin and benzylpenicillin (30). Conversely, no differences between maternal and fetal protein binding could be documented for methicillin and dicloxacillin (27). Salicylates, on the other hand, appear to have a more extensive binding to fetal than to maternal protein (31).

During pregnancy there is a gradual decrease in concentrations of maternal albumin and an increase in concentrations of fetal albumin. Consequently, at different times during pregnancy, different fetal-maternal ratios of albumin occur. At term, it appears that fetal albumin concentrations are equal or even higher than in the mother. The degree

Table 1 Antibiotics with Lower Serum Concentrations During Pregnancy and Relevant Pharmacokinetic Parameters

Drug	Elimination $t_{1/2}$	V_d	Clearance
Amikacin	↓		
Ampicillin	↓	↑	↑
Cephalosporins	↓	↓	
Erythromycin			
Gentamicin	→		
Kanamycin	→		
Methicillin	↑		
Nitrofurantoin			
Oxacillin		↑	↑

Source: From References 3, 4, and 12–18.

Table 2 Fetomaternal Concentration Ratio of Antibiotics

Drug	Fetomaternal ratio
Ampicillin	0.38–0.87
Cephalosporins	0.13–1
Clindamycin	0.4–0.5
Dicloxacillin	0.07–0.27
Fosfomycin	0.09–0.68
Gentamicin	0.21–1
Methicillin	0.83–1.43
Penicillin G	0.06–0.7
Thiamphenicol	0.3–1.5

Source: From References 3 and 19–29.

of protein binding of a drug appears to be an important determinant of the degree of placental penetration. The least protein bound drugs (e.g., ampicillin, 20%) reach higher concentrations in the fetus and in the amniotic fluid. Drugs with high protein binding (e.g., dicloxacillin, 96%) achieve higher maternal and lower fetal concentrations, as only the free fraction of the drug crosses the placental barrier. However, as additional determinants other than protein binding may play an important role in placental passage, such drugs as sulfisoxazole reach therapeutic concentrations in the fetus in spite of high protein binding.

2. Differences in pH

Fetal blood pH is slightly lower than the maternal. This pH gradient may influence the movement of drugs according to their pK_a; weak bases, with pK_a values close to the blood pH, will be mainly nonionized and consequently will easily cross the placenta, as nonionized molecules penetrate biologic membranes more quickly than ionized molecules. However, after penetration and contact with the more acidic fetal blood, these molecules are ionized as the fetal pH is less close to the pK_a. This results in an apparent fall in fetal concentrations of nonionized drug and in a subsequent concentration gradient, leading to net movement from maternal to fetal systems (32). This mechanism is commonly referred to as "ion trapping." In contrast to weak bases, ion trapping induced from fetal to maternal circulations is likely to occur with weak acids.

Other important determinants of antimicrobial transport across the placenta are water and lipid solubility, molecular weight, and the surface available for diffusion. A good example for the different effects on placental passage is the higher concentrations of trimethoprim in the fetus than in the mother, corresponding to its relatively low protein binding (42–46%), a pK_a of 6.6, and poor water solubility. Sulfamethoxazole, on the other hand, has good water solubility at physiological pH and therefore has more difficulty in crossing the lipid placental barrier. Both drugs appear to reach the amniotic fluid, and their concentration ratio there closely corresponds to that in the fetal serum (33).

Following repeated doses of antibiotics, concentrations measured in the fetus appear to be higher than following a single dose (34). It appears that repeated high bolus injections of ampicillin or gentamicin yield higher concentrations in fetal serum and amniotic fluids than a similar dose given as a continuous infusion (35). Most antimicrobial agents follow a similar pattern of transplacental transfer, and after a single intravenous dose a peak umbilical concentration is achieved within 30-60 min.

3. Fetoplacental Drug Elimination

Drug metabolism has been documented by the fetal liver as early as 7-8 weeks of pregnancy. Virtually all enzymatic processes, including phase 1 (oxidation, dehydrogenation, reduction, hydrolysis, and so on) and phase 2 (glucuronidation, methylation, acetylation, and so on) have been documented in the fetal liver (36). However, the degree of activity is very low in most cases when compared with adult liver. Similarly, drug metabolizing activity has been demonstrated in human placental tissue. However, the placentofetal unit contributes only marginally to the total elimination capacity of drugs by the maternal body. As pregnancy progresses, higher amounts of antimicrobials are excreted into the amniotic fluids through fetal urine. This process depends upon the maturation of the fetal kidney.

In general, metabolites are more polar than their parent compounds and are therefore less likely to cross the placental barrier. As a result, metabolites may accumulate in various tissues of the fetus or may be recovered from the amniotic fluid. A recent study has shown that thiamphenicol achieves higher concentrations in the umbilical vein than in the umbilical artery, reflecting some degree of extraction of the drug by the fetus, probably by renal excretion (29).

II. FETAL TOXICITY AND TERATOGENICITY DUE TO ANTIMICROBIAL DRUGS

For decades it was assumed that the placenta serves as a barrier defending the embryo and fetus from chemical or microorganic insults. In 1941, the association between the rubella virus and teratogenicity was documented (37). In 1961, the devastating teratogenic effects of thalidomide were reported (38). It is now evident that essentially all drugs and many metabolites cross the placenta to various extents. In the present medical and litiginous atmosphere, high sensitivity exists for possible toxicity or teratogenicity caused by drugs and chemicals. However, there are serious methodological problems stemming from the process of data collection that hamper our ability to judge whether a given drug is truly a teratogen.

In the next paragraphs the different approaches of data collection will be briefly discussed and their major handicaps will be mentioned. A broader discussion on these issues can be found in the texts by Heinohen et al. (39) or by Schardein (40).

A. Animal Studies

A drug is administered to pregnant animals in various stages of development, and the nature and incidence of malformations are recorded. Unlike most human studies, a dose-response curve can be established. In many cases the malformations resemble human teratogenicity (e.g., retinoic acid), whereas in others there is no correlation (e.g., coumadins).

B. Case Reports

Generally, the first notion on possible drug-associated teratogenicity is reported as a single case or a small group of cases. Many drugs that were initially incriminated as teratogens based on case reports were shown later to be innocent in larger controlled studies.

The main disadvantage in a case report is that the investigator does not know the total number of exposures to the specific drug. Let us assume, for example, that 200,000 pregnant women are treated annually with ampicillin. If 3% of all women are likely to have offspring with a major malformation (39), this means that 6000 fetuses exposed in utero to ampicillin will have malformations that are not caused by this drug. A small number of case reports on ampicillin-associated teratogenicity may distort the fact that thousands of women were exposed at the same time without any effect. Yet, a case report is an important tool if a rare drug taken by a small number of women yields a rate of teratogenicity much higher than expected in the general population. For the coumadins, valproic acid, and retinoic acid, the first concern for teratogenicity was based on case reports (40).

C. Retrospective Studies

In these studies, investigators try to answer such questions as (1) what the rate of teratogenicity is among *all* women exposed to a certain drug, and (2) what the rate of exposure is to a certain drug among *all* offspring who have a certain anomaly.

Several problems make the collection and interpretation of such data difficult. How can one be sure that all exposures are recorded? How can one rely on memory many months after the exposure (recall bias)? This is important not only with respect to the quality and quantity of the drug, but also for the time of exposure, as most teratogenic effects occur during certain stages of embryogenesis.

If a drug is extremely teratogenic (e.g., thalidomide or retinoic acid), it is likely that even a relatively small number of exposures will be associated with a high rate of malformations. On the contrary, if the teratogenicity rate is only slightly above normal figures, recall bias and incomplete cohorts may dramatically distort the conclusions.

D. Prospective Studies

In an attempt to avoid the above-mentioned shortcomings, prospective studies record all exposures in the study group and correlate them with the rate of teratogenicity. A classic example is the Collaborative Perinatal Study (39), which was executed in several centers during the 1960s and included more than 50,000 mother-child pairs. For each drug, the rate of malformations was compared to the group not exposed to the specific agent by defining the *relative risk*.

It is important to remember that the disease itself for which drugs are indicated during pregnancy may increase the risk of teratogenicity. In the Collaborative Perinatal Study, isoniazid was shown to be associated with malformations in 10 of 84 mother-child pairs, almost twice the expected rate. Theoretically, this could be related also to the tuberculosis. Retrospective analysis of 4900 exposures to isoniazid documented a rate of malformation similar to that in nonexposed pregnancies. To date it is thought that isoniazid can be safely used for prophylaxis against tuberculosis during pregnancy (40).

E. Specific Antimicrobials Causing Fetal Toxicity or Teratogenicity

In this review only drugs for which there is convincing evidence for teratogenic or toxic effects on the developing organism will be included. For many other agents there is some evidence based on case reports; however, these have not been confirmed by larger studies. Several antimicrobial agents have been shown to cause fetal toxicity similar to the toxicity association when administered postnatally.

1. Chloroquine

Chloroquine is considered by many the drug of choice for malaria, amebic hepatitis, and diskoid lupus erythematosus during pregnancy (35). This drug, if administered for long periods, may cause in children and adults cinchonism, which includes headache, vertigo, retinopathy, ototoxicity, and cardiovascular effects. Following prolonged administration throughout pregnancy, there have been several cases of cochleovestibular paresis in offspring (41,42).

2. Quinine

Similarly to chloroquine, quinine may cause cinchonism in children and adults. Auditory and optic nerve damage has been reported in fetuses exposed to toxic doses as an abortifacient. If appears, however, that when the drug is given in therapeutic doses, these toxic effects are not documented (43).

3. Primaquine

Primaquine may cause intravascular hemolysis secondary to the relative deficiency of fetal glucose-6-phosphate dehydrogenase and glutathione (44).

4. Streptomycin and Kanamycin

These two aminoglycosides have been shown to rapidly cross the placenta and to achieve high concentrations in the fetal circulation. Several cases of congenital deafness of fetuses exposed to these aminoglycosides have been reported following high doses (45). In a large survey of 391 pregnant women exposed to kanamycin, 50 mg/kg day^{-1} for prolonged periods, 2.3% of offspring had ototoxicity (9 cases) (46). No other complications or malformations were associated with these two aminoglycosides.

Gentamicin, amikacin, and tobramycin, which have largely substituted streptomycin and kanamycin for gram-negative infections, have not been shown to cause ototoxocity in the fetus. This pattern is consistent with the rate of ototoxicity in children and adults seen with these drugs compared with streptomycin and kanamycin.

5. Sulfonamides

Drugs belonging to this group readily cross the placenta, achieving fetal concentrations 70-90% of maternal. If given near term, concentrations can be detected in the neonate for several days. The main potential problem following fetal exposure to sulfonamide is competition with nonconjugated bilirubin on protein binding. During fetal life, the clearance of free bilirubin is conducted through the placenta. However, after birth, increased concentrations of nonconjugated bilirubin following its displacement by sulfonamides may cause a toxic elevation of free bilirubin, which may pass the blood-brain barrier and cause kernicterus. This complication may potentially happen following antenatal exposure to sulfonamides, as was described with postnatal exposure; such cases have not been described (46).

After being shown to be teratogenic in some animal models, several large studies have tried to define the rate of malformations caused by sulfonamides in the human fetus. Women with ulcerative colitis or Crohn's disease treated throughout pregnancy with sulfasalazine did not have a higher rate of adverse effects. Similarly, the prospective Collaborative Perinatal Project could not detect evidence of major or minor malformations in 1455 exposures in its 50,282 mother-child pairs (39).

Conversely, two retrospective studies have found higher rates of maternal usage of sulfonamides associated with teratogenicity compared with a control group (46).

6. Tetracyclines

Tetracyclines are the only group of antimicrobial agents whose fetotoxic effect has been proven beyond doubt. Consequently, they should be avoided during pregnancy. Following placental passage, they form a complex with calcium orthophosphate, which causes a permanent yellow-brown discoloration of teeth. This dental complication is not expected to occur if tetracyclines are used before months 5-6 of gestation, before calcification of deciduous teeth takes place. As the same process may involve the permanent teeth, tetracyclines should be avoided before the age of 7-8 years, when calcification of these teeth is completed (47).

As for other congenital defects, evidence is not as clear. The Collaborative Perinatal Project monitored prospectively 564 mother-child pairs exposed to various tetracyclines during the first trimester and 1944 exposures during any time in pregnancy. There was statistical evidence for minor, but not major, malformations. Associations of tetracycline with hypospadias, inguinal hernia, and hypoplasia of a limb or part of it have been pointed out; however this must be verified in further studies (39). It is impossible to tell whether the diseases for which tetracyclines were administered did not themselves increase the teratogenic risk.

During the 1960s, several cases of acute fatty degeneration of the liver were reported in pregnant women following the intravenous administration of high-dose (>2 gr/day) tetracyclines, mainly for pyelonephritis. Because of the poor maternal outcome, stillbirth and premature births were common.

7. Antifungal Agents

Both flucytosine and griseofulvin have been shown to be teratogenic in animal studies (48,49). Therefore, they are not recommended for use during pregnancy.

8. Pyrimethamine

This antimalarial agent, a folic acid antagonist, has been shown to cause teratogenicity in animals. Therefore, although its safety in humans has not been established, it is not commonly used during pregnancy.

9. Dapsone

Dapsone is used in combination with pyrimethamine to treat chloroquine-resistant falciparum malaria. This sulfone is capable of producing hemolytic anemia and methemoglobinemia, and therefore it should be used only for clear indications during pregnancy.

10. Mebendazole

Although it is very poorly absorbed from the intestine, mebendazole has been proven teratogenic and embryotoxic in animal studies and should be avoided during pregnancy (50).

REFERENCES

1. Krauer, B, Krauer, F: Drug kinetics in pregnancy. In: *Handbook of Clinical Pharmacokinetics*, Section II (M Gibaldi and L Prescott, eds.), 1983, pp. 1-17.

2. Philipson, A: Pharmacokinetics of ampicillin during pregnancy. *J. Infect. Dis. 136*: 370–376, 1977.
3. Weinstein, AJ, Gibbs, RS, Gallagher, M: Placental transfer of clindamycin and gentamicin in term pregnancy. *Am. J. Obstet. Gynecol. 124*:688–691, 1976.
4. Bernard, B, Abate, M, Thielen, PF, Attar, H, Ballard, CA, Wehnle, PF: Maternal fetal pharmacological activity of amikacin. *J. Infect. Dis. 135*:925–932, 1977.
5. Hytten, FE, Leitch, T: *The Physiology of Pregnancy*, Blackwell Scientific, Oxford, 1971.
6. Pizani, BBK, Campbell, DM, McGillivray, T: Plasma volume in normal pregnancy. *J. Obstet. Gynecol. 80*:884–887, 1973.
7. Walters, WAW, Lengling, Y: Blood volume and haemodynamics in pregnancy. In: *Obstetrics and Gynecology*, Vol. 2, Saunders, London, 1975, pp. 301–302.
8. Davidson, JM, Hytten, FE: Glomerular filtration during and after pregnancy. *J. Obstet. Gynecol. 81*:588–595, 1974.
9. Young, IM: The placenta: Blood flow and transfer. In: *Modern Trends in Physiology*, Butterworth, London, 1972, pp. 214–244.
10. Kerr, MG: Cardiovascular dynamics in pregnancy and labour. *Br. Med. Bull. 24*:19–24, 1968.
11. Ylikorkala, O, Sjostedt, E, Jarvinen, PA, Tikkanen, R, Raines, T: Trimetoprim-sulfonamide combination administered orally and intravaginally in the first trimester of pregnancy: Its absorption into serum and transfer to amniotic fluid. *Acta Obstet. Gynecol. Scand. 52*:229–234, 1973.
12. Bray, RE, Boe, RW, Johnson, WL: Transfer of ampicillin into fetus and amniotic fluid from maternal plasma in late pregnancy. *Am. J. Obstet. Gynecol. 96*:938–942, 1966.
13. Bernard, B, Barton, L, Abate, M, Ballard, CA: Maternal fetal transfer of cefazolin in the first twenty weeks of pregnancy. *J. Infect. Dis. 136*:377–382, 1977.
14. Philipson, A, Saboth, LD, Charles, D: Erythromycin and clindamycin absorption and elimination in pregnant women. *Clin. Pharmacol. Ther. 19*:68–77, 1976.
15. Good, RG, Johnson, G: The placental transfer of kanamycin in late pregnancy. *Obstet. Gynecol. 38*:60–62, 1971.
16. MacAulay, MA, Berg, SR, Charles, D: Placental transfer of methicillin. *Am. J. Obstet. Gynecol. 115*:58–65, 1973.
17. Amon, K, Amon, I, Huller, H: Verteilung und kinetik von nitrofurantoin in der fruhschwangerschaft. *Int. J. Clin. Pharmacol. Ther. Toxicol. 63*:218–222, 1972.
18. Bastert, G, Muller, WG, Wallhauser, KH, Hebauf, H: Pharmacokinetishe untersuchungen zum ubertriff von antibiotika in das fruchtwasser am enter der schwangerschaft. 3. Oxacillin. *Z. Geburtshife. Perinatol. 179*:346–355, 1975.
19. Hirsch, HA, Dreher, E, Perrochet, A, Schmid, E: Transfer of ampicillin to the fetus and amniotic fluid during continuous infusion (steady state) and by repeated single intravenous injections to the mother. *Infection 2*:207–212, 1974.
20. Croft, I, Forster, TC: Materno-fetal cephadine transfer in pregnancy. *Antimicrob Agents Chemother. 14*:924–926, 1978.
21. Barr, W, Graham, RM: Placental transmission of cephaloxidine. *J. Obstet. Gynecol. 74*:739–745, 1947.
22. Hirsch, HA, Herbet, S, Lang, R, Dettli, L, Goblinger, A: Transfer of a new cephalosporin antibiotic to the fetus and the amniotic fluid during a continuous infusion (steady state) and single repeated intravenous injections to the mother. *Anchiv für Gynakologie 216*:1–14, 1974.
23. MacAuley, MA, Abou-Sabe, M, Charles, D: Placental transfer of dicloxacillin at term. *Am. J. Obstet. Gynecol. 102*:1162–1168, 1968.
24. Ferreres, L, Paz, M, Martin, G, Gobernado, M: New studies on placental transfer of fosfomycin. *Chemotherapy (Suppl. 1)*:175–179, 1977.

25. Daubenfeld, O, Modde, H, Hirsch, HA: Transfer of gentamicin to the foetus and amniotic fluid during a steady state in the mother. *Arch. Gynecol. 217*:233–240, 1974.
26. Yoshioka, H, Monma, T, Matsudo, S: Placental transfer of gentamicin. *J. Pediatr. 80*:121–123, 1972.
27. Depp, R, Kind, AC, Kirby, WMM, Johnson, WL: Transplacental passage of methicillin and dicloxacillin into the fetus and amniotic fluid. *Am. J. Obstet. Gynecol. 107*:1054–1057, 1970.
28. Charles, D: Placental transmission of antibiotics. *J. Obstet. Gynecol. 61*:790–797, 1954.
29. Plomp, TA, Moes, RAA, Thiery, M: Placental transfer of thiamphenicol in term pregnancy. *Eur. J. Obstet. Gynecol. Reprod. Biol. 7*:383–388, 1977.
30. Tucker, GT, Boyes, RN, Bridenbaugh, PO: Binding of anilide-type local anesthetics in human plasma. II. Implications in vivo, with special reference to transplacental distribution. *Anesthesiology 33*:304–314, 1970.
31. Levy, G: Salicylate pharmacokinetics in the human neonate: In: *Basic and Therapeutic Aspects of Perinatal Pharmacology* (Morselli, PL, Garattini, S, and Sereni, F, eds.), Raven Press, New York, 1975, pp. 319–330.
32. Asling, JH, Way, EL: Placental transfer of drugs. In: *Fundamentals of Drug Metabolism and Drug Disposition* (La Du, Mandel, and Y. Way, eds.), Williams and Wilkins. Baltimore, 1972, p. 88.
33. Walter, AM, Heilmeyer, L: *Antibiotika-Fibel*, Vol. 4, Georg Thieme Verlag, Stuttgart, 1975.
34. Philipson, A: Pharmacokinetics of antibiotics in pregnancy and labour. *Clin. Pharmacokinet. 4*:297–309, 1979.
35. Chow, AW, Jewesson, PJ: Pharmacokinetics and safety of antimicrobial agents during pregnancy. *Rev. Infect. Dis. 7*:287–313, 1985.
36. Juchau, MR, Chao, ST, Omiecinski, CJ: Drug metabolism by the human fetus. In: *Handbook of Clinical Pharmacokinetics*, Section II (M Gibaldi and L Prescott, eds.), ADIS Health Sciences Press, New York, 1983, pp. 58–78.
37. Gregg, NM: Congenital cataract following German measles in the mother. *Trans. Ophthalmol. Soc. Aust. 3*:35–36, 1941.
38. McBride, WG: Thalidomide and congenital abnormalities. *Lancet 2*:1358, 1961.
39. Heinonen, OP, Slone, D, Shapiro, S: *Birth Defects and Drugs in Pregnancy*, Publishing Sciences Group, Littleton, Massachusetts, 1977.
40. Schardein, JL: *Chemically Induced Birth Defects*, Marcel Dekker, New York, 1985.
41. Matz, GJ, Naunton, RF: Ototoxicity of chloroquine. *Arch. Otolaryngol. 88*:50–52, 1968.
42. Hart, CW, Naunton, RF: The ototoxicity of chloroquine sulphate. *Arch. Otolaryngol. 80*:401–412, 1964.
43. Morgon, A, Charachon, D, Brinquier, N: Disorders of the auditory apparatus caused by embryopathy or foetopathy; prophylaxis and treatment. *Acta Otolaryngol. (Stockh.) 291 (Suppl.)*:5, 1971.
44. Adamsons, K, Jaelsson, I: The effects of pharmacologic agents upon the fetus and newborn. *Am. J. Obstet. Gynecol. 96*:437–460, 1966.
45. Assael, BM, Parini, R, Ruxoni, F: Ototoxicity of aminoglycoside antibiotics in infants and children. *Pediatr. Infect. Dis. 1*:357–365, 1982.
46. Briggs, CG, Bodendorfer, TW, Freeman, RK, Yaffe, SJ: *Drugs in Pregnancy and Lactation*, Williams and Wilkins, Baltimore, 1986.
47. Cohlan, SQ: Tetracycline staining of teeth. *Teratology 15*:127–130, 1977.
48. Schonebeck, J, Segerbrand, E: *Candida albicans* septicemia during first half of pregnancy successfully treated with 5-fluorocytoxine. *Br. Med. J. 4*:337–338, 1973.

49. Klein, MF, Beall, JR: Griseofulvin: A teratogenic study. *Science 175*:1483–1484, 1972.
50. Keystone, JS, Murdoch, JK: Mebendazole. *Ann. Intern. Med. 91*:582–586, 1979.

8

Specific Problems Associated with Drug Administration in Neonates and Infants

MARK GREENWALD AND GIDEON KOREN
The Hospital for Sick Children, and the University of Toronto, Toronto, Ontario, Canada

It is generally assumed that the intravenous route of drug administration guarantees proper delivery of the intended dose. This assumption cannot be taken for granted in the neonate and small infant. Slow infusion rates, various injection sites, variable injection volumes and different specific gravities of injected solutions are some of the factors that may influence the rate and extent of intravenous administration of antimicrobial drugs. In addition, medication errors are probably more common in this age group than is generally appreciated.

I. INFUSION RATES, DRUG VOLUMES, AND INJECTION SITES

Roberts was the first to draw attention to the importance of the infusion rate and portal of injection on the speed and completeness of drugs administered by the intravenous route (1). A full-term neonate receiving 100-140 ml water per kilogram of body weight per day generally will require an infusion rate of 10-20 ml/hr in the absence of oral intake. A preterm infant weighing less than 1 kg often will be receiving intravenous fluids at a rate of 3-5 ml/hr. Gould and Roberts have demonstrated that, at an infusion rate of 3 ml/hr, actual infusion of drug begins 160 min after injection into the system close to the reservoir and will only be completed after 12 hr (2). Drug administration will be faster when the portal for injection is closer to the neonate. This delay in the administration of a drug may compromise therapy. In addition, if serum concentrations of the drug are being monitored, accurate timing will be difficult. An attempt to increase the infusion rate is often not possible as infants in intensive care units receive an average of 10 intravenous doses per day (3) and therefore cannot tolerate an excessive infusion rate. In the original observations, injection portals were not necessarily as proximal as possible to the infant. This problem can be minimized by injecting the drug at a site as close as possible to the neonate.

Delivery of drugs to neonates should utilize pumps calibrated to accurately deliver very small volumes. If desired, these small volumes can then be infused at a rate much higher than the maintenance infusion rate, thus guaranteeing rapid delivery with only small volume of fluid delivered.

The volume in which the drug is prepared is another important factor delineated by Roberts: the higher the volume, the more time required to deliver the full dose. Consequently, flow rate in conjunction with dosage volume will dictate the time needed for full delivery of a given dose.

II. LOSS OF DRUGS WHILE CHANGING INTRAVENOUS SETS

Gould and Roberts drew attention to the fact that, owing to frequent intravenous set replacement, multiple-dose administration, and slow infusion rates in neonates, as much as 38% of the total drug doses intended may be lost in the discarded sets (2). When a drug is discontinued the physician should keep in mind the amount of drug still in the line. Flushing the set with drug-free solution or changing the set will guarantee discontinuation of the drug delivery.

III. FILTER DEVICES

Filters are often connected to the intravenous tubing in neonatal units to clean the infusion fluid of bubbles, particles, and microorganisms. However, in 1975 Wagman et al. documented the binding of antimicrobial agents to filter devices (4). In 1981, Rajchgot et al. noticed that subtherapeutic serum concentrations of gentamicin and cloxacillin

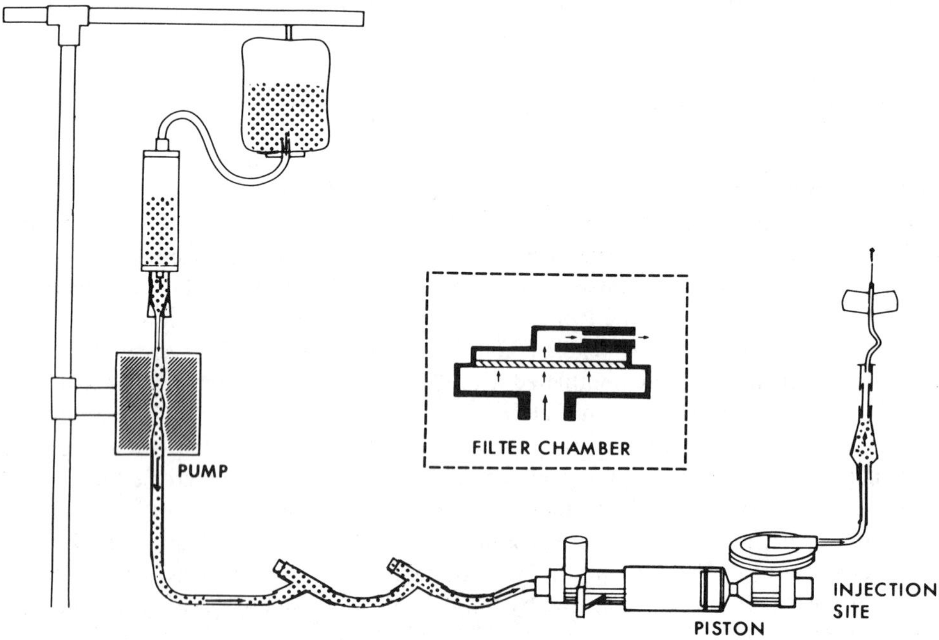

Figure 1 A combination of a slow infusion rate and injection of the drug proximal to a filter chamber may result in sequestration of the drug in the filter chamber.

were achieved in neonates receiving these drugs intravenously through a site proximal to a filter chamber (5). Subsequent analysis has shown that drugs delivered by slow infusion rates tend to be sequestered in the filter according to their specific gravity; the higher the specific gravity (e.g., cloxacillin) the more is likely the drug to stay in the filter chamber (Figure 1). Following these findings, the manufacturer devised a new filter chamber to permit full delivery of injected drugs even with slow infusion rates (Figure 2).

In order to avoid accumulation of the drug in the tubing during slow infusion rates, the dose is injected into a specially designed syringe chamber (Figure 2). Extra fluid is permitted to be drained into a small additional bag. The infusion volume first pushes the piston back to its original place; only then is the infusion fluid able to pass the unidirectional valve. This guarantees propagation of the full dose without dilution through the filter chamber. Full recovery of injected doses of gentamicin and cloxacillin can be documented in studies in vitro (6). In subsequent in vivo studies in 70 neonates serving as their own controls, we showed that concentrations produced by injecting the dose into the new device were comparable to those achieved by a direct intravenous bolus into the site nearest the neonate (7).

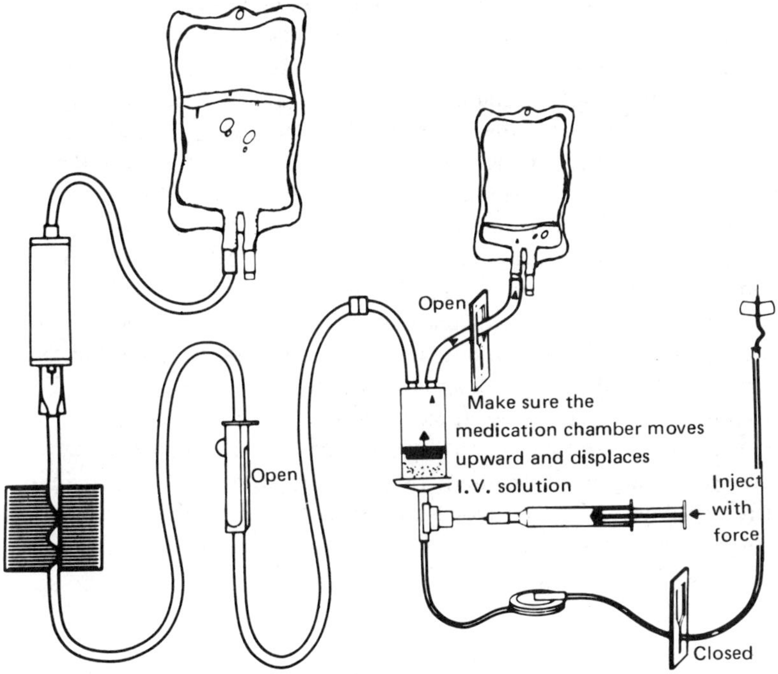

Figure 2 A newly devised filter chamber, in which the drug is injected into the specially designed syringe chamber. Extra fluid is permitted to be drained into a small additional bag. The infusion volume first pushes the piston back to its original place; only then will the infusion fluid be able to pass the unidirectional valve. This guarantees propagation of the full dose.

IV. "DILUTION INTOXICATION"

Neonates require very small doses of intravenous preparations. In order to meet the required dose it is often necessary to dilute the stock solution. For example, if a neonate requires 2.5 mg gentamicin from a stock solution of 50 mg/ml (adult preparation), then 0.05 ml is required. Because it is difficult to deal with such small injection volumes, the physician often dilutes this dose, by adding another 0.05 ml saline, for example. Here the dead space of the tuberculin syringe is filled to the 0.05-ml level. This space contains gentamicin in our example, and the addition of 0.05-ml saline "pushes" gentamicin from the dead space into the syringe; the child is likely to receive more than the intended 2.5 mg. In a recent study, Berman and his colleagues (8) demonstrated that, in the case of dilution of digoxin, the dead space would increase an intended dose of 5 μg to 12–18 μg (average, 14 μg). Thus, dilution of a very small dosage volume in order to increase accuracy ends in potential overdosing. Similarly, a case of morphine toxicity due to "dilution intoxication" has been reported (9). Roberts has calculated the effect of dilutional intoxication of several medications when prepared in the routine way (10).

V. ERRORS IN ADMINISTRATION OF DRUG DOSES

The neglected problem of errors in administration of drug doses in pediatric patients has gained some publicity in the last decade. Perlstein and his colleagues have shown that approximately 8% of the calculations of drug volumes from a stock solution is erroneous, in many cases 10-fold higher or lower than the intended dose (11). These results were confirmed in a subsequent study, showing the existance of an "accident-prone" subgroup of health personnel who tend to perform significantly more computation errors than other staff members (12). These subjects also had significantly more 10-fold errors. Although this figure of 3–6% for 10-fold calculation errors in a written test may seem excessive, a recent study from Britain reported a comparable incidence of 10-fold errors in administering intravenous acetylcysteine for acetaminophen toxicity (13).

Computational errors are not the only explanation for dosing errors. We recently reported a case of identical twins who received, because the written order was misread, two doses of 50 mg gentamicin instead of 5 mg. All appropriate staff should be aware of the appropriate dosages for neonates. A similar example is shown in Figure 3. The resultant acute renal failure took months to resolve, and it is premature to evaluate ototoxicity (14). Errors committed by parents of a sick infant are also likely to occur if the dose intended was not clearly explained (14). Pharmacy errors are less likely as pharmacists appear to be more knowledgeable and better trained in these matters than nurses and physicians (11).

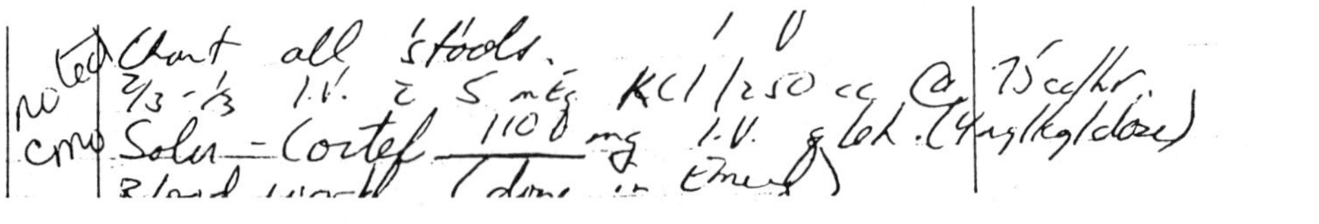

Figure 3 A 10-fold error in the dose of steroids. Notice that a letter "q" from the second line adds a zero to the dose of Solu-Cortef in the third line.

Because medication errors may result in morbidity and even mortality, various solutions to this issue have been suggested (12,14).

1. A written test for all personnel involved in the preparation of doses from stock solution; a good correlation exists between these written tests (12) and the real-life occurrence rate (14). It is suggested that staff members who fail this test will be retrained before being allowed to prepare drug doses for infants.
2. Double-checking of calculations by two staff members. Statistically, if each of them is computing the dose independently, the chance of an error should be decreased significantly; if each staff member has a 6% chance of making an error, both of them have a chance of 6% × 6% = 0.36%.
3. Use of standard tables of recommended dose and volume of stock solution of drugs given intravenously to neonates and small infants.
4. Patient-dose unit prepared by clinical pharmacists, thus obviating errors by nursing staff and doctors. Although this system increases the financial burden, pharmacists are likely to produce less errors in their computations (11).

VI. CONCLUSIONS

The common denominator of the specific problems delineated in this chapter is the very small doses of drugs given to neonates. Although these issues are not confined only to antimicrobial drugs, antibiotics by far exceed all other medications used in the nursery in terms of number of doses (3). Only well-trained personnel familiar with the appropriate doses for this age group and the effective methods to calculate them and to deliver them intravenously, will be able to guarantee optimal antimicrobial therapy to small infants.

REFERENCES

1. Roberts, RP: Intravenous administration of medication in pediatric patients: Problems and solutions. *Pediatr. Clin. North Am. 28*:23–34, 1981.
2. Goult, T, Roberts, RJ: Therapeutic problems arising from the use of intravenous route of drug administration. *J. Pediatr. 95*:465–471, 1979.
3. Aranda, JV, Cohen, S, Neims, AH: Drug utilization in a newborn intensive care unit. *J. Pediatr. 89*:315–317, 1976.
4. Wagman, GH, Bailey, JV, Weinstein, MJ: Binding of aminoglycoside antibiotics to filtration materials. *Antimicrob. Agents Chemother.* 7:316–319, 1975.
5. Rajchgot, P, Radde, JC, MacLeod, SM: Influence of specific gravity on intravenous drug delivery. *J. Pediatr. 99*:658–661, 1981.
6. Koren, G, Rajchgot, P, Good, F, Harding, E, MacLeod, SM: Improved techniques for I.V. drug delivery in children. *Am. J. IV Ther. Nutr. 10*:33–38, 1983.
7. Koren, G, Rajchgot, P, Harding, E, Perlman, M, MacLeod, SM: Evaluating a filter device used for intermittent intravenous drug delivery to newborn infants. *Am. J. Hosp. Pharm. 42*:106–108, 1985.
8. Berman, WJ, Whitman, V, Marks, KH. Inadvertent overadministration of digoxin to low-birthweight infants. *J. Pediatr. 92*:1024–1025, 1978.
9. Zenk, KE, Anderson, S: Improving the accuracy of mini-volume injections. *Infusion 7* (Jan.–Feb.), 1982.

10. Roberts, RJ: *Drug Therapy in Infants*, W. B. Saunders Co., Philadelphia, 1984, p. 30.
11. Perlstein, PH, Callison, C, White, M, et al.: Errors in drug computations during newborn intensive care. *Am. J. Dis. Child. 133*:376–379, 1979.
12. Koren, G, Barzilay, Z, Modan, M: Errors in computation of drug doses. *Can. Med. Assoc. J. 129*:721–723, 1983.
13. Mant, TGK, Tempowski, JH, Volans, GN, Talbot, JCC: Adverse reactions to acetylcysteine and effects of overdose. *Br. Med. J. 289*:217–219, 1984.
14. Koren, G, Barzilay, Z, Greenwald, M: Tenfold errors in drug administration to children: A neglected iatrogenic disease. *Pediatrics* (in press) 1986.

9

Compliance with Antimicrobial Therapy in Children

ELAINE WANG AND R. BRIAN HAYNES
McMaster University, Hamilton, Ontario, Canada

One of the important determinants of the effectiveness of any intervention that must be self-administered by the patient or parent is compliance, defined as "the extent to which a patient's behaviour, in terms of taking medications, following diets, or executing life-style changes, coincides with clinical prescriptions" (1).

I. MAGNITUDE OF THE PROBLEM

The frequency of patient compliance varies in different studies depending on the patient population studied, the methods used to promote compliance (if any), and the measurement and definition of compliance that were used. Thus, compliance rates in individuals taking antibiotics range from 7 to 89% (2-7).

II. DETERMINANTS OF COMPLIANCE

A. Social Factors

Several studies have found associations among compliance and age, sex, race, and residence (8,9). Differences observed in some studies in parental marital status, years of schooling (2), social class, and medical sophistication (10,11) have not been found consistently. Significantly better compliance was found in families with good parental relations and strong cohesiveness (9,12). Illness in other family members decreased compliance (12).

Korsch et al. examined compliance in children with renal disease who were taking immunosuppressants (12). They found that noncompliance was associated with poor self-esteem and poor socialization. In a study of contraceptive compliance, adolescent girls who were autonomous in their clinic visit (making their own appointments and paying fees themselves) were also more compliant (13).

Patient or parent knowledge of the disease and/or its treatment does not appear to influence compliance (5,6,14).

B. Therapy Factors

The complexity and duration of medication are inversely associated with compliance (15-17). The simultaneous prescription of more than one medication or the use of multiple rather than single doses adversely affects compliance (15,16).

C. Illness Factors

Low compliance has been found with the self-administered treatments that have been prescribed for all diseases studied to date and does not appear to be related to the type of illness (18). However, the patient's prior experience with illness and the perception of illness "seriousness" may modify compliance (19).

D. Factors Relating to the Physician-Patient Relationship

One study found that having a consistent physician increased compliance (3), but another study found that this decreased compliance (20). The lack of consistent relationships here likely reflects the low sophistication of current techniques for measuring the quality of patient-provider interactions. A delay in seeing patients who are attempting to make appointments and long waiting times at appointments may impair compliance. Parental understanding of the physician's instructions and the degree of their agreement with the diagnosis and proposed treatment may substantially modify compliance.

III. COMPLIANCE AND PROGNOSIS

There is a direct positive relationship between compliance and outcome that appears to be independent of the treatment prescribed, since it occurs even among patients prescribed placebos during clinical trials (4,21). Pizzo et al. (21) examined the efficacy of antibiotic prophylaxis to prevent infections and fever in cancer patients who were granulocytopenic after chemotherapy. They noted that individuals with excellent compliance did better even if they had been randomized to placebo. They suggested that patient compliance may be an important independent prognostic factor. Although this hypothesis makes intuitive sense, one must be cautious in such interpretations. Noncompliance in placebo recipients may have been related to a lack of perceived benefit, whereas a lack of compliance in drug recipients may have been due to adverse effects of the medication—two quite different "motives" for noncompliance.

IV. MEASUREMENT OF COMPLIANCE

A. Physician Impression

Physicians usually rely on their knowledge of a patient to assess that patient's compliance. Thus, few physicians measure compliance with methods that are more sophisticated than an "impression." When physician estimates of patient compliance were compared with more objective measures, these estimates were found to be inaccurate in one-third of the cases (3,6,22-24) as physicians tend to overestimate drug compliance (22). When only judgments in which physicians were most confident were analyzed, they still could not distinguish good from poor compliers (22). Even family physicians who had a long relationship with their patients identified noncompliant patients with a sensitivity of only 9% and a specificity of 87% (25). In other words, fewer than 1 in 10 noncompliant patients was identified. Furthermore, the physician's estimate of a patient's compliance was in fact no better than that which would occur by chance alone.

B. Failure to Achieve a Treatment Target

Failure to achieve a treatment target could indicate noncompliance. However, the course of the disease frequently depends on factors other than the study intervention. For example, the disease may be characterized by exacerbations and remissions; it may be triggered by environmental factors or viral infections; and its control may require a management program of which the treatment under study is only one component (26). A treatment target may be achieved if the disease was initially misdiagnosed or when full compliance to therapy is unnecessary (for example, when a small dose was adequate). Furthermore, pharmacokinetic variability, with impaired absorption or enhanced elimination of a drug, may not be easily distinguished from impaired compliance.

C. Measurement of Adverse Effects

The predictable effects that occur with certain medications suggest compliance. For example, urine becomes orange in individuals receiving rifampin (27). The absence of this change suggests noncompliance. Similarly, the skin of patients who are compliant with taking tetracycline will display a green fluorescence when viewed with a Wood's lamp (28). This form of assessment is limited to those drugs that produce clear-cut effects and may not be adequately sensitive even in those cases.

D. Pill Counts

The prescription and drug must be available through only one source to prevent counting medications from other doctors. The amount of medication apparently removed from the patient's pill containers is divided by the amount that should have been removed if the patient were fully compliant with the prescription, as indicated in the following equation:

$$\frac{\begin{array}{c}\text{Total number of pills} - \text{actual number of pills}\\ \text{Total volume of drug} - \text{volume of actual drug remaining}\end{array}}{\begin{array}{c}\text{Total number of pills} - \text{calculated number of pills}\\ \text{Volume of drug} - \text{volume of expected drug remaining}\end{array}} \times 100 = \%\ \text{Compliance}$$

The pharmacist must collaborate to ensure that the amount of drug dispensed is the amount that has been prescribed (2). Additionally, it must be emphasized that liquid measures, such as a teaspoon or a tablespoon, may vary greatly in volume (2,14). Patients must be sent reminders to return to the clinic with their medications if pill counts are performed during clinic visits. Otherwise, up to 50% of patients may not bring their drug containers (29). In some studies, home visits have been made to quantify medications kept in separate containers or shared medications (6,14,30). Pill counts cannot be performed frequently without patients knowing the purpose. Patients may discard pills once they realize the purpose of the pill count. Thus, other methods of monitoring compliance must be used after perhaps one or two such pill counts (24).

E. Drug Assays

Determination of drug concentrations in various body fluids would seem to be an objective measure of compliance. Indeed, the quantitative assay of serum concentrations of antibiotics has been used to determine drug dosages (31-33) as well as compliance. Such concentrations may vary in different individuals receiving an adequate dose because of interactions with other drugs or with food or because of individual variability in drug disposition. Such factors may yield an incorrect assessment of compliance.

The monitoring of blood concentrations requires venipuncture or capillary stick procedures, which are painful and time-consuming and may themselves reduce compliance. Urine, a more accessible specimen, has been used as an alternative to measure antibiotics (3,4,6). Research is being conducted into assays of drugs from other body fluids, such as saliva, semen, sweat, and tears (34-36).

The cost of quantitative assays prohibits their use in the routine monitoring of compliance with long-term regimens. Qualitative assays, such as a bioassay for penicillins, is one alternative (37). Similarly, incorporation of riboflavin into capsules containing a prescribed drug will cause the patient's urine to fluoresce when exposed to ultraviolet light, allowing an estimate of compliance at minimal cost (38).

Most antibiotics have a short half-life, and detection of their concentration in body fluids reflects recent rather than chronic usage. It would be possible for someone who is generally noncompliant but who takes a dose on the day of the assay to be misjudged as compliant. Gordis et al., however, have found good concordance when urine is collected at unannounced home visits compared with clinic visits (39). Drug assays compared with pill counts were found to be more sensitive of noncompliance in one study (3) but less sensitive in another study (29).

F. Self-reports

An interview may be used to assess patient compliance. The method of questioning may affect the validity of responses. For example, rather than asking "Did you take your pills?", one may get more truthful answers with, "We all have trouble remembering to take our medications sometimes. Have you missed any of your medication during the last week?" In one study of patients who were prescribed antihypertensive medications, patient self-report had a sensitivity of 50% and a specificity of 96% in detecting noncompliance when compared with the pill counts (40).

This measure overestimates compliance compared with other measures, such as pill counts or drug assays (39,41). However, interviews are unlikely to miss gross deviations in compliance (42). This method easily identifies a subset of individuals who admit to noncompliance and is very easy to utilize.

V. DIAGNOSIS OF NONCOMPLIANCE

The previous section has summarized some of the advantages and disadvantages of a number of compliance measures. Table 1 illustrates an approach for determining the most clinically relevant group of patients for compliance measurement. It is apparent that the group in whom the treatment target was not achieved and who had low compliance would benefit most from a compliance-improving intervention. The other two cells not corresponding to the ideal situation should also be attended to, but they do not result merely from lack of patient compliance.

Any patient who has missed an appointment is at high risk for noncompliance with the regimen and should be contacted promptly. Furthermore, interviewing patients will detect about half the noncompliers, at minimum cost, and allow initiation of a compliance-improving intervention for that group. Certainly, for any patient whose treat-

Table 1 Treatment Target and Compliance

	Treatment target reached?	
Compliance	Yes	No
Yes	Ideal	Misdiagnosis Wrong management
No	Overprescription	Group to be identified for compliance-improving strategies

ment response is incomplete, or who is being seen in follow-up after starting a new treatment regimen, non-threatening inquiries about noncompliance and any other difficulties encountered in taking the medication should be made as a matter of routine. These three simple maneuvers of seeking out nonattenders, watching for nonresponders, and asking all patients about their compliance will detect the majority of noncompliers. In order to identify patients who claim to be compliant but who in fact may not be, one can further investigate using pill counts or blood or urine assays for the drug.

VI. ETHICAL STANDARDS FOR APPLYING COMPLIANCE INTERVENTIONS

Because compliance is one of the means to the goal of improving health, a number of ethical prerequisites should be satisfied prior to initiating a compliance-improving program (43).

1. The disease diagnosis must be correct.
2. The disease must be nontrivial.
3. The therapy must be efficacious, that is, known to do more good than harm when taken as recommended.
4. The compliance intervention must be efficacious.
5. The patient must be an informed and willing partner in the process of achieving high compliance.

The first three of these prerequisites obviously depend upon the clinical condition being considered and the treatment prescribed for it. When low compliance is considered to be interfering with achievement of the therapeutic goal, the problem should be discussed directly with the patient in the same nonthreatening, nonjudgmental fashion, for example by asking the patient about rate of compliance. Without such a discussion, there is considerable room for confusion on the part of the patient. Furthermore, since patients have the right to refuse treatments, a candid conversation before attempting to increase compliance can avoid both contravening the patient's rights and wasting both patient and practitioner time in a futile effort.

VII. STRATEGIES TO IMPROVE COMPLIANCE

Many interventions for improving compliance have been examined. Reports of these studies have been subjected to a set of scientific and practical standards for reviewing articles on interventions to improve compliance (43). These guides require that the study had a randomized trial design, at least one credible measure of compliance, and both clinical and statistical significance. Although the majority of the cited studies refer to antibiotic management, some efficacious interventions in the management of other illnesses have been included.

In reviewing the success of various compliance interventions, a clear-cut distinction emerges between short-term and long-term treatments. Compliance with short-term treatments can be improved with clear instructions on method of administration and duration of treatment, as well as by a number of less practical maneuvers, such as special pill packaging and intramuscular injections. For longer term treatments (more than 2 weeks), the simple maneuvers are seldom sufficient. Rather, a combination of maneuvers, such as reminders, instruction, and reinforcement, must be used; these measures must be repeated as long as compliance is required. With these general principles in mind, the following studies are of high merit and interest.

VIII. COMPLIANCE IN SHORT-TERM MANAGEMENT

Two studies have shown that the addition of written instructions and an information sheet improved compliance in the use of short-term antibiotics, such as penicillin, tetracycline, and ampicillin (30,44). The study conducted by Colcher and Bass (44) showed improvement in both the compliance rate and the outcome in patients. Sharpe and Mikeal measured only the compliance level (30). Finney et al. incorporated an educational handout along with a calendar and a phone call in the middle of the regimen to improve compliance with antibiotics for otitis media (29). There was an improvement in compliance from 49% in the control group to 82% in the experimental group. A significant difference was not found in the clinical outcome measures consisting of repeat otoscopic examination and prescription of a second course of antibiotics. However, otitis media is frequently followed by an effusion despite adequate therapy. Lima and colleagues were able to improve compliance with short-term antibiotic therapy through the use of such props as a printed clock or a sticker to be affixed to the refrigerator (45). This significantly increased compliance rates from 28% in the control group to 53% in the group with the printed clock and to 60% in the group with the refrigerator sticker.

Compliance can also be improved by a simplified dosage schedule. A statistically significant improvement in compliance and respiratory function tests were found among asthmatics prescribed a long-acting theophylline preparation compared with those prescribed the usual 4 times a day schedule (46).

It would seem that the simplest ways to improve compliance with short-term medication is, first, to use written instructions and, second, to select a drug regimen that is simple and can be given infrequently.

IX. COMPLIANCE IN LONG-TERM MANAGEMENT

When primary care physicians in Toronto, Canada, were asked the methods they used to help hypertensive patients, to follow their treatment, three-quarters of them based their management on patient instruction. Less than one-third of them utilized behaviorally oriented strategies, such as frequent follow-up visits and simple dosage schedule (47). Four studies examining the role of patient instruction in compliance enhancement have not found a significant difference in the experimental compared with the control group. These studies have had sample sizes that would have been adequate to detect a clinically important benefit (48–51). Patient instruction, then, may be useful for informing patients about their illnesses and their management. It should not be the sole strategy for encouraging patient compliance in the long term.

The injection of a long-acting parenteral medication is one of the most effective methods of ensuring compliance. The use of intramuscular benzathine penicillin in the prophylaxis of rheumatic fever was examined by Feinstein and colleagues (23,52). These investigators were able to reduce the frequency of streptococcal infections by two-thirds from the incidence of between 20 and 25% in those receiving oral antibiotics.

Tuberculosis is another disorder for which antibiotics must be used for prolonged periods. Poor patient compliance with oral drug therapy is thought to be one of the major factors contributing to the relapse rate of 4% in patients with pulmonary tuberculosis living in the United Kingdom (53). The inclusion of intramuscular streptomycin is one of the methods used to improve compliance. Parenteral medications are only efficacious if patient return for follow-up, and studies showing success with such treatments also include outreach services to retrieve or visit nonattenders. Maneuvers to increase patient clinic visits, such as telephone reminders or mail reminders, also have been shown to increase compliance (54).

Other potential methods to improve patient compliance with the use of antibiotics have been examined in more detail in other illnesses (55–57). These include obtaining family support for the patient to take their medications and maneuvers directed at changes in behavior, such as the use of self-monitoring and cueing with positive reinforcement in patients who have obtained a desired outcome. In addition, contracts have been used successfully. In these, patients agree in writing to perform acts to achieve the treatment target in return for suitable rewards.

Studies in intervention to improve long-term compliance underscore the importance of using a combination of at least two strategies, including simple written instruction, contacting patients who have missed an appointment, patient feedback concerning drug concentrations and/or treatment response, and enlisting the support of family members and/or friends. All trials have shown that removal of the compliance strategy also results in deterioration in the level of compliance. Sustained improvements in compliance require sustained intervention.

Application of all compliance maneuvers requires the presence of at least one person other than the patient and is thus labor intensive. The participants in successful interventions have included physicians, nurses, pharmacists, health educators, a psychologist, and even individuals with no formal health professional training (55).

X. CONCLUSION

The prescription of efficacious antimicrobial therapy is a necessary but insufficient act to achieve the eradication of infection among most patients. Good care for patients with treatable infections must include application of efficacious maneuvers to overcome the compliance problem that afflicts the majority of patients who have been prescribed a self- or parent-administered medical regimen. This chapter has described a number of tested and validated techniques for assessing and enhancing compliance. Readers are encouraged to adopt those procedures that are best suited to their personal style and clinical circumstances. No matter what the practitioner's style and circumstances, the elements of successful compliance management include means of detecting low compliance when it occurs, ways of reducing compliance barriers, and methods of reinforcing and rewarding high compliance.

REFERENCES

1. Haynes, RB: Determinants of compliance: The disease and the mechanics of treatment. In: *Compliance in Health Care* (RB Haynes, DW Taylor, and DL Sackett, eds.), Johns Hopkins University Press, Baltimore, 1979, pp. 49-62.
2. Mattar, ME, Markello, J, Yaffe, SJ: Inadequacies in the pharmacologic management of ambulatory children. *J. Pediatr. 87*:137-141, 1975.
3. Charney, E, Bynum, R, Eldredge, D, Frank, D, MacWhinney, JB, McNabb, N, Scheiner, A, Sumpter, EA, Iker, H: How well do patients take oral penicillin? A collaborative study in private practice. *Pediatrics 40*:188-195, 1967.
4. Daschner, F, Marget, W: Treatment of recurrent urinary tract infection in children. II. Compliance of parents and children with antibiotic therapy regimen. *Acta Paediatr. Scand. 64*:105-108, 1975.
5. Leistyna, JA, MacAulay, JC: Therapy of streptococcal infections. Do pediatric patients receive prescribed oral medications? *Am. J. Dis. Child. 111*:22-26, 1966.
6. Bergman, AB, Werner, RJ: Failure of children to receive penicillin by mouth. *N. Engl. J. Med. 268*:1334-1338, 1963.
7. Mohler, DN, Wallin, DG, Dreyfus, EG: Studies in the home treatment of streptococcal disease. I. Failure of patients to take penicillin by mouth as prescribed. *N. Engl. J. Med. 252*:1116-1118, 1955.
8. Becker, MH, Drachman, RH, Kirscht, JP: Predicting mothers' compliance with pediatric medical regimens. *J. Pediatr. 81*:843-854, 1972.
9. MacDonald, ME, Hagberg, KL, Grossman, BJ: Social factors in relation to participation in follow-up care of rheumatic fever. *J. Pediatr. 62*:503-513, 1963.
10. Stewart, RB, Cluff, LE: A review of medication errors and compliance in ambulant patients. *Clin. Pharmacol. Ther. 13*:463-468, 1972.
11. Blackwell, B: The drug defaulter. *Clin. Pharmacol. Ther. 13*:841-848, 1972.
12. Korsch, BM, Fine, RN, Negrete, VF: Noncompliance in children with renal transplants. *Pediatrics 61*:872-876, 1978.
13. Litt, IF, Cuskey, WR, Rudd, S: Identifying adolescents at risk for non-compliance with contraceptive therapy. *J. Pediatr. 96*:742-745, 1980.
14. Arnhold, RG, Adebonojo, FO, Callas, ER, Callas, J, Carte, E, Stein, RC: Patients and prescriptions: Comprehension and compliance with medical instructions in a suburban pediatric practice. *Clin. Pediatr. 11*:648-651, 1970.
15. Porter, AMW: Drug defaulting in a general practice. *Br. Med. J. 1*:218-222, 1969.
16. Weintraub, M, All, WTW, Lasagna, L: Compliance as a determinant of serum digoxin concentration. *JAMA 224*:481-485, 1973.
17. Taylor, W: Compliance with antihypertensive drug therapy. *Ann. N.Y. Acad. Sci. 304*:390-403, 1978.
18. Haynes, RB: A critical review of the "determinants" of patient compliance with therapeutic regimens. In: *Compliance with Therapeutic Regimens* (DL Sackett and RB Haynes, eds.), John Hopkins University Press, Baltimore, 1976.
19. Becker, MH, Nathanson, CA, Drachman, RH: Mothers' health beliefs and children's clinic visits: A prospective study. *J. Community Health 3*:125-135, 1977.
20. Heinzelmann, F: Factors in prophylaxis behaviour in treating rheumatic fever: An exploratory study. *J. Health Hum. Behav. 3*:73-81, 1962.
21. Pizzo, PA, Robichaud, KJ, Edwards, BK, Schumaker, C, Kramer, BS, Johnson, A: Oral antibiotic prophylaxis in patients with cancer: A double-blind randomized placebo-controlled trial. *J. Pediatr. 102*:125-133, 1983.

22. Caron, HS, Roth, HP: Patients' cooperation with a drug regimen. Difficulties in identifying the noncooperator? *JAMA 203*:922–926, 1968.
23. Feinstein, AR, Wood, HF, Epstein, JA, Taranta, A, Simpson, R, Turskey, E: A controlled study of three methods of prophylaxis against streptococcal infection in a population of rheumatic children. II. Results of the first three years of the study, including methods for evaluating the maintenance of oral prophylaxis. *N. Engl. J. Med. 260*:697–702, 1959.
24. Dixon, WM, Stradling, P, Wootton, IDP: Outpatient PAS therapy. *Lancet 2*:871–872, 1957.
25. Gilbert, JR, Evans, CE, Haynes, RB, Tugwell, P: Predicting compliance with a regimen of digoxin therapy in family practice. *Can. Med. Assoc. J. 123*:119–122, 1980.
26. Wood, RE, Boat, TF, Doershuk, CF: Cystic fibrosis. *Am. Rev. Respir. Dis. 113*: 833–878, 1976.
27. Arnold, AG, Ourzon, PGD, Page, RL, Williams, SE: Non-compliance with antituberculous drugs. *Br. J. Dis. Chest 78*:295–298, 1984.
28. Litt, IF, Cluskey, WR: Compliance with medical regimens during adolescence. *Pediatr. Clin. North Am. 27*:3–155, 1980.
29. Finney, JW, Friman, PC, Rapoff, MA, Christopherson, ER: Improving compliance with antibiotic regimens for otitis media. Randomized clinical trial in a pediatric clinic. *Am. J. Dis. Child. 139*:189–195, 1985.
30. Sharpe, TR, Mikeal, RL: Patient compliance with antibiotic regimens. *Am. J. Hosp. Pharm. 31*:479–484, 1974.
31. Prober, CG, Yeager, AS: Use of the serum bactericidal titer to assess the adequacy of oral antibiotic therapy in the treatment of acute hematogenous osteomyelitis. *J. Pediatr. 95*:131–135, 1979.
32. Moore, RD, Smith, CR, Leitman, PS: The association of aminoglycoside plasma levels with mortality in patients with Gram negative bacteremia. *J. Infect. Dis. 149*: 443–448, 1984.
33. Moore, RO, Smith, CR, Leitman, PS: Association of aminoglycoside plasma levels with therapeutic outcome in Gram negative pneumonia. *Am. J. Med. 77*:657–662, 1984.
34. Leger, RM, Swanson, BN, Gerber, N: The excretion of 5,5-diphenylhydantoin in the semen of man and the rabbit: Comparison with plasma concentrations of the drug. *Proc. West. Pharmacol. Soc. 20*:69–72, 1977.
35. Peck, CC: Drug measurement in sweat: A new technique for estimating patient compliance. Talk presented at Workshop–Symposium on Compliance, Hamilton, Ontario, Canada, May 25–27, 1977.
36. Tondi, M: Compliance reliability of tear versus saliva anticonvulsant levels. *Ann. Neurol. 4*:154–155, 1978.
37. Markowitz, M, Gordis, LA: A mail-in technique for detecting penicillin in urine: Application to the study of maintenance of prophylaxis in rheumatic fever patients. *Pediatrics 41*:151–153, 1968.
38. Camfield, CS, Chaplin, S, Doyle, AB, Shapiro, SH, Cummings, C, Camfield, PR: Side effects of phenobarbital in toddlers; behavioural and cognitive aspects. *J. Pediatr. 95*:361–363, 1979.
39. Gordis, LA, Markowitz, M, Lilienfeld, AM: Studies in the epidemiology and preventability of rheumatic fever. IV. A quantitative determination of children on oral penicillin prophylaxis. *Pediatrics 43*:173–182, 1969.
40. Haynes, RB, Taylor, W, Sackett, DL, Gibson, ES, Bernholz, CD, Mukherjee, J: Can simple clinical measurements detect patient non-compliance? *Hypertension 2*:757–764, 1980.
41. Gordis, L, Markowitz, M, Lilienfeld, AM: The inaccuracy in using interviews to estimate patient reliability in taking medications at home. *Med. Care 7*:49–54, 1969.

42. Rickels, K, Briscoe, E: Assessment of dosage deviation in outpatient drug research. *J. Clin. Pharmacol. 10*:153–160, 1970.
43. Sackett, DL, Haynes, RB, Tugwell, P: *Clinical Epidemiology. A Basic Science for Clinical Medicine*, Little, Brown, Boston, 1985.
44. Colcher, IS, Bass, JW: Penicillin treatment of streptococcal pharyngitis. A comparison of schedules and the role of specific counselling. *JAMA 222*:657–659, 1972.
45. Lima, J, Nazarian, L, Charney, E, Lahti, C: Compliance with short-term antimicrobial therapy: Some techniques that help. *Pediatrics 57*:383–386, 1976.
46. Tinkleman, DG, Vanderpool, GE, Carrpell, MS: Compliance differences following administration of theophylline at six and twelve hour intervals. *Ann. Allergy 44*: 283–286, 1980.
47. Logan, AG: *Investigation of Toronto General Practitioner's Treatment of Patients with Hypertension*, Canadian Facts, Toronto, 1978.
48. Sackett, DL, Haynes, RB, Gibson, ES, et al.: Randomized clinical trial of strategies for improving medication compliance in primary hypertension. *Lancet 1*:1205–1208, 1975.
49. Shepard, DS, Foster, SB, Stason, WB, Solomon, HS, McArdle, PJ, Gallagher, SS: Cost-effectiveness of interventions to improve compliance with antihypertensive therapy. *Prev. Med. 8*:229, 1979.
50. Levine, DM, Green, LW, Deeds, SG, Chwakw, J, Russell, RP, Finlay, J: Health education for hypertensive patients. *JAMA 241*:1700–1703, 1979.
51. Swain, MA, Steckel, SB: Influencing adherence among hypertensives. *Res. Nurs. Health 4*:213, 1981.
52. Feinstein, AR, Spagnulo, M, Jonas, S, Kloth, H, Tursky, E, Levitt, M: Prophylaxis of recurrent rheumatic fever. *JAMA 206*:565–568, 1968.
53. Pearce, SJ, Horne, NW: Follow-up of patients with pulmonary tuberculosis adequately treated by chemotherapy: Is this really necessary? *Lancet 2*:641, 1974.
54. Fox, W: Compliance of patients and physicians: Experience and lessons from tuberculosis II. *Br. Med. J. 287*:101–105, 1983.
55. Haynes, RB, Sackett, DL, Gibson, ES, Taylor, DW, Hackett, BC, Roberts, RS, Johnson, AL: Improvement in medication compliance in uncontrolled hypertension. *Lancet 1*:1265–1268, 1976.
56. Logan, AG, Milne, BJ, Achber, C, Campbell, WP, Haynes, RB: Worksite treatment of hypertension by specially trained nurses: A controlled trial. *Lancet 1*:1175, 1979.
57. Nessman, DG, Carnahan, JE, Nugent, CA: Increasing compliance. Patient-operated hypertension groups. *Arch. Intern. Med. 140*:1427–1430, 1980.

Part III
Antibacterial Drugs

10
Penicillins

SUSAN M. LISBY
Children's Hospital, Columbus, Ohio

MILAP C. NAHATA
The Ohio State University, and Children's Hospital, Columbus, Ohio

Penicillin was discovered by Alexander Fleming in 1928, but it was not until 1941 that clinical trials were initiated by Florey and his colleagues (1). This was the first documented natural antibiotic, preceded only by the synthetic sulfonamides. The use of penicillin in patients with staphylococcal infections demonstrated efficacy, and the increased need for this drug could not be met by a limited supply. Refined techniques were then developed to increase the production of penicillin. It was used extensively and successfully in World War II to cure soldiers with sepsis and gas gangrene (2). In 1944, the effectiveness of penicillin in patients with syphylis was reported (3). At this time, penicillin was also recognized as a useful agent for the treatment of bacterial meningitis, but sulfonamides were still considered the drugs of choice, primarily because of the low levels of penicillin found in the cerebrospinal fluid (4). In 1950, higher doses of penicillin were used and its efficacy in patients with bacterial meningitis was established. The favorable efficacy data and the emergence of sulfonamide-resistant organisms made penicillin the drug of choice for meningococcal and pneumococcal meningitis.

I. SOURCE AND CHEMISTRY

Penicillin was first isolated from *Penicillium notatum* fermentation broths by Fleming in 1928; however, the yield of drug by this process was low. Moyer and Coghill were later able to increase the yield of penicillin by selectively growing *Penicillium chrysogenum* on improved media under submerged conditions (5). Although the production of penicillin has been attempted by biosynthetic processes, fermentation continues to be the best method for production of penicillin.

It was not until 1959 that the structure of the penicillin nucleus, 6-aminopenicillanic acid, was characterized by Batchelor and colleagues (5). The basic structure of the penicillin nucleus consists of three primary parts: (1) thiazolidine ring, (2) β-lactam ring, and (3) a side chain. The penicillin nucleus is the chief structural requirement for antimicrobial activity (6). The side chain is primarily responsible for the antibacterial spectrum and pharmacological characteristics (6). The basic structure of the penicillin nucleus and the side-chain substituents to make various penicillins are shown in Figure 1.

During the early 1950s, repository salts of penicillin were found to be stable and slightly soluble in aqueous media. Uniform and prolonged serum concentrations were obtained with these penicillins.

As the use of penicillin began to increase, penicillinase-producing strains of *Staphylococcus aureus* emerged, with the incidence of resistance increasing to almost 70% in some institutions (5). Therefore, it became a high priority to synthesize a penicillinase-resistant compound. Gourevitch and colleagues found that the presence of bulky substituents around the side-chain amide linkage could interfere with penicillinase attachment, which ultimately led to the synthesis of methicillin. The side chains of nafcillin, oxacillin,

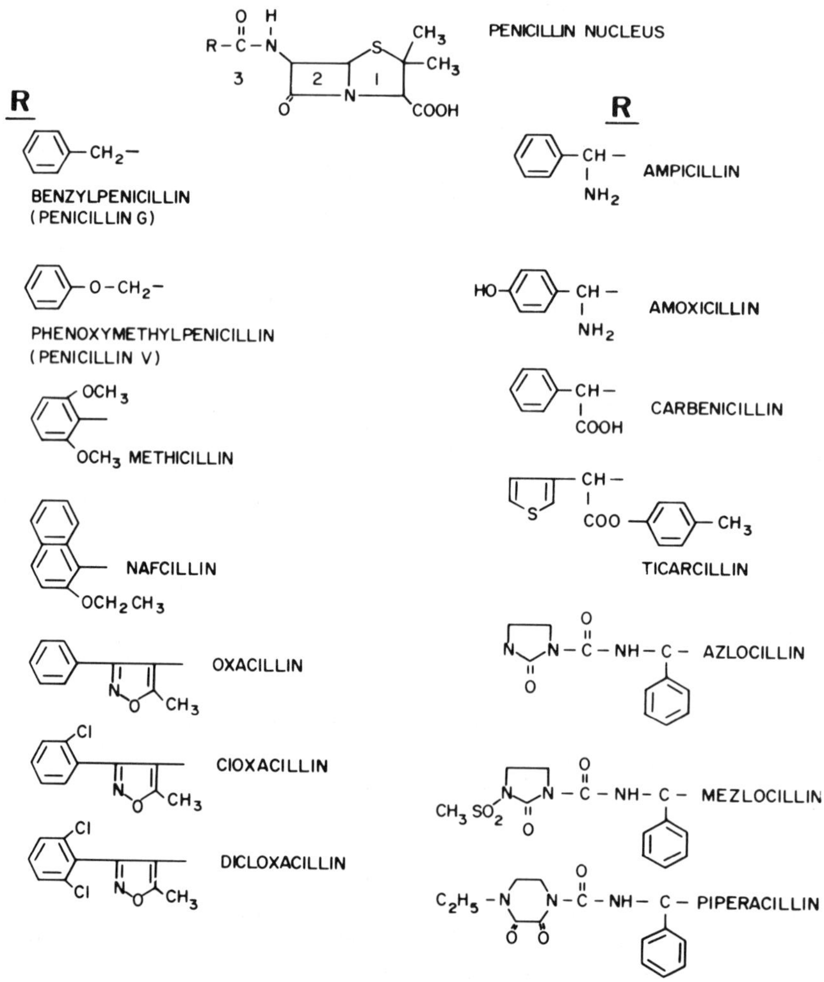

Figure 1 Chemical structures of various penicillins. These contain a thiazolidine ring (1), a β-lactam ring (2), and a side chain (3).

cloxacillin, and dicloxacillin also protect the amide linkage. The addition of chlorine molecules to oxacillin resulted in compounds with better oral absorption.

Further substitutions on the side chain led to penicillin compounds with a broader spectrum of action; the first was ampicillin. The addition of an α-amino group resulted in a broader spectrum for gram-negative microorganisms than that of penicillin G. This side chain, however, was not able to stabilize the compound against β-lactamases.

Substitution of carboxy groups on the side chain resulted in compounds that had a broader spectrum and greater activity against gram-negative organisms than ampicillin. Carbenicillin and ticarcillin were found to be effective against many strains of *Pseudomonas* species.

Piperacillin, azlocillin, and mezlocillin are the newest penicillins available, and these are structural modifications of ampicillin. Their spectrum of activity, however, is similar to that of the carboxypenicillins (carbenicillin and ticarcillin), although broader.

II. MECHANISMS OF ACTION AND RESISTANCE

Penicillins selectively inhibit the synthesis of mucopeptides in the cell wall of multiplying bacteria. This inhibitory action, however, is incomplete, and the cell continues to divide, resulting in the construction of cells with absent or defective walls. Because of the absence of the cell wall, the enzymes and osmotic forces cause the cell to lyse, thus killing the bacteria (7).

Originally, it was believed that penicillins killed susceptible bacteria by inhibiting the synthesis of peptide bonds needed for cross-linkage by inhibiting the enzyme transpeptidase (8). However, subsequent work has shown that penicillins inhibit a number of enzymes, called penicillin binding proteins (PBP), which are involved in the synthesis of the bacterial cell wall. The specific number and function of the penicillin binding proteins vary among bacterial species. The affinity of penicillin for these proteins and the ease with which the drug can reach the receptor site determine the activity of the antibiotic against the bacteria. The PBP 1, 2, and 4 appear to be most important in gram-positive organisms, whereas PBP-3 is important for many gram-negative organisms, such as *Escherichia coli* and other Enterobacteriaceae (9). In these organisms, PBP-3 participates in cell division by catalyzing a carboxypeptidase reaction. This reaction is needed for the peptidoglycan synthesis that occurs when cells divide (10).

One mechanism that certain bacteria utilize against penicillins is producing enzymes, called penicillinases or β-lactamases. These enzymes bind to the β-lactam ring of the penicillin and cause it to open, thus inactivating the drug. Most strains of *S. aureus* are resistant to penicillin owing to the production of penicillinase. Synthesis of the enzyme by *S. aureus* and other gram-positive organisms is plasmid mediated. β-Lactamase is inducible by the presence of even small amounts of penicillin (10). It is found on the surface of the cell wall, and is also an exoenzyme; therefore, it can destroy the penicillin molecule before the drug reaches the cell wall of the organism.

Semisynthetic penicillins are resistant to penicillinase and therefore are active against *S. aureus*. However, in the 1960s, reports of methicillin-resistant strains of *S. aureus* were found worldwide, and this continues to be a problem today. The mechanism of this resistance is not due to the production of penicillinase, but instead to an alteration in the binding sites of the PBP. Strains of *Staphylococcus epidermidis* and *Streptococcus pneumoniae* have also been found to be resistant to semisynthetic penicillins by this mechanism.

Like the gram-positive organisms, gram-negative bacteria also contain β-lactamases. The enzymes are located between the inner and outer membrane of the cell, a location that potentially protects the PBP. Gram-negative β-lactamases may be either chromosomally or plasmid mediated, and also may be inducible. Although the antistaphylococcal penicillins are β-lactamase stable, they have no activity against gram-negative bacteria because they are unable to penetrate the cell membrane and reach their target site.

A more recently described mechanism of resistance of gram-positive organisms to penicillin is tolerance (10). Some strains of *S. aureus* and *S. epidermidis* are able to suppress enzymes that cause autolysis when the cell wall is inhibited by penicillins. These bacteria are inhibited but not killed by the penicillin and are classified as tolerant. The minimum inhibitory concentration (MIC) may be in the normal range, but the minimum bactericidal concentrations (MBC) may be 32-fold greater than the MIC. The clinical significance of this mechanism of resistance is not known.

III. ANTIMICROBIAL ACTIVITY

Penicillins are active against a broad spectrum of microorganisms. A range of MIC values for individual drugs against common pathogens are summarized in Tables 1 and 2.

Penicillin G is active against many gram-positive organisms. Although once active against staphylococci, most strains of *S. aureus* and the coagulase-negative staphylococci are now resistant to penicillin G owing to production of penicillinases by these organisms. Most streptococci, however, remain sensitive to penicillin G. *Streptococcus pyogenes* (group A streptococci) is generally the most sensitive of the streptococci. *Streptococcus agalactiae* (group B streptococci), *Streptococcus viridans*, and group C and G β-hemolytic streptococci are also very sensitive to penicillin G. *Streptococcus pneumoniae* is generally sensitive to penicillin; however, there have been case reports of penicillin-resistant organisms in several countries (11). From March 1983 to November 1984, resistant strains of *S. pneumoniae* (serotype 19A) were isolated from nine patients at Brooklyn, New York, Veterans Administration Medical Center (11). Fully resistant strains (MIC > 1.0 μg/ml) of *S. pneumoniae*, however, are rare. From 1979 through 1984, only 1 of 3400 isolates tested by the Centers for Disease Control (CDC) were fully resistant to penicillin (MIC > 1.0 μg/ml), whereas 3.7% were partially resistant (MIC, 0.1–1 μg/ml) (11).

Enterococcal group D streptococci are less sensitive to penicillin G than other streptococci. Sensitivities are variable, and some strains are highly resistant; therefore, routine sensitivity testing is required. The nonenterococcal group D streptococci are consistently penicillin sensitive (12). Anaerobic gram-positive cocci are also susceptible to penicillin G.

Most strains of *Neisseria meningitidis* are extremely sensitive to penicillin G (13). In contrast, many strains of *Neisseria gonorrhoeae* have been less sensitive to penicillin G. When penicillin was initially used to treat gonorrhea in the late 1940s and early 1950s, the MIC of penicillin ranged from 0.003 to 0.03 units/ml (14). By the late 1950s, many strains exhibited MIC values of 0.10 units/ml or greater (15). Strains producing penicillinase represent only approximately 0.5% of the cases of gonorrhea in the United States, but they are very common in other parts of the world.

Penicillin G has activity against some gram-negative bacilli, but only at high concentrations (16). Because many antibiotics are available with greater activity, gram-negative rods are considered resistant to penicillin G.

Table 1 Minimum Inhibitory Concentrations of Natural and Semisynthetic Penicillins to Selected Bacteria

	MIC range					
Organism	Penicillin G	Penicillin V	Methicillin	Oxacillin	Nafcillin	Dicloxacillin
Staphylococcus aureus pcnase–[a]	0.006–0.4	0.006–0.08	0.01–3.1	0.1–3.1	0.1–0.8	0.05–0.3
pcnase+[b]	12.4–>200	6.3–>100	1.6–6.3	0.2–6.3	0.25–0.8	0.05–0.8
S. epidermidis pcnase–[c]	0.02–0.04	0.02–0.04	1.6	0.2	0.2	0.2
pcnase+[c]	>100	>100	3.2	0.4	0.4	0.4
Streptococcus pyogenes (group A)	0.0008–0.2	0.0015–3.2	0.2–0.4	0.04–0.1	0.02–0.2	0.006–0.2
S. agalactiae (group B)	0.005–0.04	0.0015–3.2	0.2–0.4	0.04–0.1	0.02–0.2	0.006–0.2
S. viridans	0.01–0.1	0.01–0.1	0.2–6.3	0.1–3.1	0.04–3.1	0.01–1.6
S. faecalis	1.6–2.5	6.0	>100	>100	8–>100	>100
S. pneumoniae	0.0015–0.5	0.0015–0.5	0.4	0.04–0.2	0.02–0.2	0.01–0.2
Neisseria gonorrhoeae	0.005–0.4	0.001–3.2	4.0–8.0	8–12	8–25	8–12
N. meningitidis	0.02–0.2	0.08–3.2	4.0–8.0	4.0–8.0	4.0–8.0	4.0–8.0
Hemophilus influenzae	0.05–6.3	0.2–16	6.3–25	25–50	0.1–100	25–50
Escherichia coli	12.5–>400	50–>400	>100	>100	>100	>100
Listeria monocytogenes	0.2	–	–	1.25	–	–

[a]Strains that do not produce penicillinases.
[b]Strains that produce penicillinases.
[c]Many strains now resistant to all penicillins.
Source: From References 29, 54, 57, and 72.

Table 2 Minimum Inhibitory Concentrations of Amino-, Carboxy-, and Ureidopenicillins to Selected Bacteria

Organism	MIC range						
	Ampicillin/ Amoxicillin	Amoxicillin-clavulanic acid	Carbenicillin	Ticarcillin	Mezlocillin	Azlocillin	Piperacillin
Staphylococcus aureus pcnase–[a]	0.05–0.8	0.06–8.0	1.2	1.2	0.8	0.8	0.8
pcnase+[b]	3.1–>100	0.06–8.0	Resistant	Resistant	Resistant	Resistant	Resistant
Streptococcus pyogenes	0.01–0.04	0.01–0.04	0.5–4.0	0.5–4.0	0.03–0.10	0.03–0.10	0.03–0.10
S. agalactiae	0.02–0.2	–	2–4	2–4	0.025–0.10	0.025–0.10	0.025–0.10
S. viridans	0.04–1.6	–	0.2	0.2	1.2	1.2	1.2
S. faecalis	0.12–12.5	0.5–8.0	64	64	1.0–2.0	2.0	2.0–8.0
S. pneumoniae	0.01–0.10	0.12–0.25	0.06–0.25	0.06–0.25	0.06–0.12	0.02–0.12	0.02–0.12
Neisseria gonorrhoeae	0.02–32	0.1	0.03–3.2	0.03–3.2	0.01–2.0	0.01–2.0	0.01–2.0
N. meningitidis	0.01–0.10	0.06–0.12	0.1	0.1	0.05	0.05	0.05
Hemophilus influenzae pcnase–[a]	0.01–5.0	0.06–2.0	0.5–8.0	0.5–8.0	0.25–2.0	0.50–2.0	0.25–2.0
pcnase+[b]	Resistant	0.5–2.0	Resistant	Resistant	Resistant	Resistant	Resistant
Escherichia coli	1.0–>64	1.0–>64	2–>128	2–>128	0.5–>128	4–128	0.5–128
Listeria monocytogenes	0.08–0.64	–	2.5	2.5	1.25	1.25	1.25
Klebsiella pneumoniae	1.25–>100	4.0–16.0	Resistant	64–>128	4–>128	16–>128	2–>128
Proteus mirabilis	0.5–4.0	0.5–16	0.5–16	0.5–16	0.5–16	0.5–16	0.5–16
Enterobacter cloacae	Resistant	2–>64	2–>128	2–>128	2–>128	4–>128	1–>128
Pseudomonas sp.	Resistant	Resistant	8–>128	2–>128	2–>128	4–>128	1–>128
Salmonella	4–>128	4.0	4–128	4–128	4–128	4–128	4–128
Shigella	0.5–>250	4.0	–	–	–	–	–

[a]Strains that do not produce penicillinases.
[b]Strains that produce penicillinases.
Source: From References 30–32, 90, 92, and 112.

Anaerobic gram-negative bacilli found in the respiratory tract are generally sensitive to penicillin G, however, resistant organisms have developed (17). *Bacteroides fragilis*, the most common anaerobic organism in the gastrointestinal tract, is resistant to penicillin G.

Other microorganisms sensitive to penicillin G are *Bacillus anthracis, Erysipelothrix rhusiopathiae, Pasteurella multocida*, and *Streptobacillus moniliformis* (the etiologic agent causing rat-bite fever). *Actinomyces israeli, Leptospira*, and *Clostridium* are also sensitive to penicillin G.

The antimicrobial activity of penicillin V is comparable to that of penicillin G; it is, however, less active against *Neisseria* and *Hemophilus*.

The antistaphylococcal penicillins are all similar with respect to their antimicrobial activity. The major exception is methicillin, which may be two- to threefold less active against *S. aureus*. The antistaphylococcal penicillins are active against most streptococci (with the exception of enterococcal group D streptococci); however, they are less active than penicillin G. Gram-negative organisms are resistant to the antistaphylococcal penicillins. Many gram-positive anaerobic organisms are sensitive to these agents, but the gram-negative anaerobes are not.

Since the introduction of methicillin in 1960, resistance has developed in some strains of *S. aureus* and, more commonly, *Staphylococcus epidermidis*. Resistance is often difficult to detect in vitro owing to the existence of heteroresistant populations. The resistant subpopulation often grows more slowly than the susceptible subpopulation and may be undetected if special laboratory procedures are not followed (18).

Ampicillin and amoxicillin have activity against gram-positive organisms similar to that of penicillin G. Neither agent is effective against β-lactamase-producting staphylococci. Ampicillin is more active against *Listeria monocytogenes* than penicillin G (19). The aminopenicillins have greater activity against gram-negative microorganisms than penicillin G. Many strains of *E. coli, Proteus mirabilis, Salmonella, Shigella*, and *Hemophilus influenzae* are susceptible to ampicillin and amoxicillin; however, these organisms may produce β-lactamases, rendering resistant strains (20).

The carboxypenicillins (carbenicillin and ticarcillin) have a spectrum of activity somewhat similar to that of ampicillin. These agents have less activity against gram-positive organisms than penicillin G or ampicillin. They are inactivated by β-lactamases.

The major difference between these agents and the aminopenicillins is that they have activity against certain strains of *Pseudomonas aeruginosa*. Ticarcillin is more active than carbenicillin in vitro (21). Other gram-negative organisms often susceptible to carboxypenicillins include *E. coli, P. mirabilis, Proteus vulgaris*, some Enterobacteriaceae, *Salmonella, Shigella*, and some *Serratia* species (22).

Klebsiella are resistant to both carbenicillin and ticarcillin. Ampicillin is more active against *H. influenzae* and *L. monocytogenes* than the carboxypenicillins (23). Some strains of *B. fragilis* are resistant to carbenicillin and ticarcillin. Gram-positive anaerobic organisms are generally sensitive to carboxypenicillins.

The ureidopenicillins (mezlocillin, azlocillin, and piperacillin) have an even broader antimicrobial spectrum than the carboxypenicillins. They are active against both gram-positive and gram-negative bacteria. However, these agents are subject to hydrolysis by β-lactamases and resistant strains may develop.

The ureidopenicillins have good activity against many strains of *P. aeruginosa*. Mezlocillin is approximately as active as ticarcillin, and piperacillin is about four times as active as either of these agents. Azlocillin has activity against *P. aeruginosa* approximately equal to or slightly less than that of piperacillin (24,25). Unlike the carboxypenicillins, azlocillin, mezlocillin, and piperacillin are active against some strains of *Klebsiella*. However, 40-60% of these isolates may be resistant (26,27).

The ureidopenicillins also are active against many Enterobacteriaceae, *P. mirabilis*, indole-positive *Proteus* species, and *Citrobacter diversus*. Some strains of *Serratia* are sensitive to the ureidopenicillins; however, many are resistant. Strains of *H. influenzae* and *N. gonorrhoeae* that do not produce β-lactamase are markedly sensitive to extended spectrum penicillins.

The ureidopenicillins have good activity against gram-positive organisms that do not produce β-lactamases. Penicillin G is more active against staphylococci that do not produce β-lactamase. However, the ureidopenicillins are as active as penicillin G against *S. pneumoniae* and the enterococcal group D streptococci. *B. fragilis* is generally susceptible to the ureidopenicillins, but high serum concentrations may be needed to inhibit many of these strains (28).

IV. CLINICAL PHARMACOLOGY

Clinical pharmacologic data for various penicillins are summarized in Table 3. Although presented in a format that allows comparisons of pharmacokinetic data, direct comparisons are not possible owing to the inherent differences among studies. Different patient populations, small sample sizes, and a wide range of doses studied contribute to the variability between studies, making direct comparison of pharmacokinetic data difficult. Penicillins in biologic fluids were most often measured using microbiologic methods, which are less sensitive and specific compared with chromatographic techniques.

A review of the literature reveals that limited pharmacokinetic data are available in infants and children (Table 3). Authors often failed to report volume of distribution and clearance values and presented only half-lives and peak serum concentrations. Therefore, dosage recommendations for pediatric patients are primarily based on scarce data. Dosage modifications in pediatric patients with renal and/or hepatic failure are based on pharmacokinetic data obtained from adult patients with similar disease states. No studies are available on pharmacokinetics of penicillins in children with renal and/or liver failure.

A. Benzylpenicillin (Penicillin G)

Penicillin G is commercially available for oral administration; however, the drug is rapidly destroyed by gastric acid. At pH 1-2, 50% of the administered dose is destroyed in 20 min and about one-third of the total dose is absorbed (33). Penicillin G is routinely administered by the intramuscular or intravenous routes.

After a 500-mg oral dose of penicillin G, peak concentrations in the serum are approximately 1.5-3.0 μg/ml (34). Intramuscular injection of 600,000 units of aqueous penicillin G produces peak concentrations of 6-8 μg/ml at 30 min after the injection (33). Detectable levels are found in the serum for 4-6 hr, depending on the dose administered and the renal function of the patient.

McCracken et al. studied various doses of intramuscular penicillin in newborn infants (35). Peak serum concentrations at 30-60 min after the dose were as follows: 14-24.8 μg/ml after 16,650 units/kg; 22 μg/ml after 25,000 units/kg; and 33.8-35.8 μg/ml after 50,000 units/kg. Although higher peaks were obtained with 50,000 versus 25,000 unit/kg, serum levels at 4 and 8 hr were not remarkably different (35). Peak levels after 16,650

Table 3 Pharmacokinetic Data for Various Penicillins

Drug	Route of administration	Dose	% Dose absorbed	Peak serum concentration (μg/ml)	Time to peak (hr)	Protein binding (%)	V_d	Cl_{Tb}	$t_{1/2}$ Normal renal function (hr)	$t_{1/2}$ Anuria (hr)	Patient population studied (type and age)	References
Penicillin G	PO	500 mg	20–30	1.5–2.7	–	55–60	0.35–0.4 liter/kg		0.7	6–10	–	10, 34, 42, 43
	IM	600,000 units	–	6–8	0.5	–	–	–	–	–	–	33
	IM	16,650–50,000 units/kg	–	14–35.8	0.5–1.0	–	–	–	1.4–3.2		Neonates <7 to >14 days	35, 89
Procaine penicillin G	IM	50,000 U/kg	–	5–41.9	2–12	–	–	–	–	–	Neonates	35, 36
Benzathine penicillin G	IM	2.4 million units	–	0.34–0.635 units/ml	48	–	–	–	–	–	Young adults, mean 21 years; older adults mean 75 years	38
	IM	600,000; 1.2 million units	–	0.15–0.16	24						Children <27 kg and >27 kg	37
Penicillin V	PO	250–500 mg	60	0.6–4.6	0.5–1.0	80						34, 43, 49, 50
Methicillin	IM	1–2 g	–	16–25	0.5–1.0	38	0.37–0.51		0.43	4		34, 51, 54
	IM	25 mg/kg	–	25–58	0.5–1.0	–	0.37–0.51 liter/kg	27–128 ml/min 1.73 m^{-2}	0.8–3.3	–	Premature and normal infants 1–30 days	55, 56

Table 3 (Continued)

Drug	Route of administration	Dose	% Dose absorbed	Peak serum concentration (μg/ml)	Time to peak (hr)	Protein binding (%)	V_d	Cl_{Tb}	$t_{1/2}$ Normal renal function (hr)	$t_{1/2}$ Anuria (hr)	Patient population studied (type and age)	References
Nafcillin	IM	500 mg	–	4.33–8.34	1.0	90	0.7–1.1 liter/kg		0.5–1.4	1.2–2.1	27 adults with and without renal failure	34, 43, 54, 63
	IV	37.5 mg/kg	–	48	0.5	–	0.89 liter/kg	595 ml/min 1.73 m^{-2}	0.76	–	Children, 1–163 months	65
Oxacillin	PO	500 mg	30	5–6	0.5–1.0	91			0.4–0.7	0.5–1.0		43, 54, 73, 77
	IM	20 mg/kg		47–54	1.0		0.19 liter/kg		1.2–1.6		Premature infants	
Cloxacillin	PO	500 mg	50	7–14	0.5–1.0	93	6.55 liters	155 ml/min	0.6	9.8	Adults	
Dicloxacillin	PO	500 mg	50	15–18	0.5–1.0	97	5.99 liters	110 ml/min	0.8	1–1.5	Adults	
Ampicillin	PO	500 mg	33–54	2–2.5	2.0	20	0.5 liter/kg	260 ml/min	1.5	8	Adults	43, 73, 78, 79
	PO	25 mg/kg	–	4–5	1.0						Infants	80, 82, 88
	IM	500 mg/kg	–	5–8	1.0						Adults	
	IM	50–100 mg/kg	–	35–293	0.5–1.0		0.4–0.5 liter/kg		1.7–6.2		Premature infants, neonates	
Amoxicillin	PO	500 mg	90	7.6	1–2	17	0.4 liter/kg	370 ml/min	1.0	10–15	Normals	80, 90, 96

Carbenicillin	IM	1 g	–	24	1.0	50–60	12–14 liters	130 ml/min	1–1.1	13–16	Adults	98, 99, 101
	IV	2 g	–	300	After 5-min infusion						Adults	
	IM	75 mg/kg	–	135–160	1.0				5–6		Low-birth-weight neonates <3 days	
Ticarcillin	IM	1 g	–	22	1.0	50–60	14–16 liters	130 ml/min	1.25	13–16	Adults	98, 99, 101
	IV	2 g	–	218	After 5-min infusion						Adults	
	IM	75 mg/kg	–	190	1.0		0.66–0.76 liter/kg	31 ml/min 1.73 m^{-2}	5–6		Low-birth-weight infants <7 days	
	IV	100 mg/kg		250	0.5		0.35 liter/kg	175 ml/min 1.73 m^{-2}	0.9		Children 5–13 years	
Piperacillin	IM	0.5–2 g	–	5–30	0.5–1.0	20	0.3 liter/kg	2.8–4.4 ml/min kg^{-1}	1.0	3–4	Adults	107, 108, 109, 110
	IV	2–5 g		65–450	After 15–30-min infusion						Adults	
	IV or IM	50–100 mg/kg		100–300			0.3 liter/kg	80–280 ml/min m^{-2}			Infants and children	
Mezlocillin	IV	3–5 g		270–350	After 15–30-min infusion	20	0.3 liter/kg	3.8–7.1 ml/min kg^{-1}	1.0	3–4	Adults	108, 109
	IV or IM	50–100 mg/kg		100–300			0.4 liter/kg	5–12 ml/min kg^{-1}	1.8–4.5		Neonates	
Azlocillin	IV	3–5 g		215–530	After 15–30-min infusion	40	0.2 liter/kg	1.6–2.9 ml/min kg^{-1}	1.0	5.6	Adults	108, 109
	IV or IM	50–100 mg/kg		100–300			0.2 liter/kg	1.25–1.63 ml/min kg^{-1}	2.5–4.4		Neonates	

units/kg varied with birth weight and chronological age (higher levels achieved in infants less than 6 days old). Neonates weighing less than 2000 g at birth had peak concentrations of 14-15 μg/ml; those weighing 2000-3500 g at birth had peak levels of 18-20 μg/ml (35). Lower serum concentrations can be explained by a larger volume of distribution in low-birth-weight infants.

Procaine penicillin G, 50,000 units/kg administered intramuscularly to neonates less than 1 week old (mean age, 3.6 days), resulted in sustained concentrations of 7.4-8.8 μg/ml at 2-12 hr, respectively, after the dose. At 24 hr, the mean serum concentration declined to 1.5 μg/ml (35). Serum concentrations were slightly lower in neonates greater than 7 days old. At 24 hr, the serum concentrations in this group declined to 0.4 μg/ml. Speer and colleagues (36) found higher concentrations and a wider range of peak serum concentrations (range, 7.7-41.9 μg/ml; mean, 17.1 μg/ml) 4 hr after a 50,000-unit/kg dose. At 24 hr, serum concentrations ranged from 0.2 to 5.8 μg/ml (mean, 2.1 μg/ml).

In adults, increasing the dose of procaine penicillin above 600,000 units did not increase peak concentrations substantially but prolonged the interval at which penicillin is detectable in the serum (33). To increase the peak, two injections should be given at two different body sites. After usual doses of procaine penicillin G, penicillin can be detected in the serum for 12-24 hr.

Benzathine penicillin produces lower but more sustained serum concentrations of penicillin than procaine or aqueous penicillin G. Detectable measurements are present in the serum for 3-4 weeks after an intramuscular injection. Ginsburg and co-workers (37) administered 600,000 and 1.2 million units of benzathine penicillin G to children weighing less or greater than 27 kg, respectively. Peak serum concentrations were observed at 24 hr and were similar in both groups (0.16 and 0.15 μg/ml, respectively). Serum concentrations of 0.01 μg/ml were detected in both groups 18 days after the dose. At 30 days, no penicillin was detected in the serum. However, penicillin concentrations of 0.6-12.5 μg/ml were measured in the urine from eight of nine patients. This suggested that penicillin was released from tissues as late as 30 days after the dose, but the concentration of penicillin in the serum was below the detection limit of the assay (37). Coadministration of procaine (300,000 units) and benzathine penicillin (900,000 units) to children produced higher serum concentrations for 24 hr than benzathine penicillin alone, but serum levels at 5-30 days were similar. Peak concentrations of approximately 4 μg/ml were obtained 1 hr after the dose (37).

Because penicillin G is relatively insoluble in lipid, it penetrates poorly across the blood-brain barrier. Inflammation of the meninges improves the penetration into the central nervous system by reducing the normal blood-brain barrier and by impairing the activity of the organic anion pump in the choroid plexus (34). The increased penetration of penicillin G during periods of meningeal inflammation was demonstrated by Hieber and Nelson (39) in an evaluation of 24 children with purulent meningitis. Children received 250,000 units/kg day^{-1} in six divided doses intravenously over a 15-min period. The cerebrospinal fluid-serum concentration ratio decreased from 18.4% on the first day to 9.9% on day 5 to 4.9% on day 10 of therapy. Mean penicillin concentrations in the cerebrospinal fluid (CSF) were 0.8 μg/ml on the first day and declined to 0.3 μg/ml on day 10 of therapy. Speer and co-workers (36) measured penicillin concentrations in the CSF of 25 neonates who received 50,000 units/kg of procaine penicillin G intramuscularly. None of the neonates had meningitis. Peak concentrations in the CSF at 12 hr ranged from 0.09 to 1.98 μg/ml (mean, 0.70 μg/ml). At 24 hr the mean CSF concentration was 0.12 μg/ml. Penicillin concentrations in the CSF ranged from 2.1 to 8.5% of the simultaneous serum levels (mean, 4.5%). Penicillin G concentrations in the CSF after intramuscular administration of benzathine penicillin are minimal in both adults and children (40,41).

Penicillin G is widely distributed throughout the body and has a distribution volume of 0.35-0.4 liter/kg (42). Penicillin does not penetrate well into the CSF, eye, and prostate; however, it does penetrate adequately into noncaseous abscesses, synovial fluid and joints, and the placenta (43). Penicillin is 50-60% bound to serum proteins; the actual figures reported vary depending on the analytical method used (33).

The major route of elimination of penicillin G is by the kidney, with the majority of the dose eliminated as unchanged drug. A small amount of penicillin is metabolized in the liver; penicilloic acid is the major end product (44). A small fraction of active drug is secreted into the bile. In adults, 90% of the renally excreted drug is eliminated by tubular secretion and 10% is filtered at the glomerulus. Animal research suggests that secretion occurs in the proximal tubules and a small amount may be reabsorbed in the collecting ducts (45). In newborn infants, penicillin G is eliminated primarily by glomerular filtration owing to the immaturity of the tubular secretion mechanism at this age (35). In the neonate, the half-life of penicillin G is inversely correlated with age, ranging from 3.2 hr in neonates less than 6 days old to 1.4 hr in infants greater than 2 weeks old (35). After the neonatal period, the penicillin half-life approaches that of an adult (0.7 hr). In patients with impaired renal function, the half-life of penicillin increases and may reach 6–10 hr in anuria. Bryan and Stone (46) reported penicillin clearance to decrease from 400 ml/min in normal individuals to a mean of 42.7 ml/min in seven adult anephric patients. Concurrent hepatic and renal dysfunction may prolong the half-life to a greater extent. Because it shares the anion transport system in the renal tubular cell, the administration of probenecid will inhibit tubular secretion and prolong the clearance of penicillin G (47). Clearance values are not available in pediatric patients.

B. Phenoxymethylpenicillin (Penicillin V)

Penicillin V is more acid stable than penicillin G and is therefore better absorbed (48). Approximately 60% of an oral dose is absorbed. Coadministration with food reduces the peak level to one-third, but the total amount of drug absorbed is not affected (49,50). Because of better absorption characteristics, peak serum concentrations are higher with penicillin V than with penicillin G after equal oral doses. Depending on the dose and the time of administration in relationship to ingestion of food, peak levels range from 0.6 to 4.6 μg/ml at 30-60 min after the dose. Penicillin can be detected in the serum for approximately 4 hr (51). Distribution and elimination characteristics of penicillin V are similar to those of penicillin G.

C. Semisynthetic Penicillins

1. Methicillin

Methicillin is not acid stable and is not significantly absorbed after oral administration (52). Effective serum concentrations are achieved after intramuscular administration. A 1-g dose produces a peak of 16–18 μg/ml at 30 min after the injection (52,53). Serum concentrations of 1-1.5 μg/ml are detectable at 4 hr; no drug is detected at 8 hr (54). Doubling the dose increases the peak concentration approximately twofold and prolongs the interval over which drug is detectable in the blood (54).

After a 25-mg intramuscular dose of methicillin to neonates, peak serum concentrations ranged from 25 to 58 μg/ml at 30 min to 1 hr after the dose (55,56). Low-birth-weight infants ($<$1999 g) and term infants ($>$2000 g) less than 7 days old had higher peak levels. These infants also demonstrated a smaller volume of distribution (55).

Intravenous doses of methicillin produce higher peak concentrations than equal doses administered intramuscularly. Methicillin (1 g) infused over 15 min produced levels of 26–38 μg/ml at the end of the infusion. The levels ranged from 1.2 to 3.6 μg/ml 2 hr later (57). Approximately 38% of methicillin is bound to serum proteins (51), and the drug does not readily cross the blood-brain barrier. CSF concentrations of 0.03–0.12 μg/ml have been measured when the meninges were inflamed. These concentrations are below the minimum inhibitory concentrations of methicillin for *S. aureus*. Methicillin distributes into pleural, pericardial, and ascitic fluid and joints in concentrations similar to that in the serum (58). Although only 2–3% of the dose is excreted in the bile, high concentrations are found in bile of patients with normal liver function (59).

Methicillin is primarily excreted in the urine as unchanged drug. It is removed from the body by both glomerular filtration and tubular secretion. Like penicillin, a minor amount of methicillin is metabolized in the liver (60). In adults with normal renal function, the half-life of methicillin is 0.4 hr and increases to 4 hr in anuria (43). In neonates, half-life is inversely proportional to age. Infants less than 1 week old have a half-life of 3 hr, which decreases to 1 hr by 1 month of age (55,56). Preterm infants have a slightly longer half-life than term infants of the same postnatal age (55). Children with cystic fibrosis clear methicillin faster than normal children of the same age, and therefore may require larger doses (61).

2. Nafcillin

Nafcillin is commercially available for oral administration; however, it is poorly and erratically absorbed from the gastrointestinal tract. At best, only 10–20% of the administered dose is absorbed (54).

After a 1 g intramuscular dose of nafcillin to 11 postpartum women, serum concentrations ranged from 1.56 to 50 μg/ml (mean, 7.6 μg/ml) 1 hr after the dose. At 6 hr, the mean serum concentration was 0.59 μg/ml (62). Serum concentrations may be different in other patient populations, as postpartum women often have an altered volume of distribution of drugs.

Rudnick and colleagues (63) administered a single 500-mg dose of nafcillin intramuscularly to 27 patients with and without renal failure. Peak serum concentrations 1 hr after the dose ranged from 4.33 to 8.34 μg/ml. Drug in the serum was detectable at 12 hr, and concentrations ranged from 0.03 to 0.15 μg/ml. The apparent volume of distribution ranged from 0.70 liter/kg in the severe renal failure group to 1.06 liters/kg in adult subjects with normal renal function (63). Diaz and colleagues (64) administered intravenously 25 mg/kg of nafcillin over 5–15 min to 12 adult hemodialysis patients and reported a wide variation in peak serum concentrations 15 min postinfusion (range, 3.32–332 μg/ml). Serum concentrations at 5 hr ranged from 0.6 to 2.4 μg/ml. The extreme variability in levels may have been secondary to the method of intravenous administration (64).

In children 1–163 months old, a nafcillin dose of 37.5 mg/kg given intravenously over 15 min produced a mean peak serum concentration of 48 μg/ml at 30 min after the dose (65). Serum concentrations were 1.8 μg/ml at 4 hr. The mean apparent volume of distribution (V_d) was 893 ml/kg. There was no correlation between age of the patient and pharmacokinetic values (65).

Banner et al. (66) studied the pharmacokinetics of nafcillin in 13 low-birth-weight infants (<2000 g). Neonates greater than 7 days old received 100 mg/kg day^{-1} of nafcillin in three divided doses, and those less than 7 days old received 100 mg/kg day^{-1} in two divided doses. Specific peak serum concentration values were not given, but the authors indicated that only one child had a peak of less than 80 μg/ml. Neonates less than 3 weeks old had a mean apparent volume of distribution of 326 ml/kg, and 3 infants greater than 3 weeks old had a V_d of 303 ml/kg. The large discrepancy in the values for apparent V_d obtained by Banner et al. (66) and by Feldman et al. (65) is not explainable from the information presented in both studies.

Nafcillin is 90% bound to serum proteins (43). Data on the distribution of nafcillin into the CSF are limited; however, a few case reports have suggested that nafcillin penetrates inflamed meninges adequately for the treatment of meningitis (67,68). In addition, it was shown to penetrate bone and synovial fluid (69).

Nafcillin is extensively metabolized in the liver. Although it is known that nafcillin is excreted in the bile, the percentage of the dose removed by this route is uncertain. Studies have found 8% (69), 42%, and 80% of the nafcillin dose have been recovered from the bile (70). After an intramuscular injection, approximately 19% of the nafcillin dose is eliminated in the urine if probenecid is also given (71). In adults with hepatic disease, 50% of the dose is recovered in the urine (70). Clearance of nafcillin from plasma of normal adults was reported as 584 ml/min and decreased to 163 ml/min in adults with extrahepatic obstruction (70). The half-life of nafcillin in normal adults has been reported to range from 0.5 to 1.4 hr (34,63,70). The half-life increased slightly in adults with renal failure (1.2-2.1 hr) (34,63). Adults with liver disease also have a slightly prolonged nafcillin half-life (1.2-1.7 hr). The serum half-life of nafcillin in premature neonates range from 2.23 to 5.46 hr. Total body clearance is 0.89-1.37 ml/min kg^{-1} (65). In older infants (1-164 months old), the serum half-life of nafcillin was 0.76 hr and plasma clearance was 595 ml/min 1.73 m^{-2} (65).

D. Isoxazolyl Penicillins: Oxacillin, Cloxacillin, and Dicloxacillin

Oxacillin, cloxacillin, and dicloxacillin are more acid stable than either nafcillin or methicillin and can be administered orally. The oral absorption of oxacillin, cloxacillin, and dicloxacillin is approximately 30, 50, and 50%, respectively (54). The presence of food in the stomach decreases the absorption of all three agents (72).

After a 500-mg oral dose under fasting conditions, peak serum concentrations at 30-60 min after the dose were 5-6 μg/ml for oxacillin, 7-14 μg/ml for cloxacillin, and 15-18 μg/ml for dicloxacillin (43). A dose of 20 mg/kg intramuscular oxacillin to premature infants resulted in peak serum concentrations of 47-52 μg/ml 1 hr after the injection (73).

These drugs are highly bound to serum proteins (91, 93, and 97%, respectively) (43). Although data are limited, these agents do not appear to penetrate into the CSF in adequate concentrations to treat staphylococcal meningitis. They do penetrate into synovial and pleural fluid. Sputum concentrations are variable.

Isoxazolyl penicillins are excreted by the kidney by glomerular filtration and tubular secretion. The oral dose excreted in the urine is 30, 50, and 65% for oxacillin, cloxacillin, and dicloxacillin, respectively (54). Metabolites with some antimicrobial activity are also excreted in the urine (74). In patients with normal renal function, these metabolites represent only a small fraction of the total activity in the serum. In patients with severe renal failure, active metabolites may accumulate and represent up to 50% of the penicillin activity (74).

Of the three agents, oxacillin is the most extensively metabolized, and dicloxacillin is the least. Oxacillin is partially excreted in the bile. Dicloxacillin has the longest half-life (0.8 hr), and oxacillin has the shortest (0.4-0.7 hr) (43). In patients with renal failure, the half-life of the parent compounds increases only slightly (0.5-1.0 hr for oxacillin, 0.8 hr for cloxacillin, and 1.0-1.5 hr for dicloxacillin). In premature infants less than 3 weeks old, the half-life of oxacillin is 1.2-1.6 hr (73). Patients with cystic fibrosis clear isoxazolyl penicillin faster than normal children of the same age (75,76). Pharmacokinetic data of the isoxazolyl penicillins in pediatric populations are limited.

E. Aminopenicillins

1. Ampicillin

Ampicillin is acid stable and can be administered orally; however, only 33-54% of the dose is absorbed (43). Coadministration with food delays absorption and decreases the peak serum concentration.

After a dose of 500 mg oral ampicillin to adults, peak serum concentrations of 2-2.5 μg/ml are obtained at 2 hr (78-80). Doubling the dose results in a twofold increase in serum concentrations. After a 500-mg intramuscular injection of ampicillin to adults, peak concentrations of 5-8 μg/ml are reached in 1 hr (79). Ampicillin is detectable in the serum 8 hr after the dose.

In premature infants receiving 50, 75, or 100 mg/kg, peak serum concentrations of 35-293 μg/ml were achieved at 30-60 min after an intramuscular injection (81). Infants 1-5 weeks old receiving intramuscular ampicillin, 50 mg/kg every 8 hr, had a mean peak concentration of 58 μg/ml at 30 min after the injection and a mean trough level of 2 μg/ml (81).

After oral administration of ampicillin, 25 mg/kg, to infants and children, peak serum concentrations of 4-5 μg/ml were reached at 60 min after the dose. At 6 hr after the dose, levels of 0.04-0.46 μg/ml were detected in the serum (82).

Ampicillin distributes into cerebrospinal fluid in patients with inflamed meninges. In neonates with meningitis receiving 40-70 mg/kg of ampicillin intravenously, CSF concentrations ranged from 1 to 28 μg/ml and were 11-65% of the simultaneous serum concentrations. Peak CSF concentrations were obtained 3-7 hr after intravenous administration (81). Ampicillin distributes into the exudate of acute otitis media. Adequate concentrations were detectable 80 min after an intramuscular injection (83). Ampicillin reaches concentrations in the gallbladder that are higher than simultaneous serum concentrations. Ayliffe and Davies (84) reported that ampicillin concentrations in the bile were 48 times the serum concentration at 4 hr after a single oral dose. In patients with obstruction of the cystoduct or common bile duct, ampicillin does not concentrate in the bile (85).

Ampicillin crosses the placenta and can be detected in fetal serum and amniotic fluid. A 500-mg intravenous dose given to the mother resulted in a fetal serum concentration of 6.6 μg/ml 1 hr after the dose. At 4 hr, the fetal serum concentration was only 1.2 μg/ml. In the amniotic fluid, ampicillin can be detected for a longer duration. A concentration of 1.5 μg/ml was measured at 29 hr after the dose (86). About 20% is bound to serum proteins (43). The apparent volume of distribution in adults is approximately 0.5 liter/kg (50% of body weight) (87). In premature neonates, the apparent volume of distribution ranged from 41 to 52% of total body weight (73).

Ampicillin is primarily excreted in the urine by glomerular filtration and renal tubular secretion with only a small proportion metabolized by the liver. In patients with normal renal function, ampicillin is highly concentrated in the urine. In these patients, 30% of an oral dose and 75% of an intravenous dose is excreted in the urine as unchanged drug. Probenecid prolongs the elimination and increases serum concentrations of ampicillin by competitively inhibiting tubular secretion. The serum half-life of ampicillin is 1.5 hr in patients with renal failure (88). In neonates, half-life is inversely correlated with age. In infants less than 1 week old, the half-life of ampicillin is 3.1-4.7 hr. In those 7-14 days old, the half-life is 1.7-2.8 hr, and values decrease to that of an adult after the neonatal period. Preterm infants have a slightly prolonged half-life when compared to other neonates; at less than 1 week of age they were reported to have a half-life of 4.7-6.2 hr (89). Clearance values have not been reported.

2. Amoxicillin

Amoxicillin is very similar to ampicillin except for its better absorption (90%) after oral administration. When coadministered with food, the peak serum concentration is delayed but bioavailability is not altered (90).

The peak serum concentration of amoxicillin is twice that obtained with equal doses of ampicillin; after a 500-mg oral dose of amoxicillin, the mean peak serum concentration in adults was 7.6 μg/ml (91). Because more of the dose is absorbed, a larger percentage of the dose is excreted in the urine unchanged (50-64%) compared with ampicillin. Other pharmacokinetic characteristics of amoxicillin are similar to those of ampicillin (43).

3. Amoxicillin-Clavulanic Acid (Augmentin)

The pharmacokinetics of the individual drugs in Augmentin are not significantly altered when administered as a combination drug. Some have found a slight increase in the absorption and excretion of clavulanic acid when administered with amoxicillin (91). Peak serum concentrations of clavulanic acid are reached at 40-120 min after an oral dose. After an oral dose of 250 mg, peak serum levels were 1.9-4.3 μg/ml (92). Coadministration of amoxicillin-clavulanic acid with food does not alter bioavailability of either component (92). High concentrations of both amoxicillin and clavulanic acid are obtained in the urine of patients with normal renal function after oral administration.

Oral doses of 3.3 mg/kg of clavulanic acid and 13.3 mg/kg of amoxicillin to infants and children resulted in mean peak serum concentrations of 1.5 and 5 μg/ml for clavulanic acid and amoxicillin, respectively. Peak concentrations were achieved at 60 min after the dose. Mean half-life values were 1.2 and 1.5 hr for clavulanic acid and amoxicillin (93).

4. Bacampicillin and Cyclacillin

These two are inactive drugs that must be altered before exerting their antimicrobial activity. Bacampicillin is a carboxy ester of ampicillin and is rapidly hydrolyzed in the body to ampicillin. It is more lipid soluble than ampicillin and is better absorbed in the gastrointestinal tract. Peak serum concentrations of ampicillin after an oral dose of bacampicillin are twice those obtained after doses of the parent compound. The bioavailability of bacampicillin is two to three times greater than that of ampicillin (94).

Cyclacillin, a new penicillin similar to ampicillin and amoxicillin, was found to be rapidly absorbed after oral administration. Peak serum concentrations occur at 30 min after the dose and are four times higher than those achieved with equal doses of ampicillin. Cyclacillin has a shorter half-life than ampicillin (0.59 hr) (95).

F. Carboxypenicillins: Carbenicillin and Ticarcillin

Carbenicillin and ticarcillin are not acid stable and therefore cannot be administered orally. Indanyl carbenicillin is more acid stable and lipid soluble than carbenicillin and is rapidly absorbed from the gastrointestinal tract after oral administration. Oral doses of 0.5-1.0 g indanyl carbenicillin have produced peak serum concentrations of 7-14 μg/ml at 30-120 min after the dose (97).

Carbenicillin and ticarcillin are readily absorbed after intramuscular injection. The peak serum concentrations were 24 and 22 μg/ml at 60 min after 1 g intramuscular doses of carbenicillin and ticarcillin, respectively (98). Serum concentrations at 6 hr were 4 μg/ml for carbenicillin and 6 μg/ml for ticarcillin. Ticarcillin or carbenicillin, 2 g administered intravenously over 5 min, produces peak serum concentrations: 218 μg/ml for ticarcillin and 300 μg/ml for carbenicillin. Because of the longer half-life of ticarcillin, serum concentrations of both antibiotics are similar at 2 hr after the dose (99).

Low-birth-weight neonates (<2000 g) less than 1 week old and term neonates less than 3 days of age had peak serum concentrations of 135-160 μg/ml after a dose of 75 mg/kg intramuscular carbenicillin (100). Doses of 100 mg/kg produced approximately the same peak concentrations during the rest of the neonatal period. Similarly, with ticarcillin, 75 mg/kg intramuscularly to low-birth-weight infants less than 7 days old produced a peak serum concentration of 190 μg/ml 1 hr after the dose (101). Term infants of the same age had slightly lower peak levels (160 μg/ml). Peak serum concentrations of 125 μg/ml were obtained at 1 hr after the dose in neonates 1-8 weeks old (101). An intravenous dose of 100 mg/kg to children 5-13 years old produced a peak level of 250 μg/ml at 30 min after the dose (101).

Both carbenicillin and ticarcillin are 50-60% bound to serum proteins and are distributed in an apparent volume of 12-16 liters in adults (22). The volume of distribution of ticarcillin in neonates ranged from 663 to 761 ml/kg, depending on age. Neonates less than 1 week old had a smaller distribution volume than older neonates (101). Carboxypenicillins do not penetrate the meninges under normal conditions. Although data are limited, a few case reports indicate that CSF penetration may occur in patients with meningitis (102-105). In the absence of biliary obstruction, ticarcillin and carbenicillin can be measured in bile in therapeutic concentrations (22).

Both carbenicillin and ticarcillin are found in high concentrations in the urine, with 95% of carbenicillin and 80-85% of ticarcillin excreted by this route (98,99). Of the administered dose, 10-15% ticarcillin and 5% carbenicillin is converted to penicilloic acid and excreted in the urine. The half-life of carbenicillin in adult patients with normal renal function is 60-66 min. Both carboxypenicillins have prolonged elimination $t_{1/2}$ in the presence of renal failure (13-16 hr). Urinary concentrations, however, remain relatively high unless creatinine clearance falls below 10 ml/min (106). Concomitant liver failure results in a prolonged half-life of 28-35 hr in adults (22). The addition of probenecid will increase serum concentrations and prolong the half-life owing to a decrease in the renal tubular secretion of carbenicillin and ticarcillin. Half-life is inversely correlated with postnatal age. The half-life of ticarcillin and carbenicillin in low-birth-weight infants less than 7 days old and term infants less than 3 days old was 5-6 hr. In older neonates, half-life decreased to 2-3 hr (100,101). Patients with cystic fibrosis may require higher doses due to a faster elimination of carbenicillin and ticarcillin than normal children of the same age.

G. Acylureidopenicillins: Piperacillin, Mezlocillin, and Azlocillin

The acylureidopenicillins (or extended spectrum penicillins) are not adequately absorbed in the gastrointestinal tract and must be administered parenterally. After intramuscular injection of piperacillin, peak serum concentrations occur within 30-60 min. Mean peak concentrations of 5, 13, and 30 μg/ml were obtained after 0.5-, 1.0-, and 2.0-g doses, respectively (107). Intravenous administration resulted in higher peak serum concentrations. After a 3-g and a 5-g dose of mezlocillin infused over 15-30 min, peak concentrations were 270 and 350 μg/ml, respectively. Doses of piperacillin of 2 and 5 g produced peak serum concentrations of 65 and 450 μg/ml, and 3 and 5 g of azlocillin resulted in peak concentrations of 215 and 530 μg/ml, respectively (108). In infants and children, peak concentrations after intravenous or intramuscular doses of 50-100 mg/kg of an acylureidopenicillin were approximately 100-300 μg/ml (109). Similarly, peak serum concentrations after 50-100 mg/kg IV or IM in neonates (premature and term) were approximately 100-300 μg/ml (109). Peak serum concentrations were lower after intramuscular and higher after bolus intravenous injection versus slow intravenous infusion (generally 30-min infusion).

These extended spectrum penicillins are all minimally protein bound (azlocillin, 40%; piperacillin and mezlocillin, 20%) (110). The apparent volume of distribution in adults was approximately 0.2, 0.3, and 0.4 liter/kg for azlocillin, piperacillin, and mezlocillin, respectively (42). Like other penicillins, cerebrospinal fluid penetration of the acylureidopenicillins is limited unless inflammation of the meninges occurs. In patients with meningitis, CSF concentrations were approximately 5-10% of the serum concentrations (111).

The acylureidopenicillins are primarily eliminated by renal tubular secretion and glomerular filtration. Approximately 70-90% of the dose is recovered in the urine in 24 hr (107,112). In the absence of biliary obstruction, all three agents can be detected in the bile.

These agents exhibit dose-dependent pharmacokinetics in patients with normal renal function; higher doses are cleared more slowly than lower doses. Half-life values in patients with end-stage renal disease are 5-6 hr for azlocillin and 3-4 hr for mezlocillin and piperacillin (113-117). This is significantly lower than in normal adults (1 hr) (107,118). Dosage adjustments are not needed until creatinine clearance falls below 30 ml/min.

The half-life of acylureidopenicillins in children is similar to that in adults. The values reported for piperacillin, mezlocillin, and azlocillin were 0.5-0.78 hr (117,119-121), 0.80-0.97 hr (122,123), and 0.82-1.74 hr (124-126), respectively. Neonates have a slightly longer half-life of the extended spectrum penicillins. Although data are limited, half-life values for piperacillin, mezlocillin, and azlocillin were 6.5, 1.8-4.5, and 2.5-4.4 hr, respectively (109). In the pharmacokinetic studies of the acylureidopenicillins involving neonates and children, the dosage range was not wide enough to determine whether the pharmacokinetics in this population are dose dependent. Limited studies (123,124), however, suggest that nonlinear kinetics may also occur in children. Some reports indicate that patients with cystic fibrosis require larger doses of the extended spectrum penicillins owing to rapid clearance of these drugs (120). Others have not detected a difference in the pharmacokinetics compared with other patient populations (109,124).

V. DRUG ASSAYS

The concentrations of penicillins in body fluids can be measured by microbiologic and high-performance liquid chromatographic methods. Most studies cited in this chapter have utilized microbiologic methods. These assay methods are relatively inexpensive and easy to use, but limitations include poor sensitivity and specificity. These methods also suffer from the variation in precision and accuracy of interpreting the zone of inhibition. Furthermore, if the patient is receiving concomitant antibiotics, their effect on the standard test microorganism must be excluded for proper interpretation of the antibiotic being studied.

High-performance liquid chromatographic methods are accurate, precise, sensitive, and specific for the measurement of penicillins. These methods are preferred over microbiologic assays for the determination of penicillin concentrations in biologic fluids.

VI. THERAPEUTIC INDICATIONS

Penicillins have activity against a broad spectrum of organisms and are the drugs of choice for treatment of many infections in nonallergic patients. Amoxicillin and ampicillin are effective agents in the treatment of otitis media and sinusitis due to *H. influenzae, S. pneumoniae*, and *Streptococcus pyogenes*, the most common organisms causing these infections. Oral penicillin V or intramuscular benzathine penicillin G are therapeutic agents of choice for pharyngitis and tonsillitis due to group A β-hemolytic streptococci.

Streptococcus pneumoniae is the most common organism that causes community-acquired pneumonia. If the patient is not seriously ill and the infection is present in only one lobe of the lung, patients can often be treated with oral penicillin V or intramuscular procaine penicillin G. Debilitated, immunocompromised, or seriously ill patients should be treated with intravenous penicillin G. In hospitalized patients who develop pneumonia, therapy may be altered to treat different organisms seen in nosocomial infections. Pneumonia due to *S. aureus* requires an antistaphylococcal penicillin, such as nafcillin, for adequate treatment.

Cystic fibrosis patients are often plagued with respiratory infections due to *Pseudonomas* spp. and *Staphylococcus aureus*. Although not unanimously accepted, antistaphylococcal penicillins and ticarcillin or acylureidopenicillins plus an aminoglycoside are generally indicated in this group of patients when respiratory symptoms develop.

The most common causative organisms of endocarditis are streptococci, both the *S. viridans* group and *Streptococcus bovis*. The drug of choice for this infection is parenteral penicillin G. Endocarditis due to *Streptococcus faecalis* may respond well to the synergistic action of ampicillin or penicillin plus an aminoglycoside. Endocarditis in a patient known to be an intravenous drug abuser is often caused by *S. aureus*, and parenteral nafcillin, methicillin, and oxacillin are the drugs of choice, pending sensitivity results. *Staphylococcus epidermidis* is a common cause of endocarditis in patients with artificial heart valves. Although many strains of *S. epidermidis* are resistant to antistaphylococcal penicillins, these antibiotics can be used in patients with infections due to susceptible strains.

The most common bacterial causes of meningitis are *H. influenzae, N. meningitidis*, and *Streptococcus pneumoniae* in children, and group B streptococci, *L. monocytogenes*, and enteric gram-negative rods in neonates. Bacterial meningitis in adults is most often due to *S. pneumoniae* or *N. meningitidis*. Penicillin G and ampicillin are agents of choice for all these organisms, with the exception of enteric gram-negative rods. *L. monocytogenes* and *H. influenzae* are more sensitive to ampicillin than to penicillin G. Some strains of *H. influenzae*, the most common cause of childhood meningitis, produce β-lactamase and are resistant to ampicillin. In 1981, 24% of meningitis cases due to *H. influenzae* reported to the Centers for Disease Control were resistant to ampicillin (127). Therefore, such agents as third-generation cephalosporins or chloramphenicol should be initiated empirically when meningitis due to *H. influenzae* is suspected. If culture and sensitivity results reveal an ampicillin-sensitive strain, ampicillin is the drug of choice. Ampicillin and penicillin do not effectively eradicate *N. meningitidis* or *H. influenzae* from the nares of carriers. Rifampin is required to eliminate this carrier state.

Staphylococcus aureus is a common cause of acute hematogenous osteomyelitis in both children and adults. Parenteral antistaphylococcal penicillins are the drugs of choice for initial therapy of this infection. In some patients, the antibiotic course can be completed using oral antimicrobial agents. Dicloxacillin or cloxacillin, in higher than usual doses, are suitable alternatives. In such cases, the serum activity of the antibiotic should be determined to assure adequate therapeutic levels.

Procaine penicillin G, ampicillin, and amoxicillin alone and in combination with probenecid are all effective for the treatment of uncomplicated gonorrhea. Penicillinase-producing strains of *Neisseria gonorrhoeae* have been isolated that are completely resistant to penicillin. However, these strains account for only 0.5% of the total number of cases of gonorrhea in the United States (128). In contrast, up to 50% of cases of gonorrhea in Africa and Southeast Asia are due to penicillinase-producing strains of *N. gonorrhoeae*.

Infants born to mothers with gonorrhea require prophylactic treatment with a single injection of aqueous penicillin G at birth. Neonates with untreated gonococcal ophthalmia may become blind; therefore, intravenous penicillin therapy is indicated (129). Complicated *N. gonorrhoeae* infections in neonates, such as arthritis or septicemia, also require intravenous penicillin therapy.

Penicillin G is the preferred drug for syphilis. Benzathine penicillin G is recommended for the treatment of early syphilis and also for syphilis of more than 1 year's duration. Intravenous penicillin therapy is needed to treat neurosyphilis. Penicillin G is indicated for congenital syphilis in the neonate as well.

Ampicillin and amoxicillin have been largely indicated for the treatment of urinary tract infections caused by *E. coli*; however, owing to the increasing number of strains that are resistant to ampicillin, alternative drugs may be required. Because of high concentrations of these drugs achieved in the urine, they may still be effective in eradicating the infection, even when relative resistant strains are found. Indanyl carbenicillin is the only available oral antibiotic for the treatment of urinary tract infections caused by *Pseudomonas aeruginosa*.

The carboxypenicillins and acylureidopenicillins are important agents in the management of febrile neutropenic patients. As a general rule, β-lactam antibiotics are more effective than aminoglycosides in patients with severe neutropenia (130). Studies indicate that antibiotic combinations that exhibit synergy in vitro are more effective than the antibiotic used alone or in combination regimens not known to act synergistically (131–134). Therefore, a synergistic combination of a carboxy- or acylureidopenicillin with an aminoglycoside is often indicated in this group of patients.

Antibiotic prophylaxis is another area in which penicillins are often indicated. Benzathine penicillin G is used for the prevention of recurrences of rheumatic fever (135). Penicillin V or procaine penicillin G are recommended for the prevention of endocarditis in patients with valvular heart disease (136). Procaine penicillin G, ampicillin, or amoxicillin in conjunction with probenecid provides prophylaxis against gonorrhea after sexual exposure. Similarly, benzathine penicillin G may be used for incubating syphilis if given within 24 hr after sexual contact. The use of penicillin in pregnant women or newborn infants for prophylaxis against neonatal group B streptococcal infections remains controversial (137-139).

VII. ADVERSE EFFECTS OF PENICILLINS

A. Hypersensitivity Reactions

Hypersensitivity reactions are the most common side effects of penicillins. Adverse reactions vary in intensity from a mild rash to anaphylaxis and death. Hypersensitivity reactions occur in 1-10% of patients with no history of a penicillin allergy and in 6-40% of those who previously reacted adversely to penicillin (141). A report published in 1968 estimated that life-threatening complications occur in 2-13% of all acute allergic reactions to penicillins and 3-9% of these anaphylactic reactions are fatal (142). There are no good estimates available for the incidence of penicillin hypersensitivity reactions in the pediatric population. However, children have a decreased risk of developing anaphylaxis compared with adults (143). The reasons for the lower incidence may include less exposure to β-lactams, generally reduced allergic reactivity, less vigorous antibody response, and differences in drug metabolism (144).

Penicillin is a low-molecular-weight compound and can only elicit an immune response when combined with a high-molecular-weight protein. The penicillin molecule must first be metabolically degraded, which causes the β-lactam ring to open. The opened ring reacts with tissue proteins to form the penicilloyl determinant. This is referred to as the major determinant, as approximately 95% of the degraded parent drug will be in this form. The penicilloyl determinant may also be produced from an intermediary, penicillenic acid, which is another penicillin degradation product (145). Less than 5% of penicillin is broken down by other metabolic pathways to form derivatives that are referred to as minor antigenic determinants. Both major and minor determinants are capable of eliciting an allergic reaction.

Immediate hypersensitivity reactions are due to the production of IgE antibody directed against the minor determinants and possibly in some cases to the major determinants. Accelerated and late-occurring allergic reactions are due to IgG antibody against the major determinants. IgG antibody levels against the major determinants may increase a few days after the onset of the allergic reaction, which generally corresponds to a subsiding of the reaction (146).

Penicillin allergy can manifest clinically in a number of ways, the most severe being anaphylaxis. Serum sickness, Coombs-positive hemolytic anemia, urticaria, asthma, and macular rashes are among the others. Exfoliative dermatitis and Stevens-Johnson syndrome have been associated with the use of penicillins, but these reactions are rare (10).

The likelihood of a serious allergic reaction occurring with oral penicillin agents is less than that of parenteral penicillins, although anaphylaxis has been reported after the administration of oral β-lactam antibiotics (144). The mechanisms for the difference in antigenicity of oral versus parenteral penicillin are unknown.

Patients with a history of penicillin allergy are at an increased risk of developing subsequent reactions on re-exposure to penicillins. The type of reaction and timing since the previous reaction are factors that may aid in predicting a recurrence. Patients with a history of developing anaphylaxis or exfoliative dermatitis should not be considered candidates for a rechallenge with penicillins due to the severe nature of the allergic reaction. Sensitivity to penicillins may decrease with time from the previous reaction. IgE antibodies against penicillin determinants may no longer be present in patients with a history of a penicillin allergy, and these patients can be treated with β-lactam antibiotics (147). Patients with a positive history of penicillin allergy who require penicillin therapy can be skin tested to determine if IgE antibodies are still present. However, if alternative antibiotics are available, they should be used. Pre-Pen (Kremers-Urban, Milwaukee, Wisconsin) is the only commercially available product for skin testing. It contains penicilloyl poly-L-lysine, which can detect the presence of IgE antibodies against the major determinants only. A positive test is exhibited by the production of a wheal-and-flare reaction at the site of intradermal administration. Normal saline controls should be placed simultaneously with the penicillin skin test. A negative penicillin skin test does not necessarily rule out the possibility of an anaphylactic reaction, since it does not test for the production of IgE antibody against the minor determinants. A preparation can be made from benzyl penicillin G for the detection of IgE antibodies to the minor determinants. If prepared and administered correctly, the combined use of Pre-Pen plus the benzyl penicillin G mixture should accurately predict whether IgE antibodies to penicillin are present. Penicillin skin testing can be performed in children 12 months old or greater, but there is limited information available in children younger than 1 year old. Some data suggest that infants should be capable of eliciting a wheal-and-flare reaction (143).

The cases in whom significant risks are involved in withholding therapy with β-lactam antibiotics in a penicillin-allergic patient, penicillin densensitization may be attempted. This should be performed by experienced medical staff only, and emergency equipment and medications should be readily available in the event that an anaphylactic reaction should occur.

Ampicillin is associated with a higher incidence of rash than other β-lactams, but rash may not always be an allergic manifestation. These are important to distinguish in order to avoid falsely identifying patients as penicillin allergic. The mechanism by which ampicillin causes nonallergic maculopapular rash is uncertain, but it occurs with a frequency of 5–10%. In patients also receiving allopurinol, the chance of developing rash increases to 22% (148). In patients with Epstein-Barr virus, administration of ampicillin will result in a maculopapular rash in 95–100% of cases. The reasons for the association of viral infections with ampicillin rash are not well understood. The nonallergic rash secondary to ampicillin is not necessarily an indication to stop the drug (149,150). If no additional adverse effects occur with continued administration, the rash may resolve with continued ampicillin therapy (151,152).

B. Hematologic Reactions

Neutropenia has been associated with the administration of many of the β-lactam antibiotics. The mechanism, however, is not well understood. Rouviex and colleagues (153) detected serum leukoagglutinins in eight of nine patients with neutropenia secondary to β-lactam antibiotics, suggesting an immunologically mediated mechanism. A toxic effect or dose-related mechanism has also been proposed (154). Neutropenia generally occurs after 7 days of therapy and is reversible upon immediate discontinuation of the offending agent (155).

Thrombocytopenia secondary to penicillin antibiotics has been reported but is rare (155). An immunologic mechanism has been suggested for this reaction. Platelet dysfunction has been associated with all penicillins. These agents have the ability to bind to platelet surface receptor sites, which decreases the ability of such activators as ADP, epinephrine, and arachidonic acid to bind to the platelets. This results in a prolongation of the template bleeding time but does not alter the prothrombin time (PT) or partial thromboplastin time (PTT). These adverse effects are more common with carbenicillin and ticarcillin than with mezlocillin, azlocillin, or piperacillin. The clinical significance of the reaction is not clear, but it may be an additional risk in patients with other conditions in which bleeding may be a problem (i.e., uremia, surgery, and anticoagulation therapy) (155).

Penicillins may cause hemolytic anemia due to IgG antibody directed against a penicillin-red blood cell complex. Penicillins may cause a Coombs-positive reaction in 0.1-0.5% of treated patients, but this is not always associated with hemolysis and anemia (155).

C. Central Nervous System Reactions

Central nervous system toxicity, including decreased consciousness, myoclonus, and generalized seizures, has been reported to occur after large doses of penicillin in patients with renal insufficiency (156). Reported daily doses were 25 million units or greater, and toxicity was seen 3 days or more after the start of therapy, or soon after dosage increase. Penicillin-induced seizures have been reported in both adults and children (16).

Systemic neurological reactions have been reported rarely after the administration of intramuscular procaine penicillin (157). The bizarre behavioral and neurological reactions were thought to be due to sustained concentrations of procaine in the serum.

D. Gastrointestinal Reactions

A variety of gastrointestinal reactions have been associated with the administration of penicillins. Oral penicillins may cause glossitis, stomatitis, epigastric distress, nausea, vomiting, and diarrhea (158). An often severe form of diarrhea resulting from antibiotic-induced pseudomembranous colitis may occur after continued administration of penicillin antibiotics. Most cases have been associated with ampicillin (159).

E. Hepatic Toxicity

A reversible elevation of liver enzymes may occur during therapy with any of the penicillins but is most commonly associated with carbenicillin, oxacillin, and nafcillin (160–162). The ureidopenicillins may also prove to be common offenders as their use increases. Although not consistently reported, one study found a 21% incidence of elevated serum asparate aminotransferase levels associated with piperacillin therapy (163).

F. Nephrotoxic Reactions

Renal toxicity has been reported rarely with penicillins (164–168), the most frequent being interstitial nephritis secondary to methicillin (169–179). The onset of methicillin-induced interstitial nephritis may occur 2-37 days after initiation of therapy (average, 15 days) and is generally reversible if the drug is discontinued. Progressive azotemia may result if therapy with the offending agent is continued (179). Other clinical manifestations associated with interstitial nephritis include fever, eosinophilia, hematuria, and proteinuria. Oliguria may be present. Methicillin-induced interstitial nephritis has a predilection for males and may occur at any age (179); however, the condition appears to have a milder course in children (170).

The mechanism by which methicillin causes interstitial nephritis is not understood. A delayed hypersensitivity reaction (164,180) and direct toxicity of protein-drug conjugates (178) have been suggested. Others have ruled out antibody-mediated reactions by failure to isolate antibodies from renal biopsy specimens (178). The relationship of this side effect to the dose of methicillin is controversial. Some have implicated excessive doses of methicillin as a cause of interstitial nephritis (181); others could not detect a clear dose-response relation. The true incidence of methicillin-induced interstitial nephritis is difficult to estimate from case reports. The number of methicillin-induced interstitial nephritis cases reported in the literature has declined markedly since the mid-1970s. This may reflect a decrease in the usage of methicillin and an increase in nafcillin usage, primarily owing to this side effect. In a recent prospective comparative trial of toxicities of methicillin versus nafcillin in children, urologic toxic effects occurred in 5.3% of methicillin-treated patients and in none of the nafcillin group (162). Another study involving a small number of pediatric patients showed no difference in the rate of renal toxicity of methicillin and nafcillin (182). Hemorrhagic cystitis has been reported to occur in patients receiving penicillin G (183), methicillin (184,185), carbenicillin (186), ticarcillin (187), and piperacillin (188).

G. Electrolyte Imbalance

Some penicillins may cause electrolyte disorders owing to the cation component of the salt being administered. The largest offenders, carbenicillin and ticarcillin, contain 4.7 and 6 mEg sodium per gram of drug, respectively. The ureidopenicillins contain less sodium per gram of drug (approximately 2 mEq/g). This may be an advantage for these drugs over ticarcillin and carbenicillin in patients with chronic renal failure or congestive heart failure, in whom sodium restriction is necessary.

Penicillins may induce hypokalemia by acting as nonabsorbable anions in the distal tubule of the kidney and promoting urinary potassium excretion. It has also been suggested that penicillins may cause a redistribution of potassium within the cells, thereby contributing to hypokalemia (189). Hypokalemia may be apparent as early as the second or third day of therapy (190).

H. Drug Administration-Related Side Effects

Intramuscular administration of benzathine penicillin G can cause pain at the site of injection. Deep muscle soreness and tenderness may persist for 1-3 days after the injection (191). Other rare adverse reactions associated with the intramuscular injection of benzathine or procaine penicillin G include muscle contractures, nerve injury, and abscess formation at the injection site (192). Accidental intra-arterial injection of benzathine penicillin G can lead to thrombosis and ischemic damage (193).

VIII. DRUG INTERACTIONS

A. Aminoglycosides and Penicillins

Ticarcillin, carbenicillin, mezlocillin, azlocillin, and piperacillin have all been demonstrated to inactivate aminoglycoside antibiotics (194-200). Although the exact mechanism is not known, it appears that the interaction most likely involves the nucleophilic opening of the β-lactam ring of the penicillin by an amino group of the aminoglycoside, forming a complex with no antimicrobial activity (194). The interaction occurs both in vitro and in patients with renal failure. It has been shown that such factors as drug concentration, time of contact, and temperature can influence this interaction in vitro. Therefore, aminoglycosides and penicillins should be administered separately to patients.

Inactivation of aminoglycosides does not occur in patients with normal renal function (195). Both aminoglycosides and penicillins are normally cleared faster than the time needed for the interaction to occur. In patients with renal failure, however, accumulation of both antibiotics can occur, allowing significant time for inactivation to take place. Concurrent administration of gentamicin and carbenicillin in patients with end-stage renal disease resulted in a 70% decrease in gentamicin half-life (194). In vivo inactivation of penicillins also occurs, but owing to the large difference in serum concentrations of the aminoglycoside and the penicillin, the percentage of the penicillin inactivated is insignificant.

Inactivation of aminoglycosides by penicillins may also occur in the test tube containing biologic specimens at room temperature and during refrigeration; however, this has not been shown to occur at -70°C (196). Therefore, when blood samples are obtained from patients with renal failure, aminoglycoside concentration should be measured immediately or samples frozen until the assay procedure can be performed (196). In vitro, gentamicin and tobramycin are significantly more susceptible to inactivation than amikacin or netilmicin (196,197). This also appears to be true in vivo. Blair and co-workers (194) reported that gentamicin was inactivated to a greater extent than amikacin in renal failure patients receiving carbenicillin.

B. Interactions Producing Synergy

Synergistic activity has been demonstrated in vitro for acylureidopenicillins and aminoglycosides against the Enterobacteriaceae, *Pseudomonas aeruginosa*, and *Staphylococcus aureus* (201-203). Synergistic activity may range from 50 to 90%, depending on the antibiotic combinations (205). Synergy has also been demonstrated for ticarcillin or carbenicillin in combination with aminoglycosides against *P. aeruginosa* and the Enterobacteriaceae (204,205). Both penicillin and ampicillin display synergistic activity with aminoglycosides against *Streptococcus faecalis* (206,207).

C. Interactions Producing Antagonism

In vitro antagonistic effects have been reported for cefoxitin in combination with either piperacillin or mezlocillin against *P. aeruginosa, Serratia marcescens, Enterobacter* species (excluding *Klebsiella* and *E. coli*), and indole-positive *Proteus* species. The mechanism of this antagonism is thought to be induction of β-lactamases by the cephalosporin, with resultant hydrolysis of the penicillin (108). The clinical significance of this in vitro effect has not been clearly demonstrated.

D. Interactions with Laboratory Tests

Nafcillin and methicillin have been shown to cause false-positive results in laboratory tests used to detect proteinuria (211). This has been documented with the trichloroacetic acid (TCA) method and sulfosalicylic acid test, but not with dipstick techniques. Although trichoroacetic acid and sulfosalicylic acid form insoluble salts with proteins when present in the urine, this does not appear to be the mechanism by which false-positive results occur with methicillin and nafcillin. Excessive turbidity in the test solution by methicillin and nafcillin appears to lead to a false-positive result (212).

REFERENCES

1. Fletcher, C: First clinical use of penicillin. *Br. Med. J. 289*:1721–1723, 1984.
2. Fraser, SI: Penicillin: Early trials in war casualties. *Br. Med. J. 289*:1723–1725, 1984.
3. Arnold, HL: Penicillin and early syphilis. *JAMA 251*:2011–2012, 1984.
4. Tauber, MG, Sande, MA: The impact of penicillin on the treatment of meningitis. *JAMA 251*:1877–1880, 1984.
5. Price, KE: Structure-activity relationships of semisynthetic penicillins. *Adv. Appl. Microbiol. 11*:17–75, 1969.
6. Mandell, GL, Sande, MA: Antimicrobial agents. Penicillins and cephalosporins. In: *The Pharmacological Basis of Therapeutics* (AG Gilman, LS Goodman, and A Gilman, eds.), MacMillan, New York, 1980, pp. 1126–1161.
7. Kucers, A, Bennett, NH, eds.: Penicillins. In: *The Use of Antibiotics*. Lippincott, Philadelphia, 1979, p. 21.
8. Blumberg, PM, Strominger, JL: Interaction of penicillin with the bacterial cell: penicillin-binding proteins and penicillin-sensitive enzymes. *Bacteriol. Rev. 38*: 291–335, 1974.
9. Yocum, RR, Waxman, DW, Strominger, JL: The mechanism of action of penicillin. *J. Biol. Chem. 244*:3977, 1980.
10. Neu, HC: Penicillins. In: *Antiinfective Therapy* (GL Mandell, RG Douglas, and JE Bennett, eds.), John Wiley & Sons, New York, 1985, pp. 37–75.
11. Editorial: Isolation of multiple antibiotic-resistant pneumococci. *JAMA 254*:1886, 1985.
12. Raverby, WD, Bottone, EJ, Keusch, GT: Group D streptococcal bacteremia with emphasis on the incidence and presentation of infections due to *Streptococcus bovis. N. Engl. J. Med. 289*:1400–1403, 1973.
13. Contoyiannis, P, Adamopoulos, DA: Penicillin-resistant *Neisseria meningitidis. Lancet 1*:462, 1974.
14. Reyn, A, Korner, B, Bentzon, MW: Effects of penicillin streptomycin, and tetracycline on *N gonorrhoeae* isolated in 1944 and 1957. *Br. J. Vener. Dis. 34*:227–239, 1958.
15. Sparling, PF: Antibiotic resistance in *Neisseria gonorrhoeae. Med. Clin. North Am. 56*:1133–1144, 1972.
16. Weinstein, L, Lerner, PI, Chew, WH: Clinical and bacteriologic studies of the effect of "massive" doses of penicillin G on infections caused by gram-negative bacilli. *N. Engl. J. Med. 271*:525–533, 1964.
17. Finegold, SM, George, WL, Mulligan, ME: Anaerobic infections. Part 1. *Disease-a-Month 31*:1–77, 1985.
18. Thornsberry, C, McDougal, LK: Successful use of broth microdilution in susceptibility tests for methicillin-resistant (heteroresistant) staphylococci. *J. Clin. Microbiol. 18*:1084–1091, 1983.

19. Wiggins, GL, Albritton, WL, Feeley, JC: Antibiotic susceptibility of clinical isolates of *Listeria monocytogenes. Antimicrob. Agents Chemother. 13*:854, 1978.
20. Koniforti, N, Halperin, E: Sensitivities of strains of enteropathogenic *Escherichia coli* to cephalexin and other antibiotics. *Am. J. Clin. Pathol. 64*:121, 1975.
21. Neu, HC, Garvey, GG: Comparative in vitro activity and clinical pharmacology of ticarcillin and carbenicillin. *Antimicrob. Agents Chemother. 8*:457, 1975.
22. Neu, HC: Carbenicillin and ticarcillin. *Med. Clin. North Am. 66*:61–77, 1982.
23. Sabath, LD, Stumpf, LL, Wallace, SJ, et al.: Susceptibility of *Diplococcus pneumoniae, Haemophilus influenzae* and *Neisseria meningitidis* to 23 antibiotics. *Antimicrob. Agents Chemother. 10*:53–56, 1970.
24. Wise, R, Gillett, AP, Andrews, JM, Bedford, KA: Activity of azlocillin and mezlocillin against gram-negative organisms: Comparison with other penicillins. *Antimicrob. Agents Chemother. 13*:559–565, 1978.
25. Verbist, L: Comparison of the activities of the new ureidopenicillins piperacillin, mezlocillin, azlocillin, and Bay k 4999 against gram-negative organisms. *Antimicrob. Agents Chemother. 16*:115–119, 1979.
26. Bodey, GP, Le Blanc, B: Piperacillin: In vitro evaluation. *Antimicrob. Agents Chemother. 14*:78–87, 1978.
27. Fu, KP, Neu, HC: Azlocillin and mezlocillin: New ureidopenicillins. *Antimicrob. Agents Chemother. 13*:930–938, 1978.
28. Eliopoulos, GN, Moellering, RC: Azlocillin, mezlocillin, and piperacillin: New broad-spectrum penicillins. *Ann. Intern. Med. 97*:755–760, 1982.
29. Sabath, LD: Phenoxymethylpenicillin (Penicillin V) and phenethicillin. *Med. Clin. North Am. 54*:1101–1111, 1970.
30. Bear, DM, Turck, M, Petersdorf, RG: Ampicillin. *Med. Clin. North Am. 54*:1145–1159, 1970.
31. Fuchs, PC, Barry, AL, Thornsberry, C, Gavan, TL, Jones, RN: In vitro evaluation of Augmentin by broth microdilution and disk diffusion susceptibility testing: Regression analysis, tentative interpretive criteria and quality control limits. *Antimicrob. Agents Chemother. 24*:31–38, 1983.
32. Fass, RJ: Statistical comparison of the antibacterial activities of broad-spectrum penicillins against gram-negative bacilli. *Antimicrob. Agents Chemother. 24*:156–162, 1983.
33. Fishman, LS, Hewitt, WL: The natural penicillins. *Med. Clin. North Am. 53*:1081–1099, 1970.
34. Barza, M: II. Penicillins. *Am. J. Hosp. Pharm. 34*:57–64, 1977.
35. McCracken, GH, Ginsberg, C, Chrane, DF, Thomas, ML, Horton, LJ: Clinical pharmacology of penicillin in newborn infants. *J. Pediatr. 82*:692–698, 1973.
36. Speer, ME, Mason, EO, Scharnberg, JT: Cerebrospinal fluid concentrations of aqueous procaine penicillin G in the neonate. *Pediatrics 67*:387–388, 1981.
37. Ginsburg, CM, McCracken, GH, Zweighaft, TC: Serum penicillin concentrations after intramuscular administration of benzathene penicillin G in children. *Pediatrics 69*:452–454, 1982.
38. Collart, P, Poitevin, M, Milovanovic, A, Herlin, A, Durel, J: Kinetic study of serum penicillin concentrations after single doses of benzathine and benethamine penicillins in young and old people. *Br. J. Vener. Dis. 56*:355–362, 1980.
39. Hieber, JP, Nelson, JD: A pharmacologic evaluation of penicillin in children with purulent meningitis. *N. Engl. J. Med. 297*:410–413, 1977.
40. Mohr, JA, Griffiths, W, Jackson, R, et al.: Neurosyphilis and penicillin levels in cerebrospinal fluid. *JAMA 236*:2208–2209, 1976.
41. Kaplan, JM, McCracken, GH: Clinical pharmacology of benzathine penicillin G in neonates with regard to its recommended use in congenital syphilis. *J. Pediatr. 82*:1069–1072, 1973.

42. Follath, F: Clinical pharmacokinetics of penicillins and aminoglycosides. In: *Clinical Chemotherapy Fundamentals*, Volume 1 (HP Kulmmerle, ed.), Thieme-Stratton, New York, pp. 315–334, 1983.
43. Barza, M, Weinstein, L: Pharmacokinetics of the penicillins in man. *Clin. Pharmacokinet. 1*:297–308, 1976.
44. Cole, M, Kening, MD, Hewitt, VA: Metabolism of penicillins to penicilloic acidosis and b-aminopenicillanic acid in man and its significance in assessing penicillin absorption. *Antimicrob. Agents Chemother. 3*:463, 1973.
45. Bergeron, MG, Gennari, FJ, Barza, M, Weinstein, L, Cortell, S: Renal tubular transport of penicillin G and carbenicillin in the rat. *J. Infect. Dis. 132*:374, 1975.
46. Bryan, CS, Stone, WJ: "Comparably massive" penicillin G therapy in renal failure. *Ann. Intern. Med. 82*:189, 1975.
47. Kunin, CM, Finland, M: Persistence of antibiotics in blood of patients with acute renal failure. III. Penicillin, streptomycin, erythromycin, and kanamycin. *J. Clin. Invest. 38*:1509, 1959.
48. Kucers, A, Bennett, NM, eds.: Phenoxypenicillins. In: *The Use of Antibiotics*, J. B. Lippincott, Philadelphia, 1979, pp. 55–63.
49. McCarthy, CG, Finland, M: Absorption and excretion of four penicillins, penicillin G, penicillin V, phenethicillin and phenylmercaptomethyl penicillin. *N. Engl. J. Med. 263*:315–326, 1960.
50. Cronk, GA, Wheatley, WB, Fellers, GF, Albright, H: The relationship of food intake to the absorption of potassium alpha-phenoxyethyl penicillin and potassium phenoxymethyl penicillin from the gastrointestinal tract. *Am. J. Med. Sci. 240*: 219–225, 1960.
51. Wright, AJ, Wilkowske, CJ: The penicillins. *Mayo Clin. Proc. 58*:21–32, 1983.
52. Sabath, LD, Postic, B, Finland, M: Laboratory studies on methicillin. *Am. J. Med. Sci. 244*:484, 1962.
53. Knudsen, ET, Robinson, GN: Absorption and excretion of a new antibiotic (BRL 1241). *Br. Med. J. 2*:700, 1960.
54. Neu, HC: Antistaphylococcal penicillins. *Med. Clin. North Am. 66*:51–59, 1982.
55. Sarff, LD, McCracken, GH, Thomas, ML, Horton, LJ, Threlkeld, N: Clinical pharmacology of methicillin in neonates. *J. Pediatr. 90*:1005–1008, 1977.
56. Boe, RW, Williams, CPS, Bennett, JV, et al.: Serum levels of methicillin and ampicillin in newborn and premature infants in relation to postnatal age. *Pediatrics 39*: 194–201, 1967.
57. Gilbert, DN, Sanford, JP: Methicillin: Critical appraisal after a decade of experience. *Med. Clin. North Am. 54*:1113–1125, 1970.
58. White, A, Varga, DT: Antistaphylococcal activity of sodium methicillin. *Arch. Intern. Med. 108*:671, 1961.
59. Henegar, GC, Silverman, M, Gardner, RJ, Kukral, JC, Preston, FW: Excretion of methicillin in human bile. *Antimicrob. Agents Chemother. 1*:348, 1961.
60. Kucers, A, Bennett, NM, eds.: Methicillin. In: *The Use of Antibiotics*, J. B. Lippincott, Philadelphia, 1979, pp. 64–78.
61. Yaffe, SJ, Gerbracht, LM, Mosovich, LL, Matter, ME, Danish, M, Jusko, WJ: Pharmacokinetics of methicillin in patients with cystic fibrosis. *J. Infect. Dis. 135*:828, 1977.
62. Whitehouse, AC, Morgan, JG, Schumacher, J, Hamburger, M: Blood levels and antistaphylococcal titers produced in human subjects by a penicillinase-resistant penicillin, nafcillin, compared with similar penicillins. *Antimicrob. Agents Chemother. 3*: 384–382, 1963.
63. Rudnick, M, Morrison, G, Walker, B, Singer, I: Renal failure, hemodialysis, and nafcillin kinetics. *Clin. Pharmacol. Ther. 20*:413–423, 1976.
64. Diaz, CR, Kane, JG, Parker, RH, Pelsor, FR: Pharmacokinetics of nafcillin in patients with renal failure. *Antimicrob. Agents Chemother. 12*:98–101, 1977.

65. Feldman, WE, Nelson, JD, Stanberry, LR: Clinical and pharmacokinetic evaluation of nafcillin in infants and children. *J. Pediatr. 93*:1029–1033, 1978.
66. Banner, W, Gooch, WM, Burchkar, G, Korones, SB: Pharmacokinetics of nafcillin in infants with low birth weights. *Antimicrob. Agents Chemother. 17*:691–694, 1980.
67. Ruiz DE, Warner JF: Nafcillin treatment of *Staphylococcus aureus* meningitis. *Antimicrob. Agents Chemother. 9*:554–555, 1976.
68. Kane, JG, Parker, RH, Jordan, GW, Hoeprich, PD: Nafcillin concentration in cerebrospinal fluid during treatment of staphylococcal infections. *Ann. Intern. Med. 87*: 309–311, 1977.
69. Nunes, HL, Pecora, CC, Judy, K, Rosenman, SB, Warren, GH, Martin, CM: Turnover and distribution of nafcillin in tissues and body fluids of surgical patients. *Antimicrob. Agents Chemother. 4*:237–249, 1964.
70. Marshall, JP, Salt, WB, Elam, RO, Wilkinson, GR, Schenker, S: Disposition of nafcillin in patients with cirrhosis and extrahepatic biliary obstruction. *Gastroenterology 73*:1388–1392, 1977.
71. Klein, JO, Finland, M, Wilcox, C: Nafcillin. Antibacterial action in vitro and absorption and excretion in normal young men. *Am. J. Med. Sci. 246*:10, 1963.
72. Marcy, SM, Klein, J: The isoxazolyl penicillins: Oxacillin, cloxacillin, and dicloxacillin. *Med. Clin. North Am. 54*:1127–1143, 1970.
73. Axline, SG, Yaffe, SJ, Simon, HJ: Clinical pharmacology of antimicrobials in premature infants. II. Ampicillin, methicillin, oxacillin, neomycin, and colistin. *Pediatrics 39*:97–107, 1967.
74. Thijssen, HHW, Mattie, H: Active metabolites of isoxazolypenicillins in humans. *Antimicrob. Agents Chemother. 10*:441, 1976.
75. Jusko, WJ, Mosovich, LL, Gerbracht, LM, Matter, ME, Yaffe, SJ: Enhanced renal excretion of dicloxacillin in patients with cystic fibrosis. *Pediatrics 56*:1038–1043, 1975.
76. Spino, M, Chai, RP, Isles, AF, Thiessen, JJ, Tesoro, A, Gold, R, MacLeod, SM: Cloxacillin absorption and disposition in cystic fibrosis. *J. Pediatr. 105*:829–835, 1984.
77. Nauta, EH, Mattie, H: Dicloxacillin and cloxacillin: Pharmacokinetics in healthy and hemodialysis subjects. *Clin. Pharmacol. Ther. 20*:98–108, 1976.
78. Kirby, WMM, Kind, AC: Clinical pharmacology of ampicillin and hetacillin. *Ann. N.Y. Acad. Sci. 145*:291–297, 1967.
79. Klein, JO, Finland, M: Ampicillin: Activity in vitro and absorption and excretion in normal young men. *Am. J. Med. Sci. 245*:544–555, 1963.
80. Gordon, RC, Regamey, C, Kirby, WM: Comparative clinical pharmacology of amoxicillin and ampicillin administered orally. *Antimicrob. Agents Chemother. 1*: 504–507, 1972.
81. Kaplan, JM, McCracken, GH, Horton, LJ, Thomas, ML, Davis, N: Pharmacologic studies in neonates given large dosages of ampicillin. *J. Pediatr 84*:571–577, 1974.
82. Ginsburg, CM, McCracken, GH, Thomas, ML, Clahsen, J: Comparative pharmacokinetics of amoxicillin and ampicillin in infants and children. *Pediatrics 64*:627–631, 1979.
83. Coffey, JD, Jr.: Concentration of ampicillin in exudate from acute otitis media. *J. Pediatr. 72*:693–695, 1968.
84. Ayliffe, GAJ, Davies, A: Ampicillin levels in human bile. *Br. J. Pharmacol. Chem. 24*:189–193, 1965.
85. Mortimer, PR, Mackie, DB, Haynes, S: Ampicillin levels in human bile in the presence of biliary tract disease. *Br. Med. J. 3*:88–89, 1969.

86. Bray, RE, Boe, RW, Johnson, WL: Transfer of ampicillin into fetus and amniotic fluid from maternal plasma in late pregnancy. *Am. J. Obstet. Gynecol. 96*:938–942, 1966.
87. Jusko, WJ, Lewis, GP, Schmitt, GW: Ampicillin and hetacillin pharmacokinetics in normal and anephric subjects. *Clin. Pharmacol. Ther. 16*:90, 1974.
88. Ehrnebo, M, Nilsson, SO, Boreus, LD: Pharmacokinetics of ampicillin and its prodrugs bacampicillin and pivampicillin in man. *J. Pharmacokinet. Biopharm. 7*:429, 1979.
89. McCracken, GH; Pharmacological basis of antimicrobial therapy in newborn infants. *Am. J. Dis. Child. 128*:407–419, 1974.
90. Neu, HC: Amoxicillin. *Ann. Intern. Med. 90*:356–360, 1979.
91. Adam, D, Devisser, I, Koeppe, P: Pharmacokinetics of amoxicillin and clavulanic acid administered alone and in combination. *Antimicrob. Agents Chemother. 22*: 353–357, 1982.
92. Weber, DJ, Tolkoff-Rubin, NE, Rubin, RH: Amoxicillin and potassium clavulanate: An antibiotic combination. *Pharmacotherapy 4*:122–136, 1984.
93. Nelson, JD, Kusmiesz, H, Shelton, S: Pharmacokinetics of potassium clavulanate in combination with amoxicillin in pediatric patients. *Antimicrob. Agents Chemother. 21*:681–682, 1982.
94. Ginsburg, CM, McCracken, GH, Clahsen, J, Zweighaft, TC: Comparative pharmacokinetics of bacampicillin and ampicillin suspensions in infants and children. *Rev. Infect. Dis. 3*:117–120, 1981.
95. Ginsburg, CM, McCracken, GH, Zweighaft, TC, Clahsen, JC: Comparative pharmacokinetics of cyclacillin and amoxicillin in infants and children. *Antimicrob. Agents Chemother. 19*:1086–1088, 1981.
96. Spyker, DA, Rugloski, RJ, Vann, RL, et al.: Pharmacokinetics of amoxicillin: Dose dependence after intravenous, oral, and intramuscular administration. *Antimicrob. Agents Chemother. 11*:132, 1977.
97. Knirsch, AK, Hobbs, DC, Korst, JJ: Pharmacokinetics, toleration, and safety of indanyl carbenicillin in man. *J. Infect. Dis. 127 (Suppl.)*:S105–S110, 1973.
98. Neu, HC, Garvey, GJ: Comparative in vitro activity and clinical pharmacology of ticarcillin and carbenicillin. *Antimicrob. Agents Chemother. 8*:457–462, 1975.
99. Libke, RD, Clarke, JT, Ralph, ED, et al.: Ticarcillin vs. carbenicillin clinical pharmacokinetics. *Clin. Pharmacol. Ther. 17*:441, 1975.
100. Nelson, JD, McCracken, GH: Clinical pharmacology of carbenicillin and gentamicin in the neonate and comparative efficacy with ampicillin and gentamicin. *Pediatrics 52*:801–812, 1973.
101. Nelson, JD, Kusmiesz, H, Shelton, S, Woodman, E: Clinical pharmacology and efficacy of ticarcillin in infants and children. *Pediatrics 61*:858–863, 1978.
102. Erwin, FR, Bullock, WE: Clinical and pharmacological studies of ticarcillin in gram-negative infections. *Antimicrob. Agents Chemother. 9*:94, 1976.
103. Parry, MF, Neu, HC: Ticarcillin for treatment of serious infections with gram-negative bacteria. *J. Infect. Dis. 134*:476, 1976.
104. Richardson, AE, Spittle, CR, James, KW, et al.: Experience with carbenicillin in the treatment of septicemia and meningitis. *Postgrad. Med. 44*:844, 1968.
105. Rodriguez, V, Inagaki, J, Bodey, GP: Clinical pharmacology of ticarcillin (*d*-carboxyl-3-thienmethyl-penicillin BRL 2288). *Antimicrob. Agents Chemother. 4*: 31, 1973.
106. Parry, MF, Neu, HC: Pharmacokinetics of ticarcillin in patients with abnormal renal function. *J. Infect. Dis. 133*:46, 1976.
107. Tjandramaga, TB, Mullie, A, Berbesselt, R, et al.: Piperacillin: Human pharmacokinetics after intravenous and intramuscular administration. *Antimicrob. Agents Chemother. 14*:829, 1978.

108. Drusano, GL, Schimpff, SC, Hewitt, WL: The acylampicillins: Mezlocillin, piperacillin, and azlocillin. *Rev. Infect. Dis. 6*:13–32, 1984.
109. Wilson, CB, Koup, Jr: Clinical pharmacology of extended-spectrum penicillins in infants and children. *J. Pediatr. 106*:1049–1056, 1985.
110. Rosenkranz, H, Forster, D: Comparative study of the binding of acylureidopenicillins and carbenicillin to human serum proteins. *Infection 7*:102–108, 1979.
111. Prince, AS, Neu, HC: New penicillins and their use in pediatrics. *Pediatr. Clin. North Am. 30*:3–16, 1983.
112. Meyers, BR, Hirschman, SZ, Strougo, L, Srulevitch, E: Comparative study of piperacillin, ticarcillin, and carbenicillin pharmacokinetics. *Antimicrob. Agents Chemother. 17*:608–611, 1980.
113. Leroy, A, Humbert, G, Godin, M, Fillastre, JP: Pharmacokinetics of azlocillin in subjects with normal and impaired renal function. *Antimicrob. Agents Chemother. 17*:344–349, 1980.
114. Fiegel, P, Becker, K: Pharmacokinetics of azlocillin in persons with normal and impaired renal functions. *Antimicrob. Agents Chemother. 14*:288–291, 1978.
115. Frimodt-Moller, N, Maigaard, S, Toothaker, RD, Bundtzen, RW, Brodey, MV, Craig, WA, Welling, PG, Madsen, PO: Mezlocillin pharmacokinetics after single intravenous doses to patients with varying degrees of renal function. *Antimicrob. Agents Chemother. 17*:599–607, 1980.
116. Thompson, MIB, Russo, ME, Matsen, JM, Atkin-Thor, E: Piperacillin pharmacokinetics in subjects with chronic renal failure. *Antimicrob. Agents Chemother. 19*: 450–453, 1981.
117. Wilson, CB, Koup, JR, Opheim, KE, et al.: Piperacillin pharmacokinetics in pediatric patients. *Antimicrob. Agents Chemother. 22*:442, 1978.
118. Batra, VK, Morrison, JA, Lasseter, KC, Joy, VA: Piperacillin kinetics. *Clin. Pharmacol. Ther. 26*:41–53, 1979.
119. Thirumoorthi, MC, Asmar, BI, Buckley, JA, et al.: Pharmacokinetics of intravenously administered piperacillin in preadolescent children. *J. Pediatr. 102*:941, 1983.
120. Prince, AS, Neu, HC: Use of piperacillin, a semisynthetic penicillin, in the therapy of acute exacerbations of pulmonary disease in patients with cystic fibrosis. *J. Pediatr. 97*:148, 1980.
121. Hoogkamp-Korstanje, JAA, Vanderlaag, J: Piperacillin and tobramycin in the treatment of *Pseudomonas* lung infections in cystic fibrosis. *J. Antimicrob. Chemother. 12*:175, 1983.
122. Kramer, WG, Pickering, LK, Culbert, S, et al.: Mezlocillin pharmacokinetics in pediatric oncology patients. *Antimicrob. Agents Chemother. 25*:62, 1984.
123. Pickering, LK, Kramer, WG, Armes, DA, et al.: Clinical pharmacology and efficacy of mezlocillin in pediatric patients with malignancy. *J. Antimicrob. Chemother. 9 (Suppl A)*:245, 1982.
124. Bergan, T, Mechalsen, H: Pharmacokinetics of azlocillin in children with cystic fibrosis. *Arzneimittelforsch. 29*:1955, 1979.
125. Bosso, JA, Saxon, BA, Herbst, JJ, et al.: Azlocillin pharmacokinetics in patients with cystic fibrosis. *Antimicrob. Agents Chemother. 25*:630, 1984.
126. Malmborg, AS, Alfreddsson, H, Kusoffsky, E, et al.: Azlocillin and gentamicin in respiratory tract infections with *Pseudomonas aeruginosa* in patients with cystic fibrosis. *Scand. J. Infect. Dis. 29 (Suppl.)*:64, 1981.
127. Schlech, WF, III, Ward, JI, Band, JD, Hightower, A, Fraser, DW, Broome, CV: Bacterial meningitis in the United States, 1978 through 1981. The National Bacterial Meningitis Surveillance Study. *JAMA 253*:1749–1754, 1985.

128. McCormack, WM: Penicillinase-producing *Neisseria gonorrhoea*: A retrospective. *N. Engl. J. Med. 307*:438–449, 1982.
129. Centers for Disease Control: Sexually transmitted diseases: Treatment guidelines, 1982. *Rev. Infect. Dis. 4*:S729–746, 1982.
130. Bodey, GP: Antibiotics in patients with neutropenia. *Arch. Intern. Med. 144*: 1845–1851, 1984.
131. Scott, RE, Robson, HG: Synergistic activity of carbenicillin and gentamicin in experimental *Pseudomonas* bacteremia in neutropenic rats. *Antimicrob. Agents Chemother. 10*:646–651, 1976.
132. Anderson, ET, Young, LS, Hewitt, WL: Antimicrobial synergism in the therapy of gram-negative rod bacteremia. *Chemotherapy 24*:45–54, 1978.
133. Klastersky, J, Cappel, R, Daneau, D: Clinical significance of in vitro synergism between antibiotics in gram-negative infections. *Antimicrob. Agents Chemother. 2*: 470–475, 1972.
134. Klastersky, J, Meunier-Carpenter, F, Prevost, JM: Significance of antimicrobial synergism for the outcome of gram negative sepsis. *Am. J. Med. Sci. 273*:157–167, 1977.
135. Spagnuolo, M, Pasternack, B, Taranta, A: Risk of rheumatic fever recurrences after streptococcal infections. Prospective study of clinical and social factors. *N. Engl. J. Med. 285*:641–647, 1971.
136. Kaye, D: Prophylaxis of endocarditis. In: *Infective Endocarditis* (D Kaye, ed.), University Park Press, Baltimore, 1976, pp. 245–265.
137. Gotoff, SP: Chemoprophylaxis of early onset group B streptococcal disease. *Pediatr. Infect. Dis. 3*:401–403, 1984.
138. Editorial: Prevention of early onset group B streptococcal infection in the new born. *Lancet 1*:1056–1058, 1984.
139. Paredis, A, Wong, P, Yow, MD: Failure of penicillin to eradicate the carrier state of group B streptococcus in infants. *J. Pediatr. 89*:191, 1976.
140. Roselle, GA, Bode, R, Hamilton, B, et al.: Clinical trial of the efficacy and safety of ticarcillin and clavulanic acid. *Antimicrob. Agents Chemother. 27*:291–296, 1985.
141. Sogn, DD: Penicillin allergy. *J. Allergy Clin. Immunol. 74*:589–593, 1984.
142. Idsoe, O, Guthe, T, Willcox, RR, De Weck, AL: Nature and extent of penicillin side reactions, with particular reference to fatalities from anaphylactic shock. *Bull. WHO 38*:159, 1968.
143. Sullivan, TJ: Pathogenesis and management of allergic reactions to penicillin and other beta-lactam antibiotics. *Pediatr. Infect. Dis. 1*:344–350, 1982.
144. Parker, CW: Drug allergy (three parts). *N. Engl. J. Med. 292*:511, 732, 957, 1975.
145. Parker, CW: The immunochemical basis for penicillin allergy. *Postgrad. Med. J. (Suppl.) 40*:141, 1964.
146. Sher, TH: Penicillin hypersensitivity—a review. *Pediatr. Clin. North Am. 30*:161–176, 1983.
147. Sullivan, TJ, Wedner, HJ, Shatz, GS, et al.: Skin testing to detect penicillin allergy. *J. Allergy Clin. Immunol. 68*:171, 1981.
148. Boston Collaborative Drug Surveillance Program: Excess of ampicillin rashes associated with allopurinol or hyperuricemia. *N. Engl. J. Med. 286*:505, 1972.
149. Bierman, CW, Pierson, WE, Zeitz, SJ, et al.: Reactions associated with ampicillin therapy. *JAMA 220*:1098, 1972.
150. Report of Collaborative Study Group: Prospective study of ampicillin rash. *Br. J. Med. 1*:7, 1973.

151. Almeyda, J, Levantine, A: Drug reactions. XIX. Adverse cutaneous reactions to the penicillins-ampicillin rashes. *Br. J. Dermatol. 87*:293, 1972.
152. Kerns, DL, Shera, JE, Summers, RJ, et al.: Ampicillin rash in children. *Am. J. Dis. Child. 128*:187, 1973.
153. Rouviex, B, Lassoued, K, Yittecog, D, Regnier, B: Neutropenia due to Blactamine antibodies. *Br. Med. J. 287*:1832–1834, 1981.
154. Homayouri, H, Gross, PA, Setia, U, Lynch, TJ: Leukopenia due to penicillin and cephalosporin homologues. *Arch. Intern. Med. 139*:827–828, 1979.
155. Parry, MF: Toxic and adverse reactions encountered with new beta-lactam antibiotics. *Bull. N.Y. Acad. Med. 60*:358–368, 1984.
156. Bloomer, HA, Barton, LJ, Maddock, RK: Penicillin induced encephalopathy in uremic patients. *JAMA 200*:121–123, 1967.
157. Green, RL, Lewis, JE, Kraus, SJ, et al.: Elevated plasma procaine concentrations after administration of procaine penicillin G. *N. Engl. J. Med. 291*:223–226, 1974.
158. Alanis, A, Weinstein, AJ: Adverse reactions with oral penicillins and cephalosporins. *Med. Clin. North Am. 67*:113–129, 1983.
159. Bartlett, JG: Antibiotic-associated pseudomembraneous colitis. *Hosp. Pract. 16*: 85–95, 1981.
160. Dismukes, WE: Oxacillin-induced hepatic dysfunction. *JAMA 226*:861–863, 1973.
161. Wilson, FM, Belamavic, J, Lauter, CB, et al.: Anicteric carbenicillin hepatitis. Eight episodes in four patients. *JAMA 232*:818, 1967.
162. Kitzing, W, Nelson, JD, Mohs, E: Comparative toxicities of methicillin and nafcillin. *Am. J. Dis. Child. 135*:52–55, 1981.
163. Marier, RL, Sanders, CV, Faro, S, et al.: Piperacillin v. carbenicillin in the therapy for serious infections. *Arch. Intern. Med. 142*:2000–2005, 1982.
164. Baldwin, DS, Levine, BB, McCluskey, RT, Gallo, GR: Renal failure and interstitial nephritis due to penicillin and methicillin. *N. Engl. J. Med. 279*:1245, 1968.
165. Gilbert, DN, Gourley, B, D'Agostino, A, Goodnight, SH, Worthen, H: Interstitial nephritis due to methicillin, penicillin, and ampicillin. *Ann. Allergy 28*:378, 1970.
166. Parry, MF, Ball, WD, Conte, JE, Cohen, SN: Nafcillin nephritis. *JAMA 255*:178, 1973 (letter).
167. Sohrier, RW, Bulger, RJ, Van Arsdel, PP: Nephropathy associated with penicillin and homologues. *Ann. Intern. Med. 64*:116, 1966.
168. Ruley, EJ, Lisi, LM: Interstitial nephritis and failure due to ampicillin. *J. Pediatr. 84*:878, 1974.
169. Woodroffe, AJ, Thomson, NM, Meadows, R, Lawrence, JR: Nephropathy associated with methicillin administration. *Aust. N.Z. J. Med. 4*:256, 1974.
170. Sanjad, SA, Haddad, GG, Nassar, VH: Nephropathy, an under-estimated complication of methicillin therapy. *J. Pediatr. 84*:873, 1974.
171. Olson, S, Mogens, A: Interstitial nephritis with acute renal failure following cardiac surgery and treatment with methicillin. *Acta Med. Scand. 199*:305, 1976.
172. Mayand, C, Kanfer, A, Kourilsky, O, Sraer, JD: Interstitial nephritis after methicillin. *N. Engl. J. Med. 292*:1132, 1975 (letter).
173. London, RD: Hematuria associated with methicillin therapy. *J. Pediatr. 70*:286, 1967.
174. Jensen, HA, Halveg, AB, Saunamaki, KJ: Permanent impairment of renal function after methicillin nephropathy. *Br. Med. J. 4*:406, 1971.
175. Gratton, WA: Hematuria and azotemia associated with administration of methicillin. *J. Pediatr. 64*:287, 1964.
176. Feigin, RD, Fiascone, A: Hematuria and proteinuria associated with methicillin administration. *N. Engl. J. Med. 272*:903, 1965.
177. Brauninger, GE, Remington, JS: Nephropathy associated with methicillin therapy. *JAMA 203*:125, 1968.

178. Galpin, JE, Shinaberger, JH, Stanely, TM, et al.: Acute interstitial nephritis due to methicillin. *Am. J. Med. 65*:756, 1978.
179. Ditlove, J, Weidmann, P, Bernstein, M, Massry, SG: Methicillin nephritis. *Medicine (Baltimore) 56*:483, 1977.
180. Border, WA, Lehman, DH, Egan, JD, et al.: Antitubular basement-membrane antibodies in methicillin-associated interstitial nephritis. *N. Engl. J. Med. 29*:381, 1974.
181. Feigin, RD, Van Reken, DE, Pickering, LK: Dosage in methicillin nephropathy. *J. Pediatr. 85*:734, 1974.
182. Nahata, MC, Debolt, S, Powell, DA: Adverse effects of methicillin, nafcillin and oxacillin in pediatric patients. *Dev. Pharmacol. Ther. 4*:117–123, 1982.
183. Cook, FV, Farrar, WE, Kreutner, A: Hemorrhagic cystitis and urethritis, and interstitial nephritis associated with administration of penicillin G. *J. Urol. 122*: 110–111, 1979.
184. Bracis, R, Sanders, CB, Gilbert, DN: Methicillin hemorrhagic cystitis. *Antimicrob. Agents Chemother. 12*:438–439, 1977.
185. Sarff, LD, McCracken, GH: Methicillin-associated nephropathy or cystitis. *J. Pediatr. 90*:1031–1032, 1977.
186. Chudwin, DS, Chesney, PJ, Mischler, EH, et al.: Hematuria associated with carbenicillin and other semisynthetic penicillins. *Am. J. Dis. Child. 138*:98–99, 1979.
187. Marx, CM, Alpert, SE: Ticarcillin-induced cystitis. Cross-reactivity with related penicillins. *Am. J. Dis. Child. 138*:670–672, 1984.
188. Moller, NE, Eriksen, KR, Fedderson, C, et al.: Chemotherapy against *Pseudomonas aeruginosa* in cystic fibrosis. *Eur. J. Respir. Dis. 63*:130–139, 1982.
189. Tattersall, MHN, Battersby, G, Spiers, ASD: Antibiotics and hypokalemia. *Lancet 1*:630–631, 1972.
190. Appel, GB, Neu, HC: Nephrotoxicity of antimicrobial agents. *N. Engl. J. Med. 296*: 663–670, 784–787, 1977.
191. Stollerman, GH, Rusoff, JH: Prophylaxis against group A streptococcal infections in rheumatic fever patients: Use of new repository penicillin preparations. *JAMA 150*:1571–1575, 1952.
192. Bergeson, PS, Singer, SA, Kaplan, AM: Intramuscular injections in children. *Pediatrics 70*:944–948, 1982.
193. Stroller, KP, Losey, R: Inadvertent intra-arterial injection of penicillin: An unseen danger. *Pediatrics 75*:785–786, 1985.
194. Blair, DC, Duggan, DO, Schroeder, ET: Inactivation of amikacin and gentamicin by carbenicillin in patients with end-stage renal failure. *Antimicrob. Agents Chemother. 22*:376–379, 1982.
195. Riff, LJ, Jackson, GG: Laboratory and clinical conditions for gentamicin inactivation by carbenicillin. *Arch. Intern. Med. 130*:887–891, 1972.
196. Pickering, LK, Rutherford, I: Effect of concentration and time upon inactivation of tobramycin, gentamicin, netilmicin and amikacin by azlocillin, carbenicillin, mecillinam, mezlocillin and piperacillin. *J. Pharmacol. Exp. Ther. 217*:345–349, 1981.
197. Pickering, LK, Gearhart, P: Effect of time and concentration upon interaction between gentamicin, tobramycin, netilmicin, or amikacin and carbenicillin or ticarcillin. *Antimicrob. Agents Chemother. 15*:592–596, 1979.
198. Davies, M, Morgan, JR, Anand, C: Interactions of carbenicillin and ticarcillin with gentamicin. *Antimicrob. Agents Chemother. 7*:431–434, 1974.
199. Chow, MSS, Quintiliani, R, Nightingale, CH: In vivo inactivation of tobramycin by ticarcillin. A case report. *JAMA 247*:658–659, 1982.

200. Thompson, MB, Russo, MF, Saxon, BJ, Atkinthor, E, Matsen, JM: Gentamicin inactivation by piperacillin or carbenicillin in patients with end-stage renal disease. *Antimicrob. Agents Chemother. 21*:268–271, 1982.
201. White, GW, Malow, JB, Zimelis, VM, Pahlavanzadeh, H, Panwalker, AP, Jackson, GG: Comparative in vitro activity of azlocillin, ampicillin, mezlocillin, piperacillin, and ticarcillin, alone and in combination with an aminoglycoside. *Antimicrob. Agents Chemother. 15*:540–543, 1979.
202. Perea, EJ, Nogales, MC, Aznar, J, Martin, E, Iglesias, MC: Synergy between cefotaxime, cefsulodin, azlocillin, mezlocillin and aminoglycosides against carbenicillin resistant or sensitive *Pseudomonas aeruginosa. J. Antimicrob. Chemother. 6*:471–477, 1980.
203. Bach, VT, Webb, DW, Thadepalli, H: Antimicrobial synergism of piperacillin and gentamicin against *Pseudomonas aeruginosa, Staphylococcus aureus* and *Streptococcus faecalis. Chemotherapy 26*:21–27, 1980.
204. Comber, KR, Basker, MJ, Osborne, CD, Sutherland, R: Synergy between ticarcillin and tobramycin against *Pseudomonas aeruginosa* and enterobacteriaceae in vitro and in vivo. *Antimicrob. Agents Chemother. 11*:956–964, 1977.
205. Andriole, VT: Antibiotic synergy in experimental infection with *Pseudomonas.* II. The effect of carbenicillin, cephalothin, or cephanone combined with tobramycin or gentamicin. *J. Infect. Dis. 129*:124–133, 1974.
206. Calderwood, SA, Wennersten, C, Moellering, RC, Kunz, LJ, Krogstad, DJ: Resistance to six aminoglycosidic aminocyclitol antibiotics among enterococci: Prevalence, evolution, and relationship to synergism with penicillin. *Antimicrob. Agents Chemother. 12*:401–405, 1977.
207. Gutschik, E, Jepsen, OB, Mortensen, I: Effects of combinations of penicillin and aminoglycosides on *Streptococcus faecalis*: A comparative study of seven aminoglycoside antibiotics. *J. Infect. Dis. 135*:832–836, 1977.
208. Andreoli, SP, Kleiman, MB, Glick, MR, Bergstein, JM: Nafcillin, pseudoproteinuria, and hypokalemic alkalosis. *J. Pediatr. 97*:841–842, 1980.
209. Muir, A, Hensley, WJ: Pseudoproteinuria due to penicillins, in the turbidometric measurement of proteins with trichloracetic acid. *Clin. Chem. 25*:1662, 1979.

11
Sulfonamides

MICHAEL D. REED, JAMES B. BESUNDER, AND JEFFREY L. BLUMER
Rainbow Babies and Childrens Hospital, and Case Western Reserve University School of Medicine, Cleveland, Ohio

The sulfonamides represent a diverse class of chemotherapeutic agents that have maintained a varied and often controversial position in clinical therapeutics. Until recently, either as single agents or combined in multisulfonamide preparations (i.e., "triple-sulfa"), this class of compounds has assumed a secondary therapeutic position behind the plethora of available antibiotics. Rational, fixed-dose combinations that include a sulfonamide, as well as changing patterns of certain infectious diseases, have resulted in a resurgence of interest in and use of these agents.

The discovery of sulfonamide-induced antibacterial activity in 1932 represented a major breakthrough in the treatment of infectious diseases. Prior to this time, various forms of therapy and/or materia medica were used in an attempt to successfully treat diseases of infectious origin. In 1932, Domagk of the I. G. Farbenindustrie in Germany, demonstrated that infected mice were protected by an azo dye containing a sulfonamide moiety (Prontosil) (1-3). The efficacy of Prontosil was first demonstrated in a 10-month-old infant with staphylococcal septicemia in 1933. This child was treated with Prontosil, which, based on previous animal work, was found to be metabolized in vivo to the antibacterially active sulfanilamide (4).

Domagk is primarily responsible for identifying the antibacterial activity of Prontosil, for which he received the 1938 Nobel Prize in Medicine. Over the next four decades, hundreds of sulfanilamide analogs have been developed, many of which have at one time been available for clinical use.

I. CHEMISTRY

The discovery of sulfanilamide and an understanding of sulfonamide-sulfone structure activity relationships have led to the development of five distinct and biologically diverse types of drugs, including the antibacterial sulfonamides and sulfones; antidiabetic agents or pancreatic β-cell stimulators; diuretics of the thiazide or "loop" classes; carbonic anhydrase inhibitors; and certain antithyroid agents. The relationships between structure and biologic activity of all these sulfonamide derivatives have been expertly reviewed by Maren (5). This chapter will specifically address the known structure-activity relationships relative to the antibacterial sulfonamides.

The majority of sulfonamides are insoluble in water, although their sodium salts are readily soluble. In general, the term "sulfonamides" generically denotes derivatives of sulfanilamide. The structure of sulfanilamide denoting the N_1 amide group and N_4 amino nitrogen positions and other selected sulfonamides are shown in Figure 1. Chemical substitution producing sulfonamides of varying solubility, antibacterial activity and pharmacokinetic character primarily involve the N_1 and N_4 positions. Substitution in the benzene ring generally results in inactive compounds. The N_4 amino nitrogen group is essential for the antibacterial activity of sulfonamides. Any substituent at the N_4 position must be either removed or converted in vivo to the free amine or complete loss of antibacterial activity will occur (5). The N_4-acetyl derivatives, including N_4-acetylsulfapyridine, N_4-acetylsulfadiazine, and N_4-acetylsulfamethoxazole, are devoid of any antibacterial activity (3,6,7). However, following administration of these compounds, apparent in vivo deacetylation occurs, producing antibacterially potent compounds. This reaction, as well as hepatic metabolism (see Section IV.D) may follow a recently described though poorly understood acetylation-deacetylation equilibrium (6-9).

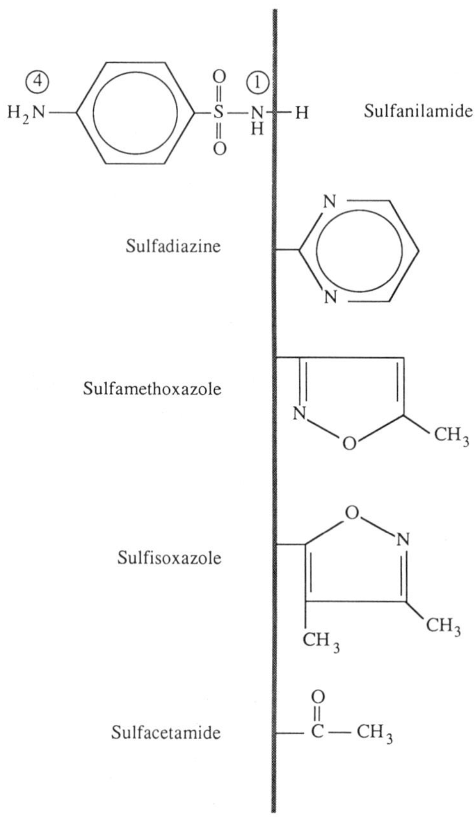

Figure 1 Structural formula for sulfanilamide and other selected sulfonamide derivatives.

As noted in Figure 1, the majority of clinically useful sulfonamides involve substitutions at the N_1 position. These substitutions usually consist of acyclic or heterocyclic derivatives, as well as 5- or 6-membered ring structures. N_1-acetyl derivatives are generally tasteless and are thus frequently used in oral liquid preparations. As mentioned above, following oral administration of N_1-acetyl derivatives, N_1-deacetylation occurs, yielding the parent antibacterially active compound (6).

Much of what is known about the structure-activity relationships of the antibacterial sulfonamides is derived from the initial work of Bell and Roblin, who evaluated the activity of 50 agents (10). Their data strongly suggested that the degree of antibacterial activity of a sulfonamide was directly related to the negative charge of the SO_2 group of an N_1-substituted derivative (i.e., the more negative the charge, the greater the antibacterial activity). This hypothesis most likely oversimplifies the multiple variables involved in the true assessment of sulfonamide structure-activity relationships (5). Despite this, it appears that most sulfonamides retain the SO_2 moiety as a result of this work.

II. MECHANISM OF ACTION

The sulfonamides exert their bacteriostatic action by competitively inhibiting bacterial folic acid synthesis (11,12). Folic acid, or more formally pteroylglutamic acid, is the precursor to tetrahydrofolic acid, a necessary coenzyme responsible for multiple metabolic reactions in vivo, including purine synthesis and pyrimidine nucleotide biosynthesis. The sulfonamides are structural analogs of para-aminobenzoic acid (PABA), thus competitively inhibiting the enzyme responsible for incorporation of PABA into dihydropteroic acid. The cell walls of sulfonamide-susceptible bacteria appear impermeable to folic acid and thus must synthesize it using PABA. In contrast, humans can absorb and utilize preformed folic acid from their diet. Since mammalian cells require preformed folic acid and are incapable of synthesizing it, sulfonamides exert no effect on these cells.

Through the years, the theory outlined here has been confirmed by multiple investigators. However, there appear to be other less well described pathways by which sulfonamides may exert their bacteriostatic action. Brown, in 1962, using a cell-free extract of *Escherichia coli*, demonstrated that sulfonamides can be utilized as alternate substrates by the enzyme systems described above, forming compounds that appear to be structural analogs of pteroic acid (13). The activity of these analogs as false precursors may render them capable of further inducing inhibitory effects upon the synthesis of folic acid. The finding of Brown may represent an alternate pathway by which sulfonamides inhibit the growth of certain bacteria or may simply reflect a minor pathway that augments the action of PABA interference.

III. ANTIMICROBIAL ACTIVITY AND RESISTANCE

The sulfonamides are broad-spectrum antibacterial agents possessing a wide range of antimicrobial activity against both gram-positive and gram-negative bacteria. Based upon the compounds' mechanism of action, these drugs are considered bacteriostatic agents inhibiting the growth of susceptible microorganisms and thus dependent upon the hosts defense mechanisms for ultimate pathogen eradication. The sulfonamides, as the first group of consistently effective systemically available chemotherapeutic agents, enjoyed widespread use following their clinical availability in both children and adults (14–16).

The extensive clinical utility of sulfonamides continued until the introduction and clinical acceptance of the antibiotics, most notably the β-lactams, tetracyclines, and chloramphenicol. During this period and beyond, marked changes in bacterial susceptibility to sulfonamides developed, particularly with respect to *Hemophilus influenzae, Neisseria meningitidis*, and *Neisseria gonorrhoeae* (3,17). A similar pattern of resistance has been observed for *Shigella flexneri* and *Shigella sonnei* (18). As a result of these changing susceptibility patterns and the advent of more potent and effective antibiotics, the sulfonamides, as single agents, have been relegated to a secondary position in infectious disease practice. Table 1 depicts comparative in vitro activity for sulfadiazine and sulfamethoxazole, two of the sulfonamides more commonly used today (19,20). These data are presented as representative of the sulfonamides as a group, although antibacterial activity may vary between different sulfa compounds as well as be epidemiologically dependent upon an individual agent's usage patterns. Acquired bacterial resistance to the sulfonamides appears to be common and is discussed in further detail below. Table 2 depicts in vitro data derived from our own institution during 1985 for sulfisoxazole compared with that for trimethoprim (21), a diaminopyrimidine frequently combined with sulfonamides for additive or synergistic activity (22-24). These data, presented for sulfisoxazole, relate to drug concentrations achievable in urine only, not blood or other body compartments.

The renewed clinical interest in the sulfonamides is primarily a result of the systematic evaluation of alternate or companion antimicrobial agents that, when combined with a sulfonamide, augment either additively or synergistically the overall antibacterial activity of each component. The polymyxins and aminoglycosides were initially shown to confer additive or synergistic activity when combined with a sulfonamide, particularly against gram-negative pathogens including *Pseudomonas aeruginosa, Serratia marcescens*, and *Proteus* spp., including L forms of *Proteus mirabilis* (17,25-28). However, the

Table 1 In Vitro Activity of Two Representative Sulfonamides Against Common Pathogens

	Minimum inhibitory concentration (μg/ml)	
Microorganism	Sulfadiazine	Sulfamethoxazole
Gram-positive		
Staphyococcus aureus	4	4
Streptococcus pneumoniae	16–32	16–32
S. faecalis	⩾128	⩾128
Nocardia asteroides	—	4
Gram-negative		
Escherichia coli	8	8
Klebsiella pneumonia	8–16	8–16
Proteus spp.	8–16	4–16
Neisseria gonorrhea	0.5–4	1–2
N. meningitidis	0.5	0.5
Salmonella typhi	2–4	2–4
Pseudomonas aeruginosa	16–32	16–32

Source: Adapted from References 19–21 and 29.

Table 2 In Vitro Activity (%) of Trimethoprim and Sulfamethoxazole Against Gram-Negative Pathogens

Microorganism, n[a]	% Susceptible: Trimethoprim ≤8 μg/ml	% Susceptible: Sulfisoxazole ≤256 μg/ml
Escherichia coli (1995)	96	80
Proteus mirabilis (384)	99	95
Serratia marcesens (118)	93	74
Morgenella morganii (39)	100	100
Pseudomonas aeruginosa (446)	3	0
Klebsiella spp. (567)	94	86
Enterobacter spp. (253)	97	91

[a]n = number of isolates.
Source: From Reference 21.

introduction of trimethoprim when combined with a sulfonamide represents a major advancement in the development of a rational and effective drug combination. Trimethoprim possesses a spectrum of antibacterial activity similar to that of the sulfonamides, although the drug is more potent. More importantly, the two drugs combined inhibit sequential steps in bacterial folate synthesis; i.e., sulfonamides inhibit the incorporation of PABA into folic acid, whereas trimethoprim prevents the reduction of dihydrofolate to tetrahydrofolate, the active agent responsible for one-carbon transfer reactions. The numerous studies on the development, in vitro activity, and clinical effectiveness of trimethoprim-sulfonamide combinations are reviewed elsewhere and are beyond the scope of this chapter (22-24).

The fixed-dose combination of trimethoprim-sulfamethoxazole was designed to combine two agents of similar pharmacokinetic characteristics in a ratio (1:5) that resulted in optimal in vivo antibiotic activity. Careful investigations have demonstrated that the concentration ratios to achieve a synergistic bactericidal effect vary with the pathogen involved, although overall, a concentration ratio of 1:19 appears optimal (29). Although these concentration relationships have been confirmed in vitro, the importance of this concentration ratio in determining the synergy of trimethoprim and sulfamethoxazole in vivo is not known. Moreover, our evaluation of the pharmacokinetics of trimethoprim-sulfamethoxazole in cystic fibrosis patients revealed serum concentration ratios that ranged from 1:25 to 1:60, with a mean steady-state serum concentration ratio of 1:42 (30). These data suggest the potential for disease alteration in drug concentration ratios that may be reflected in varying degrees of clinical effectiveness. Thus, the optimal drug ratio relationship in either blood or, more importantly, tissues relative to the pathogen involved requires more critical evaluation.

Antimicrobial resistance to sulfonamides, which was appreciated soon after their widespread clinical use, continues to be an important clinical problem. Resistance patterns vary widely and appear to relate directly to the extent of sulfonamide clinical use. Pathogens that developed resistance by the mid-1940s (i.e., group A β-hemolytic streptococci and *N. gonorrhoeae*) appear much more to be sulfonamide sensitive today (17,31, 32). In contrast, many of the Enterobacteriaceae, including *E. coli*, show resistance today, particularly in the hospital environment (20). These data primarily serve as the basis for the current restricted clinical use of sulfonamides, as single agents, for the treatment of uncomplicated lower urinary tract infections. Sulfonamide-resistant bacteria are presumed to occur by random mutation, and the resistance to many gram-negative bacteria appears to be mediated by R plasmids (3).

The exact mechanism of resistance by bacteria to sulfonamides remains unclear, although it appears to primarily involve alterations in the enzymatic processes or capacity of the bacterial cell. Woods in 1940 first suggested that certain sulfonamide-resistant bacteria were capable of synthesizing sufficient quantities of PABA to antagonize the anti-PABA effect of the drug (11). Further work by his group demonstrated the increased production of folic acid by *Staphylococcus aureus* in sulfonamide-resistant strains (33). However, it would appear from these data that other cellular enzymatic reactions are most likely involved in the development of resistance, including a mechanism to inactivate the drug and/or the development of alternative pathways for the synthesis of folic acid.

IV. CLINICAL PHARMACOLOGY

Despite their initially extensive, then varied use over the past 41/2 decades, only limited data exist describing the overall biodisposition profiles of sulfonamides in pediatric patients (9,14,17,34-38). In contrast, the pharmacokinetic properties of sulfonamides in adults have been well described in healthy volunteers and in patients with a variety of clinical disorders (6,7,17,39-41). Difficulties in the assessment of sulfonamide pharmacokinetic characteristics combined with their decreased clinical utility in pediatric patients partially explain these deficiencies in our understanding of the pharmacology of these compounds. Compounding these deficiencies are the genetic differences in hepatic metabolism ("fast" or "slow" acetylation) and renal excretion, which may be pH dependent, as well as affected by varying concentrations of parent compound and metabolite. Although frequently overlooked in pharmacological evaluations of sulfonamides, these characteristics may have a substantial impact upon a compound's pharmacokinetic profile.

A. Absorption

A plethora of sulfanilamide analogs have been and are currently available for clinical use. These agents are frequently categorized by their role in clinical medicine, i.e., poorly absorbed analogs used primarily for their ability to reduce bacterial populations within the bowel lumen; sulfonamides for topical application; and well-absorbed agents for the treatment of systemic infections.

The poorly absorbed sulfonamides, including succinylsulfathiazole and phthalysulfathiazole, are analogs conjugated at the N_4 position. Both these agents are microbiologically inactive until hydrolyzed by intestinal bacteria to the active moiety sulfathiazole. Despite the poor systemic absorption of either the parent compound or sulfathiazole, sufficient quantities (approximately $<5\%$) may be absorbed to produce untoward systemic effects. In the past, these agents were used frequently for the treatment of acute or chronic dysentery and as prophylactic agents prior to bowel surgery. The use of these agents has declined sharply with the advent of more effective treatment regimens for dysentery and the lack of evidence supporting their efficacy as surgical prophylactic agents. One poorly absorbed agent, sulfasalazine, continues to be used commonly in clinical practice, although not as a primary anti-infective agent. Sulfasalazine is broken down within the gut to sulfapyridine (which is systemically absorbed) and 5-aminosalicylate (42). The drug is primarily used as an adjuvant in the treatment of patients with ulcerative colitis and regional enteritis in which it is believed that the liberated aminosalicylate is the effective moiety (43).

The more commonly used topical sulfonamides today include silver sulfadiazine, mafenide, and the ophthalmic preparation, sulfacetamide. Silver sulfadiazine and mafenide are primarily used topically to reduce microbial colonization and as prophylaxis against infections from wounds and/or burns. Depending upon the amount of these agents applied relative to the wound or burn surface area, both sulfonamides can be absorbed systemically (44,45). Peak plasma concentrations have been observed within 2–4 hr following the application of mafenide (44). Due to the high solubility of sulfacetamide (~90 times that of sulfadiazine) and its nonirritating characteristics, this agent has been used extensively as an ophthalmic antibacterial agent. As a result of the high concentrations of sulfacetamide achieved locally upon ophthalmic instillation, the drug is most likely bactericidal against susceptible pathogens.

Sulfonamides used for the treatment of systemic infections are well absorbed by either the oral or subcutaneous route. Although early pharmacological studies performed in children provide insufficient data to critically assess absorption characteristics (14,34–37), these data suggest adequate and reproducible absorption from either route. Serum sulfonamide concentrations following oral administration in either children or adults range from 65 to 100% of those achieved following subcutaneous or intravenous administration (3,6,14,17,34–38,46–48). Peak serum concentrations are generally observed between 1 and 4 hr following oral administration (3,17,34,49,50). These ranges most likely reflect expected differences in absorption characteristics observed between oral drugs administered as a suspension in contrast to a tablet formulation, as well as physical characteristics of the specific sulfonamide (6,34,50). The oral administration of these agents as the sodium salt rather than the base generally increases their extent of absorption (51). In addition, the concomitant administration of sodium bicarbonate may increase the rate but not the total amount absorbed for certain sulfonamides (51). The presence of food in the stomach has a variable effect on sulfonamide absorption that may be related to the chemical nature of the compound. Sulfadiazine as the free base is absorbed more slowly but more completely when administered after a meal as compared with the fasting state, whereas absorption is delayed and reduced when administered as the sodium salt (51). However, these differences are minimal and do not appear to be clinically significant.

B. Protein Binding

All sulfonamides are bound, to some degree, to circulating plasma proteins. Plasma albumin is the predominate binding protein. Depending upon an individual compound's lipophilicity and pK_a, protein binding can vary between 20% (sulfadiazine) and 90+% (sulfamethazine) (Table 3). Increasing lipophilicity and/or decreasing pK_a at physiologic pH favor albumin binding (3). In general, the commonly referred to "long-acting" sulfonamides (see below) are highly (90+%) protein bound. In addition, the N_4-acetyl sulfonamide metabolites appear to be bound to a greater extent than the parent compound (3,6).

Table 3 Pharmacokinetic Parameters of Selected Sulfonamides in Adults

	$t_{1/2}$ (hr)	V_d (liter/kg)	% Protein bound
Sulfadiazine	10–15	0.36	50
N_4-acetyl	12–20	0.13	57
Sulfamethazine	2–6	0.61	90
N_4-acetyl	3–8	0.29	95
Sulfamethizole	1.5–2.5	0.35	85
N_4-acetyl	4–6	0.10	98
Sulfamethoxazole	10–12	0.17	65
N_4-acetyl	2.5–4	0.17	75
Sulfisoxazole	5–7	0.16	84–90
N_4-acetyl	16–23	0.16	84–90

Source: Adapted from Reference 6.

Early pharmacological evaluations of sulfonamides suggested concentration-dependent plasma protein binding: the lower the serum drug concentration, the greater degree of albumin binding (6,52). In patients with acute renal failure, sulfonamide protein binding may be decreased (53). This decrease in binding does not appear to result from changes in the plasma albumin concentration. In addition, certain drugs, most notably acids, have been shown to displace highly protein bound sulfonamides from their binding sites (54). Bases, on the other hand, appear to have a limited or no effect on the protein binding of sulfonamide derivatives.

C. Distribution

The sulfonamides are well distributed in body fluids and tissues. Effective antibacterial drug concentrations have been consistently documented in most body fluids, including ocular, synovial, pleural, ascitic, peritoneal, and cerebrospinal fluid (3,4,14,17,34,55-57). The volume of distribution V_d for sulfonamides varies widely, dependent upon the degree of ionization at physiologic pH and extent of metabolism and protein binding. In the adult, sulfonamide V_d values range from 0.16 to 0.61 liter/kg (Table 3). In contrast, far less specific sulfonamide V_d data are available in children. Early pharmacological evaluations of sulfonamides in children performed during the 1930s and 1940s were limited and primarily involved simple quantitation of drug concentrations in blood (14,15,34-37,46,48). Assessment of these early data would suggest similar sulfonamide V_d values in children as those observed in adults with the exception of the first year of life. During this developmental period, larger sulfonamide V_d values would be expected relative to the normal developmental changes observed in the amount and distribution of body water (58,59). This belief is supported by the more recent and vigorous pharmacological evaluations performed in children receiving either sulfamethoxazole or sulfametrole when combined with trimethoprim, as well as a few select others (38,60). Although the pharmacokinetic evaluation of one drug may be affected by the concurrent administration of a second drug, the concurrent administration of trimethoprim or erythromycin in therapeutic doses does not appear to affect the biodisposition of the sulfonamide (21,61).

D. Metabolism and Excretion

All sulfonamides are metabolized, to a varying extent, primarily in the liver. The major pathway of sulfonamide biodegradation is acetylation. Sulfonamides undergo hepatic acetylation at the N_4 atom by the enzyme *N*-acetyltransferase and possibly to a lesser extent by acetylating isoenzymes (3,41). The resulting N_4-acetylated sulfonamide metabolite possesses no antibacterial activity although it appears to retain the toxic potential of the parent compound (3,6,41). The extent to which a sulfonamide is acetylated may be related to the substituent at the N_1 atom (9). How the N_1 substituent influences acetylation at the N_4 atom remains ill defined. In addition, the rate and extent of sulfonamide acetylation may be genetically controlled in a manner similar to that observed with other drugs that undergo hepatic acetylation (41,62-65). However, in contrast to these latter agents, it has recently been demonstrated that the hepatic acetylation of sulfonamides is either a part of or a result of an acetylation-deacetylation equilibrium (9).

As has been documented for other drugs, including isoniazid and procainamide (62-65), the metabolism of sulfonamides appears to be genetically controlled (41). For some but not all sulfonamide derivatives, patients may be subdivided phenotypically into two groups—fast or slow acetylators. An individual's acetylator phenotype may be described by determining the time-dependent excretion of N_4-acetylated metabolite in urine or by evaluation of a biomodal distribution in the serum concentration-time curve for a study population. Unlike the consistent separation between fast and slow acetylators demonstrated for such drugs as isoniazid, procainamide, and hydralazine (62-65), this distinction is less clear with the sulfonamides (41).

Differences between fast and slow acetylators have been clearly described for three pyridine sulfonamide analogs, whereas no such distinction can be demonstrated for such agents as sulfamethoxazole (41). Despite early attempts to use sulfadimidine as a single agent to reflect a patient's acetylator phenotype for a series of sulfonamide compounds (66), it is clear that one agent cannot be used to demonstrate acetylation differences for all sulfonamides. These difficulties in attempts to characterize the acetylator phenotype for sulfonamides are most likely a result of an acetylation-deacetylation equilibrium that exists for the hepatic metabolism of sulfonamides (9). It would appear that the overall amount of N_4-acetylated sulfonamide produced in vivo is dependent upon the position of this metabolic equilibrium. For such drugs as sulfamethizole and sulfaethiodole, little to no N_4-acetylation can be demonstrated owing to their high rate of deacetylation, whereas substantial amounts of N_4-acetylated sulfamethizole and sulfametrole can be detected in biologic fluids because of their low rates of deacetylation (9). The exact nature of sulfonamide acetylation and/or the activity of an acetylation-deacetylation equilibrium in children remains ill defined. The majority of these data have been derived from studies performed in animals and adult subjects (6-9,41). Although these pathways partially explain the differences in the rate and extent of sulfonamide acetylation, their clinical significance is unclear.

Both parent compound and N_4-acetylated sulfonamide metabolites are primarily eliminated by the body via the kidneys ($\geqslant$90%) (3,6,7,9,17,40). Depending upon the chemical structure of the sulfonamide, these agents are excreted by tubular excretion (e.g., sulfathiazole and sulfamethizole); glomerular filtration with tubular reabsorption (e.g., sulfametrole and sulfamethoxazole); or combined tubular excretion and reabsorption (e.g., sulfaethidole and sulfisomidine). The N_4-acetylated sulfonamides are primarily excreted by tubular secretion (40,67). These data underscore the importance of renal maturation and function on the dosing of sulfonamides in children. Although only limited specific data are available on the dosing of sulfonamides in young children (9), it would appear prudent to account for normal renal maturational processes in the design of optimal dosing regimens (68-71). The influence of renal and hepatic maturation on the $t_{1/2}$ of selected sulfonamides is shown in Table 4.

Owing to the dependence upon renal elimination of parent and N_4-acetylated sulfonamide, urinary pH and flow rate may affect the rate and extent of body elimination for some sulfonamides. The influence of urinary pH and flow rate is primarily of research interest and has been extensively reviewed in adults by Hekster and Vree (6). To our knowledge, the effects of these variables upon the renal elimination of sulfonamides by children has not been evaluated, and its clinical significance relative to the currently available sulfonamides appears limited. In contrast, the solubility of both parent and metabolite in urine under pathophysiologic conditions is extremely important relative to the occurrence of sulfonamide-induced crystalluria and direct renal damage. When the concentrations of a sulfonamide and its metabolite exceed their individual pH and volume-dependent solubility in urine, sulfonamide crystals (precipitation) occur (3,6,17,72-74). Crystalluria and acute alterations in renal function were a common toxicity associated with the initial clinical use of sulfonamides (17,72-74). This preventable drug toxicity served as the basis of coadministering different sulfonamides (i.e., triple-sulfas) as each agent retained individual solubility and reduced the potential for renal complications (75). As mentioned, this adverse effect of sulfonamides is rarely observed today owing to the highly soluble nature of the currently used agents in urine of varying pH (6). However, this complication may preclude the use of sulfonamides in children who require large doses and/or chronic therapy in the presence of immature or compromised renal function.

As a result of the plethora of sulfonamide derivatives that became available clinically after the discovery of sulfanilamide, it became difficult to differentiate the pharmacological differences between these agents, necessitating a classification system. The system that was developed and is used today is based on an individual sulfonamide elimination $t_{1/2}$. This classification is shown in Table 5. It should be noted that the designation of a compound to a specific category is based upon the observed $t_{1/2}$ in adults. The actual

Table 4 Influence of Age on the Elimination Half-life ($t_{1/2}$) of Selected Sulfonamides

	Subject age				
Sulfonamide	1–7 days	1–4 weeks	1–12 months	2–7 years	Adults
Sulfadiazine	20–10	–	10	–	10–15
Sulfamethoxypyridazine	200–100	70	50	50	50
Sulfimoxole	20	12	11	–	–
Sulfisomidine	18	10	8	8	8
Sulfisoxazole	18	10	8	8	8

Source: Adapted from Reference 9.

Table 5 Classification of Sulfonamides Based Upon Elimination Half-life

Half-life $t_{1/2}$ (hr)	Common classification
≤ 4	Ultrashort acting
4–8	Short acting
8–16	Medium acting
16–60	Long acting
≥ 60	Ultralong acting

Source: Adapted from Reference 6.

apparent $t_{1/2}$ parameter estimates for selected sulfonamide derivatives in both adults and children are shown in Tables 3 and 4.

V. DETERMINATION OF SULFONAMIDES IN BIOLOGIC FLUIDS

Multiple analytic methods are available for the determination of sulfonamides and their metabolites in biologic fluids. The majority of the pharmacological data described in the literature is derived from sample quantitation using the spectrophotometric method originally described by Bratton and Marshall (76) and subsequently modified by Rieder (77). These methods allow the determination of what has been commonly referred to in the literature as free sulfonamide and total sulfonamide concentrations. Despite the previous designation of these free sulfonamide concentrations as a reflection of bacteriostatically active drug, it should be noted that these quantitations actually represent determinations of both protein-bound and unbound parent compound. The total sulfonamide concentration determined by the method of Bratton and Marshall represents the added quantitation of the sulfonamide metabolite(s). Thus, the term "free sulfonamide" in this context refers to the fraction of unmetabolized parent compound only. More recently, numerous analytic methods employing high-pressure liquid chromatography have become available (6,7,67,78). These methods accommodate small sample volumes while affording accurate and specific quantitations of parent compound and metabolite(s) in biologic fluids.

VI. THERAPEUTIC INDICATIONS

As mentioned previously, the number of therapeutic indications for sulfonamides, although many when first available, have been reduced dramatically with the development and availability of safer and more effective antimicrobial drugs. When administered systemically, the role of sulfonamide therapy today primarily involves the treatment of uncomplicated urinary tract infections or as prophylactic agents in the chronic therapy of recurrent otitis media and urinary tract infections. Other selected infectious diseases in which sulfonamides maintain a role in clinical practice include infections involving *Nocardia* species (3,79,80), and as a prophylactic agent for exposed individuals during meningococcal outbreaks when the organisms are shown to be sensitive to sulfonamides (3,17,81). However, investigators and clinicians would not consider a sulfonamide, as a single agent, the drug of first choice for the treatment of any systemic bacterial infection occurring during childhood. In contrast, ophthalmic and vaginal cream and suppository sulfonamide preparations remain a mainstay in the treatment of bacterial infections involving the eye and vagina, respectively. Topical sulfonamide creams are effective and continue to enjoy widespread use in the management of burns (44,45,82) and for umbilical cord care (83).

The renewed interest over the past two decades in the clinical use of sulfonamide preparations stems from the ability of these drugs to consistently demonstrate antibacterial synergy when combined with certain other antimicrobial agents (20). As mentioned previously in the section addressing antimicrobial activity and resistance, many antimicrobial agents, including the polymyxins, aminoglycosides, and penicillins (17,25-28), have demonstrated additive and/or synergistic activity when combined with a sulfonamide. However, the need for such combinations in clinical practice is rarely encountered today (17). More recent clinical studies with the combination of erythromycin and sulfisoxazole have demonstrated advantages over either component alone when used in the treatment of certain pediatric infections (84,85). At present, this combination is primarily used for the treatment of otitis media. In contrast, the systematic development and evaluation of sulfonamides combined with trimethoprim with a sulfonamide of similar pharmacokinetic and pharmacodynamic characteristics (23,86-88) has dramatically increased the clinical utility of sulfonamide compounds (86,88). The most frequently used combination consists of trimethoprim in a 1:5 ratio with sulfamethoxazole. This drug combination has been demonstrated to be clinically effective in the treatment of multiple childhood infections involving the skin and skin structure, upper and lower respiratory tract, and urinary tract (22,23,88-91). The combination of trimethoprim and sulfamethoxazole is at present considered the drug of first choice for the treatment of infections caused by *Pneumocystis carinii* (24). In addition, this combination may be an alternative to more established antimicrobial regimens for the treatment of gram-negative meningitis (24,92,93).

VII. UNTOWARD REACTIONS ASSOCIATED WITH SYSTEMICALLY ADMINISTERED SULFONAMIDES

Multiple adverse reactions have been associated with the clinical use of sulfonamide compounds. The overall incidence and incidence of serious untoward reactions vary depending upon the individual sulfonamide in question. In addition, adverse drug reactions appeared to occur more commonly with the earlier sulfanilamide analogs (17). Early assessment of the occurrence of adverse reactions to sulfonamides suggested overall incidence rates of 18.6, 11.9, and 6.5% in patients treated with sulfanilamide, sulfathiazole, and sulfadiazine, respectively (94). Lehr suggested that the risk of untoward effects developing in patients treated with sulfadiazine, sulfamerazine, and sulfisoxazole approximated 6, 9.5, and 8%, respectively (73). Overall, the incidence of serious drug-induced complications, including blood dyscrasias and liver or renal damage, is rare (3,20,95). Although it has been suggested that the incidence of adverse reactions may be more common with the "longer acting" sulfonamide derivatives (96-99), it is not clear if this is related to an inherent propensity to induce toxic effects by these derivatives or to their prior frequent clinical use.

The most common type of adverse drug reaction associated with sulfonamide use in children is hypersensitivity reactions. Allergic maculopapular or urticarial skin rashes, generally occurring during the second week of therapy, have been reported (20,100). Sulfonamide administration has also been associated with more serious types of hypersensitivity reactions, including erythema nodosum, erythema multiforme (Stevens-Johnson syndrome), and exfoliative dermatitis (17). The association of sulfonamide therapy and Stevens-Johnson syndrome is well described and has been suggested to occur more commonly in children compared with adults (20,97). Although the exact association of any drug as a cause of Stevens-Johnson syndrome is unclear, Stevens-Johnson syndrome associated with sulfonamides represents a serious, potentially life-threatening reaction (97,101).

The ability of therapeutic agents to displace bilirubin from albumin binding sites remains an important aspect of drug therapy in newborn infants (102,103). Although elevations in the unbound (or free) fraction of bilirubin only partially explain the propensity of sick neonates to the development of kernicterus, it is clear that these increased bilirubin concentrations are a major predisposing factor (104,105). The sulfonamides, as a class of antimicrobial agents, have been incriminated as potent competitors for bilirubin binding sites on albumin. Thus, their safety in the premature and newborn patient remains questionable. In 1956, Silverman and colleagues reported an increased mortality rate in premature infants treated with a penicillin-sulfisoxazole combination compared with oxytetracycline (106). The significant increase in mortality was associated with a significantly higher incidence of kernicterus in the infants who received the penicillin-sulfisoxazole combination. Since this communication and others (103,107-109), sulfonamide use in premature and newborn infants, as well as in mothers at term or nursing mothers, has been discouraged (103).

The exact mechanism(s) and under what physiologic conditions drugs displace bilirubin from its binding sites remain ill defined (102-105). The ability of a drug to displace bilirubin from albumin binding sites cannot be predicted based upon the chemical structure or the extent of protein binding; i.e., oxacillin displaces bilirubin, whereas methicillin and penicillin G do not; cefperazone and ceftriaxone, two β-lactam compounds extensively bound to serum albumin (>90%), do not appreciably displace bilirubin from its binding sites (103,110). Similarly, the sulfonamides display a highly variable ability to displace bilirubin and this is dependent upon the individual compound in question (103, 109,111). Such drugs as sulfisoxazole and sulfamethizole clearly compete with bilirubin for albumin binding, resulting in dramatic increases of unbound, free bilirubin concentrations (103,106,108,111), whereas sulfadiazine and sulfanilamide appear to displace little to no bilirubin, suggesting their potential clinical utility in the newborn infant (109,111). Overall, only limited data relative to bilirubin displacement exist for a small number of available sulfonamide compounds. Moreover, insufficient published information is available to clearly establish the safety or toxicity of sulfamethoxazole or sulfamethoxazole when combined with trimethoprim in the newborn patient (92). Thus, the ability of a sulfonamide or sulfonamide combination to displace bilirubin should be clearly described prior to their clinical use in premature and newborn infants.

With few exceptions, the types and overall incidence of untoward reactions to combinations of sulfonamide and trimethoprim appear similar to those observed with sulfonamides alone (22,24,112,113). The ability of trimethoprim to inhibit mammalian folate synthesis, as well as predispose patients to hematologic abnormalities, remains a controversial and unresolved issue. Hulme and Reeves (114) first suggested an association between leukopenia and trimethoprim-sulfamethoxazole administration in renal transplant patients. This observation could not be confirmed by Hall (115). A latter study by Bradley and colleagues (116) suggested a more frequent occurrence of neutropenia and thrombocytopenia in renal allograph recipients treated with trimethoprim-sulfamethoxazole and azathioprine compared with patients who received azathioprine alone. In two recent studies involving children, 72% of 17 children receiving intravenous trimethoprim-sulfamethoxazole (89) and 48% of 50 children receiving the oral combination (117) developed hematologic abnormalities (neutropenia $\leqslant$ 1500 mm^{-3} and/or thrombocytopenia $< 150{,}000$ mm^{-3}). In these studies, the hematologic abnormalities were transient and reversible. In contrast, severely malnourished children and children with cancer have benefited from trimethoprim-sulfamethoxazole without adverse hematologic effect. Overall, most investigators have found this combination to be well tolerated in children and rarely associated with serious untoward reactions (24).

VIII. DRUG INTERACTIONS

Numerous drug interactions have been associated with the administration of sulfonamide drugs. The more important of these drug-drug interactions have involved drugs infrequently used in pediatric practice, including the oral dicumarol anticoagulants (118,119) and sulfonylurea hypoglycemic agents (120,121). Other less well described interactions involving medications more commonly used in children have included phenytoin (20) and methotrexate (122). Data derived primarily from case reports have suggested that certain sulfonamides may potentiate the pharmacological effects of these compounds. The exact mechanism or mechanisms for these drug interactions remain unclear. Most investigators have suggested that these interactions are a result of competition or interference with hepatic metabolism (123) and/or displacement from albumin binding sites (124). Despite these reports, the clinical significance of these interactions is unknown but do not appear to represent a true contraindication.

IX. SUMMARY

Since their discovery and introduction into clinical medicine over 50 years ago, the sulfonamides have maintained a varied position in clinical therapeutics. Changing patterns in antibacterial activity and the introduction of safer, easier to use, and possibly more effective antibiotics have, over the years, dramatically decreased their clinical utility. This decrease in clinical use, however, has been accompanied by a return of effective in vitro antibacterial activity against many strains of formally resistant bacteria. These changes in activity in vitro and the development of rational drug combinations that include a sulfonamide (e.g., trimethoprim-sulfamethoxazole) have fostered new clinical interest in this class of compounds. Despite these developments, the sulfonamides continue to maintain a secondary therapeutic position in pediatric infectious disease practice.

REFERENCES

1. Domagk, G: Einbeitrag zur chemotherapie der bakteriellen infektionen. *Dtsch. Med. Wochenschr. 61*:250–253, 1935.
2. Domagk, G: Eine neue klasse von desinfectionsmitteln. *Dtsch. Med. Wocherschr. 61*: 829–832, 1935.
3. Mandell, GL, Sande, MA: Antimicrobial agents. In: *The Pharmacologic Basis of Therapeutics* (AG Gilman, LS Goodman, TW Rall, and F Murad, eds.), Macmillan, New York, 1985, pp. 1095–1114.
4. Fuller, AT: Is *p*-aminobenzenesulphonamide the active agent in prontosil therapy? *Lancet 1*:194–198, 1937.

5. Maren, TH: Relations between structure and biological activity of sulfonamides. *Am. Rev. Pharmacol. Toxicol. 16*:309–327, 1976.
6. Hekster, YA, Vree, TB: Clinical pharmacokinetics of sulphonamides and their N_4-acetyl derivatives. *Antibiot. Chemother. 31*:22–118, 1982.
7. Vree, TB, Hekster, YA, Damsma, JE, Van der Kleijn, E, O'Reilly, WJ: Pharmacokinetics of N_1-acetyl- and N_4-acetyl-sulphamethoxazole in man. *Clin. Pharmacokinet. 4*:310–319, 1979.
8. Vree, TB, Hekster, YA, Van der Kleijn, E: Significance of apparent half-lives of a metabolite with higher elimination rate than its parent drug. *Drug. Intell. Clin. Pharm. 16*:124–131, 1982.
9. Vree, TB, Hekster, YA, Lippens, RJJ: Clinical pharmacokinetics of sulfonamides in children: Relationship between maturing kidney function and renal clearance of sulfonamides. *Ther. Drug Monit. 7*:130–147, 1985.
10. Bell, PH, Roblin, RO, Jr.: Studies in chemotherapy. VII. A theory of the relation of structure to activity of sulfonilamide type compounds. *J. Am. Chem. Soc. 64*: 2905–2917, 1942.
11. Woods, DD: Relation of *p*-aminobenzoic acid to mechanism of action of sulphanilamide. *Br. J. Exp. Pathol. 21*:74–90, 1940.
12. Woods, DD: The biochemical mode of action of the sulphonamide drugs. *J. Gen. Microbiol. 29*:687–702, 1962.
13. Brown, GM: The biosynthesis of folic acid. II. Inhibition by sulfonamides. *J. Biol. Chem. 237*:536–540, 1962.
14. Winters, KJ, Janney, FR: Sulfadiazine: Review of its use in treatment of children. *Am. J. Dis. Child. 65*:702–711, 1943.
15. Lehr, D, Slobody, L, Greenberg, W: The use of a sulfadiazine-sulfathiazole mixture in the treatment of children. *J. Pediatr. 29*:275–285, 1946.
16. Colebrook, L, Kenny, M: Treatment of human puerperal infections and of experimental infections in mice with Prontosil. *Lancet 1*:1279–1286, 1936.
17. Weinstein, L, Madoff, MA, Samet, CM: The sulfonamides. *N. Engl. J. Med. 263*:793–800, 842–849, 900–907, 952–957, 1960.
18. Haltalin, KC, Nelson, JD: In vitro susceptibility of shigellae to sodium sulfadiazine and eight antibiotics. *JAMA 193*:705–710, 1965.
19. Bushby, SRM, Hitchings, GH: Trimethoprim, a sulphonamide potentiator. *Br. J. Pharmacol. Chemother. 33*:72–90, 1968.
20. Kucers, A, McK Bennett, N: *The Use of Antibiotics*, 3rd ed., W. M. Heinemann Medical Books, London, 1979, pp. 657–729.
21. Jacobs, MR: Department of Pathology, University Hospitals of Cleveland, unpublished observation, 1986.
22. Symposium: Trimethoprim-sulfamethoxazole. *J. Infect. Dis. 128 (Suppl.)*:S433–S816, 1973.
23. Wormser, GP, Keusch, GT, Heel, RC: Co-trimoxazole (trimethoprim-sulfamethoxazole): An updated review of its antibacterial activity and clinical efficacy. *Drugs 24*: 459–518, 1982.
24. Hughes, WT: Trimethoprim-sulfamethoxazole. *Pediatr. Clin. North Am. 30*:27–30, 1983.
25. Simmons, NA: Potentiation of inhibitory activity of colistin on *Pseudomonas aeruginosa* by sulphamethoxazole and sulphamethizole. *Br. Med. J. 3*:693–696, 1969.
26. Holmgren, J, Moller, O: Studies on the sensitivity of *Proteus mirabilis* and *Proteus vulgaris* to sulphonamide and colistin alone and in combination. *Scand. J. Infect. Dis. 2*:121–124, 1970.
27. Greenfield, S, Feingold, DS: The synergistic action of the sulfonamides and the polymyxins against *Serratia marcescens. J. Infect. Dis. 121*:555–558, 1970.

28. Montgomerie, JZ, Kalmanson, GM, Guze, LB: Synergism of polymyxin and sulfonamides in L-forms of *Staphylococcus aureus* and *Proteus mirabilis*. *Antimicrob. Agents Chemother.* *3*:523–525, 1973.
29. Bushby, SRM: Trimethoprim-sulfamethoxazole: In vitro microbiological aspects. *J. Infect. Dis. 128 (Suppl.)*:S442–S462, 1973.
30. Reed, MD, Stern, RC, Bertino, JS, Jr., Myers, CM, Yamashita, TS, Blumer, JL: Dosing implications of rapid elimination of trimethoprim-sulfamethoxazole in patients with cystic fibrosis. *J. Pediatr.* *104*:303–307, 1984.
31. Yourassowsky, E, Vanderlinden, MP, Shoutens, E: Sensitivity of *Streptococcus pyogenes* to sulphamethoxazole, trimethoprim and cotrimoxazole. *J. Clin. Pathol.* *27*:897–901, 1974.
32. Finland, M, Garner, C, Wilcox, C, Sabath, LD: Susceptibility of beta-hemolytic streptococci to 65 antibacterial agents. *Antimicrob. Agents Chemother.* *9*:11–19, 1976.
33. White, PJ, Woods, DD: The synthesis of *p*-aminobenzoic acid and folic acid by staphylococci sensitive and resistant to sulphonamides. *J. Gen. Microbiol.* *40*:243–253, 1965.
34. Forbes, GB, Perley, A, Dehlinger, J: The use of sulfamerazine in infants and children. *J. Pediatr.* *28*:24–36, 1946.
35. Clarke, GH: Sulfonamide drugs: A comparison of blood levels obtained with their administration by different routes in children. *Am. J. Dis. Child.* *73*:565–572, 1947.
36. Richmond, JB, Kravitz, H, Segar, WE: Sulfonamide dosage in early infancy. *J. Pediatr.* *36*:539–549, 1950.
37. Fichter, EG, Curtis, JA: Sulfonamide administration in newborn and premature infants. *Pediatrics.* *18*:50–57, 1956.
38. Sereni, F, Perletti, L, Marubini, E, Mars, G: Pharmacokinetic studies with a long-acting sulfonamide in subjects of different ages: A modern approach to drug dosage problems in developmental pharmacology. *Pediatr. Res.* *2*:29–37, 1968.
39. Bohni, E, Fust, B, Rieder, J, Schaerer, K, Havas, L: Comparative toxicological, chemotherapeutic and pharmacokinetic studies with sulphormethoxine and other sulphonamides in animals and man. *Chemotherapy* *14*:195–226, 1969.
40. Vree, TB, Hekster, YA, Baars, AM, Damsma, JE, Van der Kleijn, E: Pharmacokinetics of sulphamethoxazole in man. Effects of urinary pH and urine flow on metabolism and renal excretion of sulphamethoxazole and its metabolite N_4-acetylsulphamethoxazole. *Clin. Pharmacokinet.* *3*:319–329, 1978.
41. Vree, TB, O'Reilly, WJ, Hekster, YA, Damsma, JE, Van der Kleijn, E: Determination of the acetylator phenotype and pharmacokinetics of some sulphonamides in man. *Clin. Pharmacokinet.* *5*:274–294, 1980.
42. Peppercorn, MA, Goldman, P: Distribution studies of salicylazosulfapyridine and its metabolites. *Gastroenterology* *64*:240–245, 1973.
43. Klotz, U, Maier, K, Fischer, C, Heinkel, K: Therapeutic efficacy of sulfasalazine and its metabolites in patients with ulcerative colitis and Crohn's disease. *N. Engl. J. Med.* *303*:1499–1502, 1980.
44. Harrison, HN, Bales, HW, Jacoby, FJ: The absorption into burned skin of Sulfamylon acetate from 5 percent aqueous solution. *J. Trauma* *12*:994–998, 1972.
45. Ballin, JC: Evaluation of a new topical agent for burn therapy. Silver sulfadiazine (Silvadene). *JAMA* *230*:1184–1185, 1974.
46. Jorgensen, GM, McL Greeley, D: Subcutaneous administration of sodium sulfadiazine. *J. Pediatr.* *21*:325, 1942.
47. Glaser, K: One dose subcutaneous sodium sulfadiazine for acute infections. *J. Pediatr.* *28*:187–190, 1946.
48. Slobody, LB, Lehr, D, Willner, MW: Subcutaneous administration of a sulfadiazine-sulfamerazine combination in children. *Pediatrics* *2*:58–67, 1948.

49. Lewin, EB, Klein, JO, Finland, M: Trimethoprim-sulfamethoxazole: Absorption, excretion and toxicity in six children. *J. Infect. Dis. 128 (Suppl.)*:S618–S621, 1973.
50. Marks, MI, Kazemi, M, Hales, B, Neims, AH: Pharmacokinetic studies of trimethoprim-sulfamethoxazole in children with gastroenteritis. *J. Infect. Dis. 128 (Suppl.)*: S622–S625, 1973.
51. Peterson, OL, Finland, M: The effect of food and alkali on the absorption and excretion of sulfonamide drugs after oral and duodenal administration. *Am. J. Med. Sci. 204*:581–588, 1942.
52. Hawking, F: Recent work on the pharmacology of sulphonamides. *Br. Med. J. 1*: 505–509, 1945.
53. Andreason, F: Protein binding in plasma from patients with acute renal failure. *Acta Pharmacol. Toxicol. (Copenh.) 32*:417–429, 1973.
54. Anton, AH: Increasing activity of sulfonamides with displacing agents: A review. *Ann. N.Y. Acad. Sci. 226*:273–292, 1973.
55. Sabel, KG, Brandberg, A: Treatment of meningitis and septicemia in infancy with a sulphamethoxazole/trimethoprim combination. *Acta Paediatr. Scand. 64*:25–32, 1975.
56. Bruun, JN, Ostby, N, Bredesen, JE, Kierulf, P, Lunde, PNM: Sulfonamide and trimethoprim concentrations in human serum and skin blister fluid. *Antimicrob. Agents Chemother. 19*:82–85, 1981.
57. Dudley, MN, Levitz, RE, Quintiliani, R, Hickingbotham, JM, Nightingale, CH: Pharmacokinetics of trimethoprim and sulfamethoxazole in serum and cerebrospinal fluid of adult patients with normal meninges. *Antimicrob. Agents Chemother. 26*: 811–814, 1984.
58. Friis-Hansen, B: Body composition during growth: In vivo measurements and biochemical data correlated to differential anatomical growth. *Pediatrics 47 (Suppl.)*: 264–274, 1971.
59. Friis-Hansen, B: Water distribution in the foetus and newborn infant. *Acta Paediatr. Scand. 305 (Suppl.)*:7–11, 1983.
60. Siber, GR, Gorham, CC, Ericson, JF, Smith, AS: Pharmacokinetics of intravenous trimethoprim-sulfamethoxazole in children and adults with normal and impaired renal function. *Rev. Infect. Dis. 4*:566–578, 1982.
61. Desante, KA, Ryan, CF, Wallen, S, Heath, EC: Comparative bioavailability of erythromycin-sulfisoxazole combinations. *Pediatr. Infect. Dis. 5*:141–146, 1986.
62. Evans, DAP, White, TA: Human acetylation polymorphism. *J. Lab. Clin. Med. 63*: 394–403, 1964.
63. Reed, MD, Blumer, JL: Clinical pharmacology of antitubercular drugs. *Pediatr. Clin. North Am. 30*:177–193, 1983.
64. Gibson, TP, Matusik, J, Matusik, E, Nelson, HW, Wilkinson, J, Briggs, WA: Acetylation of procainamide in man and its relationship to isonicotinic acid hydrazine acetylation pehnotype. *Clin. Pharmacol. Ther. 17*:395–399, 1975.
65. Frislid, K, Berg, M, Hansteen, V, Lunde, PKM: Comparison of the acetylation of procainamide and sulfadimidine in man. *Eur. J. Clin. Pharmacol. 9*:433–438, 1976.
66. Evans, DAP: An improved and simplified method of detecting the acetylator phenotype. *J. Med. Genet. 6*:405–407, 1969.
67. Vree, TB, Hekster, YA, Damsma, JE, Tijhuis, M, Friesen, WT: Pharmacokinetics and mechanism of renal excretion of short acting sulphonamides and N_4-acetylsulphonamides in man. Structural requirements of sulphonamides for active tubular secretion. *Eur. J. Clin. Pharmacol. 20*:283–292, 1981.
68. Barne, HI, Hare, WK, McNamara, N, Hare, RS: Influence of postnatal age on kidney function of premature infants. *Proc. Soc. Exp. Biol. Med. 69*:55–67, 1948.
69. Guignard, JP, Torrado, A, DaCunha, O, Gautier, E: Glomerular filtration rate in the first three weeks of life. *J. Pediatr. 87*:268–272, 1975.

70. Leake, RD, Trygstad, CW: Glomerular filtration rate during the period of adaptation to extrauterine life. *Pediatr. Res. 11*:959–962, 1977.
71. Arant, BS: Developmental patterns of renal functional maturation in the human neonate. *J. Pediatr. 92*:705–712, 1978.
72. Barnes, JW, Kawaichi, GK: Factors influencing the formation of sulfonamide urinary concretions. *J. Urol. 49*:324–330, 1943.
73. Lehr, D: Clinical toxicology of sulfonamides. *Ann. N.Y. Acad. Sci. 69*:417–447, 1957.
74. Kruger-Thiemer, E, Bunger, P: Evaluation of the risk of crystalluria with sulfa drugs. *Proc. Eur. Soc. Study Drug Tox. 6*:185–207, 1965.
75. Lehr, D: Prevention of renal damage by use of mixtures of sulphonamides. *Br. Med. J. 2*:934–946, 1947.
76. Bratton, AC, Marshall, EK: New coupling component for sulfanilamide determination. *J. Biol. Chem. 128*:537–550, 1939.
77. Reider, J: Quantitative determination of the bacteriostatically active fraction of sulfonamides and the sum of their inactive metabolites in body fluids. *Chemotherapy 17*:1–21, 1972.
78. Vree, TB, Hekster, YA, Boars, AM, Damsma, JE, Van der Kleijn, E: Determination of trimethoprim and sulfamethoxazole (co-trimoxazole) in body fluids of man by means of high pressure liquid chromatography. *J. Chromatogr. 146*:103–112, 1978.
79. Idress, ZH, Cunningham, RJ, Wilfert, CM: Nocardiosis in children: Report of three cases and review of the literature. *Pediatrics 55*:479–484, 1975.
80. Krick, JA, Stinson, EB, Remington, JS: *Nocardia* infection in heart transplant patients. *Ann. Intern. Med. 82*:18–26, 1975.
81. Jacobson, JA, Chester, TJ, Fraser, DW: An epidemic of disease due to serogroup B *Neisseria meningitidis* in Alabama: Report of an investigation and community-wide prophylaxis with a sulfonamide. *J. Infect. Dis. 136*:104–108, 1977.
82. Lowbury, EJL, Jackson, DM, Lilly, HA, Bull, JP, Cason, JS, Davies, JWL, Ford, PM: Alternative forms of local treatment for burns. *Lancet 2*:1105–1111, 1971.
83. Speck, WT, Driscoll, JM, Polin, RA, O'Neill, J, Rosenkranz, HS: Staphylococcal and streptococcal colonization of the newborn infant. Effect of antiseptic cord care. *Am. J. Dis. Child. 131*:1005–1008, 1977.
84. Howie, VM, Ploussard, JH: Efficacy of fixed combinations of antibiotic versus separate components in otitis media. *Clin. Pediatr. 11*:205–214, 1972.
85. Ginsburg, CM, Eichenwald, HF: Erythromycin: A review of its uses in clinical practice. *J. Pediatr. 89*:872–884, 1976.
86. Salter, AJ: Trimethoprim-sulfamethoxazole: An assessment of more than 12 years of use. *Rev. Infect. Dis. 4*:196–236, 1982.
87. Bernstein, LS: Combination of trimethoprim with sulfonamides other than sulfamethoxazole. *Rev. Infect. Dis. 4*:411–418, 1982.
88. O'Brien, TF, Acar, JF, Altman, G, Blackburn, BO, Chao, L, Courtieu, A-L, Evans, DA, Guzman, M, Holmes, M, Jacobs, MR, Kent, RL, Norton, RA, Koornhof, HJ, Mederios, AA, Pasculle, AW, Surgalla, MJ, Williams, JD: Laboratory surveillance of synergy between and resistance to trimethoprim and sulfonamides. *Rev. Infect. Dis. 4*:351–357, 1982.
89. Ardati, KO, Thirumoorthi, MC, Dajani, AS: Intravenous trimethoprim-sulfamethoxazole in the treatment of serious infections in children. *J. Pediatr. 95*:801–806, 1979.
90. Smellie, JM, Greenberg, RN, Normand, ICS, Bantock, HM: Trimethoprim-sulfamethoxazole and trimethoprim alone in the prophylaxis of childhood urinary tract infections. *Rev. Infect. Dis. 4*:461–466, 1982.
91. Blumer, JL, Bertino, JS, Husak, MP: Comparison of cefaclor and trimethoprim-sulfamethoxazole in the treatment of acute otitis media. *Pediatr. Infect. Dis. 3*: 25–29, 1984.

92. Sabel, KG, Brandeburg, A: Treatment of meningitis and septicemia with sulphamethoxazole-trimethoprim combination. *Acta Paediatr. Scand. 64*:25–32, 1975.
93. Murphy, TF, Fernald, GW: Trimethoprim-sulfamethoxazole therapy for relapses of *Salmonella* meningitis. *Pediatr. Infect. Dis. 2*:465–468, 1983.
94. Long, PH: Use and abuse of chemotherapeutic and antibiotic agents. *N. Engl. J. Med. 237*:837–839, 1947.
95. Fink, HW, Smith, A: Incidence of reactions to sulfonamide drugs in infants and children. *J. Pediatr. 28*:40–48, 1946.
96. Rallison, ML, O'Brien, J, Good, RA: Severe reactions to long-acting sulfonamides. Erythema multiforme exudatium and lupus erythematosus following administration of sulphamethoxypyridazine and sulfadimethoxine. *Pediatrics 28*:908–917, 1961.
97. Carroll, OM, Bryan, PA, Robinson, RJ: Stevens-Johnson syndrome associated with long acting sulfonamides. *JAMA 195*:691–693, 1966.
98. Alarcon-Segovia, D: Drug-induced lupus syndromes. *Mayo Clin. Proc. 44*:664–681, 1969.
99. Pryles, CV: The use of sulfonamides in urinary tract infections. *Med. Clin. North Am. 54*:1077–1080, 1970.
100. Lowell, FC: Allergic reactions to sulfonamide and antibiotic drugs. *Ann. Intern. Med. 43*:333–344, 1955.
101. Beveridge, J, Harris, M, Wise, G, Stevens, L: Long-acting sulphonamides associated with Stevens-Johnson syndrome. *Lancet 2*:593, 1964.
102. Odell, GB: The dissociation of bilirubin from albumin and its clinical implications. *J. Pediatr. 55*:268–279, 1959.
103. Stern, L: Pharmacology for the pediatrician. Drug interactions part II. Drugs, the newborn infant, and the binding of bilirubin to albumin. *Pediatrics 49*:916–918, 1972.
104. Valaes, T, Gellis, SS: Is kernicterus always the definitive evidence of bilirubin toxicity? *Pediatrics 67*:940–941, 1981.
105. Cashore, WJ, Oh, W: Unbound bilirubin and kernicterus in low-birth infants. *Pediatrics 69*:481–485, 1982.
106. Silverman, WA, Anderson, DH, Blanc, WA, Crozier, DW: A difference in mortality rate and incidence of kernicterus among premature infants allotted to the prophylactic antibacterial regimens. *Pediatrics 18*:614–624, 1956.
107. Johnson, L, Sarmiento, F, Blanc, WA, Day, RL: Kernicterus in rats with inherited deficiency in glucuronyl transferase. *Am. J. Dis. Child. 97*:591–608, 1959.
108. Silverman, WA: The status of 2 year old children who had received sulfisoxazole in the neonatal period after premature birth. *Am. J. Dis. Child. 54*:741–747, 1959.
109. Brodersen, R: Bilirubin transport in the newborn infant, reviewed with relation to kernicterus. *J. Pediatr. 96*:349–356, 1980.
110. Stutman, HR, Parker, M, Marks, MI: Potential of moxalactam and other new antimicrobial agents for bilirubin-albumin displacement in neonates. *Pediatrics 75*: 294–298, 1985.
111. Brodersen, R: Competitive binding of bilirubin and drugs to human serum albumin studied by enzymatic oxidation. *J. Clin. Invest. 54*:1353–1364, 1974.
112. Glickman, R, Alvarez, S, Joubert, DW: Drug therapy reviews: Trimethoprim-sulfamethoxazole. *Am. J. Hosp. Pharm. 36*:893–906, 1979.
113. Lawson, DH, Palce, BJ: Adverse reactions to trimethoprim-sulfamethoxazole. *Rev. Infect. Dis. 4*:429–433, 1982.
114. Hulme, B, Reeves, DS: Leucopenia associated with trimethoprim-sulfamethoxazole after renal transplantation. *Br. Med. J. 3*:610–612, 1971.
115. Hall, CL: Co-trimoxazole and azathioprine: A safe combination. *Br. Med. J. 4*:15–16, 1974.

116. Bradley, PP, Warden, GD, Maxwell, JG, Rothstein, G: Neutropenia and thrombocytopenia in renal allograft recipients treated with trimethoprim-sulfamethoxazole. *Ann. Intern. Med. 93*:560–562, 1980.
117. Asmar, BI, Maqbool, S, Dajani, AS: Hematologic abnormalities after oral trimethoprim-sulfamethoxazole therapy in children. *Am. J. Dis. Child. 135*:1100–1103, 1981.
118. Sweet, J: Potentiation of warfarin by co-trimoxazole. *Br. Med. J. 3*:491, 1975.
119. Tilstone, WJ, Gray, JMB, Nimmo-Smith, RH, Lawson, DH: Interaction between warfarin and sulphamethoxazole. *Postgrad. Med. J. 53*:388–390, 1977.
120. Christensen, LK, Hansen, JM, Kristensen, M: Sulphaphenazole-induced hypoglycaemic attacks in tolbutamide-treated diabetics. *Lancet 2*:1298–1301, 1963.
121. Kristensen, M, Christensen, LK: Drug induced changes of the blood glucose lowering effect of oral hypoglycemic agents. *Acta Diabetol. Lat. 6(Suppl. 1)*:116–136, 1969.
122. Liegler, DG, Henderson, ES, Hahn, MA, Oliverio, VT: The effect of organic acids on renal clearance of methotrexate in man. *Clin. Pharmacol. Ther. 10*:849–857, 1969.
123. Lumholtz, B, Siersbaek-Nielsen, K, Skovsted, L, Kampmann, J, Hansen, JM: Sulfamethizole-induced inhibition of diphenylhydantoin, tolbutamide and warfarin metabolism. *Clin. Pharmacol. Ther. 17*:731–734, 1975.
124. Anton, AH: The effect of disease, drugs and dilution on the binding of sulfonamides in human plasma. *Clin. Pharmacol. Ther. 9*:561–567, 1968.

12
Cephalosporins

J. STEVEN LEEDER AND RONALD GOLD
The Hospital for Sick Children, Toronto, Ontario, Canada

Over the past 25 years, the cephalosporin family of antibiotics has become an increasingly important addition to the antimicrobial armamentarium of practicing clinicians. Since the introduction of cephalothin in 1962, the number of cephalosporins has proliferated rapidly, spawning three generations of compounds with similar names but with progressively broadening spectra of activity. The number of agents currently marketed, the similarity of generic and trade names, and the rapidity with which newer agents in developmental stages appear in the literature have all caused a great deal of confusion among clinicians faced with making therapeutic decisions. For these reasons, the cephalosporins have been the subject of several reviews, each attempting to clarify the relative merits of individual agents (1-6).

The good health of bathers in the polluted waters off the Sardinian coast led to the isolation of *Cephalosporium acremonium* by Guiseppe Brotzu in 1948. Extracts of this mold were subsequently found to inhibit the growth of *Staphylococcus aureus* in vitro and to successfully treat typhoid fever in humans (7). Three different products, cephalosporin P, N, and C, were isolated from cultures of this fungus, and with the determination of the structure of cephalosporin N, the similarity of these compounds to the penicillins became apparent. In 1953, the stability of cephalosporin C in dilute acid, its resistance to hydrolysis by a penicillinase from *Bacillus cereus*, and its ability to competitively inhibit the hydrolysis of benzylpenicillin by this enzyme, distinguished it from the penicillins known at that time (8). At the same time, the emergence of penicillinase-producing strains of staphylococci was becoming a serious clinical problem and the need for penicillinlike antibiotics resistant to penicillinase was perceived. Cephalosporin C was found to have limited intrinsic antibacterial activity, but cleavage of the side chain at position 7 resulted in the active nucleus 7-aminocephalosporanic acid (Figure 1). Addition of side chains at the 3 position of the dihydrothiazine ring and the 7 position of the β-lactam ring has resulted in semisynthetic compounds with greater antibacterial activity than the parent. Such manipulations (akin to the development of penicillins from 6-aminopenicillanic acid) have produced a plethora of cephalosporins with different spectra of antibacterial activity and pharmacokinetic properties.

Cephalosporin C

7-Aminocephalosporanic Acid

7-Aminopenicillanic Acid

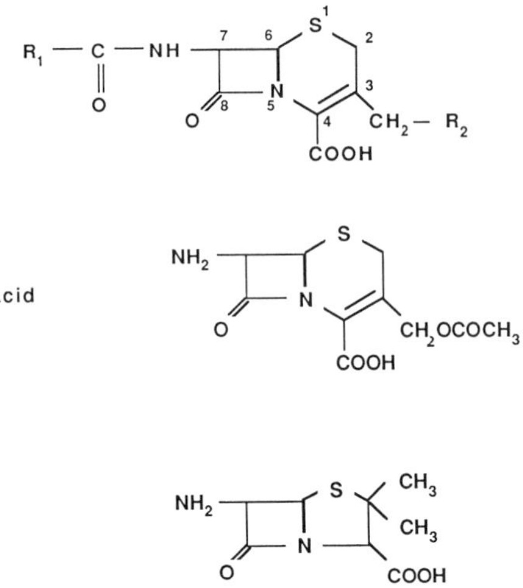

Figure 1 Structural formulas for cephalosporin C and 7-aminocephalosporanic acid, the nucleus for the synthesis of cephalosporin compounds. Included for comparison is the analogous compound used in penicillin synthesis, 7-aminopenicillanic acid.

Another two families of β-lactam antibiotics have recently been introduced into clinical practice. The cephamycins are fermentation products of *Streptomyces* sp. and can be differentiated from true cephalosporins by the presence of a methoxy group at the 7 position of the β-lactam ring (9,10). In an analogous manner to the penicillins and cephalosporins, removal of a side chain provides a nucleus from which semisynthetic congeners can be derived (Figure 2). The oxa-β-lactams are products of chemical manipulation of the 7-aminocephalosporanic acid nucleus in which the sulfur atom of the dihydrothiazine ring is replaced with an oxygen atom (11). For simplicity, the term "cephalosporin" will be used to refer to all compounds throughout this chapter.

In addition to the ease with which new cephalosporin congeners can be synthesized, such factors as the emerging and increasing resistance of gram-negative bacteria (12), as well as concern about the toxic potential of aminoglycosides, have contributed to the

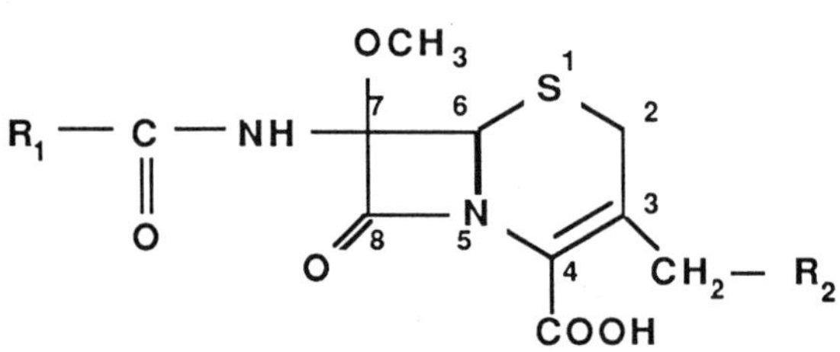

Cephamycin C

Figure 2 Structure of cephamycin C, the nucleus from which synthetic cephamycin congeners, such as cefoxitin, are derived.

increased availability, use, and perhaps overuse and abuse of this family of drugs. This chapter will outline the clinical and pharmacokinetic experience with cephalosporins in pediatric patients, with emphasis on those agents with the most potential for treating bacterial infections in this patient population.

I. Chemistry

7-Aminocephalosporanic acid (Figure 1), a product of the acid hydrolysis of cephalosporin C, has been the basis for the synthesis of many cephalosporin compounds. In general, addition of side chains at the 7 position of the β-lactam ring produces changes in antibacterial activity; modification of the 3 position of the dihydrothiazine ring alters the pharmacological properties of the compounds (13).

Classification of cephalosporins by "generation," although somewhat arbitrary, is based to a large degree on in vitro spectra of activity. Alternative criteria for classification include metabolic stability and susceptibility to β-lactamases (14). As a group, the cephalosporins are much more stable to β-lactamase attack than benzylpenicillin, but relative to newer agents, the first-generation cephalosporins (Figure 3) are relatively β-lactamase sensitive. They possess similar spectra of activity, differing for the most part in their pharmacokinetic characteristics. The thienylacetyl group of cephalothin and cephaloridine (R_1 in Figure 3) and pyridinylthiol group of cephapirin exhibit comparable antibacterial activity. However, the pyridine and methylthiadiazole substituents at the 3 position of cephaloridine and cefazolin, respectively (R_2 in Figure 3), are more metabolically

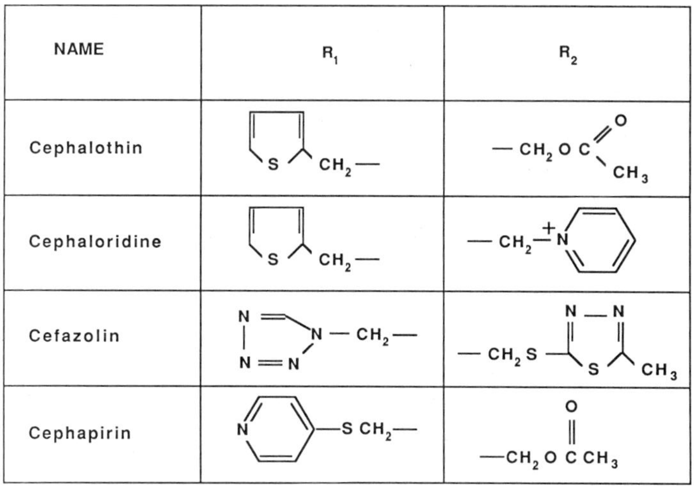

Figure 3 Chemical structures of selected first-generation cephalosporins.

stable than the acetoxymethyl groups of cephalothin and cephapirin, resulting in higher and more prolonged serum concentrations (15,16). Cephalothin is rapidly desacetylated with a consequent fivefold loss in activity against gram-negative pathogens (17).

The orally effective compounds, cephalexin, cephradine, cephaloglycine, and cefaclor, are essentially the cephalosporin counterparts of ampicillin, all having the same R_1 substituent. Analogously, cefadroxil and amoxicillin both have an α-amino *p*-hydroxyphenyl group at the 7 position of the β-lactam ring (Figure 4).

Much effort has been exerted to produce newer cephalosporins with improved stability to β-lactamases, and such chemical modification of the 7-cephalosporanic acid nucleus has produced the second-generation cephalosporins possessing extended spectra of activity against gram-negative pathogens compared with their first-generation predecessors. The introduction of two important substituents, the α-methoxy group of cefoxitin and the syn-methoximino group of cefuroxime (boxed area, Figure 5) have greatly reduced susceptibility to β-lactamases and provided the basis for future compounds with even broader spectra of activity (18-22). The increased resistance to β-lactamases associated with various substituents in the 7α position is due to steric hindrance. However, substitution of groups larger then the methoxyl group of cefoxitin results in markedly

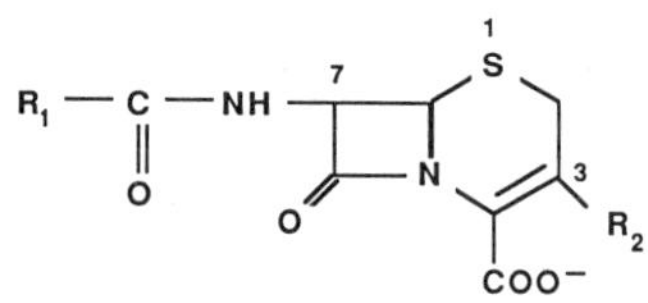

NAME	R_1	R_2
Cephalexin	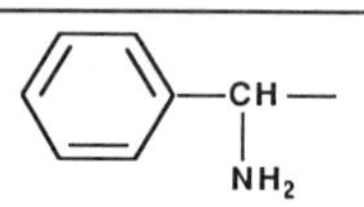	$-CH_3$
Cephradine	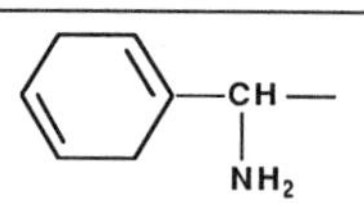	$-CH_3$
Cefadroxil	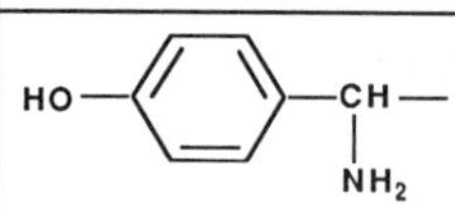	$-CH_3$
Cefaclor	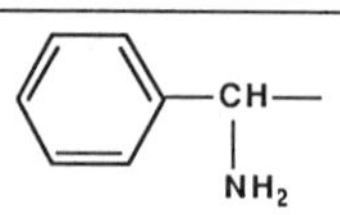	$-Cl$
Cefixime	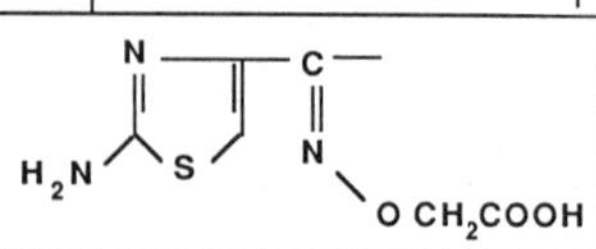	$-CH=CH_2$

Figure 4 Chemical structures of marketed and investigational oral cephalosporins.

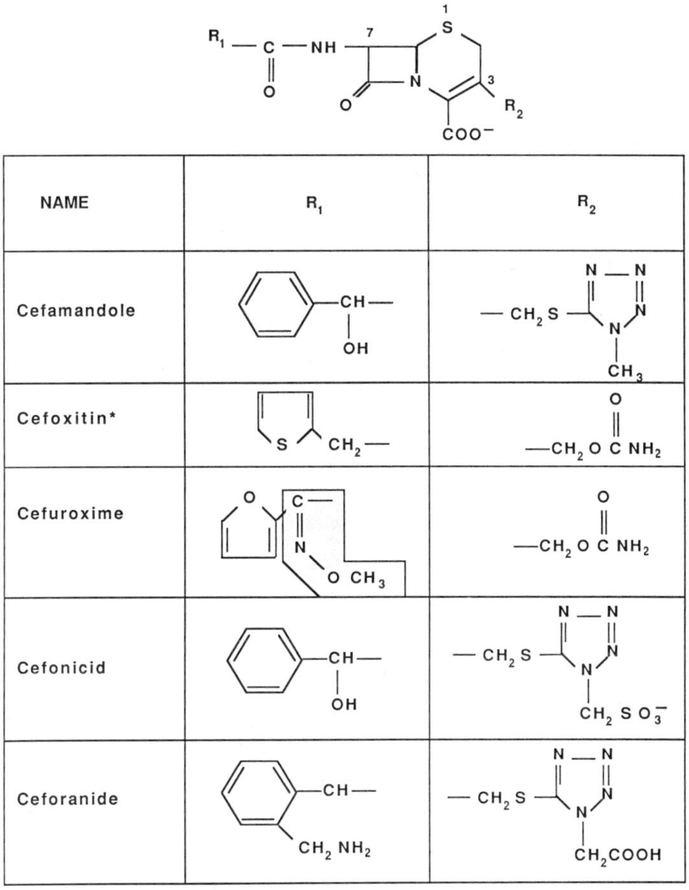

Figure 5 Structural formulas for second-generation cephalosporins and cefoxitin. Note that cefoxitin also has a methoxy ($-OCH_3$) group at position 7 of the β-lactam ring.

reduced activity (23). In addition, both cefoxitin and cefuroxime have a carbamoyl group at position 3 providing metabolic stability in vivo.

In the third-generation compounds, cefotaxime, ceftizoxime, cefmenoxime, and ceftriaxone, an aminothiazolyl side chain (boxed area, Figure 6) has been added to a syn-methoximino derivative. Since the aminothiazolyl group itself affects binding to the target enzymes inside the bacterial cells and, to some degree, entry into the periplasm but does not provide stability to β-lactamases, the combination of aminothiazolyl and methoximino groups has produced agents with further increased activity and decreased susceptibility to β-lactamase inactivation (24,25). It appears that differences in activity are minimal whether the side chain in the 3 position is an acetoxy group (cefotaxime) or a methyltetrazolethiol group (cefmenoxime) or whether only a hydrogen atom is present (26). Cleavage of the acetoxy group of cefotaxime is accompanied by loss of all activity against *Pseudomonas aeruginosa* and *Bacteroides* (27). Further metabolism of the desacetyl metabolite results in formation of a lactone ring with the carboxy group at

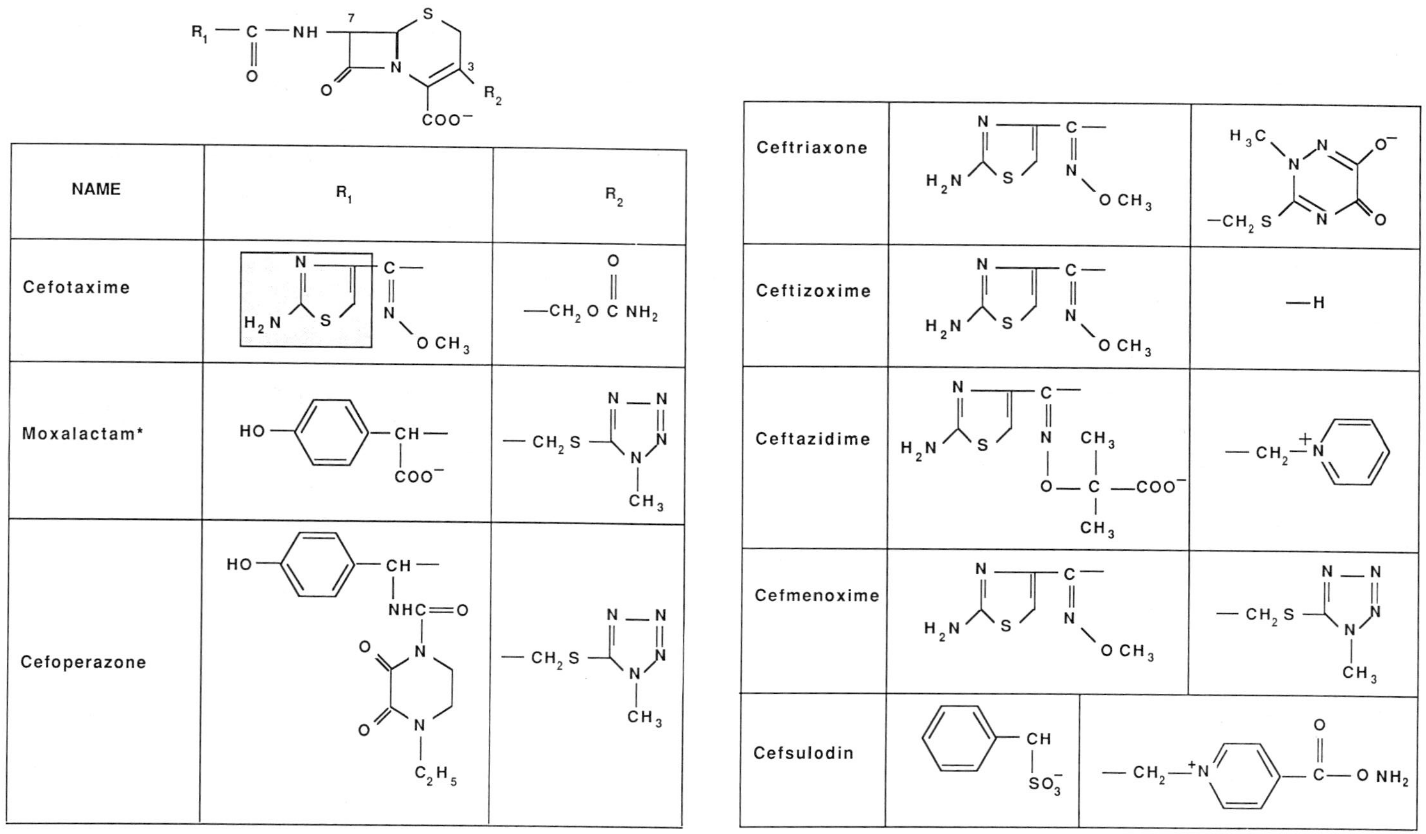

Figure 6 Structural formulas for several third-generation cephalosporins and moxalactam. Note that, for moxalactam, an oxygen atom replaces the sulfur atom at position 1 of the nucleus and a methoxy ($-OCH_3$) group is present at position 7.

position 4 of the dihydrothiazine ring. This compound has no antibacterial activity, illustrating the importance of an intact acidic carboxyl function at this position (28).

The long half-life of ceftriaxone is attributed to the presence of an enolate anion in the R_2 substituent (24). In ceftazidime, the aminothiazolyl group is attached to a 2-carboxy-2-oxypropane imino group (Figure 6), resulting in increased activity against *Pseudomonas* sp. at the price of reduced activity against gram-positive organisms and anaerobes (29,30). Analogous to piperacillin, the introduction of a 2,3-dioxopiperazine side chain into the cephalosporin nucleus yields cefoperazone, a compound with very good activity against *P. aeruginosa* and the Enterobacteriaceae. The absence of a bulky protective side chain close to the β-lactam ring, however, leaves the molecule open to β-lactamase attack (31,32). The methyltetrazolethiol side chain of cefoperazone, cefamandole, moxalactam, cefmenoxime, and cefmetazole has been associated with such side effects as disulfiramlike reactions (33) and depletion of vitamin K-dependent clotting factors (34).

In moxalactam, replacement of the sulfur atom of classic cephalosporins with oxygen is associated with an increased ability to penetrate bacteria (35), but the resultant increase in activity is offset by a relative instability to β-lactamase inactivation (11).

II. MECHANISM OF ACTION

The bactericidal activity of the cephalosporins against susceptible organisms, like that of the penicillins, is due to inhibition of cell wall synthesis. The rigid mechanical stability of the bacterial cell wall is provided by a netlike macromolecule, peptidoglycan, which is a highly cross-linked polymer of glycan chains. These glycan chains consist of alternating residues of the amino sugars *N*-acetylglucosamine (NAG) and *N*-acetylmuramic acid (NAM). Attached to each NAM residue is a short peptide chain by which adjacent glycan chains are cross-linked. The precise amino acid composition of these peptide cross-links is characteristic of the particular bacterial species. To understand the mechanism of action of the β-lactam antibiotics, one other factor concerning the composition of the bacterial cell wall is important as well. On the outside of the peptidoglycan layer of gram-negative bacteria is a lipid bilayer containing lipopolysaccharide residues. This outer membrane is not present in gram-positive bacteria and provides a barrier to diffusion for some β-lactam antibiotics. A close association between the outer membrane and peptidoglycan layers is maintained by the presence of a low-molecular-weight lipoprotein that is covalently linked to the peptidoglycan.

As currently understood, peptidoglycan biosynthesis may be considered in three stages (36). First, the uridine diphosphate (UDP) precursors UDP-NAG and UDP-NAM-pentapeptide are formed in the cytoplasm. In the second stage, the basic unit, NAG-NAM-pentapeptide, is formed and transferred to the outer surface of the cytoplasmic membrane by a membrane-bound carrier, where it is attached to a growing glycan chain. A transpeptidase enzyme links the free amino group of a neighboring peptide side chain to the fourth residue of the pentapeptide (D-alanine), releasing the fifth residue (D-alanine), thus cross-linking the peptidoglycan strands and completing the final stage (37). β-Lactams are postulated to disrupt this process by acting as structural analogs of the D-alanine-D-alanine terminal dipeptide. The transpeptidase binds the β-lactam to its active site and cleaves the β-lactam ring, resulting in a stable, inactive transpeptidase-acyl β-lactam complex (38).

β-Lactam antibiotics bind to a number of proteins associated with the bacterial cell membrane (penicillin binding proteins; PBP) that are probably the transpeptidases and other enzymes catalyzing the terminal events of cell wall synthesis (36). Some of these proteins are involved in such essential functions as cell wall division, wall elongation, septum formation, and maintenance of cell wall shape (39-41); others are not (41-43). The activity of a given β-lactam against susceptible bacteria is determined by the presence, type, and specific activity of the PBP (44). Cephalosporins, such as cephaloridine and cefsulodin, have a high affinity for PBP 1a and 1b, resulting in spheroplast formation and rapid lysis of susceptible organisms; the aminothiazolyl cephalosporins show a high affinity for PBP 3, causing long filamentous bacterial forms (25). Actual lysis of bacteria is at present thought to result from the activity of bacterial enzymes (autolysins), such as murein hydrolases. The availability of an inhibitor of these enzymes appears to be decreased by β-lactam antibiotics such that the structural integrity of the bacterial cell is destroyed by the uninhibited enzymes (45).

The nature of the substituents of β-lactam antibiotics, therefore, is important in determining their ability to bind to bacterial PBP and exert their effects on bacterial morphology. In general, the minimum inhibitory concentration (MIC) of a β-lactam reflects binding to the primary PBP target. However, permeability characteristics affect the ability of the agent to reach those targets and are also important.

III. MECHANISMS OF RESISTANCE

There are a number of mechanisms by which bacteria become resistant to the action of cephalosporins and other β-lactam antibiotics. Structural differences in the target enzymes may cause a microorganism to be intrinsically resistant to a drug (46). Resistance of this type may be acquired by mutation, but such a mechanism appears to be relatively unimportant compared with others (47).

Inability of the β-lactam agents to penetrate to their target proteins is another form of bacterial resistance (48). Only capsular macromolecules lie outside the peptidoglycan layer of gram-positive bacteria, and therefore the small β-lactam molecules have very little difficulty in reaching the PBP located on the outer surface of the cytoplasmic membrane. The surface structure of gram-negative bacteria is more complex. It consists of an outer membrane composed of a lipid bilayer containing lipopolysaccharide residues, a central peptidoglycan layer, and an inner membrane analogous to the cytoplasmic membrane of gram-positive organisms. β-Lactam antibiotics reach the periplasmic space of gram-negative bacteria by diffusing through water-filled channels of porin proteins (49-51), and thus the outer membrane serves as a impenetrable barrier to some hydrophilic β-lactams. Most resistance of this type appears to be mediated by inducible chromosomal envelope mechanisms, although some may be plasmid mediated.

An important mechanism of resistance to penicillins and cephalosporins is hydrolysis of the cyclic amide bond in the β-lactam ring by β-lactamases. Genetic control of these enzymes may be mediated by plasmid transfer or by chromosomal means (52). In gram-negative bacteria, the β-lactamases are strategically located in the periplasmic space between the inner and outer cell membranes in close proximity to the target enzymes, which are situated on the outer surface of the inner membrane. This arrangement obviously affords the organism maximum protection. Most plasmid-mediated β-lactamases act primarily as penicillinases with penicillin and ampicillin as their preferred substrates, but at least one enzyme considered to be a cephalosporinase has been isolated (53). An additional plasmid-borne enzyme is able to hydrolyze third-generation cephalosporins owing to an increased affinity of the compounds for the enzyme (54). β-Lactamases are widely distributed among bacteria, being found in gram-positive, gram-negative, and some anaerobic species (52,55,56). Although the most common plasmid-mediated β-lactamases, the TEM enzymes, are present in *Escherichia coli* and other enteric bacteria, other plasmid β-lactamases are also found in these organisms, albeit less frequently than are the TEM enzymes (52). At least four β-lactamases confined to the *Pseudomas* species have been isolated (57) but collectively occur less frequently in these species than the TEM enzymes (56). There now appear to be more than 20 known plasmid-mediated β-lactamases differing in such criteria as substrate profile, reaction with inhibitors, molecular weight, and isoelectric point (58).

Most resistance to cephalosporins, however, is due to chromosomally encoded, inducible enzymes. All members of the *Enterobacter* species and *Pseudomonas* species contain inducible β-lactamases functioning primarily as cephalosporinases but varying greatly in their affinity for β-lactam antibiotics and in the rate at which they hydrolyze these drugs (59). Clinically, treatment failure or relapse has occurred more frequently during therapy with third-generation cephalosporins than with earlier agents and has been attributed to the emergence of resistant organisms. This is often accompanied by cross-tolerance to most other β-lactam antibiotics, and in most cases, the responsible organisms are *Serratia, Enterobacter,* or *Pseudomonas* species included in the expanded spectra of the newer agents but not the spectra of the older cephalosporins (60).

Although induction of β-lactamase activity is associated with the development of bacterial resistance to β-lactam drugs, most expanded spectrum cephalosporins are resistant to hydrolysis by these enzymes (61,62). Despite their inability to hydrolyze these particular antibiotics, the drugs nevertheless are bound to the enzymes with a high affinity. Binding of these nonsubstrate molecules may prevent the subsequent binding and hydrolysis of substrate drugs, but more importantly, the level of β-lactamase expression in bacteria possessing inducible enzymes plays a role in the resistance to the newer, nonsubstrate cephalosporins (63). This method of resistance has been described as a β-lactamase directed barrier (60). In the proposed model, the uninduced state consists of only a few enzyme molecules under repressor control (64) present in the periplasmic space such that passage of substrate and nonsubstrate molecules to their penicillin binding protein targets is relatively unimpeded. β-Lactam antibiotics may interact with a cellular repressor protein such that, following induction, the number of β-lactamase molecules in the periplasmic space is markedly increased (65). Substrate drugs are bound and hydrolyzed; nonsubstrates are bound by a tight, nonhydrolytic bond, preventing access to the target proteins and subsequent lethal pharmacological effects (66). As an example of this tight binding, moxalactam inhibition of a particular cephalosporinase is characterized by the transient formation of a covalent complex resulting in stability against that enzyme. In contrast to irreversible β-lactamase inhibitors, such as clavulanic acid, the enzyme inhibition described appears to be reversible although dissociation of the covalent complex occurs over a prolonged period of time (67).

In general, the best inducers of β-lactamases are those β-lactam antibiotics that are resistant to hydrolysis (65). To date, cefoxitin is the most potent inducer and antagonizes the in vitro activity of several β-lactam agents (60). The antagonism of cefamandole and cephalothin is related to the induction of inactivating β-lactamases; that of cefuroxime, cefotaxime, cefsulodin, and moxalactam are not since the induced enzymes are incapable of hydrolyzing these agents (68,69). β-Lactamase stable cephalosporins other than cefoxitin are also able to induce enzyme activity and can be classified according to this ability. Moxalactam and cefmetazole, although somewhat less active, are included with cefoxitin as agents with high inducibility. Cefuroxime, cefotaxime, and ceftizoxime demonstrate intermediate activity, but cefoperazone and cefsulodin are relatively poor inducers of β-lactamase activity (70). It is likely that the clinical utility of a given broad-spectrum cephalosporin undergoing development will be limited by its potential to induce β-lactamase activity and the attendant emergence of bacterial resistance.

IV. ANTIBACTERIAL ACTIVITY

Classification of the cephalosporins by "generation," although somewhat arbitrary, is based on general patterns of antimicrobial activity. The first-generation cephalosporins, cephalothin and cefazolin, have good activity against most gram-positive organisms but are less active than the second-generation cephalosporins (cefamandole, cefoxitin, and cefuroxime) against Enterobacteriaceae. Third-generation cephalosporins are much more active against enteric gram-negative organisms, including β-lactamase producing strains, than their predecessors and possess some activity against *P. aeruginosa*. This expanded gram-negative activity is commonly accompanied by reduced gram-positive coverage as the third-generation compounds are generally less active than cephalothin or cefuroxime against gram-positive cocci.

A. First Generation

The first-generation cephalosporins, cephalothin, cephaloridine, cefazolin, and cephapirin, all have similar antibacterial profiles with only minor differences in activity apparent. Ranges of MIC_{90} values for representative first-generation and oral cephalosporins are compared in Table 1. At one time, a single "cephalosporin" disk was used to screen for bacterial sensitivity. Cephalothin was the first of the cephalosporins to be marketed and therefore can be considered the prototype for the first-generation compounds. It is highly active against penicillin-sensitive and penicillin-resistant *S. aureus* and *Staphylococcus epidermidis*, with minimum inhibitory concentrations (MIC) for most isolates in the 0.004–1.0 μg/ml range (71,72). Methicillin-resistant strains of *S. aureus* are usually resistant, although similarly resistant strains of *S. epidermidis* tend to remain sensitive. Cephalothin is also active against *Streptococcus pneumoniae*, and *Streptococcus pyogenes* and *viridans* are even more susceptible to the drug, with MIC $\leqslant$ 1.0 μg/ml. The group D streptococci or enterococci and *Listeria monocytogenes* are uniformly resistant to these and other cephalosporins. Cephalothin possesses only one-half to one-eighth the activity of cephaloridine against staphylococci, group A streptococci, and pneumococci but is more stable toward staphylococcal penicillinase than either cephaloridine or cefazolin (71). *Neisseria gonorrhoeae* and *Neisseria meningitidis* are very sensitive to cephalothin, with most strains inhibited by concentrations of 0.004–1.0 μg/ml. *Hemophilus influenzae* is less susceptible, although concentrations of 6 μg/ml or less will inhibit 50% of strains (MIC_{50}) (72). Similar concentrations are required to inhibit *E. coli, Proteus mirabilis, Salmonella* sp., and *Shigella* sp. Cefazolin is more active than cephalothin against *E. coli, Klebsiella*, and some strains of *Enterobacter*. Nonsusceptible species include *Enterobacter*, indole-positive *Proteus* sp., *Serratia, Acinetobacter, P. aeruginosa*, and some strains of *Bacteroides fragilis* (73).

B. Second Generation

Patterns of susceptibility to the second-generation cephalosporins are less homogeneous than for the first-generation compounds. Cefamandole is more active than cephalothin

Table 1 Range of Published MIC_{90} Values for First-generation and Oral Cephalosporins

Organism	Cephalothin	Cefazolin	Cephalexin	Cefaclor
Staphylococcus aureus	0.2–1.0	<0.05–2.0	3.1–12.5	4.0–32
S. epidermidis	0.2–1.6	0.06–1.0	3.1–32	2.0–32
Streptococcus pyogenes	<0.06–0.32	0.015–1.0	0.5–2.0	0.25–4.0
S. pneumoniae	0.06–1.5	0.005–0.78	3.1–4.0	0.5–1.6
S. faecalis	25–50	32–>128	100–>128	64
Hemophilus influenzae	0.8–40	0.12–25	3.1–>32	0.8–>32
Neisseria gonorrhoeae	3.1–4.6	1.0–8.0	2.0–32	0.25
N. meningitidis	0.8	0.5–0.8	4.0–16	0.25
Escherichia coli	8.0–>400	0.25–128	3.1–>400	1.6–>32
Klebsiella pneumonia	4.0–128	0.25–>128	6.2–25	0.8–8.0
Enterobacter cloacae	>32–>400	0.5–>128	>128	>128
Serratia marcescens	>32–>400	>128	>128	>128
Proteus mirabilis	2.0–50	1.0–128	6.2–>128	1.6–>128
P. vulgaris	>32–>400	0.5–>128	>128	>128
Salmonella sp.	2.8–50	0.8–6.2	3.1–100	0.8–2.0
Shigella sp.	16–400		3.1–12.5	0.8–8.0
Pseudomonas aeruginosa	>32–>400	>128	>128	>128
Pseudomonas sp.	>32	>128	>128	>128
Acinetobacter	>32–>100	8.0–>128		
Bacteroides fragilis	>40–>400	0.25–>128	>128	>128

Source: Compiled from References 72–125.

against *E. coli, Enterobacter* sp. (*E. cloacae* in particular), *P. mirabilis*, and indole-positive *Proteus*. In addition, 90% of *H. influenzae* strains are inhibited by concentrations (MIC_{90}) of 0.6 μg/ml (Table 2) (74,75). Most gram-positive organisms can still be considered susceptible to cefamandole, but MIC are higher than for cephalothin. *Pseudomonas* sp., *Serratia*, and *Acinetobacter* are resistant.

Cefoxitin is less active than cefamandole against gram-positive bacteria and some gram-negative microorganisms, such as *Klebsiella* and *Enterobacter* sp. but is more active against *Serratia marcescens* and indole-positive *Proteus* (73,76). MIC for cefoxitin are increased in gentamicin-resistant isolates of *S. marcescens*. A number of anaerobic bacteria are susceptible to cefoxitin at clinically attainable concentrations, and its activity against *B. fragilis*, in particular, is superior to almost all other cephalosporins, a concentration of 16 μg/ml inhibiting 90% of strains (76,77).

Cefuroxime possesses in vitro activity against staphylococci (including β-lactamase positive strains) and nonenterococcal streptococci that is comparable to that of cefamandole, and similar to both cefamandole and cefoxitin against *E. coli, Klebsiella pneumoniae, P. mirabilis*, and *Providencia* sp. (73). It is more active than cefoxitin against *Enterobacter* species but less active against *Serratia*, some indole-positive *Proteus*, and *B. fragilis* (21). Both β-lactamase producing and non β-lactamase producing strains of *H. influenzae* are susceptible to cefuroxime, with most strains inhibited at concentrations of 1 μg/ml or less. Similar activity is observed with cefamandole, but cefoxitin and cephalo-

Table 2 Range of Published MIC_{90} Values for Second-generation Cephalosporins

Organism	Cefamandole	Cefoxitin	Cefuroxime
Staphylococcus aureus	0.2–1.0	4.0–8.0	0.8–4.0
S. epidermidis	0.2–4.0	6.2–64	1.0
Streptococcus pyogenes	0.06–0.2	0.5–1.0	0.015–0.2
S. pneumoniae	0.06–0.2	0.5–1.56	0.1–0.2
S. faecalis	25–64	50–>128	>128
Hemophilus influenzae	0.4–2.0	1.6–8.0	0.5–2.0
Neisseria gonorrhoeae	0.8–4.0	0.5–0.8	0.06–0.8
N. meningitidis	0.05–0.25	0.4–1.0	0.05–4.0
Escherichia coli	1.0–128	2.0–32	4.0–16
Klebsiella pneumonia	1.0–128	2.0–25	4.0–25
Enterobacter cloacae	16–128	>128	2.0–>32
Serratia marcescens	>128	8–>128	32–>128
Proteus mirabilis	0.5–25	2.0–16	1.3–50
P. vulgaris	8–>128	3.1–16	64–>128
Salmonella sp.	6.3–12.5	2.0–3.1	2.0–6.2
Shigella sp.	25	25–100	3.3–50
Pseudomonas aeruginosa	>128	>128	>128
Pseudomonas sp.	>128	>128	>128
Acinetobacter	>128	>128	>128
Bacteroides fragilis	32–>128	8–>128	128

Source: Compiled from References 72–125.

thin are less active. Cefuroxime is superior to ampicillin against β-lactamase producing strains (78,79).

Other second-generation compounds, such as cefonicid and ceforanide, have similar spectra of activity but demonstrate activities against individual bacterial species generally less than or equal to those of cefamandole, cefoxitin, and cefuroxime (80,81). *Acinetobacter, P. aeruginosa, Pseudomonas* sp., enterococci, and *Listeria* are invariably resistant to all second-generation cephalosporins.

C. Third Generation

Compared with earlier agents, the third-generation cephalosporins possess both increased activity and increased β-lactamase stability toward many gram-negative organisms. This broader spectrum of activity, however, comes at the expense of reduced gram-positive coverage, particularly in comparison with that of the first-generation compounds. Ranges of MIC_{90} values for some of the more common third-generation cephalosporins are compared in Table 3.

Cefotaxime, the first of the most recent generation to be marketed, inhibits 90% of *S. aureus* isolates at a concentration of 4 μg/ml, approximately 10-fold less active than cephalothin (82,83). *S. epidermidis* tends to be less sensitive to cefotaxime than *S. aureus,*

Table 3 Range of Published MIC_{90} Values for Third-generation Cephalosporins

Organism	Cefotaxime	Moxalactam	Cefoperazone	Ceftazidime	Ceftriaxone	Ceftizoxime
Staphylococcus aureus	2.0–8.0	6.2–16	2.0–12.5	8.0–50	3.1–8.0	0.5–8.0
S. epidermidis	6.2–12.5	32–>128	3.1–32	16–>50	25–50	6.25–25
Streptococcus pyogenes	<0.03–0.2	0.5–2.0	0.12–1.6	0.12–0.8	0.025–0.2	0.015–0.2
S. pneumoniae	<0.03–0.1	2.0–4.0	<0.06–1.0	0.1–0.25	0.015–0.12	0.015–0.39
S. faecalis	100–>128	>128	50–>64	>128	>128	>16–>256
Hemophilus influenzae	⩽0.02–0.8	0.06–4.0	0.5–0.8	0.06–0.25	⩽0.004–0.1	⩽0.025–1.6
Neisseria gonorrhoeae	0.01–0.4	0.06–0.8	0.03–0.2	0.025–0.12	⩽0.008–0.025	0.007–1.6
N. meningitidis	0.006–0.025	0.0125–0.05		0.025	0.002–0.025	<0.008
Escherichia coli	0.125–8.0	0.1–4.0	1.0–100	0.25–2.0	0.1–1.56	0.04–0.25
Klebsiella pneumonia	0.1–0.4	<0.12–1.0	1.0–128	0.25–4.0	0.1–0.39	⩽0.025–0.1
Enterobacter cloacae	0.12–32	0.12–16	2.0–>100	0.25–50	0.5–64	0.8–>100
Serratia marcescens	0.25–>100	0.25–16	6.25–>100	0.25–3.1	0.25–50	0.12–12.5
Proteus mirabilis	0.03–0.1	0.1–4.0	0.25–64	0.06–0.125	0.02–0.1	⩽0.008–0.06
P. vulgaris	0.06–>100	0.12–32	0.25–50	0.08–0.9	0.06–3.1	0.015–6.25
Salmonella sp.	0.06–0.24	0.12–1.6	50	0.1–0.8	0.05–0.4	0.03–0.05
Shigella sp.	0.8	0.2	100	0.2–0.25	0.025–0.5	1.6
Pseudomonas aeruginosa	32–>100	32–>128	12.5–>100	2.0–12.5	16–>100	16–>128
Pseudomonas sp	32–100	>128	16–64	8.0–50	64–128	>128
Acinetobacter	100–>128	>128	8–>100	2.0–12.5	8.0–>100	4.0–25
Bacteroides fragilis	2.0–>100	0.5–50	32–>128	32–>128	50–128	3.13–25

Source: Compiled from References 72-125.

and methicillin-resistant isolates of both species are considered resistant to all third-generation cephalosporins, with MIC values exceeding 64 μg/ml (4). The activity of cefmenoxime against *S. aureus* and *S. epidermidis* is similar to that of cefotaxime and slightly greater than that of ceftriaxone, ceftizoxime, and cefoperazone. Ceftazidime is less active, and moxalactam the least active of the third-generation cephalosporins against these microorganisms (4).

Streptococcus pyogenes and *S. pneumoniae* are very sensitive to the majority of the extended spectrum cephalosporins, with MIC_{90} less than 0.5 μg/ml. The exception is moxalactam, of which concentrations in the 2-4 μg/ml range are required to inhibit 90% of strains. *Streptococcus faecalis* and *Listeria* are resistant to all the third-generation cephalosporins (4).

As a group, the third-generation cephalosporins are extremely active against *H. influenzae, N. gonorrhoeae*, and *N. meningitidis*, with MIC_{90} values less than 0.2 μg/ml and frequently below 0.05 μg/ml (84-89). Ceftriaxone is slightly more active than the others against *H. influenzae* and *N. gonorrhoeae*; ceftazidime appears to be the least active. Nevertheless, its MIC_{90} for these organisms, 0.12 μg/ml, is very easily exceeded with standard doses. *N. meningitidis* is almost universally sensitive to this group of antibiotics.

Very few differences in activity are apparent among the third-generation compounds against such microorganisms as *E. coli, K. pneumoniae, P. mirabilis, Salmonella* sp., and *Shigella* sp. The majority of these bacteria are frequently inhibited by drug concentrations below 0.5 μg/ml, although higher concentrations are required for some isolates, particularly those that are multiply drug resistant. One notable exception concerns cefoperazone, for which severalfold higher concentrations are required to inhibit *E. coli* and *K. pneumoniae* (4,84-93).

Although *E. cloacae, S. marcescens, Providencia* sp., and indole-positive *Proteus* are somewhat less sensitive to the third-generation cephalosporins than the gram-negative bacilli discussed above, similar patterns of relative activity are present. Reported MIC_{90} levels differ widely depending on the particular isolates studied (90,91), but in general, only minor differences in activity are apparent for cefotaxime, moxalactam, ceftazidime, ceftizoxime, ceftriaxone, and cefmenoxime. Cefoperazone is approximately four to eightfold less active against these organisms.

Against tested strains of *P. aeruginosa*, including β-lactamase positive and ureidopenicillin-resistant and aminoglycoside-resistant isolates, ceftazidime is the most active cephalosporin currently available, with reported MIC_{90} ranging between 0.5 and 32 μg/ml (4,91). It is also active in vitro against *Pseudomonas cepacia* (94), but most other *Pseudomonas* species are resistant. Cefoperazone, moxalactam, and cefsulodin are moderately active against *P. aeruginosa*; cefotaxime, ceftizoxime, ceftriaxone, and cefmenoxime are less active, although more active than the first- or second-generation cephalosporins. None of these antibiotics has appreciable activity against other Pseudomonads, such as *P. maltophilia*, with MIC_{90} invariably exceeding 128 μg/ml. Ceftazidime is also the most active cephalosporin against *Acinetobacter*, which are generally resistant to the other third-generation compounds at clinically achievable concentrations.

Of the third-generation cephalosporins discussed, moxalactam is the most active against *B. fragilis*, with activity similar to that of cefoxitin, but less than that of clindamycin, chloramphenicol, or metronidazole. Other anaerobic species, such as *Clostridium perfingens, Peptostreptococcus* sp., and *Fusobacterium* sp., are sensitive to the third-generation cephalosporins to varying degrees (92-96).

A number of bacterial species are consistently resistant to the third-generation cephalosporins. In addition to the methicillin-resistant *Staphylococcus aureus* and *S. epidermidis, Streptococcus faecalis* and *Pseudomonas* sp. mentioned, penicillin-resistant *S. pneumoniae, L. monocytogenes, Clostridium difficile, Campylobacter jejuni*, and *Legionella pneumophilia* are generally not susceptible to any of these antibiotics (4).

In Table 4, the relative activities of the third-generation cephalosporins against selected bacterial species are listed.

D. Oral Cephalosporins

Until recently, the orally administered cephalosporins generally shared the antibacterial spectra of the parenteral first-generation agents, albeit with a somewhat lower degree of activity. Cephalexin is active against *S. aureus*, with the majority of reported MIC_{90} values ranging between 6 and 8 μg/ml (97,98). The streptococci, with the exception of the enterococci, are also susceptible to the drug, as are some gram-negative organisms, such as *E. coli, P. mirabilis*, and *Klebsiella* sp. Only minor differences in antibacterial activity are apparent among cephalexin, cephradine, and cefadroxil. Cefaclor, on the other hand, is essentially equivalent to cephalexin and cephradine against staphylococci and

Table 4 Comparative Activities of Third-generation Cephalosporins Against Common Pathogens[a]

Organism	Most active → Least active
Staphylococcus aureus	CTX = CTZ > CTR = CPZ > CAZ > MOX
Streptococcus pyogenes	CTX = CTZ = CTR > CPZ > CAZ > MOX
S. pneumoniae	CTX = CTZ > CTR > CAZ = CPZ > MOX
S. faecalis	CTX = CTZ = CTR = CAZ = CPZ = MOX
Hemophilus influenzae	CTR > CTX = CTZ > MOX > CAZ = CPZ
Neisseria gonorrhoeae	CTR > CTX = CTZ > MOX = CPZ > CAZ
N. meningitidis	CTX = CTZ = CTR = CAZ > CPZ = MOX
Escherichia coli	CTX = CTZ = CTR = MOX > CAZ > CPZ
Klebsiella pneumonia	CTX = CTZ = CTR = MOX = CAZ > CPZ
Enterobacter cloacae	MOX > CTX = CTZ = CTR = CAZ > CPZ
Serratia marcescens	CAZ = CTZ > CTX = CTR = MOX > CPZ
Proteus mirabilis	CTR > CTX = CTZ > CAZ = MOX > CPZ
Salmonella sp.	CTX = CTZ = CTR = MOX = CAZ > CPZ
Shigella sp.	CTX = CTZ = CTR = MOX = CAZ > CPZ
Pseudomonas aeruginosa	CAZ > CPZ = MOX > CTX = CTZ = CTR
Pseudomonas sp.	CTX = CTZ = CTR = CAZ = CPZ = MOX
Acinetobacter	CAZ > CTX = CTZ = CTR = CPZ = MOX
Bacteroides fragilis	MOX = CTZ > CTX = CTR = CPZ > CAZ

[a]CTX, cefotaxime; CTZ, ceftizoxime; CTR, ceftriaxone; CAZ, ceftazidime; CPZ, cefoperazone; MOX, moxalactam.

Source: Adapted from Reference 4.

streptococci but is more active against *E. coli, P. mirabilis*, and *K. pneumoniae* (98,99). In addition, both ampicillin-resistant and ampicillin-nonresistant strains of *H. influenzae* are more susceptible to cefaclor than to these other oral cephalosporins, with the majority of isolates inhibited by a concentration of 6.25 μg/ml (100). Indole-positive *Proteus, Enterobacter, Pseudomonas*, and *Serratia* are resistant to these agents.

Cefuroxime axetil is the recently developed 1-acetoxyethyl ester prodrug of cefuroxime (101). Following oral administration, the prodrug is well absorbed from the gastrointestinal tract and de-esterified by nonspecific esterases to cefuroxime.

Most recently, a new oral cephalosporin, cefixime, possessing a spectrum of activity comparable to the third-generation cephalosporins, has become available for clinical testing. Cefixime is less active than cephalexin or cefaclor against *S. aureus* and *S. epidermidis*, similar in activity to cefaclor toward streptococci, and considerably more active than either against clinical isolates of *E. coli, K. pneumoniae, P. mirabilis, Proteus vulgaris, Providencia* sp., *Salmonella* sp., *Shigella* sp., *H. influenzae*, and *N. gonorrhoeae*. The MIC_{90} for the majority of these gram-negative organisms is below 0.5 μg/ml, the exceptions being *E. coli* (MIC_{90} = 2.5 μg/ml) and *Providencia* sp. (MIC_{90} = 0.5–1 μg/ml) (102, 103). Nonsusceptible species include *P. aeruginosa* and *Pseudomonas* sp., *Acinetobacter*, and *B. fragilis*.

V. CLINICAL PHARMACOLOGY

Clinical pharmacological data for the cephalosporins have been obtained following analysis by both microbiologic and chromatographic methods. In general, drug concentrations from clinical pharmacological studies conducted with the first- and second-generation cephalosporins were most often analyzed by microbiologic assays. Recently, there has been an increasing tendency to use more specific chromatographic techniques, although many studies continue to use bioassay methodology. As a result, pharmacokinetic data for cephalosporins with active metabolites are difficult to interpret if the drug concentrations in body fluids were measured with assays unable to distinguish between the parent compound and an active metabolite. Cephalothin, for example, is metabolized to desacetylcephalothin, which has approximately one-fifth the activity of the parent drug (17). Serum concentrations measured by bioassay, therefore, represent total activities of cephalothin and desacetylcephalothin. In addition, the proportion of each can be expected to change over the course of a pharmacokinetic study such that the combined activity against the test organism is changing as a function of time. Cephapirin and cefotaxime also have active metabolites, and pharmacokinetic data derived from microbiologic analysis for these drugs must also be interpreted with these considerations in mind.

Tables 5, 6, and 7 summarize clinical pharmacological data for a number of cephalosporins in different pediatric age groups. Direct comparisons between different studies are limited by small sample sizes, the doses studied, and inherent differences in patient populations. In particular, few pharmacokinetic data are available for the earlier cephalosporins (126).

A. Cephalothin

Cephalothin is not absorbed to an appreciable extent following oral administration, with less than 10% of an oral dose recovered in the urine. Intramuscular absorption is complete (127,128). A dose of 12.5 mg/kg IM to premature and full-term newborns produces peak

Table 5 Summary of Pharmacokinetic Data for First- and Second-generation Cephalosporins

Drug	Patient age group	$t_{1/2\beta}$ (hr)	Protein binding (%)	Distribution volume (liter/kg)	Total clearance (ml/min kg^{-1})	Renal clearance (ml/min kg^{-1})	Urinary excretion (%)	CSF Penetration (%)
First generation								
Cephalothin	Children	0.3		0.93				
	Adults	0.6	65	0.20	6.7	3.9	60	Poor
Cephapirin	Children							
	Adults	0.4	50	0.23		4.9	72	Poor
Cefazolin	Children	1.7					75	
	Adults	2.0	85	0.12	0.85	0.80	88	Poor
Second generation								
Cefamandole	Newborns	1.0		0.45				
	Infants	1.5		0.40				
	Children	1.0		0.40				
	Adults	0.8	75	0.27	3.0	2.6	75	Poor
Cefoxitin	Newborns	3.8		0.58	1.8			
	Infants	1.4		0.50	4.5		73	
	Children	0.8			6.0			
	Adults	0.8	70	0.16	4.8	4.0	85	Poor
Cefuroxime	Newborns	5.5						
	Infants	3.5		0.65	2.8			
	Children	1.2		0.65	2.8			14–18
	Adults	1.5	35	0.27	2.2	2.0	95	

Table 6 Summary of Pharmacokinetic Data for Third-generation Cephalosporins

Drug	Patient age group	$t_{1/2\beta}$ (hr)	Protein binding (%)	Distribution volume (liter/kg)	Total clearance (ml/min kg^{-1})	Renal clearance (ml/min kg^{-1})	Urinary excretion (%)	CSF Penetration (%)
Cefotaxime	Premature newborns	4.6		0.60	0.8			
	Term newborns	4.0		0.60	1.7			
	Infants	0.8		0.35	4.7	2.8	61	
	Children	1.0		0.35	4.7	2.8		
	Adults	1.1	38	0.25	4.5	2.5	60	20–30
Moxalactam	Premature newborns	7.6		0.52	16[a]			
	Term newborns	5.4		0.54	28[a]			
	Infants	1.7		0.45	31[a]			
	Children	1.6		0.30	120[a]			
	Adults	2.2	52	0.28	85[a]	77[a]	75	20–30
Cefoperazone	Premature newborns	7.5		0.53			55	
	Term newborns	4.9		0.45	0.8		37	
	Infants	2.4		0.40				
	Children	2.1		0.40	1.8			
	Adults	2.1	90	0.17	1.2	0.3	25	~5
Ceftazidime	Premature newborns	7.0		0.53	1.0			
	Term newborns	4.5		0.54	1.8			
	Infants	4.5						
	Children	2.0						
	Adults	1.8	⩽20	0.25	1.9	1.5	>90	25
Ceftriaxone	Term newborns	17.0	72	0.52	0.31		70	
	Infants	5.9		0.38	0.83	0.38	43	
	Children	4.7		0.37	0.83	0.45	52	
	Adults	7.8	95	0.15	0.23	0.11	46	17

[a]Clearance units, ml/min 1.73 m^{-2}.

Table 7 Summary of Absorption Characteristics of Oral Cephalosporins

Drug	Patient age group	Dose	Dosage form	Status	Peak concentration (mg/liter)	Time to peak (hr)	Availability (%)	$t_{1/2\beta}$ (hr)	Protein binding (%)	Urinary excretion (%)
Cephalexin	Newborns	15 mg/kg	Suspension		10.0	3.0		5.0		40
	Infants, children	15 mg/kg	Suspension	Fasting	23.4	0.5–1.0		1.0		
		15 mg/kg	Suspension	Fed	9.0	1.0		1.0		
	Adults	1000 mg	Capsule	Fasting	31.0	1.0		0.9	<10	90
		1000 mg	Capsule	Fed	20.9	2.0	90			
Cephradine	Infants, children	15 mg/kg	Suspension	Fasting	21.3	0.5		0.8		
		15 mg/kg	Suspension	Fed	9.9	0.5		1.0		
	Adults	500 mg	Capsule	Fasting	15.0	1.0	90	0.7	<20	92
		500 mg	Suspension	Fasting	19.5	0.5				
Cefadroxil	Infants, children	15 mg/kg	Suspension	Fasting	13.7	1.0		1.3		
		15 mg/kg	Suspension	Fed	11.0	1.0		1.5		
		15 mg/kg	Capsule	Fasting	12.4	2.0		1.3		
		15 mg/kg	Capsule	Fed	11.6	2.0		1.7		
	Adults	300 mg	Capsule	Fasting	10.0	1.0	94	1.4	<10	93
Cefaclor	Infants, children	15 mg/kg	Suspension	Fasting	13.1	0.5		0.6		
		15 mg/kg	Suspension	Fed	10.9	0.5		0.7		
	Adults	500 mg	Capsule	Fasting	12.4	1.0	90	1.0		
		500 mg	Capsule	Fed	6.0	2.0–3.0			25	70
Cefuroxime axetil	Infants, children	15 mg/kg	Crushed tablet	Fasting	4.6	1.5		1.3		
		15 mg/kg	Crushed tablet	Fed	6.2	2.0		1.4		
	Adults	500 mg	Tablet	Fasting	3.6	1.5	30	1.4		30
		500 mg	Tablet	Fed	4.5	2.0	40–50	1.4	33	42
Cefixime	Adults	50 mg	Not stated	Fasting	1.0	2.7	–	3.0		
		400 mg	Not stated	Fasting	3.9	4.3	–	3.1	31	20

concentrations of 20-25 μg/ml at 30 min after administration; in older infants and children aged 2.5 months to 5 years of age, the same dose achieves slightly lower concentrations of 15-17 μg/ml (129).

Limited pediatric pharmacokinetic data are available for cephalothin, although in adults, cephalothin is 65% protein bound and distributes into pleural, synovial, and ascitic fluids and broncial secretions (128,130). Atrial appendage concentrations of cephalothin ranging from 8 to 50 μg/g are reported following a single intravenous dose of 30 mg/kg to pediatric patients undergoing open-heart surgery, declining with a half-life of 30 min (131).

Penetration of cephalothin into the cerebral spinal fluid (CSF) is poor in both the absence and presence of inflamed meninges, although somewhat better under the latter conditions. CSF concentrations range between 0.16 and 0.31 μg/ml despite concurrent serum concentrations of 80-100 μg/ml (132).

Transfer of cephalothin through the placenta is rapid, with therapeutic concentrations appearing in the amniotic fluid within 15 min of intramuscular or intravenous maternal administration (129,133).

Cephalothin is rapidly metabolized in vivo and in vitro by tissue esterases to desacetylcephalothin. For reasons discussed earlier, the limited pediatric pharmacokinetic data for this drug must be interpreted with caution. Measured by high-performance liquid chromatography (HPLC), serum cephalothin concentrations in children aged 1.5-9 years decline with an estimated half-life of 18.6 min. The distribution volume is 0.93 liter/kg. Approximately 25% of an administered dose is recovered in the urine as metabolite (134). With less specific assays, the biologic half-life is reported to be approximately 30-40 min (126).

Both cephalothin and desacetylcephalothin are renally eliminated, the former by glomerular filtration and tubular secretion. Concurrent probenecid administration increases serum concentrations and reduces renal clearance of the total activity (127). Renal clearance is approximately 60% of total body clearance in adults (130). In adult patients with renal dysfunction (creatinine clearance less than 10 ml/min), the biologic half-life of cephalothin is prolonged to 3.7 hr and the clearance of desacetylcephalothin markedly impaired, resulting in metabolite accumulation (135). Hemodialysis has minimal effects on serum half-life; peritoneal dialysis is reported to reduce serum concentration by 25% (136). No data are available for pediatric patients with renal disease.

B. Cephapirin

Like cephalothin, cephapirin is poorly absorbed from the gastrointestinal tract. Intramuscular administration of 12.5- and 20-mg/kg doses to children produce peaks of 7.6 and 14.5 μg/ml, respectively (137). The drug is 45-55% protein bound and is metabolized to desacetylcephapirin, which has approximately one-half the activity of the parent compound (138). The major route of elimination, however, is the kidney, with urinary concentrations of 1600 μg/ml achieved after a 20-mg/kg intramuscular dose to children (137). Approximately 72% of an administered dose can be recovered in the urine after 6 hr (139). Serum half-life is prolonged in azotemic adults and is minimally affected by dialysis (138).

C. Cefazolin

Because of poor oral absorption, cefazolin is only administered parenterally. In patients aged 0.5-15 years, intramuscular injection of 5.0-6.25 mg/kg and 10-12.5 mg/kg produces mean peak concentrations of approximately 28 and 42 μg/ml, respectively, 0.5-1.0 hr after administration (140,141). In premature infants and newborns, intramuscular doses of 20 mg/kg produce peak concentrations of 32.0 μg/ml compared with concentrations of 54.4, 40.0, and 18.7 μg/ml in premature infants, full-term infants, and older children, respectively, receiving 50-mg/kg doses by the same route (126). The decline in peak serum concentration with age is attributed to the maturation of renal processes.

Few pharmacokinetic parameters from pediatric patients are available. The protein binding of cefazolin is approximately 85%, with a distribution volume of 0.10-0.14 liter/kg in adults (142). Penetration into the CSF is negligible regardless of the degree of meningeal inflammation (143,144). In adults with normal and diseased biliary tracts, cefazolin concentrations in bile from the gallbladder and common bile duct generally exceed concurrent serum concentrations (145). Cefazolin concentrations achieved in pus and bone from children with osteomyelitis treated with cefazolin are reported to be 9 and 3.9% of the serum concentration, respectively (146). The appearance of cefazolin in breast milk is minimal, and one study has estimated that less than 0.075% of a dose would appear in the milk on the basis of observed cefazolin concentrations in the milk of lactating mothers who received 2-g intravenous doses (147).

Cefazolin is not metabolized to an appreciable extent and is eliminated unchanged by the kidney via glomerular filtration and tubular secretion (130). High urinary concentrations of 850 and 1425 μg/ml were achieved following intramuscular doses of 6.25 and 10-12.5 mg/kg to children, respectively (140). Essentially 100% of an administered dose can be recovered in the urine within 24 hr; in children aged 6 months to 10 years, 75% of a dose can be accounted for in a 6-hr collection (148).

Estimates of cefazolin half-life in children are limited. Serum concentrations in pediatric osteomyelitis patients aged 2-16 years decline with half-lives of 1.7 and 1.8 hr after intravenous and intramuscular administration, respectively (146). These values are comparable to reported half-lives in adults with normal renal function (149). The half-life is progressively prolonged as creatinine clearance decreases in children with renal insufficiency who are not maintained on dialysis. Half-lives of 3.8-115.5 hr have been associated with reductions in creatinine clearance from 57 ml/min 1.73 m^{-2} to 1.6 ml/min 1.73 m^{-2}. In pediatric renal patients requiring regular hemodialysis, serum cefazolin concentrations measured during dialysis are reduced by 40-64% and decline with half-lives ranging between 8.3 and 29.5 hr (150). These results are similar to findings in adults with comparable degrees of renal impairment. Cefazolin is 74% absorbed after intraperitoneal instillation, and continuous ambulatory peritoneal dialysis (CAPD) accounts for approximately 20% of total body clearance in adult patients (151).

D. Second-Generation Cephalosporins

1. Cefamandole

Cefamandole is not detected in the circulation following oral dosing and is usually administered parenterally as cefamandole nafate, the sodium salt of the O-formyl ester. Hydrolysis to cefamandole is rapid and practically complete within 2 hr (152). Intramuscular administration of 17 and 33 mg/kg to newborns 11-23 days of age produces mean serum concentrations of 34.6 and 72 μg/ml, respectively, 30 min after dosing (153). Slightly lower concentrations are obtained after intramuscular dosing to older infants and children (154). The distribution volume of cefamandole is between 0.4 and 0.5 liter/kg for newborns, infants, and children (153,154), somewhat larger than the adult value of 0.25-0.30 liter/kg (128). It penetrates well into a number of tissues and body fluids, including synovial fluid, bone, gallbladder tissue and bile, pericardial fluid, and right atrial appendage (155), despite a relatively high degree (70-75%) of protein binding (156). Concentrations of 5-40 μg/ml have been achieved in joint fluid 1-4 hr after intramuscular and intravenous doses of 25 mg/kg in children with bone, joint, or soft tissue infections (157).

Cefamandole does not penetrate well into the cerebrospinal fluid (CSF) in the absence of inflamed meninges. CSF concentrations of cefamandole obtained from infants and children receiving doses of 33-37 mg/kg did not exceed 0.8 μg/ml, less than 4% of concurrent serum levels. Higher concentrations occur in the presence of meningeal inflammation but are insufficient to warrant recommendation for the treatment of central nervous system (CNS) infections (158,159).

The main route of elimination is renal, with excretion by a combination of glomerular filtration and tubular secretion. In adults with normal renal function, the renal clearance of cefamandole is reduced from 300 ml/min 1.73 m^{-2} to 80 ml/min 1.73 m^{-2} when administered with probenecid (160). Approximately 75-90% of a dose can be recovered in the urine 6 hr after an intravenous dose (156). There is no appreciable metabolism of the drug.

The half-life of cefamandole demonstrates an age-related decrease from approximately 1-2 hr in infants less than 3 months to 1 hr in children older than 1 year (154,158). The half-life in adults is approximately 50-55 min (156) and can be prolonged to 18 hr in the presence of renal dysfunction (161). Peritoneal dialysis removes cefamandole from the body very slowly, but hemodialysis is more efficient, reducing the half-life to between 2.5 and 8.0 hr during a 4 to 6-hr session.

2. Cefoxitin

Absorption of cefoxitin after intramuscular administration is rapid, with peak concentrations of 68.5 μg/ml 15 min after a 37.5-mg/kg dose to children aged 3 months to 12.6 years (162). This route is often painful, and the use of 0.5-1% lidocaine is recommended as a diluent (163). The bioavailability of intramuscular cefoxitin is estimated to be 95% and unaffected by the presence of lidocaine. A dose of 30 mg/kg infused over 15 min in infants less than 2 months of age produces concentrations of 70 μg/ml immediately post-infusion (164).

Cefoxitin is approximately 70% protein bound (16,165), although the degree of binding is reduced to 42% in adults with end-stage renal disease. High drug concentrations are attained in gallbladder tissue and bile, lung tissue, peritoneal fluid, synovial fluid, and bone (155). Cefoxitin readily crosses the placental barrier (166), but concentrations in breast milk are less than 1 μg/ml, 100-fold less than peak serum concentrations (167).

Penetration of an intact blood-brain barrier is poor even after multiple-dose administration with or without concurrent probenecid administration. Some improvement occurs with inflamed meninges, but the concentrations achieved are generally considered inadequate for clinical use (168). Doses of 75 mg/kg every 6 hr to infants and children between the ages of 4 and 57 months with meningitis produce peak CSF concentrations of 5-6 μg/ml (169).

The volume of distribution demonstrates some age dependence, decreasing from 0.58 liter/kg in newborn and premature infants studied within 2 weeks of birth (170) to 0.50 liter/kg in infants less than 2 months old (164). In comparison, adult values range from 0.16 liter/kg in subjects with normal renal function to 0.40 liter/kg in functionally anephric patients (155).

Less than 2% of cefoxitin is metabolized to an inactive decarbamoyl derivative. Elimination is primarily renal, consisting of both glomerular filtration and tubular secretion (16). Concurrent probenecid administration reduces the renal clearance by more than 50% and doubles the serum half-life but does not affect urinary recovery of the drug (171). In infants less than 2 months of age, approximately 73% of an intravenously administered dose is recovered in the urine within 8 hr, similar to the value of 80% for adults (16,155).

The serum half-life is dependent on age, averaging 3.75 hr (range, 2-6.9 hr) in premature and term newborns (170). The half-life is correlated with postnatal age owing to the tendencies of distribution volume and clearance to decrease and increase, respectively, with age. By 2 months, the half-life is 1.4 hr (164) and reaches adult values of 50 min by approximately 4 months of age (162). As expected, these developmental changes in half-life reflect the maturation of renal function. Total clearance is lowest in the premature and term newborns (0.11 liter/hr kg^{-1}) and increases to 0.27 liter/hr kg^{-1} in infants less than 2 months of age (164,170). The most rapid clearance occurs in children 3-12.6 years old (162), approximately 430 ml/min 1.73 m^{-2}, somewhat larger than the adult values of 300-340 ml/min 1.73 m^{-2} (16). Clearance is reduced to 13 ml/min 1.73 m^{-2} and the half-life prolonged to 23.5 hr in the presence of severe renal dysfunction (155). Hemodialysis shortens the half-life but peritoneal dialysis has no effect, constituting only 7.4% of the total clearance in these patients (155). No data are available for pediatric patients with renal disease.

3. Cefuroxime

Cefuroxime sodium is not appreciably absorbed after oral dosing, with less than 1% of a dose recovered in the urine (172). The acetoxyethyl ester, cefuroxime axetil, is more suitable for oral administration (see Section V.F). In infants less than 3 weeks of age, cefuroxime concentrations 30-60 min after doses of 10 mg/kg to infants less than 3 weeks of age were 15-25 μg/ml, with a tendency toward lower concentrations in older members of the group (173). Administration of 15 mg/kg IM produced similar levels at 30 min (26.6 μg/ml) in older infants aged 3 weeks to 24 months (174).

Cefuroxime is 33-41% protein bound, a relatively low degree of binding compared with other cephalosporins, such as cefamandole, cefazolin, or cefoxitin (172). It distributes into a volume approximating the extracellular space and penetrates well into bile, sputum, pleural fluid, synovial fluid, bone, pericardial fluid, atrial appendages, and middle ear effusions (175,176). The penetration of cefuroxime into the CSF is increased in the presence of inflamed meninges (173,177) and tends to decrease as meningitis resolves. In infants and children 1 month to 14 years with meningitis, cefuroxime levels in the CSF range between 1.1 and 17.1 μg/ml upon completion of an intravenous regimen of 50 mg/kg every 6 hr. CSF concentrations are estimated to be 14-18% of concurrent serum concentrations, although extreme values of 3.2 and 36.9% have been reported (177-179). There is also evidence that penetration is dose dependent. Administration of cefuroxime to pregnant women has produced detectable drug concentrations in the myometrium, amniotic fluid, placenta, and umbilical cord (180,181).

Cefuroxime is not metabolized and is excreted unchanged in the urine by glomerular filtration and tubular secretion, the latter accounting for approximately 45-50% of the renal clearance based on studies with probenecid (172). About 95% of an intravenous dose is recovered in the urine within 24 hr, the majority being excreted during the first 6 hr (172,176). The total body clearance of cefuroxime in infants and children (1 month to 6.5 years) is 195 ml/min 1.73 m^{-2} (179), somewhat higher than the renal clearance in adults with normal renal function, which ranges between 130 and 145 ml/min 1.73 m^{-2} (172,182). The half-life of cefuroxime is age-dependent, ranging from approximately 5.5 hr in 1 to 2-day-old newborns to 3–4 hr by 2 weeks of age (173). In infants and older children, the half-life is decreased to 1.0–1.5 hr (174,179), comparable to values in adults (172). When glomerular filtration falls below 20 ml/min, a marked prolongation of the cefuroxime half-life occurs accompanied by a reduction in the fraction of the dose excreted in the urine (183). The half-life is reduced from 22 hr to 3–4 hr by hemodialysis and 12–13.5 hr by peritoneal dialysis (184). Cefuroxime kinetics are unaffected by hepatic cirrhosis in the absence of ascites (185).

4. Other Second-Generation Cephalosporins

Cefonicid is unique among the second-generation cephalosporins, with a half-life of 3.5–4.4 hr in adult volunteers (186,187). Although its protein binding exceeds 95%, cefonicid achieves detectable concentrations in a number of tissues and body fluids but does not appear in breast milk (187). Elimination is primarily renal, with approximately 90% recovery in the urine after 48 hr (186). Studies with probenecid indicate that tubular secretion is the predominant renal mechanism present (187). The renal clearance is reduced from 18 ml/min to less than 0.1 ml/min in adults with end-stage renal disease maintained on hemodialysis. This is associated with a prolongation in half-life to approximately 65 hr (188). There are no available pediatric kinetic data for cefonicid.

Very limited ceforanide kinetic data exist for children. In infants and children 1 month to 17 years old, a 20-mg/kg intramuscular dose produces serum concentrations of 27–95 μg/ml 1 hr after dosing. Concentrations achieved and distribution volume appear unrelated to patient age. In contrast, the half-life in infants 1–2 years old (1.5 hr) is significantly shorter than in younger and older children in whom values are between 1.8 and 3.3 hr (189,190). In adults, the half-life is also relatively long compared with other first- and second-generation cephalosporins, averaging between 2.7 and 3.5 hr (191–193). Ceforanide demonstrates tissue penetration characteristics similar to those of cefonicid (187). It is approximately 80% protein bound and primarily eliminated renally, with 90% of a dose recovered intact in the urine (189,191). Half the renal clearance has been attributed to tubular secretion (191), although simultaneous probenecid administration does not alter any kinetic parameters. Severe renal dysfunction prolongs the half-life to approximately 25 hr, and hemodialysis removes 21–53% of a dose (193,194).

E. Third-Generation Cephalosporins

1. Cefotaxime

Interpretating cefotaxime pharmacokinetic studies is complicated by the presence of the active desacetyl metabolite. In hemolysed blood, cefotaxime is rapidly converted to desacetylcefotaxime, possibly producing misleading pharmacokinetic data when serum concentrations are subsequently analyzed, particularly since the two compounds have different kinetic properties. In addition, some bioassay test organisms are unable to differentiate between cefotaxime and its less active metabolite. For these reasons, widely disparate pharmacokinetic parameters may be obtained from apparently comparable study groups. Therefore, the kinetic parameters for cefotaxime in Table 6 are derived as much as possible from studies employing HPLC methodology.

Cefotaxime is administered only by parenteral routes. A dose of 50 mg/kg IM to neonates produces mean peak concentrations of 85-90 μg/ml approximately 10 min after injection (195). Immediately upon completion of an intravenous infusion of the same dose, concentrations of 115-120 μg/ml are achieved in newborns less than 1.5 kg and approximately 135 μg/ml in newborns greater than 1.5 kg (196). Comparable levels are seen after 50 mg/kg IV to older infants and children (197).

Cefotaxime is 30% bound to serum proteins and is widely distributed to different body tissues (4), although penetration through noninflamed meninges is negligible (198). After maternal doses of 1 g, cefotaxime activity can be detected in the cord blood, amniotic fluid, and fetus but not in breast milk (199,200).

In the presence of inflamed meninges, CSF concentrations of cefotaxime are higher and more reliable than those of the first- and second-generation cephalosporins, achieving levels that are manyfold greater than the MBC for common causative organisms of pediatric bacterial meningitis (201-204). CNS penetration of cefotaxime is correlated with the degree of inflammation, although there is no marked decline in concentration after 7-10 days of therapy and apparent resolution of the signs of inflammation (203, 204). In samples obtained 1-2 days after initiation of 50 mg/kg IV every 6 hr, the CSF-serum ratio for cefotaxime is approximately 5-10% and 20-30% at 1 and 3 hr after dosing, respectively. This appears to be a function of the rapid decline of serum concentrations and slower partitioning of the drug into the CSF. Desacetylcefotaxime penetrates more readily with CSF to serum ratios of 17-36% and 27-52% at 1 and 3 hr after dosing, respectively (197,201-204). In contrast to cefotaxime, however, penetration of the desacetyl metabolite decreases substantially, with continuing therapy only about 5% after 7 days of treatment (203). Higher degrees of CNS penetration have been reported following microbiologic analysis (203,205). In general, the degrees of penetration cited correspond to CSF cefotaxime concentrations of 4-6 μg/ml with a range of 0-30 μg/ml.

The volume of distribution of cefotaxime is age dependent, being approximately 0.6 liter/kg in premature and term newborns, 0.35 liter/kg in infants and children, and 0.25 liter/kg in adults. Likewise, the half-life and total body clearance show age-related trends that reflect the changes in renal function that accompany maturation (see Table 6). The half-life declines from 4-6 hr in premature newborns (195,196,205-207) to approximately 1 hr or less by 1 month of age, comparable to values in older children and adults (197, 208-210).

The metabolism of cefotaxime to desacetylcefotaxime constitutes 25-30% of the total body clearance. Serum concentrations of the desacetyl metabolite vary among different pediatric age groups and among individual patients but appear shortly after cefotaxime is injected, reaching peak concentrations within 1.5-2.0 hr. Serum concentrations exceeding those of cefotaxime occur by 2-4 hr and decline, with an apparent half-life of 2.1 hr in infants and children (195,196,207). Similar patterns are present in adults (209-211). Another two inactive metabolites, in which the β-lactam ring is opened, have been detected in the serum of neonates (195) and renal failure patients but are generally not found in individuals with normal renal function. Significant concentrations are present in urine, however (212,213).

Approximately 80% of a cefotaxime dose can be recovered in the urine, half as the parent compound and the remainder as desacetylcefotaxime and other inactive metabolites (209,214). The urinary elimination of cefotaxime involves both glomerular filtration and tubular secretion; concomitant administration of probenecid reduces renal clearance by almost 50% (209).

Total plasma and renal clearance and urinary recovery of intact cefotaxime are decreased in patients with severely impaired renal function (creatinine clearance less than 10 ml/min), and this is reflected in the prolonged half-life of 2.5 hr. Clearance of desacetylcefotaxime is more markedly reduced (from 235 to 2.5 ml/min in patients with creatinine clearance less than 6 ml/min), with a corresponding prolongation of the half-life to 10-23 hr. The distribution volume is not significantly affected by the degree of renal impairment (211,212,215). Hemodialysis reduces the cefotaxime half-life to about 1.5 hr and that of desacetylcefotaxime to approximately 3 hr while removing 40 and 53% of each compound, respectively (212). Cefotaxime is rapidly absorbed from the peritoneal cavity in CAPD patients but is not as efficiently removed by this process as by hemodialysis (216). The pharmacokinetics of cefotaxime are not affected by the presence of hepatic dysfunction (211).

2. Moxalactam

Moxalactam is a mixture of two epimers, R and S, with the R epimer possessing twice the in vitro activity of the S epimer (217). It is not absorbed from the gastrointestinal tract and is therefore given only parenterally. Intramuscular administration of 50 mg/kg to neonates produces peak concentrations of approximately 100 μg/ml 1.6 hr after dosing (218). The same dose infused intravenously over 10-15 min to infants and children older than 1 month results in moxalactam concentrations of 100-125 μg/ml 30 min after completion of the infusion (219,220). Comparable concentrations are achieved after similar doses in adults. The repeated administration of moxalactam does not result in accumulation of the drug (221).

Moxalactam is 52% protein bound in healthy adults but only 36% bound in sera from chronic renal failure patients (222). The protein binding of the S epimer is greater than that of the R epimer (223). Moxalactam is widely distributed throughout the body, reaching inhibitory concentrations in several tissues and fluids, including peritoneal fluid, common duct bile, bone, and others (224-226). Entry into the CSF is good in patients with bacterial meningitis, although it may be unpredictable in some (227). The average percentage penetration of moxalactam into the CSF is 20-30% compared with serum concentrations. Average CSF moxalactam concentrations 1-2 hr after a multiple dose regimen of 50 mg/kg to infants and children range from 6 to 20 μg/ml (227-229). Comparable penetration is observed in adult patients, decreasing slightly over the course of therapy (229). Mean moxalactam concentrations in breast milk are approximately 3.5 μg/ml, producing an estimated daily dose of 0.5-0.6 mg/kg to breast-fed infants (230).

The distribution volume is age related, ranging from a value of 0.52 liter/kg in neonates (218,219,221) to 0.35 liter/kg in infants and children, with the R epimer distributing into a larger volume (0.38 liter/kg) than the S epimer (0.29 liter/kg) (220,231). The volume of distribution is increased in pediatric renal failure patients to 0.64 liter/kg in an interdialytic period and to 0.82 liter/kg during hemodialysis (232). In adults with normal renal function, the distribution volume is 0.2-0.3 liter/kg (209). Slightly larger values occur in end-stage renal disease, but the increase is less dramatic than that observed in children (233-235).

Moxalactam is not appreciably metabolized and is excreted in the urine primarily by glomerular filtration. High but variable concentrations occur in urine, and renal clearance is generally 90% of total body clearance (209). In neonates weighing less than 2000 g at birth, total clearance is 16 ml/min 1.73 m^{-2}, approximately 50% that for neonates greater than 2 kg and infants less than 1 month old. Clearance is most rapid in older children (120 ml/min 1.73 m^{-2}) and gradually declines to approximately 85 ml/min 1.73 m^{-2} in adults. As a result, the serum half-life demonstrates a similar age dependence, ranging from 7.6 hr in neonates to 1.6 hr in children and approximately 2.2 hr in adults (218-222,228-232,236).

There is a direct correlation between half-life and creatinine clearance (234), and as would be expected, the elimination of moxalactam is delayed in patients with renal impairment. In both children and adults with renal dysfunction, the half-life is approximately 15-20 hr but is reduced to 3-5 hr during hemodialysis, with approximately 50% of a dose recovered in the dialysate (232,233,235). Peritoneal clearance of both the R and S epimers in CAPD patients is minimal, averaging approximately 10% of total clearance. However, both are well absorbed systemically following instillation into the peritoneal cavity, with average absolute bioavailabilities of 71 and 79%, respectively (237).

3. Cefoperazone

Like the other third-generation cephalosporins, cefoperazone is available for parenteral administration only. In infants, peak serum concentrations are achieved 15-30 min after intramuscular administration (238). Intravenous doses of 50 mg/kg generally produce serum cefoperazone concentrations between 110 and 140 μg/ml in most age groups 30 min after administration (238,239). Larger doses result in proportionally higher serum concentrations (238-241).

Cefoperazone is 90% protein bound and distributes to a number of tissues and body fluids, producing particularly high concentrations in bile with peak concentrations after a 2-g dose often exceeding 3000 μg/ml (242). The penetration of cefoperazone into the CSF is increased in the presence of meningeal inflammation but to a somewhat lesser extent than other cephalosporins. The unreliable CSF concentrations observed after single doses may be improved with multiple dosing (240,243). Single 50-mg/kg infusions of cefoperazone generally produce CSF concentrations of 1-7 μg/ml within 2-4 hr of dosing, representing about 5% of the concurrent serum concentration (239). The degree of CNS penetration following 100-mg/kg doses is similar to the lower doses, although the actual CSF concentrations are slightly higher (240).

The distribution volume in premature and term newborns ranges from 0.4 to 0.5 liter/kg and is unaffected by either birth weight or gestational age (239,244). Smaller values have been reported in infants and young children (238,240), reaching a value of 0.2 liter/kg in adults (245).

Cefoperazone is minimally metabolized and only 25-30% is excreted in the urine, suggesting, in conjunction with the high biliary concentrations observed, that the main route of elimination is via the bile. The serum half-life is longest in premature newborns less than 33 weeks gestation (9.4 hr) and approximately 7 hr in term newborns and reaches the adult value of 2.1 hr by 1 month of age (238-244). Estimates of cefoperazone total body clearance in pediatric patients are few but range between 1 and 2 ml/min kg^{-1} (240,241,243). No values are available for renal clearance, but a slightly higher percentage of cefoperazone (35-40%) is recovered in the urine of newborns compared with adults (239).

Pharmacokinetic parameters are unaffected by severe renal insufficiency or CAPD provided that hepatic function is normal (245,246). Systemic absorption from intraperitoneally administered cefoperazone ranges from 65 to 95%, with an absorption half-life of approximately 1 hr in adults (246). Peritoneal clearance of cefoperazone during CAPD represents approximately 10% of the total clearance in these patients (246).

In contrast, the half-life of cefoperazone in patients with biliary disease is prolonged to about 6 hr. Total body clearance is approximately 50% of normal, but renal clearance is unaffected (242). Analogous data in children are not available.

4. Ceftazidime

Oral absorption being negligible, ceftazidime is administered primarily by parenteral routes. In neonates, peak concentrations of 50–100 μg/ml occur 0.5–1.5 hr after intramuscular doses of 25–50 mg/kg (247,248). Intravenous infusion of 50 mg/kg to the same age group produces peak concentrations of 100–120 μg/ml immediately postdose regardless of gestational age (249). Ceftazidime is 90% bioavailable after intramuscular administration.

Ceftazidime exhibits a low degree of protein binding, less than or equal to 20% (250–252), and as for other cephalosporins, the distribution volume is age dependent, ranging from 0.5 liter/kg in premature and term newborns to 0.25 liter/kg in adults (209,248–253). The penetration into various body tissue and fluids is good, particularly for bone, bile, extravascular fluid, peritoneal fluid, and various gynecologic tissues (254–257). Although less data are available than for other third-generation cephalosporins, ceftazidime concentrations in the CSF are low (<1 μg/ml) in adult patients with normal meninges. Higher but considerably variable concentrations are seen in the presence of meningeal inflammation, representing 25–45% of concurrent serum concentrations in children and adults (253,257–260). CSF concentrations of ceftazidime following single-dose administration to infants and children 0.4–15 months of age suggest that the penetration of this drug may not be as dependent on meningeal inflammation as is that of other related compounds. In addition, the observed CSF-serum ratio demonstrates a time-dependent increase consistent with slower elimination from the CSF (260).

Ceftazidime concentrations in breast milk are higher than for other cephalosporins, reaching concentrations of 5.2 μg/ml 1 hr after and 3.8 μg/ml immediately prior to intravenous doses of 2 g administered to lactating women (261).

Ceftazidime is not metabolized but, based on studies with probenecid, is excreted unchanged in the urine, primarily by glomerular filtration (209). Greater than 90% of a single intravenous dose is recovered in the urine within 24 hr in the presence of normal renal function (250). Total body clearance is approximately 1.0 ml/min kg^{-1} in neonates $\leqslant$32 weeks gestation and 1.8 ml/min kg^{-1} in term newborns ($\geqslant$38 weeks gestation) (249) and increases with postnatal age (248). In adults, total clearance averages 1.7-2.0 ml/min kg^{-1}, very similar to that of term newborns (209,250,251). No data are available for intermediate age groups. Age-related differences in half-life parallel those seen with clearance. The half-life of 7 hr observed in premature infants is longer than that in term newborns and infants <2 months of age (4.5 hr) and infants 2-12 months old (2 hr) and than the adult value of 1.8 hr (209,247-253,260).

In adults with renal insufficiency, the half-life of ceftazidime is a function of the glomerular filtration rate, increasing to approximately 24 hr in anuric patients requiring dialysis (262-264). Hemodialysis readily removes ceftazidime from the body, reducing the half-life from 25 hr to approximately 3 hr (263). Peritoneal dialysis is less effective than hemodialysis and is associated with a half-life of 8.7 hr during a dialytic period (264). The distribution volume is relatively unaffected by the presence of renal disease (263).

The disposition of ceftazidime is also altered in adult patients with ascites. Both the half-life and distribution volume are approximately threefold greater in ascitic patients but total body clearance is unaffected. Renal clearance is reduced to 25% of that in healthy subjects, and only 15% of a dose can be recovered as unchanged drug in the urine.

5. Ceftriaxone

Available only for parenteral use, ceftriaxone administered intramuscularly is completely absorbed but associated with pain at the injection site. The pain is alleviated by the addition of 1% lidocaine, which slows the rate of absorption slightly but has no effect on the peak concentration achieved or the ultimate amount of drug absorbed (265).

Ceftriaxone pharmacokinetics in pediatric patients have been studied, most often after parenteral doses of 50 mg/kg. Intramuscular administration of this dose to neonates produces a peak serum concentration of 140 μg/ml approximately 2 hr after dosing (266). The intravenous route is more commonly employed, and the same dose also produces peak concentrations of 150 μg/ml in neonates (266,267) but higher peaks of 200 μg/ml in infants and children (268,269).

Ceftriaxone is unique among the cephalosporins in that its pharmacokinetic disposition is complicated by concentration-dependent plasma protein binding whereby the degree of binding decreases as the plasma concentrations increase over the range of 0.5-600 μg/ml. The drug is 95% protein bound at concentrations below 70 μg/ml, decreasing to values of 84% and approximately 58% at concentrations of 300 and 600 μg/ml, respectively. Albumin appears to be the major binding protein, with ceftriaxone occupying a single site per protein molecule (270).

As a result of this concentration-dependent protein binding, higher doses of ceftriaxone produce less than proportional increases in the area under the plasma concentration time curve (AUC). Proportional increases are seen, however, in the plasma concentrations of free (unbound) drug (270). The pharmacokinetic implication of this protein binding behavior is that, at higher concentrations, a larger fraction of the drug in plasma is unbound and thus available for removal from the body by the renal and nonrenal clearance mechanisms.

The protein binding of ceftriaxone shows age dependency as well. Lower protein binding of ceftriaxone is observed in neonates (72%) compared with adults, translating into a fivefold increase in the unbound drug. This is the result of a lower concentration of drug binding sites and a reduced affinity of the drug for the binding sites. As a consequence of the latter, neonatal plasma protein binding sites are less saturated than adult at comparable concentrations although the degree of affinity increases with age (271). The increase in unbound drug available for elimination is offset by the immature renal and biliary function of this age group. In infants and children under 6 years of age, ceftriaxone is 84% protein bound, less than in adults over an equivalent concentration range (272).

The clinical implications of the concentration-dependent protein binding are less clear. The tissue penetration of ceftriaxone is comparable to that of other third-generation cephalosporins, despite the high degree of plasma protein binding. Adequate concentrations are found in peritoneal fluid, blister fluid, ascites fluid, bone, bile, gallbladder wall, bile, and joint fluid (92,273). Ceftriaxone quickly reaches umbilical cord blood, the placenta, and amniotic fluid when administered to expectant mothers prior to parturition, and concentrations up to 92 μg/ml have been measured in the first voided urine of the newborn infants of these patients. Ceftriaxone also appears rapidly in breast milk, reaching concentrations of 3-4% of concurrent serum concentrations and declining with a half-life of 12-17 hr (274).

The penetration of ceftriaxone into the CNS of pediatric patients with meningitis has been determined after intravenous doses of 50-100 mg/kg. Entry is limited in aseptic meningitis (275) and in the absence of inflamed meninges (276). Mean peak ceftriaxone concentrations in the CSF are between 5 and 18 μg/ml in this dose range and generally occur 5-6 hr after dosing (275-277). There is little relationship between dose administered and degree of penetration, and CSF ceftriaxone concentrations sampled at discrete times 1-6 hr after dosing represent 5-10% of the concurrent plasma concentrations (268,269, 276-279). When diffusion into the CNS is assessed by comparison of CSF and plasma AUC, penetration is estimated to be 17% (275). Because of the relatively long terminal phase half-life, ceftriaxone concentrations manyfold greater than the MIC of infecting organisms may persist in the CNS for 12-24 hr (275,279,280).

Ceftriaxone is thought to distribute into a space equivalent to extracellular water, the volume of which per unit body surface area (5-6 liter/m^2) is independent of age (281). Correcting the apparent distribution volume $V_{d\beta}$ for surface area yields greater values for patients between 8 days and 6 years of age compared with older and younger age groups, primarily because they received larger doses per square meter than did neonates <8 days old or adults (282). The concentration-dependent protein binding discussed earlier is responsible for this dose dependency in distribution volume (270), but a recently proposed volume of distribution term (283,284) that more accurately describes the steady-state situation for a drug like ceftriaxone is nearly constant for age when corrected for body surface area (282). For comparison with other cephalosporins, the kinetic parameters of ceftriaxone found in Table 6 are corrected for body weight. Presented in this manner, the distribution volume demonstrates similar age-related trends as other cephalosporins, decreasing from 0.5 liter/kg in neonates (267,271) to 0.37 liter/kg in infants and children (268,269,272,279) and ultimately reaching the adult value of 0.15 liter/kg (285).

Ceftriaxone is eliminated by a combination of biliary and renal processes, the latter almost exclusively by glomerular filtration (270,286). The half-life is unaffected by the degree of protein binding and in all age groups studied is considerably longer than any other cephalosporin to date: 15-19 hr in neonates, 4-6 hr in infants and children, and 6-9 hr in adults (265,267-269,271,272,285). The prolonged half-life in neonates is attributed to reduced systemic clearance of the drug since both major routes of elimination are poorly developed in this age group (287). Comparison of the clearance values in Table 6 would suggest that systemic clearance is more rapid in neonates compared with adults. However, the reduced systemic clearance characteristic of neonates is more readily apparent when either clearance of the total drug (bound and unbound) is corrected for surface area or when clearance of free drug is considered regardless of the correction factor used (271). Systemic clearance is more rapid in infants and young children (268, 269,272,279,282).

The fraction of a dose excreted in the urine is also concentration dependent, with about 70% of a dose eliminated renally in newborns and decreasing with age up to 6 years. Approximately 40-50% of a dose is excreted by the kidneys in adults (282). In infants, young children, and adults, renal clearance based on total ceftraxone concentration declines during the first few hours after intravenous administration as a result of the continuous decline in the concentration of unbound drug (270,272). This is not observed in neonates because of the reduced degree of protein binding and, subsequently, the lack of an appreciable decrease in unbound drug with time (271).

The disposition of ceftriaxone is only moderately affected by renal dysfunction. The affinity of the drug for protein binding sites is reduced, resulting in a twofold increase in the concentration of unbound drug. Nevertheless, the volume of distribution is unaffected by the presence of renal disease. The half-life in functionally anephric patients is approximately double that seen in normal renal function. Hemodialysis and peritoneal dialysis do not remove a significant amount of ceftriaxone from the body (288–290).

In patients with various degrees of hepatic insufficiency, plasma protein binding is reduced, and therefore the unbound concentration of ceftriaxone increased largely as a result of reduced albumin concentrations. In addition, the affinity of drug binding is decreased in cirrhotic patients with ascites to an extent comparable to that observed in renal patients. Despite these changes, liver dysfunction has only minimal effects on various kinetic parameters, except in cirrhotic patients with ascites in whom total clearance and distribution volume of the free drug are reduced and the fractional excretion of ceftriaxone in the urine is increased.

The disposition of ceftriaxone is not altered in patients with neoplastic diseases (291).

There is little pediatric experience with other third-generation cephalosporins. Ceftizoxime and cefsulodin have been well studied in Japan but few North American data are available in children for these cephalosporins or other investigational compounds.

F. Oral Cephalosporins

Because of their structural similarities, the orally administered cephalosporins demonstrate only minor differences in their pharmacokinetic properties. Compared with the parenteral compounds, fewer pharmacokinetic data are available in pediatric patients. Absorption and disposition characteristics of the oral cephalosporins are found in Table 7.

1. Cephalexin

The oral absorption of cephalexin, in general, is rapid and complete. A review of the early literature on cephalexin reveals that absorption is delayed and peak serum levels lower in newborns and infants during the first 6 months of life, occurring around 3 hr after dosing. Peak concentrations are attained after 2 hr in infants 9–12 months old and 1 hr in children greater than 1 year of age (2). A 15-mg/kg dose of cephalexin suspension to children between the ages of 2 and 35 months produces peak concentrations of 23 μg/ml 30 min after dosing (292,293). The onset of absorption is delayed and peak concentrations lower with capsules compared with suspension and also when the drug is administered with food or milk compared with the fasting state (292,294). In the presence of food, a 15-mg/kg dose of suspension produces a peak concentration of 9 μg/ml at 1 hr and bioavailability is reduced to approximately 60% of that observed under fasting conditions (292). Bioavailability is also reduced by 40–50% in newborns (295) and infants with short bowel syndrome (296).

In adults, the suspension is also more rapidly absorbed than the capsule. Peak concentrations are proportional to the dose administered and approximately 8, 16, and 30 μg/ml, respectively, 1 hr after doses of 250 mg, 500 mg, and 1 g to fasting adult volunteers (2,297). In contrast to infant and children, coadministration of food alters the rate but not the extent of absorption when based on AUC comparisons (297,298).

Cephalexin is less than 10% protein bound at therapeutic concentrations (297) and is widely distributed throughout the body, although concentrations achieved in most tissues and fluids were not particularly high. The penetration into the CSF is limited in the absence of inflammation, and the appearance of the drug in amniotic fluid and breast milk is minimal (2,126). Cephalexin is not metabolized, and elimination is primarily renal, consisting of both glomerular filtration and tubular secretion. In adults, renal clearance is approximately 250 ml/min 1.73 m^{-2} and urinary recovery is essentially complete 6-8 hr after a single dose (297,298a). In comparison, approximately 40% of the total daily dose is excreted in newborns during a 24-hr period (295). Serum half-life data in pediatrics are very limited, but values range from approximately 5 hr in newborns to 1 hr in infants, children, and adults (2,292,298,299). The half-life is prolonged to 8.6 hr in adult renal failure patients maintained on CAPD (151) and to 15.4 hr in anephric patients (300).

2. Cephradine

Cephradine and cephalexin pharmacokinetics are almost indistinguishable in terms of half-life, elimination, urinary concentrations and urinary recovery. Under fasting conditions, peak serum concentrations, the time to peak, and extent of absorption following cephradine are very similar to cephalexin, with the sole exception the effect of food in pediatric patients. In contrast to cephalexin, the extent of absorption is reduced to a lesser degree when the oral suspension is accompanied by milk (301). This food-related effect is not as pronounced in adults. The absorption of cephradine after intramuscular administration to healthy adults is rapid, generally producing peak concentrations within 30-40 min after dosing. Absorption is slightly slower in females compared with males, particularly when injected into the gluteus maximus. Compared with the vastus lateralis and deltoid muscle groups, injection at this site in females produces peak concentrations that are lower and delayed until 2 hr after administration and reduced absorption based on AUC comparisons. Absorption characteristics in males are minimally affected by site of administration (302). Protein binding is estimated to be ⩽20%, a difference that is of little consequence in terms of distribution or elimination (2).

3. Cefaclor

The rate of cefaclor absorption is similar to that of cephalexin and cephradine although peak serum concentrations are about 50% lower than those after equivalent doses of either of these other compounds (303-305). These lower concentrations appear to be related to a pH-dependent instability (306). Doses of 10 and 15 mg/kg to infants and children produce concentrations at 30 min averaging 10.8 and 13.1 μg/ml, respectively. Administration with food reduces the 30-min concentrations by approximately 30% but does not affect the extent of absorption (303). In adults, a dose of 500 mg produces peak concentrations of 12.4 μg/ml approximately 1 hr after dosing. Postprandial administration is associated with a 50% reduction in peak concentration and a prolongation in the time to peak (2-3 hr). Concurrent probenecid administration does not affect the peak concentration attained (304).

Like cephalexin and cephradine, cefaclor is less than 20% bound to serum proteins. However, few data on tissue penetration are available. Mean peak sputum concentrations after 500-mg and 1.0-g doses are reported to be 0.4 and 0.6 μg/ml, respectively, representing approximately 3% of concurrent serum concentrations (307).

Cefaclor is renally eliminated by a combination of glomerular filtration and tubular secretion. In adult volunteers, concomitant probenecid administration prolongs the half-life from 0.8 to 1.3 hr and significantly reduces urinary concentrations (304). In the presence of normal renal function, approximately 70% of a dose is recovered in the urine after 6 hr (304,308). Serum concentrations decline with a half-life of approximately 1 hr in children and adults with normal renal function (303,304) and 3 hr in adult renal failure patients (300,304,308). Hemodialysis reduces the half-life to around 1.5 hr (309).

4. Cefadroxil

The addition of a para-hydroxyl group on the aromatic ring of cephalexin results in cefadroxil, a drug that differs from other oral cephalosporins primarily in its rate of elimination. For this reason, serum and urine concentrations are generally higher and more prolonged than with the other oral agents (293).

In infants and children, oral doses of 15-mg/kg cefadroxil suspension produce peak concentrations of approximately 14 μg/ml 1 hr after dosing (293,310). The absorption of cefadroxil administered in capsule form is slower than with the suspension, resulting in peak concentrations that are delayed until 2 hr postdose and higher serum concentrations 4 and 6 hr after ingestion. Coadministration of food (milk) has minimal effects on the absorption of cefadroxil whether administered as capsules or in suspension (293). Similar findings have been reported in adults after the administration of 300-mg capsules, with peak concentrations of 10 μg/ml occurring 1 hr after dosing and unaffected by food intake (298).

Like cefaclor, few data on tissue distribution of cefadroxil are available. Concentrations of 11.4 μg/ml and 7.4 μg/g have been reported in pleural exudate and lung tissue, respectively, 2-5 hr after single oral doses of 1000 mg. The penetration of cefadroxil into bone, muscle, and synovial fluid ranges from 23 to 43% of concurrent serum concentrations (311). Children's saliva concentrations 2 hr after 15-mg/kg doses average 0.5 μg/ml (310).

As for the other oral cephalosporins, the kidney is the major organ responsible for cefadroxil elimination. Renal clearance exceeds creatinine clearance, suggesting that a secretory process as well as glomerular filtration is involved in the renal elimination of the drug. Approximately 93% of a single oral dose is recovered in a 24-hr urine collection (312). The elimination half-life is 1.4 hr in infants, children, and adults with normal renal function (310,312). The half-life increases with progressive deterioration in renal function, reaching 22 hr in hemodialysis patients. A 6 to 8-hr hemodialysis session removes 63% of the antibiotic and reduces the half-life to 3.4 hr (312).

G. New Oral Cephalosporins

1. Cefuroxime Axetil

Cefuroxime axetil is a prodrug of cefuroxime that is rapidly de-esterified in the intestinal mucosa and absorbed as cefuroxime, thus providing an oral cephalosporin with antibacterial activity and β-lactamase stability characteristic of second-generation cephalosporins. In infants and children aged 11-68 months, peak concentrations of 5.1 μg/ml are achieved 90-120 min after the oral administration of 20-mg/kg doses of the drug prepared as crushed tablets suspended in sucrose. In contrast to cephalexin, peak concentrations are approximately 50% higher and the bioavailability 25% greater when administered simultaneously with milk. Higher serum concentrations are also observed in older children receiving cefuroxime axetil with apple sauce or milk than in the fasting state, except during the first hour after dosing. In this latter age group, the relative bioavailability of cefuroxime in fasting subjects is significantly reduced to 50 and 68% of that associated with concomitant administration of milk and applesauce, respectively. In adults, similar although less dramatic results are seen. The half-life in all age group ranges between 1.0 and 1.4 hr independently of feeding status (313).

With and without food, approximately 42 and 30%, respectively, of a dose can be recovered as cefuroxime in the urine within 12 hr of administration. The majority appears within the first 6 hr (314,315).

2. Cefixime

Although very few kinetic data are available for cefixime, it deserves mention because of its expanded spectrum of activity and resistance to β-lactamase inactivation compared with other oral cephalosporins.

When administered to healthy adults, single oral doses of 50-400 mg produce dose-dependent increases in peak concentrations ranging from 1.0 to 3.9 μg/ml, as well as linear increases in AUC. An unusual characteristic is the time dependency of the peak concentrations attained, which occur 2.7 hr after a 50-mg dose and 4.3 hr after a 400-mg dose. The half-life is 3 hr independently of dose, and 20% of an administered dose is recovered in a 24-hr urine collection (316). The drug is 31% protein bound in humans with no concentration over clinically relevant dependency of concentrations (317).

VI. TOXICITY AND ADVERSE EFFECTS

Until the advent of the extended spectrum agents, cephalosporins differed little in their propensity to cause clinically significant adverse reactions, with the sole exception of cephaloridine. Increasing use of the third-generation cephalosporins has demonstrated that side-effect profiles may, indeed, be different, particularly with respect to the occurrence of coagulopathies and Antabuse-like reactions (see Section VI.D).

A. Hypersensitivity Reactions

Hypersensitivity reactions to the cephalosporins are similar to those of the penicillins and do not appear to be more prevalent with any individual agent. Immediate reactions, such as anaphylaxis, urticaria, and bronchospasm, may occur but are less frequent than with penicillins. Maculopapular rashes, which may or may not be accompanied by fever and eosinophilia, are more common manifestations (318). Cephalosporins can form a cephaloyl compound analogous to the penicilloyl group, but it is more labile than its penicillin counterpart (319). Despite the similarities in chemical structure and degradation products, there is no consensus about the degree to which patients allergic to one class of agents will cross-react with a member of the other class. A minority of patients allergic to penicillins have positive skin tests to cephalosporins, but no skin tests that can reliably predict *a priori* allergic reactions to cephalosporins are available. Epidemiological studies suggest that cross-reactivity to cephalosporins occurs in 5-10% of penicillin-allergic patients (320). Nevertheless, administration of a cephalosporin to patients with severe immediate reactions to a penicillin should only be carried out cautiously by experienced personnel and is best avoided if possible.

A unique adverse reaction has recently been reported following the use of cefaclor in children. Reactions like those of serum sickness and erythema multiforme were reported in 1% of children (11 of 1017) given cefaclor compared with 0 of 1009 children treated with amoxicillin. Urticaria was also more frequent in the cefaclor group. These reactions were somewhat more common after the second or third course of cefaclor than after the first (321).

B. Nephrotoxicity

Cephalosporin nephrotoxicity is most often associated with cephaloridine and to a lesser degree with cephalothin. Clinical observations and experimental data in animals suggest that, in contrast to penicillin nephrotoxicity, cephaloridine nephropathy is primarily a direct toxic effect rather than a hypersensitivity phenomenon (322). Cephaloridine, like other organic anions, is taken up in the proximal tubules by a common peritubular transport pump and accumulates intracellularly. Competitive inhibition of the organic anion secretory apparatus by probenecid, penicillin G, or cephalothin reduces the cortical accumulation and nephrotoxicity of cephaloridine. The histological picture is that of acute tubular necrosis and is characterized by leukocytes and tubular cells in the urine as well as a mild albuminuria (323). The toxic moiety of the drug has not been identified. The phenomenon is dose related, doses greater than 4 g/day in adults being associated with an increased risk of nephrotoxicity (1,322). Since this drug is no longer marketed in Canada or the United States, cephaloridine-induced toxicity is no longer an important clinical concern in North America.

There is little evidence that cephalothin nephrotoxicity is a dose-related phenomenon, and features of both hypersensitivity reactions and direct toxicity have been noted in clinical cases (322). The nephrotoxic potential of newer cephalosporins currently appears to be minimal and, if present, will only surface with continued widespread use of these drugs.

C. Coagulation Defects

Of increasing concern is the high frequency of hypoprothrombinemia and bleeding associated with some of the newer cephalosporins. In particular, cefamandole, cefoperazone, and moxalactam have been implicated and, to a lesser degree, cefazolin (34,324–328). Generally, affected patients have been elderly, malnourished, or debilitated. At present, the mechanism(s) of the coagulopathy are speculative but may involve high biliary concentrations of drug that destroy vitamin K-producing intestinal bacteria and result in a deficiency of vitamin K-dependent clotting factors or interference with adenosine diphosphate-induced platelet aggregation (325,326). A third hypothesis is that the 1-methyl-5-thiotetrazole (MTT) group located at the 3 position of cefamandole, moxalactam, and cefoperazone is cleaved in vitro, inhibiting carboxylation of glutamic acid residues of preprothrombin or inactive prothrombin to γ-carboxyglutamic acid residues of the active species (327,328). Recent in vitro data suggest that both MTT and the related heterocyclic thiol 2-methyl-1,3,4-thiodiazole-5-thiol (MTD) group of cefazolin inhibit the γ-carboxylation of glutamic acid in vitro and they are both metabolized by two enzymes catalyzing thiol methylation in humans, thiopurine methyltransferase and thiol methyltransferase (329). These enzymes are under independent genetic control; thiol methylation is associated with dramatic decreases in the abilities of these compounds to inhibit the γ-carboxylation reactions. Therefore, the large, genetically controlled individual variations in the activities of these enzymes may be one factor responsible for determining susceptibility to cephalosporin-induced hypoprothrombinemia. The less frequent occurrence of cefazolin-related coagulopathy may be because it is a better substrate for the methyltransferase in vitro (329). Since a number of investigational cephalosporins, such as cefmenoxime and cefmetazole, also possess an MTT group, they may also be expected to produce this effect in susceptible patients.

Prophylactic administration of vitamin K, 10 mg/day, while on therapy, has been used with success in preventing coagulation abnormalities in adult cancer patients (330).

Vitamin K should be routinely provided to pediatric patients receiving any of these cephalosporins, particularly if clinical circumstances suggest that they are at high risk for developing coagulation problems.

D. Alcohol Intolerance

In addition to coagulation defects, a syndrome of alcohol intolerance similar to the disulfiram reaction has been reported with cephalosporins containing a methylthiotetrazole ring (331-333). The reaction is characterized by symptoms of tachycardia, facial flushing, nausea, vomiting, dizziness, and dyspnea occurring within 5-10 min of alcohol ingestion. The precise mechanism of the interaction is not known, although it appears that acetaldehyde concentrations are elevated and that the offending drugs must be present prior to alcohol ingestion for the reaction to occur (33). The methylthiotetrazole ring resembles the stereoconfiguration of disulfiram (33) and produces effects on acetaldehyde concentrations that are greater than those of the intact antibiotics (334). It is clear that not all patients who ingest alcohol while being treated with one of these β-lactamase antibiotics experience this reaction, and it is possible that the polymorphisms in methyltransferase activity discussed previously may influence an individual's susceptibility to such a reaction. Nevertheless, it would be prudent for clinicians to advise their patients to avoid alcohol while being treated with cefamandole, moxalactam, or cefoperazone. In addition, since a disulfiramlike reaction has been reported in a patient receiving moxalactam and theophylline elixir (335), suitable precautions should be exercised if the use of alcohol-containing medicinals is anticipated in pediatric patients.

E. Miscellaneous Adverse Effects

Cephalothin therapy has been associated with the development of a positive Coombs test, which may be accompanied by hemolytic anemia. This phenomenon appears to be nonimmunologic in nature, and related factors include doses of cephalothin exceeding 12 g/day, renal failure, and hypoalbuminemia (1). An isolated positive Coombs test should not require discontinuation of therapy.

Cephalosporin-induced neurotoxicity is not an issue that has received a lot of attention. A few case reports citing the neurotoxic effects of cephaloridine have been reported, but they are of little concern now that the drug is no longer marketed. Neurotoxicity attributed to newer cephalosporins is generally limited to patients with varying degrees of renal impairment in whom cephalosporin doses may have been high relative to their renal function (336-339). Associated symptoms include seizures, fluctuating levels of consciousness, paranoid delusion, headache, confusion, and nystagmus. Since most cephalosporins (except cefoperazone and ceftriaxone) are mostly renally eliminated, it would seem that appropriate dosage reduction in patients with renal dysfunction would reduce the risk of these reactions.

Alterations in the aerobic and anaerobic bowel floras are associated with several clinically relevant adverse effects, such as nonspecific diarrhea, superinfections, and the potential effect on vitamin K production discussed earlier. In general, one might expect the amount of drug available in the lower gut to be a factor influencing the degree to which the normal gut flora is altered. Diarrhea appears to be more common in patients treated with such cephalosporins as ceftriaxone and cefoperazone, which are largely excreted in the bile, compared with other cephalosporins, which are primarily renally eliminated (340-342). Nevertheless, the propensity of cephalosporins to suppress bowel flora is not solely dependent on the principal route of elimination but is more likely to reflect the increased spectrum of activity of the newer agents (341-343). No marked changes in intestinal flora were observed in one report following the oral administration of oral antibiotics, but the intestinal bacteria were greatly affected by second- and third-generation cephalosporins independent of the degree of biliary excretion (342,344). Profound effects on fecal flora are also observed in pediatric patients treated with broad-spectrum cephalosporins, with the bowel flora returning to pretreatment conditions within 5-10 days of discontinuation (344-346). Enterococcal superinfections following broad-spectrum cephalosporin therapy are perhaps the most clinically important, although fungi and *Pseudomonas* may also occur (344,347). *Candida* diaper rashes are more frequent after third-generation cephalosporins than after antibiotics with more narrow spectra of activity.

Cephalosporins have also been implicated in diarrhea associated with *C. difficile* toxin. An epidemiological study conducted in Sweden revealed that cephalosporins were second only to the lincosamides, lincomycin and clindamycin, in causing *C. difficile* toxin-related diarrhea when ranked in relation to antibiotic usage. The event occurred more frequently in elderly patients and those receiving multiple antibiotics (348).

VII. DRUG INTERACTIONS

A. Diagnostic Tests

Elevated concentrations (>600 mg/liter) of several cephalosporins can cause false-positive results if the copper reduction method (Clinitest) is used for glycosuria testing. Such concentrations are easily achievable in urine in the first few hours after parenteral doses or large oral doses of cephalosporins. Cefadroxil, cefaclor, cefamandole, ceforanide, cefoxitin, and cefotaxime but not moxalactam may interfere with this test (349). Glucose-oxidase tests (Diastix and Tes-Tape) are not affected by these agents.

When serum creatinine is determined by Jaffe's method, falsely high values may be obtained at serum cephalosporin concentrations exceeding 100 μg/ml. The alkaline picrate used in this method reacts with a number of cephalosporins, the most clinically significant being cefoxitin and cephalothin. Interference of this nature can be minimized by obtaining samples for creatinine determination at least 2 hr after an infusion. The test is unreliable in the presence of severe renal function (350,351).

B. Aminoglycosides and Loop Diuretics

Concurrent administration of the earlier cephalosporins, cephalothin and cephaloridine, with aminoglycosides has been associated with an increased risk of nephrotoxicity that may be considered synergistic (352). A similar phenomenon has been described with diuretics in animal models, but the results of such studies appear to be influenced by experimental design (321). Experience with newer cephalosporins suggests that normal doses of these agents in combinations with loop diuretics or aminoglycosides do not result in an appreciable risk of nephrotoxicity (321).

C. Other Cephalosporins

Combinations of cephalosporins may be antagonistic in terms of antibacterial activity. Cefoxitin is particularly capable of producing this effect, presumably by inducing β-lactamases in some bacterial strains that may hydrolyze concurrently administered cephalosporins (69). Since there are few circumstances requiring therapy with two cephalosporins, it would be wise to avoid such combinations.

VIII. THERAPEUTIC INDICATIONS

A. First-Generation Cephalosporins

Until the release of the new second- and third-generation drugs in the 1980s, parenteral cephalosporins were not used extensively in pediatrics (353,354). The major reasons for the limited use of first-generation drugs in children are their lack of activity against *H. influenzae* type b, their greater cost than the penicillins, and, most important, their lack of efficacy in the treatment of meningitis. The primary indication for the use of first-generation cephalosporins, such as cephalothin and cefazolin, is for the treatment of severe infections caused by staphylococci and streptococci in children who are allergic to penicillins. These drugs are useful only for skin and soft tissue infections, such as cellulitis, abscesses, pneumonia, septic arthritis, and osteomyelitis, and should not be used alone if bacterial meningitis has not been excluded (355).

B. Second-Generation Cephalosporins

Cefamandole was the first parenteral cephalosporin to be introduced with significant activity not only against gram-positive cocci but also against *H. influenzae* type b, including ampicillin-resistant strains (155). However, clinical trials demonstrated quickly that in spite of its apparent in vitro activity, cefamandole was not reliably effective in the treatment of bacterial meningitis, especially that due to *H. influenzae* (356). In addition, clinical failures of nonmeningitic infections as well as case reports of children who developed meningitis while being treated with cefamandole for pneumonia, septic arthritis, and other infections caused by *H. influenzae* have been reported (357-359). These children had no evidence of meningitis at the start of treatment. These failures of cefamandole are attributable to several factors: unreliable penetration of active drug into the cerebrospinal fluid (CSF) (155), lack of adequate stability to the β-lactamase of *Hemophilus* (360), inadequate bactericidal activity against *H. influenzae* (361), and a marked inoculum effect (362). Significantly larger amounts of cefamandole are required to kill *H. influenzae* at a concentration of 10^6 bacteria per milliliter compared with 10^4 ml^{-1}. Since many children with *Hemophilus* meningitis have bacterial concentration in the CSF of 10^6 ml^{-1} or greater, it should be no surprise that cefamandole is frequently ineffective in the treatment of meningitis. Because of these limitations and because of the availability of many other effective antibiotics, cefamandole should not be used in children.

Cefuroxime is a second-generation cephalosporin that meets the need for a single antibiotic active against the common pathogens causing severe infections in children: *Staphylococcus aureus, Streptococcus pneumoniae*, group B streptococci, *N. meningitidis*, and *H. influenzae* type b, both ampicillin-resistant and ampicillin-sensitive strains (363). Moreover, cefuroxime penetrates into the CSF in children with meningitis to produce concentrations that are at least five times greater than the amount required to kill the major causes of meningitis in children, i.e., pneumococci, meningococci, and *Hemophilus* (177-179). Cefuroxime has been compared to standard therapy and found to be at least as effective as the combination of ampicillin plus chloramphenicol in the treatment of bacterial meningitis (364,365). It can therefore be used to initiate therapy in children with meningitis rather than ampicillin and chloramphenicol, thereby avoiding the toxicity of chloramphenicol and the need to monitor chloramphenicol blood levels. Cefuroxime is also active against strains of *H. influenzae* type b that are resistant to both ampicillin and chloramphenicol. Although such strains are still rare in North America, their prevalence has reached 20-30% in parts of Europe. Cefuroxime, when used at the dose recommended to treat meningitis (200-240 mg/kg day^{-1}), is currently more expensive than ampicillin and chloramphenicol, alone or in combination. Therefore, when a sensitive strain of pneumococcus, meningococcus, or *Hemophilus* is isolated, treatment should be changed to penicillin or ampicillin.

In addition to its use in childhood meningitis, cefuroxime is very useful as initial therapy of other severe bacterial infections, such as buccal cellulitis, periorbital cellulitis, epiglottitis, pneumonia, septic arthritis, and osteomyelitis in the age group at risk of disease caused by *H. influenzae* (363,366-368). The activity of cefuroxime against *Staph. aureus, Strep. pneumoniae, Strep. pyogenes,* and *H. influenzae* permits single-drug therapy rather than combination therapy with ampicillin-chloramphenicol or cloxacillin-chloramphenicol. Moreover, for infections other than meningitis, a much lower dose of cefuroxime can be used (75 mg/kg day^{-1}), so that cefuroxime is less expensive than combination therapy and the potential toxicity of chloramphenicol is also avoided.

Cefuroxime shares with all cephalosporins a lack of activity against *L. monocytogenes* and enterococcus. In addition, it is often not sufficiently active against *E. coli* and other enteric bacteria to be used in severe infections caused by such organisms. Therefore, cefuroxime should not be used to initiate therapy of neonatal sepsis or meningitis and should not be used in clinical situations in which coliform sepsis is likely.

Reported experience with cefoxitin in children has been sparse (155). The major indication for its use is for the prevention and treatment of anaerobic infections, other than those involving the central nervous system. Cefoxitin is active against the major aerobic and anaerobic bacteria causing infections originating from the oral cavity and gastrointestinal tract, including ampicillin-resistant *Bacteroides* species. Cefoxitin is not active against *P. aeruginosa*. Because of inadequate concentrations in the CSF even when the meninges are inflamed, cefoxitin should not be used to treat patients with bacterial meningitis.

Cefoxitin has been shown to be effective in the treatment of intra-abdominal infections (155,369). In infants and young children undergoing surgery on the colon, cefoxitin provides a more convenient means of prophylaxis than such combinations as clindamycin-aminoglycoside or metronidazole-aminoglycoside.

Very little clinical experience has been reported with the other second-generation parenteral cephalosporins, ceforanide and cefonicid. Neither drug appears to offer any significant advantage over cefuroxime in terms of antibacterial spectrum, pharmacokinetic properties, or safety.

C. Third-Generation Cephalosporins

The clinical indications for the use of third-generation cephalosporins in pediatrics are still under investigation (353,354). It is clear that these very broad spectrum, highly active antibiotics should be restricted to the treatment of severe bacterial infections in hospitalized patients. They should not be used for infections likely to be caused by staphylococci, groups A and B streptococci, or pneumococci for which equally effective and much less expensive antibiotics are available. The role of these antibiotics relative to aminoglycosides in infections caused by gram-negative enteric bacilli in children remains to be determined. In compromised patients, such as neutropenic cancer patients, it is uncertain still whether any of these new agents is safe to use as single agents. It must also be remembered that, like all cephalosporins, the third-generation drugs are not active against *Listeria* or enterococci.

Cefotaxime has been shown to be as effective as ampicillin and chloramphenicol in the treatment of childhood meningitis caused by *Hemophilus, Strep. pneumoniae*, and *N. meningitidis* (370-372). It has also been shown to be effective in the treatment of gram-negative bacillary meningitis in neonates, including *Salmonella* meningitis (373,374). However, data are not yet available to determine the relative efficacy and safety of cefotaxime compared to ampicillin plus aminoglycoside in neonatal sepsis or meningitis. Since moxalactam plus ampicillin was found to be no better than ampicillin plus amikacin in neonatal meningitis (375), it is unlikely that cefotaxime will be any superior. If the clinical or bacteriologic response of the neonate to ampicillin plus aminoglycoside is inadequate, treatment with cefotaxime or other third-generation cephalosporin should be considered (376). The new cephalosporins do have a significant advantage over aminoglycosides in that CSF concentrations are sufficiently high that intraventricular therapy is unnecessary.

Cefotaxime has also been shown to be as effective as standard therapy in the treatment of other severe gram-negative rod infections in neonates and children. Experience in its use in the management of the febrile, neutropenic cancer patient is very limited. One randomized trial in adults found that cefotaxime plus amikacin was less effective than either azlocillin plus amikacin or ticarcillin plus amikacin in proven coliform bacteremia (377). However, the dose of cefotaxime used in the trial was relatively low, 100 mg/kg day^{-1}.

Cefotaxime is insufficiently active against *P. aeruginosa* or other species of *Pseudomonas* to be useful in infections caused by such organisms.

Ceftriaxone differs from the other available third-generation cephalosporins by virtue of its very long half-life. Bactericidal concentrations persist in the blood sufficiently long that severe bacterial infections have been successfully treated with once daily administration (273,378,379). Ceftriaxone has been found to be as effective as ampicillin plus chloramphenicol in the treatment of childhood meningitis. Most regimens using this drug for meningitis have employed a schedule of 50 mg/kg given every 12 hr following a loading dose of 75 mg/kg (278,380-382). Three studies have reported success using once daily administration (379,383,384). The reduced frequency of administration may result in significant cost savings compared with other new cephalosporins.

Ceftazidime differs from the above cephalosporins in being sufficiently active to be useful in the treatment of infections caused by *P. aeruginosa*. Because of its excellent penetration into the CSF, ceftazidime is the drug of choice for treatment of meningitis and brain abscess caused by *Pseudomonas* (385). Ceftazidime has also been shown to be as effective as ampicillin plus chloramphenicol in the treatment of childhood meningitis (386).

Ceftazidime has shown to be as effective as cefazolin plus tobramycin in the treatment of nonpneumococcal pneumonia in hospitalized adults (387).

Extensive experience with the use of ceftazidime in treatment of chest exacerbations in children with cystic fibrosis (CF) has accumulated (388-392). Ceftazidime was more effective than ticarcillin-tobramycin in reducing the sputum colony counts of *P. aeru-*

ginosa, but the effect persists only a few weeks after discontinuation of therapy (391). Despite superior bacteriologic results, ceftazidime was no more effective than ticarcillin-tobramycin in producing clinical improvement. The emergence of resistance to ceftazidime has not yet been a major problem in CF patients. However, because of greater cost and no greater efficacy, ceftazidime cannot be recommended as a first choice over standard therapy with the combination of an anti-pseudomonal penicillin and aminoglycoside in the management of *P. aeruginosa* infections in cystic fibrosis.

Clinical trials of monotherapy with ceftazidime in febrile, neutropenic cancer patients have recently been reviewed (393). Monotherapy is attractive because of the possibility of less toxicity than observed with standard combinations that include aminoglycosides. However, the safety and efficacy of monotherapy with ceftazidime or any other third-generation cephalosporin has yet to be confirmed. Superinfections and clinical failures caused by *Staph. aureus, P. aeruginosa*, and *Strep. faecalis* have already been reported.

Moxalactam has excellent activity against gram-negative bacilli and anaerobes. It has been shown to be as effective as standard therapy in the treatment of bacterial meningitis and other severe infections in children (394,395). However, because it is no more effective than other third-generation cephalosporins but has significantly greater problems related to the induction of bleeding disorders (see Section VI), there is little if any reason to use moxalactam.

Experience in children with other new, third-generation cephalosporins, such as cefsulodin, cefoperazone, and ceftizoxime, is extremely limited. These antibiotics and most of the other new drugs under clinical investigation do not appear to offer any substantial advantages over the third-generation cephalosporins already discussed, cefotaxime, ceftriaxone, and ceftazidime.

The very high cost of the third-generation cephalosporins is a major factor affecting their use. In addition, because of their very broad spectrum and marked activity against enteric bacteria, the third-generation cephalosporins cause significant suppression of normal bowel flora with a consequent risk of bacterial and fungal superinfections. Whether this risk is greater with cephalosporins than with standard therapy remains to be determined. Nevertheless, the new cephalosporins are of special importance in the treatment of the most common life-threatening infection of childhood: bacterial meningitis. At the present time, it appears that a number of equally effective antibiotic regimens are available for the treatment of childhood meningitis. The choice among cefuroxime, cefotaxime, ceftriaxone, ceftazidime, and ampicillin plus chloramphenicol will depend on cost, relative toxicities, and the incidence of strains of *H. influenzae* and *Strep. pneumoniae* resistant to chloramphenicol and penicillin. In most other situations, the third-generation cephalosporins should be reserved for treatment of severe infections in hospitalized children and not be used for treatment of most community acquired infections.

D. Oral Cephalosporins

The oral first-generation cephalosporins have been more popular for use in children than the parenteral forms primarily because the liquid formulations of cephalosporins have very acceptable flavors, unlike the penicillins, which are bitter and unpleasant tasting. Cephalexin can be used for oral treatment of skin and minor soft tissue infections caused by staphylococci and streptococci, such as impetigo, pyoderma, cellulitis, and pharyngitis (396). Although it is as effective as the penicillins and erythromycin in the treatment of minor staphylococcal and streptococcal infections, cephalexin has the disadvantage of being considerably more expensive. Cephalexin should not be used for the treatment of acute otitis media because of insufficient activity against most strains of *H. influenzae* (397).

Because of its reliable absorption and adequate activity, cephalexin has also been used for oral treatment of osteomyelitis and septic arthritis caused by susceptible organisms (398–400). Whenever oral therapy is used to treat severe infections, blood levels should be monitored to ensure compliance and adequate absorption (401).

Cefaclor has the advantage over cephalexin of significantly greater activity against *H. influenzae*. It has been extensively studied in comparative trials of the treatment of acute otitis media in children (402–404). It achieves satisfactory blood and middle ear fluid concentrations against the major causes of acute otitis media, namely, *Strep. pneumoniae* and *H. influenzae* and is also active against *Branhamella catarrhalis, Strep. pyogenes, Staph. aureus*, and other less common causes of otitis. Moreover, it is active against both ampicillin-resistant and ampicillin-sensitive strains of *Hemophilus* and *Branhamella*. In randomized clinical trails, cefaclor has been shown to be as effective as amoxicillin, trimethoprim-sulfamethoxazole, amoxicillin-clavulanate, and erythromycin-sulfonamide. However, because of its considerable expense compared with other antibiotics and the occurrence of a reaction like that in serum sickness and urticarial rashes in up to 3% of children (see Section VI.A), cefaclor must be considered a second line or alternative to amoxicillin, the drug of choice for acute otitis media and other upper respiratory tract infections (405).

Cefadroxil has very limited applications in pediatrics because of its high cost. Its only advantage over other oral cephalosporins is its long half-life, which permits the convenience of twice daily treatment for such conditions as streptococcal pharyngitis, otitis media, and urinary tract infections (406,407). However, penicillin V and erythromycin estolate are equally effective in treating streptococcal infections when administered twice daily (406) and trimethoprim-sulfamethoxazole is given twice daily for urinary tract infections.

The usefulness of cefuroxime will be enhanced when the oral formulation becomes available. Cefuroxime axetil, which is well absorbed after oral administration, is undergoing clinical trials. Preliminary results show it may be as well tolerated and as effective as cefaclor in the treatment of otitis media (408).

Cefixime, an oral third-generation cephalosporin with the broad-spectrum activity against gram-negative bacteria characteristic of this group of agents, is currently undergoing clinical trials in the treatment of otitis media in children. As its activity against the Enterobacteriaceae is not essential in the treatment of otitis and may be responsible for the relatively high frequency of diarrhea reported in preliminary studies in adults, it is questionable that cefixime should be used for respiratory tract infections caused primarily by *Strep. pneumoniae* and *H. influenzae*. The major therapeutic indication for cefixime and other oral third-generation cephalosporins is more likely to be in the management of complicated urinary tract infections and for oral therapy of other gram-negative enteric infections.

REFERENCES

1. Weinstein, L, Kaplan, K: The cephalosporins. Microbiological, chemical, and pharmacological properties and use in chemotherapy of infection. *Ann. Intern. Med.* *72*:729–739, 1970.

2. Nightingale, CH, Greene, DS, Quintiliani, R: Pharmacokinetics and clinical use of cephalosporin antibiotics. *J. Pharm. Sci. 64*:1899–1927, 1975.
3. Thompson, RL: The cephalosporins. *Mayo Clin. Proc. 52*:625–630, 1977.
4. Neu, HC: The in vitro activity, human pharmacology, and clinical effectiveness of new β-lactam antibiotics. *Annu. Rev. Pharmacol. Toxicol. 22*:599–642, 1982.
5. Garzone, P, Lyon, J, Yu, VL: Third-generation and investigational cephalosporins. I. Structure-activity relationships and pharmacokinetic review. *Drug. Intell. Clin. Pharm. 17*:507–515, 1983.
6. Garzone, P, Lyon, J, Yu, VL: Third-generation and investigational cephalosporins. II. Microbiologic review and clinical summaries. *Drug Intell. Clin. Pharm. 17*:615–622, 1983.
7. Abraham, EP: The cephalosporins. *Pharmacol. Rev. 14*:473–500, 1962.
8. Abraham, EP: A glimpse of the early history of the cephalosporins. *Rev. Infect. Dis. 1*:99–105, 1979.
9. Stapley, EO, Jackson, M, Hernandez, S, Zimmerman, SB, Currie, SA, Mochales, S, Mata, JM, Woodruff, HB, Hendlin, D: Cephamycins, a new family of β-lactam antibiotics. I. Production by actinomycetes including *Streptomyces lactamdurans* sp. n. *Antimicrob. Agents Chemother. 2*:122–131, 1972.
10. Miller, TW, Goegelman, RT, Weston, RG, Putter, I, Wolf, FJ: Cephamycins, a new family of β-lactam antibiotics. II. Isolation and chemical characterization. *Antimicrob. Agents Chemother. 2*:132–135, 1972.
11. Yoshida, T: Structure function relationships of 1-oxacephems and moxalactam. In: New beta-lactam antibiotics: A review from chemistry to clinical efficacy of the new cephalosporins. *Symp. Frontiers Pharmacol. 1*:23–33, 1981.
12. Finland, M: Emergence of antibiotic resistance in hospitals, 1935–1975. *Rev. Infect. Dis. 1*:4–21, 1979.
13. Huber, FM, Chauvette, RR, Jackson, BG: Preparative methods for 7-aminocephalosporanic acid and 6-aminopenicillanic acid. In: *Cephalosporins and Penicillins* (EH Flynn, ed.), Academic Press, New York, 1972, pp. 27–73.
14. O'Callaghan, CH: Description and classification of the newer cephalosporins and their relationships with the established compounds. *J. Antimicrob. Chemother. 5*: 635–671, 1979.
15. Rattie, E, Ravin, L: Pharmacokinetic interpretations of blood levels and urinary excretion data for cefazolin and cephalothin after intravenous and intramuscular administration in humans. *Antimicrob. Agents Chemother.* 7:606–613, 1975.
16. Schrogie, JJ, Rogers, JD, Yeh, KC, Davies, RO, Holmes, GI, Skeggs, H, Martin, CM: Pharmacokinetics and comparative pharmacology of cefoxitin and cephalosporins. *Rev. Infect. Dis. 1*:90–98, 1979.
17. Wick, WE: In vitro and in vivo comparison of cephalothin and desacetylcephalothin. *Antimicrob. Agents Chemother. 1965*:870–875, 1966.
18. Christensen, B, Ruswinkle, L, Cama, L: The design of new drugs that resist microbial inactivation. *Rev. Infect. Dis. 1*:64–72, 1979.
19. Richmond, M: Factors influencing the antibacterial activity of beta-lactam antibiotics. *J. Antimicrob. Chemother. 4(Suppl. B)*:15–32, 1978.
20. Stapley, E, Birnbaum, J, Miller, A, Wallick, W, Handlin, D, Woodruff, H: Cefoxitin and cephamycins: Microbial studies. *Rev. Infect. Dis. 1*:73–89, 1979.
21. Neu, H, Fu, K: Cefuroxime, a beta-lactamase-resistant cephalosporin with a broad spectrum of gram-positive and gram-negative activity. *Antimicrob. Agents Chemother. 13*:657–664, 1978.
22. O'Callaghan, CH: Structure-activity relations and β-lactamase resistance. *Philos. Trans. R. Soc. Lond. 289*:197–205, 1980.
23. Firestone, RA, Schelechow, N, Johnston, DBR, Christensen, BG: Substituted penicillins and cephalosporins. II. C-6(7)-alkyl derivatives. *Tetrahedron Lett.* 375–378, 1972.

24. Dürckheimer, W, Blumbach, J, Heymes, R, Schrinner, E, Seeger, K: Chemistry and structure-activity relationships in the aminothiazole cephalosporin series. In: New beta-lactam antibiotics: A review from chemistry to clinical efficacy of the new cephalosporins. *Symp. Frontiers Pharmacol. 1*:3–21, 1981.
25. Curtis, NAC, Orr, D, Ross, GW, Boulton, MG: Affinities of penicillins and cephalosporins for the penicillin-binding proteins of *Escherichia coli* K-12 and their antibacterial activity. *Antimicrob. Agents Chemother. 16*:533–539, 1979.
26. Nakano, H, Kumiya, T. The development of ceftizoxime, a new parenteral cephalosporin. In: *β-Lactam Antibiotics: Mode of Action, New Developments, and Future Prospects* (M Salton and GD Shockman, eds.), Academic Press, New York, 1981, pp. 415–428.
27. Neu, HC: Antibacterial activity of desacetylcefotaxime alone and in combination with cefotaxime. *Rev. Infect. Dis 4(Suppl.)*:S374–S378, 1982.
28. Reeves, DS, White, LO, Holt, HA, Bahari, D, Bywater, J, Boax, RP: Human metabolism of cefotaxime. *J. Antimicrob. Chemother. 6(Suppl. A)*:93–101, 1980.
29. Verbist, L, Verhaegen, J: GR 20263: A new aminothiazolyl cephalosporin with high activity against *Pseudomonas* and *Enterobacteriaceae. Antimicrob. Agents Chemother. 17*:807–812, 1980.
30. Hamilton-Miller, JMT, Brumfitt, W: Activity of ceftazidime (GR 20263) against nosocomially important pathogens. *Antimicrob. Agents Chemother. 19*:1067–1069, 1981.
31. Neu, HC, Fu, KP, Aswakopee, N, Aswakopee, P, Kung, E: Comparative activity and β-lactamase activity of cefoperazone, a piperazine cephalosporin. *Antimicrob. Agents Chemother. 16*:150–157, 1979.
32. Saikawa, I, Mitsuhashi, S: Studies on new beta-lactam antibiotics having 2,3-dioxopiperazine group: Piperacillin and cefoperazone. In: *β-Lactam Antibiotics: Mode of Action, New Developments, and Future Prospects* (M Salton and GD Shockman, eds.), Academic Press, New York, 1981, pp. 353–360.
33. Buening, MK, Wold, JS: Ethanol-moxalactam interactions in vivo. *Rev. Infect. Dis. 4(Suppl.)*:S555–S563, 1982.
34. Weitekamp, MR, Aber, RC: Prolonged bleeding times and bleeding diathesis associated with moxalactam administration. *JAMA 249*:69–71, 1983.
35. Sawai, T, Matsuba, K, Tamura, A, Yamagishi, S: The bacterial outer membrane permeability of β-lactam antibiotics. *J. Antibiot. 32*:59–65, 1979.
36. Spratt, BG: The mechanism of action of penicillin. *Sci. Prog. 65*:101–128, 1978.
37. Wise, EM, Park, JT: Penicillin: Its basic site of action as an inhibitor of a peptide cross-linking reaction in cell wall mucopeptide synthesis. *Proc. Natl. Acad. Sci. USA 54*:75–81, 1965.
38. Tipper, DJ, Strominger, JL: Mechanism of action of penicillins: A proposal based on their structural similarity to acyl-D-alanyl-D-alanine. *Proc. Natl. Acad. Sci. USA 54*:1133–1141, 1965.
39. Spratt, BG: Distinct penicillin-binding proteins involved in the division, elongation and shape of *Escherichia coli. Proc. Natl. Acad. Sci. USA 72*:2999–3003, 1975.
40. Spratt, BG: Temperature sensitive cell division mutants of *Escherichia coli* with thermolabile penicillin-binding proteins. *J. Bacteriol. 131*:293–305, 1977.
41. Suzuki, H, Nishimura, Y, Hirota, Y. On the process of cell division in *Escherichia coli*: A series of mutants of *E. coli* altered in the penicillin-binding proteins. *Proc. Natl. Acad. Sci. USA 75*:664–668, 1978.
42. Iwaya, M, Strominger, JL: Simultaneous detection of D-alanine carboxypeptidase IB-C and penicillin-binding component IV in a mutant of *Escherichia coli* K12. *Proc. Natl. Acad. Sci. USA 74*:2980–2984, 1977.
43. Matsuhashi, M, Takagaki, Y, Maruyama, IN, Tamaki, S, Nishimura, Y, Suzuki, H, Ogin, U, Hirota, Y: Mutants of *Escherichia coli* lacking in highly penicillin-sensitive

D-alanine carboxypeptidase activity. *Proc. Natl. Acad. Sci. USA 74*:2976–2979, 1977.
44. Spratt, BG: Biochemical and genetic approaches to the mechanism of action of penicillin. *Philos. Trans. R. Soc. Lond. Biol. 289*:273–283, 1980.
45. Tomasz, A: From penicillin-binding proteins to the lysis and death of bacteria: A 1979 view. *Rev. Infect. Dis. 1*:434–467, 1979.
46. Utsui, Y, Yokota, T: Role of an altered penicillin protein in methicillin- and cephem-resistant *Staphylococcus aureus*. *Antimicrob. Agents Chemother. 28*:397–403, 1985.
47. Tomasz, A: Penicillin binding proteins: Their role in beta-lactam action and resistance. In: *Contemporary Issues in Infectious Diseases*, Vol. 1, *New Dimensions in Antimicrobial Therapy* (RK Root and MA Sande, eds.), Churchill Livingstone, New York, 1984, pp. 1–16.
48. Zimmerman, W, Rosselet, S: Function of the outer membrane of *Escherichia coli* as a permeability barrier to beta-lactam antibiotics. *Antimicrob. Agents Chemother. 12*:368–372, 1977.
49. DiRienzo, JM, Nakamura, K, Inouye, M: The outer membrane proteins of gram-negative bacteria: Biosynthesis, assembly and function. *Annu. Rev. Biochem. 47*: 481–532, 1978.
50. Kobayashi, Y, Takahaski, T, Nakae, T: Diffusion of beta-lactam antibiotics through liposome membranes containing purified porins. *Antimicrob. Agents Chemother. 22*:775–780, 1980.
51. Jaffe, A, Chabbert, YA, Semonin, O: Role of porin proteins Omp F and Omp L in the permeation of beta-lactams. *Antimicrob. Agents Chemother. 22*:942–948, 1982.
52. Sykes, RB, Matthew, M: The β-lactamases of Gram-negative bacteria. *J. Antimicrob. Chemother. 2*:115–157, 1976.
53. Levesque, R, Roy, PH: Mapping of a plasmid pLQ3 from *Achromobacter* and cloning of its cephalosporinase gene in *Escherichia coli*. *Gene 18*:69–75, 1982.
54. Kliebe, C, Nies, BA, Meyer, JF, Tolxdorff-Neutzling, RM, Weidemann, B: Evolution of plasmid-coded resistance to broad-spectrum cephalosporins. *Antimicrob. Agents Chemother. 28*:302–307, 1985.
55. Leung, T, Williams, JD. β-Lactamases of subspecies of *Bacteroides fragilis*. *J. Antimicrob. Chemother. 4 (Suppl. B)*:47–54, 1978.
56. Matthew, M: Plasmid-mediated β-lactamases of Gram-negative bacteria: Properties and distribution. *J. Antimicrob. Chemother. 5*:349–358, 1979.
57. Jacoby, GA, Matthew, M: The distribution of β-lactamase genes on plasmids found in *Pseudomonas*. *Plasmid 2*:41–47, 1979.
58. Medeiros, AA, Cohenford, M, Jacoby, GA: Five novel plasmid-determined β-lactamases. *Antimicrob. Agents Chemother. 27*:715–719, 1985.
59. Jack, GW, Richmond, MHA: A comparative study of eight distinct β-lactamases synthesized by gram-negative bacteria. *J. Gen. Microbiol. 61*:43–61, 1970.
60. Sanders, CC, Sanders, WE, Jr.: Emergence of resistance during therapy with the newer β-lactam antibiotics: Role of inducible β-lactamases and implications for the future. *Rev. Infect. Dis. 5*:639–648, 1983.
61. Sanders, CC, Moellering, RC, Jr., Martin, RR, Perkins, RL, Strike, DG, Gootz, TD, Sanders, WE, Jr.: Resistance to cefamandole: A collaborative study of emerging clinical problems. *J. Infect. Dis. 145*:118–125, 1982.
62. Richmond, MH: The β-lactamase stability of a novel β-lactam antibiotic containing a 7α-methoxyoxacephem nucleus. *J. Antimicrob. Chemother. 6*:445–453, 1980.
63. Seeberg, AH, Tolxdorff-Neutzling, RM, Weidemann, B: Chromosomal β-lactamases of *Enterobacter cloacae* are responsible for resistance to third-generation cephalosporins. *Antimicrob. Agents Chemother. 23*:918–925, 1983.
64. Gootz, TD, Sanders, CC, Goering, RV: Resistance to cefamandole: Derepression of

beta-lactamase by cefoxitin and mutation in *Enterbacter cloacae. J. Infect. Dis. 146*:34–42, 1982.
65. Gootz, TD, Sanders, CC: Characterization of β-lactamase induction in *Enterobacter cloacae. Antimicrob. Agents Chemother. 23*:91–97, 1983.
66. Sanders, CC: Inducible β-lactamases and non-hydrolytic resistance mechanisms. *J. Antimicrob. Chemother. 13*:1–3, 1984.
67. Murakami, K, Yoshida, T: Covalent binding of moxalactam to cephalosporinase of *Citrobacter freundii. Antimicrob. Agents Chemother. 27*:727–732, 1985.
68. Waterworth, PM, Emmerson, AM: Dissociated resistance among cephalosporins. *Antimicrob. Agents Chemother. 15*:497–503, 1979.
69. Sanders, CC, Sanders, WE Jr., Goering, RV: In vitro antagonism of beta-lactam antibiotics by cefoxitin. *Antimicrob. Agents Chemother. 21*:968–975, 1982.
70. Minami, S, Yotsuji, A, Inoue, M, Mitsuhashi, S: Induction of β-lactamase by various β-lactam antibiotics in *Enterobacter cloacae. Antimicrob. Agents Chemother. 18*: 382–385, 1980.
71. Farrar, WE, O'Dell, NM: Comparative beta-lactamase resistance and anti-staphylococcal activities of parenterally and orally administered cephalosporins. *J. Infect. Dis. 137*:490–493, 1978.
72. Chang, TW, Weinstein, L: In vitro biological activity of cephalothin. *J. Bacteriol. 85*:1022–1027, 1963.
73. Verbist, L: Comparison of the antibacterial activity of nine cephalosporins against Enterobacteriaceae and nonfermentative gram-negative bacilli. *Antimicrob. Agents Chemother. 10*:657–663, 1976.
74. Neu, HC: Cefamandole, a cephalosporin antibiotic with an unusually wide spectrum of activity. *Antimicrob. Agents Chemother. 6*:177–182, 1974.
75. Griffith, RS, Black, HR, Brier, GL, Wolny, ID: Cefamandole: In vitro activity and clinical pharmacokinetics. *Antimicrob. Agents Chemother. 10*:814–823, 1976.
76. Neu, HC: Cefoxitin, a semisynthetic cephamycin antibiotic: Antibacterial spectrum and resistance to hydrolysis by gram-negative beta-lactamases. *Antimicrob. Agents Chemother. 6*:170–176, 1974.
77. Cuchural, G, Jacobus, N, Gorbach, SL, Tally, FP: A survey of *Bacteroides* susceptibility in the United States. *J. Antimicrob. Chemother. 8(Suppl. D)*:27–31, 1981.
78. Eykyn, S, Jenkins, C, King, A, Phillips, I: Antibacterial activity of cefuroxime, a new cephalosporin antibiotic compared with that of cephaloridine, cephalothin, and cefamandole. *Antimicrob. Agents Chemother. 9*:690–695, 1976.
79. Jones, RN, Fuchs, PC, Gavan, TL, Gerlach, EH, Barry, AL, Thornsberry, C: Cefuroxime, a new parenteral cephalosporin: Collaborative in vitro susceptibility comparison with cephalothin against 5,887 clinical bacterial isolates. *Antimicrob. Agents Chemother. 12*:47–50, 1977.
80. Actor, P, Uri, JV, Zajac, I: SKF 75073, new parenteral broad-spectrum cephalosporin with high and prolonged serum levels. *Antimicrob. Agents Chemother. 13*: 784–790, 1978.
81. Jones, RN, Thornsberry, C, Barry, AL, Fuchs, PC, Gavan, TL, Gerlach, EH: Bl-S786, a new parenteral cephalosporin. II. In vitro antimicrobial activity comparison with six related cephalosporins. *J. Antibiot. 30*:583–592, 1978.
82. Hamilton-Miller, JMT, Brumfitt, W, Reynolds, AV: Cefotaxime (HR 756), a new cephalosporin with exceptional broad spectrum activity in vitro. *J. Antimicrob. Chemother. 4*:437–444, 1978.
83. Masuyoshi, S, Arai, S, Miyamoto, M, Mitsuhashi, S: In vitro antimicrobial activity of cefotaxime, a new cephalosporin. *Antimicrob. Agents Chemother. 18*:1–8, 1980.
84. Hinkle, AM, Leblanc, BM, Bodey, GP: In vitro evaluation of cefoperazone. *Antimicrob. Agents Chemother. 17*:423–427, 1980.

85. Chow, AW, Bartlett, KH: Comparative in vitro activity of ceftazidime (GR 20263) and other β-lactamase stable cephalosporins against anaerobic bacteria. *J. Antimicrob. Chemother. 8(Suppl. B)*:91–95, 1981.
86. Neu, HC, Meropol, NJ, Fu, KP: Antibacterial activity of ceftriaxone (Ro 13-9904), a β-lactamase-stable cephalosporin. *Antimicrob. Agents Chemother. 19*:414–423, 1981.
87. Fu, KP, Neu, HC: Antibacterial activity of ceftizoxime, a β-lactamase-stable cephalosporin. *Antimicrob. Agents Chemother. 17*:583–590, 1980.
88. Greenwood, D, Pearson, N, Eley, A, O'Grady, F: Comparative in vitro activities of cefotaxime and ceftizoxime (FK 749): New cephalosporins with exceptional potency. *Antimicrob. Agents Chemother. 17*:397–401, 1980.
89. Stamm, JM, Girolami, RL, Shipkowitz, NL, Bower, RR: Antibacterial activity of cefmenoxime (SCE-1365). *Antimicrob. Agents Chemother. 19*:454–460, 1981.
90. Angehrn, P, Probst, PJ, Reiner, R, Then, RL: Ro 13-9904, a long-acting broad-spectrum cephalosporin: In vitro and in vivo studies. *Antimicrob. Agents Chemther. 18*:913–921, 1980.
91. Neu, HC, Labthavikul, P: Antibacterial activity and β-lactamase stability of ceftazidime, an aminothiazolyl cephalosporin potentially active against *Pseudomonas aeruginosa. Antimicrob. Agents Chemother. 21*:11–18, 1982.
92. Richards, DM, Heel, RC, Brogden, RN, Speight, TM, Avery, GS: Ceftriaxone: A review of its antibacterial activity, pharmacological properties and therapeutic use. *Drugs 27*:469–527, 1984.
93. Richards, DM, Heel, RC: Ceftizoxime: A review of its antibacterial activity, pharmacological properties and therapeutic use. *Drugs 29*:281–329, 1985.
94. Fleming, PC, Knie, B: Activity of ceftazidime against *Pseudomonas aeruginosa* from bacteraemic and fibrocystic patients. *J. Antimicrob. Chemother. 8(Suppl. B)*: 169–173, 1981.
95. Richards, DM, Brogden, RN: Ceftazidime: A review of its antibacterial activity, pharmacological properties and therapeutic use. *Drugs 29*:105–161, 1985.
96. Carmine, AA, Brogden, RN, Heel, RC, Romankiewicz, JA, Speight, TM, Avery, GS: Moxalactam (Latamoxef): A review of its antibacterial activity, pharmacokinetics and therapeutic use. *Drugs 26*:279–333, 1983.
97. Eykyn, S, Jenkins, C, King, A, Phillips, I: Antibacterial activity of cefamandole, a new cephalosporin antibiotic, compared with that of cephaloridine, cephalothin and cephalexin. *Antimicrob. Agents Chemother. 3*:657–661, 1973.
98. Bill, NJ, Washington, JA: Comparison of in vitro activity of cephalexin, cephradine and cefaclor. *Antimicrob. Agents Chemother. 11*:470–474, 1977.
99. Sanders, CC: In vitro studies with cefaclor, a new oral cephalosporin. *Antimicrob. Agents Chemother. 12*:490–497, 1977.
100. Sinai, R, Hammerberg, S, Marks, MI, Pai, CH: In vitro susceptibility of *Hemophilus influenzae* to sulfamethoxazole-trimethoprim and cefaclor, cephalexin and cephradine. *Antimicrob. Agents Chemother. 13*:861–864, 1978.
101. Harding, SM, Williams, PEO, Ayrton, J: Pharmacology of cefuroxime as the 1-acetoxyethyl ester in volunteers. *Antimicrob. Agents Chemother. 25*:78–82, 1984.
102. Kamimura, T, Kojo, H, Matsumoto, Y, Mine, Y, Goto, S, Kuwahara, S: In vitro and in vivo antibacterial properties of FK 027, a new orally active cephem antibiotic. *Antimicrob. Agents Chemother. 25*:98–104, 1984.
103. Neu, HC, Chin, N-X, Labthavikul, P: Comparative in vitro activity and β-lactamase stability of FR 17927, a new orally active cephalosporin. *Antimicrob. Agents Chemother. 26*:174–180, 1984.
104. Jones, R, Fuchs, P, Gavan, T, Gerlach, E, Barry, A, Thornsberry, C: BL-S786, a new parenteral cephalosporin. I. A collaborative in vitro susceptibility comparison

to cephalothin against 5,762 clinical bacterial isolates. *J. Antibiot. (Tokyo) 30*: 576–582, 1977.

105. Brumfitt, W, Kosmidis, J, Hamilton-Miller, JMT, Gilchrist, JNG: Cefoxitin and cephalothin: Antimicrobial activity, human pharmacokinetics, and toxicology. *Antimicrob. Agents Chemother. 6*:290–299, 1974.
106. Actor, P, Guarini, J, Uri, J, Dickson, J, Pauls, JF, Weisbach, JA: Disk susceptibility studies with cefazolin and cephalothin. *Antimicrob. Agents Chemother. 5*: 63–67, 1974.
107. Motley, M, Shadomy, S: In vitro studies with cefazolin. *Antimicrob. Agents Chemother. 6*:856–861, 1974.
108. Jones, RN, Fuchs, PC: Comparison of in vitro antimicrobial activity of cefamandole and cefazolin with cephalothin against over 8000 clinical bacterial isolates. *Antimicrob. Agents Chemother. 9*:1066–1069, 1976.
109. Tally, FP, Jacobus, NV, Barza, M: In vitro activity and serum protein-binding of cefaclor. *J. Antimicrob. Chemother. 5*:159–165, 1979.
110. Bodey, GP, Fainstein, V, Hinkle, AM: Comparative in vitro study of new cephalosporins. *Antimicrob. Agents Chemother. 20*:226–230, 1981.
111. Counts, GW, Turck, M: Antibacterial activity of a new parenteral cephalosporin—HR 756: Comparison with cefamandole and ceforanide. *Antimicrob. Agents Chemother. 16*:64–68, 1979.
112. Van Landuyt, HW, Pyckavet, M: In vitro activity of cefotaxime against cephalothin-resistant clinical isolates. *Antimicrob. Agents Chemother. 16*:109–111, 1979.
113. Mouton, RP, Bongaerto, GPA, Van Gestal, M: Comparison of activity and beta-lactamase stability of cefotaxime with those of six other cephalosporins. *Antimicrob. Agents Chemother. 16*:757–760, 1979.
114. Neu, HC, Aswakopee, N, Fu, KP, Aswakopee, P: Antibacterial activity of a new 1-oxa cephalosporin compared with that of other β-lactam compounds. *Antimicrob. Agents Chemother. 16*:141–149, 1979.
115. Barza, M, Tally, FP, Jacobus, NV, Gorbach, SL: In vitro activity of LY127935. *Antimicrob. Agents Chemother. 16*:287–292, 1979.
116. Verbist, L: Comparison of in vitro activities of eight β-lactamase-stable cephalosporins against β-lactamase-producing gram-negative bacilli. *Antimicrob. Agents Chemother. 19*:407–413, 1981.
117. King, A, Warren, C, Shannon, K, Phillips, I: In-vitro antibacterial activity of cefoperazone, a piperazine cephalosporin. *J. Antimicrob. Chemother. 8*:107–113, 1981.
118. Bint, A, Yeoman, P, Kilburn, P, Anderson, R, Stansfield, E: In vitro activity of ceftazidime compared with that of other cephalosporins. *J. Antimicrob. Chemother. 8(Suppl. B)*:47–51, 1981.
119. Knothe, H, Dette, GA: The in vitro activity of ceftazidime against clinically important pathogens. *J. Antimicrob. Chemother. 8(Suppl. B)*:33–41, 1981.
120. Shannon, K, King, A, Warren, C, Phillips, I: In vitro antibacterial activity and susceptibility of the cephalosporin Ro 13-9904 to beta-lactamases. *Antimicrob. Agents Chemother. 18*:292–298, 1980.
121. Shelton, S, Nelson, JD, McCracken, GH: In vitro susceptibility of gram-negative bacilli from pediatric patients to moxalactam, cefotaxime, Ro 13-9904 and other cephalosporins. *Antimicrob. Agents Chemother. 18*:476–479, 1980.
122. Kamimura, T, Matsumoto, Y, Okada, N, Mine, Y, Nishida, M, Goto, S, Kuwahara, S: Ceftizoxime (FK 749), a new parenteral cephalosporin: In vitro and in vivo antibacterial activities. *Antimicrob. Agents Chemother. 16*:540–548, 1979.
123. Tsuchiya, K, Kondo, M, Kida, M, Nakao, M, Iwahi, T, Yumiko, N, Takeuchi, M, Nozaki, Y: Cefmenoxime (SCE-1365), a novel broad-spectrum cephalosporin: In

vitro and in vivo antibacterial activities. *Antimicrob. Agents Chemother. 19*:56–65, 1981.
124. Schell, RF, Smith, BR, Lefrock, JL, Francisco, MA: Antimicrobial activity of cefmenoxime compared with those of other cephalosporins. *Antimicrob. Agents Chemother. 23*:774–777, 1983.
125. Bauernfeind, A: An evaluation of the activity of cephalosporins against *Pseudomonas aeruginosa. J. Antimicrob. Chemother. 8(Suppl. B)*:111–117, 1981.
126. Brogard, JM, Comte, F, Pinget, M: Pharmacokinetics of cephalosporin antibiotics. *Antibiot. Chemother. 25*:123–162, 1978.
127. Klein, JO, Eickhoff, TC, Tilles, JG, Finland, M: Cephalothin: Activity in vitro, absorption and excretion in normal subjects and clinical observations in 40 patients. *Am. J. Med. Sci. 248*:640–656, 1964.
128. Nightingale, CH, French, MA, Quintiliani, R: Cephalosporins. In: *Applied Pharmacokinetics* (WE Evans, JJ Schentag, and WJ Jusko, eds.), Applied Therapeutics, Inc., San Francisco, 1980, pp. 240–274.
129. Sheng, KT, Huang, NN, Promadhattavedi, V: Serum concentrations of cephalothin in infants and children and placental transmission of the antibiotic. *Antimicrob. Agents Chemother. 1964*:200–206, 1965.
130. Kirby, WMM, Regamey, C: Pharmacokinetics of cefazolin compared with four other cephalosporins. *J. Infect. Dis. 128(Suppl.)*:S341–S346, 1973.
131. Green, ER, Subramanian, S, Faden, H, Quintiliani, R, NIghtingale, CH: A comparison of the penetration characteristics of cephapirin and cephalothin into right atrial appendage, muscle, fat, and pericardial fluid of pediatric patients undergoing open-heart operation. *Ann. Thorac. Surg. 31*:155–160, 1981.
132. Vianna, NJ, Kaye, D: Penetration of cephalothin into the spinal fluid. *Am. J. Med. Sci. 254*:216–220, 1967.
133. MacAulay, MA, Charles, D: Placental transfer of cephalothin. *Am. J. Obstet. Gynecol. 100*:940–946, 1968.
134. Rolewicz, TF, Mirkin, BL, Cooper, MJ, Anders, MW: Metabolic disposition of cephalothin and desacetylcephalothin in children and adults: Comparison of high-performance liquid chromatographic and microbial assay procedures. *Clin. Pharmacol. Ther. 22*:928–935, 1977.
135. Nilsson-Ehle, I, Nilsson-Ehle, P: Pharmacokinetics of cephalothin: Accumulation of its deacetylated metabolite in uremic patients. *J. Infect. Dis. 139*:712–716, 1979.
136. Perkins, RL, Smith, EJ, Saslaw, S: Cephalothin and cephaloridine: Comparative pharmacodynamics in chronic uremia. *Am. J. Med. Sci. 257*:116–124, 1969.
137. Gordon, RC, Barrett, FF, Clark, DJ, Yow, MD: Laboratory and pharmacologic studies of BL-P-1322 (cephapirin sodium) in children. *Curr. Ther. Res. 13*:398–406, 1971.
138. McCloskey, RV, Terry, EE, McCracken, AW, Sweeny, MJ, Forland, MF: Effect of hemodialysis and renal failure on serum and urine concentrations of cephapirin sodium. *Antimicrob. Agents Chemother. 1*:90–93, 1972.
139. Khan, AJ, Pryles, CV: Clinical and pharmacological evaluation of cephapirin sodium (BL-P-1322) in infants and children. *Curr. Ther. Res. 15*:198–204, 1973.
140. Pickering, LK, O'Connor, DM, Anderson, D, Bairan, AC, Feigin, RD, Cherry, JD: Clinical and pharmacologic evaluation of cefazolin in children. *J. Infect. Dis. 128 (Suppl.)*:S407–S414, 1973.
141. Gold, JA, McKee, JJ, Ziv, DS: Experience with cefazolin: An overall summary of pharmacologic and clinical trials in man. *J. Infect. Dis. 128(Suppl.)*:S415–S421, 1973.

142. Regamey, C, Gordon, RC, Kirby, WMM: Cefazolin vs cephalothin and cephaloridine. A comparison of their clinical pharmacology. *Arch. Intern. Med. 133*:407–410, 1974.
143. Reller, LB, Karney, WW, Beaty, HN, Holmes, KK, Turck, M: Evaluation of cefazolin, a new cephalosporin antibiotic. *Antimicrob. Agents Chemother. 3*:488–497, 1973.
144. Thys, JP, Vanderkelen, B, Klastersky, J: Pharmacological study of cefazolin during intermittent and continuous infusion: A crossover investigation in humans. *Antimicrob. Agents Chemother. 10*:395–398, 1976.
145. Ram, MD, Watanatittan, S: Levels of cefazolin in human bile. *J. Infect. Dis. 128 (Suppl.)*:S361–S363, 1973.
146. Tetzlaff, TR, Howard, JB, McCracken, GH, Jr., Calderon, E, Larrondo, J: Antibiotic concentrations in pus and bone of children with osteomyelitis. *J. Pediatr. 92*:135–140, 1978.
147. Yoshioka, H, Cho, K, Takimoto, M, Maruyama, S, Shimizu, T: Transfer of cefazolin into human milk. *J. Pediatr. 94*:151–152, 1979.
148. Khan, AJ: Clinical and laboratory evaluation of cefazolin: A new cephalosporin antibiotic in pediatric patients. *Curr. Ther. Res. 15*:727–733, 1973.
149. Levison, ME, Levison, SP, Ries, K, Kaye, D: Pharmacology of cefazolin in patients with normal and abnormal renal function. *J. Infect. Dis. 128 (Suppl.)*:S354–S357, 1973.
150. Hiner, LB, Baluarte, HJ, Polinsky, MS, Grushkin, AB: Cefazolin in children with renal insufficiency. *J. Pediatr. 96*:335–339, 1980.
151. Bunke, CM, Aronoff, GR, Brier, ME, Sloan, RS, Luft, FC: Cefazolin and cephalexin kinetics in continuous ambulatory peritoneal dialysis. *Clin. Pharmacol. Ther. 33*:66–72, 1983.
152. Wold, JS, Joost, RR, Black, HR, Griffith, RS: Hydrolysis of cefamandole nafate to cefamandole in vivo. *J. Infect. Dis. 137 (Suppl.)*:S17–S24, 1978.
153. Agbayani, MM, Khan, AJ, Kemawikasit, P, Rosenfeld, W, Salazar, D, Kumar, K, Glass, L, Evans, HE: Pharmacokinetics and safety of cefamandole in newborn infants. *Antimicrob. Agents Chemother. 15*:674–676, 1979.
154. Chang, CT, Khan, AJ, Agbayani, MM, Jhaveri, R, Amin, I, Evans, HE: Pharmacokinetics and safety of cefamandole in infants and children. *Antimicrob. Agents Chemother. 14*:838–841, 1978.
155. Sanders, CV, Greenberg, RN, Marier, RL. Cefamandole and cefoxitin. *Ann. Intern. Med. 103*:70–78, 1985.
156. Neu, HC: Comparison of the pharmacokinetics of cefamandole and other cephalosporin compounds. *J. Infect. Dis. 137 (Suppl.)*:S80–S87, 1978.
157. Thirumoorthi, MC, Dajani, DS, Vincent, CV, Maurer, MJ: Pharmacology, safety and efficacy of cefamandole in childhood infections. *Antimicrob. Agents Chemother. 20*:21–24, 1981.
158. Walker, SH, Gahol, VP: Pharmacokinetics of cefamandole in infants and children. *Antimicrob. Agents Chemother. 14*:315–317, 1978.
159. Steinberg, EA, Overturf, GD, Baraff, LJ, Wilkins, J: Penetration of cefamandole into spinal fluid. *Antimicrob. Agents Chemother. 11*:933–935, 1977.
160. Mellin, H-E, Welling, PG, Madsen, PO: Pharmacokinetics of cefamandole in patients with normal and impaired renal function. *Antimicrob. Agents Chemother. 11*:262–266, 1977.
161. Meyers, BR, Hirschman, SZ: Pharmacokinetics of cefamandole in patients with renal failure. *Antimicrob. Agents Chemother. 11*:248–250, 1977.
162. Feldman, WE, Moffitt, S, Sprou, N: Clinical and pharmacokinetic evaluation of parenteral cefoxitin in infants and children. *Antimicrob. Agents Chemother. 17*:669–674, 1980.

163. Sonneville, PF, Albert, KS, Skeggs, H, Gentner, H, Kwan, KC, Martin, CM: Effect of lidocaine on the absorption, disposition and tolerance of intramuscularly administered cefoxitin. *Eur. J. Clin. Pharmacol. 12*:273–279, 1977.
164. Regazzi, MB, Chirico, G, Cristiani, D, Rondini, G, Rondanelli, R: Cefoxitin in newborn infants. A clinical and pharmacokinetic study. *Eur. J. Clin. Pharmacol. 25*: 507–509, 1983.
165. Schrogie, JJ, Davies, RO, Yeh, KC, Rogers, JD, Holmes, GI, Skeggs, H, Martin, CM: Bioavailability and pharmacokinetics of cefoxitin sodium. *J. Antimicrob. Chemother. 4(Suppl. B)*:69–78, 1978.
166. Dubois, M, Delapierre, D, Chanteux, L, Demonty, J, Lambotte, R, Kramp, R, Dresse, A: A study of the transplacental transfer and the mammary excretion of cefoxitin in humans. *J. Clin. Pharmacol. 21*:477–483, 1981.
167. Dresse, A, Lambotte, R, Dubois, M, Delapierre, D, Kramp, R: Transmammary passage of cefoxitin: Additional results. *J. Clin. Pharmacol. 23*:438–440, 1983.
168. Liu, C, Hinthorn, DR, Hodges, GR, Harms, JL, Couchonnal, G, Dworzack, DL: Penetration of cefoxitin into human cerebrospinal fluid: Comparison with cefamandole, ampicillin, and penicillin. *Rev. Infect. Dis. 1*:127–131, 1979.
169. Feldman, WE, Moffitt, S, Manning, NS: Penetration of cefoxitin into cerebrospinal fluid of infants and children with bacterial meningitis. *Antimicrob. Agents Chemother. 21*:468–471, 1982.
170. Roos, R, von Hattingberg, HM, Belohradsky, BH, Marget, W: Pharmacokinetics of cefoxitin in premature and newborn infants studied by continuous serum level monitoring during combination therapy with penicillin and amikacin. *Infection 8*:301–306, 1980.
171. Vlasses, PH, Holbrook, AM, Schrogie, JJ, Rogers, JD, Ferguson, RK, Abrams, WB: Effect of orally administered probenecid on the pharmacokinetics of cefoxitin. *Antimicrob. Agents Chemother. 17*:847–855, 1980.
172. Foord, RD: Cefuroxime: Human pharmacokinetics. *Antimicrob. Agents Chemother. 9*:741–747, 1976.
173. Renlund, M, Pettay, O: Pharmacokinetics and clinical efficacy of cefuroxime in the newborn period. *Proc. R. Soc. Med. 70(Suppl. 9)*:175–178, 1977.
174. Sorin, M, Ghnassia, JC, Demerleire, F, Saudubray, JM: Pharmacokinetics and clinical study of cefuroxime in infants. *Proc. R. Soc. Med. 70(Suppl. 9)*:179–182, 1977.
175. Bergogne-Berezin, E, Even, P, Berthelot, G, Pierre, J: Cefuroxime: Pharmacokinetic study in bronchial secretions. *Proc. R. Soc. Med. 70(Suppl. 9)*:34–37, 1977.
176. Daikos, GK, Kosmidis, J, Stathakis, C, Anyfantis, A, Plakoutsis, T, Papathanassiou, B: Bioavailability of cefuroxime in various sites including bile, sputum and bone. *Proc. R. Soc. Med. 70(Suppl. 9)*:38–41, 1977.
177. Sirinavin, S, Chiemchanya, S, Visudhipan, P, Lolekha, S: Cefuroxime treatment of bacterial meningitis in infants and children. *Antimicrob. Agents Chemother. 25*: 273–275, 1984.
178. Schaad, UB, Krucko, J, Pfenninger, J: An extended experience with cefuroxime therapy of childhood bacterial meningitis. *Pediatr. Infect. Dis. 3*:410–416, 1984.
179. del Rio, MA, Chrane, DF, Shelton, S, McCracken, GH, Jr., Nelson, JD: Pharmacokinetics of cefuroxime in infants and children with bacterial meningitis. *Antimicrob. Agents Chemother. 22*:990–994, 1982.
180. Craft, I, Mullinger, BM, Kennedy, MRR: Placental transfer of cefuroxime. *Br. J. Obstet. Gynecol. 88*:141–145, 1981.
181. Bousfield, P, Browning, AK, Mullinger, BM, Elstein, M: Cefuroxime: Potential use in pregnant women at term. *Br. J. Obstet. Gynecol. 88*:146–149, 1981.
182. Goodwin, CS, Dash, CH, Hill, JP, Goldberg, AD: Cefuroxime pharmacokinetics

after a short infusion and in vitro activity against hospital pathogens. *J. Antimicrob. Chemother. 3*:253–261, 1977.

183. Bundtzen, RW, Toothaker, RD, Nielson, OS, Madsen, PO, Welling, PG, Craig, WA: Pharmacokinetics of cefuroxime in normal and impaired renal function: Comparison of high-pressure liquid chromatography and microbiological assays. *Antimicrob. Agents Chemother. 19*:443–449, 1981.
184. Local, FK, Munro, AJ, Kerr, DNS, Sussman, M: Pharmacokinetics of intravenous and intraperitoneal cefuroxime in patients undergoing peritoneal dialysis. *Clin. Nephrol. 16*:40–43, 1981.
185. Okolicsanyi, L, Venuti, M, Orlando, R, Xerri, L, Pugina, M: Pharmacokinetic studies of cefuroxime in patients with liver cirrhosis. *Arzneimittelforsch. 32*:777–782, 1982.
186. Barriere, SL, Hatheway, GJ, Gambertoglio, JG, Lin, ET, Conte, JE, Jr.: Pharmacokinetics of cefonicid, a new broad-spectrum cephalosporin. *Antimicrob. Agents Chemother. 21*:935–938, 1982.
187. Tartaglione, TA, Polk, RE: Review of the new second generation cephalosporins: Cefonicid, ceforanide, and cefuroxime. *Drug Intell. Clin. Pharm. 19*:188–198, 1985.
188. Blair, AD, Maxwell, BM, Forland, SC, Jacob, L, Cutler, RE: Cefonicid kinetics in subjects with normal and impaired renal function. *Clin. Pharmacol. Ther. 35*: 798–803, 1984.
189. Dajani, AS, Thirumoorthi, MC, Bawdon, RE, Buckley, JA, Pfeffer, M, van Harken, DR, Smyth, RD: Pharmacokinetics of intramuscular ceforanide in infants, children and adolescents. *Antimicrob. Agents Chemother. 21*:282–287, 1982.
190. Thirumoorthi, MC, Buckley, JA, Vincent, CV, Kobos, D, Dajani, AS: Efficacy and safety of ceforanide in the treatment of childhood infections. *Pediatr. Infect. Dis. 2*:377–380, 1983.
191. Smyth, RD, Pfeffer, M, Glick, A, van Harken, DR, Hottendorf, GH: Clinical pharmacokinetics and safety of high doses of ceforanide (BL-S786R) and cefazolin. *Antimicrob. Agents Chemother. 16*:615–621, 1979.
192. Estey, EH, Weaver, SS, Le Blanc, BM, Brown, N, Ho, DH, Bodey, GP: Ceforanide kinetics. *Clin. Pharmacol. Ther. 30*:398–403, 1981.
193. Hawkins, SS, Alford, RH, Stone, WJ, Smyth, RD, Pfeffer, M: Ceforanide kinetics in renal insufficiency. *Clin. Pharmacol. Ther. 30*:468–474, 1981.
194. Hess, JR, Berman, SJ, Boughton, WH, Sugihara, JG, Musgrave, JE, Wong, EGC, Siemsen, AM: Pharmacokinetics of ceforanide in patients with end stage renal disease on hemodialysis. *Antimicrob. Agents Chemother. 17*:251–253, 1980.
195. de Louvois, J, Mulhall, A, Hurley, R: The safety and pharmacokinetics of cefotaxime in the treatment of neonates. *Pediatr. Pharmacol. 2*:275–284, 1982.
196. McCracken, GH, Jr., Threlkeld, NE, Thomas, ML: Pharmacokinetics of cefotaxime in newborn infants. *Antimicrob. Agents Chemother. 21*:683–684, 1982.
197. Trang, JM, Jacobs, RF, Kearns, GL, Brown, AL, Wells, TG, Underwood, FL, Kluza, RB: Cefotaxime and desacetylcefotaxime pharmacokinetics in infants and children with meningitis. *Antimicrob. Agents Chemother. 28*:791–795, 1985.
198. Kosmidis, J, Stathakis, C, Mantopoulos, K, Pouriezi, T, Papathanassiou, B, Daikos, GK: Clinical pharmacology of cefotaxime penetration into bile, sputum, bone and including cerebrospinal fluid. *J. Antimicrob. Chemother. 6(Suppl. A)*:145–152, 1980.
199. Kafetzis, DA, Lazarides, CV, Siafas, CA, Georgakopoulos, PA, Papadatos, CJ: Transfer of cefotaxime in human milk and from mother to foetus. *J. Antimicrob. Chemother. 6(Suppl. A)*:135–141, 1980.
200. Pierre, J, Bergogne-Berezin, E, Ravina, J, Vernant, D: Étude du passage transplacentaire du céfotaxime. *Nouv. Presse Med. 10*:587–589, 1981.

201. Asmar, BI, Thirumoorthi, MC, Buckley, JA, Kobos, DM, Dajani, AS: Cefotaxime diffusion in cerebrospinal fluid of children with meningitis. *Antimicrob. Agents Chemother. 28*:138–140, 1985.
202. Wells, TG, Trang, JM, Brown, AL, Marmer, BC, Jacobs, RF: Cefotaxime therapy of bacterial meningitis in children. *J. Antimicrob. Chemother. 14(Suppl. B)*:181–189, 1984.
203. Bégué, P, Floret, D, Mallet, E, Raynaud, EJ, Safran, C, Sarlangues, J, Teyssier, G: Pharmacokinetics and clinical evaluation of cefotaxime in children suffering with purulent meningitis. *J. Antimicrob. Chemother. 14(Suppl. B)*:161–165, 1984.
204. Humbert, G, Leroy, A, Nair, SR, Cherubin, CE: Concentrations of cefotaxime and the desacetyl metabolite in serum and CSF of patients with meningitis. *J. Antimicrob. Chemother. 13*:487–494, 1984.
205. Kafetzis, DA, Brater, DC, Kapiki, AN, Papas, CV, Dellagrammaticas, H, Papadatos, CJ: Treatment of severe neonatal infections with cefotaxime. Efficacy and pharmacokinetics. *J. Pediatr. 100*:483–489, 1982.
206. von Hattingberg, HM, Marget, W, Belohradsky, BH, Roos, R: Pharmacokinetics of cefotaxime in neonates and children: Clinical aspects. *J. Antimicrob. Chemother. 6(Suppl. A)*:113–118, 1980.
207. Baird-Lambert, J, Doyle, PE, Thomas, D, Cvejic, M, Buchanan, N: Pharmacokinetics of cefotaxime in neonates. *J. Antimicrob. Chemother. 13*:471–477, 1984.
208. Kafetzis, DA, Brater, DC, Kanarios, J, Sinaniotis, CA, Papadatos, CJ: Clinical pharmacology of cefotaxime in pediatric patients. *Antimicrob. Agents Chemother. 20*:487–490, 1981.
209. Lüthy, R, Blaser, J, Bonetti, A, Simmen, H, Wise, R, Siegenthaler, W: Comparative multiple-dose pharmacokinetics of cefotaxime, moxalactam and ceftazidime. *Antimicrob. Agents Chemother. 20*:567–575, 1981.
210. Fu, KP, Aswakopee, P, Ho, I, Matthijssen, C, Neu, HC: Pharmacokinetics of cefotaxime. *Antimicrob. Agents Chemother. 16*:592–597, 1979.
211. Wise, R, Wright, N, Wills, PJ: Pharmacology of cefotaxime and its desacetyl metabolite in renal and hepatic disease. *Antimicrob. Agents Chemother. 19*:526–531, 1981.
212. Ings, RMJ, Fillastre, JP, Godin, M, Leroy, A, Humbert, G: The pharmacokinetics of cefotaxime and its metabolites in subjects with normal and impaired renal function. *Rev. Infect. Dis. 4(Suppl.)*:S379–S391, 1982.
213. Reeves, DS, White, LO, Holt, HA, Bahari, D, Bywater, MJ, Bax, RP: Human metabolism of cefotaxime. *J. Antimicrob. Chemother. 6(Suppl. A)*:93–101, 1980.
214. Coombes, JD: Metabolism of cefotaxime in animals and humans. *Rev. Infect. Dis. 4(Suppl.)*:S325–S332, 1982.
215. Matzke, GR, Abraham, PA, Halstenson, CE, Keane, WF: Cefotaxime and desacetyl cefotaxime kinetics in renal impairment. *Clin. Pharmacol. Ther. 38*:31–36, 1985.
216. Albin, HC, Demotes-Mainard, FM, Bouchet, JL, Vincon, GA, Martin-Dupont, C: Pharmacokinetics of intravenous and intraperitoneal cefotaxime in chronic ambulatory peritoneal dialysis. *Clin. Pharmacol. Ther. 38*:285–289, 1985.
217. Wise, R, Wills, PJ, Bedford, KA: Epimers of moxalactam: In vitro comparisons of activity and stability. *Antimicrob. Agents Chemother. 20*:30–32, 1981.
218. de Louvois, J, James, J, Mulhall, A: Latamoxef and the newborn. *Arch. Dis. Child. 59*:346–350, 1984.
219. Schaad, UB, McCracken, GH, Jr., Threlkeld, N, Thomas, ML: Clinical evaluation of a new broad-spectrum oxa-beta-lactam antibiotic, moxalactam, in neonates and infants. *J. Pediatr. 98*:129–136, 1981.
220. Reed, MD, Aranoff, SC, Meyers, CM, Husak, MP, Bertino, JS, Jr., Blumer, JL: Developmental pharmacokinetics of moxalactam. *Antimicrob. Agents Chemother. 24*:383–387, 1983.

221. Latif, R, Thirumoorthi, MC, Buckley, JA, Kobos, DM, Aravind, MK, Kauffman, RE, Dajani, AS: Pharmacokinetic and clinical evaluation of moxalactam in infants and children. *Dev. Pharmacol. Ther. 3*:222–231, 1981.
222. Peterson, LR, Bean, B, Fasching, CE, Korchik, WP, Gerding, DN: Pharmacokinetics, protein binding, and extravascular distribution of moxalactam in normal and renal failure patients. *Antimicrob. Agents Chemother. 20*:378–381, 1981.
223. Yamada, H, Ichihashi, T, Hirano, K, Kinoshita, H: Plasma protein binding and urinary excretion of R(−) and S(−) epimers of an arylmalonylamino 1-oxacephem. I. In humans. *J. Pharm. Sci. 70*:112–113, 1981 (letter).
224. Shimada, J, Ueda, Y: Moxalactam–absorption, excretion, distribution and metabolism. *Rev. Infect. Dis. 4(Suppl.)*:S569–S580, 1982.
225. Wittmann, DH, Schassan, H-H: Distribution of moxalactam in serum, bone, tissue fluid, and peritoneal fluid. *Rev. Infect. Dis. 4(Suppl.)*:S610–S616, 1982.
226. Muellar, O, Fabricius, K, Krueger, E, Rueckert, U: Pharmacokinetics and clinical efficacy of moxalactam in biliary tract infections. *Rev. Infect. Dis. 3(Suppl.)*: S688–S691, 1982.
227. Thirumoorthi, MC, Buckley, JA, Aravind, MK, Kauffman, RE, Dajani, AS: Diffusion of moxalactam into the cerebrospinal fluid in children with bacterial meningitis. *J. Pediatr. 99*:975–979, 1981.
228. Kaplan, SL, Mason, EO, Jr., Garcia, H, Kvernland, SJ, Loiselle, EM, Anderson, DC, Mintz, AA, Fergin, RD: Pharmacokinetics and cerebrospinal fluid penetration of moxalactam in children with bacterial meningitis. *J. Pediatr. 98*:152–157, 1981.
229. Modai, J, Wolff, M, Lebas, J, Meulemans, A, Manuel, C: Moxalactam penetration into cerebrospinal fluid in patients with bacterial meningitis. *Antimicrob. Agents Chemother. 21*:551–553, 1982.
230. Miller, RD, Keegan, KA, Thrupp, LD, Brann, J: Human breast milk concentrations of moxalactam. *Am. J. Obstet. Gynecol. 148*:348–349, 1984.
231. Nahata, MC, Durrell, DC, Barson, WJ: Moxalactam epimer kinetics in children. *Clin. Pharmacol. Ther. 31*:528–532, 1982.
232. Kaplan, SL, Berry, PL, Mason, EO, Jr., Kramer, WG: Pharmacokinetics of moxalactam in anuric children and during hemodialysis. *Pediatr. Pharmacol. 3*:29–36, 1983.
233. Leroy, A, Humbert, G, Fillastre, JP: Pharmacokinetics of moxalactam in subjects with normal and impaired renal function. *Antimicrob. Agents Chemother. 19*: 965–971, 1981.
234. Lam, M, Manion, CV, Czerwinski, AW: Pharmacokinetics of moxalactam in patients with renal insufficiency. *Antimicrob. Agents Chemother. 19*:461–464, 1981.
235. Jacobsen, EJ, Zahrowski, JJ, Nissenson, AR: Moxalactam kinetics in hemodialysis. *Clin. Pharmacol. Ther. 30*:487–490, 1981.
236. Romagnoli, MF, Flynn, K, Siber, GR, Goldmann, DA: Moxalactam pharmacokinetics in children. *Antimicrob. Agents Chemother. 22*:47–50, 1982.
237. Morse, G, Janicke, D, Cafarell, R, Piontek, K, Apicella, M, Jusko, WJ, Walshe, J: Moxalactam epimer disposition in patients undergoing continuous ambulatory dialysis. *Clin. Pharmacol. Ther. 38*:150–156, 1985.
238. Varghese, M, Khan, AJ, Kumar, K, Rosenfeld, W, Schaeffer, HA, Evans, HE: Pharmacokinetic evaluation of cefoperazone in infants. *Antimicrob. Agents Chemother. 28*:149–150, 1985.
239. Rosenfeld, WN, Evans, HE, Batheja, R, Jhaveri, RC, Vohra, K, Khan, AJ: Pharmacokinetics of cefoperazone in full-term and premature neonates. *Antimicrob. Agents Chemother. 23*:866–869, 1983.
240. Chartrand, SA, Marks, MI, Johnston, JT, Frederick, DF, Scribner, RK: Cefoperazone pharmacokinetics in acute childhood meningitis. *J. Pediatr. 103*:991–995, 1983.

241. Bosso, JA, Chan, GM, Matsen, JM: Cefoperazone pharmacokinetics in preterm infants. *Antimicrob. Agents Chemother. 23*:413–415, 1983.
242. Kemmerich, B, Lode, H, Borner, K, Belmega, D, Jendroschek, T, Koeppe, P, Goertz, G: Biliary excretion and pharmacokinetics of cefoperazone in humans. *J. Antimicrob. Chemother. 12*:27–37, 1983.
243. Cable, D, Overturf, G, Edralin, G: Concentrations of cefoperazone in cerebrospinal fluid during bacterial meningitis. *Antimicrob. Agents Chemother. 23*:688–691, 1983.
244. Phillips, JB, III, Braune, K, Ravis, W, Cassady, G, Dillon, H: Pharmacokinetics of cefoperazone in newborn infants. *Pediatr. Pharmacol. 4*:193–197, 1984.
245. Bolton, WK, Scheld, WM, Spyker, DA, Sande, MA: Pharmacokinetics of cefoperazone in normal volunteers and subjects with renal insufficiency. *Antimicrob. Agents Chemother. 19*:821–825, 1981.
246. Keller, E, Jansen, A, Pely, K, Hoppe-Seyler, G, Schollmeyer, P: Intraperitoneal and intravenous cefoperazone kinetics during continuous ambulatory peritoneal dialysis. *Clin. Pharmacol. Ther. 35*:208–213, 1984.
247. Bocazzi, A, Rizzo, M, Caccamo, ML, Assael, BM: Comparison of the concentrations of ceftazidime in the serum of newborn infants after intravenous and intramuscular administration. *Antimicrob. Agents Chemother. 24*:955–956, 1983.
248. Mulhall, A, de Louvois, J: The pharmacokinetics and safety of ceftazidime in newborn infants. *J. Antimicrob. Chemother. 15*:97–103, 1985.
249. McCracken, GH, Jr., Threlkeld, N, Thomas, ML: Pharmacokinetics of ceftazidime in newborn infants. *Antimicrob. Agents Chemother. 26*:583–584, 1984.
250. Harding, SM, Monro, AJ, Thornton, JE, Ayrton, J, Hogg, MIJ: The comparative pharmacokinetics of ceftazidime and cefotaxime in healthy volunteers. *J. Antimicrob. Chemother. 8(Suppl. B)*:263–272, 1981.
251. Kemmerich, B, Warns, H, Lode, H, Borner, K, Koeppe, P, Knothe, H: Multiple-dose pharmacokinetics of ceftazidime and its influence on fecal flora. *Antimicrob. Agents Chemother. 24*:333–338, 1983.
252. Leeder, JS, Spino, M, Isles, AF, Tesoro, AM, Gold, R, MacLeod, SM: Ceftazidime disposition in acute and stable cystic fibrosis. *Clin. Pharmacol. Ther. 36*:355–362, 1984.
253. Low, DC, Bissenden, JG, Wise, R: Ceftazidime in neonatal infections. *Arch. Dis. Child. 60*:360–364, 1985.
254. Wittman, DH, Schassan, H-H, Kohler, F, Seibert, W: Pharmacokinetic studies of ceftazidime in serum, bone, bile, tissue fluid and peritoneal fluid. *J. Antimicrob. Chemother. 8(Suppl. B)*:293–297, 1981.
255. Daschner, FD, Peterson, EE, Just, H-H, Hillemans, HG: Penetration of ceftazidime into serum, myometrium, endometrium, salpinges and subcutaneous tissue. *J. Antimicrob. Chemother. 12(Suppl. A)*:247–249, 1983.
256. Benoni, G, Arosio, E, Raimondi, MG, Apolloni, E, Passarella, E, Lechi, A, Velo, GP: Distribution of ceftazidime in ascitic fluid. *Antimicrob. Agents Chemother. 25*:760–763, 1984.
257. Walstad, RA, Hellum, KB, Blika, S, Dale, LG, Fredriksen, T, Myhre, KI, Spencer, GR: Pharmacokinetics and tissue penetration of ceftazidime: Studies on lymph, aqueous humour, skin blister, cerebrospinal and pleural fluid. *J. Antimicrob. Chemother. 12(Suppl. A)*:275–282, 1983.
258. Modai, J, Vittecoq, D, Decazes, JM, Wolff, M, Meulemans, A: Penetration of ceftazidime into the cerebrospinal fluid of patients with bacterial meningitis. *Antimicrob. Agents Chemother. 24*:126–128, 1983.
259. Fong, IW, Tomkins, KB: Penetration of ceftazidime into the cerebrospinal fluid of patients with and without evidence of meningeal inflammation. *Antimicrob. Agents Chemother. 26*:115–116, 1984.

260. Blumer, JL, Aronoff, SC, Myers, CM, O'Brien, CA, Klinger, JD, Reed, MD: Pharmacokinetics and cerebrospinal fluid penetration of ceftazidime in children with meningitis. *Dev. Pharmacol. Ther. 8*:219–231, 1985.
261. Blanco, JD, Jorgensen, JH, Castaneda, YS, Crawford, SA: Ceftazidime in human breast milk. *Antimicrob. Agents Chemother. 23*:479–480, 1983.
262. Ackerman, BH, Ross, J, Tofte, RW, Rotschafer, JC: Effect of decreased renal function on the pharmacokinetics of ceftazidime. *Antimicrob. Agents Chemother. 25*: 785–786, 1984.
263. Leroy, A, Leguy, F, Borsa, F, Spencer, GR, Fillastre, JP, Humbert, G: Pharmacokinetics of ceftazidime in normal and uremic patients. *Antimicrob. Agents Chemother. 25*:638–642, 1984.
264. Tourkantonis, A, Nicolaidis, P: Pharmacokinetics of ceftazidime in patients undergoing peritoneal dialysis. *J. Antimicrob. Chemother. 12 (Suppl. A)*:263–267, 1983.
265. Patel, IH, Weinfeld, RE, Konikoff, J, Parsonnet, M: Pharmacokinetics and tolerance of ceftriaxone in humans after single-dose intramuscular administration in water and lidocaine diluents. *Antimicrob. Agents Chemother. 21*:957–962, 1982.
266. Mulhall, A, de Louvois, J, James, J: Pharmacokinetics and safety of ceftriaxone in the neonate. *Eur. J. Pediatr. 144*:379–382, 1985.
267. McCracken, GH, Jr., Siegel, JD, Threlkeld, N, Thomas, M: Ceftriaxone pharmacokinetics in newborn infants. *Antimicrob. Agents Chemother. 23*:341–343, 1983.
268. Steele, RW, Eyre, LB, Bradsher, RW, Weinfeld, RE, Patel, IH, Spicehandler, J: Pharmacokinetics of ceftriaxone in pediatric patients with meningitis. *Antimicrob. Agents Chemother. 23*:191–194, 1983.
269. Gould Chadwick, E, Yogev, R, Shulman, ST, Weinfeld, RE, Patel, IH: Single-dose ceftriaxone pharmacokinetics in pediatric patients with central nervous system infections. *J. Pediatr. 102*:134–137, 1983.
270. Stoeckel, K, McNamara, PJ, Brandt, R, Plozza-Nottebrock, H, Ziegler, WH: Effects of concentration-dependent plasma protein binding on ceftriaxone kinetics. *Clin. Pharmacol. Ther. 29*:650–657, 1981.
271. Schaad, UB, Hayton, WL, Stoeckel, K: Single dose ceftriaxone kinetics in the newborn. *Clin. Pharmacol. Ther. 37*:522–528, 1985.
272. Schaad, UB, Stoeckel, K: Single-dose pharmacokinetics of ceftriaxone in infants and young children. *Antimicrob. Agents Chemother. 21*:248–253, 1982.
273. Harrison, CJ, Welch, D, Marks, MI: Ceftriaxone therapy in pediatric patients. *Am. J. Dis. Child. 137*:1048–1051, 1983.
274. Kafetzis, DA, Brater, DC, Fanourgakis, JE, Voyatzis, J, Georgakopoulos, P: Ceftriaxone distribution between maternal blood and fetal blood tissues at parturition and between blood and milk postpartum. *Antimicrob. Agents Chemother. 23*:870–873, 1983.
275. Martin, E, Koup, Jr., Paravicini, U, Stoeckel, K: Pharmacokinetics of ceftriaxone in neonates and infants with meningitis. *J. Pediatr. 105*:475–481, 1984.
276. Latif, R, Dajani, AS: Ceftriaxone diffusion into cerebrospinal bluid of children with meningitis. *Antimicrob. Agents Chemother. 23*:46–48, 1983.
277. del Rio, M, McCracken, GH, Jr., Nelson, JD, Chrane, D, Shelton, S: Pharmacokinetics and cerebrospinal bactericidal activity of ceftriaxone in the treatment of pediatric patients with bacterial meningitis. *Antimicrob. Agents Chemother. 22*: 622–627, 1982.
278. Steele, RW, Bradsher, RW: Comparison of ceftriaxone with standard therapy for bacterial meningitis. *J. Pediatr. 103*:138–141, 1983.
279. Reed, MD, Rekate, HL, Aronoff, SC, Myers, CM, Blumer, JL: Single-dose plasma and cerebrospinal fluid pharmacokinetics of ceftriaxone in infants and children. *Clinical Pharmacy 2*:558–563, 1983.

280. Bryan, JP, Rocha, H, da Silva, HR, Taveres, A, Sande, MA, Scheld, WM: Comparison of ceftriaxone and ampicillin plus chloramphenicol for the therapy of acute bacterial meningitis. *Antimicrob. Agents Chemother. 28*:361–368, 1985.
281. Friis-Hansen, B: Body water compartments in children: Changes during growth and related changes in body composition. *Pediatrics 28*:169–181, 1961.
282. Hayton, WL, Stoeckel, K: Age-associated changes in ceftriaxone pharmacokinetics. *Clin. Pharmacokinet. 11*:76–86, 1986.
283. McNamara, PJ, Gibaldi, M, Stoeckel, K: Volume of distribution terms for a drug (ceftriaxone) exhibiting concentration-dependent protein binding. I. Theoretical considerations. *Eur. J. Clin. Pharmacol. 25*:399–405, 1983.
284. McNamara, PJ, Gibaldi, M, Stoeckel, K: Volume of distribution terms for a drug (ceftriaxone) exhibiting concentration-dependent protein binding. II. Physiological significance. *Eur. J. Clin. Pharmacol. 25*:407–412, 1983.
285. Luderer, JR, Patel, IH, Durkin, J, Schneck, DW: Age and ceftriaxone kinetics. *Clin. Pharmacol. Ther. 35*:19–25, 1984.
286. Arvidsson, A, Alván, G, Angelin, B, Borgå, O, Nord, CE: Ceftriaxone: Renal and biliary excretion and effect on the colon microflora. *J. Antimicrob. Chemother. 10*:207–215, 1982.
287. Assael, BM: Pharmacokinetics and drug distribution during postnatal development. *Pharmacol. Ther. 18*:159–192, 1982.
288. Ti, T-Y, Fortin, L, Kreeft, JH, East, DS, Ogilvie, RI, Somerville, PJ: Kinetic disposition of intravenous ceftriaxone in normal subjects and patients with renal failure on hemodialysis or peritoneal dialysis. *Antimicrob. Agents Chemother. 25*:83–87, 1984.
289. Patel, IH, Sugihara, JG, Weinfeld, RE, Wong, EGC, Siemsen, AW, Berman, SJ: Ceftriaxone pharmacokinetics in patients with various degrees of renal impairment. *Antimicrob. Agents Chemother. 25*:438–442, 1984.
290. Kowalsky, SF, Echols, RM, Parker, MA: Pharmacokinetics of ceftriaxone in subjects with renal insufficiency. *Clinical Pharmacy 4*:177–181, 1985.
291. Salvador, P, Smith, RG, Weinfeld, RE, Ellis, DH, Bodey, GP: Clinical pharmacology of ceftriaxone in patients with neoplastic diseases. *Antimicrob. Agents Chemother. 23*:583–588, 1983.
292. McCracken, GH, Jr., Ginsburg, CM, Clahsen, JC, Thomas, ML: Pharmacologic evaluation of orally administered antibiotics in infants and children: Effect of feeding on bioavailability. *Pediatrics 62*:738–743, 1978.
293. Ginsburg, CM: Comparative pharmacokinetics of cefadroxil, cefaclor, cephalexin and cephradine in infants and children. *J. Antimicrob. Chemother. 10(Suppl. B)*: 27–31, 1982.
294. Tetzlaff, TR, McCracken, GH, Jr., Thomas, ML: Bioavailability of cephalexin in children: Relationship to drug formulations and meals. *J. Pediatr. 92*:292–294, 1978.
295. Boothman, R, Kerr, MM, Marshall, MJ, Burland, WL: Absorption and excretion of cephalexin by the newborn infant. *Arch. Dis. Child. 48*:147–150, 1973.
296. Menardi, G, Guggenbichler, JP: Bioavailability of oral antibiotics in children with short-bowel syndrome. *J. Pediatr. Surg. 19*:84–86, 1984.
297. Griffith, RS: The pharmacology of cephalexin. *Postgrad. Med. J. 59(Suppl. 5)*: 16–27, 1983.
298. Pfeffer, M, Jackson, A, Ximenes, J, De Menzes, JP: Comparative human oral clinical pharmacology of cefadroxil, cephalexin and cephradine. *Antimicrob. Agents Chemother. 11*:331–338, 1977.
298a. Brogard, JM, Pinget, M, Dorner, M, Lavillaureix, J: Determination of cefalexin pharmacokinetics and dosage adjustments in relation to renal function. *J. Clin. Pharmacol. 15*:666–673, 1975.

299. Marget, VW, Daschner, F: Untersuchungen zur Anwendung von Cephalexin im Kindesalter. *Arzneimittelforsch. 19*:1956–1958, 1969.
300. Spyker, DA, Thomas, BL, Sande, MA, Bolton, WK: Pharmacokinetics of cefaclor and cephalexin: Dosage nomograms for impaired renal function. *Antimicrob. Agents Chemother. 14*:172–177, 1978.
301. Ginsburg, CM, McCracken, GH, Jr.: Pharmacokinetics of cephradine suspension in infants and children. *Antimicrob. Agents Chemother. 16*:74–76, 1979.
302. Vukovich, RA, Brannick, LJ, Sugerman, AA, Neiss, ES: Sex differences in the intramuscular absorption and bioavailability of cephradine. *Clin. Pharmacol. Ther. 18*:215–220, 1975.
303. McCracken, GH, Jr., Ginsburg, CM, Clahsen, JC, Thomas, ML: Pharmacokinetics of cefaclor in infants and children. *J. Antimicrob. Chemother. 4*:515–521, 1978.
304. Santoro, J, Agarwal, BN, Martinelli, R, Wenger, N, Levison, ME: Pharmacology of cefaclor in normal volunteers and patients with renal failure. *Antimicrob. Agents Chemother. 13*:951–954, 1978.
305. Korzeniowski, OM, Scheld, WM, Sande, MA: Comparative pharmacology of cefaclor and cephalexin. *Antimicrob. Agents Chemother. 12*:157–162, 1977.
306. Fogelsong, MA, Lamb, JW, Dietz, JV: Stability and blood level determinations of cefaclor, a new oral cephalosporin antibiotic. *J. Antimicrob. Chemother. 13*:49–52, 1978.
307. Simon, C, Gutzemeier, U: Serum and sputum levels of cefaclor. *Postgrad. Med. J. 55(Suppl. 4)*:30–34, 1979.
308. Bloch, R, Szwed, JJ, Sloan, RS, Luft, FC: Pharmacokinetics of cefaclor in normal subjects and patients with chronic renal failure. *Antimicrob. Agents Chemother. 12*:730–732, 1977.
309. Spyker, DA, Gober, LL, Scheld, WM, Sande, MA, Bolton, WK: Pharmacokinetics of cefaclor in renal failure: Effects of multiple doses and hemodialysis. *Antimicrob. Agents Chemother. 21*:278–281, 1982.
310. Ginsburg, CM, McCracken, GH, Jr., Clahsen, JC, Thomas, ML: Clinical pharmacology of cefadroxil in infants and children. *Antimicrob. Agents Chemother. 13*: 845–848, 1978.
311. Quintiliani, R: A review of the penetration of cefadroxil into human tissue. *J. Antimicrob. Chemother. 10(Suppl. B)*:33–38, 1982.
312. Leroy, A, Humbert, G, Godin, M, Fillastre, JP: Pharmacokinetics of cefadroxil in patients with impaired renal function. *J. Antimicrob. Chemother. 10(Suppl. B)*: 39–46, 1982.
313. Ginsburg, CM, McCracken, GH, Jr., Petruska, M, Olson, K: Pharmacokinetics and bactericidal activity of cefuroxime axetil. *Antimicrob. Agents Chemother. 28*: 504–507, 1985.
314. Harding, SM, Williams, PEO, Ayrton, J: Pharmacology of cefuroxime as the 1-acetoxyethyl ester in volunteers. *Antimicrob. Agents Chemother. 25*:78–82, 1984.
315. Sommers, DK, Van Wyk, M, Williams, PEO, Harding, SM: Pharmacokinetics and tolerance of cefuroxime axetil in volunteers during repeated dosing. *Antimicrob. Agents Chemother. 25*:344–347, 1984.
316. Brittain, DC, Scully, BE, Hirose, T, Neu, HC: The pharmacokinetic and bactericidal characteristics of oral cefixime. *Clin. Pharmacol. Ther. 38*:590–594, 1985.
317. Bialer, M, Tonelli, AP, Kantrowitz, JD, Yacobi, A: Serum protein binding of a new oral cephalosporin, CL 284,635, in various species. *Drug Metab. Dispos. 14*:132–136, 1986.
318. Sanders, WE, Johnson, JE, Taggart, JG: Adverse reactions to cephalothin and cephapirin. *N. Engl. J. Med. 290*:424–429, 1974.
319. Levine, BB: Antigenicity and cross-reactivity of penicillins and cephalosporins. *J. Infect. Dis. 128(Suppl.)*:S364–S366, 1973.

320. Petz, LD: Immunologic cross-reactivity between penicillins and cephalosporins: A review. *J. Infect. Dis. 137(Suppl.)*:S74–S79, 1978.
321. Levine, LR: Quantitative comparison of adverse reactions to cefaclor vs. amoxicillin in a surveillance study. *Pediatr. Infect. Dis. 4*:358–361, 1985.
322. Barza, M: The nephrotoxicity of cephalosporins: An overview. *J. Infect. Dis. 137(Suppl.)*:S60–S73, 1978.
323. Tune, BM: Relationship between the transport and toxicity of cephalosporins in the kidney. *J. Infect. Dis. 132*:189–194, 1975.
324. Dupuis, LL, Paton, TW, Suttie, JW, Thiessen, JJ, Rachlis, A: Cefazolin-induced coagulopathy. *Clin. Pharmacol. Ther. 35*:237, 1984.
325. Bang NU, Tessler, SS, Heidenreich, RO, Marks, CA, Mattler, LE: Effects of moxalactam on blood coagulation and platelet function. *Rev. Infect. Dis. 4(Suppl.)*: S546–S554, 1982.
326. Quintiliani, R: Bleeding disorders associated with newer cephalosporins. *Clinical Pharmacy 2*:360–361, 1983.
327. Smith, CR, Lipsky, JJ: Hypoprothrombinemia and platelet dysfunction caused by cephalosporin and oxalactam antibiotics. *J. Antimicrob. Chemother. 11*:496–499, 1983.
328. Lipsky, JJ, Lewis, JC, Novick, WJ: Production of hypoprothrombinemia by moxalactam and 1-methyl-5-thiotetrazole in rats. *Antimicrob. Agents Chemother. 25*: 380–381, 1984.
329. Kerremans, AL, Lipsky, JJ, Van Loon, J, Gallego, MO, Wenshilboum, RM: Cephalosporin-induced hypoprothrombinemia: Possible role for thiol methylation of 1-methyltetrazol-5-thiol and 2-methyl-1,3,4-thiadaizole-thiol. *J. Pharmacol. Exp. Ther. 235*:382–388, 1984.
330. Fainstein, V, Bodey, GP, McCredie, KB, Keating, MJ, Estey, EH, Bolivar, R, Elting, L: Coagulation abnormalities induced by β-lactam antibiotics in cancer patients. *J. Infect. Dis. 148*:745–750, 1983.
331. Portier, H, Chalopin, JM, Freysz, M, Tanter, Y: Interaction between cephalosporins and alcohol. *Lancet 2*:263, 1980.
332. Drummer, S, Hauser, WE, Remington, JS: Antabuse-like effect of β-lactam antibiotics. *N. Engl. J. Med. 303*:1417–1418, 1980.
333. McMahon, FG: Disulfiram-like reaction to a cephalosporin. *JAMA 243*:2397, 1980.
334. Buening, MK, Wold, JS, Israel, KS, Kammer, RB: Disulfiram-like reaction to β-lactams. *JAMA 245*:2027, 1981.
335. Brown, KR, Guglielmo, BJ, Pons, VG, Jacobs, RA: Theophylline elixir, moxalactam and a disulfiram reaction. *Ann. Intern. Med. 97*:621–622, 1982.
336. Murray, G: Toxic paranoid reaction to cephalothin. *Drug Intell. Clin. Pharm. 8*: 71, 1974.
337. Yost, RL, Lee, JD, O'Leary, JP: Convulsions associated with sodium cefazolin: A case report. *Am. Surg. 43*:417–420, 1977.
338. Gardner, ME, Fritz, WL, Hyland, RN: Antibiotic-induced seizures: A case report attributed to cefazolin. *Drug Intell. Clin. Pharm. 12*:268–271, 1978.
339. Bechtel, TP, Slaughter, RL, Moore, TD: Seizures associated with high cerebrospinal fluid concentrations of cefazolin. *Am. J. Hosp. Pharm. 37*:271–273, 1980.
340. Arvidsson, A, Alván, G, Angelin, B, Borgå, O, Nord, CE: Ceftriaxone: Renal and biliary excretion and effect on the colon microflora. *J. Antimicrob. Chemother. 10*:207–215, 1982.
341. Nilsson-Ehle, I, Nord, CE, Ursing, B: Ceftriaxone pharmacokinetics and effect on microflora in patients with acute bacterial meningitis. *Scand. J. Infect. Dis. 17*: 77–82, 1985.
342. Sakata, H, Fujita, K, Yoshioka, H: The effect of antimicrobial agents on the fecal flora of children. *Antimicrob. Agents Chemother. 29*:225–229, 1986.

343. Bodey, GP, Fainstein, V, Garcia, I, Rosenbaum, B, Wong, Y: Effect of broad-spectrum cephalosporins on the microbial flora of recipients. *J. Infect. Dis. 148*: 892–897, 1983.

344. Sunakawa, K, Akita, H, Iwata, S, Sato, Y: Clinical superinfection and its attendant symptomatic changes in pediatrics. *Infection 13(Suppl. 1)*:S103–111, 1985.

345. Lambert-Zechovsky, N, Bingen, E, Proux, MC, Aujard, Y, Mathieu, H: Influence de la céfopérazone sur la flore fécale de l'enfant. *Pathol. Biol. (Paris) 32*:439–442, 1984.

346. Bourillon, A, Brackman, D, Boussougant, Y, de Paillerets, F: Cefotaxime effects on the intestinal flora of the newborn. *Dev. Pharmacol. Ther. 7(Suppl. 1)*144–149, 1984.

347. Jones, RN: Gram-positive superinfections following beta-lactam chemotherapy: The significance of the enterococcus. *Infection 13(Suppl. 1)*:S81–S88, 1985.

348. Aronsson, B, Möllby, R, Nord, CE: Antimicrobial agents and *Clostridium difficile* in acute enteric disease: Epidemiologic data from Sweden 1980–1982. *J. Infect. Dis. 151*:476–481, 1985.

349. Kowalsky, SF, Wishnoff, FG: Evaluation of potential interaction of new cephalosporins with Clinitest. *Am. J. Hosp. Pharm. 39*:1499–1501, 1982.

350. Hyneck, ML, Berardi, RR, Johnson, RM: Interference of cephalosporins and cefoxitin with serum creatinine determination. *Am. J. Hosp. Pharm. 38*:1348–1352, 1981.

351. Saah, AJ, Koch, TR, Drusano, GL: Cefoxitin falsely elevates creatinine levels. *JAMA 247*:205–206, 1982.

352. Foord, RD: Cephaloridine, cephalothin and the kidney. *J. Antimicrob. Chemother. 1(Suppl.)*:119–133, 1975.

353. McCracken, GH, Nelson, JD: The third generation cephalosporins and the pediatric practitioner. *Pediatr. Infect. Dis. 1*:123–125, 1982.

354. Moellering, RC: Ceftazidime: A new broad spectrum cephalosporin. *Pediatr. Infect. Dis. 4*:390–394, 1985.

355. Norris, SM: The cephalosporin antibiotic agents. II. First- and second-generation agents. *Infect. Control 4*:577–582, 1984.

356. Steinberg, EA, Overturf, GD, Wilkins, J, Baraff, LJ, Streng, JM, Leedom, JM: Failure of cefamandole in treatment of meningitis die to *Haemophilus influenzae* type b. *J. Infect. Dis. 137*:S180–S186, 1978.

357. Hart, MH, Cherry, JD: Cefamandole failure in *Haemophilus influenzae* endocarditis. *Pediatr. Infect. Dis. 4*:694–696, 1985.

358. Chartrand, SA, Marks, MI, Roberts, R, et al.: Development of *Haemophilus influenzae* meningitis in patients treated with cefamandole. *J. Pediatr. 98*:1003–1005, 1981.

359. Aronoff, SC, Thomford, W, Berlino, JS, et al.: Development of meningitis during therapy with cefamandole. *Pediatrics 67*:727–728, 1981.

360. Azimi, PH, Chase, PA: The role of cefamandole in the treatment of *Haemophilus influenzae* infections in infants and children. *J. Pediatr. 98*:995–1000, 1981.

361. Bergeron, MG, Claveau, S, Simard, P: Limited in vitro activity of cefamandole against 100 beta-lactamse- and non-beta-lactamase-producing *Haemophilus influenzae* strains: Comparison of moxalactam, chloramphenicol, and ampicillin. *Antimicrob. Agents Chemother. 19*:101–105, 1981.

362. Syriopoulou, VP, Scheifele, DW, Sack, CM, Smith, AL: Effect of innoculum size on the susceptibility of *Haemophilus influenzae* to beta-lactam antibiotics. *Antimicrob. Agents Chemother. 17*:516–517, 1979.

363. Nelson, JD: Cefuroxime: A cephalosporin with unique applicability to pediatric practice. *Pediatr. Infect. Dis. 2*:394–396, 1983.

364. Yogev, R: Advances in diagnosis and treatment of childhood meningitis. *Pediatr. Infect. Dis. 4*:321–325, 1985.
365. Swedish Study Group: Cefuroxime versus ampicillin and chloramphenicol for the treatment of bacterial meningitis. *Lancet 1*:295–299, 1982.
366. Nelson, JD, Kusmiesz, H, Shelton, S: Cefuroxime therapy for pneumonia in infants and children. *Pediatr. Infect. Dis. 1*:159–163, 1982.
367. Nelson, JD, Bucholz, RW, Kusmiesz, H, et al.: Benefits and risks of sequential parenteral-oral cephalosporin therapy for suppurative bone and joint infections. *J. Pediatr. Orthoped. 2*:255–262, 1982.
368. Wood, C, Rue, Y, (eds.): *Cefuroxime Update*, International Congress and Symposium Series No. 38. Grune and Stratton, New York, 1981.
369. Neu, HC: Cefoxitin: An overview of clinical studies in the United States. *Rev. Infect. Dis. 1*:233–239, 1979.
370. Lapointe, J-R, Beliveau, C, Chicoine, L, Joncas, JH: A comparison of ampicillin-cefotaxime and ampicillin-chloramphenicol in childhood bacterial meningitis: An experience in 55 patients. *J. Antimicrob. Chemother. 14(Suppl. B)*:167–180, 1984.
371. Jacobs, RF, Wells, TG, Steele, RW, Yamauchi, T: A prospective randomized comparison of cefotaxime vs ampicillin and chloramphenicol for bacterial meningitis in children. *J. Pediatr. 107*:129–133, 1985.
372. Kobayashi, Y, Morikawa, Y, Haruta, T: Clinical evaluation of cefotaxime in treatment of purulent meningitis in children. *Clin. Ther. 4*:89–110, 1981.
373. Naqvi, SH, Maxwell, MA, Dunkle, LM: Cefotaxime therapy of neonatal gram-negative bacillary meningitis. *Pediatr. Infect. Dis. 4*:499–502, 1985.
374. Lecour, H, Seara, A, Miranda, AM, Cordeiro, J, Sarmento, J: Treatment of 160 cases of acute bacterial meningitis with cefotaxime. *J. Antimicrob. Chemother. 14 (Suppl. B)*:195–202, 1984.
375. McCracken, GH, Threlkeld, N, Mize, S, Baker, CJ, Kaplan, SL, Fainezicht, I, Feldman, WE, Schaad, U: Moxalactam therapy for neonatal meningitis due to Gram-negative enteric bacilli. *JAMA 252*:1427–1432, 1984.
376. McCracken, GH: Management of neonatal meningitis, 1984. *J. Antimicrob. Chemother. 14(Suppl. B)*:23–31, 1984.
377. Klastersky, J, Glauser, MP, Schimpf, SC, Zinner, SH, Gaya, H: Prospective randomized comparison of three antibiotic regimens for empirical therapy of suspected bacteremic infection in febrile granulocytopenic patients. *Antimicrob. Agents Chemother. 29*:263–270, 1986.
378. Higham, M, Cunningham, FM, Teele, DW: Ceftriaxone administered once or twice a day for treatment of bacterial infections of childhood. *Pediatr. Infect. Dis. 4*: 22–26, 1985.
379. Yogevm, R, Shulman, ST, Chadwick, EG, Davis, AT, Glogowski, W: Once daily ceftriaxone for central nervous system infections and other serious pediatric infections. *Pediatr. Infect. Dis. 5*:298–303, 1986.
380. del Rio, MA, Chrane, D, Shelton, S, McCracken, GH, Nelson, JD: Ceftriaxone versus ampicillin and chloramphenicol for treatment of bacterial meningitis in children. *Lancet 1*:1241–1244, 1983.
381. Aronoff, SC, Reed, MD, O'Brien, CA, Blumer, JL: Comparison of the efficacy and safety of cetriaxone to ampicillin/chloramphenicol in the treatment of childhood meningitis. *J. Antimicrob. Chemother. 13*:143–151, 1984.
382. Barson, WJ, Miller, MA, Brady, MT, Powell, DA: Prospective comparative trial of ceftriaxone vs. conventional therapy for treatment of bacterial meningitis in children. *Pediatr. Infect. Dis. 4*:362–368, 1985.
383. Martin, E: Once-daily administration of ceftriaxone in the treatment of meningitis and other serious infections in children. *Eur. J. Clin. Microbiol. 2*:509–515, 1983.

384. Congeni, BL, Bradley, J, Hammerschlag, MR: Safety and efficacy of once daily ceftraixone for the treatment of bacterial meningitis. *Pediatr. Infect. Dis. 5*:293-297, 1986.
385. Fong, IW, Tomkins, KB: Review of *Pseudomonas aeruginosa* meningitis with special emphasis on treatment with ceftazidime. *Rev. Infect. Dis.* 7:604-612, 1985.
386. Rodriguez, WJ, Khan, WN, Gold, B, Feris, J, Puig, J, Sturla, C: Ceftazidime in the treatment of meningitis in infants and children over one month of age. *Am. J. Med. 79(Suppl. 2A)*:52-61, 1985.
387. Mandell, LA, Nicolle, LE, Ronald, AR, Duperval, R, Robson, HG, Feld, R, Vincelette, J, Fong, I: A multicentre prospective randomized trial comparing ceftazidime with cefazolin/tobramycin in the treatment of hospitalized patients with non-pneumococcal pneumonia. *J. Antimicrob. Chemother. 12(Suppl. A)*:9-20, 1983.
388. Mastella, G, Agostini, M, Barlocco, G, et al.: Alternative antibiotics for the treatment of *Pseudomonas* infections in cystic fibrosis. *J. Antimicrob. Chemother. 12(Suppl. A)*:297-311, 1983.
389. Heilesen, AM, Permin, J, Koch, C, et al.: Treatment of chronic *Pseudomonas aeruginosa* infection in cystic fibrosis patients with ceftazidime and tobramycin. *Scand. J. Infect. Dis. 15*:271-276, 1983.
390. Padoan, R, Brienza, A, Crossignani, RM, et al.: Ceftazidime in treatment of acute pulmonary exacerbations in patients with cystic fibrosis. *J. Pediatr. 103*:320-324, 1983.
391. Gold, R, Overmeyer, A, Knie, B, Fleming, PC, Levison, H: Controlled trial of ceftazidime vs. ticarcillin and tobramycin in the treatment of acute respiratory exacerbations in patients with cystic fibrosis. *Pediatr. Infect. Dis. 4*:172-177, 1985.
392. Blumer, JL, Stern, RC, Klinger, JD, Yamashita, TS, Meyers, CM, Blum, A, Reed, MD: Ceftazidime therapy in patients with cystic fibrosis and multiply-drug-resistant *Pseudomonas. Am. J. Med. 79(Suppl. 2A)*:37-46, 1985.
393. Pizzo, PA, Tahler, M, Hathorn, J, et al.: New beta-lactam antibiotics in granulocytopenic patients. *Am. J. Med. 79(Suppl. 2A)*:75-82, 1985.
394. Kaplan, SL, Mason, EO, Kvernland, SJ, Loiselle, EM, Feigin, RD: Moxalactam treatment of serious infections primarily due to *Haemophilus influenzae* type b in children. *Pediatrics 71*:187-191, 1983.
395. Kaplan, SL, Mason, EO, Mason, SK, Catlin, FI, Lee, RT, Murphy, M, Feign, RD: Prospective comparative trial of moxalactam versus ampicillin or chloramphenicol for treatment of *Haemophilus influenzae* type b meningitis in children. *J. Pediatr. 104*:447-453, 1984.
396. Griffith, RS, Black, HR: Cephalexin. *Med. Clin. North Am. 54*:1229-1244, 1970.
397. Stechenberg, BW, Anderson, D, Chang, MJ, et al.: Cephalexin compared to ampicillin treatment of otitis media. *Pediatrics 58*:532-536, 1976.
398. Jackson, MA, Nelson, JD: Etiology and medical management of acute suppurative bone and joint infections in pediatric patients. *J. Pediatr. Orthoped. 2*:313-323, 1982.
399. Walker, SH: Staphylococcal osteomyelitis in children: Success with cephaloridin-cephalexin therapy. *Clin. Pediatr. 12*:98-100, 1983.
400. Tetzlaff, TR, McCracken, GH, Nelson, JD: Oral antibiotic therapy for skeletal infections. *J. Pediatr. 92*:485-490, 1978.
401. Nelson, JD: Oral antibiotic therapy for serious infections in hospitalized patients. *J. Pediatr. 92*:175-176, 1978.
402. Giebink, GS, Batalden, PB, Russ, JN, Le, CT: Cefaclor vs amoxicillin in treatment of acute otitis media. *Am. J. Dis. Child. 138*:287-292, 1984.

403. Marchant, CD, Shurin, PA, Turcyzk, VA, et al.: A randomized controlled trial of cefaclor compared with trimethoprim-sulfamethoxazole for treatment of acute otitis media. *J. Pediatr. 105*:633–638, 1984.
404. Odio, CM, Kusmiesz, H, Shleton, S, Nelson, JD: Comparative treatment trial of augmentin versus cefaclor for acute otitis media with effusion. *Pediatrics 75*: 819–826, 1985.
405. Wald, ER, Reilly, JS, Casselbrant, M, et al.: Treatment of acute maxillary sinusitis in childhood: A comparative study of amoxicillin and cefaclor. *J. Pediatr. 104*: 297–302, 1984.
406. Ginsburg, CM, McCracken, GH, Steinberg, JB, et al.: Treatment of group A streptococcal pharyngitis in children. *Clin. Pediatr. 21*:83–88, 1982.
407. Puhakka, H, Virolainen, E, Eskola, J, Holm, S: Cefadroxil in the treatment of acute otitis media in children. *J. Antimicrob. Chemother. 10(Suppl. B)*:99–103, 1982.
408. Rodriguez, WJ, Chhabra, OP, Guarinello, AP, et al.: Cefuroxime axetil vs cefaclor in acute otitis media with effusion. *Pediatr. Res. 20*(966):319A, 1986.

13
Aminoglycosides

STUART M. MacLEOD
McMaster University, Hamilton, Ontario, Canada

It would be difficult to overestimate the importance of aminoglycosides in pediatric infectious disease. Gram-negative infections are a common occurrence, including the septicemia and meningitis of the newborn period, necrotizing enterocolitis of premature infants, the bacteremia-septicemia of the immunosuppressed, osteomyelitis in the normal child, and gram-negative pneumonia and septicemia in the patient with cystic fibrosis. Although treatment of some of these conditions may soon be undertaken with newer antibiotics, such as the third-generation cephalosporins, it appears likely that aminoglycosides will continue to be widely used, at least for the foreseeable future, possibly in combination with other potent antibiotics (1,2).

I. HISTORY

Schatz et al. (3) isolated streptomycin in 1944 after studying more than 10,000 organisms (4). The antibiotic was a product of *Streptomyces griseus*, the productive strain being found in a diagnostic culture from a chicken's throat (4). Streptomycin became established as a mainstay of antitubercular therapy and has maintained that role to the present day. Its activity against gram-negative and gram-positive organisms was too variable to permit widespread use, although it was shown to have synergistic activity with penicillin against *Enterococcus* and was thus widely used for the treatment of bacterial endocarditis. Streptomycin was followed in the developmental sequence by neomycin, which proved too nephrotoxic for systemic use (5). The complex of kanamycins A, B, and C was isolated in 1957 (6), and the commercial preparation, which contained primarily kanamycin A, was used extensively in the 1960s. Use declined mainly because of the development of resistance and recognition of the lack of activity against *Pseudomonas aeruginosa*. Gentamicin, originally discovered in 1963 (7), is active against most enteric bacteria and *P. aeruginosa*, although variable resistance among the latter species has been described (4). There are many components of the gentamicin group, but the commonly available preparation contains C_1, C_{1A}, and C_2 (4). As the use of gentamicin became more widespread in the 1970s there was concern about increasing resistance by *P. aeruginosa* and also about ototoxicity and nephrotoxicity associated with gentamicin use. Another two aminoglycosides, tobramycin and netilmicin, have been widely marketed with the hope of increased efficacy and reduced toxicity. A kanamycin derivative, amikacin, has been developed with the objective of reducing the susceptibility to degradation by enzymes elaborated by gram-negative organisms. The various claims of relative safety and efficacy remain contentious in some cases, but it is apparent that gentamicin, tobramycin, and amikacin are at present the preferred antipseudomonal drugs and tobramycin and amikacin appear to be less nephrotoxic than other aminoglycosides. Although netilmicin was shown to be less nephrotoxic than gentamicin and tobramycin in animal studies, this advantage has not been supported by subsequent clinical experience. It does appear that netilmicin may be less ototoxic than other aminoglycosides. Although other aminoglycosides have been developed by the pharmaceutical industry, it is not clear that they will reach the market at a time of concern over drug toxicity, with a resulting focus on the development of less toxic alternatives to aminoglycoside treatment.

II. CHEMISTRY

A detailed review of the pharmaceutical chemistry of aminoglycosides is beyond the scope of this chapter, but the subject is well reviewed at a level of clinical relevance in *Antibiotic and Chemotherapy* (4). As discussed in that text, the important members of this group are characterized by aminosugars joined by glycosidic linkages to aminocyclitols. It is suggested that a more correct name for these compounds would be aminoglycosidic aminocyclitols. The interested reader is referred to *Antibiotic and Chemotherapy* (4) for a full discussion of the chemical characteristics of the various members of the aminoglycoside group.

The structure of gentamicin is shown in Figure 1, including the structural modifications found in minor components A, B, and B_1, as well as the substituent groups of C_1, C_{1a}, and C_2, the components found in commercially available gentamicin. It is noteworthy that some of the congeners show differing antimicrobial activity. For example,

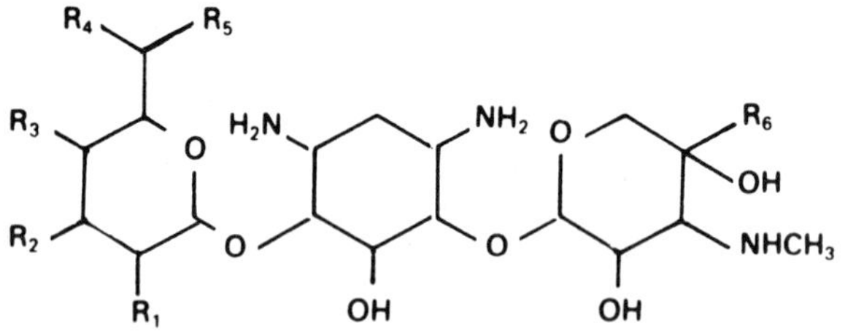

GENTAMICIN	R_1	R_2	R_3	R_4	R_5	R_6
A	NH_2	OH	OH	H	OH	H
B	OH	OH	OH	H	NH_2	CH_3
C_1	NH_2	H	H	CH_3	$NHCH_3$	CH_3
C_{1a}	NH_2	H	H	H	NH_2	CH_3
C_2	NH_2	H	H	CH_3	NH_2	CH_3
B_1	OH	OH	OH	CH_3	NH_2	CH_3
X	NH_2	OH	OH	H	OH	CH_3

Figure 1 Gentamicin: Chemical structures of congeners.

gentamicin A has markedly reduced activity against *Staphylococcus aureus* and *Escherichia coli* and also lacks antipseudomonal action (4). Gentamicin X is active against *Trichomonas vaginalis* and *Entamoeba histolytica* (4).

With respect to toxicity, it has been suggested that renal damage may correlate with the number of amino groups present in the aminoglycoside structure although this relationship does not stand up well to analysis. It has also been hypothesized that free amino groups may be associated with cochlear toxicity and methylamine functions may be associated with vestibular toxicity. For example, neomycin B, with four free amino groups and two methylamine groups, is nephrotoxic and has cochlear toxicity much more marked than its vestibular toxicity. Neomycin A, with three amino groups and one methylamine group, is much less toxic both to kidneys and to the 8th nerve. Streptomycin, with only two free amino groups, is relatively nonnephrotoxic, but so is kanamycin with four free amino groups. Gentamicin also has four free amino groups and is more nephrotoxic than either streptomycin or kanamycin. Structure-activity relationships appear complicated, and it is unlikely that discrepancies in toxicity or effectiveness can readily be explained on the basis of structural difference. Analysis is further complicated because common preparations often contain more than one component, as discussed in the case of gentamicin.

Of greater importance may be the ability of aminoglycosides to displace calcium from biologic membranes, an action related to their polycationic state in vivo. The aminoglycosides vary in this capacity, and the displacement from phospholipid binding sites is also influenced by acidity and by local calcium concentration. The exact structure-activity relationship is not understood, but it is possible that these actions may predict the ability of aminoglycosides to inhibit some intracellular enzymes. It is possible that nephrotoxicity or ototoxicity may be greater when the affinity of the aminoglycoside for calcium binding sites is higher. In the studies of Lullmann and Vollmer, the least nephrotoxic aminoglycosides, streptomycin and amikacin, showed a lower affinity for calcium binding sites in phosphatidylserine monolayers than did more nephrotoxic drugs, such as neomycin, gentamicin, or sisomicin (8).

III. MECHANISM OF ACTION

Aminoglycosides have a bactericidal action that starts with inhibition of protein synthesis. The antibacterial efficacy appears to be concentration dependent, and the speed of bacterial killing can be enhanced fourfold by a tenfold increase in antibiotic concentration.

An oxygen-dependent active transport system is necessary in susceptible bacteria for cell wall or membrane penetration by aminoglycosides (9). Anaerobes are generally resistant to aminoglycosides because they lack the oxygen-dependent transport system; a similar failure of penetration has also been described in some other bacterial species as an explanation for resistance (10).

At an intracellular level, aminoglycosides bind to the 30S subunit of the bacterial polyribosome at the A site or site of aminoacyl transfer RNA binding. In some cases, they may block initiation of synthesis of a protein chain; in others a misreading of the genetic code may result with the eventual synthesis of nonfunctional proteins. The synthesis of incorrect proteins may result in cellular malfunction and eventual death. It is possible that the ability of aminoglycosides to bind to lipids at calcium binding sites may be important as a determinant of antibacterial effects as well as of organ toxicity. Clearly, there are differences among aminoglycosides in their antibacterial efficacy and toxic effects, and there must be subtle differences among them in mechanism of action.

IV. ANTIMICROBIAL ACTIVITY

As noted, the aminoglycosides have achieved therapeutic prominence mainly because of their activity against gram-negative enteric bacteria. Most important pathogens have minimal inhibitory concentrations (MIC) well within the safely achievable concentration range, with the exception of *P. aeruginosa*, which is relatively resistant to kanamycin and slightly less sensitive to netilmicin than to gentamicin, tobramycin, and amikacin. The MIC for some common pathogens are shown in Table 1. It is noteworthy that anaerobes are resistant to aminoglycosides (see above) and gram-positive organisms other than *S. aureus* and *Staphylococcus epidermidis* are relatively resistant. Absolute MIC figures vary considerably from study to study, but the pattern is consistent with that shown in Table 1.

Table 2 summarizes the relative efficacy of selected aminoglycosides against some common pathogens. This comparison is drawn from numerous sources and represents an apparent consensus on relative activity as accepted in our institution in 1986.

Table 1 Antibiotic Spectrum of Various Aminoglycosides Against Organisms Lacking Known Aminoglycoside-Modifying Enzymes

		Mean MIC (μg/ml)				
Organism	No. of strains	Tobramycin	Gentamicin C	Sisomicin	Netilmicin	Amikacin
Escherichia coli	10	0.7	0.6	0.4	0.5	2.0
Klebsiella pneumoniae	10	0.7	0.8	0.4	0.5	1.7
Enterobacter aerogenes	10	1.2	0.7	0.7	0.5	1.7
E. cloacae	10	1.6	1.4	0.9	0.4	2.5
Serratia marcescens	10	2.8	1.5	1.9	3.0	2.0
Proteus mirabilis	8	0.4	0.5	0.4	0.8	1.2
P. vulgaris	6	0.4	0.4	0.2	0.4	1.0
P. morgani	10	0.3	0.4	0.2	0.7	0.9
P. retgeri	7	0.7	0.8	0.6	1.0	0.9
Providencia stuartii	10	3.5	3.7	2.6	5.7	1.2
Salmonella sp.	9	0.8	0.7	0.4	0.6	1.6
Pseudomonas aeruginosa	10	0.4	2.3	0.9	7.0	3.0
Staphylococcus aureus	9	0.2	0.3	0.2	0.3	1.1
S. epidermidis	4	0.06	0.08	0.05	0.06	0.5

Source: Modified from Leitner and Price (122).

Table 2 Relative Efficacy of Selected Aminoglycosides

Organism(s)	Relative effectiveness[a]
Escherichia coli	GNS > AT > K
Enterobacter aerogenes	G > NS > AT > K
Klebsiella aerogenes	N > S > AGT > K
Proteus sp.	S > GN > T > AK
Providencia sp.	AK > G > NT
Pseudomonas aeruginosa[b]	ST > G > AN
Serratia marcescens	G > ANS > T > K
Gram-positive species	S > GNATK

[a]S = sisomicin, N = netilmicin, G = gentamicin, A = amikacin, T = tobramycin, K = kanamycin.
[b]Susceptible strains.

Table 3 shows the aminoglycoside susceptibility of selected enterobacteriaceae isolated from a series of North American nurseries in the period 1973-1978 and from patients in the neonatal meningitis cooperative study (1971-1978) reported by Siegel and McCracken (11).

Synergism occurs variably but has been shown in vitro for aminoglycosides used in combination with carbenicillin, ticarcillin, piperacillin, third-generation cephalosporins, and thienamycin against *P. aeruginosa, Pseudomonas cepacia, E. coli*, the *Klebsiella-Enterobacter-Serratia* group, *Acinetobacter, Providencia*, and *Aeromonas hydrophila* (12,13). In some cases the effects of aminoglycoside and supplementary antibiotics are additive, and this has been shown for group C streptococci, *Streptococcus viridans, Staph. aureus, Pseudomonas maltophilia*, and *Nocardia asteroides* (12). It has generally proved more difficult to confirm synergy, as demonstrated in vitro through intact animal studies or through clinical testing. A full review of this topic is not possible here; however, the probability of clinically significant synergy resulting from combination therapy with aminoglycosides is generally accepted for enterococcal infections, including endocarditis, for tuberculosis, for staphylococcal infections (synergy with cloxacillin or vancomycin), for pseudomonal septicemia, or for gram-negative sepsis in an immunocompromised host (14,15). Young (16) has reported synergistic effects of amikacin and cefsulodin in the treatment of intraperitoneal *P. aeruginosa* infection in a mouse model. Shulman and Yogev have presented similar data in support of in vivo synergy between amikacin and *N*-formidoyl thienamycin in septic neutropenic infant rats (12).

Antagonism of aminoglycoside effect may be seen both in vivo and in vitro if the aminoglycoside is allowed to interact with high concentrations of penicillins. This effect is particularly well described for carbenicillin and ticarcillin, which are used in high dosage (concentrations). A similar physical-chemical interaction has been described between aminoglycosides and heparin in vitro (17).

Table 3 Aminoglycoside Susceptibilities of Selected Enterobacteriaceae Isolated from Eight North American Nurseries (1973–1978) and from Neonatal Meningitis Cooperative Study Patients (1971–1978)

	Ampicillin $\leqslant 10\mu g/ml$	Kanamycin $\leqslant 15\mu g/ml$	Amikacin $\leqslant 15\mu g/ml$	Gentamicin $\leqslant 5\mu g/ml$	Netilmicin $\leqslant 5\mu g/ml$
Escherichia coli					
Nurseries	1034/1221[a] (85)[b]	1170/1221 (96)	1210/1221 (99)	1163/1221 (95)	1208/1221 (99)
Meningitis	71/87 (82)	76/86 (88)	83/85 (98)	78/80 (98)	22/23 (96)
Klebsiella-Enterobacter					
Nurseries	82/534 (15)	495/534 (93)	529/534 (99)	517/534 (97)	528/534 (99)
Meningitis	15/31 (48)	28/29 (97)	32/32 (100)	28/30 (93)	22/24 (92)

[a]Total number of organisms susceptible per total number of organisms tested.
[b]Cumulative percentage of susceptible organisms
Source: Reprinted from Reference 11 (with permission).

V. RESISTANCE TO AMINOGLYCOSIDES

From the time of their introduction, concern has been expressed about the possible emergence of resistance to these important antibiotics. For the most part, in the clinical setting this fear has proven exaggerated, although development of resistance can readily be shown for many organisms tested in vitro. In vivo, some protection against the emergence of resistance may be afforded by the extremely rapid bactericidal action of aminoglycosides against most susceptible strains of bacteria (16). The extensive killing of the target organism results in a prolonged postantibiotic effect that discourages the development of resistance. Of particular concern has been the apparent change in susceptibility of gram-negative organisms with prolonged use. In a baseline study involving 14 participating hospitals, Gerding and Larson (18) reported that 1.4% of 14,851 gram-negative isolates were resistant to amikacin but 8.4% of 17,727 were resistant to gentamicin and 6.0% of 11,814 were resistant to tobramycin. In this study there followed a period of 12-78 months in which amikacin was used as the first-line aminoglycoside in the participating hospitals. During that period there was a slight increase in the incidence of a resistance to amikacin to 1.7% of 94,935 isolates; gentamicin resistance fell to 7.0% of 94,755 isolates and tobramycin resistance fell to 5.3% of 82,994 isolates. Clearly, there are shifts in the pattern of aminoglycoside sensitivity depending on the frequency of use, but these changes are apparently less dramatic than previously expected on the basis of clinical experience in the 1970s, when increasingly frequent reports of hospital outbreaks of infection caused by resistant gram-negative bacilli suggested that gentamicin and tobramycin might become ineffective in the 1980s.

Several mechanisms may be involved in the development of resistance to aminoglycosides.

1. Alterations may occur at the level of bacterial polyribosomes such that lessening affinity for the aminoglycoside or a change in the nature of the interaction between the drug and the aminoacyl transfer RNA binding site occurs.
2. As noted, some organisms lack the oxygen-dependent transport mechanism necessary for active uptake of aminoglycosides. Treatment may select impermeable strains or enhance the growth of impermeable mutants. At least one study (12) suggests this as the most important mechanism of resistance to amikacin among isolates in a pediatric hospital. Reduced permeability usually results in multiple aminoglycoside resistance (i.e., cross-resistance)
3. An increasingly large number of enzymes have been described with capability of catalyzing the inactivation of aminoglycosides by acetylation, adenylation, and phosphorylation (4). The aminoglycosides differ in their susceptibility to inactivation by such modifications, with amikacin the most stable and gentamicin the least stable among the aminoglycosides commonly used for treatment of gram-negative sepsis (4). Genes controlling the elaboration of these inactivating enzymes are transferred as plasmids or R factors.

Development of resistance to the killing effects of aminoglycosides may be encouraged by suboptimal dosing or by dosing intervals that greatly exceed the period of postantibiotic effect. It has been shown that combinations of aminoglycosides with other bactericidal antibiotics, such as ticarcillin or piperacillin, will reduce the emergence of resistance among gram-negative bacilli (13). Resistance among anaerobic bacteria is determined by their lack of the oxygen-dependent active transport mechanism (9).

VI. CLINICAL PHARMACOLOGY

A variety of aminoglycosides is available commercially or has been the subject of pre-clinical scientific studies; however, comment here will be restricted to those in wide clinical use: streptomycin, neomycin, gentamicin, tobramycin, amikacin, and netilmicin. Although such drugs as framycetin are important for topical therapy and neomycin is used as a nonabsorbable antibacterial to alter bowel flora, they will not be discussed specifically in the section that follows. Similarly, spectinomycin, which is an amino-cyclitol used sometimes in the treatment of *Neissereia gonorrhoeae*, will not receive direct comment although it may occasionally warrant use in adolescent medicine.

A. Routes of Administration and Absorption

Aminoglycosides are used topically for the treatment of superficial otic and ophthalmic infections, and endophthalmitis may be treated with aminoglycosides given locally or, in the case of infections confined to the anterior chamber, by systemic administration. Adequate aminoglycoside concentrations can only be achieved in the vitreous humor with direct injection of 0.5 mg of gentamicin or tobramycin. Gentamicin and tobramycin can also be given by subconjunctival or subtenon injection in a dose of 20–40 mg (4). The aminoglycosides are active against *S. aureus* and *P. aeruginosa*, the major pathogens at this site. The MIC for *S. aureus* is in the range of 0.2–1 μg/ml and the MIC for *P. aeruginosa* is 1–8 μg/ml (4).

Aminoglycosides may also be used topically as 0.1% ointment for the treatment of superficial skin infections caused by organisms likely to be susceptible. It has been suggested that absorption of aminoglycosides may occur after the use of topical sprays in a dose of 15 mg/kg per day in premature infants (19). Such a dose given concomitantly with systemic aminoglycosides has been reported to cause deafness in a premature infant (20). It has also been suggested that aminoglycoside absorption is likely to be enhanced following application to extensively burned areas or to skin surfaces disrupted by such conditions as epidermolysis bullosum.

Absorption is negligible following oral administration of aminoglycosides although serum concentrations as high as 10 μg/ml have been described after administration of 10–15 mg of gentamicin to infants with necrotizing enterocolitis (21). Neomycin and other aminoglycosides are used orally to reduce bowel flora, particularly in the treatment of patients with hepatic encephalopathy or in preparation for bowel surgery. In this setting systemic absorption does not seem to occur. Similarly, absorption after inhalation therapy with aminoglycosides for gram-negative pneumonia or cystic fibrosis is insignificant and serum concentrations usually associated with toxicity or efficacy have not been observed.

All available aminoglycosides are well absorbed following intramuscular injection, but most administration now is by the intravenous route. In the neonatal intensive care unit, close attention must be paid to the drug delivery system in order to assure predictable intravenous administration of the aminoglycoside and attainment of therapeutic serum concentrations following low infusion rates (22).

B. Distribution

Aminoglycosides may be used in pregnancy for the treatment of intrauterine infections or tuberculosis, and a number of studies have documented transplacental transfer of the antibiotic (23-25) with achievement of cord or fetal concentrations sufficient to cause toxicity. Maternal serum concentrations may be lower than anticipated because of the expansion of extracellular fluid volume that occurs during pregnancy. Cord blood concentrations have been found in the range 15-70% of those in maternal serum (11). Ototoxicity has been described in newborns following maternal administration of streptomycin for treatment of tuberculosis (26).

Concentrations attained in preterm infants have been shown to vary considerably from the normal observed in adult studies. The toxic range for gentamicin in neonates has not been precisely defined (27), but there is general agreement that trough concentrations should not exceed 2-3 μg/ml and an attempt should be made to maintain peak levels lower than 8-10 μg/ml (28,29).

As a general rule, infants requiring gentamicin have been treated with 2.5 mg/kg given twice daily (30); however, several studies have documented that in infants below 35 weeks of gestational age such a dose may result in trough and peak levels above the putative therapeutic range (27,31). This observation has been confirmed by our own studies (32); neonates who had lower gestational age and/or a lower birth weight achieved higher trough and peak gentamicin levels in response to equal doses, as shown in Figure 2.

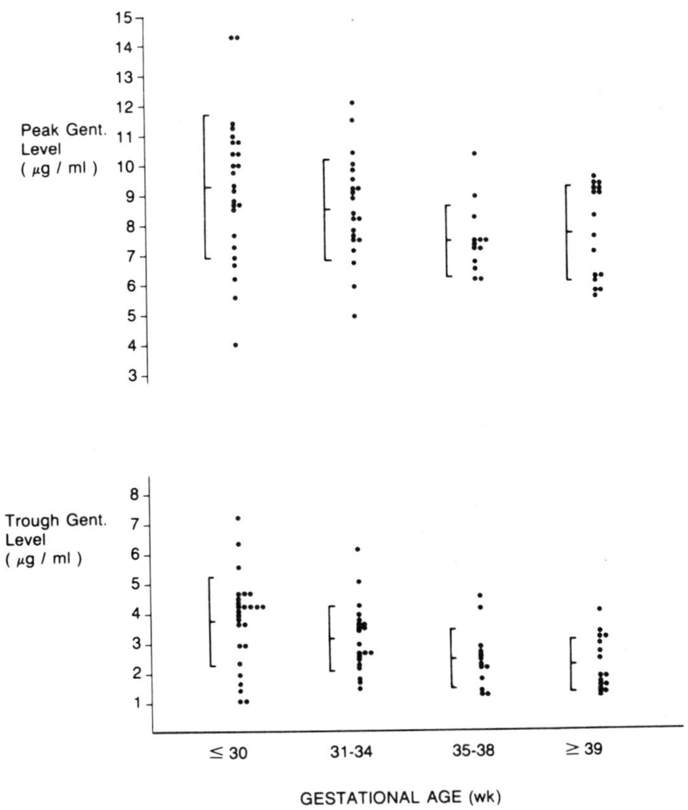

Figure 2 The influence of birth weight on gentamicin levels in 76 neonates treated with 5.0 ± 0.2 mg/kg per day. Each bar shows mean ± 1 SD.

Children of <35 weeks gestational age and/or weighing <1.2 kg were shown to have mean trough gentamicin levels higher than 3 μg/ml when treated with 5 mg/kg per day. There is a strong correlation between gestational age and birth weight, and consideration of either or both parameters is necessary in the evaluation of gentamicin concentrations and the prediction of response to dosage adjustment (31,32).

Mortality is high in normal and preterm infants with meningitis treated with systemic aminoglycosides; this is usually attributed to poor penetration of the blood-brain barrier (33) even though the barrier is reported to be more permeable in the immediate newborn period (34) and in the presence of infection (35). In contrast, it has been reported by Yogev and Kolling (36) that aminoglycoside cerebrospinal fluid (CSF) concentrations 25% of corresponding serum concentrations may be found in patients receiving treatment for shunt-associated ventriculitis. There is continuing debate over the advisability of intraventricular aminoglycoside use. McCracken has reported significant increases in mortality with intraventricular gentamicin therapy in newborns with meningitis (37), but Wright et al. found an improved cure rate in selected cases of neonatal meningitis treated with intraventricular amikacin (38).

We have recently reported studies of CSF pharmacokinetics of tobramycin in a 2-year-old child (39). Following the insertion of an intraventricular catheter to treat excessive intracranial pressure, we had the opportunity to successively monitor serum and CSF concentrations of four different drugs. Tobramycin, like other aminoglycosides, penetrates the CSF only to a limited extent when given intravenously, but our results suggested that the redistribution of this drug from the CNS back to the systemic circulation may be a relatively more active process. Despite the presence of an open intraventricular catheter, 34% of a tobramycin dose could be recovered from the urine. It may be that the apparent slow penetration of tobramycin into the CSF is augmented by a faster CSF clearance of the drug. The conjunction of these two factors may therefore explain the low CSF concentrations achieved with intravenous tobramycin. The very high concentrations of tobramycin (1000 mg/liter) produced by a 5-mg intraventricular injection suggest that, if there is a portal of access, CSF concentrations should be monitored to enhance safety and efficacy (39).

Another consideration relevant to the distribution of aminoglycosides is the effect of the underlying infection. Bergeron has recently reviewed the changes of antibiotic tissue concentration with acute infection and has shown that aminoglycoside penetration of target tissues is generally increased (35). For example, in rat studies, cortical concentrations of gentamicin in control kidneys were found to be 50% lower than those observed in the presence of acute pyelonephritis after single or chronic dosing (35). Concentrations achieved in joint fluid and ascitic or peritoneal fluid during infection are also anticipated to fall within the putative therapeutic range following achievement of adequate serum concentrations (40).

Phillips and Milner reported gentamicin and neomycin tissue levels found at necropsy in 20 preterm and 2 term infants. They found relatively high aminoglycoside concentrations in kidney, as would be expected. Concentrations in lung were in the putative therapeutic range, but concentrations in heart, muscle, and brain were variable but generally low (41). Binding of aminoglycosides to plasma protein is <20% for all members of the group, and this is not an important determinant of drug distribution. Severe burns or the presence of extensive ascites with or without peritoneal infection may also influence serum concentrations of aminoglycosides. Such conditions have the effect of greatly increasing extracellular fluid volume, and hence the volume of distribution of the aminoglycoside is enhanced. In these circumstances, serum concentration will prove unpredictable and monitoring of serum concentrations as a guide to dosing becomes essential (42,43).

C. Metabolism

The aminoglycosides do not undergo significant biotransformation in vivo apart from the enzyme-catalyzed modification described under mechanisms of bacterial resistance. Such alteration to form inactive derivatives only occurs in the presence of appropriate resistant organisms.

D. Excretion

Most studies have shown a close relationship between glomerular filtration and aminoglycoside clearance (44). All members of the aminoglycoside group appear to undergo filtration at the glomerulus followed by tubular uptake in the proximal convoluted tubular cell (see below). Tubular secretion or release into the systemic circulation may occur subsequently and account for the prolonged terminal half-life described by Schentag (45). There may be considerable interindividual variation in the residency time of aminoglycosides in the proximal convoluted tubular cell, and it has been suggested by Schentag that there may be a group of individuals who are especially suspectible to aminoglycoside nephrotoxicity because of their retention of the nephrotoxin in the deep tissue compartment (45).

Of particular interest is the handling of aminoglycoside by the newborn since both glomerular filtration and tubular function are diminished at birth and full maturation can only be expected to develop over the first year of life (46-58). Koren et al. have examined these relationships in a recent study and have shown the elimination half-life of gentamicin to be dependent on clearance (32). Elimination half-life is the product of the equation $t_{1/2} = Vd \times 0.693/Cl$; therefore it is possible that alterations in the distribution volume of gentamicin may cause changes in the serum concentration profile of the aminoglycosides. Interestingly, Koren's studies showed a surprisingly consistent distribution volume of gentamicin independent of gestational age or birth weight (32). Conversely, gentamicin clearance was significantly lower in infants weighing 1 kg or less than in the remainder of the group weighing 1-1.5 kg. The stratification of clearance, half-life, and concentrations on the basis of birth weight appears to be more satisfactory than stratification according to gestational age over or under 30 weeks (32). Since almost all neonates having birth weights less than 1 kg are also less than 30 weeks of gestational age, it seems advisable to use a 1-kg limit as the breakpoint. The pharmacokinetic data presented by Koren et al. suggest that preterm infants with birth weights less than 1 kg should receive smaller amounts of gentamicin (and probably other aminoglycosides) than those given to neonates of higher birth weight.

At steady state, the serum concentration will depend upon dose and clearance according to the equation serum concentration = dose/clearance. Therefore, the daily dose in infants of birth weight <1 kg should be reduced according to the relative proportion of their clearance (mean, 31 ml/kg hr^{-1} in Koren's study) to the clearance in infants of birth weight >1 kg (mean, 39 ml/kg hr^{-1}). This suggests a 20% reduction of their daily dose to 3.5-4 mg/kg per day or, alternatively, a prolongation of their dose interval so that 2.5 mg/kg is given every 16-18 hr. Because gentamicin concentrations were not shown to exceed the putative therapeutic range even in most very low birth weight infants, Koren has recommended an increase in the dosage interval in order to permit more time for drug elimination and attainment of lower trough concentrations (32).

Unfortunately, aminoglycoside dosing cannot readily be adjusted on the basis of objective measurement of renal function in the newborn since reliable determination of creatinine clearance is impossible. Schwartz et al. (59) have recently suggested a simple method for the estimation of glomerular filtration rate in term infants during the first year of life. This method will not, however, solve our greater problems with low-birth-weight infants, as suggested. The most prudent clinical course is adoption of a conservative dosing regime (see below) followed by therapeutic drug monitoring. In fact, renal function can be assessed on the basis of serum aminoglycoside concentration measurement (44).

Urinary acidity may influence the antibacterial activity of some aminoglycosides, particularly streptomycin, used in the treatment of renal tuberculosis, but it does not appear to be a major determinant of urinary excretion (60).

At least three studies have examined the effect of exchange transfusion in neonates on gentamicin concentrations and have concluded that a significant reduction occurs in the immediate posttransfusion period (21-62% reduction in gentamicin concentration) (61-63). The calculation of a 62% reduction in gentamicin concentration during exchange transfusion made by Kliegman et al. (61) was questioned by Green, who recalculated Kliegman's data and concluded that gentamicin removal by exchange transfusion was relatively minor (64). Hemodialysis has been reported in adults to clear gentamicin at a rate equal to 60% of creatinine clearance, but peritoneal dialysis is capable of clearing only 20% of a gentamicin dose within 36 hr (4).

A further important question in pediatrics is the relative clearance of aminoglycosides in patients with cystic fibrosis. Many antibiotics have been found to show lower serum concentrations than anticipated after conventional dosing in cystic fibrosis patients (65-67). Similar findings have been described for aminoglycosides (68-71), although the magnitude of the effect seems generally less than that described for such antibiotics as cloxacillin and ceftazidime (64-66). The most careful study on the pharmacokinetic behavior of aminoglycosides in cystic fibrosis is that of Levy et al. (72). This study suggested an increase of approximately 20% in aminoglycoside total body clearance in patients with cystic fibrosis, but the observation could not be explained on the basis of enhanced renal clearance. Clinical experience suggests that cystic fibrosis patients will tolerate higher doses of aminoglycosides in the treatment of their gram-negative pneumonias. A dosage of 7.5-10 mg/kg per day of gentamicin or tobramycin is commonly used in our institution, and putatively toxic serum concentrations are rarely seen at that dosage level. This is strong presumptive evidence of enhanced renal excretion or altered distribution of aminoglycosides in these patients.

VII. THERAPEUTIC DRUG MONITORING

It is understandable that such drugs as aminoglycosides, having a narrow margin of safety, would be viewed as legitimate targets for therapeutic drug monitoring with the object of reducing toxicity. Pursuit of this goal was hampered in the past by lack of assays that were sufficiently sensitive for application to small pediatric sample sizes, especially those available in neonatology. The bioassays in common use until 10 years ago also suffered from a lack of specificity, a particularly important failing when the assay was applied in patients who were likely to be receiving other antibiotics in addition to the aminoglycoside that was the target of measurement.

The past decade has seen the introduction of a number of highly specific and sensitive aminoglycoside assays, all suitable for employment in pediatrics and in neonatology. The detail of available assay methodology is described elsewhere in this volume, but the competition among analytic methods is being won in the modern hospital setting by the nonradioisotopic immunoassay techniques. Such assays are highly specific and sensitive and can be carried out on sample volumes of 50 μl or less. The initial cost of equipment and subsequent reagent costs may be high, but the demands on laboratory personnel are minor even with heavy utilization and the training time for new technicians is brief.

The indications for therapeutic drug monitoring are described in Table 4, and for the most part these do not require elaboration. In essence, therapeutic drug monitoring is indicated whenever distribution of the aminoglycoside is likely to be unpredictable because of physiologic or pathophysiologic variation (73). We should, however, be cautious in our expectations of the predictive value of aminoglycoside concentration measurements (74). At extremes we may be led to anticipate toxicity or therapeutic failure, but it is impossible, especially in neonatology or in the presence of such disease states as burns and cystic fibrosis, to define accurately a therapeutic range within which antibacterial efficacy will be assured without risk of toxicity.

It has been a common experience in therapeutic drug monitoring to find that concentrations are subtherapeutic rather than falling within the putative toxic range. Such a finding in our neonatal intensive care unit led us into a detailed investigation of the drug delivery system and eventually allowed us to achieve more reliable intravenous dosing with aminoglycosides in low-birth-weight infants (22,75). The question is frequently raised as to correlation of toxicity with high peak concentrations in serum or with failure of troughs to fall below a particular concentration. This issue has never been resolved either in pediatric or in adult medical practice. Common sense would suggest that investigations focused on pharmacokinetic performance as a predictor of toxicity encounter

Table 4 Pediatric Therapeutic Drug Monitoring: Aminoglycosides

General indications
Therapy beyond 5 days
Uncertain clinical response
High fever
Atypical body constituency, e.g., obesity, expanded extracellular fluid, low birth weight
Specific indications
Renal impairment
Rapidly changing renal function
Hemodialysis
Chronic ambulatory peritoneal dialysis
Prematurity
Burns
Cystic fibrosis
Therapeutic failure
Signs of nephrotoxicity
Signs of ototoxicity

difficulty because the best correlation is likely to be found with concentrations in the target tissue for toxicity. Tissue concentrations vary widely in response to a multitude of host factors, including genetic determinants, disease state, and mode of drug dosing (e.g., intermittent bolus versus continuous infusion), so we should not be surprised to find an obscure relationship between serum concentration and eventual toxicity (76). There seems little merit given this unclear association in frequent monitoring of both peak and trough concentrations of aminoglycosides. When monitoring is indicated for any of the reasons shown in Table 4, it should be sufficient to measure troughs when the monitoring is aimed at avoidance of toxicity and peaks when aimed at the assurance of antibacterial efficacy. It may be prudent to measure both peak and trough during at least one dosing cycle, usually after the third dose in children or during the third day of therapy in newborns. A steady-state concentration should be achieved after 4–5 half-lives have elapsed unless there is a rapid change in renal function or in the disease state that originally necessitated treatment.

VIII. THERAPEUTIC INDICATIONS

The use of aminoglycosides in hospitalized children with proven or suspected infections is immense. The most common indications for aminoglycoside therapy are

1. Proven or suspected neonatal sepsis
2. Cystic fibrosis
3. Severe burns
4. Proven or suspected infection in an immunocompromised patient
5. Tuberculosis

As discussed earlier, the available aminoglycosides have comparable spectra of antibacterial activity, with a few exceptions. Only streptomycin and kanamycin are sufficiently active against *Mycobacterium tuberculosis* to be used in therapy (4). Amikacin and netilmicin may be active against some of the enterobacteriaceae otherwise resistant to aminoglycosides, and there is less likely to be resistance of *P. aeruginosa* to amikacin. It has been suggested that tobramycin is more active than gentamicin against *P. aeruginosa*, but this difference does not seem to be of major clinical significance. Gentamicin has been reported to be more effective than other aminoglycosides against *Serratia marcescens* (77).

A recent extensive review of *Klebsiella* bacteremia in an adult general hospital showed that 99% of isolates were sensitive to amikacin at a concentration of 8 μg/ml and while 76 and 85% were sensitive to gentamicin and tobramycin, respectively, at concentrations of 4 μg/ml. In contrast, 100% of isolates were susceptible to the third-generation cephalosporins cefotaxime and ceftazidime (78).

Aminoglycosides are a mainstay of therapy for acute infective pulmonary exacerbations in children with cystic fibrosis. Many of the pulmonary isolates are of organisms sensitive to aminoglycosides, especially *P. aeruginosa*. Attempts have been made to control chronic pseudomonal colonization with inhaled aminoglycosides as well as with intermittent intensive parenteral therapy. Studies in our hospital have suggested that short-term inhaled tobramycin therapy does not result in significant chronic reduction in quantitative sputum cultures for *P. aeruginosa* nor does it yield significant systemic concentrations of aminoglycoside with the attendant risk of organic toxicity (79).

Oncology practice in a pediatric setting has changed over the past two decades with a shift to longer survival and ultimate confrontation with infective complications. A recent report from the Memorial Sloan Kettering Cancer Center (80) suggested that 54% of deaths in children with acute leukemia stem directly from infective complications and another 14% result from hemorrhage combined with infection. The leading causes of sepsis in patients with leukemia and lymphoma are *E. coli, P. aeruginosa*, and *Klebsiella* species, causing 23.6, 14.9, and 10.8%, respectively, of all major infective episodes. For all these organisms an aminoglycoside should be part of the first-line therapy in the face of life-threatening sepsis. Studies of varied therapeutic approaches, including the use of combinations of aminoglycosides with β-lactam antibiotics, double β-lactam combinations, and monotherapy with a third-generation cephalosporin, such as ceftazidime, have not yet resulted in displacement of the aminoglycoside β-lactam combination as the standard therapy for febrile neutropenic patients (80).

The use of aminoglycosides in neonatology is also widespread. At least 75% of the low-birth-weight infants passing through our neonatal intensive care unit receive at least one course of aminoglycoside therapy for proven or suspected gram-negative sepsis or meningitis. The choice of aminoglycoside for use in neonatology does not appear to be critically important. Efficacy seems similar for gentamicin, tobramycin, amikacin, or netilmicin, but we have shown the possibility of minimized nephrotoxic risk with amikacin compared with gentamicin or tobramycin (29). McCracken (37) has warned against the risk of increased mortality when gentamicin is given intrathecally to low-birth-weight infants despite the persistence of considerable mortality (approximately 30%) when gentamicin and ampicillin are given intravenously. Aminoglycosides are also first-line therapy for necrotizing enterocolitis (NEC) although the choice among members of the group again seems relatively unimportant. Gentamicin has been given orally in the treatment of NEC in a dose of 10–15 mg/kg per day and has been shown to yield a serum concentration above 10 μg/ml in the presence of that disease (11,21).

Although tuberculosis has assumed a role of lesser importance in modern industrialized countries, it remains a major scourge of the pediatric age group in developing countries. Streptomycin is an integral part of all short-course or intermittent therapy regimens as well as of more conventional treatments. In developing countries, where a series of treatments may be tried without success because of suboptimal compliance, it should be remembered that 8th nerve toxicity from streptomycin is likely to correlate with cumulative dose so that the second- and third-line treatment regimens should not automatically include streptomycin if a therapeutic and potentially toxic dose (e.g., dosage equivalent to 60 g of streptomycin for a normal adult) has already been given.

Aminoglycosides also have a role in the treatment of infection with atypical mycobacteria, some of which at least are more susceptible to amikacin than to other members of the group (77).

IX. DOSING GUIDELINES

Most clinical pharmacologists are wary of rigid dosing guidelines, especially for such drugs as aminoglycosides with considerable interindividual pharmacokinetic variation, which is even more marked in low-birth-weight neonates (32,52,55–58,81–93). Dosing rules must be viewed as a general guideline to be modified in accordance with individual requirements, as indicated by some objective measure, such as therapeutic drug monitoring or assessment of serum killing titer for the organism causing infection. It is a reasonable

Table 5 Dosage Guidelines for Gentamicin and Tobramycin

	Initial G/T dose				
Age	Normal renal function	Mild impairment[a]	Moderate impairment[a]	Severe impairment	Hemodialysis
		CrCl > 50 ml/min 1.73 m^{-2}	CrCl 10–50 ml/min 1.73 m^{-2}	CrCl < 10 ml/min 1.73 m^{-2}	NA
Preterm neonates ≤ 1 kg	3.5 mg/kg IV every 24 hr	3.5 mg/kg IV every 24–36 hr	3.5 mg/kg IV every 36–48 hr	3.5 mg/kg IV every 48–72 hr	
Preterm neonates ≥ 1 kg and full term	5.0 mg/kg per day IV divided every 12 hr	2.5 mg/kg IV every 12–18 hr	2.5 mg/kg IV every 18–36 hr	2.5 mg/kg IV every 36–72 hr	NA
Infants and children	7.5 mg/kg per day IV or IM divided every 8 hr (maximum, 300 mg/day prior to serum concentration monitoring)	1.9–2.5 mg/kg IV or IM every 8–12 hr	1.25–2.5 mg/kg IV or IM every 12–24 hr	0.6–2.5 mg/kg IV or IM every 24–48 hr	1.25–1.75 mg/kg IV postdialysis
Adults	3 mg/kg per day IV or IM divided every 8 hr (maximum, 300 mg/day prior to serum concentration monitoring)	0.75–1 mg/kg IV or IM every 8–12 hr	0.5–1 mg/kg IV or IM every 12–24 hr	0.25–1 mg/kg IV or IM every 24–48 hr	0.5–0.7 mg/kg IV postdialysis

[a]Patients should first receive one dose per normal renal function guidelines as a loading dose. Further dosing should proceed as described and adjusted according to serum concentrations.

Table 6 Recommended Guidelines for Amikacin Dosing

Renal function	Dose
Normal	
Neonates (including low-birth-weight infants)	15 ng/kg per day divided every 12 hr
Older children	15 ng/kg per day divided every 8 hr
Impaired[a]: creatinine clearance ml/min 1.73 m^{-2}	
50–80	5 mg/kg every 8 hr
10–50	5 mg/kg every 12 hr
<10	5 mg/kg every 12–24 hr

[a]Or refer to nomogram in Reference 94.

objective to attempt to attain killing titers at a peak of 1:8 (i.e., an eightfold dilution of serum will still show cidal activity against the test organism). The dosing guidelines in Table 5 for gentamicin and tobramycin, Table 6 for amikacin, and Table 7 for netilmicin are intended to indicate a suitable starting point for aminoglycoside therapy. In most complicated cases further dosage individualization will be necessary.

X. TOXICITY

As highlighted in much of the foregoing description, the clinical use of aminoglycosides is marked by a balancing of therapeutic benefit versus the risk of dose-related toxicity. Toxicity that is not dose related does occur (see Table 8) but is not normally of great clinical significance. Hypersensitivity reactions are seen in up to 5% of aminoglycoside recipients. Aplastic anemia, agranulocytosis, and a bleeding diathesis secondary to a circulating factor V antagonist have been rarely recorded, especially after streptomycin. In contrast, the dose-related toxicities are common, especially when inadequate attention has been paid to individualization of aminoglycoside dosage in the face of changing renal

Table 7 Recommended Guidelines for Netilmicin Dosing

Renal function	Dose
Normal	
Neonates (including low-birth-weight infants)	5 mg/kg per day divided every 12 hr
Newborn infants 1–4 weeks of age	7.5 mg/kg per day divided every 8 hr
Older children	5.5–8.0 mg/kg per day divided every 8 hr
Impaired: Creatinine clearance (ml/min 1.73 m^{-2})	
50–80	2.5 ng/kg every 8–12 hr
10–50	2.5 ng/kg every 12–24 hr
<10	2.5 ng/kg every 24–48 hr

Table 8 Adverse Reactions to Aminoglycosides

Not dose related
Hypersensitivity reactions: fever, rash, eosinophilia
Aplastic anemia, granulocytopenia
Bleeding diathesis, secondary circulating factor V antagonist (associated with streptomycin)
Dose related
Nephrotoxicity
8th nerve toxicity
Neuromuscular blockade

function (95). The effect of dosing regimen on toxicity has been well reviewed by Thompson (96).

Neuromuscular blockade is the least common of the dose-related toxicities but may be seen as a life-threatening apnea, especially in low-birth-weight infants who have received a general anesthetic with the use of additional neuromuscular blocking agents. Severe hypocalcemia may also predispose patients to this toxicity. For the most part, enhanced neuromuscular blockade is a theoretical risk unlikely to be of clinical significance with the newer aminoglycosides used in safe dosage. The potency of aminoglycosides as neuromuscular blockers is less than 1% that of tubocurarine.

XI. NEPHROTOXICITY

Aminoglycosides undergo glomerular filtration and are subsequently taken up by the proximal tubular cell, possibly by both an active (the basic amino acid transport system) and a passive (endocytosis) process although the occurrence of active transport is contentious (60,97,98). Within the proximal tubular cell the aminoglycosides are heavily concentrated in the lysosomes (up to 100-fold higher concentration than found in serum at corresponding times), where they appear to bind to neutral lipids, possibly displacing calcium from its binding sites in the process. Once the drug is concentrated at an intracellular site it appears to produce rapid morphological change followed by prolonged residence in the proximal convoluted tubular cell. Investigations of renal tubular transport and intrarenal distribution of aminoglycosides have been well reviewed by Whelton (60) and by Morin et al. (97,99). The relationship between aminoglycoside accumulation in lysosomes and the ultimate cell damage is unclear. The aminoglycosides are able to inhibit some lysosomal enzymes, and this probably accounts for the ultrastructural changes seen on electron microscopy: the appearance of cytosegrosomes and myeloid bodies, the products of organelle disruption, and the accumulation of electron-dense polar lipids. It is possible that the aminoglycosides exert their toxic effects by binding to lipids in such a way as to alter the lipid environment necessary for enzyme function. Whether altered enzyme function leads directly to cell death through overloading of the lysosome or leads indirectly to alteration of the lysosomal membrane has not been determined (97).

The ability of aminoglycosides to cause proximal convoluted tubular cell damage is beyond dispute. A major part of the literature on the pediatric use of aminoglycosides is concerned with the adjustment of therapeutic dosing to minimize renal damage (27,29,

100–103) and with the altered distribution of aminoglycosides in the presence of parenchymal disease or of other nephrotoxic drugs. None of this will be reviewed here. On the basis of both animal and clinical studies it can be concluded that all aminoglycosides produce some degree of renal damage that may be detectable only with measurements more sensitive than those normally applied to the study of renal function. Sensitive markers of lysosomal integrity (*N*-acetylglucosaminidase) or brush-border function (β_2-microglobulin or alanine aminopeptidase) have been used by us and others (29,101–107) to study drug-induced nephrotoxicity.

If enzymuria (NAG) is accepted as the most sensitive marker available of lysosomal status, which seems central to the question of aminoglycoside-induced renal damage, we would conclude that gentamicin is more nephrotoxic than tobramycin, which is in turn slightly more nephrotoxic than amikacin when any of these aminoglycosides are used for the treatment of proven or suspected gram-negative sepsis in patients in the neonatal intensive care unit. The differences identified are probably not of major clinical significance, and the choice of amikacin on this basis is only warranted in infants deemed to be at high risk of renal impairment (29).

It has been suggested that newborn infants are less susceptible to aminoglycoside nephrotoxicity than are older children or adults, but this is difficult to substantiate from the limited studies available (101–103). Certainly our studies suggest that the occurrence of lysosomal damage in newborns exposed to aminoglycoside therapy does occur. Studies of aminoglycoside nephrotoxicity in newborn rats suggest that damage equivalent to or greater than that seen in adults occurs following aminoglycoside exposure, but recovery may be more rapid once therapy is stopped (108).

The risk factors suggested as important determinants of aminoglycoside-induced renal damage are reviewed in Table 9. Of these, those listed as probable, including sodium-volume depletion and cumulative dosage with chronic therapy, are most likely to predict renal damage. These issues have been provocatively reviewed by Moench and Smith (76).

It is important to highlight the conflicting evidence on serum concentration as a predictor of renal damage following aminoglycoside therapy. Although high concentrations are often found in association with renal damage, it is not easy to determine a causal relationship. Koren et al. recently showed that gentamicin clearance can be used as an index of renal function in the newborn (44), and it seems likely that the elevation of gentamicin observed in "toxic" patients reflects rather than predicts toxicity within the narrow therapeutic range.

Table 9 Risk Factors for Renal Toxicity of Aminoglycosides

Probable	Possible
Host factors	
Na^+ depletion	Age
Dehydration	Prior renal impairment
K^+ depletion	Varied tissue accumulation
Drug factors	
Cumulative dosage	High serum concentrations
Drug interactions	Continuous infusion

Source: Adapted from Reference 76.

XII. OTOTOXICITY

Early experience with dihydrostreptomycin, streptomycin, and neomycin was sufficient to convince practitioners that aminoglycosides were significantly ototoxic. In fact, dihydrostreptomycin was withdrawn from antitubercular use because of cochlear toxicity and neomycin was restricted to use topically and by the nonabsorbed oral route. It has always been difficult, especially in pediatrics, to obtain a precise estimate of the incidence of aminoglycoside-induced vestibular or cochlear toxicity because of the blurred limits of causality attributable to drug or to pre-existing disease. The consensus among studies of aminoglycoside-associated ototoxicity seems to set the incidence at about 2%, although transient changes in vestibular function or auditory acuity are probably more common than this in the treated population (109–111).

The mechanism by which aminoglycosides damage the inner ear is not known with certainty, but animal studies have shown the killing of hair cells in the organ of Corti in a fashion analogous to that causing damage seen in renal proximal convoluted tubular cells. It has been suggested that aminoglycosides bind to a lipid receptor (possibly phosphatidylinositol phosphate or phosphatidylinositol diphosphate) (112,113). It is possible that local enzyme activity is inhibited because of disruption of the lipid environment essential to some enzyme functions.

Of particular concern in pediatric practice is the effect of aminoglycosides on otic development in premature newborns; the medical literature has seen a recent reawakening of dispute on this issue, perhaps because of the availability for the first time of non-ototoxic drugs, such as third-generation cephalosporins, for the therapy of gram-negative sepsis. Although these drugs are expensive, it has been suggested that they might replace aminoglycosides in the neonatal intensive care unit, a decision with important implications since almost 75% of low-birth-weight infants in our hospital receive aminoglycosides at some time for the treatment of proven or suspected gram-negative infection.

In 1981, Eviatar and Eviatar (114) reported a 7% increase of sensorineural hearing loss in 43 infants receiving aminoglycosides but found no cases among 276 healthy newborns. A more extensive prospective study with untreated neonatal intensive care unit survivors as controls was reported by Finitzo-Hieber et al. in 1985 (115). These authors carried out a long-term assessment of 149 infants ranging in gestational age from 27 to 42 weeks (50 received amikacin, 49 received netilmicin, and 51 were untreated). A single case of sensorineural hearing loss was detected in each group using auditory evoked potential measures at 6 weeks and 7, 12, and 18 months postterm. It was concluded that, although the overall incidence of hearing impairment in these infants was 2%, there was no significant difference in risk relative to control associated with treatment with either aminoglycoside.

On the basis of this study it has been suggested editorially that aminoglycosides do not "contribute substantially to the prevalence of deafness in infants surviving intensive care" (111). Such a conclusion may be premature (115), since the Finitzo-Hieber study lacked sufficient statistical power to detect reliably a 4% increase of aminoglycoside-induced ototoxicity in a population of high-risk infants. Furthermore, it is likely that amikacin is less nephrotoxic than other aminoglycosides in this age group (29) and netilmicin is reported to be less ototoxic than other aminoglycosides in adults (77). Certainly aminoglycosides can be used with caution in high-risk newborns, but it would be imprudent to ignore completely the chance of the augmented risk of ototoxicity. The problems associated with the assessment of age-related changes in the drug effect on sensorineural hearing have been reviewed by Brummett and Jackson (117).

Ototoxicity is not an overwhelming concern in older children, although it is part of the risk-benefit analysis to be made whenever aminoglycoside therapy is contemplated. In children with cystic fibrosis who often receive high-dose aminoglycoside therapy, we have been impressed by the infrequent occurrence of toxicity either to kidneys or to the 8th nerve.

Aminoglycosides may be categorized on the basis of their propensity to cause vestibular or cochlear damage. Streptomycin and gentamicin are more likely to cause vestibular toxicity, but tobramycin and netilmicin have almost equal effects on vestibular and cochlear portions of the 8th nerve. All the other aminoglycosides in common use are more likely to produce a reduction in auditory acuity if any ototoxicity occurs. It has been suggested that netilmicin is the least nephrotoxic of available aminoglycosides, but objective confirmatory studies are lacking (77). From animal studies it appears that cell damage in the organ of Corti is permanent, but clinically there is a possibility of considerable recovery, especially from vestibular damage, in which external cuing may compensate for the drug-induced disability.

XIII. DRUG INTERACTIONS INVOLVING AMINOGLYCOSIDES

Considering the wide use of these drugs, reports of clinically significant interactions have been surprisingly rare. Of course there are interactions featuring antibacterial synergy, which are desirable, as discussed above. Other welcome interactions include the putative ability of sodium loading or amiloride treatment to reduce aminoglycoside uptake and toxicity in the renal proximal convoluted tubule. Interactions associated with enhanced toxicity are listed in Table 10. It is of course possible that interaction will occur with any concomitantly administered drug that has the ability to cause neuromuscular blockade, renal toxicity, or ototoxicity.

Table 10 Clinically Significant Drug Interactions with Aminoglycosides

Putative interacting drug(s) or drug classes	Nature of interaction
Amiloride	Reduced uptake of aminoglycoside in proximal renal tubule and reduced nephrotoxicity
Amphotericin B	Additive nephrotoxicity
Cephalothin/cephaloridine	Enhanced nephrotoxicity and ototoxicity
Cisplatinum	Additive nephrotoxicity
Indomethacin	Reduced renal clearance (118)
Loop diuretics	Enhanced ototoxicity
Furosemide	
Ethacrynic ac.	
Neuromuscular blocking agents	Enhanced N/M blockage especially in LBW infants
Penicillins, especially carbenicillin/ticarcillin	Physicochemical interaction in vivo or in vitro to reduce aminoglycoside effect (119,120)
Vancomycin	Enhanced nephrotoxicity (121)

XIV. SUMMARY

The pharmaceutical industry has actively sought replacements for the aminoglycosides almost from the time of their introduction. The vigor of this search was determined by appropriate medical concern over the narrow margin of safety associated with aminoglycoside therapy. Pediatricians have every reason to be wary of the potential for nephrotoxic and ototoxic complications when their patients, particularly those with severe infection or multisystemic disease, receive aminoglycosides. That aminoglycosides are still prominent in the management of pediatric infectious disease is also indicative of their value as antimicrobial agents. They will not easily be replaced by third-generation cephalosporins or complicated multiple-drug regimens. For the foreseeable future, pediatricians will need to remain well informed about the safety and efficacy of available aminoglycosides. With prudent use these agents will remain a valuable part of the therapeutic armamentarium. This chapter has attempted a presentation of the core knowledge essential for their optimal use.

REFERENCES

1. Siengenthaler, WE, Bonatti, A, Luthy, R: Aminoglycoside antibiotics in infectious diseases. An overview. *Am. J. Med. 80*(Suppl. 6b):2–14, 1986.
2. Chadwick, EG, Yogen, R, Shulman, ST: Combination antibiotic therapy in pediatrics. *Am. J. Med. 80*(Suppl. 6B):166–171, 1986.
3. Schatz, A, Bugle, E, Waksman, SA: Streptomycin, a substance exhibiting antibiotic activity against gram positive and gram negative bacteria. *Proc. Soc. Exp. Biol. Med. 55*:66–69, 1944.
4. Garrod, LP, Lambert, HP, O'Grady, F: *Antibiotic and Chemotherapy*, 5th ed., Churchill-Livingstone, New York, 1981.
5. Waksman, SA, Le Chevalier, HA: Neomycin, a new antibiotic active against streptomycin-resistant bacteria including tuberculous organisms. *Science 109*:305–307, 1949.
6. Umezawa, H, Veda, M, Maeda, K: Production and isolation of a new antibiotic, kanamycin. *J. Antibiot. (Tokyo)* Series A *10*:181–188, 1957.
7. Weinstein, M, Luedemann, G, Oden, E, Wagman, GH: Gentamicin, a new broad spectrum antibiotic complex. *Antimicrob. Agents Chemother. 3*:1–7, 1963.
8. Lullmann, H, Vollmer, B: An interaction of aminoglycoside antibiotics with Ca binding to lipid monolayers and to biomembranes. *Biochem. Pharmacol. 31*:3769–3773, 1982.
9. Bryan, LE: Mechanisms of aminoglycoside antibiotic resistance in anaerobic bacteria. *Antimicrob. Agents Chemother. 15*:7–13, 1979.
10. Noone, P: Use of antibiotics: Aminoglycosides. *Br. Med. J. 2*:549–552, 613–614, 1978.
11. Siegel, JD, McCracken, GB: Aminoglycosides in pediatrics. In: *The Aminoglycosides* (A Whelton and HC Neu, eds.), Marcel Dekker, New York, 1982, pp. 527–535.
12. Shulman, ST, Yogev, R: Treatment of pediatric infections with amikacin as first line aminoglycoside. *Am. J. Med. 79*(Suppl. 1A):43–50, 1985.
13. Baltch, AL, Smith, RP: Combinations of antibiotics against *Pseudomonas aeruginosa. Am. J. Med. 79*(Suppl. 1A):8–16, 1985.
14. Sande, MA, Irwin, RG: Penicillin-aminoglycoside synergy in experimental streptococcus bacilliary endocarditis. *J. Infect. Dis. 129*:572–576, 1974.

15. Sande, MA, Courtney, K: Nafcillin gentamicin synergism in experimental staphylococcal endocarditis. *J. Lab. Clin. Med. 88*:118–124, 1976.
16. Young, LS: Use of aminoglycosides in immunocompromised patients. *Am. J. Med. 79*(Suppl. 1A):21–27, 1985.
17. Jackson, GG: Present status of aminoglycoside antibiotics and their safe, effective use. *Clin. Ther. 1*:200–215, 1977.
18. Gerding, DN, Larson, TA: Aminoglycoside resistance in gram negative bacilli during increased amikacin use. *Am. J. Med. 79*(Suppl. 1A):1–7, 1985.
19. Lewis, HE: Deafness and topical antibiotic sprays. *Lancet 1*:1400, 1985.
20. Morrell, P, Hey, E, Mackee, I, Rutter, N, Lewis, M: Deafness in preterm babies associated with topical antibiotic spray containing neomycin. *Lancet 1*:1167–1168, 1985.
21. Miranda, J, Schimmel, M, Mimms, G, Spinelli, W, Driscoll, J, James, L, Rosen, T: Gentamicin absorption during prophylactic use for necrotizing enterocolitis. *Dev. Pharmacol. Ther. 7*:303–306, 1984.
22. Rajchgot, P, Radde, IC, MacLeod, SM: Influence of specific gravity on intravenous drug delivery. *J. Pediatr. 99*:658–661, 1981.
23. Kauffman, RE, Morris, JA, Azarnoff, DL: Placental transfer and fetal urinary excretion of gentamycin during constant rate maternal infusion. *Pediatr. Res. 9*: 104–107, 1975.
24. Yashmika, H, Monma, T, Matsuda, S: Placental transfer of gentamycin. *J. Pediatr. 80*:121–123, 1972.
25. Bernard, B, Garcia-Cazares, SJ, Ballard, C: Tobramycin: Maternal-fetal pharmacology. *Antimicrob. Agents Chemother. 11*:688–694, 1977.
26. Robinson, G Cambon, K: Hearing loss in infants of tuberculous mothers treated with streptomycin during pregnancy. *N. Engl. J. Med. 271*:949–951, 1964.
27. Mulhall, A, De Louvois, J, Hurley, R: Incidence of potentially toxic concentrations of gentamicin in the neonate. *Arch. Dis. Child. 58*:897–900, 1983.
28. Taylor, WJ, Finn, AL: *Individualizing Drug Therapy*, Gross, Townsend, Frank, Inc., New York, 1981.
29. Rajchgot, P, Prober, CG, Soldin, S, Perlman, M, Good, F, Harding, E, Klein, J, MacLeod, SM: Aminoglycoside-related nephrotoxicity in the premature newborn. *Clin. Pharmacol. Ther. 35*:394–401, 1984.
30. McCracken, GH, Nelson, JD: *Antimicrobial Therapy for Newborns*, Grune & Stratton, New York, 1977.
31. Szefler, SJ, Wynn, RJ, Clarke, DF, Buckwald, S, Shen, D, Schentag, JJ: Relationship to gentamicin serum concentrations to gestational age in preterm infants. *J. Pediatr. 97*:312–315, 1980.
32. Koren, G, Leeder, JS, Harding, E, Jacques, D, MacLeod, SM: Optimization of gentamicin therapy in very low birth weight infants. *Pediatr. Pharmacol. 5*:79–87, 1985.
33. Swartz, MN: Intraventricular use of aminoglycosides in the treatment of gram negative bacillary meningitis: Conflicting views. *J. Infect. Dis. 143*:293–295, 1981.
34. Boreus, LO: Distribution. In: *Principles of Pediatric Pharmacology*, Churchill-Livingston, New York, 1982, pp. 46–74.
35. Bergeron, MG: Tissue penetration of antibiotics. *Clin. Biochem. 19*:90–100, 1986.
36. Yogev, R, Kolling, WM: Intraventricular levels of amikacin after intravenous administration. *Antimicrob. Agents Chemother. 20*:583–586, 1981.
37. McCracken, GH, Mize, SG, Threlkfeld, N: Intraventricular gentamicin therapy in gram negative bacillary meningitis. *Lancet 1*:787–791, 1980.
38. Wright, PF, Kaiser, AB, Bowman, CM, McKee, KJ, Trujillo, H, McGee, ZA: The pharmacokinetics and efficacy of an aminoglycoside administered into the cerebral ventricles in neonates. *J. Infect. Dis. 143*:141–147, 1981.

39. Koren, G, Lavi, S, Greenwald, M, Roifman, C, Leeder, JS, Gelfand, EW, MacLeod, SM: Cerebrospinal fluid pharmacokinetics of tobramycin, ceftazidime, phenobarbitone and phenytoin in a child. *Clin. Pharmacokinet. 10*:371–375, 1985.
40. Neu, HC: Pharmacology of aminoglycosides. In: *The Aminoglycosides* (A Welton and HC Neu, eds.), Marcel Dekker, New York, 1982, pp. 125–142.
41. Phillips, AM, Milner, RD: Tissue concentrations of netilmicin and gentamicin in neonates. *J. Infect. Dis. 149*:474, 1984.
42. Sawchuk, RJ, Zaske, DE: Pharmacokinetics and dosing regimens which utilize multiple intravenous infusions: Gentamicin in burn patients. *J. Pharmacokinet. Biopharm. 4*:183–195, 1976.
43. Sawchuk, RJ, Zaske, ED, Cipolle, RJ, Wargin, WA, Strate, RG: Kinetic model for gentamicin dosing with the use of individual patient parameters. *Clin. Pharmacol. Ther. 21*:362–369, 1977.
44. Koren, G, James, A, Perlman, M: A simple method for the estimation of glomerular filtration rate by gentamicin pharmacokinetics during routine drug monitoring in the newborn. *Clin. Pharmacol. Ther. 38*:680–685, 1985.
45. Schentag, JJ: Aminoglycoside pharmacokinetics as a guide to therapy and toxicology. In: *The Aminoglycosides* (A Whelton and HC Neu, eds.), Marcel Dekker, New York, 1982, pp. 143–167.
46. McCracken, GH, West, NR, Horton, LJ: Urinary excretion of gentamicin in the neonatal period. *J. Infect. Dis. 123*:257–262, 1971.
47. Arant, B: Developmental pattern of renal functional maturation in the human neonate. *J. Pediatr. 92*:705–712, 1978.
48. Braunlich, H: Kidney development: Drug elimination mechanisms. In: *Drug Disposition During Development* (PL Morselli, ed.), Spectrum Publications, New York, 1977, p. 89.
49. Leave, RD, Trysfad, CW: Glomerular filtration rate during the period of adaptation to extrauterine life. *Pediatr. Res. 11*:959–962, 1977.
50. Miranda, JC, Schimmel, MM, James, LS, Spinelli, W, Rosen, TS: Gentamicin kinetics in the neonate. *Pediatr. Pharmacol. 5*:57–61, 1985.
51. Noordwien, B, Hook, JB: Developmental aspects of renal pharmacology. *Pharmacol. Ther. 17*:85–110, 1982.
52. McCracken, GH, Jones, LG: Gentamicin in the neonatal period. *Am. J. Dis. Child. 120*:524–533, 1970.
53. Siegel, JD, McCracken, GH, Thomas, ML, Threlkeld, N: Pharmacokinetic properties of netilmicin in newborn infants. *Antimicrob. Agents Chemother. 15*:246–253, 1979.
54. Edgren, B, Karna, P, Sciamanna, D, Dolanski, E: Gentamicin dosing in the newborn. *Dev. Pharmacol. Ther. 7*:263–272, 1984.
55. Hindmarsh, K, Nation, R, Williams, G, John, E, French, J: Pharmacokinetics of gentamicin in very low birth weight preterm infants. *Eur. J. Clin. Pharmacol. 24*:649–653, 1983.
56. Husson, C, Chevalier, J, Jezequel, M, Mathe, J, Costil, J, Aymard, P: Pharmacokinetic study of gentamicin in preterm and term neonates. *Dev. Pharmacol. Ther. 7*(Suppl. 1):125–129, 1984.
57. Kasik, JW, Jenkins, S, Leuschen, MP, Nelson, RM: Postconceptional age and gentamicin elimination half-life. *J. Pediatr. 106*:502–505, 1985.
58. Landers, S, Berry, P, Kearns, G, Kaplan, S, Rudolph, A: Gentamicin disposition and effect on development of renal function in the very low birth weight infant. *Dev. Pharmacol. Ther. 7*:285–302, 1984.
59. Schwartz, GJ, Feld, LG, Langford, DJ: A simple estimate of glomerular filtration rate in full term infants during the first year of life. *J. Pediatr. 104*:849–854, 1984.

60. Whelton, A: Renal tubular transport and intrarenal aminoglycoside distribution. In: *The Aminoglycosides* (A Whelton and HC Neu, eds.), Marcel Dekker, New York, 1982, pp. 191–122.
61. Kliegman, RM, Bertino, JS, Fanaroff, AA, Gavan, TL, Speck, WT: Pharmacokinetics of gentamicin during exchange transfusions in neonates. *J. Pediatr. 96*:927–930, 1980.
62. Yakatan, G, Smith, R, Leff, R, Kay, J: Pharmacokinetic considerations in exchange transfusions in neonates. *Clin. Pharmacol. Ther. 24*:90–94, 1978.
63. Fuquay, D, Koup, J, Epstein, M, Smith, A: Effect of exchange transfusion on serum gentamicin concentrations. *Dev. Pharmacol. Ther. 3*:214–221, 1981.
64. Green, TP: Gentamicin elimination during exchange transfusion. *J. Pediatr. 98*: 507–508, 1981.
65. Spino, M, Chai, R, Isles, A, Tesoro, AM, Gold, R, MacLeod, SM: Cloxacillin absorption and disposition in cystic fibrosis. *J. Pediatr. 105*:829–835, 1984.
66. Leeder, JS, Spino, M, Isles, AF, Tesoro, AM, Gold, R, MacLeod, SM: Ceftazidime disposition in acute and stable cystic fibrosis. *Clin. Pharmacol. Ther. 36*:355–362, 1984.
67. Schacter, SH, Spino, M, Isles, AF, Tesoro, AM, Prober, C, MacLeod, SM, Thiessen, JJ: Pharmacokinetics of cefoperazone in patients with cystic fibrosis and healthy volunteers. Proc. 13th Int. Cong. on Chemother (Vienna) (KH Spitzy and K Karrer, eds.), 1983, Part 103, pp. 45–49.
68. Michaelsen, H, Bergan, T: Pharmacokinetics of netilmicin in children with and without cystic fibrosis. *Antimicrob. Agents Chemother. 19*:1029–1031, 1981.
69. Kelly, HW, Menendez, R, Fan, L, Murphy, S: Pharmacokinetics of tobramycin in cystic fibrosis. *J. Pediatr. 100*:318–321, 1983.
70. Kearns, GL, Hillman, BS, Wilson, JT: Dosing implications of altered gentamicin disposition in patients with cystic fibrosis. *J. Pediatr. 100*:312–318, 1982.
71. Finkelstein, E, Hall, K: Aminoglycoside clearance in patients with cystic fibrosis. *J. Pediatr. 94*:163–164, 1979.
72. Levy, J, Smith, A, Koup, J, Williams-Warren, J, Ramsey, B: Disposition of tobramycin in patients with cystic fibrosis: A prospective controlled study. *J. Pediatr. 105*: 117–124, 1984.
73. Zasje, DE, Cipolle, RJ, Strate, RJ: Gentamicin dosage requirements: Wide interpatient variations in 242 surgery patients with normal renal function. *Surgery 87*: 164–169, 1980.
74. Brahams, D: Dosage of gentamicin and monitoring of blood levels. *Lancet 1*:1395–1396, 1986.
75. Koren, G, Rajchgot, P, Harding, E, Perlman, M, MacLeod, SM: Evaluating a filter device used for intermittent intravenous drug delivery to newborn infants. *Am. J. Hosp. Pharm. 42*:106–110, 1985.
76. Moench, TR, Smith, CR: Risk factors for aminoglycoside nephrotoxicity. In: *The Aminoglycosides* (A Whelton and HC Neu, eds.), Marcel Dekker, New York, 1982, pp. 401–418.
77. Eichenwald, HF: Antimicrobial therapy in infants and children: Update 1976–1985. Part II. *J. Pediatr. 107*:337–345, 1985.
78. de la Torre, M, Romero-Vivas, J, Guerrero, A, Meseguer, M, Bouza, E: *Klebsiella* bacteremia: An analysis of 100 episodes. *Rev. Infect. Dis. 7*:143–150, 1985.
79. Stephens, D, Garey, N, Isles, A, Levison, H, Gold, R: Efficacy of inhaled tobramycin in the treatment of pulmonary exacerbations in children with cystic fibrosis. *Pediatr. Infect. Dis. 2*:209–211, 1983.
80. Brown, AE: Management in the febrile neutropenic patient with cancer: Therapeutic considerations. *J. Pediatr. 106*:1035–1042, 1985.

81. Leff, RD, Roberts, RJ: Aminoglycoside dosage in pediatric patients: Considerations regarding pharmacokinetic based dose adjustment in patients requiring high versus low dose therapy. *Dev. Pharmacol. Ther. 3*:242–250, 1981.
82. Nahata, MC, Powell, DA, Durrell, DE, Miller, MC, Glazer, JP: Effect of gestational age and birth weight on tobramycin kinetics in newborn infants. *J. Antimicrob. Chemother. 14*:59–65, 1984.
83. Nahata, MC, Powell, DA, Durrell, DE, Miller, MA, Glazer, JP: Intrapatient variation in tobramycin kinetics in low birth weight infants during first postnatal week. *Eur. J. Clin. Pharmacol. 26*:647–649, 1984.
84. Arbeter, A, Saccar, C, Eisner, S, Sarni, E, Yaffe, S: Tobramycin sulfate elimination in premature infants. *J. Pediatr. 103*:131–135, 1983.
85. Granati, B, Assael, B, Chung, M, Montini, C, Parini, R, Pollatzon, P, Gagliardi, L, Radwanski, E, Rubaltelli, F: Clinical pharmacology of netilmicin in preterm and term newborn infants. *J. Pediatr. 106*:664–669, 1985.
86. Lanad, J, Dominguez-Gil, A, Dominguez-Gil, AA, Malaga, S, Crespo, M, Nuno, F: Modification in the pharmacokinetics of amikacin during development. *Eur. J. Clin. Pharmacol. 23*:155–160, 1982.
87. Prober, CG, Yeager, AS, Arvin, AM: The effect of chronologic age on the serum concentration of amikacin in full term and premature infants. *J. Pediatr. 98*:636–640, 1981.
88. Rusconi, F, Parini, R, Cananna, G, Assael, B: Monitoring of amikacin in the neonate. *Ther. Drug Monit. 5*:179–183, 1983.
89. Cookson, B, Tripp, J, Leung, T, Williams, J: Evaluation of amikacin dosage regimes in the low and very low birthweight newborn. *Infect 8*(Suppl. 3):S239–S242, 1980.
90. Kumor, KM, McDonald, JM, Lietman, PS: Effect of "high-dose" amikacin in children. *Dev. Pharmacol. Ther. 7*:368–376, 1984.
91. Vugelstein, B, Kowarski, A, Lietman, P: The pharmacokinetics of amikacin in children. *J. Pediatr. 91*:333–339, 1977.
92. Zarowitz, BJ, Wynn, RJ, Buckwald, S, Szefler, SJ: High gentamicin trough concentrations in neonates of less than 28 weeks gestational age. *Dev. Pharmacol. Ther. 5*:68–75, 1982.
93. Hendriksson, P, Svenningsen, N, Juhlin, I, Haeger, K: Netilmicin in moderate to severe infections in newborns and infants: A study of efficacy, tolerance and pharmacokinetics. *Scand. J. Infect. Dis. (Suppl.) 23*:155–159, 1980.
94. Sarubbi, FA, Hull, JH: Amikacin serum concentrations: Preductions of levels and dosage guidelines. *Ann. Intern. Med. 89*:612–618, 1978.
95. McCracken, GH: Aminoglycoside toxicity in infants and children. *Am. J. Med. 80*(Suppl. 63):172–178, 1986.
96. Thompson, WL: Aminoglycoside dosing regimens once daily, thrice or continuous administration. In: *The Aminoglycosides* (A Whelton and HC Neu, eds.), Marcel Dekker, New York, 1982, pp. 489–495.
97. Morin, JP, Fillastre, JP: Aminoglycoside-induced lysosomal dysfunctions in kidneys. In: *The Aminoglycosides* (A Whelton and HC Neu, eds.), Marcel Dekker, New York, 1982, pp. 303–324.
98. Silverblatt, F, Kuehn, C: Autoradiography of gentamicin uptake by the rat proximal tubule cell. *Kidney Int. 15*:335–345, 1979.
99. Morin, JP, Viotte, G, Vandewalle, A, Van Hoof, F, Tulkens, P, Fillastre, JP: Gentamicin-induced nephrotoxicity: A cell biology approach. *Kidney Int. 18*:583–590, 1980.
100. Sirinavin, S, McCracken, GH, Nelson, JD: Determining gentamicin dosage in infants and children with renal failure. *J. Pediatr. 86*:331–334, 1980.

101. Tessin, I, Bergmark, J, Hiesche, K, Jagenburg, R, Trollfors, B: Renal function of neonates during gentamicin treatment. *Arch. Dis. Child. 57*:758–760, 1982.
102. Adelman, RD, Zakauddin, S: Urinary enzyme activities in children and neonates receiving gentamicin therapy. *Dev. Pharmacol. Ther. 1*:325–332, 1980.
103. Itsarayoungyuen, S, Riff, L, Schauf, V, Hamilton, L, Ottembiak, J, Vidyasager, D: Tobramycin and gentamicin are equally safe for neonates: Results of a double-blind randomized trial with quantitative assessment of renal function. *Pediatr. Pharmacol. 2*:143–155, 1982.
104. Deance, N, Price, RG, Robinson, D, Stirling, JL: β-Galactosidase, β-glucosidase and *N*-acetyl-β-glucosaminidase in human kidney. *Clin. Chim. Acta 24*:189–197, 1969.
105. Kunin, CM, Chesney, RW, Craig, WA, England, AC, De Angelis, C: Enzymuria as a marker of renal injury and disease: Studies of *N*-acetyl-β-glucosaminidase in the general population and in patients with renal disease. *Pediatrics 62*:751–760, 1978.
106. Lockwood, TD, Bosmann, HB: The use of urinary *N*-acetyl-β-glucosaminidase in human renal toxicology. I. Partial biochemical characterization and excretion in humans and release from the isolated perfused rat kidney. *Toxicol. Appl. Pharmacol. 49*:1–14, 1979.
107. Jones, BR, Bhalla, RB, Mladek, J, Kaleya, RN, Cralla, RJ, Alcock, NW, Schwartz, MK, Young, CW, Reidenberg, MM: Comparison of methods of evaluation nephrotoxicity of cis-platinum. *Clin. Pharmacol. Ther. 27*:557–562, 1980.
108. MacLeod, S, Sturgess, J, Mahon, W: Gentamicin nephrotoxicity after subchronic dosing: Comparison between 1 week and 10 week old rats. Proc First World Conf on Clin Pharmacol Ther (London) A0365, (P Turner and C Padgham, eds.), MacMillan (London), 1980.
109. Barza, M, Lauermann, M: Why monitor serum levels of gentamicin. *Clin. Pharmacokinet. 3*:202–215, 1978.
110. Assael, BM, Parini, R, Rusconi, F: Ototoxicity of aminoglycoside antibiotics in infants and children. *Pediatr. Infect. Dis. 1*:357–365, 1982.
111. Editorial: Deafness in low birth weight infants: Is it avoidable? *Lancet 1*:1373–1374, 1985.
112. Schacht, J: Isolation of an aminoglycoside receptor from guinea pig inner ear tissues and kidney. *Arch. Otorhinolaryngol. 224*:129–134, 1979.
113. Stockhorst, E, Schacht, J: Radioactive labelling of phospholipids and proteins by cochlear perfusion in the guinea pig and the effect of neomycin. *Acta Otolaryngol. (Stockh.) 83*:401–409, 1977.
114. Eviatar, L, Eviatar, A: Aminoglycoside ototoxicity in the neonatal period. *Otolaryngol. Head Neck Surg. 89*:818–821, 1981.
115. Finitzo-Hieber, T, McCracken, G, Brown, K: Prospective controlled evaluation of auditory function in neonates given netilmicin or amikacin. *J. Pediatr. 106*:129–136, 1985.
116. Davey, P: Aminoglycosides and neonatal deafness. *Lancet 2*:612, 1985.
117. Brummett, RE, Jackson, RT: Age related changes influencing the effects of drugs on sensoneural hearing. *Pharmacol. Ther. 26*:209–219, 1984.
118. Zarfin, Y, Koren, G, Maresky, D, Perlman, M, MacLeod, S: Possible indomethacin-aminoglycoside interaction in preterm infants. *J. Pediatr. 106*:511–513, 1985.
119. McLaughlin, JE, Reeves, DS: Clinical and laboratory evidence for inactivation of gentamicin by carbenicillin. *Lancet 1*:261–264, 1971.
120. Davies, M: Interactions of carbenicillin and ticarcillin with gentamicin. *Antimicrob. Agents Chemother. 7*:431–434, 1975.
121. Odio, C, McCracken, GH, Nelson, JD: Nephrotoxicity associated with vancomycin-aminoglycoside therapy in term children. *J. Pediatr. 105*:491–493, 1984.
122. Leitner, F, Price, KE: Aminoglycosides under development. In: *The Aminoglycosides* (A Whelton and HC Neu, eds.), Marcel Dekker, New York, 1982, pp. 29–64.

14
Vancomycin

JOHN F. MILLIKEN
The Hospital for Sick Children, Toronto, Ontario, Canada

Few other compounds in medicine have come from such humble beginnings and achieved such a record of clinical efficacy as has vancomycin. Shortly after the introduction of penicillin into the armamentarium of infectious disease therapeutics, *Staphylococcus aureus* developed a clinically significant resistance to that compound. As a result of that clinical pressure, Eli Lilly and Company developed a program to find a compound that would be therapeutically effective and safe for the treatment of severe staphylococcal infections. In the early 1950s, a missionary collected a soil sample while walking along a jungle path in Borneo and sent it to his friend Dr. E. C. Kornfeld at Lilly. The soil sample contained *Streptomyces orientalis*, which elaborates an active compound that was bactericidal against all staphylococci with which it was tested (1,2).

Further in vitro work established that this new substance, compound 05865, did not induce resistance by the staphylococcus (3). Animal toxicities were found to be acceptable, and the compound was released for studies in human disease. The early preparations "were obtained by using picric acid precipitations" (1) and contained visible impurities, which earned it the nickname of Mississippi Mud. Because of its ability to vanquish the severe infections caused by this vexing organism, compound 05865 became "vancomycin." Owing to its then significant side effects of thrombophlebitis, fevers, rigors, and rashes, the semisynthetic penicillins and cephalosporins were met with great relief by patients and their physicians, and this new product was replaced in the early 1960s by these equally effective and better tolerated compounds.

Vancomycin is now enjoying a renaissance due to the ability of the same *Staphylococcus* to resist the compounds that had previously relegated it to the pharmaceutical back burner. It is also finding new applications as medical technology has advanced the frontiers of neonatology and oncology. Advances in these and other areas have provided help for patients in whom severe morbidity is caused by previously inocuous opportunistic organism that are now resistant to most antibiotics except vancomycin.

I. CHEMISTRY

Chemically, vancomycin is one of a small group of glycoprotein antibiotics that are obtained from the species *Actinomyces*. This group is composed of vancomycin, ristocetin, avoparcin, actinoidin, actaplanin, A35512, and teichomycin A2 (4). Only the first and last members of this group are used in the treatment of human disease. All these compounds share a similar structure as a tricyclic glycopeptide, except that vancomycin contains only five aromatic rings and all of the others contain seven (4). The definitive structure of the vancomycin molecule was finally reported in 1978 (5). The structure was deduced from x-ray diffraction studies done on a crystalline degradation product CDP-1 (see Figure 1). Until that time, crystallization of the parent compound had not been achieved.

The molecule has undergone a small number of attempts to enhance its efficacy as an antibiotic by altering its structure. No modification has been able to improve on the bactericidal activity of the parent compound. Loss of the vancosamine disaccharide results in only minimal loss of activity (6), but the substitution of the amide group in the asparagine substituent causes complete loss of bactericidal activity (7,8).

An unusual property of this compound is its ability to chelate ionic metals, such as copper and iron. This property is exploited as part of the purification process. It is not known if chelation of these or any other metals serves as part of the mode of action of its antibacterial activity. This property has not been noted to cause any adverse reactions, nor has it been employed as a therapeutic chelator for iron overdose (6).

II. PROPOSED MECHANISMS OF ACTION

There are three proposed mechanisms of action of vancomycin on gram-positive bacteria. The first and most widely supported is that of inhibition of cell wall synthesis. Other modes of action include the alteration of the permeability of the cell membrane and the selective inhibition of RNA synthesis. The evidence for these proposals will be reviewed.

With the elucidation of the three-dimensional structure of the vancomycin molecule came the in vitro support for the exact mechanism of binding of vancomycin to cell wall

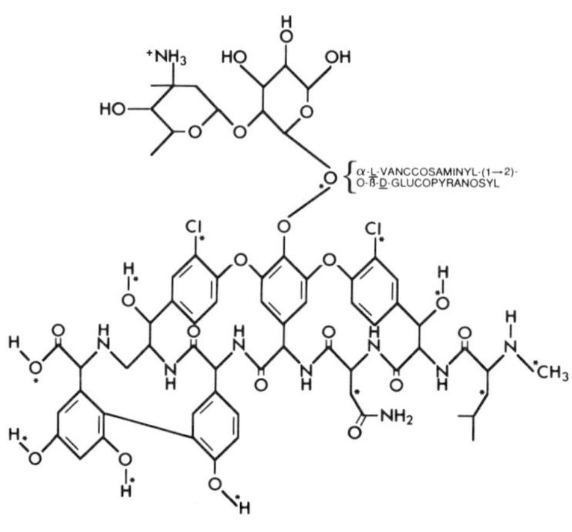

Figure 1 Vancomycin.

constituents. Consequently, the mechanism of the interruption of cell wall synthesis could be postulated. Vancomycin easily penetrates through the cell wall of the gram-positive organisms. This does not occur with the gram-negative organisms as their outer membrane of lipopolysaccharide phospholipid-protein is protective (4).

Vancomycin and its group of glycoprotein antibiotics differ from the lactams in that they exert their effect in the second stage of cell wall synthesis. The lactams (penicillins) work by interrupting the terminal transpeptidation reaction in the third phase of cell wall synthesis (9). Vancomycin readily penetrates into the cytosol (10,11). Once inside the cell, the vancomycin molecule forms a complex with acyl-D-ala-D-ala terminus of the UDP-*N*-acetylmuramylpentapeptide. The complex is formed by the acyl-D-ala-D-ala terminus fitting into a "cleft" on the surface of the vancomycin molecule. Binding within the cleft is accomplished by the formation of five hydrogen bonds as the molecule folds around the dialanyl terminus (4). Under normal conditions, in the absence of vancomycin, this cell wall building block is transported across the cell membrane via a phospholipid carrier (12,13). In the presence of vancomycin, the phospholipid-bound pentapeptide accumulates within the cell as a result of inhibition of the glycopeptide synthetase system (13). In the rapidly dividing cell, therefore, cell wall synthesis is blocked. It has been proposed that the block in synthesis occurs as a result of steric hindrance caused by the presence of the vancomycin-pentapeptide complex (4,14,15).

Vancomycin has also been shown to inhibit the synthesis of the cell membrane, although this occurs after the termination of cell wall production. With the cessation of cell wall synthesis, it is proposed that the above-mentioned intracellularly accumulated "wall" substrates would interfere with the mechanisms of membrane synthesis (11). The contribution of inhibition of membrane synthesis to the killing effect of vancomycin is unknown.

A third mechanism of action was proposed in 1959 (18). At that time it was demonstrated that within 1 hr after the addition of vancomycin to an in vitro suspension of *S. aureus* there was a complete inhibition of synthesis of ribonucleic acid when compared with controls. There was no change noted in the simultaneous synthesis of bacterial protein or DNA. As such, it is not clear how this effect would fit into an explanation for the bactericidal activity of the drug. This effect has not since been demonstrated.

III. ANTIMICROBIAL ACTIVITY AND RESISTANCE

Vancomycin has enjoyed a constant antimicrobial effect against almost all gram-positive organisms since its discovery 30 years ago. During that time, there has been no increase in resistance among the susceptible organisms. Vancomycin is bactericidal against multiplying bacteria (19), except that its effect against the enterococci is only bacteriostatic (10). This remarkable record may well be explained by the hypothesis that it has multiple modes of action.

Staphylococcal infection is probably the greatest indication for treatment with this agent. Resistant species were found initially in the 1950s (20). These strains represent the highest median minimal inhibitory concentration (MIC) in Table 1. Since that time, only twice have resistant strains of staphylococci been isolated (21,22). There appears to be no difference in MIC between the methicillin sensitive and resistant strains (see Table 1). Tolerance has been described for both *S. aureus* and *Staphylococcus epidermidis* against vancomycin (32). The clinical significance of this phenomenon is unknown.

Table 1 Antimicrobial Effects of Vancomycin

Organism	Strains	Range of MIC (mg/liter)			Reference
		MIC_{50}	MIC_{90}	MIC_{100}	
Staphylococcus aureus	734			⩽1.0	10
Methicillin sensitive	616	0.25–10			14
	156	1.0	1.0		23
	29	1.6	3.2		24
	20	0.25	0.5		25
Methicillin resistant	537	0.5–2.0			14
	60	1.0	2.0		23
	14	1.6	3.2		24
	10	1.0	1.0		25
S. epidermidis	488			⩽2.0	10
	73	1.0	2.0		23
	19	3.2	3.2		24
	10	2.0	2.0		25
Methicillin sensitive	554	1.0–8.0			14
Methicillin resistant	172	1.56–6.3			14
Other CNS[a]	404	0.78–4.0			14
	87	1.6–3.2	1.6–3.2		24
Streptococcus pneumoniae	7			⩽1.0	10
	217	0.04–1.0			14
	18	0.5	0.5		23
Multiple resistance[b]	6	0.25			14
Relatively Penicillin resistant	10	0.5	0.5		26
Penicillin resistant	7		0.4–0.8		27
	4	0.25			28
	7	⩽0.5			25

	[illegible]	[illegible]			14
	18	0.5	0.5		23
	10	0.25	0.5		25
Group B streptococcus	335	.06–1.6			14
	18	0.5	1.0		23
	10	0.5	0.5		25
Groups C and G	6	0.06			14
	10	0.5	0.5		25
S. bovis	32			⩽2.0	10
	96	0.5–0.63			14
Enterococcus	927			⩽4.0	10
	673	1.6–8.0			14
	98	1.6	3.2		24
	97	1.0	2.0		25
Viridans streptococci	118	0.625–1.0			14
	21			⩽1.0	10
Penicillin resistant	10	0.5	0.5		25
Diphtheroids	137	⩽0.04–0.8			14
Listeria monocytogenes	3			⩽1.0	10
	33	2.5–⩽5.0			14
	10	1.0	1.0		25
Clostridium difficile	227	0.78–2.0			14
	5	1.6	3.2		24
	111		1.0	4.0	29
C. perfringens	49	0.39–0.8			14
	3	3.2	6.4		24
	50	0.33			30
Neisseria sp.		0.5–5.0			31
Bacillus anthracis		0.5–5.0			31

[a]CNS = coagulase-negative staphylococci. [b]Multiply drug resistant *Streptococcus pneumoniae*.

An organism is defined as being sensitive if the MIC for vancomycin is ≤5 mg/liter. At The Hospital for Sick Children in Toronto, we have established our sensitivities' "break point" for vancomycin at 6 mg/liter. With that break point, we have isolated only two strains of vancomycin-resistant, coagulase-negative staphylococci (CNS) during the past 2 years. Because of the ongoing increase in the population at risk for invasive CNS as well as the number of blood cultures with these organisms, microbiology laboratories will have to maintain a diligent search for the presence of resistant strains.

All strains of *Streptococcus pneumoniae* groups A (pyogenes), C, and D are sensitive to vancomycin (see Table 1). Group B streptococci (*S. agalactiae*, GBS1) are very sensitive except a strain found in 1964 with MIC > 100 mg/liter. Since that time, there have been no isolates of GBS identified that are resistant to vancomycin (19,23,29). Owing to the bacteriostatic effect on enterococci, this organism may not be sensitive to vancomycin alone. Resistance has also been reported with strains of *Streptococcus bovis, mutans, viridans*, and *Leuconostoc* (14,33,34).

Listeria monocytogenes and diphtheroids appear to be sensitive in vitro to vancomycin (Table 1). Clostridial species are by and large a sensitive group. Note should be made of the following points: *Clostridium ramosum* carries a median MIC of 6.2 mg/liter (19). *Clostridium difficile* is uniformly sensitive. *Clostridium perfringens* can have a marked tolerance for vancomycin (30). *Actinomyces* and lactobacilli are organisms that should not be considered sensitive until formal sensitivity testing has been carried out on a clinical isolate (14,19).

IV. SYNERGY, INDIFFERENCE, AND ANTAGONISM

Much work has been done on demonstrating the in vitro effects of different combinations of antibiotics with vancomycin on various organisms. The results of some of this work are presented in Table 2 (15-17). Note should be made of the fact that in one study

Table 2 Effect of Antibiotic Combinations with Vancomycin Against Various Organisms

Organism	Antibiotic with vancomycin	Effect
Staphylococcus aureus	Aminoglycoside	Synergism
	Rifampin	Synergism/antagonism/indifference
	Fusidic acid	Indifference
S. epidermidis	Aminoglycoside	Synergism/indifference
	Cephalosporin	Synergism/antagonism
	Rifampin	Synergism/antagonism/indifference
	Aminoglycoside + rifampin	Synergism (16)
	TMP–SMX	Indifference (17)
Enterococci	Aminoglycoside	Synergism
	Rifampin	Indifference
Viridans streptococci	Aminoglycoside	Synergism
Streptococcus bovis	Aminoglycoside	Synergism
Group G	Aminoglycoside	Synergism

Source: From Reference 15 (except as noted).

(35) the combination of vancomycin and rifampin selected out the rifampin-resistant strains in one-half of the strains tested. A word of caution is pertinent with regard to the clinical interpretation of these data. Many of these results are determined using non-standardized techniques giving varying results (36). Although the in vitro literature for the combination of vancomycin and rifampin against the staphylococci appears to be confused, various clinical studies have found it to be an effective combination (37-41).

V. CLINICAL PHARMACOLOGY

Vancomycin is available as an oral preparation, characterized by a disagreeable taste (42). There is little if any absorption from the gastrointestinal tract (10,43-45). Following oral administration, the drug can be detected in the urine of patients with normal renal function (46). An anephric child developed a serum concentration of 34 mg/liter while being treated with oral vancomycin for pseudomembranous colitis (47). In this situation, serum concentrations should be monitored. Otherwise, the drug is not absorbed and reaches the colon in adequate concentrations (45,46,48) (Table 3).

Intramuscular injection of this compound is reported to be exceedingly painful and would mitigate against its administration via that route (10,43,46).

Intraperitoneal injection of vancomycin has been shown to be an effective treatment for gram-positive peritonitis (49,50). Kinetics of this compound when given intraperitoneally are not well documented in children. When given via this route, there will be systemic absorption of approximately 55-65% of the administered dose after 6 hr. Multiple

Table 3 Vancomycin Concentration (mg/liter) in Various Body Fluids with Simultaneous Serum Vancomycin Concentrations

Body fluid	No. patients	Mean fluid vancomycin	Mean serum vancomycin	Fluid-serum ratio
Aqueous humor	5	⩽0.78	14.0	<0.06
Ascitic fluid				
Single dose	11	2.3	6.2	0.37
Multiple dose	3	6.7	8.6	0.78
Bile	16	2.3	6.4	0.36
CSF				
Uninflamed meninges	11	0	6.3	0.0
Meningitis	10	3.9	NA	0.18
Pericardial fluid				
Single dose	11	2.3	6.2	0.37
Multiple dose	3	6.7	8.6	0.78
Peritoneal dialysate	6	0-5.0	5-25	
	4	2.2	8.0-35	
Pleural fluid	14	2.9	7.3	0.40
Synovial fluid	6	5.7	7.0	0.81
	1	10.3	8.0	1.30

Source: Modified from Reference 43.

studies have also demonstrated that peritoneal dialysis does not significantly alter the serum half-life of the drug in patients with reduced renal function (43,51).

There are no reports of systemic absorption when vancomycin is given intrathecally (43).

Almost all of an intravenously administered dose of vancomycin is eliminated in an unaltered form by renal excretion. There is a small body of evidence that the compound also has a minor route of excretion via a hepatic metabolic pathway (52). This pathway is hypothesized as a result of evidence of elimination in the anephric patient. The compound is found in the bile as well as in the feces (48) of patients given the drug intravenously.

The data for pharmacokinetics of vancomycin given intravenously suffer from the fact that there is no standardized approach to dosing, infusion time, time to draw samples, or assays used to determine concentrations. This is more especially true for younger infants and neonates (see Tables 4 and 5). The intravenous dose is rapidly distributed into a large volume of distribution, with an elimination half-life of 6–10 hr in the small premature infant. The half-life appears to be inversely proportional to the post-conceptual age or weight of the patient. This is the result of immaturity of the neonatal kidney (56). Figures 2 and 3 document the maturational changes of vancomycin pharma-

Table 4 Vancomycin Pharmacokinetics in Infants and Children

Group	No.	Mean age and weight	Dose (mg/kg)	Infusion time (min)	Mean peak[a] (μg/ml)	Mean trough[b] (μg/ml)	Assay[c]	Reference
Premature								
Single dose	7	3.3 days, 1.23/kg	10	30	17	9	MB	48
	7	4.7 days, 1.57/kg	15	30	25	10	MB	48
Full term								
Single dose	7	2.6 days, 3.07/kg	15	30	30	12	MB	
Multiple dose	5	<8 days	15 twice a day	30	53.8	21.7	FPI	53
	6	>8 days	15 three times a day	30	42.4	10.0	FPI	
Infants	33	>1 month	10 four times a day	30	33.3	6.1	FPI	53
Single dose	12	3.1 month	10	60	26	5.9	MB	
	4	4.3 month	15	60	28	5.2	MB	53
	5	4 years		60	32.5	3.0	MB	

[a]Serum level drawn immediately after the dose.
[b]Serum level drawn at 6 hr or immediately prior to the next dose.
[c]MB = microbiologic assay. FPI = flourescence polarization immunoassay.

Table 5 Vancomycin Elimination Kinetics[a]

Group	No.	Dose (mg/kg)	Mean weight (kg)	Infusion time (min)	V_d (ml/kg)	$T_{1/2\beta}$ (hr)	SD or SS	Reference
Premature	7	10	1.23	30	736	9.8	SD	48
	7	15	1.57	30	706	5.9	SD	48
	3		<1.0	30	970	9.9	SS	54
	6		>1.0	30	450	2.6	SS	54
Full term	7	15	3.07	30	690	6.7	SS	48
	3			60	352	9.1	SS	55
	11			60	410	4.3	SS	55
	12	10	4.9	60	595	4.1	SD	48
	4	15	5.2	60	964	4.1	SD	48
Children	5	15	15.5	60	818	2.4	SD	48
	6	10	27	30	538	2.2	SD	48

[a] V_d = volume of distribution; SS = steady state; SD = single dose.

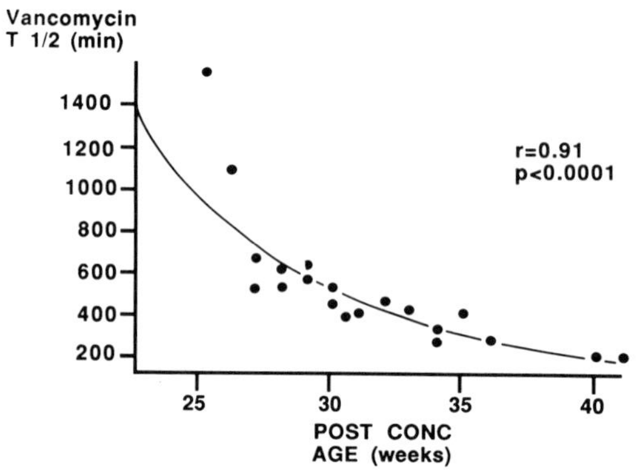

Figure 2 Maturational changes in vancomycin elimination $t_{1/2}$ in preterm infants.

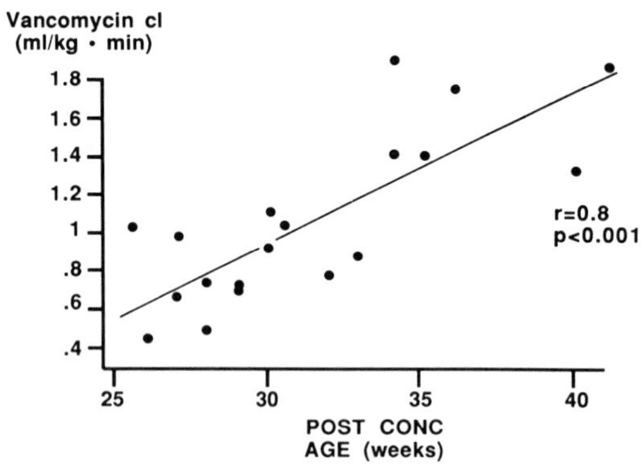

Figure 3 Maturational changes in vancomycin systemic clearance in preterm infants.

Table 6 Recommended Doses and Dose-Intervals of Vancomycin for Preterm Infants in Order to Maintain a Steady-State Peak of 30 mg/liter and Trough of 6 mg/liter

Postconceptional age (weeks)	<27	27–30	31–36	>37
Body weight (gr)	<800	800–1200	1200–2000	>2000
Daily dose (mg/kg)	18	24	36	45
Dose interval (hour)	36	24	12/18	12
Dose per injection (mg/kg)	27	24	18/27	22.5

cokinetics in preterm infants. Consequently, dose schedule should be modified, as shown in Table 6 (56).

The drug is made available in vials containing 500 mg for reconstitution for intravenous use and in screw-top containers of 1 g each for administration as an oral solution (package insert).

VI. DRUG ASSAYS

Of the techniques available to the clinical laboratory for the measurement of serum concentrations of vancomycin, five methods have recently been compared (57): a bioassay, high-pressure liquid chromatography (HPLC), fluorescence polarization immunoassay (FPIA), radioimmunoassay (RIA), and fluorescence immunoassay (FIA). These assays utilize serum volumes ranging from 0.5 ml (HPLC) to 100 μl (FIA), making them applicable to drug monitoring for the smallest neonates. Of the test systems studied, the FPIA was considered to be the most precise, easiest to run as a "stat" or batch test, automated, and to have a shorter turnaround time when compared with the other four systems. The FIA was found to be too imprecise for clinical use, but the other four were comparable in their precision.

VII. THERAPEUTIC INDICATIONS

Its 30 years of continuous efficacy against gram-positive organisms has allowed vancomycin to carve out a fairly specific niche in the treatment of infectious diseases (see Table 7). The prophylactic uses of this compound are finding new and varied applications. Traditional use for bacterial endocarditis prophylaxis in the penicillin-allergic patient is still recommended. In the same category of patient, vancomycin is also recommended for prosthetic implant surgery. There is a considerable literature on its use as an orally administered agent in the prophylaxis of life-threatening infections in the patient who is immunosuppressed as a result of induction chemotherapy for an underlying malignancy or preparation for a transplantation procedure. These studies have been carried out in adults; vancomycin in combination with other orally administered antimicrobials is not currently recommended as a prophylactic regimen in children. Ongoing studies are encouraging for the prevention of dental plaque and carries as well as hemodialysis graft infection. It is hoped that further study will allow the reduction of the incidence of these two important conditions. Vancomycin has been shown to be ineffective for the prevention of ventriculoperitoneal shunt infections.

Vancomycin is recommended in the treatment of severe staphylococcal infections in the penicillin- or cephalosporin-allergic host and in the presence of a resistant organism or in a patient who is clinically failing to respond to standard therapy. The empirical treatment of hospital-acquired infection in which methicillin-resistant strains are found and staphylococci are a diagnostic consideration will depend on the sensitivities of the hospital strain(3) as well as the toxic potential of combined antimicrobial therapy in a given patient.

Except for the treatment of the coagulase-negative staphylococcal endocarditis, vancomycin should be reserved for the patient with an allergy to the lactam antibiotics. For *Staph. aureus* or *Streptococcus viridans* endocarditis, vancomycin can be used as a single agent for treatment. Occasionally, rifampin will have to be added to this treatment regimen. For *Strep. bovis* endocarditis, vancomycin can be used alone or with the

Table 7 Indications for Use of Vancomycin

Indications	Penicillin allergic	Vein oral[a]	Combined with other antibiotic	Reference
Prophylactic				10, 42, 45, 58–60
Bacterial endocarditis	+	V	+	
Prosthetic implant procedure	+	V		
[Remission-induction for neutropenic cancer patients]	+	O		
[Dental carious disease, paste or gel]		O		
[Hemodialysis graft infections]		V		
Therapeutic				
Severe staphylococcal infections				10, 30, 61–67
Lactam allergic	+	V		
Methicillin-resistant *S. aureus*		V		
Coagulase-negative staphylococci		V		
Failure to respond to other agents		V		
Endocarditis				10, 30, 41, 45, 60, 68–75
Viridans streptococci	+	V		

Staphylococcus aureus	+	V		
S. epidermidis		V	+	
Group D streptococci	+	V	+	
Streptococcus bovis	+	V		
Diphtheroids	+	V		
Central nervous system infection				10, 31, 40, 75–82
Proximal ventriculoperitoneal shunt infections		V	+	
Meningitis		V		
Methicillin-resistant staphylococci				
Lactam-allergic patient, anaphylactic type				
Failure of prior treatment				
Central venous catheter infections		V	+	75, 83, 84
Staphylococcal peritonitis		V/IP		10, 49–51, 75
Acute staphylococcal ileocolitis		O		10, 45, 85
Clostridium difficile toxin-associated enterocolitis		O		10, 44, 45, 49, 75, 85–94

[a]IP = intraperitoneal.
Brackets indicate potential prophylactic applications in children.

addition of streptomycin if dosing intervals are prolonged to every 12 hr. For prosthetic valve endocarditis, in which disease caused by coagulase-negative staphylococci and diphtheroids are of prime concern, vancomycin should be combined with rifampin and gentamicin. Because vancomycin is bacteriostatic against the enterococcus, it must be used in combination with an aminoglycoside in treating endocarditis caused by this organism. For culture-negative endocarditis, consideration must be given to the combination of vancomycin and gentamicin in the penicillin-allergic patient and in the patient who fails to respond to penicillin and an aminoglycoside. A single case report showed that vancomycin was ineffective in the treatment of group B streptococcal endocarditis (68). In all cases of bacterial endocarditis, the serum inhibitory and killing levels must be followed and used to help guide therapy. Whenever vancomycin is used in combination with an aminoglycoside, serum concentrations and renal function must be rigorously followed.

To date, antimicrobial therapy for cerebrospinal fluid (CSF) shunt infection can only be considered part of a regimen that includes the replacement of the infected shunt. It is clear that vancomycin has its place in the treatment of gram-positive shunt infections and usually in combination with rifampin and/or trimethoprim-sulfa methoxazole. Combination therapy should be instituted as the CSF penetration of vancomycin is poor in uninflamed meninges. Intraventricular treatment appears to be effective, but this treatment with vancomycin is still considered investigational. As there are no chemical preservatives in any preparations of vancomycin, concern for a chemical ventriculitis is not warranted from that source. When vancomycin is dissolved in 5% dextrose and physiologic saline, the resulting pH is approximately 4.0, requiring an adjustment into the physiologic range. This maneuver may be beyond the capabilities of a community hospital pharmacy.

Indications for the use of vancomycin in the treatment of meningitis include meningitis caused by methicillin-resistant staphylococci, failure of prior treatment with a first choice drug, and staphylococcal meningitis in a patient with a known penicillin allergy of the anaphylactic type.

In the patient with a central venous line and a presumed bacteremia, vancomycin and an aminoglycoside have been recommended as empirical treatment because of the association of coagulase-negative staphylococci and plastic foreign bodies. Lack of clinical response and/or persistent positive blood cultures mandate the prompt removal of the offending line. More clinical trials need to be undertaken to determine the best agents and duration of therapy in order to realize the full potential of nonsurgical salvage of these lines.

Toxin-mediated enterocolitis caused by *C.* difficile is effectively treated by the oral administration of low dose (125 mg every 6 hr in adults, 15-20 mg/kg day^{-1} in children) vancomycin. Both oral and parenteral administration of vancomycin have resulted in concentrations of the drug in the feces of symptomatic children well in excess of the bactericidal concentration of the organism. There are inherent problems with this treatment that are very pertinent to the pediatrician. The first is that there are effective alternatives to vancomycin for mild to moderate disease. Metronidazole has been found to be as effective when directly compared with vancomycin. The relapse rate is no different. Second, the cost of treatment with metronidazole is approximately 5% of the vancomycin cost. Finally, vancomycin is known to have a disagreeable taste and therefore makes compliance difficult even for hospitalized patients. These considerations suggest that vancomycin be reserved for the severe end of the spectrum of this disease.

VIII. TOXICITY

The list of toxic or adverse effects associated with the use of vancomycin can be divided into four broad categories: ototoxicity, nephrotoxicity, infusion-related or histamine release response, and miscellaneous effects.

Recent publications regarding adverse effects in laboratory animals (guinea pigs, mice, rats, cats, and dogs) have yielded no evidence of ototoxicity (95,96). In a careful review of the published evidence concerning ototoxicity caused by vancomycin, Brummett found little or no clear-cut support for such an association (97). If this effect does in fact occur, it is thought to be extremely rare. A recent retrospective review of 100 courses of therapy with vancomycin given over 8 years revealed no evidence for auditory toxicity (98). In reports of vancomycin-associated hearing loss, there have been other events in the patient's course to explain the noted deficit. Prominent findings in clinical reports concerning ototoxicity and vancomycin include renal impairment without dosage adjustment and serum concentrations in the toxic range, concommittent use of an aminoglycoside, especially streptomycin, and a pre-existing eighth nerve deficit (99). A case report of eighth nerve injury has been reported with peak serum concentrations of less than 50 mg/liter. Trough concentrations were reported as high as 32 mg/liter. There was improvement in the hearing deficit with reduction of the dose alone (100). Prospective studies have failed to demonstrate an ototoxic effect of the drug (99). As it is wise to consider vancomycin as a possible etiology when clinical hearing loss occurs and to discontinue its use in that instance, a further recommendation to seek other explanations and to document serum concentrations should carry greater weight.

The association of nephrotoxicity with the use of vancomycin appears to be as nebulous as that for ototoxicity. Since the early 1970s, the incidence of nephrotoxicity has greatly diminished. This decrease is postulated to be the result of greater purification of the compound. Additionally, there is evidence that renal transplant recipients do not suffer deterioration in their renal function as a result of vancomycin therapy (101). In an above-mentioned series (98), 5% of the patients receiving vancomycin alone developed evidence of renal impairment manifested as an increase in their serum creatinine concentration. All the patients involved had peak serum vancomycin concentrations of 49–76 μg/ml and/or trough concentrations of 39–65 μg/ml prior to the change in their renal function. A return to normal renal function required an adjustment in dose, not necessarily the discontinuation of the drug. This work would suggest that the effect on renal function is related to the serum concentration and to the duration of therapy with the drug (99).

Of greater concern to the clinician is the apparent synergistic nephrotoxicity when vancomycin is combined with an aminoglycoside. The incidence of reduction of renal function is approximately 35% in patients on both compounds (98). This association has been observed in children (102), and normal renal function returned after cessation of treatment in the cases reported. Careful monitoring of the serum concentrations of both compounds and periodic evaluation of renal function is indicated for patients in whom treatment with vancomycin and an aminoglycoside is used simultaneously.

The immediate reaction of the "red man" syndrome appears to be a dose-related phenomenon in that it occurs as a result of rapid infusion of the drug and therefore of rapid increase in serum concentration. This reaction is manifest most commonly as flushing and a macular or maculopapular rash of the neck, face, trunk, and extremities, occurring during or shortly after the intravenous administration of the drug. The reaction is thought to be caused by a systemic release of histamine, which can lead to the development of the rash, hypotension, tachycardia, and occasionally shock and cardiac arrest.

A 2-year-old child receiving a 25-mg/kg dose intravenously over a period of 10 min succumbed as a result of hypotension and a cardiac arrest (103). In an animal model, this reaction can be blocked by the prior administration of an antihistamine. In human volunteers, the release of histamine is not observed when the administered dose is given over a 60-min infusion time or in a dilute solution $\leqslant$ 10 mg/ml. It is therefore recommended that the drug be given in dilute solution (2.5–5 mg/ml) and over a minimum infusion time of 60 min (99). Pertinent risk factors include the rate of administration and its administration during general anesthesia (96,103–106). It is important to recognize this reaction for two reasons. First, it can be avoided by decreasing the rate of administration or, theoretically, by pretreating with antihistamines. Second, this is not a manifestation of an allergic reaction and the drug can still be given in the future if sensitivity testing indicates that therapy with vancomycin is required.

Miscellaneous reactions consist of phlebitis, which occurs in up to 13% of patients; fever, which is transient; chills, nausea, anaphylaxis, and neutropenia with recovery on cessation of the drug; and eosinophilia (98,99).

IX. CONTRAINDICATIONS

Contraindications for the use of vancomycin are important to remember because, although rare, they can cause significant morbidity. This compound should not be given via the intramuscular route because of the severe pain this causes. Systemic infection should not be treated via the enteral route as it is not absorbed. The drug should not be given when the serum concentration is known to be in the toxic range; there are reports of associated audio- and nephrotoxicity, especially in the patient receiving simultaneous aminoglycoside treatment. It should not be used in patients in whom there is a known history of previous serious allergic event (107).

X. DRUG INTERACTIONS

Vancomycin is an acidic compound with a pH of 2.5–4.5 when reconstituted in water. As a result, vancomycin should not be mixed or given simultaneously with any alkaline substance as this may cause a precipitate to form. Commonly used therapeutic agents that may precipitate when mixed with vancomycin include heparin, ticarcillin, aminophylline, amobarbital sodium, dexamethasone sodium phosphate, hydrocortisone sodium succinate, methicillin sodium, pentobarbital sodium, phenobarbital sodium, phenytoin sodium, secobarbital sodium, sodium bicarbonate, sulfisoxizole diolamine, vitamin B complex with C, and warfarin sodium (107).

REFERENCES

1. Griffith, RS: Vancomycin use—an historical review. *J. Antimicrob. Chemother. 14 (Suppl D)*:1–5, 1984.
2. Banner, W, Ray, CG: Vancomycin in perspective. *Am. J. Dis. Child. 138*:14–16, 1984.

3. Zeigler, DW, Wolfe, RN, McGuire, JM: Vancomycin a new antibiotic. II. In vitro antibacterial studies. In: *Antibiotics Annual 1955–1956*, Medical Encyclopedia, Inc., New York, 1956, pp. 612–618.
4. Barna, JCJ, Williams, DH: The structure and mode of action of glycopeptide antibiotics of the vancomycin group. *Annu. Rev. Microbiol. 38*:339–357, 1984.
5. Sheldrick, GM, Jones, PG, Kennard, O, Williams, DH, Smith, GA: Structure of vancomycin and its complex with acetyl-D-alanyl-D-alanine. *Nature 271*:223–225, 1978.
6. Marshal, FJ: Structure Studies on Vancomycin. *J. Med. Chem. 8*:18–22, 1965.
7. Pfeiffer, RR: Structural features of vancomycin. *Rev. Infect. Dis. 3 (Suppl.)*:S205–S209, 1981.
8. Harris, CM, Harris, TM: Structure of the glycopeptide antibiotic vancomycin. Evidence for an asparagine residue in the peptide. *J. Am. Chem. Soc. 104*:4293–4295, 1982.
9. Weinstein, L: The penicillins. In: *The Pharmacological Basis of Therapeutics* (LS Goodman and A Gilman, eds.), Macmillan, New York, 1985, pp. 1116–1117.
10. McHenry, MC, Gavan, TL: Vancomycin. *Pediatr. Clin. North Am. 30*:31–47, 1983.
11. Jordan, DC: Effect of vancomycin on the synthesis of the cell wall and cytoplasmic membrane of *Staphylococcus aureus. Can. J. Microbiol. 11*:390–393, 1965.
12. Garrod, LP, Lambert, HP, O'Grady, F: Modes of action. In: *Antibiotic and Chemotherapy*, Churchill Livingstone, Edinburgh, 1981, pp. 251–261.
13. Anderson, JS, Matsuhashi, M, Haskin, MA, Strominger, JL: Lipid phosphoacetylmuramyl-pentapeptide and lipid-phosphodisaccharide-pentapeptide: Presumed membrane transport intermediates in cell wall synthesis. *Proc. Natl. Acad. Sci. USA 53*: 881–889, 1965.
14. Watanakunakorn, C: Mode of action and in vitro activity of vancomycin. *J. Antimicrob. Chemother. 14(Suppl. D)*:7–18, 1984.
15. Watanakunakorn, C: Mechanism of action: In vitro antimicrobial spectrum and clinical use of vancomycin. Symposium on vancomycin, November 2, 1985, Atlanta, Georgia. Sponsored by Eli Lilly & Company (to be published).
16. Bingen, E, Lambert-Zechovsky, N, et al.: In vitro optimal combination against methicillin-resistant staphylococcal epidermidis isolated in children with staphylococcal septicemia. Program and Abstracts of the Twenty-fifth ICAAC, Abstract 1056, 1985, p. 287, American Society for Microbiology, Washington, D.C.
17. Walsh, TJ, Auger, FA, et al.: Activity of trimethoprim-sulfamethoxazole in combination with vancomycin, rifampin, and novobiocin against methicillin-resistant *Staphylococcus aureus*. Program and Abstracts from the Twenty-fifth ICAAG, Abstract 1057, 1985, p. 287, American Society for Microbiology, Washington, D.C.
18. Jordan, DC, Innis, WE: Selective inhibition of ribonucleic acid synthesis in *Staphylococcus aureus* by vancomycin (letter). *Nature 184*:1894–1895, 1959.
19. Watanakunakorn, C: The antibacterial action of vancomycin. *Rev. Infect. Dis. 3 (Suppl.)*:S210–S215, 1981.
20. Petersdorf, RG, Curtin, JA, Bennett, IL: The sensitivity of two hundred strains of hemolytic staphylococcus to a series of antibiotics. *Arch. Intern. Med. 100*:927–936, 1957.
21. Klastersky, J, Beumer, J, Daneau, D: Bacteriophage types and antibiotic susceptibility of *Staphylococcus aureus. Appl. Microbiol. 22*:1000–1007, 1971.
22. Richmond, AS, Simberkoff, MS, Schaefler, S, Rahal, JJ: Resistance of *Staphylococcus aureus* to semi-synthetic penicillins and cephalothin. *J. Infect. Dis 135*:108–112, 1977.
23. Verbist, L, Tjandramaga, B, et al.: In vitro activity and human pharmacokinetics of teicoplanin. *Antimicrob. Agents Chemother. 26*:881–886, 1984.

24. Varaldo, PE, Debbia, E, Schito, GC: In vitro activity of teichomycin and vancomycin alone and in combination with rifampin. *Antimicrob. Agents Chemother. 23*: 402–406, 1983.
25. Eliopoulos, GM, Thauvin, CT, Gerson, B, Moellering, RC: In vitro activity and mechanism of action of A21978Cl, a novel cyclic lipopeptide antibiotic. *Antimicrob. Agents Chemother. 27*:357–362, 1985.
26. Jackson, MA, Shelton, S, Nelson, JD, McCracken, GH: Relatively penicillin-resistant pneumococcal infections in pediatric patients. *Pediatr. Infect. Dis. 3*:129–132, 1984.
27. Liu, HH, Tomasz, A: Penicillin tolerance in multiply drug-resistant natural isolates of *Streptococcus pneumoniae. J. Infect. Dis. 152*:365–372, 1985.
28. Jacobs, MR, Koornhof, HJ, et al.: Emergence of multiply resistent pneumococci. *N. Engl. J. Med. 299*:735–740, 1978.
29. Eickoff, TC, Klein, JO, Daly, AK, Ingall, D, Finland, M: Neonatal sepsis and other infections due to group B beta hemolytic streptococci. *N. Engl. J. Med. 271*:1221–1228, 1964.
30. Jung, WK: Susceptibility of 50 isolates of *Clostridium perfringens* to cefotaxime, fosfomycin, penicillin G, and vancomycin; variable tolerance for vancomycin. *Chemotherapy 29*:99–103, 1983.
31. Gump, DW: Vancomycin of treatment of bacterial meningitis. *Rev. Infect. Dis. 3 (Suppl.)*:S289–S292, 1981.
32. Watanakunakorn, C: Antibiotic tolerance of *Staphylococcus epidermidis. Scand. J. Infect. Dis. 17*:59–61, 1985.
33. Schlaes, DM, Marini, J, Jacobs, MR: Infection caused by vancomycin-resistant *Streptococcus sanguis*. II. *Antimicrob. Agents Chemother. 25*:527–528, 1984.
34. Buu-Hoi, A, Branger, C, Acar, JF: Leuconostoc: An opportunistic pathogen resistant to vancomycin. In: *Program and Abstracts of the Twenty-Fifth Interscience Conference on Antimicrobial Agents and Chemotherapy* (ICAAC), Abstract 1083, 1985, p. 291, American Society for Microbiology, Washington, D.C.
35. Lowy, FD, Chang, DS, Lash, PR: Synergy of combinations of vancomycin, gentamicin, and rifampin against methicillin-resistant, coagulase-negative staphylococci. *Antimicrob. Agents Chemother. 23*:932–934, 1983.
36. Bayer, AS, Morrison, JO: Disparity between time-killed and checkerboard methods for determination of in vitro bactericidal interactions of vancomycin plus rifampin versus methicillin-susceptible and -resistant *Staphylococcus aureus. Antimicrob. Agents Chemother. 26*:220–223, 1984.
37. Van der Auwera, P, Thys, KP, Meunier-Carpentier, F, Klastersky, J: The combination of oxacillin and rifampin in staphylococcal infections: A review of laboratory and clinical studies of the Institut Jules Bordet. *J. Antimicrob. Chemother. 13 (Suppl. C)*:31–42, 1984.
38. Faville, RJ, Zaske, DE, Kaplan, EL, Crossly, K, Sabath, LD, Quie, PG: *Staphylococcus aureus* endocarditis: Combined therapy with vancomycin and rifampin. *JAMA 240*:1963–1965, 1978.
39. Yogev, R: Cerebrospinal fluid shunt infections: A personal view. *Pediatr. Infect. Dis. 4*:113–118, 1985.
40. Gardner, P, Leipzig, T, Phillips, P: Infections of central nervous system shunts. *Med. Clin. North Am. 69*:297–314, 1985.
41. Sande, MA, Scheld, WM: Combination antibiotic therapy of bacterial endocarditis. *Ann. Intern. Med. 92*:390–395, 1980.
42. Kaplan, EL: Vancomycin in infants and children: A review of pharmacology and indications for therapy and prophylaxis. *J. Antimicrob. Chemother. 14(Suppl. D)*: 59–66, 1984.
43. Moellering, RC: Pharmacokinetics of vancomycin. *J. Antimicrob. Chemother. 14 (Suppl. D)*:43–52, 1984.

44. Weinstein, L: Antimicrobial agents; vancomycin. In: *The Pharmacological Basis of Therapeutics* (LS Goodman and A Gilman, eds.), Macmillan, New York, 1985, pp. 1192–1193.
45. Cunha, BA, Ristuccia, AM: Clinical usefulness of vancomycin. *Clinical Pharmacy 2*: 417–424, 1983.
46. Moellering, RC, Krogstad, DJ, Greenblatt, DJ: Pharmacokinetics of vancomycin in normal subjects and in patients with reduced renal function. *Rev. Infect. Dis. 33 (Suppl.)*:S230–235, 1981.
47. Thompson, CM, Long, SS, Gilligan, PH, Prebis, JW: Absorption of oral vancomycin—possible associated toxicity. *Int. J. Pediatr. Nephrol. 4*:1–4, 1983.
48. Schaad, UB, McCracken, GH, Nelson, JD: Clinical pharmacology and efficiency of vancomycin in pediatric patients. *J. Pediatr. 96*:119–126, 1980.
49. McClung, MR: Peritonitis in children receiving continuous ambulatory peritoneal dialysis. *Pediatr. Infect. Dis. 2*:328–332, 1983.
50. Powell, D, San Luis, E, Calvin, S, McDaid, T, Potter, D: Peritonitis in children undergoing continuous ambulatory peritoneal dialysis. *Am. J. Dis. Child. 139*:29–32, 1985.
51. John, CA, Zimmerman, SW, Rogge, M: The pharmacokinetics of antibiotics used to treat peritoneal dialysis-associated peritonitis. *Am. J. Kidney Dis. 4*:3–17, 1984.
52. Rotschafer, JC, Crossley, K, Zaske, DE, Mead, K, Sawchuck, RJ, Solem, LD: Pharmacokinetics of vancomycin: Observations in 28 patients and dosage recommendations. *Antimicrob. Agents Chemother. 22*:391–394, 1982.
53. Mercier, JC, Bingen, E, Lambert-Zechovsky, N, et al.: Assessment of serum vancomycin levels in neonates and children with severe staphylococcal infection. Presented at the Twenty-fourth Interscience Conference on Antimicrobial Agents and Chemotherapy, Washington, D.C., October 8–10, 1984, American Society for Microbiology, Washington, D.C.
54. Kramer, WG, Gross, JR, Kaplan, SL, Mason, EO: Vancomycin pharmacokinetics in premature infants. *Pediat. Pharmacol. 5*(1):17–22.
55. Israele, V, McCracken, GH, Threlkeld, N, Darabi, A: Pharmacokinetics of vancomycin in young infants. Presented at the Twenty-fifth Interscience Conference on Antimicrobial Agents and Chemotherapy, Minneapolis, Minnesota, September 29–October 2, 1985.
56. James, A, Koren, G, Milliken J, Soldin, S, Prober, C: Vancomycin pharmacokinetics and dose recommendations for preterm infants. *Antimicrob. Agent Chemother. 31*: 52–54, 1987.
57. Pfaller, MA, Krogstad, DJ, et al.: Laboratory evaluation of five assay methods for vancomycin: Bioassay, high pressure liquid chromatography, fluorescence polarization immunoassay, and fluorescence immunoassay. *J. Clin. Microbiol. 20*:311–316, 1984.
58. Shulman, ST, Armen, DP, Bisno, AL, et al.: Prevention of bacterial endocarditis. A statement for health professionals by the committee on rheumatic fever and bacterial endocarditis of the council on cardiovascular diseases in the young of the American Heart Association. *Am. J. Dis. Child. 139*:232–235, 1985.
59. Fivush, BA, Bock, GH, Guzzetta, PC, Salcedo, JR, Roley, EJ: Vancomycin prevents polytetraflouroethylene graft infections in pediatric patients receiving chronic hemodialysis. *Am. J. Kidney Dis. 5*:120–123, 1985.
60. Newsom, SWB: The treatment of endocarditis by vancomycin. *J. Antimicrob. Chemother. 14(Suppl. D)*:79–84, 1984.
61. Schaad, UB, Nelson, JD, McCracken, GH: Pharmacology and efficacy of vancomycin for staphylococcal infections in children. *Rev. Infect. Dis. 3(Suppl.)*:S282–288, 1981.
62. Kirby, WMM: Vancomycin therapy in severe staphylococcal infections. *Rev. Infect. Dis. 3(Suppl.)*:S236–S239, 1981.

63. Kirby, WMM: Vancomycin therapy of severe staphylococcal infections. *J. Antimicrob. Chemother. 14(Suppl. D)*:73–78, 1984.
64. Markowitz, N, Saravolatz, L, Pohlod, D, et al.: Comparative efficacy and toxicity of trimethoprim-sulfamethoxazole vs vancomycin in the therapy of *S. aureus* infection. Presented at the Twenty-fifth Interscience Conference on Antimicrobial Agents and Chemotherapy, Minneapolis, Minnesota, September 29–October 2, 1985, American Society for Microbiology, Washington, D.C.
65. Klastersky, J, Coppens, L, van der Auwera, P, Meunier-Carpentier, F: Vancomycin therapy of oxacillin-resistant *Staphylococcus aureus* infections. *J. Antimicrob. Chemother. 11*:361–367, 1983.
66. Sheagren, JN: *Staphylococcus aureus*: The persistent pathogen. *N. Engl. J. Med. 310*:1437–1442, 1984.
67. Friedman, LE, Brown, AE, Miller, DR, Armstrong, D: *Staphylococcus epidermidis* septicemia in children with leukemia and lymphoma.
68. Geraci, JE, Wilson, WR: Vancomycin therapy for infective endocarditis. *Rev. Infect. Dis. 3(Suppl.)*:S250–S258, 1981.
69. Kuckers, A: Vancomycin. *J. Antimicrob. Chemother. 14*:564–567, 1984.
70. Stanton, BF, Baltimore, RS, Clemens, JD: Changing spectrum of infective endocarditis in children. Analysis of 26 Cases, 1970–1979. *Am. J. Dis. Child. 138*:720–725, 1984.
71. Durack, DT, Kaplan, EL, Bisno, AL: Apparent failures of endocarditis prophylaxis: Analysis of 52 cases submitted to a national registry. *JAMA 250*:2318–2322, 1983.
72. Geraci, JE: Vancomycin. *Mayo Clin. Proc. 52*:631–634, 1977.
73. Siegel, JD: Bacterial endocarditis in infants and children: Incidence and pathogenesis. *Pediatr. Infect. Dis. 2 (Suppl.)*: S41–S43 1983.
74. Bayer, AS, Lam, K: Vancomycin and rifampin in experimental endocarditis due to methicillin-resistant *Staphylococcus aureus*—in vitro–in vivo correlations. Presented at the Twenty-fourth Interscience Conference of Antimicrobial Agents and Chemotherapy, Washington, D.C., October 8–10, 1984, American Society for Microbiology, Washington, D.C.
75. Fekety, R: Vancomycin. *Med. Clin. North Am. 66*:175–181, 1982.
76. Idio, C, McCracken, GH, Nelson, JD: CSF shunt infections in pediatrics. *Am. J. Dis. Child. 138*:1103–1108, 1984.
77. Nelson, JD:Cerebrospinal fluid shunt infections. *Pediatr. Infect. Dis. 3(Suppl.)*: S30–32, 1984.
78. Yogev, R: Cerebrospinal fluid shunt infections: A personal view. *Pediatr. Infect. Dis. 4*:113–118, 1985.
79. Vichyanond, P, Olson, LC: Staphylococcal CNS infections treated with vancomycin and rifampin. *Arch. Neurol. 41*:637–639, 1984.
80. Bayston, R, Barnicoat, M, Cudmore, RE, et al.: The use of intraventricular vancomycin in the treatment of CSF shunt associated ventriculitis. *Z. Kinderchir. 39 (Suppl. 2)*:111–113, 1984.
81. Frame, PT, McLaurin, RL: Treatment of CSF shunt infections with intrashunt plus oral antibiotic therapy. *J. Neurosurg. 60*:354–360, 1984.
82. Howard, MA, Grady, MS, Park, TS, Lank, KM, Scheld, WM: Pharmacokinetics following intraventricular vancomycin in hydrocephalic rats. Presented at the Twenty-fifth Interscience Conference on Antimicrobial Agents and Chemotherapy, Minneapolis, Minnesota, September 29–October 2, 1985, American Society for Microbiology, Washington, D.C.
83. Peters, G, Pulverer, G: Pathogenesis and management of *Staphylococcus epidermidis* "plastic" foreign body infections. *J. Antimicrob. Chemother. 14(Suppl. D)*:67–71, 1984.
84. Winston, DJ, Dudnick, DV, Chapin, M, Ho, WG, Gale, RP, Martin, WJ: Coagulase-negative staphylococcal bacteremia in patients receiving immunosuppressive therapy. *Arch. Intern. Med. 143*:32–36, 1983.

85. Fekety, R, Silva, J, Armstrong, J, et al.: Treatment of antibiotic-associated enterocolitis with vancomycin. *Rev. Infect. Dis. 3(Suppl.)*:S273–S281, 1981.
86. Bartlett, JG: Treatment of antibiotic-associated pseudomembranous colitis. *Rev. Infect. Dis. 6(Suppl. 1)*:S235–S241, 1984.
87. Fekety, R, Silva, J, Buggy, B, Deery, HG: Treatment of antibiotic-associated colitis with vancomycin. *J. Antimicrob. Chemother. 14(Suppl. D)*:97–102, 1984.
88. Fekety, R, Silva, J, Deery, G, Buggy, B: Comparative efficacy of low vs high dose oral vancomycin (125 or 500 mg four times per day) in treatment of adults with antibiotic-associated *Clostridium difficile* colitis. Presented at the Twenty-fourth Interscience Conference on Antimicrobial Agents and Chemotherapy, Washington, D.C., October 9–12, 1984, American Society for Microbiology, Washington, D.C.
89. Ellis, ME, Mandal, BK, Dunbar, EM, Bundell, KR: *Clostridium difficile* and its cytotoxin in infants admitted to hospital with infectious gastroenteritis. *Br. Med. J. [Clin. Res.] 288*(6416):524–526, 1984.
90. Han, VK, Sayed, H, Chance, GW, Brabyn, DG, Shaheed, WH: An outbreak of *Clostridium difficile* necrotizing enterocolitis: A case for oral vancomycin therapy? *Pediatrics 71*:935–941, 1983.
91. Teasley, DG, Olson, MM, Gerhard, RL, et al.: Prospective randomized trial of metronidazole versus vancomycin for *Clostridium difficile* associated diarrhoea and colitis. *Lancet 2*:1044–1046, 1983.
92. Walters, BH, Roberts, R, Stafford, R, Seneviratne, E: Relapse of antibiotic associated colitis: Endogenous persistence of *Clostridium difficile* during vancomycin therapy. *Gut 24*:206–212, 1983.
93. Trnka, YM, Lamont, JT: *Clostridium difficile* colitis. *Adv. Intern. Med. 29*:85–107, 1984.
94. Dupuis, L: Vancomycin: Is the renaissance justifiable? *Drug Inform. Bull.* (The Hospital for Sick Children, Toronto) *2*:1–5, 1985.
95. Brummett, RE: Effects of antibiotic-diuretic interactions in the guinea pig model of ototoxicity. *Rev. Infect. Dis. 3(Suppl.)*:S216–S223, 1981.
96. Wold, JS, Turnipseed, SA: Toxicology of vancomycin in laboratory animals. *Rev. Infect. Dis. 3(Suppl.)*:S224–S229, 1981.
97. Brummett, RE: Ototoxicity of vancomycin. Symposium on Vancomycin, Novenber 2, 1985, Atlanta, Georgia. Sponsored by Eli Lilly & Co. (to be published).
98. Farber, BF, Moellering, RC: Retrospective study of the toxicity of preparations of vancomycin from 1974 to 1981. *Antimicrob. Agents Chemother. 23*:138–141, 1983.
99. Cooper, GL, Given, DB: *Vancomycin: A Comprehensive Review of 30 Years of Clinical Experience*. Parker Row Publishers, Inc. USA, March, 1986.
100. Traber, PG, Levine, P: Vancomycin ototoxicity in a patient with normal renal function. *Ann. Intern. Med. 95*:458, 1981.
101. Appel, GB, Neu, HC: The nephrotoxicity of antimicrobial agents. *N. Engl. J. Med. 296*:722–728, 1977.
102. Odio, C, McCracken, GH: Nephrotoxicity associated with vancomycin-aminoglycoside therapy in four children. *J. Pediatr. 105*:491–493, 1984.
103. Mayhew, JF, Deutsch, S: Cardiac arrest following administration of vancomycin. *Can. Anaesth. Soc. J. 32*:65–66, 1985.
104. Pau, AK, Khakoo, R: Red-neck syndrome with slow infusion of vancomycin. *N. Engl. Med. 313*:756–757, 1985.
105. Garrelts, JC, Peterie, JD: Vancomycin and the red man's syndrome. *N. Engl. J. Med. 312*:245, 1985.
106. Odio, C, Mohs, E, et al.: Adverse reactions to vancomycin used as prophylaxis for CSF shunt procedures. *Am. J. Dis. Child. 138*:17–19, 1984.
107. Letter from Robert Kammer, M.D., Clinical Investigation and Regulatory Affairs, Lilly Research Laboratories, Indianapolis, Indiana, May 1986.

15
Tetracyclines

DANIEL A. GOLDSTEIN
The Hospital for Sick Children, Toronto, Ontario, Canada

I. INTRODUCTION

Aureomycin, the first tetracycline, was introduced into clinical medicine in 1948. As the first wide-spectrum, orally-administered antibiotic, it represented a significant therapeutic advance over the other available antibiotics; penicillin and streptomycin (1). Aureomycin (chlortetracycline) is the product of the bacterium *Streptomyces aureofaciens* and was named for its golden color. Terramycin (oxytetracycline), produced by *Strep. rimosus*, was introduced in 1950, and tetracycline in 1957. Although tetracycline is also a bacterial product, it is produced largely by chemical modification of chlor- and oxytetracycline. Further modification resulted in the introduction of demeclocycline (demethylchlortetracycline), methacycline, doxycycline, minocycline, and several analogs which are not commonly in clinical use: clomocycline, limecycline, and rolitetracycline.

The introduction of other antibiotics, the emergence of resistance, and the realization that tetracyclines could produce significant dental pathology in children have substantially limited the role of tetracyclines. Some discussion of this interesting group of compounds is merited, however, because of their frequent use for venereal and other infections in the older child and adolescent, their wide spectrum, and their low cost.

II. STRUCTURE AND STRUCTURE-FUNCTION RELATIONSHIPS

The generally available tetracyclines and their respective structures are shown in Table 1. The fundamental four-ring structure is essential to antimicrobial activity and is present in all currently available tetracyclines. Modification at positions other than 5, 6, and 7 generally diminishes or abolishes antimicrobial activity (2). The activity and the spectrum of side effects are generally similar for all of the tetracycline analogs with the exception of minocycline (see below). The newer tetracyclines, doxy- and minocycline, are more lipophilic and are excreted less rapidly than the older analogs.

All of the older tetracyclines suffer from poor solubility. This has resulted in the use of hydrochloride or sulfate salts for most clinical applications. In addition, chlortetra-

Table 1 Structure of the Tetracycline Antibiotics

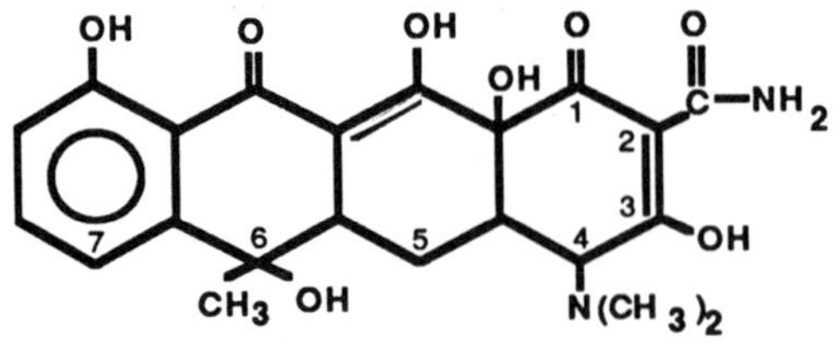

Congener	Substituent at position 5	6	7
Chlortetracycline			Cl
Oxytetracycline	OH,H		
Methacycline	OH,H	$=CH_2$	
Demeclocycline		OH,H	Cl
Doxycycline	OH,H	CH_3,H	
Minocycline		H,H	$N(CH_3)_2$

cycline is unstable in solution, particularly at neutral to alkaline pH (1). The solubility, stability, and low pH of these analogs has ceased to be of clinical significance because the intravenous forms of these drugs have been largely supplanted by newer tetracyclines or by alternative antibiotics.

The tetracycline antibiotics exert a reversible bacteriostatic effect in diverse species of bacteria via the inhibition of protein synthesis (2). The precise mechanism is currently a matter of debate, but a noncovalently mediated interference with the 30S subunit of the bacterial ribosome appears to result either in the direct failure of tRNA binding to the ribosome (3) or to inability of elongation factor Tu (required for tRNA binding) to interact appropriately with the ribosome (4). In either case, the further elongation of proteins currently undergoing synthesis is prohibited. The resistance of eukaryotic cells to tetracyclines is believed to be the result of structural differences in one or more components of the protein synthetic mechanism, since the drugs appear to freely enter mammalian cells and inhibit intracellular pathogens, such as *Chlamydia* and *Rickettsia*. The mechanism of action has recently been reviewed in great detail (2).

III. MICROBIAL SENSITIVITY AND RESISTANCE

The tetracyclines are truely broad-spectrum agents. Their in vitro spectrum, currently limited to some extent by the emergence of resistance, includes gram-positive cocci and bacilli, gram-negative diplococci, some gram-negative bacilli, *Mycoplasma, Chlamydia*, spirochetes, Rickettsiae, and atypical mycobacteria. Only the fungi are uniformly resistant to tetracyclines.

Mechanisms of resistance to tetracyclines have been extensively investigated, with a review by Chopra in 1985 (2). Only a brief summary of the extensive work in this field will be presented here, with emphasis on the clinically significant resistance patterns of particular organisms.

The first recognition of acquired resistance to tetracycline came in the early 1950s in studies of *Staphlococcus aureus* (5). Plasmid-mediated resistance has since been recognized in a variety of gram negative and gram positive organisms. These include *Bacillus* species, *Bacteroides, Campylobacter, Escherichia coli, Hemophilus influenzae, Pseudomonas aeruginosa, Proteus* species, *Providentia* species, *Salmonella, Shigella, Staphlococci, Streptococci* (including anaerobic strep), and *Vibrio cholerae* (2). The Enterobacteriaceae have been extensively studied (2), with documentation of at least five major plasmid types carrying multiple genes for tetracycline resistance on transposable elements. In addition to inducibility, these gene complexes are known to undergo amplification under selective pressure, resulting in an increased number of gene copies per plasmid (2) and/or an increased number of plasmids per organism (6).

Chromosomally mediated resistance, possibly due to incorporation of plasmid sequences into the genome, is also reported. This occurs in *E. coli* (7), *Bacillus subtilis* (8), *Neisseria gonorrhoeae* (9), and possibly *S. aureus* (2).

Studies on the ultimate location of these gene products indicate that membrane or cytoplasmic proteins are modified individually or in combination by the various plasmids. The precise mechanism by which these proteins result in resistance is unknown, but decreased accumulation of antibiotic has been demonstrated in resistant organisms as a result of decreased uptake (10), increased efflux (11,12), or a combination of these factors. A degree of ribosomal resistance may be present in some species as well (13) but does not appear to be the sole mechanism of resistance in any nonmycoplasmal species to date (12).

In vivo, bacterial resistance arises rapidly in humans (14-17) and animals (18,19) receiving tetracyclines. Long-term administration in animals results in the selection of organisms that are not only resistant but also possess growth characteristics that allow them to survive for prolonged periods in the absence of selective antibiotic pressure (19,20).

The antibiotic sensitivities of clinically relevant pathogens are shown in Table 2. Other pathogens that are generally considered susceptible to tetracycline include *Donovan's bacillus, Treponema pallidum, Borrelia* species, *Chlamydia, Rickettsia* (see Table 5), and *Francisella tularensis*. In vitro sensitivity studies are lacking for these organisms. Very little information has been obtained for agents other than tetracycline, minocycline, and doxycycline. In general, all the other agents are equivalent to tetracycline (21). For more extensive information, the reader should refer to the review by Atkinson (24).

A number of trends are observable in the susceptibility data. Most evident is the acquisition of resistance among previously sensitive species of gram-negative enteric bacilli. Significant resistance is also evident in streptococci and in multiply resistant staphylococci. This latter trend has been followed carefully in Great Britain and seems to parallel trends in tetracycline utilization (37-39). The emergence of clinically important resistance among *H. influenzae* and pneumococci was also noted in the 1970s (40,41). Resistance continues to be problematic, particularly among organisms responsible for nongonococcal urethritis (42-44), and the need for local or isolate specific sensitivities is becoming increasingly evident.

Another trend is the generally superior activity of minocycline against many organisms that have developed resistance to tetracycline, or even to doxycycline. These include methicillin-resistant staphlococci (23), *Propionibacterium* species (26), some gram-negative rods (21,22), *Legionella* (32), and *Hemophilus ducrei* (31). Unfortunately, this phenomenon is largely seen at concentrations in excess of those clinically attainable or is of too small a magnitude to be generally useful, particularly in view of the high incidence of side effects seen with minocycline.

Table 2 Susceptibilities of Clinically Important Pathogens to Tetracycline Group Antibiotics

Organism	No.	Date	Tetracycline Range	Tetracycline MIC$_{50}$	Tetracycline MIC$_{90}$	Doxycycline Range	Doxycycline MIC$_{50}$	Doxycycline MIC$_{90}$	Minocycline Range	Minocycline MIC$_{50}$	Minocycline MIC$_{90}$	Reference
Gram-positive cocci												
Hemolytic streptococci	13	1951				Chlortetracycline: range, 0.25–1.0						5
Streptococci group A	63	1968	0.19–0.50	0.78		0.09–25	0.39		0.09–25	0.39		21[a]
S. pyogenes		1978	1.6–>100	3.19		0.39–>100	1.6		0.39–12.5	0.78		22
S. viridans spp.		1951				Chlortetracycline: range, 0.2–10						5
		1968	3.9–100	3.1		0.09–50	0.39		0.09–50	0.39		21[a]
Nonhemolytic streptococci	23	1951				Chlortetracycline: range, 0.2–2.5						5
Streptococci group B	12	1968	1.6–50	1.6		0.78–25	0.78		0.39–100	0.39		21[a,b]
Streptococci group C	3	1968	6.3–12.5	6.3		0.78–1.6	1.6		0.39–0.78	0.78		21[a]
Streptococci group D	3	1968	1.6	1.6		0.78	0.78		0.39–0.78	0.78		21[a]
S. faecalis	5	1951				Chlortetracycline: range, 2–50						5
	36	1968	6.3–>100	>100		1.6–>100	50		1.6–>100	100		21[a]
S. pneumoniae		1951				Chlortetracycline: range, 0.5–1						5
	35	1968	0.19–3.1			0.04–0.39	0.19		0.04–0.78	0.09		21
		1978	0.2–100	0.8		0.1–12	0.2		0.1–25	0.2		22
Staphylococcus aureus	67	1951				Chlortetracycline: range, 0.07–10						5
	56	1968	1.6–>100	3.1		0.39–>100	1.6		0.39–12.5	0.78		21[a]
Methicillin resistant	13	1974	Resistant			Resistant				2	4	23[c]
Methicillin sensitive	13	1974		0.5	>10			2.0			0.5	23[c]
Penicillin resistant	169	1975		84% Sensitive (<4)						84% Sensitive (<2)		28[c]
Gram-positive bacilli												
Bacillus cereus		1968	0.78	0.78		0.19–0.39	0.39		0.19–0.78	0.19		21[a]

B. anthracis			0.12–5									24
Corynebacterium diphtheriae	14	1971	0.4–0.8		0.8							24
	133	1982		86% Resistant at 32								25[d]
Lactobacillus spp.	21	1975		1.6	25		1.2	8.4		0.33	—	26
Lysteria monocytogenes	10	1978	0.25–1									24
Propionibacterium spp.	75	1975		0.9	25		0.3	6.2		<0.16	2.5	26
Gram negative, enteric												
Campylobacter jejuni		1983				<0.5–32	<0.5	8				27
Enterobacter spp.	7	1975							1 of 7 sensitive			28
Enterobacter aerogenes		1968	6.3–50	25		12.5–25	25		6.3–12.5	12.5		21[a]
E. cloacae		1968		>500			>500			>500		21[a]
Escherichia coli	40	1951				Chlortetracycline: range, 1.0–25						5
	48	1968	3.1–500	12.5		1.6–500	12.5		3.1–500	6.3		21[a]
	126	1975							28 of 126 sensitive			28
E. coli, enterotoxigenic		1983				0.5–32	2	32				27
Klebsiella		1968	6.3–500	50		6.3–300	50		3.1–500	25		21[a]
Proteus spp.	57	1951				Chlortetracycline: range, 2–200						5
Proteus mirabilis	34	1968		>100			>100			>100		21[a]
Proteus spp.	124	1975							8 of 124 sensitive			28
Providentia spp.	3	1968		>100			>100			>100		21[a]
Pseudomonas aeruginosa	21	1951				Chlortetracycline: range, 20–250						5
	15			200			300			100		21[a]
Pseudomonas pseudomallei	64		0.8–12	<1.6	>3.1							24
Salmonella typhosa		1951				Chlortetracycline: range, 1–6						5
Salmonella spp.		1983				0.5–64	2	64				27

Table 2 (Continued)

Organism	No.	Date	Tetracycline Range	Tetracycline MIC_{50}	Tetracycline MIC_{90}	Doxycycline Range	Doxycycline MIC_{50}	Doxycycline MIC_{90}	Minocycline Range	Minocycline MIC_{50}	Minocycline MIC_{90}	Reference
Serratia spp.	4	1968		200			200			25		21[a]
Shigella			1.6–>500	100		1.6–500	100		1.6–500	100		22
		1983				0.5–32	4	16				27
Yersinia enterocolitica	14	1983				0.5–2	<0.5	<0.5				27
Y. pestis			0.2–0.5									24
Vibrio cholerae	14	1977	0.1–1.4		<1.4							24
V. parahemolyticus	9	1983				<0.5	<0.5	<0.5				27
Gram negative, nonenteric												
Brucella melitensis	98	1982	<0.05	<0.05	<0.05							29
Hemophilus influenzae	15	1968	3.1–12.5	6.3		1.6–6.3	1.6		1.6–6.3	3.1		21[a]
			0.8–3.1	1.6		0.8–3.1	1.6		0.8–3.1	1.6		22
	21	1978	0.13–32		1.0							24
Hemophilus spp. (respiratory)		1975		0.5	12					0.22	<2	30
Hemophilus ducrei		1982	0.25–32	8	16	0.12–8	1	4	0.008–4	0.5	2	31
Legionella pneumophilia		1980		>16	>16		4	8		2	4	32
Neisseria gonorrhoeae		1951				Chlortetracycline; range, 0.25–1						5
	25	1968	0.39–6.3	0.78		0.09–3.1	0.39		0.19–3.1	0.39		21[a]

		1982		0.10	0.25		0.06	0.22	0.02	0.11		33
N. meningitidis			0.3–3.1	0.8		0.8–6	1.6		0.8–1.6	1.6		22
Anaerobic organisms												
Aerobacter aerogenes	21	1951				Chlortetracycline: range, 1–50						5
Bacteroides spp.	176			9	>25		3	>10		2.5	10	26
Clostridium perfringes	17					Chlortetracycline: range, 1–50						5
Clostridium spp.	29	1975		6.25	>25		0.62	>10		0.38		26
Fusobacterium spp.	19	1975		0.8	9		0.6	<10		<0.16	<10	26
Peptostreptococcus spp	119	1975		1.8	>25		0.62	10		0.27	7	26
Miscellaneous organisms												
Chlamydia spp			0.5–4	2		0.5–4			0.5–4			22
Mycoplasma pneumoniae			1.6–3.1	1.6		1.6	1.6		1.6	1.6		22
Ureaplasma urealyticum	52	1984							0.125–32	0.25	16	34
Mycobacterium cheloniae		1982	1–>64	2	16	0.5–>64	0.5	32	0.5–>64	0.5	16	35[e]
M. fortuitum		1982	4–16	8	16	0.5–32	8	32	0.5–16	4	16	35[e]
M. marinum	19	1981	1–16	4	16	1–4	2	4	1–8	4	4	36
Actinomyces spp.	74	1976	0.25–8		1.0							24

[a]Reference includes data for chlor-, demeclo-, oxy-, and methacycline.
[b]MIC for six sensitive strains only.
[c]Data derived from graphs.
[d]Local endemic resistance.
[e]Broth method. Plate method varies significantly.

IV. PHARMACOKINETICS

The pharmacokinetic data for the tetracyclines are, at best, incomplete. Many of the available data were obtained using biologic assays for activity, with subsequent correction to serum concentration. Data regarding protein binding are particularly variable because of the marked dependency of these measurements on sample handling and analysis techniques. Nonetheless, the data are sufficiently complete to allow some useful generalizations and to permit rational dosing. Pharmacokinetic data for the clinically useful tetracyclines are shown in Table 3. Except as noted below, all this information is derived from adults.

A. Absorption

The bioavailability of tetracyclines varies with the individual analog and with the conditions under which absorption takes place. The location of absorption is probably the duodenum and proximal ileum (45). The bioavailability of the older tetracyclines is in the range of 60–90%. Food has a marked effect on tetracycline itself and a lesser effect on the other analogs. Doxycycline and minocycline are better than 90% absorbed, with minimal food effects. Iron interferes markedly with the absorption of all tetracyclines, but calcium salts diminish the absorption of only the older analogs. When administered with milk, doxycycline and minocycline have a 20–30% reduction in bioavailability, in contrast to the 65% reduction reported with tetracycline (51).

Time to peak concentration is 1–3 hr for all the tetracyclines (45,46). The older tetracyclines generally have peak concentrations of 2–4 μg/ml and trough levels of 1–2 μg/ml when given in the usual oral therapeutic doses. With intravenous dosing, peak levels are of the order of 6–10 μg/ml. Doxycycline and minocycline levels are about half those of older tetracyclines, but these analogs are correspondingly more active.

Plasma time-concentration curves tend to be broadened by enterohepatic recirculation or by other mechanisms so that sharp peaks and strictly linear decay are rarely seen with oral dosing. Depending upon the analog used, 20–80% of a given dose may be found in the feces. Because of biliary excretion, high fecal recovery does not necessarily reflect poor absorption.

There are no adequate absorption data in children. Minocycline may be less well adsorbed in 8- to 12-year-old ill children than in adults (52), but the data are not sufficient to distinguish alterations in absorption from alterations in distribution and excretion.

B. Protein Binding

Protein binding data for the various tetracycline derivatives are shown in Table 3. Binding varies from 20 to 95% for the various analogs, with doxycycline and minocycline the most avidly bound. These protein binding effects are not of major clinical importance, but variations in protein binding probably account for some of the differences in urinary recovery. Hypoalbuminemia may result in an apparent lowering of serum concentrations for highly bound analogs. This does complicate measurement, but it should be noted that the concentration of free antibiotic in the blood will be unaffected by protein binding at steady state.

Table 3 Pharmacokinetics of the Tetracycline Antibiotics

Drug	Bioavailability (%)	Effect of[a]			Protein binding (%)	Half-life (hr)	Urinary excretion (%)	Adult dose (46)		Pediatric dose, PO (46)
		Food	Ca	Fe				PO	IV	
Tetracycline	77 (22)	++	++	++	55–60 (22) 24–31 (45)	6–10 (46,47)	60 (49)	250–500 mg every 6 hr	500 mg every 6 hr	6–12 mg/kg every 6 hr
Chlortetracycline	30–40 (46)				48–70 (45)	6–9 (46)	15 (46)	250–500 mg every 6 hr	500 mg every 6 hr	6–12 mg/kg every 6 hr
Oxytetracycline	58 (22)	+	++	++	25–35 (22) 20–30 (45)	6–9 (46)	40 (46)	250–500 mg every 6 hr	500 mg every 6 hr	6–12 mg/kg every 6 hr
Methacycline	95 (22)					10–16 (46,47)	40 (46) 52 (49) 18–38 (48)	300 mg every 12 hr	—	6 mg/kg every 12 hr
Demeclocycline	66 (22)	+	++	++	80–90 (22)	10–16 (46,47)	40 (46) 46 (49) 38–56 (48)	300 mg every 12 hr	—	6 mg/kg every 12 hr
Doxycycline	93 (22)	+/−	+	++	80–85 (22)	15–20 (46) 8–14 (47) 10–21 (50)	30 (46) 39 (49) 38–49 (48)	100 mg every 12 hr	100–200 mg every 12 hr	2 mg/kg every 12 hr
Minocycline	98 (22)	+/−	+	++	80–85 (22) 76 (48)	15–20 (46) 9 (48)	12 (49) 9 (48)	100 mg every 12 hr	100–200 mg every 12 hr	2 mg/kg every 12 hr

[a]Reduction in bioavailability: +/– = <20%, + = 20–30%, ++ = >30%.

C. Distribution

The tetracycline antibiotics distribute well into body tissues and fluids, with the notable exception of cerebrospinal fluid (CSF). Overall volumes of distribution are reported as 0.9-2 liters/kg (45).

Concentrations of drug in gastrointestinal tissue and appendix appear to be greater than in the serum, and hepatobiliary concentrations exceed the serum concentration for all the tetracyclines (48,53). Stool concentrations are, accordingly, quite high. Penetration into the prostate, ovary, uterus, and bladder is good (48). With doxycycline, prostatic fluid concentrations averaging 60% of serum levels can be rapidly attained (54). Epididymal concentrations in dogs are equivalent to those in serum (55). Renal tissue concentrations depend upon the analog chosen, but urinary concentrations are high for all tetracyclines. Doxycycline concentrations are satisfactory in kidney (22).

CSF penetration (with inflammation) is variable, being 10% of serum levels for tetracycline and oxytetracycline, 25% for doxycycline, and 15% for minocycline (22). Brain tissue and intraocular concentrations are, in contrast, quite good (48).

Sputum concentrations, even with minocycline or doxycycline, are only about 20% of serum concentrations (22,48), and equilibration with serum concentrations requires 48 hr (53,56). Salivary concentrations of minocycline are excellent, but other tetracyclines seem to enter saliva only poorly. Thyroid, breast, skin, and lymph node concentrations of tetracycline are also excellent.

D. Elimination

The elimination characteristics of the tetracyclines are outlined in Table 3. Elimination of an intravenous dose is usually described adequately by a linear (first-order) model. Half-life and renal excretion vary significantly among the analogs.

Tetracycline, chlortetracycline, and oxytetracycline have half-lives of 6-10 hr and are dosed on a 6-hr interval. Chlortetracycline is notable for having only 15% urinary recovery, being excreted into the bile unchanged and as metabolites. The nature of the metabolites has not been investigated in detail. Chlortetracycline can be administered without dosage adjustment in renal failure (57).

Methacycline and demeclocycline have half-lives of 10-16 hr and are dosed on a 12-hr interval. They are largely excreted unchanged into the urine, with over 90% of demeclocycline recovered over a 4-day interval (58).

Doxycycline and minocycline have half-lives ranging from 15 to 21 hr and are also dosed on a 12-hr interval. In spite of the high urinary recovery of doxycycline (35%) and minocycline (10%), neither of these antibiotics accumulates to a significant extent in renal failure (59-61). This is attributed to a compensatory increase in nonrenal clearance owing to increased hepatic metabolism, decreased enterohepatic recirculation, or some other unknown mechanism.

There has been only minimal investigation of tetracycline kinetics in childhood. Lymecycline, which is not currently in use, was investigated in newborn infants. As might be expected, the half-life was prolonged in newborns owing to decreased renal clearance. The volume of distribution was also smaller in infants (62), reflecting known differences in body composition. Minocycline kinetics was investigated in 8 to 12-year-old Asian Indian children with a variety of disease states and nutritional deficiencies (52). Overall serum concentrations were lower than expected. The data suggest that more rapid excretion and poor absorption may both play a role in this effect.

The above findings with minocycline probably cannot be entirely attributed to age. Studies of adults with poor nutritional status indicate an increased rate of elimination due to increased renal clearance, decreased volume of distribution, and reduced bioavailability (62).

In spite of the association of acute fatty liver of pregnancy with the use of tetracycline during gestation, the excretion rate and liver-plasma ratio in healthy pregnant women appear to be unchanged from those in nonpregnant female controls (64).

V. PREPARATIONS

The available preparations of tetracycline antibiotics are shown in Table 4. Intravenous preparations often contain additives, such as procaine or sodium metabisulfite, which are capable of producing significant side effects. Many of the oral preparations contain phosphate or other binders of divalent cations in an attempt to improve bioavailability.

Table 4 Commercially Available Tetracycline Preparations[a]

Tetracycline	Tablet, 250, 500 mg
	Capsule, 250, 500 mg
	Suspension, 125 mg in 5 ml
	IV, 250, 500 mg
	Also topical and ophthalmic
Chlortetracycline[b]	Capsule, 50, 100, 250 mg
	Suspension, 125 mg in 5 ml
	IV, 500 mg
	Also topical and ophthalmic
Oxytetracycline	Tablet, 250 mg
	Capsule, 250 mg
	Suspension, 125 mg in 5 ml
	IV, 500 mg
	Also topical, ophthalmic, vaginal
Methacycline	Capsule, 150, 300 mg
	Suspension, 75 mg in 5 ml
Demeclocycline	Tablet, 75, 150, 300 mg
	Suspension, 75 mg in 5 ml
Doxycycline	Capsule, 100 mg
	Suspension, 25 mg in 5 ml
	IV, 100 mg (as hyclate)
Minocycline	Capsule, 50, 100 mg
	Also topical

[a]Rolitetracycline is also available for intravenous use in Canada.
[b]Chlortetracycline only available in topical forms in North America.

Table 5 Clinical Indications for Tetracycline Antibiotics

Treatment of first choice[a]	Effective but alternative therapy is preferred
Pasturella tularensis (tularemia)	*Neisseria gonorrhoeae* (gonorrhea)
Brucellosis	*Streptococcus pneumoniae*
Pseudomonas pseudomallei (melioidosis)	*Bacillus anthracis* (anthrax)
Vibrio cholerae (cholera)	*Erysipelothrix insidiosa* (erysipelas)
Mycoplasma pneumoniae	*Escherichia*, some strains
Rickettsial infections	*Hemophilus influenzae* (respiratory infections)
Rocky Mountain spotted fever	*H. ducrei* (chancroid)
Murine typhus	*Pasturella pestis* (plague, with streptomycin)
Epidemic typhus	*Malleomyces mallei* (glanders)
Rickettsialpox	*Clostridium tetani*
Q fever	*C. welchii*
Borrelia (relapsing fever)	*Treponema pallidum* (syphilis)
Psitticosis	
Lymphogranuloma venereum	
Granuloma inguinale	
Inclusion conjunctivitis	
Nocardia asteroides (minocycline)	
Lyme disease (68)	
Atypical *Mycobacteria* (some strains)	
Miscellaneous clinical indications	
Prophylaxis for traveler's diarrhea (69)	
Chronic bronchitis (?) (70)	
Acne (topical or parenteral) (71–73)	
Pleural or pericardial sclerosis (74)	
Inappropriate antidiuretic hormone secretion (demeclocycline) (75)	

[a]Not recommended in children under 8 years owing to risk of tooth discloration or deformity.

VI. DRUG ASSAYS

Serum concentration measurements have not assumed great importance in the current use of tetracyclines. Assay systems for tetracyclines include biologic, chromatographic, and fluorometric techniques. Biologic assays are performed for the occasional clinical application (65). A sensitivity of 1 μg/ml is possible with serum samples of 200 μl or less. When determining the sensitivity of slowly growing organisms, such as *Mycobacteria*, it should be recognized that tetracyclines undergo significant spontaneous degradation when assay times exceed 24 hr (36).

Highly sensitive high-pressure liquid chromatographic assays are available but are complicated by difficulty in extraction, drug instability, and the need for special chromatographic media (66). Fluorescent assays, which take advantage of the fluorescence so characteristic of this group of drugs, can provide exquisite sensitivity on serum or tissue samples. Sample sizes for these methods are also usually 200 μl or less, but the infrequent need for serum concentrations and the complexity of these assays has relegated them to use in clinical research.

VII. THERAPEUTIC INDICATIONS

The therapeutic indications for tetracycline antibiotics are listed in Table 5. As noted, many of these indications are not pertinent in the child less than 8 years of age because of the risk of dental damage. Additional infections, such as diphtheria, are often treated with tetracycline in underdeveloped nations because of the ready availability and low cost of the drug. In developed nations, tetracyclines see their greatest use in the treatment of chronic bronchitis, acne, and sexually transmitted diseases.

VIII. ADVERSE REACTIONS

A. Allergic and Immunologic

Anaphylactic reactions to tetracyclines appear to be extremely rare, and lesser acute allergic reactions,such as exanthems, occur infrequently (76). Other immunologically mediated sequelae include isolated cases of systemic lupus following degraded tetracycline (77), asthma in a tetracycline worker (78), pulmonary infiltrates with eosinophilia (PIE syndrome) due to tetracycline (79) and minocycline (80), and immune hemolytic anemia due to tetracycline (81).

B. Gastrointestinal

Patients receiving tetracyclines frequently complain of dose-related nausea, dyspepsia, and vomiting (76). The incidence of significant gastric complaints ranges from 15 to 50% (76,82,83), with vomiting in 2-3% of cases. Frank esophageal ulceration or gastritis may occur (84). These effects appear to be due to the direct corrosive action of tetracyclines. Adhesion of a capsule or tablet directly to mucosal surfaces may contribute to local corrosive effects. This has been studied in the cat, in which lymecycline appears to have less corrosive effect than doxycycline or oxytetracycline (84).

Fatty degeneration of the liver is seen in animals and humans receiving large doses of parenteral tetracycline, chlortetracycline, and oxytetracycline. Frank liver failure with jaundice, associated azotemia, encephalopathy, and death may occur (85). Intravenous doses of 2 g/day or more are generally required to induce hepatic changes in adults

(85–88). Early in the clinical use of tetracyclines, it became evident that tetracycline use during pregnancy was associated with an increased risk of fatty degeneration. Unfortunately, the pathophysiology of fatty liver of pregnancy has not been elucidated and the role of tetracyclines in precipitating or exacerbating this condition remains unclear. Many of the reported cases have initially suffered from pre-eclampsia or pyelonephritis. Renal compromise, with retention of tetracycline, may have contributed to the pathophysiology in these cases. At least one patient had typical hepatic findings on autopsy without a recent course of tetracyclines but with positive bone fluorescence, leading to the speculation that sequestered tetracycline in bone or other tissues may lead to fatty degeneration due to increased calcium mobilization during pregnancy (85).

Isolated pancreatitis has been reported following tetracycline therapy by mouth (89). Acute fatty liver is frequently associated with pancreatic changes ranging from mild elevations of amylase to frank necrotic pancreatitis (85–87).

C. Dental and Skeletal

The occurrence of irreversible dental discloration and enamel dysplasia following intrauterine or childhood exposure to tetracyclines has severely limited the use of these antibiotics in pediatrics. By age 8, the anterior teeth are usually calcified to the extent that cosmetic effects following tetracycline are not noticeable (90). Intravenous therapy during gestation or in the immediate perinatal period will often result in cosmetically unacceptable outcomes. Severely affected infants (deep pigmentation) represented 46% of 50 tetracycline-exposed infants studied by Wallman and Hilton (91), and many of these infants had enamel dysplasia and tooth deformity. This effect was dose related, and oxytetracycline appeared to produce a lower frequency (1 of 8) and severity of pigmentation.

Outside the perinatal period there is a dose-related darkening of teeth in children receiving tetracycline or demeclocycline (90). Although the average discoloration resulting from a single course of therapy was imperceptible, a few children suffered unacceptable cosmetic effects following a single course of therapy. There was no enamel hypoplasia noted in these children, most of whom had undergone multiple courses of therapy. Doxycycline given intravenously during the perinatal period to 25 children resulted in mild pigmentation without dysplasia in one infant (92). In contrast, minocycline has recently been reported to cause irreversible adult-onset distal tooth staining (93). Deposi- of an iron-minocycline complex is thought to be responsible for this effect, which is not reported with other tetracyclines. Many months of exposure are usually required to produce this effect, but it has resulted from a 4-week course of therapy.

The dental outcome following tetracycline exposure in childhood clearly depends upon dose, timing, route of administration, and the specific tetracycline analog chosen. It seems highly unlikely that a single course of doxycycline given after the perinatal period would result in significant dental effects. Doxycycline may prove to be the drug of choice for a limited number of rickettsial or borrileal infections in childhood because of the risks associated with chloramphenicol, but efficacy studies are lacking.

Effects on bone growth have been documented in premature infants, in whom fibular growth rate is retarded during therapy with tetracycline (94). Growth rate returns to normal following therapy. No effect on bone physiology has been documented in the older child or adult.

D. Nervous System

The most disturbing nervous system toxicity associated with tetracyclines is the development of increased intracranial pressure. This complication was first noted in infants (95, 96) and subsequently was recognized in adults (97). Bulging fontanelle, papilledema, headache, irritability, vomiting, and diplopia may occur. Cerebrospinal fluid chemistry and cytology generally remain normal, and the syndrome has resolved completely in all reported cases. The mechanism of this side effect, its absolute frequency, and the relative susceptibility of infants and children cannot be determined from the available literature.

Subjective weakness is occasionally reported with the older tetracyclines. Intravenous tetracycline causes increased weakness in myasthenia gravis and briefly potentiates curare-induced neuromuscular blockade, probably because of chelation of calcium (76). There is an isolated report of myopathy following 2 months of tetracycline therapy (98).

Minocycline seems to be unique in the high incidence of neurological complaints associated with its use for the prophylaxis of meningococcal carriers. Dizziness, true vertigo, nausea, vomiting, and weakness were common complaints within 3 days of onset of therapy. Significant neurovestibular toxicity was seen in 75-90% of subjects (82,83, 99). There is no clear relationship between the development of symptoms and either dose or serum concentrations (82). Symptoms generally resolve within 48 hr of discontinuing the drug (83). Because of these side effects, minocycline is no longer recommended for meningococcal prophylaxis.

E. Renal

Tetracyclines can produce acute nephrotoxicity when administered with methoxyflurane or in association with acute fatty liver. In addition, older tetracyclines have been reported to exacerbate renal failure in patients having chronic renal disease (100–102). In most cases this is limited to an increase in the blood urea nitrogen (BUN) concentration without concomitant changes in serum creatinine or in creatinine clearance. Rare patients have demonstrated a significant reversible loss of glomerular filtration associated with tetracycline (100) and demeclocycline (101). Minocycline, which does not accumulate in renal failure, nevertheless results in an increase in BUN. These isolated BUN changes are believed to be the result of antianabolic effects (i.e., increased urea load) rather than a true nephrotoxic effect (103). Doxycycline does not appear to result in renal dysfunction or to interfere with anabolic activity (104) and can be used with impunity in renal failure. Mild elevations in BUN have also been noted in patients receiving tetracyclines and diuretics concurrently (105).

Nephrogenic diabetes insipidus can be produced with demeclocycline (106) but not with the other tetracyclines. This effect has been useful in the treatment of patients having inappropriate secretion of antidiuretic hormone (75). Minocycline has been reported to cause interstitial nephritis (107). The consumption of degraded tetracycline is associated with the development of a reversible Fanconi syndrome with proteinuria, aminoaciduria, glycosuria, and renal potassium wasting. This may be associated with serious illness due to fluid and electrolyte imbalances (108). Experimentation in rats indicates that anhydro-4-epi-tetracycline, which forms spontaneously from tetracycline, is responsible for this phenomenon (109).

F. Dermatologic and Pigmentary Changes

Dermatologic complaints related to tetracyclines are largely limited to fixed drug eruptions and photosensitivity. Contact dermatitis has been reported (76). Fixed eruptions are rare, with 11 new cases reported in a review by Jolly et al. in 1978 (110). Photosensitivity, including photo-onycholysis, is not a major clinical problem with tetracycline therapy, but this may only reflect the limited sun exposure of many North Americans. Photosensitization probably can occur following any of the tetracyclines but is most commonly reported with demeclocycline (111). Doxycycline may be more phototoxic than minocycline (111). Photo-onycholysis, which may or may not be preceded by recognized photodermatitis and which may be months delayed in appearance, is reported with demeclocycline, doxycycline, and tetracycline (112).

Pigmentary changes following tetracycline therapy have been reported. Tissues other than skin, particularly the thyroid, may be affected (76). Minocycline seems to cause pigmentary changes more frequently than other tetracyclines, possibly because of its lipophilicity. Pigmentation of sites of skin inflammation (113), pigmented conjunctival cysts (114), and "black thyroid" (115,116) have been reported with minocycline. Thyroid function does not appear to be adversely affected.

G. Infectious and Immunosuppressive

Alterations of normal oral, gastrointestinal, and vaginal flora may occur with the use of tetracyclines. Although antibiotic-associated colitis has not been reported, the possibility should probably not be discounted entirely. Monilial infections of the female genital tract occur frequently, and oral candidiasis sometimes occurs following therapy with tetracyclines (76).

Doxycycline, minocycline, and demeclocycline have been shown to interfere with the in vitro oxidative burst metabolism of human polymorphonuclear leukocytes (117). Photoactivation enhances this effect (118). The more lipophilic tetracyclines (doxy-, mino-, demeclo-, and methacycline) also appear to suppress in vitro mitogen responsiveness (119). The clinical significance of these observations is unknown.

H. Carcinogenesis and Teratogenicity

No carcinogenic effect has been attributed to the tetracyclines. Teratogenic associations with tetracyclines, other than bone and tooth effects, are rare and have not been investigated sufficiently to establish a causal relationship (120).

IX. CONTRAINDICATIONS

The absolute contraindications to tetracyclines include pregnancy or lactation, age less than 8 years, and known hypersensitivity to tetracyclines (46). The contraindication in pregnancy reflects the hazards of dental malformation in the fetus as well as the risk of maternal hepatic dysfunction. It has been argued that, in children, the benefit of short courses of tetracyclines may outweigh the risk of tooth staining and the hazards of chloramphenicol in rickettsial disorders or in Lyme arthritis, but these issues remain to be resolved. Severe renal failure is a contraindication to tetracyclines other than chlortetracycline, doxycycline, and possibly minocycline (57,59-61). All tetracyclines should be used with caution in hepatic disease. Although minocycline has been shown not to accumulate in hepatic failure (121), experience is limited.

The need for bactericidal activity, as in endocarditis, is a relative contraindication to tetracyclines. Bacteriostatic agents in general may interfere with the activity of bactericidal agents, and tetracycline has been shown clinically to interfere with the response to penicillin in meningococcal carrier states (122).

X. DRUG INTERACTIONS

Pharmacokinetic and pharmacodynamic interactions with tetracyclines have been demonstrated. The absorption of tetracycline group antibiotics is substantially reduced in the presence of calcium, magnesium, or aluminum. Antacid or cathartic preparations containing these ions have been shown to chelate tetracyclines in vitro (123–125) and to decrease the bioavailability in vivo (126–129). Exogenous calcium sources, such as milk, have also been shown to inhibit absorption (127,130). In addition, antacids may interfere with capsule dissolution (131).

Ferrous sulfate interferes with the bioavailability of tetracyclines (132), including doxycycline and minocycline (130). The interference was eliminated by administration of the iron more than 3 hr prior to or 2 hr after the administration of tetracyclines (133). Similarly, bismuth subsalicylate (Pepto-bismol) reduces the availability of doxycycline by 50% when given 2 hr before, but not 2 hr after, a doxycycline dose (134). Copper, nickel, cobalt, zinc, and manganese also complex in vitro with tetracyclines (125), but in vivo investigations of bioavailability are lacking.

The use of excipients that precipitate metal ions, such as citrate or phosphate, produces a statistically significant improvement in bioavailability in a number of preparations, but this effect is probably not of clinical significance (135).

Several anticonvulsants appear to enhance doxycycline excretion. Phenobarbital reduced the mean half-life to 11.1 hr (control, 15.3 hr) (136), carbamazepine to 8.4 hr, and phenytoin to 7.2 hr (137) in adult volunteers. Therapeutic failure on the basis of this interaction has not been documented, but adjustment of doxycycline dose and interval may be needed when patients are receiving these medications. It is tempting to speculate that this interaction is the result of induction of the cytochrome P_{450} system. However, cimetidine (an inhibitor of P_{450} activity) does not influence the elimination of tetracycline (129). This may reflect the lesser contribution of hepatic metabolism to the elimination of tetracycline or the presence of multiple cytochromes.

Pharmacodynamic interaction between chlortetracycline and penicillin, with antagonism of clinical response to the bactericidal effects of penicillin, has been demonstrated in military recruits treated for pneumococcal meningitis (122).

Other interactions include the combination of methoxyflurane and tetracycline, which appears to be particularly nephrotoxic (138). Antibiotic-induced alterations in bowel flora can affect the bioavailability or disposition of many drugs. Although this has not been demonstrated with the tetracyclines, caution should be used when tetracyclines are coadministered with digoxin or with warfarin-related drugs (46).

REFERENCES

1. Garrod, PL, Lambert, HP, O'Grady, F: *Antibiotic and Chemotherapy*, E. & S. Livingstone, New York, 1981, pp. 169–182.
2. Chopra, I: Mode of action of the tetracyclines and the nature of bacterial resistance to them. In: *The Tetracyclines*, Handbook of Experimental Pharmacology, Vol. 78 (JJ Hlavka and JH Boothe, eds.), Springer-Verlag, New York, 1985.

3. Hognauer, G, Turnowsky, F: The effects of streptomycin and tetracycline on codon-anticodon interactions. *FEBS Lett. 26*:185–188, 1972.
4. Smythies, JR, Benington, F, Morin, RD: On the molecular mechanism of the action of the tetracyclines. *Experientia 28*:1253–1255, 1972.
5. Altmeier, WA, Culbertson, WR: Chloramphenicol (chloromycetin) and aureomycin in surgical infections. *JAMA 145*:449–457, 1951.
6. Nordstrom, K, Ingram, LC, Lundback, A: Mutations in R factors of *Escherichia coli* causing an increased number of R factor copies per chromosome. *J. Bacteriol. 110*: 562–569, 1972.
7. Chopra, I, Howe, TGB: Bacterial resistance to tetracyclines. *Microbiol. Rev. 42*: 707–724, 1978.
8. Williams, G, Smith, I: Chromosomal mutations causing resistance to tetracycline in *Bacillus subtilis. Mol. Gen. Genet. 177*:23–29, 1979.
9. Warner, PF, Zubrzycki, LJ, Chila, M: Polygenes and modifier genes for tetracycline and penicillin resistance in *Neisseria. J. Gen. Microbiol. 117*:103–110, 1980.
10. Young, TW, Hubball, SJ: R factor mediated resistance to tetracycline in *Escherichia coli* K-12. An R factor with a mutation to temperature sensitive tetracycline resistance. *Biochem. Biophys. Res. Commun. 70*:117–124, 1976.
11. Ball, PR, Shales, SW, Chopra, I: Plasmid mediated tetracycline resistance in *Escherichia coli* involves increased efflux of the antibiotic. *Biochem. Biophys. Res. Commun. 93*:74–81, 1980.
12. McMurry, I, Petrucci, RE, Levy, SB: Active efflux of tetracycline encoded by four genetically different tetracycline resistance determinants in escherichia coli. *Proc. Natl. Acad. Sci. USA 77*:3974–3977, 1980.
13. Chabbert, YA, Scavizzi, MR: Chelocardin-inducable resistance in *Escherichia coli* bearing R plasmids. *Antimicrob. Agents Chemother. 9*:36, 1976.
14. Datta, N, Faiers, MC, Reeves, DS, Brumfitt, W, Orskov, F, Orscov, I: R factors in *Escherichia coli* in faeces after oral chemotherapy in general practice. *Lancet 1*:312–315, 1975.
15. Guinee, PAM, Ungeuto, NR, Van Leeuwen, WJ: *Escherichia coli* with transferable resistance in patients treated with tetracycline for long periods of time. *Ned. Tijdschr. Geneesk. 115*:998–1000, 1971.
16. Hartley, CL, Richmond, MH: Antibiotic resistance and survival of *Escherichia coli* in the alimentary tract. *Br. Med. J. 4*:71–74, 1975.
17. Sompolinsky, D, Yaron, V, Alkan, WJ: Microbial changes in the human fecal flora following the administration of tetracyclines and chloramphenicol. *Am. J. Proctol. 18*:471–478, 1967.
18. Howe, K, Linton, AH, Osborne, AD: The effect of tetracycline on the coliform gut flora of broiler chickens with special reference to antibiotic resistance and O-serotypes of *Escherichia coli. J. Appl. Bacteriol. 41*:453–464, 1976.
19. Linton, AH, Howe, K, Osborne, AD: The effects of feeding tetracycline, nitrovin, and quindoxin on the drug resistance of coli aerogenes bacteria from calves and pigs. *J. Appl. Bacteriol. 38*:255–275, 1975.
20. Linton, AH, Handley, B, Osborne, AD: Fluctuations in *Escherichia coli* O-serotypes in pigs throughout life in the presence and absence of antibiotic treatment. *J. Appl. Bacteriol. 44*:285–298, 1978.
21. Steigbigel, NH, Reed, CW, Finland, M: Susceptibility of common pathogenic bacteria to seven tetracycline antibiotics. *Am. J. Med. Sci. 255*:179–195, 1968.
22. Neu, HC: A symposium on the tetracyclines: A major reappraisal. *Bull. N.Y. Acad. Med. 54*:141–155, 1978.
23. Minuth, JN, Holmes, TM, Musher, DM: Activity of tetracycline, doxycycline, and minocycline against methicillin susceptible and methicillin resistant staphylococci. *Antimicrob. Agents Chemother. 6*:411–414, 1974.

24. Atkinson, BA: Species incidence and trends of susceptibility to antibiotics in the United States and other countries. In: *Antibiotics in Laboratory Medicine* (V Lorian, ed.), Williams and Wilkins, Baltimore, 1986.
25. Rockhill, BC, Sumar, MD, Hadiputranto, H, Siregar, SP, Muslihun, B: Tetracycline resistance of *Corynebacterium diphtheriae* isolates from diphtheria patients in Jakarta, Indonesis. *Antimicrob. Agents Chemother. 21*:842–843, 1982.
26. Chow, AW, Patten, V, Guze, LB: Comparative susceptibility of anaerobic bacteria to minocycline, doxycycline, and tetracycline. *Antimicrob. Agents Chemother. 7*: 46–47, 1975.
27. Carlson, JR, Thornton, SA, Dupont, HL, West, AH, Mathewson, JJ: Comparative in vitro activity of ten antimicrobial agents against bacterial enteropathogens. *Antimicrob. Agents Chemother. 24*:509–513, 1983.
28. Candoza, C, Ellner, PD: Difference in susceptibility of enterobacteriaciae and penicillin resistant *Staphlococcus aureus* to tetracycline and minocycline. *Antimicrob. Agents Chemother.* 7:227–228, 1975.
29. Guttierres-Altes, A, Dias-Encisco, M, Penagarch, P, Campos-Bueno, A: In vitro activity of *n*-formidoyl thienamycin against 82 isolates of *brucella melitenses* compared with cefoxitin, rifampin, tetracycline, and co-trimoxazole. *Antimicrob. Agents Chemother. 21*:501–503, 1982.
30. Wood, MJ, Farrel, W, Kattan, S, Williams, JD: Activity of minocycline and tetracycline against respiratory pathogens related to blood levels. *J. Antimicrob. Chemother. 1*:323–331, 1975.
31. Bilgeri, YR, Ballard, RC, Duncan, MO, Mauff, AC, Koornhof, HJ: Antimicrobial susceptibility of 103 strains of *Hemophilus ducreyi* isolated in Johannesburg. *Antimicrob. Agents Chemother. 22*:686–688, 1982.
32. Edelstein, PH, Meyer, RD: Susceptibility of *Legionella pneumophila* to twenty antimicrobial agents. *Antimicrob. Agents Chemother. 18*:403–408, 1980.
33. Liebowitz, LD, Ballard, RC, Koornhof, HJ: In-vitro susceptibility and cross resistance of South African isolates of *Neisseria gonorrhoeae* to 14 antimicrobial agents. *Antimicrob. Agents Chemother. 22*:598–603, 1982.
34. Maghlhaes, M, Veras, A: Minocycline resistance among clinical isolates of Ureaplasma urealyticum. *J. Infect. Dis. 149*:117, 1984.
35. Swensen, JM, Thornsberry, C, Silcox, VA: Rapidly growing mycobacteria: Testing of susceptibility to 34 antimicrobial agents by broth dilution. *Antimicrob. Agents Chemother. 22*:186–192, 1982.
36. Wallace, RJ, Wiss, K: Susceptibility of *Mycobacterium marinum* to tetracyclines and aminoglycosides. *Antimicrob. Agents Chemother. 20*:610–612, 1981.
37. Dadswell, JV: Survey of the incidence of tetracycline resistant hemolytic streptococci between 1958 and 1965. *J. Clin. Pathol. 20*:641–642, 1967.
38. Rees, TA: Decline in frequency of isolation of tetracycline resistant beta-hemolytic streptococci from ear, nose, and throat 1967–71. *Lancet 1*:938–939, 1971.
39. White, AB, et al. (ad-hoc study group on antibiotic resistance): Tetracycline resistance in pneumococci and group A streptococci. *Br. Med. J. 1*:131–133, 1977.
40. Howard, AJ, Hince, CJ, Williams, JD, et al. (ad-hoc study group on antibiotic resistance): Antibiotic resistance in *Streptococcus pneumoniae* and *Hemophilus influenzae. Br. Med. J. 1*:1657–1660, 1978.
41. Hansman, D: *Haemophilus influenzae* type B resistant to tetracycline isolated from children with meningitis. *Lancet 2*:893–896, 1975.
42. Spaepen, MS, Knudsin, RB, Horne, HW: Tetracycline resistant T-mycoplasmas (Ureaplasma urealyticum) from patients with a history of reproductive failure. *Antimicrob. Agents Chemother. 9*:1012–1018, 1976.
43. Stimson, JB, Hale, KJ, Bowie, WR, Holmes, KK: Tetracycline resistant *Ureaplasma*

urealyticum: A cause of persistant nongonococcal urethritis. *Ann. Intern. Med. 94*: 192–194, 1981.

44. Maghlhaes, M, Veras, A: Minocycline resistance among clinical isolates of *Ureaplasma urealyticum*. *J. Infect. Dis. 149*:117, 1984.
45. Kunin, CM, Finland, M: Clinical pharmacology of the tetracycline antibiotics. *Clin. Pharmacol. Ther. 2*:51–69, 1961.
46. Bochner, F, Carruthers, G, Kampmann, J, Steiner, J: *Handbook of Clinical Pharmacology*, Little, Brown, Boston, 1983, pp. 383–386.
47. Doluisio, JT, Dittert, LW: Influence of repetitive dosing of tetracyclines on the biologic half life in serum. *Clin. Pharmacol. Ther. 10*:690–701, 1969.
48. MacDonald, H, Kelly, RG, Allen, ES, Nobel, JF, Kanegis, LA: Pharmacokinetic studies on minocycline in man. *Clin. Pharmacol. Ther. 14*:852–861, 1973.
49. Steigbigel, NH, Reed, GW, Finland, M: Absorption and excretion of five tetracycline analogs in young men. *Am. J. Med. Sci. 255*:296–312, 1968.
50. Rosenblatt, JE, Barrett, JE, Brodie, JL, Kirby, WMM: Comparison of in vitro activity and clinical pharmacology of doxycycline with other tetracyclines. In: *Antimicrobial Agents and Chemotherapy* (GL Hobby, ed.), American Society for Microbiology, Ann Arbor, Michigan, 1966, pp. 134–140.
51. Leyden, JJ: Absorption of minocycline hydrochloride and tetracycline hydrochloride. *J. Am. Acad. Dermatol. 12*:308–312, 1985.
52. Vasuki, K, Seth, V, Ghai, OP: Serum minocycline kinetics in children. *Indian J. Med. Res. 71*:764–767, 1980.
53. MacCulloch, D, Richardson, RA, Alwood, GK: The penetration of doxycycline, oxytetracycline, and minocycline into sputum. *N.Z. Med. J. 80*:300–302, 1974.
54. Oosterlink, W, Wallijn, E, Wjindaele, JJ: The concentration of doxycycline in human prostate gland and its role in the treatment of prostatitis. *Scand. J. Infect. Dis. (Suppl.) 9*:85–88, 1976.
55. Warner, JJ, Turner, BI, Alford, RH, Rhamy, RK: The clinical implications of epididymal levels of tetracycline. *Invest. Urol. 19*:92–93, 1981.
56. Ruhen, RW, Tandon, MK: Minocycline, doxycycline, and tetracycline levels in serum and bronchial secretions of patients with chronic bronchitis. *Pathology 7*: 193–197, 1975.
57. Kunin, CM, Rees, SB, Merril, JP, Finland, M: Persistence of antibiotics in blood of patients with acute renal failure, tetracycline and chlortetracycline. *J. Clin. Invest. 38*:1487–1491, 1959.
58. Sweeny, WM, Dornbush, AS, Hardy, SM: Antibiotic action in urine and feces after oral and intravenous administration of demethylchlortetracycline. *N. Engl. J. Med. 263*:620–624, 1960.
59. Alestig, K: Studies on doxycycline during IV and oral treatment with reference to renal function. *Scand. J. Infect. Dis. 5*:193–198, 1973.
60. Heany, D, Eknoyan, G: Minocycline and doxycycline kinetics in renal failure. *Clin. Pharmacol. Ther. 24*:233–239, 1978.
61. Sklenar, I, Spring, P, Dettli, L: One dose and multiple dose kinetics of minocycline in patients with renal disease. *Agents Actions 7*:369–377, 1977.
62. Serini, F, Perletti, L, Manfreidi, N, Marini, A: Tissue distribution and urinary excretion of a tetracycline derivative in newborn and older infants. *Pediatrics 67*:299–305, 1965.
63. Raghuram, TC, Krishnaswamy, K: Tetracycline kinetics in undernourished subjects. *Int. J. Clin. Pharmacol. Ther. Toxicol. 19*:409–413, 1981.
64. Whalley, PJ, Martin, FG, Adams, RH, Combes, B: Tetracycline disposition in normal pregnancy. *Obstet. Gynecol. 28*:103–110, 1966.
65. Edberg, SC: The measurement of antibiotics in human body fluids: Techniques and significance. In: *Antibiotics in Laboratory Medicine* (V Lorian, ed.), Williams and Wilkins, Baltimore, 1986.

66. Rouan, MC: Antibiotic monitoring in body fluids. *J. Chromatogr. 340*:361–400, 1985.
67. Ory, EM: The tetracyclines. In: *Antimicrobial Therapy* (BM Kagen, ed.), W. B. Saunders, Philadelphia, 1974, p. 99.
68. Steere, AC, Hutchinson, GJ, Rhan, DW, Sigal, LH, Craft, JE, DeSanna, ET, Malawista, SE: Treatment of the early manifestations of Lyme disease. *Ann. Intern. Med. 99*:22–26, 1983.
69. Freeman, LD, Hooper, DR, Lathen, DF, Nelson, DP, Harrison, WO, Anderson, DS: Brief prophylaxis with doxycycline for the prevention of traveller's diarrhea. *Gastroenterology 84*:276–280, 1983.
70. Nicotra, MB, Rivera, M, Awe, RJ: Antibiotic therapy of acute exacerbations of chronic bronchitis. *Ann. Intern. Med. 97*:18–21, 1982.
71. Hubble, CG, Hobbs, ER, Rist, MT, White, JW: Efficacy of minocycline compared with tetracycline in treatment of acne vulgaris. *Arch. Dermatol. 118*:989–992, 1982.
72. Poulos, ET, Tedesco, FJ: Acne vulgaris—double blind trial comparing tetracycline and clindamycin. *Arch. Dermatol. 112*:974–976, 1976.
73. Blaney, DJ, Cook, CH: Topical use of tetracycline in the treatment of acne. *Arch. Dermatol. 112*:971–973, 1976.
74. Zaloznik, AJ, Oswald, SG, Langin, M: Intrapleural tetracycline in malignant pleural effusions—a randomized study. *Cancer 51*:752–755, 1983.
75. Cherrill, DA, Stote, RM, Birge, JR, Singer, I: Demeclocycline treatment in the syndrome of inappropriate antidiuretic hormone secretion. *Ann. Intern. Med. 83*:654–656, 1975.
76. Hoigne, R, Keller, H, Sonntag, R: Penicillins, cephalosporins, and tetracyclines. In: *Meyler's Side Effects of Drugs*, 10th ed. (MNG Dukes, ed.), Elsevier, New York, 1984, pp. 446–491.
77. Sulkowski, SR, Haserick, JR: Simulated systemic lupus erythematosus from degraded tetracycline. *JAMA 189*:178–180, 1964.
78. Menon, MPS, Das, AK: Tetracycline asthma—a case report. *Clin. Allergy 7*:285–290, 1977.
79. Ho, D, Tashkin, DP, Bein, ME, Sharma, O: Pulmonary infiltrates with eosinophilia associated with tetracycline. *Chest 76*:33–36, 1979.
80. Otero, M, Goodpasture, HC: Pulmonary infiltrates and eosinophilia from minocycline. *JAMA 250*:2602, 1983.
81. Simpson, MB, Pryzbylik, J, Innis, B, Denham, MA: Hemolytic anemia after tetracycline therapy. *N. Engl. J. Med. 312*:840–842, 1985.
82. Gump, DW, Ashikaga, T, Fink, TJ, Radin, AM: Side effects of minocycline: Different dosage regimens. *Antimicrob. Agents Chemother. 12*:642–646, 1977.
83. Fanning, WL, Gump, DW: Distressing side effects of minocycline hydrochloride. *Arch. Intern. Med. 136*:761–762, 1976.
84. Carlborg, B, Densert, O, Lundqvist, C: Tetracycline induced esophageal ulcers. A clinical and experimental study. *Laryngoscope 93*:184–187, 1983.
85. Dowling, HF, Lepper, MH: Hepatic reactions to tetracycline. *JAMA 188*:307–309, 1964.
86. Wenk, RE, Gebhardt, FC, Bhagavan, BS, Lustgarten, JA, McCarthy, EF: Tetracycline associated fatty liver of pregnancy, including possible pregnancy risk with chronic dermatologic use of tetracycline. *J. Reprod. Med. 26*:135–141, 1981.
87. Kunelis, CT, Peters, JL, Edmondson, HA: Fatty liver of pregnancy and its relationship to tetracycline therapy. *Am. J. Med. 38*:359–377, 1965.
88. Peters, RL, Edmondson, HA, Mikkelsen, WP: Tetracycline induced fatty liver in non-pregnant patients. *Am. J. Surg. 113*:622–632, 1967.
89. Elmore, MF, Rogge, JD: Tetracycline-induced pancreatitis. *Gastroenterology 81*: 1134–1136, 1981.

90. Grossman, ER, Walcheck, A, Freedman, H: Tetracyclines and permanent teeth: The relation between dose and tooth color. *Pediatrics 17*:567–570, 1971.
91. Wallman, IS, Hilton, HB: Teeth pigmented by tetracycline. *Lancet 1*:827–829, 1962.
92. Forti, G, Benincori, C: Doxycycline and the teeth. *Lancet 1*:782, 1969.
93. Poliak, SC, Digiovanna, JJ, Gross, EG, Gantt, G, Peck, GL: Minocycline associated tooth discoloration in young adults. *JAMA 254*:2930–2933, 1985.
94. Cohlan, SQ, Bevelander, G, Tiamsic, T: Growth inhibition of prematures receiving tetracycline. *Am. J. Dis. Child. 105*:453–461, 1963.
95. Fields, JP: Bulging fontanel: A complication of tetracycline therapy in infants. *J. Pediatr. 58*:74–76, 1961.
96. Wilson, SGF, Dally, WJ: Meningeal irritation due to tetracycline administration. *Arch. Dis. Child. 41*:691–692, 1966.
97. Walters, BNJ, Gubbay, SS: Tetracycline and benign intracranial hypertension: Report of five cases. *Br. Med. J. 282*:19–20, 1981.
98. Sinclair, D, Phillips, C: Transient myopathy apparently due to tetracycline. *N. Engl. J. Med. 307*:821–822, 1983.
99. Drew, TH, Altman, R, Black, K, Goldfield, M: Minocycline for prophylaxis of infection with *Neisseria meningitides*: High rate of side effects in recipients. *J. Infect. Dis. 133*:194–198, 1976.
100. George, CRP, Evans, R: Tetracycline toxicity in renal failure. *Med. J. Aust. 1*: 1271–1273, 1971.
101. Miller, PD, Linas, SL, Schrier, RW: Plasma demeclocycline levels and nephrotoxicity. *JAMA 243*:2513–2518, 1980.
102. George, CRP, Guinness, MDG, Lark, DJ, Evans, RA: Minocycline toxicity in renal failure. *Med. J. Aust. 1*:640–641, 1973.
103. Shils, ME: Some metabolic aspects of tetracyclines. *Clin. Pharmacol. Ther. 3*: 321–339, 1962.
104. Stenbaek, O, Myhre, E, Berdal, BP: The effect of doxycycline on renal function in patients with advanced renal insufficiency. *Scand. J. Infect. Dis. 5*:199–202, 1973.
105. Boston Collaborative Drug Surveillance Program: Tetracycline and drug attributed rises in blood urea nitrogen. *JAMA 220*:377–379, 1972.
106. Castell, DO, Sparks, HA: Nephrogenic diabetes insipidus due to demethylchlortetracycline hydrochloride. *JAMA 193*:237–239, 1965.
107. Walker, RG, Thompson, NM, Dowling, JP, Ogg, CS: Minocycline-induced acute interstitial nephritis. *Br. Med. J. 1*:524, 1979.
108. Cleveland, WW, Adams, WC, Mann, JB, Nyhan, WL: Acquired Fanconi syndrome following degraded tetracycline. *J. Pediatr. 66*:333–342, 1965.
109. Lowe, MB, Tapp, E: Renal damage caused by anhydro-4-epi-tetracycline. *Arch. Pathol. 81*:362–364, 1966.
110. Jolly, HW, Sherman, IJ, Carpenter, CL, Nesbitt, LT, Meek, TJ: Fixed drug eruptions to tetracyclines. *Arch. Dermatol. 114*:1484–1485, 1978.
111. Frost, P, Weinstein, GD, Gomez, EC: Phototoxic potential of minocycline and doxycycline. *Arch. Dermatol. 105*:681–683, 1972.
112. Frank, SB, Cohen, HJ, Minkin, W: Photo-onycholysis due to tetracycline hydrochloride and doxycycline. *Arch. Dermatol. 103*:520–521, 1971.
113. Fenske, NA, Millns, JL, Greer, KE: Minocycline induced pigmentation at sites of cutaneous inflamation. *JAMA 244*:1103–1105, 1980.
114. Messmer, E, Font, RL, Sheldon, G, Murphy, D: Pigmented conjunctival cysts following tetracycline/minocycline therapy. *Opthalmology (Rochester) 90*:1462–1468, 1983.
115. Billano, RA, Ward, WQ, Little, WP: Minocycline and black thyroid. *JAMA 249*: 1887, 1983.
116. Madeiros, LJ, Federman, M, Silverman, ML, Balogh, K: Black thyroid associated with minocycline therapy. *Arch. Pathol. Lab. Med. 108*:268–269, 1984.

117. Glette, J, Sandberg, S, Hopen, G. Solberg, CO: Influence of tetracycline on human polymorphonuclear leukocyte function. *Antimicrob. Agents Chemother. 25*:354-357, 1984.
118. Glette, J, Sandberg, S, Haneberg, B, Solberg, CO: Effect of tetracyclines and UV light on oxygen consumption by human leukocytes. *Antimicrob. Agents Chemother. 26*:489-492, 1984.
119. Potts, RC, MacConnachie, A, Brown, RA, Gibbs, JH, Robertson, AJ, Hassan, HAA, Swanson Beck, J: Some tetracycline drugs suppress mitogen-stimulated lymphocyte growth but others do not. *Br. J. Clin. Pharmacol. 16*:127-132, 1983.
120. Briggs, GG, Bodendorfer, TW, Freeman, RK, Yaffe, SJ: *Drugs in Pregnancy and Lactation*. Williams and Wilkins, Baltimore, 1983, pp. 344-348.
121. Devine, LF, Johnson, DP, Hageman, CR, Pierce, WE, Rhode, SL, Pekinpaugh, RO: The effect of minocycline on meningococcal nasopharyngeal carrier state in Naval personnel. *Am J. Epidemiol. 93*:337-345, 1971.
122. Lepper, MH, Dowling, HF: Treatment of pneumococcal meningitis with penicillin compared to penicillin and aureomycin. *AMA Arch. Intern. Med. 88*:489-494, 1951.
123. Lambs, L, Brion, M, Berthon, G: Metal ion-tetracycline interactions in biological fluids. Part 3. Formation of mixed metal ternary complexes of tetracycline, doxycycline, and minocycline with calcium and magnesium, and their involvement in the bioavailability of these antibiotics in blood plasma. *Agents Actions 14*:743-749, 1984.
124. Price, KE, Zolli, Z, Atkinson, JC, Luther, HG: Antibiotic inhibitors. Part II. Studies on the inhibitory actions of selected divalent cations for tetracycline. *Antibiot. Chemother. 7*:689, 1957.
125. Albert, A, Rees, CW: Avidity of the tetracyclines for the cations of metals. *Nature (Lond.) 177*:433-434, 1956.
126. Sweeny, WM, Hardy, SM, Dornbush, AC, Ruegger, JM: Absorption of tetracycline in human beings affected by certain excipients. *Antibiot. Med. 4*:642-656, 1957.
127. Price, KE, Zolli, Z, Atkinson, JC, Luther, HG: ANtibiotic inhibitors. I. The effect of certain milk constituents. *Antibiot. Chemother. 7*:672-688, 1957.
128. Harcourt, RS, Hamburger, M: The effect of magnesium sulfate in lowering tetracycline blood levels. *J. Lab. Clin. Med. 50*:464-468, 1957.
129. Garty, M, Hurwitz, A: Effect of cimetidine and antacids on gastrointestinal absorption of tetracyclines. *Clin. Pharmacol. Ther. 28*:203-207, 1980.
130. Leyden, JJ: Absorption of minocycline hydrochloride and tetracycline hydrochloride. Effect of food, milk, and iron. *J. Am. Acad. Dermatol. 12*:308-312, 1984.
131. Myazakis, Inoue, H, Nadai, T: Effect of antacids on the dissolution of minocycline and demethylchlortetracycline from capsules. *Pharmazie 36*:482-484, 1981.
132. Neuvonen, PJ, Gothoni, G, Hackman, R, Bjorksten, K: Interference of iron with the absorption of tetracyclines in man. *Br. Med. J. 4*:532-534, 1970.
133. Gothoni, G, Neuvonen, PJ, Mattila, M, Hackman, R: Iron-tetracycline interaction: Effect of time interval between doses. *Acta Med. Scand. 191*:409-411, 1972.
134. Ericson, CD, Feldman, S, Pickering, LK, Cleary, TG: Influence of subsalicylate bismuth on absorption of doxycycline. *JAMA 247*:2266-2267, 1982.
135. Kunin, CM, Finland, M: Clinical pharmacology of the tetracycline antibiotics. *Clin. Pharmacol. Ther. 2*:51-69, 1960.
136. Neuvonen, PJ, Pintilla, O: Interaction between doxycycline and barbiturates. *Br. Med. J. 1*:535-536, 1974.
137. Pentilla, O, Neuvonen, PJ, Aho, K, Lehtovaara, R: Interaction between doxycycline and some anti-epileptic drugs. *Br. Med. J. 2*:470-472, 1974.
138. Kuzoku, EY: Methoxyflurane, tetracyclines, and renal failure. *JAMA 211*:1162-1164, 1970.

16
Chloramphenicol

MICHAEL J. RIEDER
The Hospital for Sick Children, Toronto, Ontario, Canada

Chloramphenicol has enjoyed waning and waxing popularity since the time of its introduction into clinical practice and has been the stimulus for a great deal of debate, scholarly speculation, and rhetoric (1-6). The falling into and out of favor of the drug has coincided with the changing spectrum of microbial illness and our expanding knowledge of the action, kinetics, metabolism, and toxicity of the agent (7).

Chloramphenicol was first described by Ehrlich and co-workers in 1947 as an antibiotic secreted by *Streptomyces venezuela*, a soil bacterium found in mulched soil near Caracas, Venezula (8). In 1948, a similar organism taken from a compost heap in Illinois was found to produce the same agent (9). This drug was isolated and characterized by Bartz during that year and given the name *chloramphenicol* (10). This new antibiotic proved remarkably effective in treating an outbreak of typhus in Bolivia and Mexico (11, 12). Chloramphenicol was efficatious when used to treat patients initially diagnosed as having scrub typhus who were subsequently found to have typhoid fever (13,14). Chloramphenicol was found to have activity against gram-positive and gram-negative bacteria and *Rickettsia*, thus constituting the first truly "broad-spectrum" antibiotic. A method of synthetic preparation on an industrial scale was developed, and the antibiotic rapidly entered widespread clinical use (15,16).

Its synthetic mode of preparation made it inexpensive and plentiful; indeed, it is the only antibiotic prepared solely by chemical synthesis for commercial use. The drug was soon used extensively; however, the recognition of severe adverse effects, especially bone marrow suppression and the "gray baby" syndrome, led to a precipitous decline in the use of chloramphenicol (17-43).

Impetus to this decline was given by the development of alternate antibiotic agents, such as the semisynthetic penicillins (6). However, in 1974, reports of *Hemophilus influenzae* type b resistant to ampicillin began to appear in the literature (44-46). The increased incidence of disease caused by these strains led to the use of chloramphenicol as a first-line antibiotic in the treatment of presumptive bacterial meningitis in children, as well as in other cases of invasive *H. influenzae* disease (47). This has been facilitated by our burgeoning knowledge of the pharmacokinetics, metabolism, and therapeutic drug

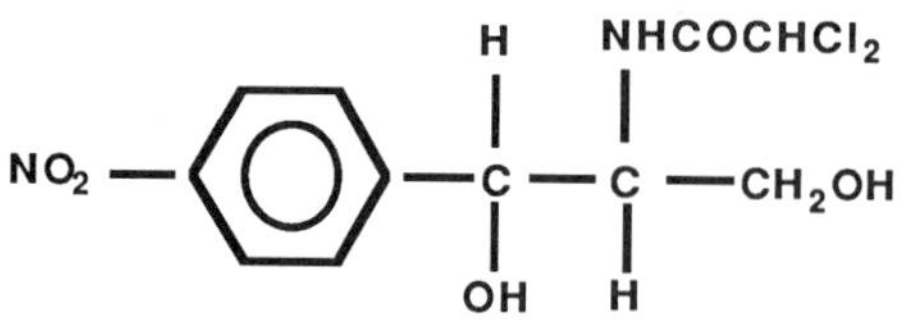

Figure 1 Chloramphenicol.

monitoring implications of chloramphenicol (6,7). The development of alternate agents for the therapy of invasive *Hemophilus* disease in recent years has led to a decline in the use of chloramphenicol (48,49).

I. CHEMISTRY

Chloramphenicol is a lipid-soluble compound that is composed of an aromatic nitro moiety with an alaphatic side chain (Figure 1) (50). The chemical structure is D (-)-threo-2-dichloracetamide-1-*p*-nitrophenyl-1,3-propanediol (15). This agent is very stable at room temperature if protected from light and will remain unchanged over a pH range from 0.4 to 9.5 is unaffected by boiling in water, is very soluble in ethanol (400 mg/ml), and is only slightly soluble in water (2-4 mg/ml) (10). The drug itself is a yellowish white powder with an extremely bitter taste. In water, the drug has a pH of 5.5.

Of the four isomers of chloramphenicol that have been synthesized, none is more active than natural chloramphenicol (51). A series of compounds in which the nitro group is reduced was synthesized in an attempt to lessen its toxicity; however, all were less active than chloramphenicol (51). One derivative of the basic structure is in clinical use in continental Europe; it is thiamphenicol, in which the nitro group at the para position of the aromatic ring is substituted with a sulfonylmethyl group (Figure 2) (52).

Investigators in the 1950s were able to increase the solubility of chloramphenicol by forming esters between chloramphenicol and palmitic acid or a succinate group at the 3-carbon position of the propanediol side chain (3,6). These esters are more water soluble than chloramphenicol itself; they are used to prepare chloramphenicol palmitate oral suspension and the intravenous preparation of chloramphenicol succinate. These esters are biologically inactive and must undergo in vivo hydrolysis to liberate active chloramphenicol (4-7,50,52,53).

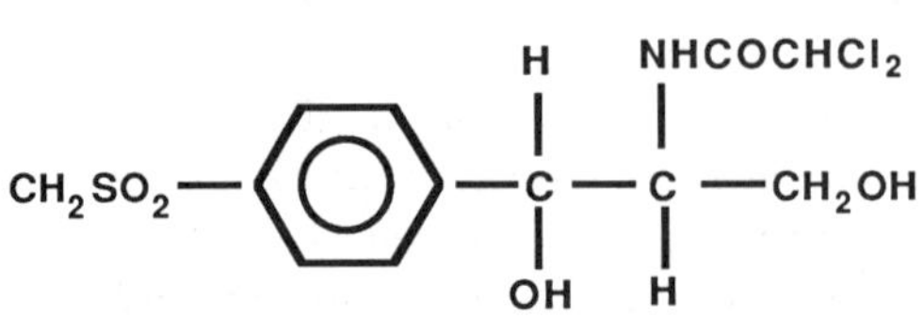

Figure 2 Thiamphenicol.

II. MECHANISM OF ACTION

Chloramphenicol acts by inhibition of protein synthesis in the bacterial ribosome (3,5,7). It has been shown to inhibit peptidyltransferase in the microorganism's 50S ribosome (54). Inhibition of this enzyme blocks polypeptide formation in the ribosomes without producing irreversible damage to the cell (55). The eukaryotic 70S ribosome in mitochondria is similar to the bacterial 50S ribosome; chloramphenicol has been shown to be capable of inhibiting mitochondrial protein synthesis in eukaryotic cells, including human cells (56).

This inhibition of protein synthesis is responsible for chloramphenicol's bacteriostatic action on most susceptible organisms (5). It is of importance to note that chloramphenicol is bacteriocidal in vitro against most strains of *H. influenzae, Streptococcus pneumoniae*, and *Neisseria meninigiditis* (57). Whether the mechanism of action is different from that displayed by chloramphenicol against other microbes is unknown (5). However, chloramphenicol has been shown to be concentrated in polymorphonuclear leukocytes, which may be important in in vivo killing of *H. influenzae* at the cellular level (58).

III. ANTIMICROBIAL ACTIVITY AND RESISTANCE

Chloramphenicol has a broad spectrum of antimicrobial activity (Table 1). It is active against all aerobic bacteria, with the exception of *Pseudomonas aeruginosa* and indole-positive *Proteus* species (5,7,50). However, many gram-negative organisms have wide variations in susceptibility within individual species (50,59).

Chloramphenicol will inhibit most anaerobes at a concentration of 20 μg/ml or less (60). It is active against *Rickettsia, Chlamydia*, certain mycoplasmas, and the mollusous phase of schistosomiasis (61-63). It is inactive against fungi, viruses, mycobacterium, and protozoa (45,62).

Bacterial resistance to chloramphenicol has classically occurred by the acquisition of an R plasmid that encodes for the enzyme chloramphenicol acetyltransferase (64). This enzyme, which requires acetylcoenzyme A as a substrate, acetylates the hydroxyl group on the aliphatic side chain (65). This has been found in gram-negative bacteria, including *H. influenzae*. It is linked to tetracycline resistance and may coexist on the plasmid with β-lactamase mediated ampicillin resistance (64-67). These have included both nonencapsulated and type b strains (50,67-72). Widespread use of chloramphenicol in the Far East has also lead to the development of strains of *Salmonella typhimurium* resistant to chloramphenicol, ampicillin, and trimethoprim-sulfamethoxazole (71). Although the determinant may be the same, it is known that the plasmid coding for resistance in *H. influenzae* is different from the plasmid coding for resistance in *S. typhimurium*.

Nonenzymatic mechanisms of resistance also exist. Decreased cellular permeability in *Escherichia coli* and *Pseudomonas* has been described (73). *E. coli* mutants with ribosomal insensitivity to chloramphenicol have been found, as well as *H. influenzae* isolates from sputum that demonstrate nonenzymatic resistance to chloramphenicol (50,74).

Thiamphenicol is less active than chloramphenicol against both gram-positive and gram-negative bacteria, giving it a very small therapeutic window for many common pathogens; the minimum inhibitory concentration (MIC) required for these organisms is

Table 1 Chloramphenicol Minimum Inhibitory Concentrations

Bacteria	MIC_{25}[a]	MIC_{50}	MIC_{75}	MIC_{95}
Gram-positive				
Staphylococcus aureus		5		12.5
S. epidermidis				3.2
Streptococcus pyogenes	3.2		6.3	
S. pneumoniae	2.1	2.4		3.8 (MIC_{90})
S. faecalis	2.5	100		
Streptococcus D (nonenterococcus)			1.9	7.8
Gram-negative				
Neisseria gonorrhoeae				<5
N. meningitidis			1	2
Brucella species	0.6		2.5	
Campylobacter fetus	0.81		1.6	3.1
Enterobacter species		5	20	
Escherichia coli		5	25	
Hemophilus ducrei	0.25		0.5	
H. influenzae		0.5		1
Klebsiella pneumoniae		5	10	
Legionella pneumophilia				0.5
Proteus species	5	10	20	
Proteus mirabilis		12		
P. vulgaris	0.8		3	
Pseudomonas species		<25		
Pseudomonas aeruginosa	<25 (MIC_{10})			
Salmonella species			5	10
Salmonella typhosa		3.1		
Serratia marcescens		32 (MIC_{40})		
Shigella species			10	
Shigella flexneri		0.8		1.6
Anaerobes				
Bacteroides species		3.1		12.5
Bacteroides fragilis			3.1	12.5
Clostridium perfingens				3.2
Clostridium species		1.6	3.1	
Mycoplasma pneumoniae			0.8	

[a]Percentage of strains inhibited at various μg/ml concentrations of chloramphenicol (59).

greater than the serum level at which hematopoiesis is inhibited in a dose-related fashion (51). An important exception to this is that thiamphenicol is as active against *Streptococcus pyogenes, H. influenzae, N. meningitidis,* and *S. pneumoniae* as chloramphenicol (51). There is complete cross-resistance with chloramphenicol via chloramphenicol acetyltransferase, albeit with the enzyme having a somewhat lower affinity for thiamphenicol than it does for chloramphenicol (51).

IV. CLINICAL PHARMACOLOGY

Chloramphenicol is an unusual drug in that the absorption and bioavailability of the active moiety may be better in most patients when the drug is given orally rather than by the intravenous route (50,74–77). The reasons for this are detailed in Figure 3. Chloramphenicol as administered to patients is available in three forms: crystalline chloramphenicol, an oral suspension of chloramphenicol palmitate, or an intravenous solution of chloramphenicol succinate (7,50). Crystalline chloramphenicol (the preparation used to manufacture chloramphenicol capsules) can be absorbed directly from the gastrointestinal tract, but chloramphenicol palmitate must first be hydrolyzed before active chloramphenicol can be absorbed (79). Similarly, the intravenous solution of chloramphenicol succintate must undergo hydrolysis so that free (and, thus, active) chloramphenicol can be liberated into the blood (6). Accordingly, it is best to consider the clinical pharmacology of these three preparations separately.

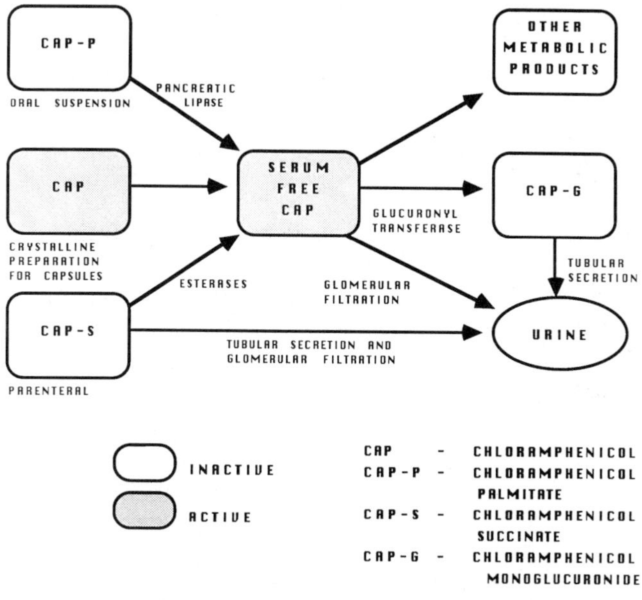

Figure 3 Metabolism of chloramphenicol. (Modified from Dajani and Kauffman, the renaissance of chloramphenicol, *Pediat. Clin. North Am. 28*:195, 1981.)

A. Crystalline Chloramphenicol

Crystalline chloramphenicol is absorbed unaltered from the gastrointestinal tract. The absorption of a poorly water soluble compound, such as chloramphenicol, is proportional to its dissolution, which in turn is affected by the size and aggregation of the primary particles (51). Preparations with large particles may have only a quarter of the bioavailability of preparations with smaller particles (80). Peak concentrations after an oral dose in adults are reached in 2-3 hr; with a 7 mg/kg dose, these reach 8-13 μg/ml, rising to 15-25 μg/ml with a 30-mg/kg dose (80). Absorption of fine particles of crystalline chloramphenicol from the gastrointestinal tract is virtually 100% (51). The usual desired serum concentration of serum free chloramphenicol is between 10 and 20 μg/ml. This is true regardless of the route by which chloramphenicol is given.

Approximately 53% of plasma chloramphenicol is bound to protein in healthy adults free of hepatic disease (81). Plasma protein binding has been found to be lower in patients with hepatic cirrhosis (42%) and in premature neonates (32%) (81). In keeping with its high lipid solubility, chloramphenicol is well distributed throughout the body. It achieves cerebrospinal fluid concentrations 50-60% of simultaneously determined serum concentrations (82). Concentrations in brain tissue can reach nine times that of a paired blood concentration (83). It also penetrates polymorphonuclear leukocytes, the kidney, liver, aqueous and vitreous humors, bile, pleural fluid, urine, stool, saliva, sputum, and across the placenta (5,84). It is present in breast milk (85). The concentrations present in many of these fluids, such as saliva, are too variable to be predictive of serum levels (84).

Only 13% of circulating chloramphenicol is excreted unchanged, 10% into the urine and 3% into the bile (86-88). The remainder of the drug is excreted after hepatic glucuronidation by the hepatic enzyme glucuronyltransferase (87). Glucuronic acid is conjugated with chloramphenicol at the primary alcohol on carbon 3 of the propanediol side chain. This is then secreted into the urine by the renal tubules (87). A small amount of chloramphenicol is metabolized into other metabolites, such as chloramphenicol base (this lacks the dichloroacetanide group) and a glycolic metabolite, in which the two chlorine atoms are replaced by a single hydroxyl group (89). This last metabolite is found primarily in neonates and retains some degree of antimicrobial activity (50,89). The metabolic pathways other than glucuronidation may be of some importance in the idiosyncratic toxicity of chloramphenicol, a point we will return to later (6).

An appreciation of hepatic chloramphenicol glucuronlytransferase is critical in understanding the tragedy of the "gray baby" syndrome (see Section VIII.B) that occurred in newborn nurseries in the late 1950s (90). When data from this event were analyzed, it became clear that the affected infants excreted much less chloramphenicol monoglucuronide than expected (91). Subsequently, it has been determined that glucuronyltransferase is present in small amounts prenatally. This activity rises rapidly postnatally, reaching adult levels in rats by day 10 of postnatal life (91). This is a separate pathway than that used to glucuronate bilirubin. This reduced ability to conjugate active (and, hence, potentially toxic) chloramphenicol to an inactive (and nontoxic) glucuronic conjugate put the neonate at high risk for the cardiovascular calamity referred to as the gray baby syndrome, a consequence of elevated serum concentrations of chloramphenicol. The half-life of crystalline chloramphenicol in adult volunteers is 2--5 hr (80). This is not significantly altered by renal failure but may be considerably prolonged in patients with hepatic disease (80,81). Although there is a general correlation between elevated serum bilirubin values and diminished clearance of chloramphenicol, there is wide interpatient variation. Attempts to directly relate the results of hepatic function tests with chloramphenicol metabolism in individual patients have been unsuccessful (81,93). Renal failure decreases the clearance of inactive metabolites of chloramphenicol as well as that of the prodrug chloramphenicol succinate.

B. Chloramphenicol Succinate

Chloramphenicol for intravenous use is prepared as a solution of chloramphenicol succinate. This is a biologically inactive prodrug that must be hydrolyzed to free chloramphenicol to be active. The lung and kidney contain esterases that can convert chloramphenicol succinate to free chloramphenicol. However, the majority of hydrolysis occurs in the liver, where hepatic esterase is the primary enzyme responsible for liberating chloramphenicol by ester hydrolysis (94). This enzyme has been shown to have considerably lower activity in fetuses and neonates than in older children and adults (94,95).

Table 2 details the results of pharmacokinetic investigations of chloramphenicol succinate. It has long been apparent that some patients have indeterminate half-lives while on intravenous therapy with chloramphenicol (82,95,101). This is the result of highly variable urinary loss of the prodrug by tubular secretion and variable rates of hydrolysis of the ester to yield the active drug (98–100). Thus, the loss of average quantities of 33% of prodrug significantly reduced the bioavailability of intravenous chloramphenicol versus oral chloramphenicol and even more so in certain patients, in whom up to 80% of the prodrug could be lost (6,50,77,78,98–100). The half-life of chloramphenicol succinate in adults is approximately 1 hr, but it can vary from 20 min to 3 hr in infants and toddlers. After hydrolysis, the chloramphenicol is dealt with by the metabolic pathways described above. Table 3 details the studies available to date. The half-life is approximately 1½ hr in adults, but it may be longer in younger patients, especially premature infants (50,95). There is also very wide interpatient variability in half-life, with up to a 20-fold difference noted in some studies (82). Prolongation of the half-life from 10 to 36 hr has been demonstrated in low-birth-weight and premature infants (95,104). There is no significant difference in volume of distribution between infants and older children (50). Rajchgot and his co-workers have studied the use of a loading dose of chloramphenicol in newborns (105). They found that all newborns who received a loading dose had serum levels in the therapeutic range within the first 12 hr of therapy, but nearly half of the infants treated conventially had subtherapeutic serum levels during this same time period (105). Patients on long-term therapy have been shown to have decreased serum concentrations of chloramphenicol after 1–2 weeks of therapy (106). The desired serum concentration of free chloramphenicol is from 10 to 20 μg/ml.

Peak chloramphenicol concentrations are attained at approximately 90 min after an intravenous dose; at this time and immediately before the next dose are the best times to collect serum for therapeutic drug monitoring. It is possible to estimate clearance from one concentration drawn at 6 hr after the first dose if meticulous attention is paid to the details of drug administration (107).

Chloramphenicol succinate has also been administered by the intramuscular route. In 1970, Du Pont et al. demonstrated that oral administration produced higher serum levels than did intramuscular administration (108). When we consider the knowledge we have since gained on the metabolism of chloramphenicol, this should come as no surprise. Field trials of intramuscular chloramphenicol in Africa have produced clinical results

Table 2 Chloramphenicol Succinate Pharmacokinetics

Mean age (range)	% Dose in urine	Half-life (hr)	V_d (liter/kg)	References
Adults	32	0.25,[a] 1.6[b]		Glazko et al., 1977 (96)
Adults	13 (2–56)	1.2	0.3	Slaughter et al., 1980 (97)
4 years (2 months to 20 years)	31 (7–43)	2.7	2.1	Nahata and Powell, 1981 (98)
2 years (3 days to 16 years)	33 (6–80)	0.7	0.36[c]	Kauffman et al., 1981 (99)
1.7 years (12 days to 7 years)	42 (13–82)	0.4	0.4	Sack et al., 1982 (100)

[a] α Estimate.
[b] β Estimate.
[c] Calculated; Co = dose/V_d.

Table 3 Chloramphenicol Pharmacokinetics[a]

Age range	Half-life (hr)	V_d (liter/kg)	Reference
1 day to 11 years	5.9 (0.8–17.8)		Friedman et al., 1979 (82)
1 month to 6 years	3.9 (2.1–8.3)	1.39 (0.8–2.1)	Sack et al., 1980 (102)
3 months to 12 years	4.1	0.51	Pickering et al., 1980 (103)
Adults	1.7 (1–2.5)	0.55 (0.4–1)	Slaughter et al., 1980 (97)
1 day to 8 weeks	10–36[b] 5.5–15.7[c]		Glazer et al., 1980 (95), low-birth-weight infants
5–23 months	4	1.19	Yogev et al., 1981 (78)
2 months to 20 years	4 (2–7.8)	0.71 (0.25–2)	Nahata and Powell, 1981 (98)
3 days to 16 years	5.1 (1.7–12)		Kauffman et al., 1981 (99)
12 days to 7 years	4.6	1.12	Sack et al., 1982 (100)
1–30 days	16.1		Rajchgot et al., 1983 (104), premature infants

[a]Free chloramphenicol kinetics after administration of chloramphenicol succinate.
[b]At 1–8 days of age.
[c]At 11 days to 8 weeks of age.

Table 4 Chloramphenicol Palmitate Pharmacokinetics[a]

Age range	Half-life (hr)	Time to C_{max} (hr)	Reference
1 day	27.1	12	Weiss et al., 1960 (91)
1–12 years	4.9	2	
3 months to 12 years		2	Pickering et al., 1981 (103)
5–23 months	6.5	2.25	Yogev et al., 1981 (78)
2 months to 7 years	5.1		Tuomanen et al., 1981 (75)
6 months to 6 years	N 2.8 M 3.7	N 1.5 M 2.5	Eriksson et al., 1983 (115)
6–60 months	N 3.3 M 6.8		Mehta, 1983 (116)
3 days to 32 weeks	3 and 6[b]	4	Shankaran and Kauffman, 1984 (117)

[a]N = normal nutrition; M = protein-energy malnutrition.
[b]Half-lives only could be determined in two neonates.

equivalent to standard therapy (109). Shann et al. have shown in a nonrandomized trial from New Guinea that chloramphenicol succinate has equivalent bioavailability when given intramuscularly or intravenously (110,111).

C. Chloramphenicol Palmitate

Chloramphenicol palmitate is a water-soluble ester formed by the esterification of the fatty acid palmitic acid with chloramphenicol (53). It is thought that this is hydrolyzed to palmitate and chloramphenicol by pancreatic lipase, a theory supported by in vitro experimental work as well as the improved bioavailability of chloramphenicol palmitate in children with cystic fibrosis treated with pancreatic extracts (112-114). The pharmacokinetics of this compound are shown in Table 4.

The usual half-life of chloramphenicol palmitate in toddlers and older children is 5 hr (75,100). There is considerable variation in the half-life of chloramphenicol following administration as the palmitate ester, depending on the age of the patient. This may be prolonged to a modest degree (6 hr), to a considerable degree (up to 27 hr in 1-day-old infants), or indeterminately (100,117). The extreme variability in absorption by neonates demonstrated by Shankaran and Kauffman is in contrast to the excellent absorption displayed in older children (75,77,78,103,117). Children suffering from protein-energy malnutrition also display erratic absorption and prolonged half-lives, which may be twice that of age-matched controls who have been adequately nourished (115,116). This suggests that, although chloramphenicol palmitate is an excellent agent for the majority of patients who can tolerate oral medications, neonates and children with protein-energy malnutrition should receive the drug parenterally. Peak concentrations for the purposes of therapeutic drug monitoring are attained at approximately 2 hr after an oral dose. Concentrations should be obtained when patients are switched from intravenous to oral therapy because of the potential for higher serum concentrations when on oral therapy. The desired serum concentration of free chloramphenicol is from 10 to 20 μg/ml.

Table 5 Chloramphenicol Preparations

Formulation	Dosage form	Concentration
Crystalline chloramphenicol	Optic, ophthalmic, cutaneous, capsules	5 mg/ml, 10 mg/g, 50, or 100, or 250 g
Chloramphenicol palmitate	Oral suspension	30 mg/ml
Chloramphenicol succinate	Intravenous	100 mg/ml

Trade names

Chloromycetin (Canada, USA, UK)	Kemicetin (UK)
Novophenicol, Chloroptin, Fenicol, Novophenicol (Canada)	Aquamycetin, Chloromsoar (Federal Republic of Germany)
Amphicol, Opthoclor (USA)	Sintomicetine, Tifomycine (France)

Source: From References 50, 51, and 115.

V. PREPARATIONS AND DOSAGE

The dose of chloramphenicol (Table 5) has traditionally been 100 mg/kg day^{-1} given every 6 hr (119). The recommended dose for newborn infants is 25 mg/kg day^{-1} at 6 hr intervals, and the dose for infants older than 2 weeks of age has been recommended as 50 mg/kg day^{-1} every 6 hr (90). It is now clear that these dosages should be somewhat modified (6).

The neonate, as previously mentioned, is at special risk from infection because of the baby's precarious immunologic status (33). It is essential to implement effective therapy as soon as possible when infection is suspected. The use of chloramphenicol as a common drug in the newborn nursery is unlikely, but on the occasions when it is used it is traditionally given in the dosages described above. As Lietman has shown, this results in optimal serum levels in only one-third of patients (90). Further, it takes four half-lives to reach a reasonably steady state. When we consider the wide variations in half-lives seen among newborns (Table 3), then we must reconsider our initial approach. It seems appropriate, given the findings of Rajchgot et al., to initiate chloramphenicol therapy in the neonate with a loading dose of 20-25 mg/kg and then to continue therapy with a dose of 25 mg/kg day^{-1} with a dose given every 6 hr (90,105). Infants from 2 weeks to 6 months of age should be treated with 50 mg/kg day^{-1} of chloramphenicol (6).

In the older child, the current recommendation of 100 mg/kg day^{-1} will yield supratherapeutic, i.e., potentially toxic, serum levels in nearly half the patients thus treated (6). Kauffman and Tuomanen and their colleagues have recommended that therapy be initiated at a dose of 75 mg/kg day^{-1}, as this rarely yields subtherapeutic concentrations and also rarely results in supratherapeutic concentrations (75,77). However, a caution underlying all these dosage recommendations is that in all cases the serum concentration must be monitored during chloramphenicol therapy (6,7,120,121).

Therapy should be via the intravenous route for neonates and children with protein-energy malnutrition (115-117). It should also be via this route for children unable to tolerate oral medication or with circulatory instability. In older children and adults, therapy may be changed to the oral route after the patient is stable (6,75,77). It is necessary to monitor serum concentrations at this time, as it may be necessary to reduce the dosage when changing from intravenous to oral chloramphenicol.

VI. DRUG ASSAYS

Therapeutic drug monitoring is very helpful in providing optimal therapy (122,123). The earliest method to quantitate serum chloramphenicol relied on the reduction of the aromatic nitro group to an amine; a colored product was produced by diazotization (124, 125). This assay cross-reacts with a variety of other substances in serum and does not distinguish between prodrug, active drug, and metabolites. Accordingly, it is not a useful method at the present time. A bioassay specific for active drug using a marine organism, *Beneckea natriegens*, has been developed (126). It has a reasonably short turn around time (within 4 hr); however, it does not provide any information about the prodrug and is unable to distinguish between the drug and some of its metabolites, such as the glycolic metabolite found in neonates, that have some degree of antimicrobial activity (50,126). The possibility of detecting a nonchloramphenicol antibiotic also exists. Enzymatic assays with chloramphenicol acetyltransferase have been developed; these are specific and rapid, as well as using small sample volumes (a consideration of particular import in pediatrics) (127,128). These systems require expensive equipment and facilities for disposal of radioisotopes. Numerous high-pressure and high-performance liquid chromatographic techniques have been developed for the assay of both chloramphenicol and chloramphenicol succinate (129–133). These, like the enzymatic assay, require small sample volumes (on the order of 50 μl), are very specific, and have short turnaround times. They do not involve the use of radioisotopes. As with the enzymatic assays, operator expertise and expensive equipment are needed. An additional advantage of the chromatographic methods is that they are capable of quantifying the prodrug chloramphenicol succinate. These last two methods, enzymatic and chromatographic, have equivalent errors, accuracy, and precision (134). The preferred method would depend on local expertise; nonetheless, the ability to quantitate chloramphenicol succinate and the potential for the identification of chloramphenicol metabolites make the chromatographic methods very attractive for kinetic studies, and the ability to quantitate chloramphenicol and chloramphenicol succinate simultaneously can be useful in the clinical environment.

It has been argued that it is unnecessary to monitor levels in patients other than neonates and that other indices of dose-related toxicity, such as anemia or reticulocytopenia, are acceptable to monitor for toxicity (135). However, it is difficult to accept this judgement when rapid, precise assays are available (6,7,50).

VII. THERAPEUTIC INDICATIONS

The development of new semisynthetic penicillins and cephalosporins has considerably reduced the first-line indications for chloramphenicol (Table 6) (119). Since the emergence of ampicillin-resistant strains of *H. influenzae* in the mid-1970s, chloramphenicol has been recommended for the empirical treatment of putative bacterial meninigitis in infants and children as well as in the therapy of invasive *Hemophilus* disease while awaiting sensitivity results. However, strains of *H. influenzae* resistant to chloramphenicol have been described. In addition, the variable kinetics and toxicity associated with chloramphenicol necessitate monitoring serum concentrations. Numerous small trials have demonstrated similar clinical efficacy and safety between the newly developed third-generation cephalosporins and standard therapy (136–141). The third-generation cephalosporins have the advantage of single-agent therapy without the necessity for therapeutic drug monitoring. These new cephalosporins are gaining in use for this indication and are likely to do so through the 1980s and 1990s (48,144).

Table 6 Indications for Chloramphenicol

By organism	By disease
Hemophilus influenzae systemic infections	Central nervous system infections
Typhoid fever	Meningitis
Invasive *Salmonella* infections	Ventriculitis
Anaerobic infections	Brain abscess
Rickettsial infections	Intra-abdominal abscess
	Bacterial ophthalmitis
	Chronic granulomatous disease

Chloramphenicol remains very useful for the treatment of brain abcess; its penetration into cerebral tissue is superior to that of any other antibiotic (83). Central nervous system infections, such as pneumococcal or meningococcal meningitis, in patients with allergies to these agents, represent situations in which chloramphenicol is an ideal drug.

Additionally, chloramphenicol remains the drug of choice in the treatment of typhoid fever and other invasive salmonella infections, although the development of resistant strains has made suspectability testing an essential part of therapy (71,145). In children below the age of 9 years and in pregnant women, in whom the use of tetracycline is contraindicated, it is the drug of choice for rickettsial infections (6). Chloramphenicol is useful in the patient with serious infections, such as bacterial meningitis, who is allergic to the penicillins and cephalosporins. Its ability to penetrate polymorphonuclear leukocytes may make it helpful in chronic granulamatous disease, although this is not well established (58).

Chloramphenicol remains very useful for the treatment of anaerobic infection of many types, particularily intra-abdominal abcesses (144,146,147). Chloramphenicol has also been found to be useful in elevating the white blood cell count in a case of chronic neutropenia, a somewhat surprising event given its well-known bone marrow toxicity (148).

Chloramphenicol has widespread use in developing countries because of its low cost and wide spectrum of activity. Intramuscular use has the advantage of being cheaper in terms of supplies and staff time and safer from the standpoint of possible overhydration (109-111). Intramuscular administration is contraindicited in patients with hemorrhagic disorders or circulatory instability and is obviously of little value to patients who require an intravenous line for other reasons (111).

VIII. TOXICITY

Chloramphenicol has acquired notoriety among antibiotics because of its well-described toxicities (2).

A. Blood Dyscrasias

Aplastic anemia has been reported after chloramphenicol use since shortly after its introduction into clinical practice (17-24,149,150). This lead to recommendations that its use be restricted to the treatment of life-threatening infections, a very sensible recommendation given the trivial indications for which it was frequently prescribed (18,19,24). Chloramphenicol has had two types of blood dyscrasias attributed to it (25). The first is a maturational arrest in the bone marrow, a common and apparently dose-related event that occurs in essentially all patients receiving chloramphenicol when they achieve serum concentrations exceeding 30–40 μg/ml (25,151). Erythrocyte vacuolization and reticulocytopenia occur, the earliest changes being elevations in plasma transferrin saturation as iron utilization decreases (152). Anemia, leukopenia, or thrombocytopenia may result. These changes are reversible on cessation of chloramphenicol therapy (25). Essentially everyone who attains a high enough level of chloramphenicol will manifest this event while on therapy (25).

The second type of blood dyscrasia described is an aplastic anemia. This is an idiosyncratic phenomenon, apparently has no relation to total drug dose and usually occurs weeks to months after the cessation of chloramphenicol therapy (18-21,25). It is characterized by pancytopenia; the bone marrow may be hypo- to hypercellular (25). The mortality for this disease has been estimated to be at least 50%; Best (18) and Wallerstein et al. (19) have noted a slight preponderance of females among patients with this disorder. A clustering of cases in the first decade of life has been noted by Welch et al. (21) and Yunis and Bloomberg (25), which may reflect the pattern of chloramphenicol utilization. The incidence of this disorder is difficult to state with precision, but it is estimated to occur with an incidence ranging from 1 per 20,000 to 1 per 200,000 (18,19,21,25). These figures are at best approximations; the initial calculations by Wallerstein et al., for example, were performed by using the number of cases of aplastic anemia in the state of California related to chloramphenicol as the numerator and an average number of doses estimated by dividing the amount of chloramphenicol sold for human use by an estimated usual therapeutic course was used as the denominator (19). This could grossly over- or underestimate the true incidence per dose because of the wide variations possible in the denominator. It should be emphasized that there have been few epidemiologically sound studies performed to address the true incidence of this complication as opposed to complications of other antibiotics (153,154). The mechanism of this frightening complication is uncertain. Several theories have been advocated. In 1967, Holt proposed that rare enzyme-producing bacteria converted chloramphenicol to a toxin (155). This was offered as an explanation for the infrequent occurrence of aplastic anemia cases reported in association with parenteral chloramphenicol therapy. However, this theory has now been discarded in favor of alternative explanations.

In 1969, Dameshak described aplastic anemia occurring in identical twins exposed to chloramphenicol and postulated that a genetic metabolic defect, perhaps unmasked by chloramphenicol, lead to damage to the bone marrow stem cell elements (156). Yunis suggested that the p-nitrophenyl group is metabolized to a reactive intermediate in certain individuals and then exerts toxic effects on the bone marrow (157). Another theory advanced was that pre-existing marrow damage was necessary for the drug to cause aplastic anemia, based on studies of mice pretreated with busulfan prior to chloramphenicol challenge (158). The vast majority of chloramphenicol is metabolized to a monoglucuronide (36). However, a small portion of total chloramphenicol is metabolized by pathways affecting the dichloracetyl and p-nitrophenyl groups; these pathways may have an important role in the idiosyncratic bone marrow aplasia caused by chloramphenicol. The dichloracetyl group is oxidatively dehalogenated by two pathways; the first is a cytochrome P_{450}-mediated pathway that produces an hydroxylacetamido derivative or chloramphenicol oxamic acid (159,160). A reactive intermediate with a single chlorine atom is produced during these reactions (159,160). The second pathway yields chloramphenicol oxamic acid and a 2-amino metabolite by the actions of aldehyde dehydrogenase and an amidase, respectively, on chloramphenicol, which is first converted to chloramphenicol aldehyde by glutathione transferase.

The p-nitrophenyl group is degraded by cytochrome P_{450}, yielding p-nitroso, amine, and hydroxylame metabolites (161). Irreversible inhibition of DNA synthesis in human bone marrow has been demonstrated by Yunis (161). Toxicity thought to be due to cytochrome P_{450}-generated metabolites has been indirectly demonstrated for other compounds, such as the aromatic anticonvulsants (162,163).

This mechanism has not been directly proven, but there is considerable in vitro and indirect evidence supporting it (161). A reported case of fatal aplastic anemia following dose-related toxicity indicates that the classification and mechanisms outlined above may not be as clear-cut as it seems (26).

Thiampenicol, which has a sulfomethyl group where chloramphenicol has a nitro group, regularly produces dose-related maturational arrest and has received much attention because idiosyncratic aplastic anemia has not been reported with this agent after 16 million courses of therapy (51,52). It is wise to be somewhat sceptical about such claims, as previous claims—such as the reported Israeli immunity to chloramphenicol-induced aplastic anemia—have been proven invalid on more careful investigation (51). Nonetheless, in vitro toxicity studies have demonstrated different mechanisms of toxicity for human bone marrow for thiamphenicol and the nitroso derivative of chloramphenicol, the latter causing breaks in double-stranded DNA (164). Thiamphenicol exhibits a greater degree of dose-related maturational arrest of hematopoiesis than does chloramphenicol (51).

The majority of cases of aplastic anemia associated with chloramphenicol therapy have been described after oral administration (144,155,165). It was believed that idiosyncratic aplastic anemia occurred only after the drug was used orally (2,155). However, reported cases of aplastic anemia after both topical ophthalmic and parenteral use indicate that this situation is probably one of utilization rather than biology (4,166-168).

B. The "Gray Baby" Syndrome

The blood dyscrasias described were joined by the description of another significant toxicity in the late 1950s. Vasomotor collapse followed by death in some cases and, in some cases in which the drug had been stopped, by recovery and survival, had been noted among patients treated with chloramphenicol for typhoid fever (27-31). This had usually been attributed to the disease, although the possibility of the drug being contributory to the patient's deterioration had been considered (27). In 1959, Sutherland described a syndrome of cardiovascular collapse occurring in three neonates receiving large doses of chloramphenicol for the treatment of presumed infections (32). The suspicion of drug toxicity was soon confirmed by a series of interesting clinical and epidemiologic observations. The newborn infant, especially the premature newborn, represents an immunocompromised host (33). Investigators working on reducing the toll of infections among both full-term and premature newborns had initiated a series of trials of prophylactic antibiotic use in the late 1950s. Shortly after the initiation of these studies, it was noted that the newborns in the study groups treated with chloramphenicol plus or minus other antibiotics had a considerable increase in mortality from the control groups (34-37). Indeed, Burns and his co-workers noted a threefold increase in deaths among their infant patients treated with chloramphenicol (34). During this same period, epidemiologists discovered facts supporting these observations.

The infant mortality rate in the United States had steadily decreased since the mid-1930s. However, in 1957, there was an increase in the figure from 26.0 deaths per 1000 live births in 1956 to 26.3 deaths per 1000 live births in 1957 (38). This stimulated epidemiologic investigations of the problem, which revealed that inadequate perinatal care and the use of excess dosages of chloramphenicol in newborns, especially premature newborns, were directly related to the rising infant mortality (39). The clinical picture of cardiovascular collapse, termed the "gray baby" syndrome or the "gray sickness" by the clinicians caring for these infants, was strikingly similar, consisting of initial vomiting or regurgitation followed by a diminished sucking reflex. This was followed by rapid, irregular respirations and abdominal distension. Loose, greenish stools were often passed. Periods of cyanosis were noted, which swiftly progressed to a bodywide ashen color.

Flaccidity and hypothermia were then noted. The infants frequently deteriorated and died within 3 days of the onset of symptoms (34). Recovery occurred in some babies whose chloramphenicol had been stopped, usually over 1 or 2 days after the time of the drug's discontinuation (34). The gray baby syndrome has since been noted in older children, adolescents, and adults treated with chloramphenicol (40–43).

Since Sutherland's insightful description of the syndrome in 1959, it has become clear through the work of Weiss, Young, and Lietman and their co-workers that the newborn is at special risk for the development of this grave adverse reaction because of the limited capacity of the newborn liver to detoxify free chloramphenicol by glucuronidation, leading to elevated serum concentrations of chloramphenicol (30,89–92). However, although the newborn is at special risk for this devastating illness, it has also been reported in toddlers, older children, adolescents, and adults who have therapeutically and sometimes inadvertently been given large doses of chloramphenicol that have resulted in extremely elevated serum concentrations (40–43). In the majority of adult cases, this has been due to gross overdoses (43). Serum concentrations of chloramphenicol have generally been in the range of 70–250 μg/ml in cases of the gray syndrome (5,6).

Smith and Weber described the advent of the gray syndrome as heralded by lactic acidosis unresponsive to bicarbonate therapy followed by mild hepatocellular dysfunction, which is followed in 6–12 hr by cardiovascular collapse (50). ECHO cardiography during the acute phase of the gray syndrome has demonstrated biventricular dilation with a reduced left ventricular shortening fraction (169). Hemodynamic monitoring of two patients with the gray baby syndrome demonstrated reduced oxygen consumption in both cases; in one case the reduced oxygen consumption preceded the development of cardiogenic shock and it was concomitant with evidence of cardiogenic shock in the second case (170). Unexplained metabolic acidosis has been reported as a presenting feature of the chloramphenicol-related gray syndrome (171).

The mechanism of this syndrome is uncertain. However, it seems clear that the short time course over which the syndrome evolves makes it unlikely that disruption of mitochondrial protein biogenesis is responsible for this disorder (51). Experimental work with isolated perfused newborn pig hearts have demonstrated inhibition of stage 3 respiration—that is, oxygen consumption in the presence of exogenous adenosine diphosphate—in a fashion suggesting that the mechanism of the gray syndrome may be due to interference with carbohydrate metabolism by impairing the aspartate-malate shuttle at the level of the α-ketoglutarate-malate exchange transport mechanism (172). Some patients with this syndrome will recover if the drug is withdrawn (34). In patients who have received inadvertent overdoses, both exchange transfusions and charcoal column hemoperfusion have been used in attempts to reduce the body's burden of free chloramphenicol (173–175). It is controversial as to how well exchange transfusion will work in the routine management of patients with an overdose of a nonpolar, lipid-soluble drug that distributes freely throughout body tissues; charcoal hemoperfusion has been demonstrated to decrease serum chloramphenicol levels (173–175). However, despite an impressive reduction in serum chloramphenicol levels in one patient so treated, the patient did not survive the overdose (175).

C. Other Adverse Effects

Oral administration of chloramphenicol has been associated with nausea, vomiting, diarrhea, metallic aftertaste, and glossitis (4,176). Laferriere and Marks reported that vomiting is less common if chloramphenicol is given before meals (5). Chloramphenicol is a rare cause of antibiotic-associated colitis (177). Mucosal candidiasis has been reported in association with oral chloramphenicol therapy (75). Hepatitis has been reported in two patients with chronic granulomatous disease of childhood while they were receiving chloramphenicol. It has been recommended that liver function be monitored in patients with this disorder who are taking chloramphenicol (178,179). It is difficult to justify monitoring liver function tests in patients who do not have chronic granulomatous disease or hepatic disease while on chloramphenicol therapy (180).

Patients on prolonged courses of chloramphenicol have developed encephalopathy, optic neuritis, and peripheral neuritis (181,182). These adverse effects were reversible after cessation of drug therapy. Arrested hair and physical growth have been reported in a child with cystic fibrosis treated with chloramphenicol (183).

Experimental models have demonstrated delayed wound healing and impaired antibody synthesis, but the clinical significance of these observations is unknown (184–187). Vesicular and maculopapular reactions have been reported (4). Three patients with Mediterranean-type glucose-6-phosphate dehydrogenase deficiency have been reported to undergo hemolysis while on treatment with chloramphenicol for typhoid fever (188). There was severe hemolysis noted while the patients were receiving chloramphenicol and actively infected. When these patients were given chloramphenicol after their infections had resolved, there was mild hemolysis. In patients with oriental-type glucose-6-phosphate dehydrogenase deficiency, in vitro testing has not demonstrated any difference in the survival of erythrocytes exposed to chloramphenicol over controls (189).

IX. CONTRAINDICATIONS

There are very few absolute contraindications to chloramphenicol. It should not be used in patients who have demonstrated anaphylaxis to the agent, but this is a very rare disorder (190). It may be more dangerous to use in patients with previous marrow damage and should be avoided in patients who have a family history of reactions to chloramphenicol (158,166). Chloramphenicol has not been shown to be associated with major or minor fetal malformations if used during pregnancy, but caution should be exercised in the use of this agent in women near term, as babies born to mothers on chloramphenicol therapy at the time of delivery have been reported to be at risk for the gray baby syndrome (191). Although the concentrations of chloramphenicol achieved in breast milk are too low to yield the gray baby syndrome in infants breast-fed by women on chloramphenicol therapy, the theoretical risk of idiosyncratic aplastic anemia and the potential problems with the infant's bowel flora that may result from exposure of the infant to even small doses of chloramphenicol suggest that chloramphenicol should not be used during lactation (191). As previously noted, neonates and patients with serious hepatic disease are at increased risk of developing dose-related toxicity (81,90,93).

X. INTERACTIONS

Chloramphenicol has inhibitory effects on a variety of drug oxidation pathways involving cytochrome P_{450} (192–194). It has been shown to impair the biotransformation of tolbutamide, phenytoin, and dicumarol in humans (195). It has been demonstrated that phenobarbital will lower serum chloramphenicol concentrations when given concurrently with chloramphenicol, presumably by induction of drug-metabolizing enzymes (196).

Patients who were on concurrent treatment with phenytoin and chloramphenicol had elevations in serum chloramphenicol concentrations, presumably by inhibition of drug-metabolizing enzymes (196). All the phenytoin-treated patients in the study by Krausinski and co-workers who were given chloramphenicol therapy demonstrated toxic peak chloramphenicol concentrations during the course of treatment (196).

Prober has reported that concurrent therapy with rifampin decreased serum chloramphenicol concentrations in two children receiving intravenous therapy for *H. influenzae* meningitis (198). As this combination is frequently used in order to eradicate the nasopharyngeal carriage of *H. influenzae* in children with invasive *Hemophilus* disease, this may be an interaction of considerable importance (47). Additionally, rifampin has been demonstrated both experimentally and clinically to induce the drug-metabolizing enzymes of such agents as warfarin, digitonin, tolbutamide, and phenytoin (199). Acetaminophen has been reported by Buchanan and Moodley to prolong the half-life of chloramphenicol in children with kwashiorkor and in adults given an intravenous dose of acetaminophen (200). However, Kearns and co-workers in a study of oral acetaminophen administration to febrile children receiving chloramphenicol therapy found no difference in chloramphenicol pharmacokinetics between the children who received acetaminophen and those who did not (201). The adults studied were given intravenous acetaminophen as opposed to the oral doses used by Kearns; this may have contributed to the conflicting results (201).

Chloramphenicol has been reported to have an antagonistic action when used with ampicillin against species of enteric gram-negative bacteria to which it is bacteriostatic (202,203). For bacteria to which it is bacteriocidal, chloramphenicol is synergistic to other bacteriocidal antibiotics (51,202).

REFERENCES

1. Dunne, M, Herxheimer, A, Newman, M, Ridley, H: Indications and Warnings about chloramphenicol. *Lancet 2*:788–782, 1973.
2. Polin, HB, Plaut, ME: Chloramphenicol. *N.Y. State Med. J. 77*:378–381, 1977.
3. Meissner, HC, Smith, AL: The current status of chloramphenicol. *Pediatrics 64*: 348–356, 1979.
4. Feder, HM, Osier, C, Maderzao, EG: Chloramphenicol: A review of its use in clinical practice. *Rev. Infect. Dis. 3*:479–491, 1981.
5. Laferriere, CI, Marks, MI: Chloramphenicol: Properties and clinical use. *Pediatr. Infect. Dis. 1*:257–264, 1982.
6. Kauffman, RE: The role of chloramphenicol in pediatric therapy. In: *Developmental Pharmacology* (SM MacLeod, AB Okey, and SP Spielberg, eds.), Alan R. Liss, Inc., New York, 1983, pp. 315–327.
7. Dajani, AS, Kauffman, RE: The renaissance of chloramphenicol. *Pediatr. Clin. North Am. 28*(1):195–202, 1981.
8. Ehrlich, J, Bartz, QR, Smith, RM, et al.: Chloromycetin, a new antibiotic from a soil actinomycete. *Science 106*:417–419, 1947.
9. Gottlieb, D, Battachyrra, PK, Anderson, HW, et al.: Some properties of an antibiotic obtained from a species of streptomyces. *J. Bacteriol. 55*:409, 1948.
10. Bartz, QR: Isolation and characterization of chloromycetin. *J. Biol. Chem. 17*:445–450, 1948.
11. Payne, EH, Knandt, JA, Polacios, S: Treatment of epidemic typhus with chloromycetin. *J. Trop. Med. 51*:68, 1948.
12. Smadel, JE, Leon, AP, Levy, HL, Jr., et al.: Chloromycetin in the treatment of patients with typhus fever. *Proc. Soc. Exp. Biol. Med. 68*:12, 1948.

13. Woodward, TE, Smadel, JE, Levy, HL, Jr., et al.: Preliminary report on the beneficial effect of chloromycetin in the treatment of typhoid fever. *Ann. Intern. Med. 28*:131–134, 1948.
14. Smadel, JE: Chloramphenicol (chloromycetin) in the treatment of infectious diseases. *Am. J. Med. 7*:671, 1949.
15. Rebstock, MC, Crooks, HM, Jr., Controulis, J, et al.: Chloramphenicol (chloromycetin). *J. Am. Chem. Soc. 71*:2458–2475, 1949.
16. Bell, WE: Infections of the brain and spinal cord. In: *The Practice of Pediatric Neurology*, 2nd ed. (KF Swaiman and FS Wright, eds.), C. V. Mosby, Toronto, 1983, pp. 659–675.
17. Smith, KM, Condit, PK, Proctor, RL, Satcher, V: Fatal aplastic anemia: An epidemiological study of its relationship to the drug chloramphenicol. *J. Chron. Dis. 17*:899–914, 1964.
18. Best, WR: Chloramphenicol-associated blood dyscrasias. *JAMA 201*:99–106, 1967.
19. Wallerstein, RD, Condit, PK, Kasper, CK, et al.: Statewide study of chloramphenicol therapy and fatal aplastic anemia. *JAMA 208*:2041–2050, 1969.
20. Lewis, CN, Putnam, LE, Hendricks, LE, et al.: Chloramphenicol (chloromycetin) in relation to blood dyscrasas with observations on other drugs. *Antibiot. Chemother. 2*:601–609, 1952.
21. Welch, H, Lewis, CN, Kerland, I: Blood dyscrasias, a nationwide survey. *Antibiot. Chemother. 4*:609–613, 1954.
22. Welch, H, Lewis, CN, Weinstein, HI, Beckman, BB: Severe reactions to antibiotics. *Antibiot. Med. Clin. Ther. 4*:800–805, 1957.
23. Fraumeni, JF: Bone marrow depression induced by chloramphenicol or phenylbutazone: Leukemia and other sequelae. *JAMA 201*:150–156, 1967.
24. Bottinger, LE, Westerholm, B: Drug-induced blood dyscrasias in Sweden. *Br. Med. J. 3*:339–343, 1973.
25. Yunis, AA, Bloomberg, GR: Chloramphenicol toxicity: Clinical features and pathogenesis. *Prog. Hematol. 4*:138–159, 1967.
26. Daum, RS, Cohen, DL, Smith, AL: Fatal aplastic anemia following apparent "dose-related" chloramphenicol toxicity. *J. Pediatr. 94*:403–406, 1979.
27. Patel, JC, Barkin, PD, Modi, CJ: Chloramphenicol in typhoid fever: Preliminary report of clinical trials in six cases. *Br. Med. J. 2*:908, 1949.
28. Arya, BP: Hypothermia with chloramphenicol. *Lancet 1*:970, 1950.
29. Chatterjee, PK, Roy, BB: Vasomotor collapse after chloramphenicol. *Br. Med. J. 2*:1334, 1950.
30. Stephens, PR: Unsuccessful treatment of typhoid fever with chloramphenicol. *Lancet 1*:731, 1950.
31. Marmion, DE: Treatment of typhoid fever with chloramphenicol: Clinical study of 330 cases of enteric fever treated in Egypt. *Trans. R. Soc. Trop. Med. Hyg. 46*:619, 1952.
32. Sutherland, JM: Fatal cardiovascular collapse of infants receiving large amounts of chloramphenicol. *Am. J. Dis. Child. 97*:761–767, 1959.
33. Prober, CG: Treatment of bacterial infections in the neonate. *Clin. Invest. Med. 8*: 368–370, 1985.
34. Burns, LE, Hodgman, JE, Cass, AB: Fatal circulatory collapse in premature infants receiving chloramphenicol. *N. Engl. J. Med. 261*:1318–1321, 1959.
35. Kent, SP, Wideman, GL: Prophylactic antibiotic therapy in infants born after premature rupture of membranes. *JAMA 171*:1199–1203, 1959.
36. Lambdin, MA, Waddell, WW, Birdsong, M: Chloramphenicol toxicity in the premature infant. *Pediatrics 25*:935–940, 1960.
37. Lischner, H, Seligman, SJ, Krammer, A, Parmalee, AH, Jr.: An outbreak of neonatal

deaths among term infants associated with administration of chloramphenicol. *J. Pediatr. 59*:21–34, 1961.
38. Hunt, EP, Chenoweth, AD: Recent trends in infant mortality in the United States. *Am. J. Public Health 51*:190–207, 1961.
39. Buetow, KC: An epidemiological approach to the problem of rising neonatal mortality in Baltimore. *Am. J. Public Health 51*:217–227, 1961.
40. Craft, AW, Brocklebank, JT, Hey, EN, Jackson, RH: The "grey toddler." Chloramphenicol toxicity. *Arch. Dis. Child. 49*:235–237, 1974.
41. Morton, K: Chloramphenicol overdose in a six-week old infant. *Am. J. Dis. Child. 102*:430, 1961.
42. Brown, RT: Chloramphenicol toxicity in an adolescent. *J. Adolesc. Health Care 3*: 53, 1982.
43. Thompson, WL, Anderson, SE, Jr., Lipsky, JJ, Lietman, PS: Overdoses of chloramphenicol. *JAMA 234*:149–150, 1975.
44. Thomas, WJ, McReynolds, JW, Mock, CR, Bailey, DW: Ampicillin-resistant *Haemophilus influenzae* meningitis. *Lancet 1*:313, 1974.
45. Gunn, BA, Woodall, JB, Jones, JF: Ampicillin-resistant *Haemophilus influenzae. Lancet 2*:845, 1974.
46. Centers for Disease Control: Ampicillin-resistant *Haemophilus influenzae* meningitis—Texas. *Morbid Mortal. Weekly Rep. 23*:29, 1974.
47. American Academy of Pediatrics: *Report of the Committee on Infectious Diseases* (Red Book), 19th ed., pp. 105–107, 1982.
48. McCracken, GH: New concepts in the management of infants and children with meningitis. *Pediatr. Infect. Dis. 2*:S51–55, 1983.
49. Rhodes, HH, Johnson, CM: Antibiotic therapy for severe infections in infants and children. *Mayo Clin. Proc. 58*:158–164, 1983.
50. Smith, AL, Weber, A: Pharmacology of chloramphenicol. *Pediatr. Clin. North Am. 30*(1):209–236, 1983.
51. Garrod, LP, Lambert, HP, O'Grady, F: Chloramphenicol. In: *Antibiotic and Chemotherapy* (LP Garrod, HP Lambert, F O'Grady, eds.), Churchill Livingstone, New York, 1981, pp. 155–168.
52. Ferrari, V: Introductory address—salient features of thiamphenicol. *Sex. Transmit. Dis. 11*:336–339, 1984.
53. Ross, S, Burke, FG, Rice, GC: The use of chloromycetin palmitate in infants and children: A preliminary report. *Antibiot. Chemother. 2*:299–207, 1952.
54. Pongs, O, Bald, R, Erdmann, VA: Identification of chloramphenicol-binding protein in *Escherichia coli* ribosomes by affinity labelling. *Proc. Natl. Acad. Sci. USA 70*: 2229–2233, 1979.
55. Cundliffe, E, McQuillen, K: Bacterial protein synthesis: The effects of antibiotics. *J. Mol. Biol. 30*:137, 1967.
56. Lietman, PS: Pharmacologic effects on developing enzyme systems. *Fed. Proc. 31*: 62–64, 1972.
57. Rahal, JJ, Jr., Simberkoff, MS: Bacteriocidal and bacteriostatic action of chloramphenicol against meningeal pathogens. *Antimicrob. Agents Chemother. 16*:13–18, 1979.
58. Jacobs, RF, Wilson, CB, Laxton, JG, et al.: Cellular uptake and intracellular activity of antibiotics against *Haemophilus influnzae* type b. *J. Infect. Dis. 145*:152–159, 1982.
59. Atkison, BA: Species incidence, trends of susceptibility to antibiotics in the United States and minimum inhibitory concentrations. In: *Antibiotics in Laboratory Medicine*, 2nd ed. (V Lorian, ed.), Williams and Wilkins, Baltimore, 1985, pp. 1074–1077.

60. Brown, WJ, Waati, PE: Susceptibility testing of clinically isolated anaerobic bacteria by an agar dilution technique. *Antimicrob Agents Chemother 17*:629–635, 1980.
61. Denny, FW, Clyde, WA, Jr., Glezer, WB: *Mycoplasma pneumoniae* diseases: Clinical spectrum, pathophysiology, epidemiology and control. *J. Infect. Dis. 123*:74–92, 1971.
62. McLean, IW, Jr., Schwab, JL, Hillegas, AB, et al.: Susceptibility of micro-organisms to chloramphenicol (chloromycetin). *J. Clin. Invest. 28*:953–963, 1949.
63. Warren, KS, Weisberger, AS: Supression of schistosomiasis in snails by chloramphenicol. *Nature 209*:422–423, 1966.
64. Mendelman, PM, Doroshow, CA, Gandy, SL, et al.: Plasmid-mediated resistance in multiply resistant *Haemophilus influenzae* type b causing meningitis: Molecular characterization of one strain and review of the literature. *J. Infect. Dis. 150*:30–39, 1984.
65. Shaw, WV: Comparative enzymology of chloramphenicol resistance. *Ann. N.Y. Acad. Sci. 182*:234, 1971.
66. Roberts, MC, Swenson, C, Orvens, L, et al.: Characterization of chloramphenicol resistant *Haemophilus influenzae. Antimicrob. Agents Chemother. 18*:610–618, 1980.
67. Hansman, D: Multiple drug resistance in *Haemophilus influenzae* type b. *Med. J. Aust. 142*:536–537, 1985.
68. Uchiyama, N, Greene, GR, Kitts, DB, Thrupp, LD: Meningitis due to *Haemophilus influenzae* type b resistant to chloramphenicol and ampicillin. *J. Pediatr. 97*:421–424, 1980.
69. Sills, JA, MacMahon, P, Hull, E, Fitzgerald, T: *Haemophilus influenzae* type b resistant to chloramphenicol and ampicillin. *Br. Med. J. 286*:722, 1983.
70. Centers for Disease Control: Ampicillin and chloramphenicol resistance in systemic *Haemophilus influenzae* disease. *Mortal. Morbid. Weekly Rep. 33*:35–37, 1984.
71. Lamb, VA, Mayhall, CG, Spodora, AC, et al.: Outbreak of *Salmonella typhimurium* gastroenteritis due to an imported strain resistant to ampicillin, chloramphenicol and trimethoprim-sulfamethoxazole in a nursery. *J. Clin. Microbiol. 20*:1076–1079, 1984.
72. Azeman, P, Stull, T, Roberts, M, et al.: Rapid detection of chloramphenicol resistance in *Haemophilus influenzae. Antimicrob. Agents. Chemother. 20*:168–170, 1981.
73. Sompolinsky, D, Samara, Z: Mechanisms of high-level resistance to chloramphenicol in different *Escherichia coli* variants. *J. Gen. Microbiol. 50*:55, 1968.
74. Baughman, G, Fehenstalk, S: Chloramphenicol resistance mutation in *Escherichia coli* which maps in the major ribosomal protein gene cluster. *J. Bacteriol. 137*:1315, 1979.
75. Tuomanen, EI, Powell, KR, Marks, MI, et al.: Oral chloramphenicol in the treatment of *Haemophilus influenzae* meningitis. *J. Pediatr. 99*:968–974, 1981.
76. Check, WA: Oral chloramphenicol for bacterial meningitis: Effective and safe. *JAMA 244*:1883–1884, 1980.
77. Kauffman, RE, Thirumoorthi, MC, Buckley, JA, et al.: Relative bioavailability of intravenous chloramphenicol succinate and oral chloramphenicol palmitate in infants and children. *J. Pediatr. 99*:963–967, 1981.
78. Yogev, R, Kolling, WM, Williams, T: Pharmacokinetic comparison of intravenous and oral chloramphenicol in patients with *Haemophilus influenzae* meningitis. *Pediatrics 67*:656–660, 1981.
79. Glazko, AJ, Dill, WA, Kazenko, A, et al.: Physical factors affecting the rate of absorption of chloramphenicol esters. *Antibiot. Chemother. 8*:516, 1958.
80. Glazko, AJ, Kindel, AW, Alegnani, WC, et al.: An evaluation of the absorption

characteristics of different chloramphenicol preparations in normal human subjects. *Clin. Pharmacol. Ther. 9*:472, 1968.
81. Koup, JP, Lau, AH, Brodsky, B, Slaughter, RL: Chloramphenicol pharmacokinetics in hospitalized patients. *Antimicrob. Agents Chemother. 15*:653–657, 1979.
82. Friedman, CA, Lovejoy, FC, Smith, AL: Chloramphenicol disposition in infants and children. *J. Pediatr. 95*:1071–1072, 1979.
83. Kramer, PW, Griffith, RS, Campbell, RL: Antibiotic penetration of the brain: A comparative study. *J. Neurosurg. 31*:295–302, 1969.
84. Koup, JP, Lau, AH, Brodsky, B, Slaughter, RL: Relationship between serum and saliva chloramphenicol concentrations. *Antimicrob. Agents Chemother. 15*:658–661, 1979.
85. Havelka, J, Hejzlar, M, Popov, V, et al.: Excretion of chloramphenicol in human milk. *Chemotherapy 13*:204–207, 1968.
86. Kunin, CM, Glazko, AJ, Finland, M: Persistance of antibiotics in blood of patients with acute renal failure. II. Chloramphenicol and its metabolic products in the blood of patients with severe renal disease or hepatic cirrhosis. *J. Clin. Invest. 38*: 1498, 1959.
87. Glazko, AJ, Wolf, LM, Dill, WA, et al.: Biochemical studies on chloramphenicol (chloromycetin). *J. Pharmacol. Exp. Ther. 96*:445, 1949.
88. Glazko, AJ, Dill, WA, Rebstock, MC: Biochemical studies on chloramphenicol (chloromycetin). *J. Biol. Chem. 183*:679, 1950.
89. Dill, WA, Thompson, EM, Fiskens, RA, Glazko, AJ: A new metabolite of chloramphenicol. *Nature 185*:535–536, 1960.
90. Lietman, PS: Chloramphenicol and the neonate—1979 view. *Clin. Pharmacol. 6*:151–162, 1979.
91. Weiss, CF, Glazko, AJ, Weston, JK: Chloramphenicol in the newborn infant: A physiologic explanation of its toxicity when given in excessive doses. *N. Engl. J. Med. 262*:787–794, 1960.
92. Young, WS, Lietman, PS: Chloramphenicol glucuronyl transferase: Assay, ontogeny and inducibility. *J. Pharmacol. Exp. Ther. 204*:203–211, 1978.
93. Azzollini, F, Gazzangia, A, Lodu, E, et al.: Elimination of chloramphenicol and thiamphenicol in subjects with cirrhosis of the liver. *Int. J. Clin. Pharmacol. Ther. Toxicol. 6*:130, 1972.
94. Yamakawa, T, Itoh, S, Onishi, S, et al.: Developmental changes in hepatic esterase activity towards chloramphenicol succinate and its Michaelis-Menton constant of liver, kidney and lung in humans. *Dev. Pharmacol. Ther. 7*:205–212, 1984.
95. Glazer, JP, Danish, MA, Plotkin, SA, Yolfe, SJ: Disposition of chloramphenicol in in low birth weight infants. *Pediatrics 66*:573–578, 1980.
96. Glazko, AJ, Dill, WA, Kinkel, AW, et al.: Absorption and excretion of parenteral doses of chloramphenicol sodium succinate (CMS) in comparison with oral doses of chloramphenicol (CM). Presented at 78th Annual Meeting, American Society for Clinical Pharmacology and Therapeutics, Dallas, Texas, 1977.
97. Slaughter, RL, Peeper, JA, Cerra, FB, et al.: Chloramphenicol sodium succinate kinetics in critically ill patients. *Clin. Pharmacol. Ther. 28*:69–77, 1980.
98. Nahata, MC, Powell, DA: Bioavailability and clearance of chloramphenicol after intravenous chloramphenicol succinate. *Clin. Pharmacol. Ther. 30*:368–372, 1981.
99. Kauffman, RE, Miceli, JN, Strebel, L, et al.: Pharmacokinetics of chloramphenicol and chloramphenicol succinate in infants and children. *J. Pediatr. 98*:315–320, 1981.
100. Sack, CM, Koup, JR, Opheim, KE, et al.: Chloramphenicol succinate kinetics in infants and young children. *Pediatr. Pharmacol. 2*:93–103, 1982.
101. Friedman, CA, Lovejoy, FC, Smith, AL: Chloramphenicol kinetics in infants and children. *Pediatr. Res. 12*:405, 1978.

102. Sack, CM, Koup, JR, Smith, AL: Chloramphenicol pharmacokinetics in infants and young children. *Pediatrics 66*:574–584, 1980.
103. Pickering, LK, Hoecker, JL, Kramer, WG, et al.: Clinical pharmacology of two chloramphenicol preparations in children: Sodium succinate (intravenous) and palmitate (oral) esters. *J. Pediatr. 96*:757–761, 1981.
104. Rajchgot, P, Prober, C, Soldin, S, et al.: Chloramphenicol pharmacokinetics in the newborn. *Dev. Pharmacol. Ther. 6*:305–314, 1983.
105. Rajchgot, P, Prober, CG, Soldin, S, et al.: Initiation of chloramphenicol therapy in the newborn infant. *J. Pediatr. 101*:1018–1021, 1982.
106. Nahata, M, Powell, DA: Chloramphenicol serum concentration falls during chloramphenicol succinate dosing. *Clin. Pharmacol. Ther. 33*:308–313, 1983.
107. Koup, JR, Sack, CM, Smith, AL, et al.: Rapid estimation of chloramphenicol clearance in infants and children. *Clin. Pharmacokinet. 6*:83–88, 1981.
108. Du Pont, HL, Hornich, RB, Weiss, CF, et al.: Evaluation of chloramphenicol acid succinate therapy of induced typhoid fever and Rocky Mountain spotted fever. *N. Engl. J. Med. 282*:53–57, 1970.
109. Puddicombe, JB, Wali, SS, Greenwood, BM: A field trial of a single intramuscular injection of long-acting chloramphenicol in the treatment of meningococcal meningitis. *Trans. R. Soc. Trop. Med. Hyg. 78*:399–403, 1984.
110. Shann, F, Linnemann, V, Mackenzie, A, et al.: Absorption of chloramphenicol sodium succinate after intramuscular administration in children. *N. Engl. J. Med. 313*:410–414, 1985.
111. Anonymous: Intramuscular or intravenous antibiotics? *Lancet 1*:660–662, 1984.
112. Glazko, AJ, Dill, WA, Kazenko, A, et al.: Physical factors affecting the rate of absorption of chloramphenicol esters. *Antibiot. Chemother. 8*:516, 1958.
113. Doug, J, De Roeck, A: Hydrolysis and absorption of chloramphenicol palmitate. *J. Pharm. Belg. 20*:475, 1965.
114. Palmer, J, Kieth, J, Haung, N: Absorption of chloramphenicol palmitate in patients with cystic fibrosis. *CF Club 21*:82, 1980.
115. Eriksson, M, Paalzow, L, Balme, P, Mariam, TW: Chloramphenicol pharmacokinetics in Ethiopian children of differing nutritional status. *Eur. J. Clin. Pharmacol 24*:817–823, 1983.
116. Mehta, S: Drug disposition in children with protein energy malnutrition. *J. Pediatr. Gastr. Nut. 2*:407–417, 1983.
117. Shankaran, S, Kauffman, RE: Use of chloramphenicol palmitate in neonates. *J. Pediatr. 104*:q113–116, 1984.
118. Krogh, CME: *Compendium of Pharmaceuticals and Specialities*, 20th ed., Canadian Pharmaceutical Association, Ottawa, 1985, pp. 121–124.
119. Samale, MA, Mandel, GL: Chloramphenicol. In: *Pharmacological Basis of Therapeutics* (AG Gilman, LS Goodman, TW Rall, and F Murad, eds.), Macmillan, New York, 1985, pp. 1179–1184.
120. Rajchgot, P, Prober, CG, Soldin, S, et al.: Toward optimization of therapy in the neonate. *Clin. Pharmacol. Ther. 33*:551–555, 1983.
121. Rajchgot, P: Neonatal drug monitoring and drug delivery systems. *Clin. Invest. Med. 8*:371–377, 1985.
122. Boreus, LO: The role of therapeutic drug monitoring in childhood. *Pediatr. Pharmacol. 3*:145–148, 1983.
123. Rosin, H, Crea, A, Forster, J: The benefits of drug monitoring in patients with bacterial disease, e.g., chloramphenicol monitoring. *Pediatr. Pharmacol. 3*:175–180, 1983.
124. Glazko, AJ, Wolf, LM, Dill, WA: Biochemical studies on chloramphenicol (chloromycetin). *Arch. Biochem. 23*:411, 1949.

125. Mason, EO, Kaplan, SL, Baker, CJ, et al.: Modification of the colourimetric assay for chloramphenicol in the presence of bilirubin. *Antimicrob. Agents Chemother. 15*:544, 1979.
126. Bannatyne, R, Cheung, R: Chloramphenicol bioassay. *Antimicrob. Agents Chemother. 16*:43–45, 1979.
127. Smith, AL, Smith, DH: Improved enzymatic assay of chloramphenicol. *Clin. Chem. 24*:1452, 1978.
128. Robison, LR, Seligsohn, R, Lerner, SA: Simplified radioenzymatic assay for chloramphenicol. *Antimicrob. Agents Chemother. 13*:25, 1978.
129. Koup, JP, Brodsky, B, Lau, A, et al.: High-performance liquid chromatographic assay of chloramphenicol in serum. *Antimicrob. Agents Chemother. 14*:439–444, 1978.
130. Petersdorf, SH, Raisys, VA, Opheim, HE: Micro-scale method for liquid-chromatographic determinants of chloramphenicol in serum. *Clin. Chem. 25*:1300–1302, 1979.
131. Aravind, MK, Miceli, JN, Kauffman, RE, et al.: Simultaneous measurement of chloramphenicol and chloramphenicol succinate by high-pressure liquid chromatography. *J. Chromatogr. 221*:176–181, 1980.
132. Velagopudi, R, Smith, RV, Ludden, TM, et al.: Simultaneous detection of chloramphenicol and chloramphenicol succinate in plasma using high-performance liquid chromatography. *J. Chromatogr. 228*:423, 1982.
133. Soldin, SJ, Golas, CL, Prober, CG, et al.: Measurement of chloramphenicol and its succinate ester by high performance liquid chromatography: *Clin. Appl. Clin. Chem. 285*:1549, 1982.
134. Pickering, LK, Hoecker, JL, Kramer, WG, et al.: Assays for chloramphenicol compared: Radio-enzymatic, gas chromatographic with electron capture and gas chromatographic-mass spectrometric. *Clin. Chem. 25*:300, 1979.
135. Ekblad, H, Ruushanen, O, Lindberg, R, Iisalo, E: The monitoring of serum chloramphenicol levels in children with severe infections. *J. Antimicrob. Chemother. 15*: 489–494, 1985.
136, Del Rio, MD, Chrane, D, Shelton, S, et al.: Cetriaxone versus ampicillin and chloramphenicol for treatment of bacterial meningitis in children. *Lancet 1*:1241–1244, 1983.
137. Steele, RW, Bradsher, RW: Comparison of ceftriaxone with standard therapy for bacterial meningitis. *J. Pediatr. 103*:138–141, 1983.
138. Congeni, BL: Comparison of cetriaxone and traditional therapy of bacterial meningitis. *Antimicrob. Agents Chemother. 25*:40–44, 1984.
139. McMohn, AA, Sowa, MA, Ryn, DM: Evaluation of cefatazadine. Ampicillin and chloramphenicol in experimental *Haemphilus influenzae* type b meningitis. *J. Antimicrob. Chemother. 13*:437–445, 1984.
140. Aronoff, SC, Reed, MD, O'Brian, CA, Blumer, JL: Comparison of the efficacy and safety of ceftriaxone to ampicillin/chloramphenicol in the treatment of childhood meningitis. *J. Antimicrob. Chemother. 13*:143–151, 1984.
141. Sakata, Y, McCracken, GH, Jr., Thomas, ML, Olson, KD: Pharmacokinetics and therapeutic efficacy of imipenin, ceftazidin and cefriaxone in experimental meningitis due to an ampicillin and chloramphenicol-resistant strain of *Haemophilus influenzae* type b. *Antimicrob. Agents Chemother. 25*:29–32, 1984.
142. Jacobs, RF, Wells, TG, Steele, RW, Yamauchi, T: A prospective randomized comparison of cefataxime versus ampicillin and chloramphenicol for bacterial meningitis in children. *J. Pediatr. 107*:129–133, 1985.
143. McCracken, GH, Jr.: New developments in the management of children with bacterial meningitis. *Pediatr. Infect. Dis. 3*:S32–34, 1984.

144. Gleckman, RA: Warning-chloramphenicol may be good for your health. *Arch. Intern. Med. 135*:1125–1126, 1975.
145. Hook, EW: Typhoid fever today. *N. Engl. J. Med. 310*:116–118, 1982.
146. Harding, GKM, Buchwald, FJ, Ronald, AR, et al.: Prospective, randomized comparative study of clindamycin, chloramphenicol and ticarcillin, each in combination with gentamicin, in therapy for intraabdominal and female genital tract sepsis. *J. Infect. Dis. 142*:384–392, 1980.
147. Fanconi, S, Seger, RA, Willi, U, et al.: Oral chloramphenicol therapy for multiple liver abcesses in hyperimmunglobulinemia E syndrome. *Eur. J. Pediatr. 142*:292–295, 1984.
148. Adams, GR, Pearson, HA: Chloramphenicol-responsive chronic neutropenia. *N. Engl. J. Med. 309*:1039–1041, 1981.
149. Cooperative Study Group for Aplastic and Refractory Anaemias: Toxic etiology of aplastic anemia. *Sex. Transm. Dis. 11*:343–346, 1984.
150. Aksoy, M, Erden, S, Dincol, G, et al.: Aplastic anemia due to chemicals and drugs: A study of 108 patients. *Sex. Transm. Dis. 11*:347–350, 1984.
151. Scott, JL, Finegold, SM, Belkin, GA, Lawrence, JS: A controlled double-blind study of the hematologic toxicity of chloramphenicol. *N. Engl. J. Med. 272*:1132, 1965.
152. Rubin, D, Weisberger, AS, Botti, RE, Storaozli, JP: Changes in iron metabolism in early chloramphenicol toxicity. *J. Clin. Pharmacol. 37*:1286, 1958.
153. Rudolph, AE, Price, EV: Penicillin reactions among patients in venereal disease clinics. A national survey. *JAMA 223*:499–501, 1973.
154. Weinstein, L: Perspectives in infectious diseases. *N.Y. State J. Med. 76*:1836, 1976.
155. Holt, R: The bacterial degradation of chloramphenicol. *Lancet 1*:1259–1260, 1967.
156. Dameshak, W: Chloramphenicol aplastic anemia in identical twins—a clue to pathogenesis. *N. Engl. J. Med. 281*:42–43, 1969.
157. Yunis, AA: Chloramphenicol-induced bone marrow suppression. *Semin. Hematol. 10*:225–234, 1973.
158. Morley, A, Trainor, K, Renes, J: Residual marrow damage: Possible explanation for idiosyncrasy to chloramphenicol. *Br. J. Haematol. 32*:525–531, 1976.
159. Bella, DD: Biological properties of chloramphenicol as related to structural features: From classical knowledge to future developments. In: *Safety Problems Related to Chloramphenicol and Thiamphenicol Therapy* (Y Najean, G Tognoni, and A Yunis, eds.), Raven Press, New York, 1981, pp. 31–42.
160. Krishno, G, Aykac, J, Siegel, D: Recent studies on the mechanisms of chloramphenicol activation responsible for aplastic anemia. In: *Safety Problems Related to Chloramphenicol and Thiamphenicol Therapy* (Y Najean, G Tognoni, and A Yunis, eds.), Raven Press, New York, 1981, pp. 5–16.
161. Yunis, AA: Chloramphenicol toxicity and the role of the *p*-nitro in aplastic anemia. In: *Safety Problems Related to Chloramphenicol and Thiamphenicol Therapy* (Y Najean, G Tognoni, and A Yunid, eds.), Raven Press, New York, 1983, pp. 17–30.
162. Gerson, WT, Fine, DG, Spielberg, SP, Sensenbremmer, CC: Anticonvulsant-induced aplastic anemia; increased susceptibility to toxic drug metabolites in vitro. *Blood 6*: 889–893, 1983.
163. Spielberg, SP: In vitro assessment of pharmacogenetic susceptibility to toxic drug metabolites in man. *Fed. Proc. 43*:2308–2313, 1984.
164. Yunis, AA: Differential in vitro toxicity of chloramphenicol, nitroso-chloramphenicol and thiamphenicol. *Sex. Transm. Dis. 11*:340–342, 1984.
165. Matthews, SJ, Shawver-Matthews, S: Chloramphenicol toxicity—oral versus intravenous administration. *J. Pediatr. 97*:869, 1980.

166. Rosenthal, RI, Blackman, A: Bone marrow hypoplasia following use of chloramphenicol eye drops. *JAMA 191*:148–149, 1965.
167. Pickering, LK, Cleary, TG, Kohl, SK: Chloramphenicol toxicity—oral versus intravenous administration (reply). *J. Pediatr. 97*:869–870, 1980.
168. Fraunfelder, FT, Bagley, GG, Kelly, DJ: Fatal aplastic anemia following topical administration of ophthalmologic chloramphenicol. *Am. J. Ophthalmol. 93*:356–360, 1982.
169. Fripp, RR, Carter, MC, Werner, J, et al.: Cardiac function and acute chloramphenicol toxicity. *J. Pediatr. 103*:487–490, 1983.
170. Wilkinson, JD, Pollack, MM, Costello, J: Chloramphenicol toxicity: Hemodynamic and oxygen utilization effects. *Pediatr. Infect. Dis. 4*:69–72, 1985.
171. Evans, LS, Kleiman, MB: Acidosis as a presenting feature of chloramphenicol toxicity. *J. Pediatr. 108*:475–477, 1986.
172. Werner, JC, Whitman, V, Schuler, HG, et al.: Acute myocardial effects of chloramphenicol in newborn pigs; a possible insight into the grey baby syndrome. *J. Infect. Dis. 152*:344–350, 1985.
173. Mauer, SM, Chavers, BM, Kjellstrand, CM: Treatment of an infant with severe chloramphenicol intoxication using charcoal-column hemoperfusion. *J. Pediatr. 96*:136–139, 1980.
174. Stevens, DC, Kleiman, MB, Lietman, PS: Exchange transfusion in acute chloramphenicol toxicity. *Br. Clin. Lab. Observ. 99*:651–653, 1981.
175. Freundlich, M, Cynamon, H, Tamer, A, et al.: Management of chloramphenicol intoxication in infancy by charcoal hemoperfusion. *J. Pediatr. 103*:485–490, 1983.
176. Phadke, MV, Joshi, VS, Naik, SG: Toxicity of chloramphenicol in children. *J. Indian Med. Assoc. 37*:26–30, 1961.
177. Bartlett, JG: Antibiotic-associated pseudomembranous colitis. *Rev. Infect. Dis. 1*: 530–539, 1979.
178. Casale, TB, Macher, AM, Fauci, AS: Complete hematologic and hepatic recovery in a patient with chloramphenicol hepatic-pancytopenia syndrome. *J. Pediatr. 101*: 1025, 1982.
179. Casale, TB, Macher, AM, Fauci, AS: Do we really need to monitor liver function in patients receiving chloramphenicol (reply)? *J. Pediatr. 103*:342, 1983.
180. Feder, HM, Jr.: Do we really need to monitor liver function in patients receiving chloramphenicol? *J. Pediatr. 103*:341–342, 1983.
181. Levine, PH, Regelson, W, Holland, JF: Chloramphenicol-associated encephalopathy. *Clin. Pharmacol. Ther. 11*:194–198, 1970.
182. Joy, RJT, Scaletter, R, Sodee, DB: Optic and peripheral neuritis: Probable effect of prolonged chloramphenicol therapy. *JAMA 173*:1731–1734, 1960.
183. Kapp, JP, Arora, B, Sibingo, MS: Depression of erythropoiesis, physical growth and hair growth by chloramphenicol in a three-year old child with cystic fibrosis. *Clin. Pediatr. 16*:64–66, 1977.
184. Caulfield, JB, Burke, JF: Inhibition of wound healing by chloramphenicol. *Arch. Pathol. 92*:119–125, 1971.
185. Damert, GJ, Sohule, PG: Effect of chloramphenicol on in vitro function of lymphocytes. *J. Infect. Dis. 139*:220–224, 1979.
186. Kaplan, SS, Finch, S: Studies on the mechanism of chloramphenicol impairment of human leucocyte function (34778). *Proc. Soc. Exp. Biol. Med. 134*:287–290, 1970.
187. Weisberger, AS: Mechanisms of action of chloramphenicol. *JAMA 209*:97–103, 1969.
188. McCaffrey, RP, Halstead, CH, Wahab, MFA, Robertson, RP: Chloramphenicol-induced hemolysis in caucasian glucose-6-phosphate dehydrogenase deficiency. *Ann. Intern. Med. 74*:722–726, 1971.

189. Chan, TK, Chesteman, CN, Macfadyean, AJ, Todd, D: The survival of glucose-6-phosphate dehydrogenase-deficient erythrocytes in patients with typhoid fever on chloramphenicol therapy. *J. Lab. Clin. Med.* *77*:177–184, 1971.
190. Drexel, H, Kirchmair, W, Dientsl, F: Anaphylactic shock after intravenous chloramphenicol. *Milit. Med.* *123*:756, 1981.
191. Anonymous: Chloramphenicol. In: *Drugs in Pregnancy and Lactation* (GG Briggs, TW Brodendor, RK Freeman, and SJ Yaffe, eds.), Williams and Wilkins, Baltimore, 1983, pp. 62–63.
192. Dixon, RL, Fonts, JR: Inhibition of microsomal drug metabolising pathways by chloramphenicol. *Biochem. Pharmacol.* *11*:715–720, 1962.
193. Grogan, DE, Lane, M, Smith, FE, et al.: Interactions of flavins and chloramphenicol with microsomal enzyme systems. *Biochem. Pharmacol.* *21*:3131–3144, 1972.
194. Adams, HR, Issacson, E, Masters, BBS: Inhibition of hepatic microsomal enzymes by chloramphenicol. *J. Pharmacol. Exp. Ther.* *203*:388–396, 1977.
195. Christensen, LK, Skovsted, L: Inhibition of drug metabolism by chloramphenicol. *Lancet* *2*:1397–1399, 1969.
196. Krausinski, K, Kusmeisz, H, Nelson, JD: Pharmacologic interactions among chloramphenicol, phenytoin and phenobarbital. *Pediatr. Infect. Dis.* *1*:232–235, 1982.
197. Adams, HR: Pharmacodynamic actions of antimicrobial agents in host cell membranes. *J. Am. Vet. Med. Assoc.* *185*:1127–1130, 1984.
198. Prober, CG: Effect of rifampin on chloramphenicol levels. *N. Engl. J. Med.* *312*:1127–1130, 1984.
199. Kay, L, Kampman, JP, Svendsen, TL, et al.: Influence of rifampicin and isoziazid on the kinetics of phenytoin. *Br. J. Clin. Pharmacol.* *20*:323–326, 1985.
200. Buchanan, N, Moodley, GP: Interaction between chloramphenicol and paracetamol. *Br. Med. J.* *2*:367, 1979.
201. Kearns, GL, Bocchini, JA, Jr., Brown, RD, et al.: Absence of a pharmacokinetic interaction between chloramphenicol and acetaminophen in children. *J. Pediatr.* *107*:134–139, 1985.
202. Asmar, BI, Dajani, AS: Ampicillin-chloramphenicol interaction against enteric gram-negative organisms. *Pediatr. Infect. Dis.* *2*:39–42, 1983.
203. Stowe, CM: Antimicrobial drug interactions. *J. Am. Vet. Med. Assoc.* *185*:1137–1141, 1984.

17
Macrolide Antibiotics

CHARLES M. GINSBURG
University of Texas Health Science Center at Dallas, Dallas, Texas

The macrolide ("large-ring") antibiotics are a class of chemical compounds characterized by a multimembered lactone ring to which single or multiple ketones and amino sugars are attached. Members of this class include erythromycin, troleandomycin, josamycin, and rosamycin. Although each of these agents has been tested in humans and has been approved for clinical use, only erythromycin has achieved widespread clinical usage in infants and children.

Erythromycin is derived from a strain of *Streptomyces erytheus*, an acetinomycete that was first isolated over 30 years ago from soil collected in the Phillipine Archipelago (1). Over the years, there have been a variety of chemical modifications to the basic macrocyclic lactone nucleus of erythromycin (Figures 1 and 2). These alterations were designed to produce analogs with enhanced bioavailability and a smaller incidence of adverse effects than the parent compound. Currently, there are two parenteral (gluceptate and lactiobionate) and four oral forms of erythromycin (base, stearate, ethylsuccinate, and estolate) that are approved for clinical use. Additionally, "acid-resistant" coatings of various types have been applied to erythromycin base to produce enteric-coated formulations. Neither of the parenteral preparations is used with any frequency in infants and children.

I. CHEMISTRY

Erythromycin base is a bitter, basic (pK_a = 8.6) white crystalline compound that is relatively insoluble in water but readily soluble in organic acids. The drug is relatively stable at 4°C but rapidly loses antimicrobial activity at higher temperatures. Following oral administration, erythromycin base is susceptible to gastric acid inactivation, and this leads to erratic absorption and inconsistent serum and tissue concentrations (2-4). The stearate, a salt, and the ethylsuccinate, an ester, are more resistant to the effects of gastric secretion than is the base; the estolate, a salt of a strong acid, is not displaced by the weaker gastric acids and, therefore, is more resistant to inactivation than the other oral compounds (5-12).

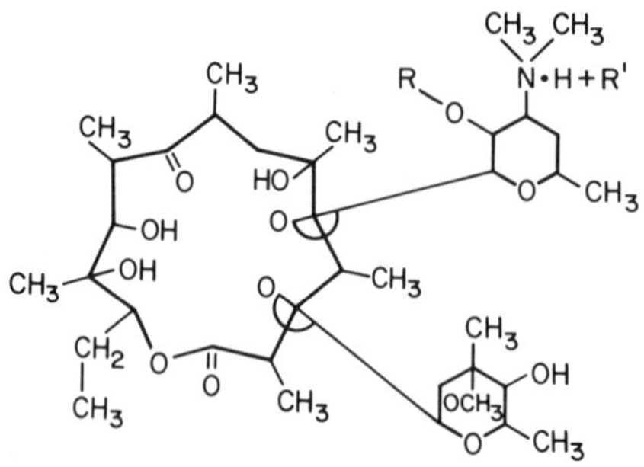

Figure 1 Chemical structure of the macrocylic lactone nucleus of erythromycin.

	R	R
Erythromycin Base	H	
Erythromycin Stearate	H	$C_{17}H_{35}COO$
Erythromycin Estolate	CH_2CH_2CO	$C_{12}H_{25}O5O_3$
Erythromycin Ethyl Succinate	$CH_2CH_2OOCCH_2$	CH_2COO

Figure 2 Oral analogs of erythromycin.

II. MECHANISM OF ACTION

Macrolide antibiotics exert their antimicrobial activity at the 50S bacterial ribosome (13, 14). The precise mechanism of their action is not entirely understood; however, these agents appear to disrupt the functional cycle of the microbe by binding specific ribosomal subunits. The specificity of action of the drug at these sites inhibits peptide bond formation without altering the nucleic acid cycle. As such, there is a potential for competitive interference at the ribosomal site; therefore, erythromycin and other members of the macrolide group of antibiotics may inhibit the antimicrobial activity of chloramphenicol, lincomycin, and other agents that target the 50S ribosomal subunits (14). Resistance to erythromycin or other macrolides may occur when microbes undergo mutational changes in the ribosomal subunit that result in altered binding sites.

III. ANTIMICROBIAL ACTIVITY

The activity of erythromycin against a variety of bacterial strains is shown in Table 1. In vitro, erythromycin is most active against gram-positive bacteria, including many strains of β-lactamase-producing *Staphylococcus aureus*. Although the Enterobacteriaciae are generally resistant to erythromycin, some gram-negative bacilli, such as *Hemophilus influenzae* and species of *Neisseria*, have varying degrees of susceptibility to the drug. Strains of *Neisseria gonorrhoeae* are generally susceptible to concentrations of 0.1 μg/ml or less.

Most anaerobic bacteria, particularly those inhabiting the oropharyngx, are susceptible to erythromycin. Approximately 50% of strains of *Bacteroides fragilis* are inhibited by concentrations of erythromycin of 3.12 μg/ml or less. Erythromycin is active against

Table 1 In Vitro Activity of Erythromycin

Organism	Minimal inhibitory concentration (μg/ml) Mean (MIC_{50})	Range
Streptococcus pneumoniae	0.03	0.003–0.4
Corynbacterium diphtheriae	0.1	0.003–3.12
Campylobacter jejuni	0.12	0.1–100
Streptococcus pyogenes	0.04	0.007–0.62
Legionella pneumophilia	0.2	0.0625–0.5
Staphylococcus aureus	0.4	0.005–100
Clostridium tetani	0.6	0.2–0.7
C. perfringens	0.5	0.5–3.12
Corynebacterium acnes	0.48	0.006–0.78
Bacteroides fragilis	0.78	0.096–25
Peptostreptococcus sp.	0.19	0.024–0.39
Hemophilus influenzae	3.12	0.1–6.25
Bordetella pertussis	0.29	0.02–1.56
Neisseria gonorrhoeae	0.1	0.004–6.25
N. meningitidis	3.12	0.20–6.25
Mycoplasma pneumoniae	0.0125	0.006–0.025
Brucella	5.0	0.3–10.0
Escherichia coli	100	12.5–100
Shigella	100	25–100
Salmonella	100	12.5–100
Klebsiella pneumoniae	100	3.12–100
Pseudomonas	100	100

some microaerophilic to anaerobic organisms; however, the range of inhibitory concentrations for these organisms is large. Strains of *Campylobacter jejuni* are generally susceptible to erythromycin. The susceptibility of *Mycobacteria* to erythromycin is highly variable; strains of *Mycobacterium scrofulaceum*, *Mycobacterium kansasii*, and *Mycobacterium terrae* are generally susceptible to concentrations of the drug that can be achieved in blood and tissue; others, such as *Mycobacterium fortuitum*, are uniformally resistant. Yeasts and fungi are also resistant to erythromycin.

IV. CLINICAL PHARMACOLOGY

Erythromycin passes readily into most tissue and body fluids (15-24), with the exception of cerebrospinal fluid, where, even in the presence of meningeal irritation, the concentrations of drug are subtherapeutic for susceptible bacteria. Like other members of the macrolide class, erythromycin is concentrated in the liver, where demethylation to des-*N*-methyl erythromycin takes place by a microsomal system requiring cytochrome P_{450}.

Excretion of orally administered erythromycin occurs primarily into the bile and feces. For reasons that are unclear, the amount of biliary excretion of erythromycin base exceeds that of the estolate (18). Only 3–5% of an orally administered dose of erythromycin is excreted in the urine, with excretion solely dependent on glomerular filtration (24). There are few data on the excretion of erythromycin or any of the macrolide antibiotics in infants and children with compromised renal function; however, in anuric adults the serum half-life of these agents is not significantly affected, increasing from 1.6 to approximately 5 hr.

A. Erythromycin Base

There are few data on the pharmacokinetics of erythromycin base in infants and children. Because the instability of the drug in gastric secretions leads to erratic absorption and inconsistent serum concentrations, various acid-resistant coatings have been applied to the base to enhance absorption and bioavailability. In the only pharmacological study of erythromycin enteric-coated base in infants and children, Ginsburg and associates found peak plasma concentrations of erythromycin of 3–4 μg/ml at 2–3 hr following the oral administration of 15 mg/kg doses of erythromycin enteric-coated base administered in a mixture of applesauce and water or applesauce and milk (25). The mean concentrations of erythromycin in serum at 4 and 6 hr after administration were larger in patients who received the drug with water than with milk. By 8 hr, the last sample period, erythromycin was detectable in all sample specimens from both groups of patients in concentrations ranging from 0.06 to 1.68 μg/ml (Figure 3).

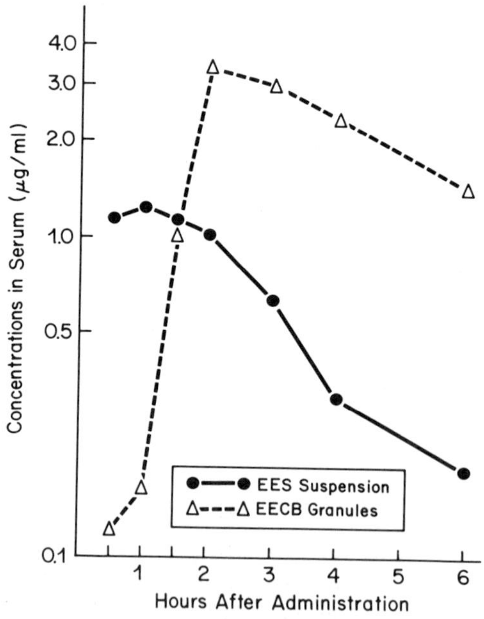

Figure 3 Serum concentrations of erythromycin following erythromycin ethylsuccinate suspension (15 mg/kg) and erythromycin coated base granules (15 mg/kg). (Reprinted with permission from *Pediatric Infectious Disease*.)

In crossover studies comparing erythromycin enteric-coated base and erythromycin ethylsuccinate suspension administered in applesauce to infants and children, there were significant differences in the bioavailability of the two preparations (25). The time to peak serum concentrations was longer after erythromycin enteric-coated base than after ethylsuccinate suspension; however, the mean peak serum concentrations of erythromycin were three to fourfold larger and the area under the curve (AUC) was approximately 200% greater following erythromycin enteric-coated base than after erythromycin ethylsuccinate. The delayed time to peak following the erythromycin base is undoubtedly a reflection of the delayed absorption of the erythromycin enteric-coated base from the gastrointestinal tract.

There are no pharmacological studies with erythromycin ethylsuccinate in newborn infants; however, Patamasucon and colleagues studied the pharmacokinetics of erythromycin ethylsuccinate suspension after single and multiple doses in infants younger than 4 months of age (26). After a 10 mg/kg dose of erythromycin ethylsuccinate suspension, peak serum concentrations of 1.1 μg/ml of erythromycin occurred 1 hr after ingestion and drug was detectable in serum in concentrations of 0.5 μg/ml or greater for up to 6 hr (Figure 4). Aside from the delay in the time to peak in infants who received multiple doses of the drug, there were no significant differences in the peak serum concentrations, elimination half-lives, or AUC values between the infants who were studied after single and multiple doses. McCracken and colleagues reported similar findings in a study of the pharmacology of erythromycin ethylsuccinate suspension in fasting and nonfasting children (27). In these studies, the serum concentrations of erythromycin after 15 mg/kg doses of erythromycin ethylsuccinate suspension in nonfasting patients were from 30 to 80% greater than those observed in children who received the drug on an empty stomach. Furthermore, the mean serum concentrations were larger at all time intervals from 0.5 to 6 hr in patients who received the drug with infant formula. This is reflected in the larger area under the curve values in fasting (4.8 μg/ml-hr) than nonfasting (2.4 mg/ml-hr)

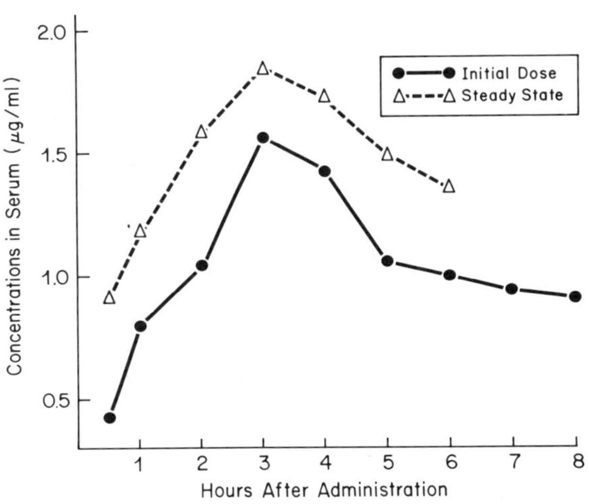

Figure 4 Serum concentrations of erythromycin after erythromycin estolate suspension (10 mg/kg). (Adapted from Patamasucon, P, et al.: *Antimicrob. Agents Chemother. 19*: 736, 1981.)

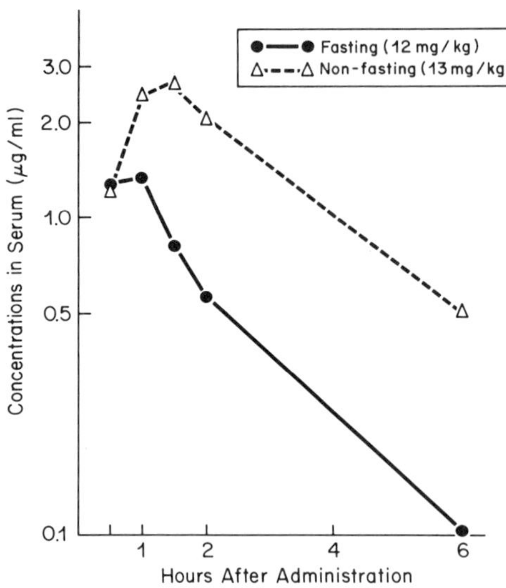

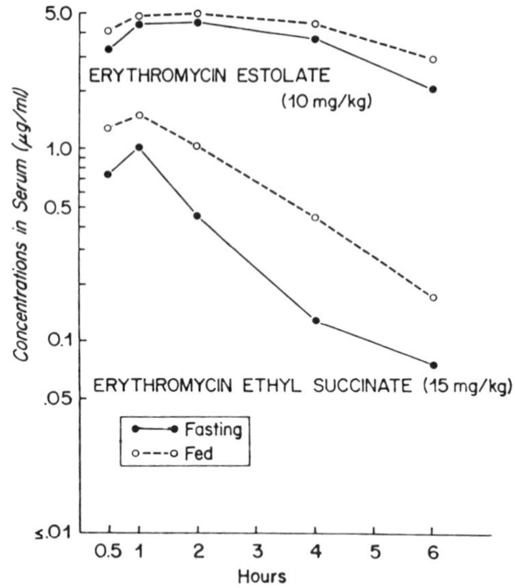

Figure 5 Serum concentrations of erythromycin following erythromycin ethylsuccinate granules. (Adapted from Coyne, TC, et al.: *J. Clin. Pharmacol. 18*:194, 1978.)

Figure 6 Serum concentrations of erythromycin after erythromycin estolate (10 mg/kg) and erythromycin ethylsuccinate (15 mg/kg). (Reprinted with permission from *Annals of Otology, Rhinology and Laryngology 90*:37, 1981.)

patients. Coyne and associates studied the pharmacokinetics of erythromycin ethylsuccinate administered in the form of granules (28). Following ingestion of 13 mg/kg doses, peak concentrations of erythromycin in serum occurred at 1 hr in fasting children and at 2 hr in children who ingested the drug with a meal consisting of infant formula, soda crackers, and applesauce (Figure 5). In these studies, the serum concentrations were significantly larger at 1.5, 2, and 6 hr and the area under the curve was 300% larger in children who ingested the granules with food compared with those who received the drug in a fasting state. The authors concluded that erythromycin ethylsuccinate granules should be administered in the presence of food to achieve maximum bioavailability.

B. Erythromycin Estolate

Erythromycin estolate suspension is rapidly absorbed following oral administration and produces larger concentrations in serum than do the other oral forms of erythromycin (27). Burns and Hodgman studied the pharmacokinetics of erythromycin estolate after single and multiple doses in 87 low-birth-weight infants who weighed from 1500 to 2500 g (29). After 10 mg/kg doses of erythromycin estolate delivered by nasogastric tube, mean peak concentrations of 1.8 and 1.2 μg/ml of erythromycin occurred at 2 hr in infants weighing 1500–2001 g and 2001–2500 g, respectively. Erythromycin was present in the serum of all patients in concentrations ranging from 0.03 to 3.45 μg/ml at 6 hr after the dose. By 12 hr, 43% of the serum samples contained concentrations of erythromycin of 0.5 μg/ml or greater; however, by 24 hr there was no drug detectable in the serum of any of the infants. The pharmacokinetics of the estolate were independent of birth weight and age. Furthermore, the investigators found no evidence of accumulation of erythromycin estolate in the serum of another group of low-birth-weight infants of the same age who received multiple doses of erythromycin estolate over an 8-day period. Although there are no similar data on the pharmacokinetics of erythromycin estolate in term infants, Patamasucon and colleagues compared the pharmacokinetics of erythromycin estolate and erythromycin ethylsuccinate in young infants (mean age, 29 days) who were receiving erythromycin ethylsuccinate or erythromycin estolate for treatment for chlamydial conjunctivitis (26). Following 10 mg/kg doses of the drugs, peak concentration of 1.8 and 1.3 μg/ml occurred in the serum of patients who received erythromycin estolate and erythromycin ethylsuccinate, respectively. After the first hour following ingestion, the concentrations of erythromycin in serum were significantly larger, at all time intervals, in patients who received erythromycin estolate; the AUC value for the estolate was three to fourfold larger than that of the ethylsuccinate. Similar differences between the two formulations were observed by McCracken et al. in studies performed in older infants and children who were studied in crossover fashion in the fasting and nonfasting state (27). In this latter study, the dose of the ethylsuccinate (15 mg/kg) was 50% greater than that of the estolate (10 mg/kg); however, the serum concentrations of erythromycin following the ethylsuccinate were only 20-25% of those achieved with the estolate (Figure 6). Coadministration of the erythromycin estolate in milk did not affect serum concentrations. By contrast, the serum concentrations in nonfasting patients who received the ethylsuccinate were 30-80% greater than those observed in patients who received the drug while fasting.

V. CONCENTRATIONS OF ERYTHROMYCIN IN BODY FLUIDS

A. Placental Transfer

Kiefer and associates obtained cord blood and amniotic fluid samples from infants born to mothers who received a single and multiple doses of erythromycin in dosages ranging from 200 to 800 mg (30). Following single doses of erythromycin administered to the mother 2 hr prior to delivery or cesarean section, only 1 of 18 cord blood and none of the amniotic fluid samples contained measurable antimicrobial activity (Figure 7). It is difficult, however, to evaluate these data since 38% of the maternal blood specimens had no antimicrobial activity detectable in their serum at the time of delivery. By contrast, erythromycin was detectable in the maternal serum of all patients who received multiple 800 mg doses of erythromycin estolate; erythromycin was detectable in the cord blood of 8 of these 12 infants.

Philapson et al. administered single and multiple oral doses of erythromycin base or erythromycin estolate to pregnant women who were undergoing therapeutic abortions (31) (Figure 8). They reported that the mean concentrations of erythromycin in fetal blood at 4 hr after administration of an oral dose to the mother was 0.02 μg/ml after a single dose and 0.6 μg/ml after multiple doses. The mean maternal erythromycin serum concentrations at the time of the abortions were 1.41 and 3.48 μg/ml in women who received single and multiple doses, respectively. The difference in the serum concentrations that were observed after single and multiple doses also occurred in fetal tissues. After a single dose of erythromycin, drug was detectable in the fetal liver but not in any of the other fetal tissues that were studied. By contrast, all of the fetal tissues, including brain and bone, had detectable antimicrobial activity after multiple doses of the drug were administered to the mother. The largest concentrations of erythromycin occurred in

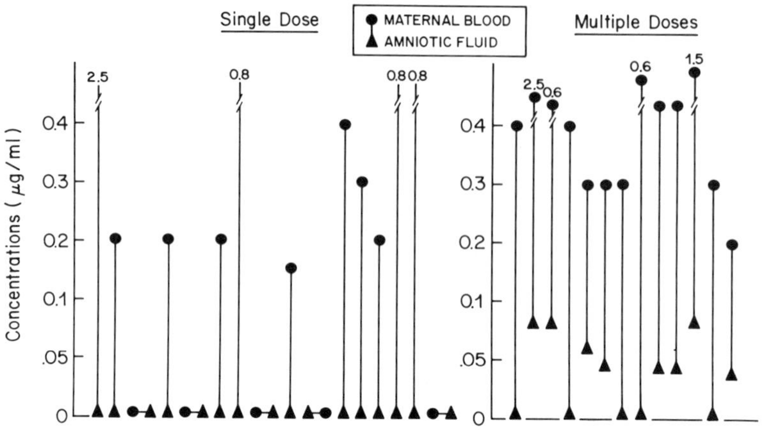

Figure 7 Concentrations of erythromycin in maternal blood and amniotic fluid after erythromycin estolate. (Adapted from Kiefer, L, et al.: *Am. J. Obstet. Gynecol. 69*:174, 1955. Reprinted with permission from *Pediatric Infectious Disease*.)

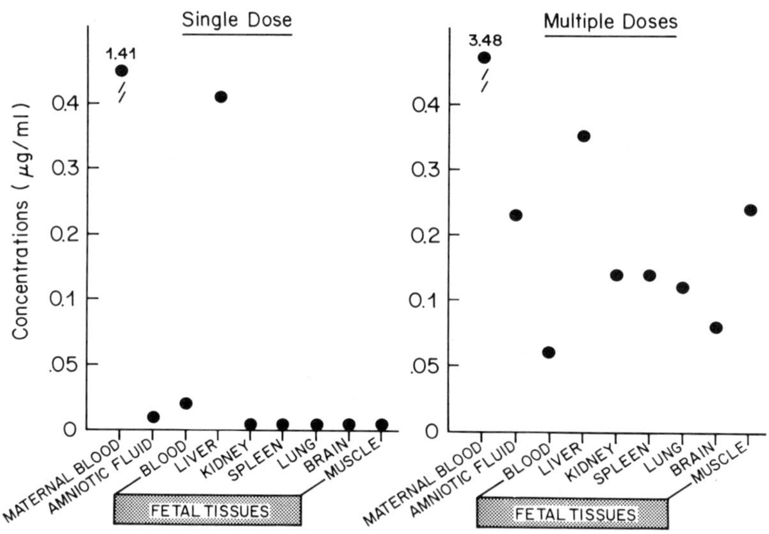

Figure 8 Concentrations of erythromycin in fetal tissues in relation to concentrations in maternal blood after 500 mg doses of erythromycin estolate. (Adapted from Philapson, A, Sabath, LD, Charles, D: *N. Engl. J. Med. 288*:1218, 1973. Reprinted with permission from *Pediatric Infectious Disease*.)

the liver, where the mean concentrations were approximately 10% of the maternal serum concentrations and fivefold larger than in fetal serum.

B. Tonsils

There are limited data available on the concentrations of erythromycin achieved in tonsillar tissue of children after ingestion of one of the oral formulations of erythromycin. Ginsburg and associates studied serum and tonsillar concentrations of erythromycin after single and multiple doses of erythromycin ethylsuccinate (15 mg/kg) and erythromycin estolate (10 mg/kg) in children who were undergoing tonsillectomy (32). The tonsil concentrations of erythromycin following the estolate ranged from 0.3 to 2.3 μg/ml and those of the ethylsuccinate were from nondetectable to 1.3 μg/ml. The concentrations of erythromycin in serum and tonsil found after one or many doses of the estolate were significantly greater than those obtained after single or multiple doses of the ethylsuccinate (Figure 9). Additionally, the concentrations of drug in tonsil after multiple doses of either suspension were larger than those obtained after a single dose.

C. Tears

McCracken et al. measured tear concentrations of erythromycin in infants who were receiving erythromycin estolate or erythromycin ethylsuccinate for the treatment of skin and soft tissue infection (27). In these studies, erythromycin was present in tears throughout the 6-hr study period, and in many instances the concentration of drug in the tears exceeded those in the blood. The tear levels did, however, parallel the concentrations in

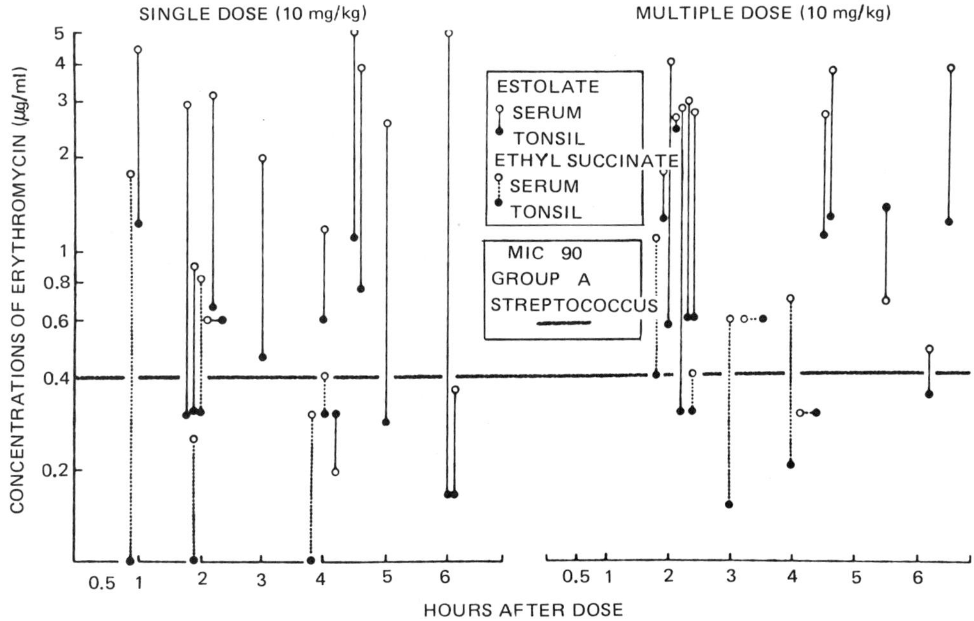

Figure 9 Concentrations of erythromycin in serum and tonsils after single and multiple doses of erythromycin estolate and erythromycin ethylsuccinate. (Reprinted with permission from *J. Pediatr.*)

the serum; 18 of 22 tear samples (82%) from estolate-treated patients contained ≥ 1 μg/ml of drug but only 11 of 25 (44%) ethylsuccinate-treated patients had similar levels. The tear concentrations of both erythromycin preparations were unaffected by concomitant milk and drug administration.

Patamasucon et al. found that 69% of tear specimens from infants who received erythromycin for treatment of chlamydial conjunctivitis had larger erythromycin concentrations than the highest serum concentrations measured in the patient (26). Although the mean tear concentration (2.7 μg/ml) of erythromycin exceeded the mean serum concentrations (1.29 μg/ml) in ethylsuccinate-treated patients, this was not the case in patients who received the estolate. In this latter group, the mean concentrations in the two body fluids were similar. Overall, the mean tear concentrations between the estolate- and ethylsuccinate-treated patients were not significantly different.

D. Middle Ear Fluid

Although various forms of erythromycin, particularly ethylsuccinate and erythromycin estolate, have been used alone and in combination for the treatment of infants and children with otitis media for the past two decades, there is a limited amount of information available on the concentration of erythromycin that is achieved in the middle ear fluids.

Bass and associates administered 12.5 mg/kg doses of erythromycin ethylsuccinate and erythromycin estolate to infants and children with acute otitis media and measured the concentrations of erythromycin in middle ear fluid 2 hr postingestion (33). In these studies, the concentrations of erythromycin ranged from less than 0.07 to 1.2 μg/ml following the ethylsuccinate and from 1.68 to 8.0 μg/ml after the estolate. The mean concentration at 2 hr was 0.84 and 4.18 μg/ml for patients who received ethylsuccinate and estolate, respectively. In another study performed in children with acute purulent otitis media, Ginsburg et al. reported that the concentrations of erythromycin were larger in middle ear fluid and serum at 1-2 hr in patients who received erythromycin estolate compared with those who received equimolar doses (15 mg/kg) of erythromycin ethylsuccinate suspension (Figure 10) (34). All estolate-treated patients and six of eight ethylsuccinate-treated patients had concentrations of drug in middle ear fluid in excess of the MIC_{90} for strains of *H. influenzae*. Nelson and associates measured the concentration of erythromycin in the middle ear fluid of children with middle ear effusions who were undergoing surgery for implantation of tympanostomy tubes (35). Approximately 45 min after ingesting 10 mg/kg doses of either erythromycin ethylsuccinate or erythromycin estolate in suspension form, erythromycin was detectable in the middle ear fluid of all patients. The mean concentration of the estolate was substantially larger (1.95 μg/ml) than that of the ethylsuccinate (0.31 μg/ml). The levels were in excess of the minimum inhibitory concentrations for *S. pneumoniae* and *Staphylococcus pyogenes* but smaller than those required for treatment of most infections caused by *H. influenzae*.

E. Saliva

Based on the hypothesis that the antimicrobial concentration in saliva might accurately reflect the concentration of drug in the middle ear fluid and, thus, provide investigators with a noninvasive method for determining middle ear concentrations of antibiotics, Ginsburg and associates studied the salivary concentrations of a number of orally administered antimicrobials (27,34). Following 10 and 15 mg/kg doses of erythromycin

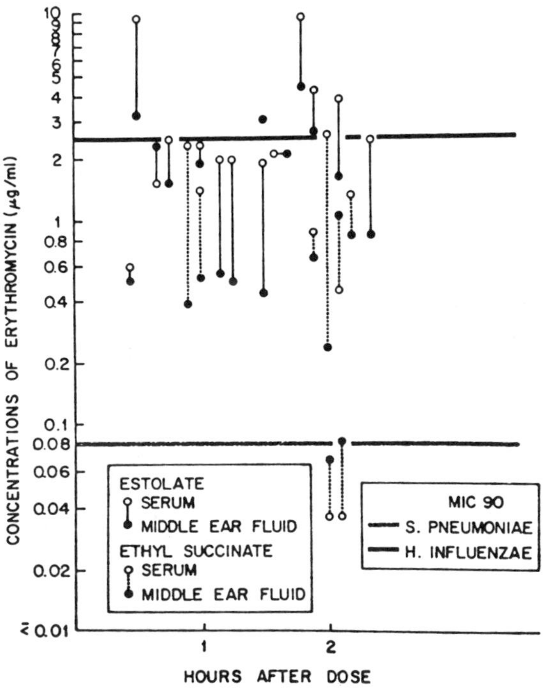

Figure 10 Middle ear fluid concentrations of erythromycin after 15 mg/kg doses of erythromycin estolate and erythromycin ethylsuccinate. (Reprinted with permission from *Annals of Otology, Rhinology and Laryngology 90*:36, 1981.)

estolate and erythromycin ethylsuccinate suspensions, respectively, concentrations of erythromycin of ⩾0.1 μg/ml were detected in 80–88% of salivary samples. The levels exceeded the MIC values for most pneumococci (0.01–0.2 μg/ml) and group A streptococci (0.02–0.2 μg/ml) but were smaller than the MIC values for most strains of *H. influenzae*. In these studies, the concentrations of erythromycin in saliva were unaffected by the feeding status of the infant and, despite the marked disparity in the serum concentrations in the AUC values of the two formulations, the salivary concentrations after both drugs were comparable. Unfortunately, however, the concentrations in saliva did not correlate accurately with the concentrations in the middle ear fluid.

In these crossover studies, designed to determine if the salivary concentrations of drug following ingestion of pediatric suspensions might represent a residuum of the orally administered suspension rather than reflecting active penetration of the drug into saliva, concentrations of erythromycin in saliva of adult patients who ingested the ethylsuccinate were larger, at all time intervals, in patients who ingested suspension or chewed tablets than in those who swallowed the tablets intact (27). The concentrations of drug in the saliva of patients who swallowed the tablet were similar to those found in infants who ingested the drug in suspension form. By contrast, none of the volunteers who ingested erythromycin estolate in capsule form had drug detectable in their saliva 1 hr postingestion. This, undoubtedly, represents delayed absorption from the gastrointestinal tract rather than failure of the drug to penetrate in the salivary secretions since erythromycin was detectable in all salivary samples at 4 hr. The percentage of patients who had erythromycin detectable in their saliva at 4 hr following ingestion of the solid formulation was larger following the estolate (10 of 10; 100%) than the ethylsuccinate (2 of 7; 28.5%).

VI. CLINICAL USES

Since its introduction in 1952, the clinical efficacy of erythromycin has been proven repeatedly against various gram-positive infections. Both penicillin-sensitive and penicillin-resistant *S. aureus* infections (meningitis, osteomyelitis, furuncles, pneumonia, bacteremia, endocarditis) have been successfully treated with the drug. However, emerging resistance and the formulation of penicillinase-resistant penicillins, cephalosporins, and clindamycin has diminished these indications.

Streptococcus A pyogenes infections (pharyngitis, scarlet fever, and erysipelas) are very sensitive to erythromycin, and the drug is widely used in children allergic to penicillins suffering from these conditions. Similarly, the drug may be considered in the prophylaxis of rheumatic fever in penicillin-allergic children. Erythromycin has been employed for intropartum therapy of vertical transmission of group B *Streptococcus*. The drug is effective in the treatment of pneumococcal pneumonia and meningitis, although currently penicillins or cephalosporins are the first-choice drugs for these indications.

In some cases of subacute bacterial endocarditis caused by *Streptococcus viridans*, erythromycin administered intravenously has been shown to be effective. Complete eradication of diptheria bacillus was shown in cases of carrier state treated with erythromycin orally. Erythromycin may be considered in the treatment of *Clostridium tetani* infections in combination with the antitoxin.

Atypical pneumonia caused by *Mycoplasma pneumoniae* may be treated effectively with erythromycin. Similarly, the drug is used for treatment of pregnant women with evidence of genital mycoplasma. Erythromycin is an effective substitute for penicillins in the case of gonorrheal infections.

VII. TOXICITY

Erythromycin has been regarded as one of the safest antimicrobials that is administered to infants and children (36). Anaphylactoid and other hypersensitivity reactions are exceedingly uncommon (37). Kuder reported skin eruptions or other possible allergic reactions in only 0.5% of 20,525 patients who received erythromycin estolate or proprionyl erythromycin (38). The most common adverse reaction associated with the oral erythromycin preparations is gastrointestinal distress. Nausea, vomiting, and epigastric pain have been reported to occur with varying frequency after ingestion of all forms of erythromycin. The adverse gastrointestinal symptoms appear to be dose related. Ginsburg et al. reported a 45% incidence of gastrointestinal complaints in children who were treated with 25 mg/kg doses of erythromycin ethylsuccinate for group A streptococcal pharyngitis (46). By contrast, only 5% of patients who received 15 mg/kg doses of erythromycin estolate had gastrointestinal symptoms. Although it has been suggested that gastrointestinal complaints can be attenuated or eliminated in adults if the oral erythromycins are administered with food, there are no data in children to confirm or refute this observation (39).

Ototoxicity, manifested by sudden bilateral sensorineural hearing loss, has been reported in adults who have received erythromycin (22,40). The majority of cases have occurred in patients who are in their fifth or sixth decade who have received the drug intravenously or in dialysate solution. Hearing loss generally in the range of 30–80 dB occurs during the first few days of administration of drug and, in many instances, is associated with dosages in excess of 4 g/day. In all reported cases, there was prompt return of auditory function within days to weeks after discontinuation of the drug. The mechanism for the auditory dysfunction is not known.

Hepatotoxicity is the most severe and well publicized of the adverse reactions caused by erythromycin (41). Signs and symptoms of erythromycin-induced hepatotoxicity generally occur 2–3 weeks into a course of therapy in patients who have not previously received erythromycin. By contrast, patients who have had erythromycin in the recent past will generally have onset of symptoms within 1–2 days after initiation of therapy. The clinical characteristics of the syndrome are fairly topical. Patients complain of nausea and epigastric pain; in some instances, the pain and physical findings are so severe that they mimic acute cholecytitis or an acute intra-abdominal process. Approximately 50% of patients have fever and higher chemical evidence of hepatic dysfunction. Eosinophilia, often in excess of 500 cells mm^{-3}, occurs in approximately two-thirds of patients.

These hepatotoxic reactions were thought to be unique for the estolate preparations; however, in recent years it has become apparent that all forms of erythromycin, including the base, are capable of producing this syndrome (41). Although the precise incidence of this hypersensitivity reaction is not known, it is estimated to occur in 0.1% of children and 0.25% of adults who are treated with erythromycin (42). Available evidence suggests that the syndrome is exceedingly rare in prepubertal children (36,43).

Fortunately, the clinical and laboratory abnormalities associated with erythromycin hepatotoxicity subside rapidly after discontinuation of the drug. Erythromycin should not be administered to any patient who has previously had clinical or biochemical evidence of hepatic dysfunction secondary to administration of erythromycin.

VIII. PHARMACOLOGICAL INTERACTIONS

Erythromycin and other members of the macrolide class have been reported to produce clinically significant pharmacological interactions with theophylline, carbamazepine, warfarin, digitalis, ergotamine, and methyl prednisolone (42). The interaction between erythromycin and theophylline has been that most thoroughly documented (44). Concomitant administration of these drugs has resulted in theophylline toxicity in children and adults presumably because of competitive inhibition by erythromycin for the binding site in the cytochrome P_{450} oxidase system. This results in increased body fluid concentrations of theophylline. Similar mechanisms have been proposed to explain the neurological toxicity that has occurred in patients who have received carbamazepine and erythromycin concurrently (45). In these instances, patients manifest dizziness, diplopia, drowsiness, headache, ataxia, and dysarthria as a result of the decreased hepatic metabolism of carbamizine. Within hours after discontinuing erythromycin, plasma concentrations of carbamazine decrease and toxic symptoms resolve. The mechanisms for the interaction between the macrolides and methyl prednisolone and warfarin are less well understood but also seem to be secondary to decreased hepatic metabolism of the drugs.

REFERENCES

1. McGuire, JM, Bunch, RL, Anderson, RC, et al.: "Ilotycin." A new antibiotic. *Antibiot. Chemother. 2*:1064–1065, 1952.
2. Smith, JW, Dyke, RW, Griffith, RS: Absorption following oral administration of erythromycin. *JAMA 151*:805–810, 1953.
3. Griffith, RS: Blood levels and clinical results with erythromycin. In: *Antibiotics Annual, 1954–1955*, (H Welch and F Marti-Ibanz, eds.), Medical Encyclopedia, Inc., New York, p. 269, 1955.
4. Josselyn, LE, Sylvester, JC: Absorption of erythromycin. *Antibiot. Chemother. 3*: 63–66, 1953.
5. Josselyn, LE, Edincoff, C, Sylvester, JC: Absorption of erythromycin. III. Various pharmaceutical forms. In: *Antibiotics Annual, 1954–1955* (H Welch and F Marti-Ibanez, eds.), Medical Encyclopedia, Inc., New York, p. 279, 1955.
6. Griffith, RS, Black, HR: Comparison of the blood levels obtained after single and multiple doses of erythromycin estolate and erythromycin stearate. *Am. J. Med. Sci. 243*:69–74, 1964.
7. Griffith, RS: Comparison of antibacterial activity in the sera of subjects ingesting propionyl erythromycin and propionyl erythromycin lauryl sulfate. *Antimicrob. Agents Annu.* 192–201, 1961.
8. Hirsch, HA, Pryles, CV, Finland, M: Effect of food on absorption of a new form of erythromycin propionate. *Am. J. Med. Sci. 239*:198–202, 1960.
9. Stephens, VC, Conine, JW, Murphy, HW: Esters of erythromycin. IV. Alkyl sulfate salts. *J. Am. Pharm. Assoc. 48*:620–622, 1959.
10. Lee, CC, Anderson, RC, Stephens, VC: Further studies on propionyl erythromycin ester lauryl sulfate. *Antibiot. Chemother. 11*:110–117, 1961.
11. Wick, WE, Mallet, GE: New analysis for the therapeutic efficacy of propionyl erythromycin and erythromycin base. *Antimicrob. Agents Chemother.* 410, 1968.
12. Stephens, VC, Pugh, CT, Davis, NE, et al.: A study of behavior of propionyl erythro mycin in blood by a new chromatographic method. *J. Antibiot. 22*:551–557, 1969.
13. Oleinick, NL, Corcoran, JW: Two types of binding of erythromycin to ribosomes from antibiotic-sensitive and resistant *Bacillus subtilis* 168, *J. Biol. Chem. 244*:727–735, 1969.
14. Taubman, SB, Jones, NR, Young, FE, Corcoran, JW: Sensitivity and resistance to erythromycin in *Bacillus subtilis* 168: The ribosomal binding of erythromycin and chloramphenicol. *Biochem. Biophys. Acta 123*:438–440, 1966.
15. Heilman, FR, Herrel, WE, Wellman, WE, Geraci, JE: Some laboratory and clinical observations on a new antibiotic, erythromycin (Ilotycin). *Proc. Staff Meet. Mayo Clin. 27*:285–304, 1952.
16. Borski, AA, Pulaski, EJ, Kimbrough, JC, Fusillo, MH: Prostatic fluid, semen, and prostatic tissue concentration of the major antibiotics following intravenous administration. *Antibiot. Chemother. 4*:905–910, 1954.
17. Winningham, DG, Nemoy, NJ, Stamey, TA: Diffusion of antibiotics from plasma into prostatic fluid. *Nature 219*:139–143, 1968.
18. Hammond, JB, Griffith, RS: Factors affecting the absorption and biliary excretion of erythromycin and two of its derivatives in humans. *Clin. Pharmacol. Ther. 2*: 308–312, 1961.
19. Bass, JW, Steele, RW, Wiebe, RA, Dierdorff, EP: Erythromycin concentrations in middle ear exudates. *Pediatrics 48*:417–422, 1971.
20. Smith, CB, Friedewald, WT, Chanock, RM: Shedding of *Mycoplasma pneumoniae* after tetracycline and erythromycin therapy. *N. Engl. J. Med. 276*:1172–1175, 1967.

21. Ginsburg, CM, McCracken, GH, Culbertson, MC: Concentrations of erythromycin in serum and tonsil: Comparison of the estolate and ethyl succinate preparations. *J. Pediatr. 89*:1011–1013, 1976.
22. Nolan, J, Lyle, W: Erythromycin in aqueous humor. *Trans. Ophthalmol. Soc. UK 96*:338–340, 1976.
23. Axelsson, A, Brorson, JE: The concentration of antibiotics in sinus secretions. *Oto-Rino-Laryngol. 83*:323–331, 1974.
24. Griffith, RS, Johnstone, DM, Smith, JW: The distribution and secretion of erythromycin following intravenous injection. In: *Antibiotics Annual, 1953-1954* (H Welch and F Marti-Ibanez, eds.), Medical Encyclopedia, Inc., New York, p. 496, 1955.
25. Ginsburg, CM, McCracken, GH, Petruska, M, Olson, U: Pharmacokinetics of erythromycin enteric coated base in children. Manuscript in preparation.
26. Patamasucon, P, Kaojaren, S, Kusmiesz, H, Nelson, JD: Pharmacokinetics of erythromycin ethylsuccinate and estolate in infants under 4 months of age. *Antimicrob. Agents Chemother. 19*:736–739, 1981.
27. McCracken, GH, Ginsburg, CM, Clahsen, J, Thomas, ML: Pharmacologic evaluation of orally administered antibiotics in infants and children: Effect of feeding on bioavailability. *Pediatrics 62*:738–743, 1978.
28. Coyne, TC, Shum, S, Chun, AHC, et al.: Bioavailability of erythromycin ethyl succinate in pediatric patients. *J. Clin. Pharmacol. 18*:194–202, 1978.
29. Burns, L, Hodgman, J: Studies of prematures given erythromycin estolate. *Am. J. Dis. Child. 106*:280–286, 1963.
30. Kiefer, L, Rubin, A, McCoy, JB, Foltz, EL: The placental transfer of erythromycin. *Am. J. Obstet. Gynecol. 69*:174–177, 1955.
31. Philapson, A, Sabath, LD, Charles, D: Transplacental passage of erythromycin and clindamycin. *N. Engl. J. Med. 288*:1219–1221, 1973.
32. Ginsburg, CM, McCracken, GH, Culbertson, MD: Concentrations of erythromycin in serum and tonsil: Comparison of the estolate and ethylsuccinate suspensions. *J. Pediatr. 89*:1011–1013, 1976.
33. Bass, JW, Steele, RW, Wiebe, RA, Dierdorff, EP: Erythromycin concentrations in middle ear exudates. *Pediatrics 48*:417–422, 1971.
34. Ginsburg, CM, McCracken, GH, Nelson, JD: Pharmacology of oral antibiotics used for treatment of otitis media and tonsillopharyngitis in infants and children. *Ann. Otol. 90*:37–43, 1981.
35. Nelson, JD, Ginsburg, CM, McCelland, O, et al.: Concentrations of antimicrobial agents in middle ear fluid, saliva and tears. *Int. J. Pediatr. Otorhinolaryngol. 3*: 326–334, 1981.
36. Ginsburg, CM, Eichenwald, HF: Erythromycin: A review of its uses in pediatric practice. *J. Pediatr. 89*:872–874, 1976.
37. Pigatto, PD, Riboldi, A, Riva, F, et al.: Fixed drug eruption to erythromycin. *Acta Derm. Venereol. (Stockh.) 64*:272–273, 1984.
38. Kvder, HV: Proprionyl erythromycin: A review of 20,525 case reports for side effect data. *Clin. Pharmacol. Ther. 1*:604–609, 1960.
39. Bechtol, LD, Bessent, CT, Perual, MB: The influence on food on absorption of erythromycin esters and enteric-coated erythromycin in single dose studies. *Curr. Ther. Res. 25*:618–625, 1979.
40. Haydon, RC, Thelin, JW, Davis, WE: Erythromycin ototoxicity: Analysis and conclusions based on 22 case reports. *Otolaryngol. Head Neck Surg. 92*:678–684, 1984.
41. Eichenward, HF: Adverse reactions to erythromycin. *J. Pediatr. Infect. Dis. 5*: 147–150, 1986.

42. *Fed. Register 47*:2247, 1982.
43. Ginsburg, CM: A prospective study on the incidence of liver function abnormalities in children receiving erythromycin estolate, erythromycin ethylsuccinate or penicillin V for treatment of pneumonia. *J. Pediatr. Infect. Dis. 5*:151–154, 1986.
44. Murray, MD, Brown, BK: Theophylline-erythromycin interaction in an infant. *Clin. Pharmacol. 1*:107–111, 1982.
45. Goulden, KJ, Camfield, P, Dooley, JM, et al.: Severe carbamazepine intoxication after coadministration of erythromycin. *J. Pediatr. 109*:135–137, 1986.
46. Ginsburg, CM, McCracken, GH, Crow, SD: Erythromycin therapy for Group A streptococcal pharyngitis: Results of a study of estolate and ethylsuccinate formulations. *Am. J. Dis. Child. 138*:536–539, 1984.

18
The Lincosamides

GIDEON KOREN
The Hospital for Sick Children, and the University of Toronto, Toronto, Ontario, Canada

Lincomycin was introduced in 1962 (1,2). It is produced by the actinomycete *Streptomyces lincolnensis*, which was isolated in earth from Lincoln, Nebraska. Clindamycin, a derivative of lincomycin, was first reported in the literature in 1967 (3). Gradually it has replaced its parent drug owing to its better absorption and superior antibacterial activity.

I. CHEMISTRY

Figure 1 shows the chemical structure of the lincosamides. Structurally, these agents are dissimilar from any other antibiotic. Both lincomycin and clindamycin are derivatives of the amino acid *trans*-L-4-*N*-propylhygrinic acid and are supplied as hydrochlorides, which are water and methanol soluble. The free base of lincomycin (pK_a = 7.6) is soluble in both water and most organic solvents. The molecular weight of the hydrochloride is 461. Clindamycin hydrochloride is only sparsely soluble at neutral pH and is too irritating to be used parenterally. Its pK_a is 7.45. Consequently, it is the inactive phosphate form that is used parenterally; this form is rapidly hydrolyzed to free palmitate clindamycin. The bitter taste of clindamycin hydrochloride is detected at concentrations as low as 8 μg/ml in water.

Recently, a series of analogs of clindamycin has been described in which the naturally occurring 5-membered cyclic amino acid amide portion of the molecule was replaced by a 4-, 6-, or 7-membered ring. The most promising compound is pirlimycin, in which the ring consists of six members as well as some additional changes (Fig. 2). This structural modification results in lower toxicity and higher antibacterial activity in preliminary animal studies (4).

II. MECHANISM OF ANTIBACTERIAL ACTIVITY

Lincosamides inhibit bacterial protein synthesis by binding to the 50S subunit of the ribosome (5,6). This action closely resembles the mechanism of erythromycin and chloramphenicol despite their different structures.

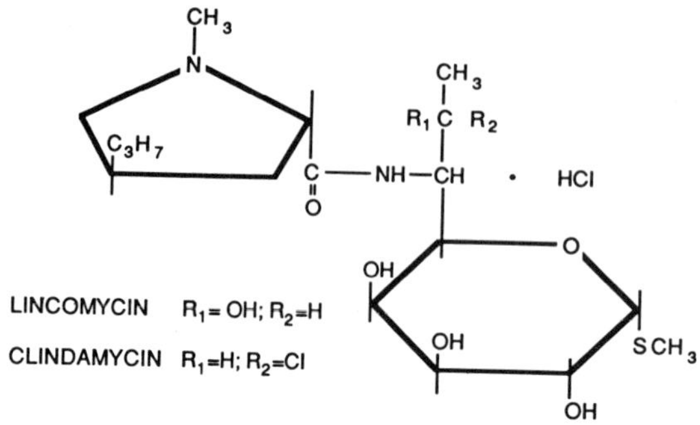

Figure 1 Chemical structure of the lincosamides.

Recent studies have documented that contact of *Streptococcus pyogenes, Staphylococcus aureus*, or *Bacteroides fragilis* with clindamycin, at concentrations below those that inhibit growth, potentiate complement-mediated opsonization of the bacteria by leukocytes (7). This effect was associated with a greater and more rapid deposition of C3 on the bacterial cell surface (7). These observations suggest that clindamycin may affect bacterial growth even at concentrations below the minimum inhibitory concentration (MIC) by potentiating phagocytosis. Animal experiments supporting these in vitro studies have shown that the presence of subinhibitory concentrations of clindamycin prevents the production of bacterial exotoxins and enhances the infiltration of polymorphonuclear leukocytes (7).

The lincosamides are very effective against most strains of staphylococci, streptococci, and pneumococci (8-21). Most strains of streptococci are inhibited by <0.7 μg/ml of lincomycin and <0.09 μg/ml of clindamycin. Most staphylococci are inhibited by 0.5 μg/ml lincomycin and 0.1 μg/ml of clindamycin (Table 1). However, methicillin-resistant strains may not be sensitive to lincosamides. Some erythromycin-resistant strains of staphylococci are also resistant to the lincosamides.

An important characteristic of the lincosamides is their high degree of activity against anaerobes, especially the cocci and gram-negative rods (22-36). Their effect on clostridia

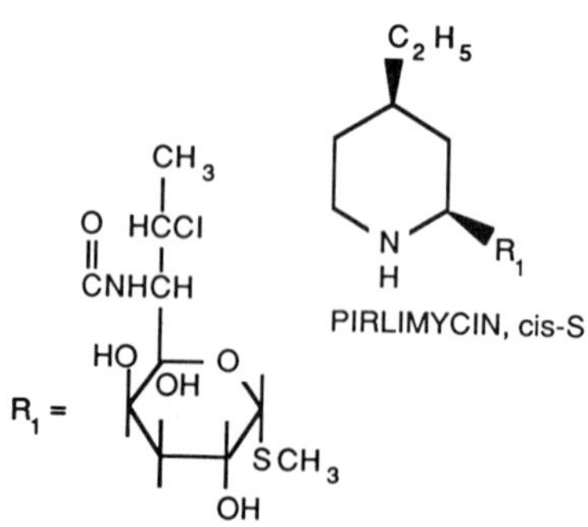

Figure 2 Chemical structure of pirlimycin.

Table 1 Distribution of Lincosamides in Various Tissues

Agent	Dose	Patients	Tissue	Concentration (μg/ml)	Reference
Lincomycin	600 mg IM every 6 hr	Adults	Hip capsule	9.4 (<0.2–32.0)	91
			Synovial fluid	5.4 (2.8–8.1)	
			Calcaneous bone	7.2 (<0.2–53.8)	
			Cortical bone	5.4 (0.2–8.1)	
Lincomycin HCl	600 mg IM X 1	Adults	Serum	6.3	97
			Synovial fluid	1	
	600 mg IM	Adults	Bone	1.96	98
			Serum	3.2	
Clindamycin HCl	600 mg IM X 3	Adults	Calcaneous bone	3.77 (0.77–6.75)	93
			Cortical bone	3.87 (1.15–9.59)	
Clindamycin phosphate	300 mg X 3	Adults	Bone	2.63	89
			Serum	7.33	
Clindamycin HCl	300 mg X 4	Adults	Bone	0.65	90
			Serum	3.13	
Clindamycin	150 mg X 1	Adults	Synovial fluid	2.18	87
			Serum	2.06	
	300 mg X 1		Synovial fluid	3.85	88
			Serum	3.06	
	150 mg X 5		Synovial fluid	5.0	
			Serum	3.6	
Lincomycin HCl	600 mg IM every 12 hr	Adults	Pleural fluid	5.9	99
			Serum	9.6	
	500 mg PO every 8 hr	Adults	Pleural fluid	1.3	
			Serum	2.9	

Table 1 (Continued)

Agent	Dose	Patients	Tissue	Concentration (μg/ml)	Reference
Clindamycin HCl	150 mg X 14		Serum	9.3	88
			Pleural fluid	1.3–22.1	
Lincomycin HCl	600 mg X 1	Adults	Serum	35.1	95
			CSF, meningitis	9.2	
	600 mg X 1	Adults	Serum	14.2	95
			CSF, no meningitis		
Clindamycin phosphate	50 mg/kg day^{-1}	Children, 1 month to 9 years	CSF	0.31 (detectable in 3 of 7 children)	85
			Blood	16.91	
Clindamycin HCl	150 mg X 5	Adults	Prostate	1.7	88
			Serum	1.6	
Clindamycin HCl	150 mg X 12	Adults	Semen	2.6	88
			Serum	2.9	
Lincomycin HCl	100 mg PO, single	Adults	Serum	6.1	47
			Ascites	22.0	
Lincomycin HCl	Total 2.4 gr IM	Adults	Serum	20.4	96
			Aqueous humor	1.3	
Lincomycin HCL	75 mg subconjunctivally	Adults	Aqueous humor	Peak 30–135; detectable for 12 hr	92
Clindamycin HCl	150 mg X 4	Adults	Aqueous humor	Nil	94

	300 X 4			0.19	
Lincomycin HCl	600 mg IV	Adults	Serum	8.8	47
			Bile	67	
Clindamycin HCl	300 mg X 4	Adults	Serum	3.13	86
			Bile duct bile	26.2	
			Gallbladder	41.3	
Clindamycin HCl	300 mg X 1	Adults	Erythrocytes	0.96	88
			Serum	4.78	
Lincomycin HCl	500 mg every 12 hr, 12 doses	Adults	Serum	1.32	47
			Human milk	1.28	
Clindamycin	300 mg every 6 hr	Adults	Human milk	0.7–1.8	
	600 mg every 6 hr		Human milk	2.1–3.8	
Lincomycin HCl		Adults and infants	Maternal peak serum	3.5–12.5	100
			Fetal CSF	0–3.8	
			Cord blood	0.3–2.7	
Clindamycin	Single oral dose, 450 mg	Adults and infants	Fetal blood	0.32	101
			Peak maternal serum	5.16	
	Multiple (4–20) oral doses (450 mg)		Fetal blood	0.7	
			Peak maternal serum	6.3	

is variable, with *Clostridum sporogenes* and *Clostridium tertium* more resistant and *Clostridium perfringens* and *Clostridium tetani* more sensitive.

Only some *Bacteroides* species are sensitive to lincomycin, whereas most of them are sensitive to clindamycin.

Recent studies have demonstrated that *C. perfringens*, proprionibacteria anaerobic cocci, and curved rods were susceptible to clindamycin. Most *Clostridium difficile* strains and fusobacteria were also susceptible to the drug. In addition, clindamycin has shown excellent activity against *B. fragilis* and other *Bacteroides* sp. (37).

Dual clindamycin-erythromycin resistance of *Bacteroides* sp. was first recognized in 1976, and transferable resistance was reported in 1979 (38,39). Two clindamycin resistance transfer factors, PBFTM10 and PIP410, have been characterized. Local outbreaks of clindamycin resistance have been reported in the United States and Europe; however, the resistance rate remained steady at a rate of 5% among *B. fragilis* and 1% among other *Bacteroides* sp. (40).

This relatively low resistance rate may reflect the relative restricted use of the drug (41).

Gram-negative bacilli, including *Neisseria gonorrhoeae* and *Neisseria meningitidis* are resistant to both lincosamides (8,10,12,13-20,42-45). The same is true for all viruses and fungi.

In general, despite a very similar range of antibacterial activity, clindamycin is more active than lincomycin against all strains. The lincosamides have complete cross-resistance. Resistance to some strains of *S. aureus* can be induced in vitro by erythromycin. Conversely, the lincosamides themselves may induce resistance against certain strains of *S. aureus*. In some cases, a few days' treatment with lincomycin may produce resistance of *Streptococcus viridans* or other strains of streptococcus.

Recently, a new derivative of the lincosamides, pirlimycin, has been described, which has an in vitro antibacterial activity nearly identical to that of clindamycin (Figure 2). This compound has been shown to be 2–20 times more active than clindamycin when administered experimentally to mice infected with strains of *Staph. aureus, Strep. pyogenes, Streptococcus pneumoniae, B. fragilis*, and *Plasmodium berghli* (4).

III. PHARMACOKINETICS

Before discussing in detail lincosamide pharmacokinetics, it should be mentioned that the published data are based upon on a bioassay that does not distinguish between clindamycin and its bioactive metabolites (2,46). Although it is assumed that the main metabolites, *N*-demethylclindamycin and clindamycin sulfoxide do not contribute significantly to plasma concentrations, the relative proportion of these metabolites after oral, intramuscular, and intravenous administration or in different age groups or disease states are not known. Moreover, the kinetic profile of the inactive clindamycin phosphate, which is the intravenous prodrug, is not known.

A. Absorption

The absorption of lincomycin following an oral dose is rapid but incomplete. Bioavailability ranges from 20 to 35% (13–15). Food appears to impair both the rate and extent of lincomycin absorption. Peak serum concentrations achieved following a meal are only about one-half of concentrations attained if the drug is administered to fasting subjects. Lincomycin absorption appears to be similar in children and adults.

The absorption of clindamycin depends on several factors. Oral clindamycin palmitate is hydrolyzed rapidly by the gut before being absorbed, and the ester form cannot be identified in the serum (45,48). Both the palmitate ester and hydrochloride salt have comparable patterns of absorption, with bioavailability exceeding 80%. The hexadecylcarbonate ester has reduced bioavailability compared with the other preparations. Clindamycin absorption is comparable after single and multiple dosing and after administration of capsules or tablets (49).

Clindamycin phosphate, which is used intramuscularly or intravenously, is hydrolyzed relatively slowly (46,48). Unhydrolyzed clindamycin phosphate concentrations of 1-2 μg/ml can be identified 30-60 min after administration. As a result of this delayed hydrolysis, peak plasma concentrations are achieved after only 1 hr in children and 3 hr in adults. It appears that peak concentrations are more rapidly attained in more physically active individuals. Comparison of different clindamycin preparations with respect to bioavailability is complicated as different studies have used different parameters, mainly peak or area under concentration-time curve, for evaluation of rate or extent of absorption. In general, it appears that oral bioavailability is almost complete and is not influenced by the presence of food in the gut (14,17,49,50), although the rate of absorption is slower after a meal. Table 2 summarizes correlation between lincosamide doses and resultant peak plasma concentrations in children and adults. It should be mentioned that although peak (C_{max}) and the time to peak (T_{max}) are commonly used to compare the absorption of different preparations of a drug, their values are dependent not only upon the extent and rate of absorption, but also on distribution and elimination (see Chapter 3).

B. Distribution

Both lincosamides are widely distributed in the body following oral, intramuscular, or intravenous administration. The calculated distribution volume for lincomycin equals roughly the total body water (54). For clindamycin V_d is between 44 and 79 liters 1.73 m^{-2} (50-55). Although data with respect to distribution volume in children are limited, it appears that in newborns and small infants the V_d is larger than in older children and adults (50-52). This trend, however, has to be evaluated very carefully as different studies have used different methodologies for the calculation of V_d. Lincomycin is not found in very high concentrations in any particular organ. Clindamycin is 50 times more lipid soluble than lincomycin, which accounts for its wide distribution. Most data on the distribution of lincosamides in various tissues are derived from adult patients (Table 2).

Clindamycin is reported to have protein binding between 60 and 94%, the value for lincomycin being 72-82% (53). Both lincosamides are highly bound to the glycoprotein component of the globulin fraction of the serum. Clindamycin binding appears to be concentration dependent. At 1 μg/ml 93% of the drug is protein bound, whereas at 100 μg/ml only 68% is bound. Lincomycin protein binding is pH dependent: 82% at pH 8.5 and negligible at pH 3.6.

Both lincomycin and clindamycin have relatively low penetration into the cerebrospinal fluid (CSF). Clindamycin concentrations in primates are 10-25% of those of the serum. Measured concentrations in brain tissue were very low or absent even during trauma, when cerebral blood flow increased. During meningitis, lincomycin concentrations in CSF are approximately 40% of serum values (13,47,56).

Table 2 Correlation Between Lincosamide Dose and Serum Concentrations

Agent	Route	Dose (mg)	Time-to-peak T_{max} (hr)	Peak C_{max} (μg/ml)	Population
Lincomycin HCl	Oral	250 6 hr	4	2–7	Adults
		500 6 hr			
Lincomycin HCl	IM	200		3.5–4.2	Adults
		600	1–2	8–18	
Clindamycin	IM	300	1.5–3	3.17–6.56	Adults
		600			
Clindamycin hydrochloride	Oral	150	1.06 ± 0.37	2.84 ± 0.65	Adults
		300	0.91 ± 0.38	3.44 ± 0.87	
		450	0.76 ± 0.31	5.58 ± 1.26	
Clindamycin phosphate	IM	117 m^{-2}	1	9	Children, 2 months to 11 years
		150 m^{-2}	1	9	
Clindamycin palmitate	Oral	4/kg	4	5.4	Infants, 2 months
Clindamycin hydrochloride	Oral	30/kg	1.5	6.1	Infants, 3–14 months
Clindamycin hydrochloride	Oral	2/kg	0.56 ± 0.25	2.26 ± 0.77	Children, 8–11 years
Clindamycin phosphate	IV	15/kg day		5.2–13.7	Preterm infants
Clindamycin phosphate	IV	17.9–40/kg day		16.6–69.2	Preterm infants, full-term infants <4 weeks, infants >4 weeks
Clindamycin phosphate	IM	116 m^{-2}	2	2.88	Adults
		173 m^{-2}	2.6		
Clindamycin hydrochloride	Oral	150 mg	0.86 ± 0.53	2.8 ± 1.26	Adults
Clindamycin palmitate	Oral	150 mg	1.16 ± 0.24	2.05 ± 0.66	Adults
Clindamycin hydrochloride	Oral	150 mg	0.7–2	1.55–2.32	Adults
Lincomycin hydrochloride	Oral	600 mg		12.8	Normal adults
				24.4	Severe renal failure
				42	Intermittent hemodialysis
				42.8	Intermittent hemodialysis

Source: Data from References 46, 48, 50–52, 54, 59, 63, 65, 66, 102, and 103.

Clindamycin has recently been shown to be concentrated within neutrophils and alveolar macrophages to levels 50-fold in excess of extracellular concentrations (41,57). Lincosamides have been shown to attain high concentrations in bone capsule and synovial fluids. It appears, however, that there is differential penetration according to the nature of the bone. Concentrations in bone marrow are comparable to those in serum; spongy bone has 50–75% whereas compact bone 0–15% of that in the serum (Table 1). Following subconjunctival injection of lincomycin, high concentrations can be found in the aqueous 1–2 hr after the injection and is still detected after 12 hr. Also, very high concentrations can be detected in the bile and saliva after parenteral administration.

Both lincosamides are well distributed into the cord serum and amniotic fluids. Also, human milk attains significant levels of both lincomycin and clindamycin even after the first oral doses. Both lincosamides achieve significant concentrations in peritoneal and pleural fluids, prostate, and semen.

C. Elimination

Both lincosamides are eliminated mainly by the liver, with renal excretion of the parent drug contributing a small portion of total body clearance. Although the precise metabolic products of lincomycin have not been elucidated, it is known that less than 10% of an oral dose and 10–50% of intramuscular or intravenous dose can be recovered unchanged from the urine (13–15,47,48). That 4–14% of a parenteral dose of lincomycin can be recovered from stool and that high concentrations are attained in bile indicate that some elimination occurs by bile excretion or transport through the intestinal wall (15). Elimination rate of lincomycin is prolonged in cases of hepatic insufficiency (58), probably reflecting an impaired rate of metabolic elimination. Patients with renal insufficiency have prolonged half-lives of lincomycin and higher serum concentrations (59). It has been recommended that the dose should be decreased to 25–30% in these patients. Peritoneal dialysis and hemodialysis do not appear to change these parameters. It is conceivable, however, that this observation reflects, at least in part, an analytic problem. Bioassay does not differentiate between lincomycin and bioactive metabolites. It is therefore possible that the renally excreted metabolites accumulate during azotemia.

Clindamycin is metabolized by the liver to *N*-demethylclindamycin and clindamycin sulfoxide. These metabolites are excreted by the kidney and biliary system. Only negligible amounts of clindamycin can be recovered unchanged in the urine or feces. The elimination rate of the drug is prolonged and peak concentrations are increased in patients with impaired hepatic function. The distribution volume of clindamycin in these patients is unchanged, whereas clearance rate is slower (60,61). There is a slight prolongation of clindamycin $T_{1/2}$ (62,63) in patients with renal failure. However, any pharmacokinetic data on clindamycin elimination should be interpreted cautiously. The bioassay using *Sarcina lutea* does not distinguish between clindamycin itself and *N*-demethylclindamycin (three times more active) and clindamycin sulfoxide (seven times less active). During normal renal function, serum concentrations of the metabolites are negligible as their elimination $T_{1/2}$ is shorter than the parent drug. As these metabolites are renally excreted, they may accumulate and yield erroneous pharmacokinetic parameters during azotemia. This may explain higher concentrations of clindamycin in patients with uremia immediately after the end of infusion, with prolonged elimination period (64).

It appears that $T_{1/2}$ in children is comparable, in the range of 2 months to 11 years [mean, 2.41 and 3.43 hr according to Kauffmann (52) and 1.89 ± 0.82 hr according to De Haan (50)], to adult values (0.78–4.76 hr) (46,50,55,65).

Several recent studies have assessed the developmental aspects of clindamycin disposition in newborn infants. Bell and his colleagues (51) studied the disposition characteristics of the drug in infants less than 1 year of age. Concentrations were measured during steady-state conditions. Mean serum elimination $T_{1/2}$ was significantly longer in preterm infants (8.68 hr) than in full-term infants (3.6 hr) during the first 4 weeks of life ($p <$ 0.01). In full-term infants, $T_{1/2}$ remained unchanged during the first year of life. These differences in elimination $T_{1/2}$ could be attributed to the reduced clearance rate of clindamycin in younger (or lower weight) infants. Infants > 4 weeks of postnatal age had significantly increased clearance than either preterm or full-term infants younger than 4 weeks (1.6 vs. 0.29 and 0.68 liter/hr). In addition, the prolonged hydrolysis of clindamycin phosphate ester may also affect elimination $T_{1/2}$ of the drug.

Renal excretion of clindamycin expressed as the fraction of drug dose that appeared in the urine during a dosing interval was 16% in preterm infants < 4 weeks of age, 14.4% in full-term infants < 4 weeks, and 22.8% in infants > 4 weeks of age. Based on these differences in clearance of clindamycin, the authors recommended that in infants > 4 weeks or 3.5 kg, intravenous clindamycin dosage be 20 mg/kg day^{-1} in four divided doses. In preterm infants < 4 weeks the dose should be reduced to 15 mg/kg day^{-1} in three divided doses. Term infants > 1 week of age may receive 20 mg/kg day^{-1} in four doses.

In three preterm infants, the reduced dose of 15 mg/kg day^{-1} was tested, yielding peak concentrations between 5.2 and 13.7 μg/ml and trough between 0 and 3.8 μg/ml.

We studied the pharmacokinetics of clindamycin administered intravenously to a group of 12 preterm infants treated for suspected or proven necrotizing enterocolitis or anaerobic infections (66). In 7 infants studied after 2-6 days of therapy, middose interval serum concentrations attained after doses of 17.9-44 mg/kg day^{-1} (mean, 31.3 ± 18.2) ranged from 12.75 to 40 μg/ml (mean, 23.1 ± 8.3). Peak serum concentrations ranged from 16.6 to 69.2 μg/ml. There was a positive correlation between dose and steady-state concentrations. Each dose increment of 1 mg/kg day^{-1} resulted in an approximate incremental concentration of 1 μg/ml. Elimination $T_{1/2}$ ranged from 3.5 to 9.75 hr (mean, 6.3 ± 2.1 hr). The clearance rate of clindamycin ranged from 22.2 to 134.9 ml/kg hr^{-1} (mean, 61.6 ± 31.6 ml/kg hr^{-1}). Clearance rate was not lower and $T_{1/2}$ not longer (3.79-8 hr) in 4 neonates with renal insufficiency than in patients with normal renal function.

IV. TOXICITY

Approximately 5-20% of patients receiving lincomycin have been reported to develop diarrhea. Recent studies have shown that clindamycin at gut concentrations occurring during therapeutic use cause malabsorption of water and electrolytes in the human, which may contribute to the diarrhea occurring during clindamycin therapy in the absence of pseudomembranous colitis (67). During the first years of clinical usage of clindamycin it was associated with less diarrhea than was lincomycin. However, soon a significantly more serious gastrointestinal side effect, pseudomembranous colitis, emerged in association with clindamycin. A careful evaluation of the literature reveals that, long before Cohen et al. described the first cases of clindamycin-associated colitis (68), a similar syndrome was described with lincomycin, including fever, leukocytosis, abdominal pain, and severe bloody or mucous diarrhea (69-72). These signs may appear during or after the course of clindamycin. They are usually associated with oral but may occur with parenteral administration of the drug. The disease appears to be more prevalent in the elderly; however, it has been described in children (73). The severity of the diarrhea varies from mild and self-limited to severe and fatal. Fatalities are usually secondary to profound shock and dehydration. Sigmoidoscopic examination reveals erythematous mucosa with edema and white or yellow raised plaques several millimeters in size. Histologically, ulceration and inflammation lead to the formation of a pseudomembrane.

Although precise incidence of this condition is not clear, it is believed to be more frequent than the 1 in 50,000 courses of treatment reported by the manufacturer (74).

It appears that this serious complication is not dose or duration dependent; it generally continues for up 2 weeks but may persist for months. Recurrences have been described. The mechanism of the toxicity is not known. In some patients the colitis is preceded by the more common diarrhea, but not in every case. Although it is conceivable that, being a potent antibiotic, clindamycin significantly changes intestinal flora, causing emergence of a more potent bacterium, this premise has not been fully proven. Larson and Price proposed that a toxin produced by *C. difficile* is causing the clinical picture (75). This suggestion has been coupled by animal studies showing that vancomycin could ameliorate colitis due to clindamycin-resistant *C. difficile* (76). Recent studies have documented the presence of *C. difficile* in drug-related diarrhea following other antibiotics, such as ampicillin, cephalosporins, and aminoglycosides (77).

Additional adverse effects of the lincosamides involve the liver, neuromuscular system, heart, skin, and hematopoietic system.

Parenteral administration of clindamycin phosphate may cause elevation of SGOT, SGPT, and serum alkaline phosphatase but not of bilirubin. Although in most cases there is no further evidence of serious hepatic injury, biopsy in a young man treated for staphylococcal endocarditis has shown evidence of hepatic injury that had substantially resolved within 2 weeks (78). A rapid intravenous infusion of clindamycin may cause arrhythmia and even cardiac arrest. These changes have been attributed to the structural similarity of the drug to quinidine, and the currently recommended infusion rate is no more than 50 mg/kg hr^{-1}.

Both lincosamides depress neuromuscular transmission by a postsynaptic action in a transient fashion (79,80). When given after curare the lincosamides may decrease neuromuscular transmission and thus prolong postanesthetic respiratory depression. About 10% of cases treated with lincosamides have skin rashes; rarely skin involvement may be severe, with full blown Stevens-Johnson syndrome. Thrombocytopenia, granulocytopenia, and anaphylactoid reactions have been described.

V. CLINICAL INDICATIONS

As mentioned above, clindamycin has almost completely substituted for lincomycin owing to its better oral bioavailability and more effective antibacterial action. It is useful as an alternative drug to penicillins and cephalosporins in gram-positive infections, especially those due to *S. aureus* (56,81,82). In both children and adults, clindamycin has shown excellent results in treating streptococcal pharyngitis, gram-positive otitis, pyoderma, and pneumonia. Clindamycin has been proven highly effective in staphylococcal septicemia and acute or chronic osteomyelitis because of its good bone penetration (56).

Based on its high efficacy against anaerobic bacteria, clindamycin may be used for both prophylaxis and treatment of such infections, especially *B. fragilis*. Both intra-abdominal infections and sepsis, including female genitourinary tract, can be effectively treated with clindamycin (82).

There is increasing evidence for involvement of oral anaerobic bacteria in cervical lymphadenitis and peritonsilar, retropharyngeal, and parapharyngeal abscesses. Chronic suppurative otitis media caused by anaerobes may be complicated by osteitis of adjacent bones. Although most of these infections can be effectively treated with penicillins, clindamycin may serve as a powerful agent, especially when anaerobes or *S. aureus* is involved (81).

In the treatment of nosocomial pneumonia and in lower respiratory tract infections in immunocompromised patients, in whom a need for antibiotics with a broader antimicrobial spectrum may exist, clindamycin may be a possible alternative to penicillin. This is especially relevant when staphylococcal pneumonia is strongly suspected. Whereas in aspiration pneumonia penicillin appears to be the preferred therapy, clindamycin has been clearly documented as a superior choice in primary lung abscesses (82).

In the treatment of severe abdominal and female pelvic infections, clindamycin has been shown to be superior to cephalothin, cefamandole, and cefoperazone and equivalent to cefoxitin and metronidazole (83).

Mixed staphylococcal and anerobic infections in skin, subcutaneous tissue, bone, and joints are primary indications for clindamycin. *Staphylococcus epidermidis* infections, including septicemia and endocarditis, should not be treated with clindamycin because of a high rate of resistance (57).

The topical use of clindamycin to treat acne vulgaris was proven equivalent to oral tetracycline. The topical use was not associated with side effects (84).

REFERENCES

1. Mason, DJ, Dietz, A, Deboer, C: Lincomycin, a new antibiotic. I. Discovery and biological properties. In: *Antimicrobial Agents and Chemotherapy–1962*, American Society for Microbiology, Ann Arbor, Michigan, 1963, pp. 554–559.
2. Herr, RR, Bergy, ME: Lincomycin, a new antibiotic. II. Isolation and characterization. In: *Antimicrobial Agents and Chemotherapy–1962*, American Society for Microbiology, Ann Arbor, Michigan, 1963, pp. 560–564.
3. Magerlein, BJ, Binkenmeyer, RD, Kagan, F: Chemical modification of lincomycin. In: *Antimicrobial Agents and Chemotherapy–1966*, American Society for Microbiology, Ann Arbor, Michigan, 1967, pp. 727–736.
4. Birkenmeyer, RD, Kroll, SJ, Lewis, C, Stern, KF, Zurenko, GE: Synthesis and antimicrobial activity of clindamycin analogues: Pirlimycin, a potent antibacterial agent. *J. Med. Chem. 27*:216–223, 1984.
5. Josten, JJ, Allen, PM: The mode of action of lincomycin. *Biochem. Biophys. Res. Commun. 14*:241–245, 1964.
6. Chang, FN, Sih, CJ, Weisblum, B: Lincomycin, an inhibitor of aminocyl SRIA binding to ribosomes. *Proc. Natl. Acad. Sci. USA 55*:431–438, 1966.
7. Gemmell, CG: Clindamycin and its action on the susceptibility of pathogenic bacteria to phagocytosis. *Scand. J. Infect. Dis. (Suppl.) 43*:17–23, 1984.
8. Barber, M, Walerwarth, PM: Antibacterial activity of lincomycin and pristinamycin: A comparison with erythromycin. *Br. Med. J. 2*:603–606, 1964.
9. Benner, EJ, Adams, AP: Unusual resistance of *Staphylococcus aureus* to lincomycin and 7-chlorolincomycin. In: *Antimicrobial Agents and Chemotherapy–1969*, American Society for Microbiology, Ann Arbor, Michigan, 1970, pp. 100–103.
10. Fass, RJ, Saslaw, S: Clindamycin: Clinical and laboratory evaluation of parenteral therapy. *Am. J. Med. Sci. 263*:368–382, 1972.
11. Geddes, AM, Bridgwater, FAJ, Williams, DN, Oon, J, Grimshaw, GJ: Clinical and bacteriological studies with clindamycin. *Br. Med. J. 2*:703–704, 1970.

12. Garrison, DW, DeHaan, RM, Lawson, JB: Comparison of in vitro antibacterial activities of 7-chloro 7-deoxylincomycin, lincomycin and erythromycin. In: *Antimicrobial Agents and Chemotherapy–1967*, American Society of Microbiology, Ann Arbor, Michigan, 1968, pp. 397–400.
13. Kaplan, K, Chew, WH, Weinstein, L: Microbiological, pharmacological and clinical studies of lincomycin. *Am. J. Med. Sci. 250*:137–146, 1965.
14. McGehee, RF, Jr., Smith, CB, Wilcox, C, Finland, M: Comparative studies of antibacterial activity in vitro and absorption and excretion of lincomycin and clindamycin. *Am. J. Med. Sci. 256*:279–292, 1968.
15. McCall, CE, Steigbigel, NH, Finland, M: Lincomycin: Activity in vitro and absorption and excretion in normal young men. *Am. J. Med. Sci. 254*:144–155, 1967.
16. Lewis, C, Clapp, HW, Grady, JE: In vitro and in vivo evaluation of lincomycin, a new antibiotic. In: *Antimicrobial Agents and Chemotherapy–1962*, American Society for Microbiology, Ann Arbor, Michigan, 1963, pp. 570–582.
17. Meyers, BR, Kaplan, K, Weinstein, L: Microbiological and pharmacological behavior of 7-chlorolincomycin. *Appl. Microbiol. 17*:653–657, 1969.
18. Oppenheimer, S, Tuck, M: Laboratory and clinical evaluation of 7-deoxylincomycin. *Am. J. Med. Sci. 256*:314–321, 1968.
19. Monnier, J, Bourse, R: Antistophylococcal activity of lincomycin. *Chemotherapia 12*:1–000, 1967.
20. Phillips, L, Fernandes, R, Warren, C: In vitro comparison of erythromycin, lincomycin and clindamycin. *Br. Med. J. 2*:89–90, 1970.
21. Shadomy, S, Bruce, JL, Kannan, MM: Effect of inoculum size on in vitro susceptibility testing with lincomycin. *Appl. Microbiol. 16*:1663–1668, 1968.
22. Bartlett, JG, Sutter, VL, Finegold, SM: Treatment of anaerobic infections with lincomycin and clindamycin. *N. Engl. J. Med. 287*:1006–1010, 1972.
23. Bodner, SJ, Koenig, MG, Treanor, LL, Goodman, JS: Antibiotic susceptibility testing of bacteroides. *Antimicrob. Agents Chemother. 2*:52–56, 1972.
24. Finegold, SM, Harada, NE, Miler, LG: Lincomycin: Activity against anaerobes and effect on normal human fecal flora. In: *Antimicrobial Agents and Chemotherapy–1965*, American Society for Microbiology, Ann Arbor, Michigan, 1966, pp. 659–667.
25. Fass, RJ, Scholand, JF, Hodges, GR, Saslow, S: Clindamycin in the treatment of serious anaerobic infections. *Ann. Intern. Med. 78*:853–859, 1973.
26. Ingham, HR, Selkon, JB, Codd, AA, Hale, JH: The effect of carbon dioxide on the sensitivity of *Bacteroides fragilis* to certain antibiotics in vitro. *J. Clin. Pathol. 23*: 254–258, 1970.
27. Ingham, HR, Selkon, JB, Codd, AA, Hale, JH: A study in vitro of the sensitivity to antibiotics of *Bacteroides fragilis. J. Clin. Pathol. 21*:432–436, 1968.
28. Kislak, JW: The susceptibility of *Bacteroides fragilis* to 24 antibiotics. *J. Infect. Dis. 125*:295–299, 1972.
29. Lerner, PI: Susceptibility of *Actinomyces* species to lincomycin and as 7-halogenated analogues. In: *Antimicrobial Agents and Chemotherapy–1968*, American Society for Microbiology, Ann Arbor, Michigan, 1969, pp. 461–464.
30. Lerner, PI: Susceptibility of *Actinomyces* to cephalosporine and lincomycin. In: *Antimicrobial Agents and Chemotherapy–1967*, American Society for Microbiology, Ann Arbor, Michigan, 1968, pp. 730–735.
31. Martin, WJ, Gardner, M, Washington, JA: II. In vitro antimicrobial susceptibility of anaerobic bacteria isolated from clinical specimens. *Antimicrob. Agents Chemother. 1*:148–154, 1972.
32. Nastro, LJ, Finegold, SM: Bactericidal activity of five antimicrobial agents against *Bacteroides fragilis. J. Infect. Dis. 126*:104–107, 1972.
33. Pien, FD, Thompson, RL, Martin, WJ: Clinical and bacteriologic studies of anaerobic Gram-positive cocci. *Mayo Clin. Proc. 47*:251–257, 1972.

34. Sapiro, FL, Kwok, YY, Sutter, VL, Finegold, SM: Standardized antimicrobial disk susceptibility testing of anaerobic bacteria: In vitro susceptibility of *Clostridium perfringens* to nine antibiotics. *Antimicrob. Agents Chemother. 2*:320–322, 1972.
35. Thornton, GF, Cramer, JA: Antibiotic susceptibility of *Bacteroides* species. In: *Antimicrobial Agents and Chemotherapy–1970*, American Society for Microbiology, Ann Arbor, Michigan, 1971, pp. 509–513.
36. Wilkins, TD, Holderman, LV, Abramson, JJ, Moore, WEC: Standardized single-disc method for antibiotic susceptibility testing of anaerobic bacteria. *Antimicrob. Agents Chemother. 1*:451–456, 1972.
37. Salaki, JS, Block, R, Tally, FP, Kislak, JW: *Bacteroides fragilis* resistant to clindamycin. *Am. J. Med. 60*:426–428, 1976.
38. Dornbusch, K, Olsson-Liljequist, B, Nord, CE: Antibacterial activity of new-beta lactam antibiotics on cefoxitin-resistant strains of *Bacteroides fragilis. J. Antimicrob. Chemother. 6*:207–216, 1980.
39. Tally, FP, Chahural, GJ, Jr., Bieluch, VM, Jacobus, NV, Halamy, MH: Clindamycin resistance to anaerobic bacteria. *Scand. J. Infect. Dis. (Suppl.) 43*:34–43, 1984.
40. Nord, CE, Olsson-Liljequist, B: Antimicrobial susceptibility of anaerobic bacteria in Sweden in 1983. *Scand. J. Infect. Dis. (Suppl.) 43*:44–49, 1984.
41. Nordbring, F: Aspects of the clinical use of clindamycin. *Scand. J. Infect. Dis. (Suppl.) 43*:89–90, 1984.
42. Cooper, RG, Gibbs, MH: The antibiotic sensitivity of *Bordetella* in South Australia. *Med. J. Aust. 2*:843, 1967.
43. Kutscher, E, Southern, PM, Jr., Sanford, JP: Clinical significance of lincomycin-resistant *Neisseria gonorrhoeae*. In: *Antimicrobial Agents and Chemotherapy–1968*, American Society for Microbiology, Ann Arbor, Michigan, 1969, pp. 331–334.
44. Matsen, JM: In vitro study of clindamycin and five other lincomycin analogs against strains of *Haemophilus influenzae. J. Lab. Clin. Med. 77*:378–383, 1971.
45. Phillips, I, Ridley, M, Rimmer, D, Lynn, R, Warren, C: In vitro activity of twelve antibacterial agents against *Neisseria gonorrhoeae. Lancet 1*:263–265, 1970.
46. De Haan, RM, Metzler, CM, Schellenberg, D, Van den Bosch, WD: Pharmacokinetic studies of clindamycin phosphate. *J. Clin. Pharmacol. 13*:190–209, 1973.
47. Medina, A, Fisk, EN, Hjelt-Harvey, J, Brown, CD, Prijat, A: Absorption, diffusion and secretion of a new antibiotic, lincomycin. In: *Antimicrobial Agents and Chemotherapy–1963*, American Society for Microbiology, Ann Arbor, Michigan, 1964, pp. 189–196.
48. Metzler, CM, De Haan, R, Schellenberg, D, Van den Bosch, WD: Clindamycin dose-bioavailability relationships. *J. Pharm. Sci. 62*:591–598, 1973.
49. Wagner, JG, Novak, E, Palel, NC, Chidesler, CG, Lummes, WL: Absorption, excretion and half life of clindamycin in normal adult males. *Am. J. Med. Sci. 256*:25–37, 1968.
50. De Haan, RM, Metzler, CM, Schellenberg, D, Van den Bosch, WD, Masson, EL: Pharmacokinetic studies of clindamycin hydrochloride in humans. *Int. J. Clin. Pharmacol. 6*:105–119, 1972.
51. Bell, MJ, Shackelford, P, Smith, R, Schroeder, K: Pharmacokinetics of clindamycin phosphate in the first year of life. *J. Pediatr. 105*:482–486, 1984.
52. Kaufman, RE, Shoeman, DW, Han Wan, S, Azarnoff, DL: Absorption and excretion of clindamycin-2-phosphate in children after intramuscular injection. *Clin. Pharmacol. Ther. 13*:704–709, 1973.
53. Sokolski, WT: Plasma protein-binding studies with lincomycin and clindamycin. *Proc. Ann. Meet. Am. Sci. Microb.*, 1975.
54. Ma, P, Lim, M, Nodine, JH: Human pharmacological studies of lincomycin, a new antibiotic for Gram-positive organisms. In: *Antimicrobial Agents and Chemo-*

therapy–1963, American Society for Microbiology, Ann Arbor, Michigan, 1964, pp. 183–188.

55. Novak, E, Vitti, TG, Panzer, JD, Schlagel, C, Hearron, MS: Antibiotic tolerance and serum levels after intravenous administration of multiple large doses of lincomycin. *Clin. Pharmacol. Ther. 12*:793–797, 1971.
56. Lerner, PI: Penetration of cephalothin and lincomycin into the cerebrospinal fluid. *Am. J. Med. Sci. 257*:125–131, 1969.
57. Hedstrom, SA: Clindamycin as an anti-staphylococcal agent—indications and limitations. *Scand. J. Infect. Dis. (Suppl.) 43*:62–66, 1984.
58. Bellamy, HM, Jr., Bates, BB, Reinarz, JA: Lincomycin metabolism in patients with hepatic insufficiency: Effect of liver disease on lincomycin serum concentrations. In: *Antimicrobial Agents and Chemotherapy–1966*, American Society for Microbiology, Ann Arbor, Michigan, 1967, pp. 36–41.
59. Reinarz, JA, McIntosh, DA: Lincomycin excretion in patients with normal renal function, severe azotemia and with hemodialysis and peritoneal dialysis. In: *Antimicrobial Agents and Chemotherapy–1965*, American Society for Microbiology, Ann Arbor, Michigan, 1966, pp. 232–238.
60. Avant, GR, Schenker, S, Alford, RH: The effect of cirrhosis on the disposition and elimination of clindamycin. *Am. J. Dig. Dis. 20*:223–230, 1975.
61. Hinthorn, DR, Baker, LH, Romig, DA: Use of clindamycin in patients with liver disease. *Antimicrob. Agents Chemother. 9*:498–501, 1976.
62. Peddie, BA, Dann, E, Bailey, RR: The effect of impairment of renal function and dialysis on the serum and urine levels of clindamycin. *Aust. N.Z. J. Med. 5*:198–202, 1975.
63. Eastwood, JB, Gower, PE: A study of the pharmacokinetics of clindamycin in normal subjects and patients with chronic renal failure. *Postgrad. Med. J. 50*:710–712, 1974.
64. Joshi, AM, Stein, RM: Altered serum clearances of intravenously administered clindamycin phosphate in patients with uremia. *J. Clin. Pharmacol. 14*:140–144, 1974.
65. Forist, AA, De Haan, RM, Metzler, CM: Clindamycin bioavailability from clindamycin 2-palmitate and clindamycin 2-hexadecylcarbonate in man. *J. Pharmacokinet. Biopharm. 1*:89–98, 1973.
66. Koren, G, Zarfin, Y, Maresky, D, Spiro, T, MacLeod, SM: Pharmacokinetics of intravenous clindamycin in newborn infants. *Pediatr. Pharmacol.* 1986 (in press).
67. Spiller, RC, Higgins, BE, Frost, PG, Silk, DBA: Inhibition of jejunal water and electrolyte absorption by therapeutic doses of clindamycin in man. *Clin. Sci. 67*: 117–120, 1984.
68. Cohen, LE, McNeill, CJ, Wells, RF: Clindamycin-associated colitis. *JAMA 223*: 1379–1380, 1973.
69. Clinical Abstracts: Lincomycin, Kalamazoo, Michigan. The Upjohn Co., 1968, p. 21.
70. Kaplan, K, Weinstein, L: Lincomycin. *Pediatr. Clin. North Am. 15*:131–139, 1968.
71. Bennet, EJ, Tellman, WH: Pseudomembraneous colitis as a sequel to oral lincomycin therapy. *Am. J. Gastroenterol. 54*:55–58, 1970.
72. Ecker, JA, Williams, RG, McKittrick, JE, Failing, JF: Pseudomembraneous enterocolitis—an unwelcome gastrointestinal complication of antibiotic therapy. *Am. J. Gastroenterol. 54*:214–228, 1970.
73. Stanley, RJ, Tedesco, FJ: Antibiotic-associated pseudomembraneous colitis. *CRC Crit. Rev. Clin. Radiol. Nucl. Med.* September 10, 255–277, 1976.
74. Frankel, RI: Clindamycin-efficacy and toxicity. *West. J. Med. 122*:526–530, 1975.
75. Larson, HE, Price, AB: Pseudomembranous colitis: Presence of clostridial toxins. *Lancet 2*:1312–1314, 1977.
76. Bartlett, JG, Gorbach, S: Treatment of aspiration pneumonia and primary lung abscess. Penicillin G vs clindamycin. *JAMA 234*:935–937, 1975.

77. Silva, J, Fekety, R, Werk, C, Ebright, J, Cudmore, M, Batts, D, Syrfamaki, C, Lubeno, J: Inciting an etiologic agent of colitis. *Rev. Infect. Dis. 6 (Suppl. 1)*:5214–5228, 1984.
78. Elmore, M, Rissing, JP, Rink, L, Brooks, GF: Clindamycin-associated hepatotoxicity. *Am. J. Med. 57*:627–630, 1974.
79. Rubbo, JT, Gergis, SD, Sokoll, MD: Comparative neuromuscular effects of lincomycin and clindamycin. *Anesth. Analg. (Cleve.) 56*:329–332, 1977.
80. Samuelson, RJ, Glesecke, AH, Kallus, FT, Stanley, VF: Lincomycin-curare interaction. *Anaesth. Analg. (Cleve.) 54*:103–105, 1975.
81. Lundberg, C, Heimdahl, A, Nord, CE: Clindamycin in the upper respiratory tract infections. *Scand. J. Infect. Dis. (Suppl.) 43*:50–55, 1984.
82. Schreiner, A: Use of clindamycin in lower respiratory tract infections. *Scand. J. Infect. Dis. (Suppl.) 43*:56–61, 1984.
83. Gorbach, SL: Current experience with clindamycin in the treatment of abdominal and female pelvic infections. *Scand. J. Infect. Dis. (Suppl.) 43*:82–88, 1984.
84. Braathen, LR: Topical clindamycin versus oral tetracycline and placebo in acne vulgaris. *Scand. J. Infect. Dis. (Suppl.) 43*:71–75, 1984.
85. DA 50–441. Antibiotic report SS Cleocin Phosphate, First Quarterly Report, p 10/00612.
86. Soles, JEL, Sutcliffe, M, O'Grady, F: Excretion of clindamycin in the bile of patients with biliary tract disease. *Chemotherapy 19*:11–15, 1973.
87. Platt, MA, Roth, H: Penetration of clindamycin into synovial fluid. *Clin. Pharmacol. Ther. 11*:577–580, 1970.
88. Panzer, JD, Brown, DC, Epstein, WL, Lipson, RL, Mahaffey, HW, Atkinson, WH: Clindamycin in various body tissues and fluids. *J. Clin. Pharmacol. 12*:259–262, 1972.
89. Nicholas, P, Meyers, BR, Levy, RN, Hirschman, SZ: Concentration of clindamycin in human bone. *Antimicrob. Agents Chemother. 8*:220–221, 1975.
90. Vocek, V, Hjzlar, M, Slovk, M, Pavlansky, R: Penetration of clindamycin into bone in man: A preliminary report. *Chemotherapy 17*:22–25, 1972.
91. Parsons, RL, Beavis, JP, Hossack, GA, Paddock, GM: Plasma, bone, hip capsule, synovial and drain fluid concentrations of lincomycin during total hip replacement. *Br. J. Clin. Pharmacol. 4*:433–437, 1977.
92. Boyle, GL, Lichtig, ML, Leopold, JH: Lincomycin levels in human ocular fluids and serum following subconjunctival infection. *Am. J. Ophthalmol. 71*:1303–1306, 1971.
93. Schurman, DJ, Johnson, BL, Finerman, G, Amstutz, HC: Antibiotic bone penetration. Concentrations of methicillin and clindamycin phosphate in human bone taken during total hip replacement. *Clin. Orthop. 11*:142–146, 1975.
94. Panzer, JD, Atkinson, WH: Final report—Dalacin C. Intraocular penetration study, 1969.
95. Rimmer, DMD, Soles, JEL: Lincomycin and clindamycin. *Antibiot. Chemother. 25*: 204–216, 1978.
96. Becker, EF: The intraocular penetration of lincomycin. *Am. J. Ophthalmol. 67*: 963–965, 1969.
97. Deodhar, SD, Russell, F, Dick, WC, Nuki, G, Buchanan, WW: Penetration of lincomycin ("Lincocin") and clindamycin ("Dalacin C") into the synovial cavity in rheumatoid arthritis. *Curr. Med. Res. Opin. 1*:108–115, 1972.
98. Vacek, V, Hejzlar, M, Pavlansky, R: Penetration of lincomycin into bone in man. Proc 5th Int Congr Chemother, Vol. 1, 1967, pp. 345–353.
99. Thomas, PA, Jolly, PC: Lincomycin diffusion into pleural drainage fluid of post thoracotomy patients. *Am. Rev. Respir. Dis. 96*:1044–1048, 1967.

100. Duignan, NM, Andrews, J, Williams, JD: Pharmacological studies with lincomycin in late pregnancy. *Br. Med. J. 3*:75–78, 1973.
101. Philipson, A, Sabath, LD, Charles, D: Transplacental passage of erythromycin and clindamycin. *N. Engl. J. Med. 288*:1219–1221, 1973.
102. Shibata, K, Itoh, T, Fujii, M, Shinagawa, N, Nishi, H, Muramatsu, T: Laboratory and clinical studies of clindamycin 2-palmitate in surgical practice. *Jpn. J. Antibiot. 26*:389–392, 1973.
103. Unertl, K, Doschner, FD, Marget, W: A semiautomatic microtube dilution method for determining antibiotic blood concentrations. *Chemotherapy 20*:331–338, 1974.
104. Smith, JA, Morgan, JR, Rachlis, AR, Rapsin, FR: Clindamycin in human breast milk. *Can. Med. Assoc. J. 112*:806, 1975.

19
Rifampin

ITAMAR SHALIT
Tel Aviv Medical Center, Sackler School of Medicine, Tel Aviv, Israel

In 1957, in the Dow-Lepetit Research Laboratory in Milan, Italy, a new class of antimicrobial compounds—the rifamycin complex— was extracted from fermentation broths of *Nocardia mediterranei* (1). Named after the popular French movie, *Rififi,* the rifamycin complex was found to contain several distinct antibacterial compounds, the most active of which was rifamycin B.

Further studies and chemical modifications led to the introduction of rifamycin SV in 1961 (2). This compound was extremely active against *Mycobacterium tuberculosis* and gram-positive bacteria but was not well absorbed orally. It took 4 years more and many interim modifications of rifamycin SV before rifampin (or rifampicin, according to the European nomenclature) was introduced, displaying broader antibacterial spectrum, better oral absorption, and favorable pharmacokinetic properties (3). In 1968, rifampin became available for routine therapeutic use.

I. CHEMISTRY

Rifampin is 3-(4-methylpiperazinyliminomethyl)rifamycin SV. Its structure is illustrated in Figure 1.

Rifampin is an "inner-salt" (zwitterion) with a molecular weight of 823 daltons and a melting point of 185°C. It is a tasteless brick-red crystalline powder, slightly soluble in water, acetone, alcohol, and ether and readily soluble in ethyl acetate, methyl alcohol, and chloroform. Solubility in aqueous solutions is increased at low pH (4). The drug displays remarkable diffusion through lipids (5).

As a dry powder, rifampin is stable at 25°C for more than 5 years. In aqueous solution, at room temperature, it loses 20% of its potency within 10 hr (4). However, when a suspension of 1% w/v of rifampin is commercially prepared as a simple syrup, the drug is stable for 4 weeks at room temperature and 6 weeks at 2-8°C (6).

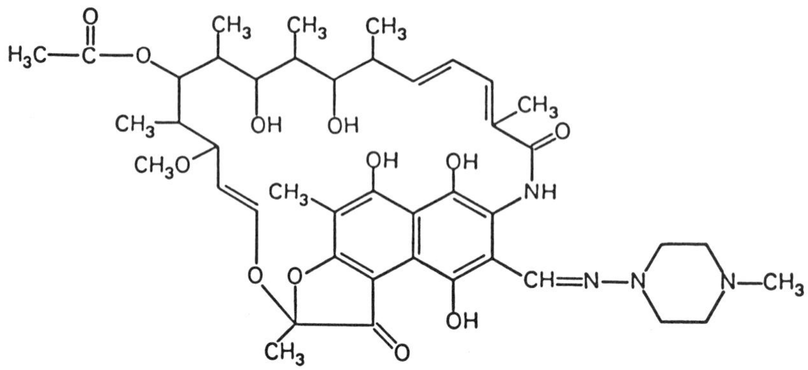

Figure 1 Rifampin.

II. MECHANISM OF ACTION

Rifampin's mode of activity has been studied extensively in gram-positive and gram-negative bacteria, as well as in mycobacteria, viruses, and mammalian and tumor cells (7). In 1967, Hartmann et al. (8) demonstrated that rifampin inhibits RNA synthesis in *Escherichia coli* by binding to the bacterial enzyme, DNA-dependent RNA polymerase. Similar findings were subsequently reported in a variety of bacteria. Later studies have further defined the mode of antibacterial activity of this drug (9).

The lipid-soluble rifampin penetrates into the bacterial cytoplasm, where each molecule binds to one molecule of the β subunit of the bacterial enzyme, DNA-dependent RNA polymerase (molecular weight $\approx$ 150,000) (10). The high affinity of rifampin to the enzyme is demonstrated by the low equilibrium constant K of the rifampin-enzyme complex ($K = 10^{-9}$ M at 37°C) (11). The binding of rifampin to the enzyme interferes with the transcription of DNA to RNA by blocking the chain initiation process of RNA synthesis (9), presumably by allosteric interference of the rifampin-enzyme complex (12). The low concentrations of rifampin required to inhibit bacterial RNA polymerase correlate with the low minimal inhibitory concentration (MIC) of the drug against gram-positive bacteria. The higher MIC values encountered for gram-negative bacteria are due to reduced penetration of the drug into such organisms (13).

Mammalian cells also contain DNA-dependent RNA polymerase; however, the mammalian enzyme is practically insensitive to rifampin and is not inhibited by concentrations 10,000-fold higher than those that inhibit the bacterial enzyme (13). Hence, clinically relevant concentrations of rifampin that kill a wide variety of microorganisms do not inhibit the RNA synthesis of human host cells.

The antifungal activity of rifampin is dependent upon the concomitant use of amphotericin B (14). Medoff et al. have postulated that amphotericin B activity results in alteration in the permeability barrier of the fungal surface membrane, which in turn facilitates rifampin penetration. Once inside the fungal cell, rifampin selectively inhibits the synthesis of certain types of ribosomal RNA (15). Although not fully characterized, the mechanism of inhibition is believed to be different from RNA polymerase inhibition in bacterial cells (14,15).

Bacterial resistance to rifampin is most often due to a one-step mutation, leading to a change in amino acid sequence in the β subunit of the bacterial RNA polymerase (16). It has been shown that a change in one amino acid renders the enzyme less sensitive to the drug and results in bacterial resistance (17). Other modes of acquiring resistance, such as alteration in permeability, have not been clearly demonstrated in relation to rifampin.

III. ANTIMICROBIAL ACTIVITY AND RESISTANCE

Rifampin is a broad-spectrum antimicrobial agent. It inhibits and kills a wide variety of microorganisms, including gram-positive and gram-negative bacteria, mycobacteria, *Chlamydia*, rickettsiae, and (in combination with amphotericin B) fungi. Its antiviral activity in vitro usually requires high concentrations, which are not clinically relevant (18). Table 1 summarizes the minimal inhibitory concentration (MIC) of rifampin against

Table 1 Minimum Inhibitory Concentration of Rifampin

Organism	MIC_{90} (μg/ml)[a]	MIC, range (μg/ml)
Staphylococcus aureus	0.015	0.008–0.015
S. epidermidis	0.015	0.004–0.015
Streptococcus Group A	0.12	0.03–0.12
Streptococcus Group B	1	0.25–1
Streptococcus faecalis	8	1–8
S. viridans	0.12	0.03–8
S. pneumoniae	4.0	0.06–32[b]
Hemophilus influenzae	1	0.5–64
H. ducreyi	⩽0.015	⩽0.015
Neisseria gonorrhoeae	0.5	0.06–2
N. meningitidis	0.5	0.015–1
Listeria monocytogenes	0.25	⩽0.12–0.25
Legionella pneumophila	0.03	0.015–0.03
Legionella spp.	NA	0.03–0.25
Chlamydia trachomatis	NA	0.005–0.007
Mycobacterium tuberculosis	NA	0.005–0.2
M. kansasii	NA	0.1–1.0
M. marinum	NA	0.64–2.5
M. ulcerans	NA	0.005–0.2
M. avium-intracellulare	NA	2–>20
M. fortuitum	>64	16–>64
M. chelonei	>64	>64
M. leprae	0.3	0.3
Escherichia coli	16	8–16
Klebsiella pneumoniae	32	16–32
Enterobacter spp.	64	8–64
Citrobacter spp.	32	32

Table 1 (Continued)

Organism	MIC_{90} (μg/ml)[a]	MIC, range (μg/ml)
Proteus mirabilis	8	4–8
P. vulgaris	32	8–32
Morganella morganii	32	8–32
Providencia rettgeri	32	8–64
P. stuartii	16	4–16
Serratia marcescens	32	32–64
Flavobacterium meningosepticum	1.25	0.6–1.25
Acinetobacter spp.	8	4–16
Pseudomonas aeruginosa	64	32–>64
Pseudomonas spp.	32	4–>64
Clostridium difficile	<1	<1
Bacteroides fragilis	NA	0.26[c]
Brucella spp.	NA	0.15–25
Rickettsia prowazeki	0.01	0.008–0.01
Reference strains[d]	MIC, mode (μg/ml)	
Staphylococcus aureus ATCC 29213	0.015	0.008–0.06
S. aureus ATCC 25923	0.03	0.015–0.12
Streptococcus faecalis ATCC 29212	2	1–2
Escherichia coli ATCC 25922	16	8–16
Pseudomonas aeruginosa ATCC 27853	64	32–64

[a]NA = data not available.
[b]Including multiple antibiotic-resistant strains from South Africa.
[c]Range not reported.
[d]Each figure derived from 12 independent MIC determinations for each strain.
Source: Data compiled from References 7 and 19–23.

various microorganisms. Rifampin is highly active against gram-positive organisms. Staphylococci, including methicillin-resistant strains, and most streptococci are highly susceptible, with the exception of *Streptococcus faecalis*, which is only moderately sensitive. Among four multiresistant *Streptococcus pneumoniae* strains obtained from South Africa, three had MIC of 4 μg/ml and one had MIC of 32 μg/ml (24). *Bacillus anthracis* and *Clostridium* spp. are susceptible, but *Nocardia* are resistant (25,26).

Among the gram-negative bacteria, the most susceptible organisms in vitro are *Legionella* spp., *Listeria monocytogenes, Hemophilus ducreyi, Hemophilus influenzae, Neisseria gonorrhoeae*, and *Neisseria meningitidis. Brucella* spp., *Flavobacterium meningosepticum*, and *Bacteroides fragilis* are also susceptible in vitro.

Proteus, Acinetobacter, and *Salmonella* spp. are intermediately sensitive to rifampin, whereas most other Enterobacteriaceae and nonfermentative gram-negative bacilli are insensitive (MIC_{90} = 16–64 μg/ml).

Among the mycobacteria, *M. tuberculosis, Mycobacterium leprae*, and most strains of *Mycobacterium kansasii, Mycobacterium marinum* (*balnei*), and *Mycobacterium ulcerans* are highly susceptible; whereas most *Mycobacterium avium-intracellulare, Mycobacterium fortuitum* and *Mycobacterium chelonei* strains are resistant.

Other susceptible microorganisms include *Chlamydia trachomatis, Chlamydia psittaci*, and *Rickettsia prowazekii* (20,21). Anecdotal reports indicate that such protozoa as *Naegleria fowleri* and *Pneumocystis carinii* are also susceptible to rifampin (27,28).

A. Bacterial Resistance

Mutants resistant to rifampin can be elicited both in vitro and in vivo among most bacterial species that are usually sensitive to the drug. Resistance occurs as a result of a one-step mutation leading to alteration in the bacterial enzyme, DNA-dependent RNA polymerase, rendering it much less sensitive to rifampin activity (16).

The rate of appearance of rifampin-resistant mutants among isolates of *M. tuberculosis* has been studied both in vitro and in vivo (29–31). It was shown that naturally occurring resistant mutants are rarely encountered (estimated mutation frequency of 10^{-10}) (29). However, when tubercle bacilli are exposed to rifampin in vitro or when isolates are obtained from patients treated with rifampin as a single drug, the frequency of mutation increases ($\approx 10^{-7}$) (32). In one study, 5 of 11 patients with tuberculosis treated with rifampin alone developed rifampin-resistant isolates within 3 months (30). Similar observations have been reported in patients with *M. kansasii* and *M. leprae* infections treated with rifampin as a single agent (33,34).

The use of rifampin monotherapy has also been associated with rapid emergence of resistant mutants in nonmycobacterial infections (25,35,36), including those due to *Staphylococcus aureus, Streptococcus pyogenes, Strep. pneumoniae*, and *N. meningitidis* (estimated frequency of mutants = 10^{-7}), as well as in *E. coli* (estimated rate of 10^{-8}). The development of resistance to rifampin is usually not associated with the development of resistance to other antibiotics.

In an attempt to avoid the rapid emergence of bacterial resistance to rifampin, it is generally not prescribed as a single agent. Indeed, the addition of isoniazid to rifampin has reduced the emergence of resistant tubercle bacilli (37). This combination has since become the most useful chemotherapeutic regimen for pulmonary tuberculosis. Similarly, combining fusidic acid or novobiocin with rifampin decreases the emergence of rifampin-resistant staphylococci (38), and subinhibitory concentrations of erythromycin or oxytetracycline inhibit the emergence of rifampin-resistant *Chlamydia* in vitro (21). It should be noted, however, that rifampin-resistant mutants emerge even when the drug is used in combination with other antimicrobials, as demonstrated by the appearance of resistant staphylococci in patients treated with a combination of rifampin and vancomycin (39,40).

B. Activity with Other Antimicrobial Agents

Many studies have examined potential synergy between rifampin and a wide variety of antimicrobial agents against various strains of microorganisms. In vitro synergy commonly has been demonstrated. Some studies also have purported to demonstrate enhanced in vivo activity (39,41,42). One such area of investigation is the antistaphyoococcal activity of rifampin in combination with various antistaphylococcal drugs, including vancomycin, β-lactams, aminoglycosides, and erythromycin (43–47). Staphylococcal strains that have been tested include methicillin-sensitive and methicillin-resistant isolates (41,48). The results of these studies have been inconsistent; although many have demonstrated synergism, others have demonstrated antagonism. The conflicting results are most probably due to the different methods utilized (i.e., checkerboard analysis vs. time-kill curve techniques). This is further supported by two recent studies that report discordant results of checkerboard testing vs. time-kill curves in assessing the antistaphylococcal activity of vancomycin plus rifampin (49) and cloxacillin plus rifampin (50).

The antistaphylococcal efficacy of rifampin-containing combinations have been studied in cases of endocarditis (including prosthetic valve-associated infections), central nervous system shunt infections, and chronic osteomyelitis (48,51,52). Enhanced clinical efficacy has been reported in most cases, despite a few instances of demonstrable in vitro antagonism. It should be emphasized, however, that clinical experience is based mainly on small retrospective series, with few comparative prospective analyses (41).

Another extensively studied combination is that of rifampin plus trimethoprim. These drugs have been found to be additive or synergistic against streptococci, *Proteus* spp., and many other enterobacteriaceae, nonfermentative gram-negative bacilli, and *B. fragilis* (53,54). In addition, the frequency of emergence of rifampin-resistant mutants is markedly decreased in the presence of subinhibitory concentrations of trimethoprim (53,54).

The combination of nalidixic acid and rifampin was found to be synergistic against various gram-negative bacteria in vitro (55). Novobiocin enhanced rifampin activity against *Salmonella typhi* isolates, including multiresistant strains (56). In a recent clinical study, the addition of rifampin to penicillin for the treatment of group A streptococcal pharyngitis improved the clinical and bacteriologic cure rates over those of penicillin alone (57). The triple combination of ticarcillin, tobramycin, and rifampin has been found synergistic against *Pseudomonas aeruginosa* (58). This combination has been used successfully in a few anecdotal cases of severe, refractory *Pseudomonas* infection (59).

Rifampin used in combination with amphotericin B is reported to be more effective than either drug alone when tested in vitro against a wide variety of fungi, including various strains of *Candida, Histoplasma, Cryptococcus, Coccidioides, Aspergillus, Blastomyces*, and *Rhizopus* (60-66). Clinical experience with this combination is limited to a few anecdotal case reports (67-69). The results of animal studies have been inconsistent. In murine models of histoplasmosis, blastomycosis, and aspergillosis, the combination was more effective than either drug alone (65,70), whereas no enhanced activity was found in murine models of candidiasis and coccidioidomycosis, despite in vitro synergy (71,72).

Antagonism between rifampin and other antimicrobials is uncommon. As was previously mentioned, few in vitro studies have demonstrated antagonism between rifampin and vancomycin, oxacillin, or trimethoprim against staphylococci (43,44), however, conflicting results are reported by other investigators or when a different in vitro method is used (41,49,50).

In vitro antagonism was also reported between rifampin and ampicillin against isolates of *L. monocytogenes* (73). In contrast, the combination of penicillin and rifampin proved to be as effective as penicillin alone (without antagonism) in a rabbit model of *Listeria* meningitis (74).

IV. PHARMACOKINETICS

A. Data From Adults

Most data on rifampin absorption, distribution, and elimination are from adult studies. Following oral administration, rifampin is almost completely absorbed from the gastrointestinal tract. The absorption rate is mainly affected by gastric pH and food intake. Acidification of gastric juice with histamine injection results in serum concentrations twice as high as those observed after alkalinization with sodium bicarbonate (75), whereas food intake prior to rifampin ingestion results in delayed absorption with a reduction in peak serum concentration attained (76). In one study, the mean peak serum concentration was 6.6 μg/ml attained 4 hr after a 600-mg dose administered with food. This compared with a mean peak concentration of 8.8 μg/ml attained 2 hr after a dose administered in the fasting state (77). In addition to the above factors, simultaneous administration of para-aminosalicylic acid also interferes with rifampin absorption, leading to both lower peak serum concentrations and a delay in attaining this peak (78).

Following absorption from the gastrointestinal tract, rifampin is transported to the liver via the portohepatic circulation and undergoes deacetylation in hepatocytes (79). Desacetylrifampin is biologically active but to a lesser extent than rifampin and is transferred more rapidly into the bile, competing with bilirubin for excretion (79). Elimination of the drug in the bile is followed by reabsorption from the intestinal tract (enterohepatic circulation). Desacetylrifampin is reabsorbed at a much slower rate than the native drug, and most of the metabolite is excreted in the feces. Approximately 60% of a single rifampin dose is eliminated from the body by this route (20).

In addition to the major metabolic pathway of deacetylation, there is evidence for a glucuronidation process, which also takes place in the hepatocytes. This process appears to be of little pharmacokinetic significance (79).

The rate of excretion for rifampin and its metabolites into the bile is limited, and a transport maximum T_m has been demonstrated (79). The T_m in adults is reached at doses of 300–450 mg; if the excretory capacity is exceeded, plasma concentrations of rifampin rise, and consequently, urine concentrations rise as well. These phenomena are best demonstrated by measuring the peak serum concentration of rifampin following administration of increasing oral doses of the drug. Doubling the oral dose from 150 to 300 mg results in a corresponding increase in peak serum concentration from 2 to 4 μg/ml. Further doubling of rifampin dose to 600 mg is followed by a more than twofold increase in serum concentration (to $\simeq$10 μg/ml), and additional increase to a dosage of 1200 mg produces a disproportionately high serum peak of 32 μg/ml (79).

The mean peak serum concentration of rifampin in adults following a standard 600-mg oral dose is 9–10 μg/ml, the range, derived from several reports, being 3.2-32 μg/ml (76,80,81). The mean trough concentration 24 hr after this dose is 0.78 μg/ml (80). The calculated area under the time-concentration curve (AUC) following a 600-mg dose is in the range of 45-65 μg/ml hr^{-1} according to various studies (77,82,83). Time to peak concentration T_{max} is approximately 2 hr after administration (range, 1–4 hr) and varies between subjects as well as in a given subject (76,79,81).

The biologic half-life of rifampin increases with the dose, from a mean value of 2.6 hr for a 300-mg dose and 3.3 hr for 600 mg to 5.1 hr for 900 mg (76). This phenomenon is most likely due to the above-mentioned transport maximum T_m for biliary excretion of rifampin.

The volume of distribution (V_d) of rifampin is calculated to be 160% of body weight (112 liters for a 70-kg adult) (84). The fraction of the drug bound to plasma protein is approximately 75–80%, primarily to albumin (smaller drug fractions are bound to gammaglobulin and fibrinogen) (76). Protein binding is reversible and relatively weak. The affinity value would suggest a percentage of free rifampin in the order of 15–20%.

Pharmacokinetic data are summarized in Table 2. Following administration of repeated daily doses of rifampin there is a 40% decrease in the biologic half-life of the drug

Table 2 Pharmacokinetic Parameters of Rifampin[a]

	Peak serum level (μg/ml)		Trough serum level (μg/ml, 24 hr)		T_{max} (hr)		$T_{1/2}$ (hr),	AUC (μg/ml hr^{-1}),	V_d;	Protein binding (%),
	Mean	Range	Mean	Range	Mean	Range	range	range	mean[b]	range
Adults	9	3.2–32	0.78	0–3.5	2	1–4	3.3–3.9	45–65	160	75–80
Infants and children	10.7	4.6–17.2			1		2.9	56		
Neonates	6				8					

[a]Following a single oral dose of 600 mg to adults and 10 mg/kg to neonates and children.
[b]Percentage of body weight.
Source: Data compiled from References 76, 77, and 79–84.

within the first 2 weeks (32,76). A concomitant decrease in peak serum concentration is observed as well (76,79). These changes are due to gradual increases in the formation and biliary excretion of desacetylrifampin, which are induced by rifampin itself. The self-induced increase in hepatic metabolism (a cytochrome oxidase P_{450}-coupled process) is most pronounced during the first 6 days of rifampin administration and reaches a plateau during the second week of therapy (79).

The major route of rifampin elimination from the body is via bile excretion with fecal elimination. Antibacterial activity appears in the bile 1-2 hr after oral administration and gradually increases, reaching a plateau after 4-6 hr. Most of the antibacterial activity is due to desacetylrifampin (approximately 300 μg/ml, 4-6 hr after a 600-mg dose) (79). Over 60% of the administered dose is eventually eliminated in the feces.

Renal clearance of rifampin in normal adults is calculated to be 30.2 ± 3.6 ml/min 1.73 m^{-2}. On average, the renal clearance of rifampin corresponds to 12.2% of the glomerular filtration rate. Urinary excretion of rifampin correlates closely with serum concentration. Peak urine concentrations are reached 6 hr after an oral dose and are reported to be 150 μg/ml, 250 μg/m, and 450 μg/ml following oral administration of 150, 300, and 600 mg of rifampin, respectively. Approximately 13% of a 150-mg dose, 17% of a 300-mg dose, and 24% of a 600-mg dose have been recovered in the urine during the first 12 hr following drug administration (76).

Following repeated daily administration of rifampin, with resulting decrease in peak serum concentration and biologic half-life, there is a corresponding decrease in urinary concentration and recovery rate (85). In addition, the fraction of desacetylrifampin in the urine, accounting for ≃ 50% of urinary bioactivity on day 1 of therapy, is markedly reduced after the first week of therapy (79). An additional metabolite, formylrifampicin, accounts for about 10% of the antibacterial activity in the urine after oral administration. This metabolite is thought to be formed spontaneously in the urine (76).

B. Pharmacokinetics in Infants and Children

There are few studies regarding rifampin pharmacokinetics in infants and children. Acocella et al. (86) found that a single oral dose of 10 mg/kg given to infants resulted in a mean peak serum concentration of 3.5 μg/ml. This corresponded to one third of the concentration achieved in adults given the same dose. In contrast, the T_{max}, $t_{1/2}$, and rate of urinary excretion in these infants were similar to adult values, indicating that the differences in peak concentration may be related to larger total body water compartment in young infants and not to altered absorption or excretion of the drug.

McCracken et al. (82) have studied the pharmacokinetics of rifampin following a single oral dose of 10 mg/kg in infants and children 6-58 months of age. The mean peak serum concentration was 10.7 ± 0.81 μg/ml with a T_{max} of 1 hr and a $t_{1/2}$ of 2.9 hr. The calculated area under the serum concentration-time curve was 56 μg/ml hr^{-1}. These data are comparable to the corresponding values previously reported in adults receiving an oral dose of 600 mg.

In newborns, rifampin pharmacokinetic data differ from those obtained in infants and children. In one study (86), single oral doses of 10 mg/kg yielded a mean peak serum concentration of 6 μg/ml and T_{max} of 8 hr, accompanied by a corresponding delay in urinary excretion. When repeated daily doses of rifampin were administered to newborns, higher peaks (12 μg/ml), shorter T_{max} (2 hr); and increased AUC and urinary excretion were elicited on day 3 of therapy compared with day 1. These data suggest accumulation of the drug in newborns. The differences in kinetic data observed in newborns are probably due to a less efficient elimination of the drug through the bile and imply that doses of 10 mg/kg should not be exceeded (or even reduced) in this age group (76,86).

C. Parenteral Rifampin

Rifampin is mainly used as an oral drug; however, in Europe, an intravenous formulation is licensed and available for clinical use. Nitti et al. (83) studied the pharmacokinetics of rifampin in a small series of adults following 300-, 450-, and 600-mg doses, given intravenously at a constant rate over 180 min. Following the 300-mg dose, a mean peak serum concentration of 4.05 ± 2.05 μg/ml was observed with a corresponding $t_{1/2}$ of 2.13 ± 0.03 hr and a calculated AUC of 17.6 ± 6.7 μg/ml hr^{-1}. The 600-mg dose yielded a mean peak of 13.53 ± 1.43 μg/ml, $t_{1/2}$ of 2.85 ± 0.3 hr, and an AUC of 64.1 ± 5.8 μg/ml hr^{-1}. Overall, these data resemble those obtained in adults after oral administration of similar doses.

D. Distribution in the Body

Rifampin is readily distributed into various tissues and body compartments. This is due to the favorable lipid-water partition ratio of rifampin, which accounts for its capacity to cross biologic membranes.

High rifampin concentrations, exceeding serum concentrations by severalfold, are attained in the bile (300–400 μg/ml, 6 hr after a 600-mg dose), urine (up to 450 μg/ml 6 hr after a 600-mg dose), and liver (36 μg/ml following a 450-mg dose) (79,87,88). Concentrations of rifampin exceeding simultaneous serum levels are also demonstrated in lung, gallbladder wall, stomach wall, and extracellular fluid (87,88).

Concentrations as high as 12 μg/ml have been measured in the sputum of tuberculosis patients treated daily with a 900-mg dose (90). In children, mean salivary concentrations of 1.7 μg/ml (range, 0.54–7.2 μg/ml) were measured 2 hr after a 10-mg/kg dose; whereas tear concentrations reached a peak of 7.7 μg/ml, similar to serum levels (82).

Therapeutic concentrations of rifampin have also been demonstrated in pus obtained from abdominal abscesses (91), caseous material from tuberculous lesions (92), breast milk, aqueous humor, pleural effusion, and prostatic tissue (79,80,89). Therapeutic concentrations of rifampin are also found in bone. In one study, bone concentrations of 3.35 ± 0.75 μg/g were obtained after a single 600-mg dose, with a corresponding serum concentration of 8.67 ± 1.77 μg/ml (110).

Penetration of rifampin into the cerebrospinal fluid (CSF) increases in the presence of meningeal inflammation. Concentrations in the range of 0–0.5 μg/ml were attained in normal CSF after oral rifampin doses, whereas four- to eightfold higher concentrations were demonstrated when the meninges were inflamed (93). Therapeutic concentrations in the CSF have also been documented in cases of tuberculous meningitis (94,95). In one series of 10 patients with tuberculous meningitis, the peak CSF concentrations following a dose of 300 mg twice a day were 0.18–1.37 μg/ml (95). In two cases of neonatal *Flavobacterium* meningitis, peak CSF concentrations of 0.85 and 1.1 μg/ml were documented following the intramuscular administration of rifamycin SV (the parent compound of rifampin) (96).

Owing to its high lipid solubility, rifampin penetrates well into various cells, including intact polymorphonuclear leukocytes and macrophages. The drug readily kills viable intraphagocytic bacteria, such as *E. coli* and *S. aureus* (97), and could, therefore, be utilized in disorders of intracellular bacterial killing, such as chronic granulomatous disease (98).

An unusual aspect of rifampin's wide distribution in body compartments is the color it may impart to various body fluids. The urine, feces, tears, CSF, saliva, and sweat of patients may have an orange-red discoloration. Soft contact lenses may be permanently stained by rifampin, and patients should be warned of this possibility (99).

E. Rifampin Kinetics in Hepatic and Renal Impairment

In patients with various hepatic diseases, there is an overall decrease in biliary excretion of the drug. Conditions associated with increased portocaval shunting (e.g., cirrhosis) result in an increase in the amount of drug that bypasses the liver. In diseases characterized by hepatic parenchymal damage (e.g., hepatitis), there is a decrease in production of desacetylrifampin, and in biliary atresia, there is significant reduction in biliary excretion of rifampin and its metabolites. These conditions are therefore accompanied by increases in the serum concentrations of unchanged drug and a concomitant prolongation of biologic half-life (76). In a study comparing patients with cirrhosis to normal controls, rifampin serum concentrations 8 hr after a 600-mg dose were two- to threefold higher in the patients, and mean biologic half-life in the patients was 5.4 hr compared with 2.8 hr in controls (100). It should be emphasized that the nature of the liver disease (i.e., acute or chronic) does not seem to affect the observation of reduced hepatic rifampin clearance, and patients with acute viral hepatitis display pharmacokinetic findings similar to those with chronic hepatitis and cirrhosis (101).

Renal clearance of rifampin is reduced in patients with impaired renal function. However, this phenomenon is not associated with a clinically significant accumulation of rifampin in the serum (76,102). Studies have suggested that elimination of the drug by hemodialysis and peritoneal dialysis does not warrant alterations in dosage (76,103). Therefore, the usual recommended dosages of rifampin are suitable for dialysis patients.

V. PREPARATIONS OF RIFAMPIN

Rifampin is available in the United States and Canada for oral use only. In Europe and some other countries, an intravenous preparation is available as well. In North America, the intravenous preparations are available on an emergency basis. Oral preparations include capsules of 150 and 300 mg and syrup containing 100 mg in 5 ml.

Rifampin is also available in preparations containing fixed combinations of rifampin and isoniazid: 100 mg isoniazid + 150 mg rifampin and 150 mg isoniazid + 300 mg rifampin.

The usual adult dosage is 600 mg or 8–12 mg/kg, given once daily either 1 hr before or 2 hr after a meal. In patients with hepatic impairment, doses of 8 mg/kg or lower are usually recommended (4,6). In infants and children, the recommended dosage is 10–20 mg/kg day, to a maximum 600 mg/day, administered as above. The higher dosage should be exployed in more severe infections, including those of the central nervous system (104). In neonates, a dosage of 10 mg/kg given once daily is recommended (104).

For prophylaxis of adult meningococcal contracts, 600 mg is given twice daily for 2 days. Children aged 1 month to 12 years should receive 10 mg/kg twice daily for 2 days, and infants under the age of 1 month are given 5 mg/kg twice daily for 2 days (104).

For prophylaxis of *H. influenzae* type b contacts, a single daily dose of 20 mg/kg should be given for 4 days (maximum daily dose, 600 mg) (105). Some authorities recommend a prophylactic daily dose of 10 mg/kg for infants less than 1 month of age (105).

VI. DRUG ASSAYS

Several methods are available for the determination of rifampin concentrations in a variety of body fluids. The most widely used is the agar disk diffusion bioassay method (106) using *Sarcina lutea* ATCC 9341 as a test organism. *Bacillus subtilis* ATCC 6633 has also been employed for urinary bioassay. Virtually any form of fluid or tissue can be assayed by this method, provided that an appropriate control and a pretreatment sample are available. The sample size required for adequate examination may be as low as 100 μl, and the minimum concentration of rifampin that can be measured precisely is 0.2 μg/ml (106,107).

The bioassay method has certain limitations. It cannot distinguish between rifampin and its biologically active metabolite, desacetylrifampin. In addition, bioassay cannot be accurately performed if the patient is being treated concurrently with an antibiotic to which the test organism is sensitive. When a penicillinase-sensitive penicillin is used with rifampin, the latter may be assayed after adding penicillinase to the agar.

Other methods, less frequently utilized, include spectrophotometry, an adequate technique for urinary assay that does not distinguish the drug from its metabolites (108). Thin-layer chromatography can distinguish the parent compound from its metabolites but is only suitable when high concentrations are present (109).

An additional method that is rapid, precise, and relatively simple is high-pressure liquid chromatography (HPLC) (107). Rifampin and its two metabolites (desacetylrifampin and formylrifampin) can be readily distinguished by this method. The amount of sample required is 50 μl, but amounts as low as 20 μl may be sufficient. The time necessary for completion of HPLC is short (approximately 30 min), and concomitant use of other antibiotics does not interfere with the test. The lower limit of accurate detection is 0.5 μg/ml (107). This method is highly suitable for the determination of rifampin and its metabolites in serum and urine.

VII. THERAPEUTIC INDICATIONS

A. Tuberculosis

Rifampin, in combination with isoniazid, is the standard therapy for active pulmonary tuberculosis. This regimen has been shown to be more effective than combinations of formerly used antituberculosis drugs, leading to more rapid sterilization of sputum, fewer side effects, and ability to employ shorter courses of therapy (111,112). Rifampin-containing regimens are also indicated for the treatment of extrapulmonary tuberculosis, including skeletal, urinary tract, miliary, and meningeal disease (104). The drug has also been used successfully in conjunction with other antituberculous drugs in cases of *M. kansasii* and *M. marinum* infections, as well as some instances of atypical mycobacterial lymphadenitis in children (113,114).

B. Leprosy

Rifampin is highly effective against *M. leprae*. It is more rapidly bactericidal than the sulfone drugs and is effective against sulfone-resistant strains (115). Currently, the World

Health Organization recommends the use of rifampin and clofazimine in combination with dapsone for the treatment of patients with multibacillary leprosy. In cases of paucibacillary disease, the combination of dapsone with intermittent rifampin is indicated (116).

C. Prophylaxis of Meningococcal and *H. influenzae* Contacts

Rifampin is recommended as the drug of choice for prophylaxis of close contacts of patients with meningococcal meningitis or meningococcemia (104). The drug has been shown to erradicate meningococci from the nasopharynx in approximately 90% of carriers. The emergence of rifampin-resistant meningococci has been reported on rare occasions following a short course of rifampin prophylaxis (117).

Rifampin is also recommended for prophylaxis of household contacts of children with invasive *H. influenzae* disease when there is a household member younger than 49 months (105). The need for rifampin prophylaxis among day-care center contacts of the index case is controversial, although most experts advise its use when two or more cases of invasive disease have occurred among day-care attendees within a 60-day period (105). (For dosage regimens, see page 383-4). As with meningococci, the emergence of rifampin-resistant *H. influenzae* was rarely encountered following a 4-day regimen of rifampin prophylaxis (118).

In addition to the approved indications discussed above, rifampin has been advocated as a useful adjunct for the treatment of many other infections. In many instances, the supporting data are derived from small series or retrospective analyses, and in most cases, additional prospective comparative studies are needed before definite recommendations can be established. The following conditions fall into this category:

1. Endocarditis

The combination of rifampin with vancomycin or an antistaphylococcal penicillin may be useful in the treatment of staphylococcal endocarditis in patients who fail to respond to β-lactams or vancomycin alone (119,120). The combination is particularly useful (1) if therapeutic failure occurs in patients with prosthetic valve infection; (2) for cases complicated by myocardial or peripheral abscesses; (3) if the staphylococcal isolate is tolerant to β-lactams or vancomycin (48,121-123).

2. Osteomyelitis

Rifampin in combination with other antistaphylococcal agents, such as β-lactams, vancomycin, or carboxyquinoline derivatives, has been shown in small series to be effective in the treatment of chronic staphylococcal osteomyelitis that is refractory to standard therapy (52,124,125). Larger series and long-term follow-up are required before further recommendations can be established.

3. Central Nervous System Shunt Infections

A few pediatric patients with staphylococcal CNS shunt infections have demonstrated prompt clinical and bacteriologic response to vancomycin-rifampin combinations (51, 126). In at least one case, prior vancomycin therapy had been unsuccessful (51). As with prosthetic valve endocarditis, rifampin may be useful in staphylococcal infections associated with indwelling foreign bodies.

4. Staphylococcal Carrier State

Rifampin alone or in combination with other antistaphylococcal drugs markedly reduces the nasal carriage of *S. aureus* (127). This mode of therapy has proven useful in interrupting nosocomial outbreaks of methicillin-resistant staphylococcal infections (128) and reduced the rate of infection in cases of recurrent furunculosis (122).

5. Streptococcal Pharyngitis

In a prospective comparative study, rifampin added to penicillin V resulted in improved clinical and bacteriologic outcome in children with streptococcal pharyngitis when compared with penicillin V alone (57). In another prospective study, rifampin plus benzathine penicillin G was superior to the latter in eradicating group A streptococci from chronic carriers (129). Rifampin added to penicillin may therefore be beneficial in selected cases of culture-positive, recurrent streptococcal pharyngitis and in colonized individuals who have had rheumatic fever or are household contacts of such patients (57).

6. Multiple-Antibiotic Resistant *S. pneumoniae*

The rare cases of meningitis due to multiple-antibiotic resistant pneumococci that have been encountered in South Africa, Australia, Canada, and the United States present a unique therapeutic problem. The South African strains were sensitive to rifampin, and two cases of meningitis (one each from Australia and the United States) were successfully treated with rifampin-containing regimens (130,131). In South Africa, rifampin plus fusidic acid were successfully used to eradicate such strains (132). Based on these data, it seems warranted to use rifampin-containing regimens in the rare outbreaks of multiresistant pneumococcal infections.

7. Brucellosis

Rifampin alone or in combination with tetracycline or trimethoprim-sulfamethoxazole has been used successfully in patients with various forms of brucellosis (23,133). In addition, there is some evidence that rifampin-containing regimens are associated with lower relapse rates (23). At present, rifampin should probably be considered in cases of endocarditis, osteomyelitis, and neurological disease caused by *Brucella* for whom prolonged therapy and good tissue penetration are desired.

8. *Legionella* Infections

Legionella pneumophila and a few other *Legionella* species are highly susceptible to rifampin in vitro (19). Based on experimental animal models and several case reports (134,135), the combination of rifampin and erythromycin is currently recommended for the treatment of severe *Legionella* infection that is refractory to erythromycin alone (134).

9. Chronic Granulomatous Disease (CGD)

The unique ability of rifampin to penetrate into polymorphonuclear cells and kill intracellular staphylococci was demonstrated in granulocytes obtained from healthy subjects as well as those with CGD (136). The reported clinical efficacy of rifampin in CGD patients with persistent staphylococcal abscesses (98) should encourage additional clinical trials of rifampin-containing regimens in this disease.

10. Chlamydia

The 1% rifampin eye ointment, applied three times per day for 6-7 weeks, is effective in the treatment of sexually transmitted chlamydial inclusion conjunctivitis (137). In children, this preparation is beneficial for treating hyperendemic trachoma when applied twice daily for 6 weeks; its efficacy is comparable to that of oxytetracycline ointment (138).

11. Leishmaniasis

Data accumulated from the literature regarding over 100 patients treated with rifampin for cutaneous leishmaniasis indicate that the drug is beneficial in most cases (23). Therapeutic failures are uncommon. Prospective comparitive studies are underway to further assess the efficacy and dosing regimens for rifampin in this disease.

12. Neonatal Meningitis due to *F. meningosepticum*

This rare neonatal infection is caused by an unusually resistant microorganism and associated with high mortality in this age group (23,96). The bacteria are sensitive to rifampin in vitro, and a few cases of neonatal meningitis have been treated successfully with rifampin in combination with other agents, without major side effects (96,139). In view of the rarity and severity of such infections in such patients, it is difficult to conduct well-controlled, comparative studies. At present, it seems reasonable to include rifampin in the initial therapy of neonatal meningitis due to *Flavobacterium.*

13. Fungal Infections

Despite multiple reports of in vitro synergy between amphotericin B and rifampin against various fungal strains, in vivo studies are limited and controversial (60,65,71,72). Clinical data regarding therapeutic efficacy are derived from anecdotal case reports, and prospective studies will be needed to weigh the clinical potential of rifampin-amphotericin B combinations.

14. Urinary Tract Infections

The combination of rifampin with trimethoprim displays excellent antibacterial activity in vitro against most pathogens associated with urinary tract infection (53,54). Clinical studies have established favorable pharmacokinetic and therapeutic properties as well (140). At present, rifampin-trimethoprim combinations should probably be reserved for those patients with chronic or recurrent urinary tract infection, due to resistant microorganisms, for whom alternative treatment is unavailable.

15. Miscellaneous Infections

Anecdotal case reports have been published on successful therapy against a variety of refractory infections in the past 15 years, using rifampin alone or in combination. These include instances of invasive staphylococcal infections treated with rifampin alone or in combination with tetracyclines or aminoglycosides (141,142); *Pneumocystis carinii* pneumonia in infants treated with rifampin alone (28); shigellosis treated with rifampin alone and in combination; and a variety of gram-negative infections, including those due to *Pseudomonas aeruginosa*, successfully treated with rifampin-aminoglycoside combinations (59,143,144). These reports are anecdotal and will require additional confirmation.

VIII. TOXICITY

The adverse effects of rifampin are related to the duration of therapy and dosage. Short-term therapy, such as that given for meningitis prophylaxis, is associated with mild, transient, non-life-threatening side effects (118,145); children are affected with the same frequency as adults (145).

Various adverse reactions, usually mild in nature, have been encountered during prolonged daily therapy; however, in many instances, the drug had been given in combination with other agents, such as isoniazid. This poses difficulty in assessing the toxicity of each individual agent.

Therapeutic regimens based on intermittent administration of rifampin (given once or twice weekly) are associated with an increased incidence and severity of side effects (146,147). This is particularly true with higher doses of the drug (1200 mg per dose or higher) (148). The adverse reactions associated with such regimens are most probably due to an immunologic reaction, as illustrated by the demonstration of rifampin-dependent antibodies in the circulation of such patients (149). The antibodies are most commonly of the IgM class, but IgG, IgA, and IgE antibodies have also been detected (146).

It is postulated that rifampin given chronically on a daily basis is accompanied by immunologic tolerance to the drug, whereas during intermittent therapy, there is a repeated "booster" effect, leading to accumulation of rifampin-dependent antibodies that in turn participate in the formation of circulating immune complexes or other immune-mediated reactions (146,147,150). Hypersensitivity reactions similar to those observed during intermittent therapy have also been encountered in noncompliant patients (who take the drug irregularly) and cases in whom rifampin has been reinstituted following past treatment (4,151). The various adverse effects of rifampin can be categorized according to body system.

A. Skin

Cutaneous manifestations occur in up to 5% of patients and are usually manifested as a mild to moderate erythematous or maculopapular rash that may be accompanied by conjunctival irritation, lacrimation, stomatitis, or glossitis (146,147). Such reactions can be minimized if rifampin is taken with meals. More severe manifestations, such as urticaria and intense pruritus are most often associated with intermittent rifampin therapy (151, 152). Generally, dermatologic side effects occur early in the course of therapy and are transient in nature. Interruption of therapy is rarely indicated (151).

Two cases of drug-related pemphigus have responded to discontinuance of therapy. In one case, no additional treatment was required, and the other responded to corticosteroids (153).

In the uncommon event of acute rifampin overdose, there is an orange-red discoloration of the skin. Such patients are referred to as "lobster red" or "red man" syndrome (154).

B. Gastrointestinal Tract

Gastrointestinal side effects occur in up to 2% of patients, are rarely serious, and consist of anorexia, nausea, mild abdominal pain, pyrosis, and, less commonly, vomiting and diarrhea (146,151). Symptoms begin shortly after administration of the drug and can be ameliorated by giving rifampin during or immediately after meals.

Pseudomembranous colitis has been rarely attributed to rifampin (155,156). In some cases, however, other antimicrobial agents had been given as well (156). Antibiotic-associated colitis has been observed in hamsters after repeated exposure to the drug. Isolates of *Clostridium difficile* recovered from the colonic contents of these animals were highly resistant to rifampin, in contrast to strains isolated prior to rifampin administration (157). The results of this study suggest that colitis may be due to selection of rifampin-resistant *C. difficile.*

C. Liver

Most available data regarding rifampin hepatotoxicity are derived from series of patients who were not treated with rifampin alone (37,158-160). Early studies in experimental animals and humans given rifampin alone failed to demonstrate hepatotoxicity by liver biopsy (146).

The most common form of hepatic impairment is mild, transient, clinically inapparent elevation of serum bilirubin, alkaline phosphatase, and aminotransferases that occurs early in the course of treatment in 5-14% of patients (100,146,147). In most instances, abnormal tests spontaneously return to normal despite continuation of rifampin therapy (146).

Hepatitis is an uncommon complication of rifampin-containing regimens and has been reported in less than 1% of rifampin recipients (4). If hepatitis occurs, the drug should be discontinued. Rifampin may be resumed cautiously, with careful monitoring of liver function, once hepatic function tests have returned to normal (151).

The combination of isoniazid and rifampin seems to result in an increased risk of hepatotoxicity compared with either drug alone (159,161). In a retrospective study conducted by the Centers for Disease Control, 3.3% of children treated with isoniazid and rifampin demonstrated hepatotoxic reactions, similar to the rate observed in adults (159). Earlier reports indicating a significantly higher incidence of hepatotoxicity among children were usually associated with higher isoniazid dosages, coadministration of other potentially hepatotoxic drugs, or use in the setting of tuberculous meningitis (162-164).

Fatal hepatotoxicity is very rare. In a retrospective analysis conducted in 1973, 16 deaths associated with jaundice were identified among over 500,000 rifampin recipients (37). Increased risk for severe hepatic impairment appears in alcoholics, individuals with associated systemic disease (e.g., renal and hepatic), and those given other potentially hepatotoxic drugs concurrently (146,151,158,162). In such patients, the need for rifampin therapy should be carefully assessed and, if utilized, should be followed by close monitoring of hepatic function.

D. Central Nervous System

Dizzyness, drowziness, headache, and visual disturbance are uncommon side effects of rifampin therapy (4,37) and have been reported in children as well as adults (145). There have been a few anecdotal case reports of adults who have experienced more severe reactions, such as ataxia and confusional state associated with hallucinations and delusions (165). Acute rifampin overdose has not usually been associated with significant central nervous system manifestations (154).

E. Hematologic

Serious hematologic side effects have been reported following intermittent administration of rifampin and have been associated with the formation of rifampin-dependent antibodies (146–151,166). The principal manifestations have been immune thrombocytopenic purpura (166) and hemolytic anemia (167). In several cases, other hypersensitivity reactions, such as hypotension, shortness of breath, and renal failure, have been encountered as well. Isolated cases of agranulocytosis and eosinophilia have also been related to rifampin administration (168,169).

The occurrence of thrombocytopenic purpura, hemolytic anemia, or agranulocytosis should lead to prompt withdrawal of rifampin. The drug should not be administered again to such patients, since readministration is likely to cause recurrence of symptoms (146, 151,170). Reinstitution of rifampin therapy to patients who were previously treated uneventfully with the drug should be carried out cautiously, since hypersensitivity reactions may accompany the second course. The drug is best started in low dosage, with gradual increase to full dose. Hematologic as well as hepatic and renal parameters should be followed closely in such cases (151).

F. Renal

Light-chain proteinuria can be detected in many patients receiving rifampin, usually without apparent ill effect (171). In some cases, however, reversible renal failure has complicated proteinuria that developed in the setting of dehydration (172).

Acute renal failure is a rare complication of rifampin therapy. Most cases were reported in patients treated intermittently, rarely during daily administration (7,173,174). In many cases, rifampin-dependent antibodies could be demonstrated in the serum and renal biopsy findings consisted of glomerular complement deposition with resulting inflammation and glomerular destruction (146). In a few instances, the histopathologic changes were characteristic of drug-induced interstitial nephritis (172,175). In each case of rifampin-induced renal failure, the drug has been promptly discontinued; however, in several instances, hemodialysis was required before renal function returned to normal. Subjects who have experienced renal toxicity from rifampin should not receive the drug again.

G. The "Flu Syndrome" and Respiratory Manifestations

The "flu syndrome" consists of episodic headache, malaise, fever, and bone pains beginning 1–2 hr after a rifampin dose and subsiding after approximately 12 hr (146,152). Symptoms reappear with each successive dose. The flu syndrome is immunologically mediated and associated with circulating rifampin-dependent antibodies. Women and the elderly are most often affected, particularly those given high and intermittent dosages of rifampin (146). Reducing the individual doses and reversion to daily dosage will alleviate symptoms in most cases.

Dyspnea and wheezing are rarely encountered in rifampin recipients and may accompany the flu syndrome (176). Rarely, such patients have experienced more severe reactions, such as hypotension or shock (151). Respiratory side effects should be managed in a similar manner to the flu syndrome.

H. Immunosuppressive Effects of Rifampin

Various in vitro and in vivo studies have demonstrated immunosuppressive effects associated with rifampin. The most consistent findings have been diminution in lymphoblastic transformation by phytohemagglutinin and reaction to tuberculin (both in vivo and in vitro) (177–179). Humoral immune responses are less consistently affected by rifampin. Thus far, there has been no evidence of adverse clinical effects associated with rifampin-induced immunologic alteration (146,180).

I. Teratogenic Effects

Rifampin has been reported to cross the placental barrier and attain therapeutic concentrations in fetal tissues (6,90,181); however, the effects of the drug on the human fetus are largely unknown. In rats and mice, high oral doses of rifampin given to the pregnant animal result in an increase in congenital malformations, primarily spina bifida and cleft palate (182). In one report from the Ciba and Lepetit companies, the incidence of malformations among the offspring of 226 women treated with rifampin during pregnancy was 4.3%, compared with 1.8% for infants exposed to tuberculosis and 6.5% for those exposed to other antituberculosis drugs (182). In view of the potential teratogenic effect of rifampin, the drug should not be used during pregnancy, even as prophylaxis against meningococcal infection; however, its therapeutic use in cases of severe tuberculous infection during pregnancy may be justified (122,182).

J. Effects on Vitamin D Metabolism

Rifampin has been noted to reduce the serum concentration of 25-hydroxycholecalciferol. No alterations in 1,25-dihydroxycholecalciferol or parathyroid hormone are seen, however (183). In a few cases, osteomalacia was attributed to prolonged use of rifampin (184). No controlled data are currently available regarding the clinical effects of rifampin on skeletal growth, bone metabolism, or vitamin D metabolism in the pediatric age group.

K. Acute Rifampin Overdosage

As of 1985, eight well-documented instances of rifampin overdosage have been reported in the literature (154). Of these, three were fatal, in each case complicating alcohol abuse. The common clinical features were an orange-red skin discoloration (lobster red or red man) and similar discoloration of urine, sweat, feces, tears, and plasma. Other clinical features included gastrointestinal symptoms, pruritus, angioedema, and obtundation (154). Mild, transient elevation of hepatic enzymes and bilirubin was noted in most patients. Despite high serum rifampin concentrations in one of the patients, serum half-life and urinary clearance were well within the range noted following therapeutic dosage. The treatment of acute rifampin overdosage includes gastric lavage, administration of activated charcoal, and intensive supportive measures. There is no known specific antidote.

In summarizing the above data from the viewpoint of the pediatrician, one should note that rifampin can be considered a rather safe drug for use in infants and children if the drug is not given intermittently and a daily dosage of 10–20 mg/kg is not exceeded. Overall, side effects are not common and are usually mild and self-limited. Attention should be paid to children with pre-existing hepatic impairment and those receiving other potentially hepatotoxic agents. Close monitoring of liver function tests is warranted in such cases. In newborn infants, assay of serum concentrations may prove useful because of the potential for accumulation of rifampin in this age group.

IX. CONTRAINDICATIONS

Rifampin is contraindicated in patients with known hypersensitivity to the drug. Cross-allergy occurs only with other rifamycins (4,6).

Rifampin should be discontinued and not reinstituted in patients experiencing the following adverse effects (presumably due to drug hypersensitivity): renal insufficiency, thrombocytopenic purpura, hemolytic anemia, and hypotension. In addition, the drug should not be readministered to those who have experienced rifampin-associated agranulocytosis (167,168).

Rifampin should be avoided in patients with jaundice and should be used with caution in those with impaired liver function, especially if isoniazid or other potentially hepatotoxic agents are given concomitantly (151,159,162). Liver function tests should be monitored closely in such patients and the drug discontinued if signs of hepatotoxicity appear (151).

Rifampin usage is best avoided during pregnancy. It may be considered, however, in pregnant women with severe tuberculous infection (122,182).

Rifampin is not recommended for intermittent therapy owing to the increased risk of severe side effects. A possible exception is the once-a-month rifampin regimen used for lepromatous patients, which has not been associated with an increased incidence or severity of side effects (115). Patients and parents should be advised against intentional or accidental interruption of the daily dosage regimen. If rifampin is to be reinstituted after a period of interruption, it should be given with caution. Some authors recommend restarting with a 75-mg dose followed by a gradual increase to the full dosage (151).

X. DRUG INTERACTIONS

Interactions of rifampin with other drugs can be divided into two main categories: (1) drug interactions affecting rifampin pharmacokinetics, and (2) drug interactions in which rifampin exerts an effect on the kinetics of other drugs.

The main drug in the first category is para-aminosalicylic acid (PAS). Coadministration of PAS and rifampin results in a delayed absorption of rifampin owing to the adsorption of rifampin by bentonite, the principal excipient of aminosalicylic acid granules. It is recommended, therefore, that administration of PAS and rifampin be separated by 8–12 hr (78).

Another drug, probenecid, has been reported to increase serum rifampin concentration when given 30 min prior to rifampin dose (185); however, in a larger subsequent study these observations could not be confirmed (186).

Simultaneous administration of rifampin and ketoconazole to a child suffering from mycobacterial infection and tinea capitis was associated with a significant decrease in serum concentrations of both drugs (187). Although it was suggested that ketoconazole interfered with rifampin absorption, the exact mechanism has not been elucidated.

The second category of drug interactions is based on rifampin's ability to induce the hepatic enzymes responsible for drug metabolism. Administration of rifampin causes proliferation of the smooth endoplasmic reticulum of hepatocytes and results in an increase in the cytochrome P_{450} content in the liver (188,189). This in turn is associated with increased oxidative enzymatic activity in the hepatocytes and is directly related to the enhanced rate of hepatic metabolism of various drugs (188,190).

The facilitated drug metabolism exerted by rifampin is manifested by decreased half-life and reduced peak serum concentrations and area under the concentration-time curve (AUC) of certain drugs. Significant clinical effects may result from insufficient drug concentrations (191-194).

The main drugs affected by the concomitant use of rifampin include the following.

A. Corticosteroids

The mean plasma clearance of prednisolone has been reported to increase by 45% in patients treated concomitantly with rifampin; the AUC decreased by a mean of 66% (195). Renal transplant patients treated with corticosteroids to prevent rejection have experienced decreased renal function when given rifampin (196). Similarly, a child with nephrotic syndrome became unresponsive to corticosteroids after rifampin was started (197). In another report, adrenal crisis was precipitated by rifampin in two patients with Addison's disease receiving cortisone replacement therapy (191). These observations have led several authors to the conclusion that corticosteroid dosage should be doubled or tripled in patients treated concomitantly with rifampin (191,195).

B. Digitoxin

Greater than 50% reduction in serum digitoxin concentrations have been reported following rifampin administration. In addition, a significant decrease in digitoxin half-life, from a mean of 8.2 days to 4.5 days, has been demonstrated (198). In a few cases, the resulting subtherapeutic digitoxin concentrations were associated with acute heart failure (199). A similar event has also been reported in a patient treated with digoxin (200). Cardiac glycoside concentrations should therefore be monitored carefully and drug dosage modified accordingly to assure therapeutic levels in patients treated concomitantly with rifampin.

C. Chloramphenicol

Prober has recently reported two children with *H. influenzae* meningitis in whom chloramphenicol concentrations were reduced to subtherapeutic levels while prophylactic rifampin was given concomitantly (201). This observation raises the question of appropriate timing for rifampin prophylaxis in index cases treated with chloramphenicol for invasive *H. influenzae* infections. A possible solution may involve starting rifampin administration immediately after chloramphenicol has been discontinued. Alternatively, chloramphenicol dosage should be increased and serum concentrations monitored when rifampin is given concurrently.

D. Oral Contraceptives

The reduced efficacy of oral contraceptives, evidenced by increased pregnancy rate, breakthrough bleeding, spotting, and alteration in the menstrual cycle, has been reported in women treated concurrently with rifampin (192,198). These observations were supported by pharmacokinetic studies demonstrating decreased serum half-life and increased clearance of the estrogenic compounds and progesterone component of oral contraceptives in rifampin-treated women (202,203)

E. Methadone

Rifampin administration to opiate addicts treated with methadone has been associated with increased withdrawal symptoms (194). A marked increase in total body clearance of methadone was documented in these cases. Increased methadone dosage is indicated in order to avoid withdrawal symptoms in patients treated with both drugs.

F. Additional Drugs

Those drugs affected similarly by rifampin include quinidine, verapamil, oral hypoglycemics (tolbutamide and chlorpropamide), warfarin, ketoconazole, dapsone, and hexobarbital (187,190,193,198,204-207). In each case, increased dosage was required to attain therapeutic levels of the drug, and discontinuation or replacement of rifampin (e.g., by isoniazid) resulted in reversal of the adverse pharmacokinetic effect within 1 week.

Biliary excretion of bilirubin is competitively inhibited by administration of rifampin (76). This may be important in neonates with pre-existing hyperbilirubinemia, although in the few cases with transient elevation of bilirubin reported in the literature, no adverse clinical effects have been recognized (96).

Administration of rifampin may also interefere with the interpretation of some laboratory tests. The Bromsulphalein (BSP) test will yield falsely high values owing to competitive inhibition of its excretion by rifampin (100). Bioassays for vitamin B_{12} and folate concentrations may be affected by rifampin administration, since the indicator organism used in these tests is sensitive to the latter (208). To overcome this problem, a nonbioassay or rifampin-resistant organism should be employed.

REFERENCES

1. Sensi, P: History of the development of rifampin. *Rev. Infect. Dis. 5(Suppl.)*:S402–S406, 1983.
2. Sensi, P, Gallotta, R, Greco, AM, Gallo, GG: Rifomycin. XV. Activation of rifomycin B and rifomycin O. Production and properties of rifomycin S and rifomycin SV. *Farmaco [Sci.] 16*:165–180, 1961.
3. Maggi, N, Pasqualucci, CR, Ballotta, R, Sensi, P: Rifampicin: A new orally active rifamycin. *Chemotherapia 11*:285–292, 1966.
4. Rifampicin. In: Martindale.*The Extra Pharmacopoeia*, 28th ed. (EF Reynolds, ed.), Pharmaceutical Press, London, 1982, pp. 1577–1582.
5. Mandell, GL: Interaction of intraleukocytic bacteria and antibiotics. *J. Clin. Invest. 52*:1673–1679, 1973.
6. Medical Economics Company: Rifadin. In: *Physicians' Desk Reference*, 39th ed. Oradell, New Jersey, 1985, pp. 1382–1383.
7. Farr, B, Mandell, GL: Rifampin. *Med. Clin. North Am. 66*:157–168, 1982.
8. Hartmann, G, Honikel, KO, Knusel, F, Nuesch, J: The specific inhibition of the DNA-directed RNA synthesis by rifamycin. *Biochim. Biophys. Acta 145*:843–844, 1967.
9. Johnston, DE, McClure, WR: Abortive initiation of in vitro RNA synthesis on bacteriophage λ DNA polymerase. In: *RNA Polymerase* (Losick R, Chamberlin M, ed.), Cold Spring Harbor Laboratory, Cold Spring Harbor, New York, 1976, pp. 413–428.
10. Wehrli, W, Staehelin, M: Interaction of rifamycin with RNA polymerase. In: *RNA Polymerase and Transcription*, Proceedings of the First Lepetit Colloquim (L. Silvestri, ed.), North-Holland, Amsterdam, 1970, pp. 65–70.
11. Wehrli, W: Kinetic studies of the interaction between rifampicin and DNA-dependent RNA polymerase of *Escherichia coli*. *Eur. J. Biochem. 80*:325–330, 1977.

12. McClure, WR, Cech, CL: On the mechanism of rifampicin inhibition of RNA synthesis. *J. Biol. Chem. 253*:8949–8956, 1978.
13. Wehrli, W: Rifampin: Mechanisms of action and resistance. *Rev. Infect. Dis. (Suppl.) 5*:S407–S411, 1983.
14. Medoff, G: Antifungal action of rifampin. *Rev. Infect. Dis. (Suppl.) 5*:S614–S619, 1983.
15. Medoff, G. Kobayashi, GS, Kwan, CN, et al.: Potentiation of rifampicin and 5-fluorocytosine as antifungal antibiotics by amphotericin B. *Proc. Natl. Acad. Sci. USA 69*:196–199, 1972.
16. Di Mauro, D, Snyder, L, Marino, P, et al.: Rifampicin sensitivity of the components of DNA-dependent RNA polymerase. *Nature 222*:533–537, 1979.
17. Ovchinnikov, A, Monastyrskaya, GS, Gubanov, VV, et al.: Primary structure of *Escherichia coli* RNA polymerase. Nucleotide substitution in the β subunit gene of the rifampin resistant rpoB255 mutant. *MGG 184*:536–538, 1981.
18. Subak-Sharpe, JH, Timbury, MC, Williams, JF: Rifampin inhibits the growth of some mammalian viruses. *Nature 222*:341–345, 1969.
19. Thornsberry, C, Hill, BC, Swenson, JM, McDougal, LK: Rifampin: Spectrum of antibacterial activity. *Rev. Infect. Dis. (Suppl.) 5*:S412–S417, 1983.
20. Rifampicin (Rifampin). In: *The Use of Antibiotics*, 3rd ed. (A Kucers and N McBennett, eds.), J. B. Lippincott, Philadelphia, 1979, pp. 552–584.
21. Jones, RB, Ridgway, GL, Boulding, S, Hunley, KL: In vitro activity of rifamycins alone and in combination with other antibiotics against *Chlamydia trachomatis*. *Rev. Infect. Dis. (Suppl.) 5*:S556–S561, 1983.
22. Plummer, FA, Nsanze, H, D'Costa, LJ, et al.: Short-course and single-dose antimicrobial therapy for chancroid in Kenya: Studies with rifampin alone and in combination with trimethoprim. *Rev. Infect. Dis. (Suppl.) 5*:S565–S572, 1983.
23. Conti, R, Parenti, F: Rifampin therapy for brucellosis, *Flavobacterium* meningitis and cutaneous leishmaniasis. *Rev. Infect. Dis. (Suppl.) 5*:S600–S605, 1983.
24. Jacobs, MR, Mithal, Y, Robins-Browne, RM, et al.: Antimicrobial susceptibility testing of pneumococci: Determination of Kirby-Bauer breakpoints for penicillin G, erythromycin, clindamycin, tetracycline, chloramphenicol and rifampin. *Antimicrob. Agents Chemother. 16*:190–197, 1979.
25. Kunin, CM, Brandt, D, Wood, H: Bacteriologic studies of rifampin, a new synthetic antibiotic. *J. Infect. Dis. 119*:132–137, 1969.
26. Tanzil, HOK, Chatim, A, Utomo, RR, Harun, H: Sensitivity of various species of *Nocardia* to rifampin in vitro. *Am. Rev. Respir. Dis. 105*:455–456, 1972.
27. Thong, YH, Rowan-Kelly, B, Shepherd, C, Ferrante, A: Growth inhibition of *Naegleria fowleri* by tetracycline, rifampicin, and miconazole. *Lancet 2*:876, 1977.
28. Szychowska, Z, Prandota-Schoepp, A, Chabudzinska, S: Rifampicin for *Pneumocystis carinii* pneumonia. *Lancet 1*:935, 1983.
29. Stottmeier, VD: Emergence of rifampin resistant mycobacterium tuberculosis in Massachusetts. *J. Infect. Dis. 133*:88–90, 1976.
30. Baronti, A, Lukinovich, N: A pilot trial of rifampicin in tuberculosis. *Tubercle 49*: 180–185, 1968.
31. McClatchy, JK, Waggoner, RF, Lester, W: In vitro susceptibility of mycobacteria to rifampin. *Am. Rev. Respir. Dis. 100*:234–236, 1969.
32. Mandell, GL, Sande, M: Antimicrobial agents (continued). In: *The Pharmacological Basis of Therapeutics*, 7th ed. (LS Goodman and A Gilman, eds.), Macmillan, New York, 1985, pp. 1202–1205.
33. Davidson, PT, Waggoner, R: Acquired resistance to rifampicin by *Mycobacterium kansasii*. *Tubercle 57*:271–273, 1976.
34. Jacobson, RR, Hastings, RC: Rifampin-resistant leprosy. *Lancet 2*:1304–1305, 1976.

35. Eickhoff, TC: In vitro and in vivo studies of resistance to rifampin in meningococci. *J. Infect. Dis. 123*:414–420, 1971.
36. McCabe, WR, Lorian, V: Comparison of the antibacterial activity of rifampicin and other antibiotics. *Am. J. Med. Sci. 256*:255–265, 1968.
37. Radner, DB: Toxicologic and pharmacologic aspects of rifampin. *Chest 64*:213–216, 1973.
38. Jensen, K: Methicillin-resistant staphylococci. *Lancet 2*:1078, 1968.
39. Acar, JF, Goldstein, FW, Duval, J: Use of rifampin for the treatment of serious staphylococcal and gram-negative bacillary infections. *Rev. Infect. Dis. (Suppl.) 5*: S502–S506, 1983.
40. Simon, GL, Smith, RH, Sande, MA: Emergence of rifampin-resistant strains of *Staphylococcus aureus* during combination therapy with vancomycin and rifampin: A report of two cases. *Rev. Infect. Dis. (Suppl.) 5*:S507–S508, 1983.
41. Van Der Auwera, P, Meunier-Carpentier, F, Klastersky, J: Clinical study of combination therapy with oxacillin and rifampin for staphylococcal infections. *Rev. Infect. Dis. (Suppl.) 5*:S515–S522, 1983.
42. Karchmer, AW, Archer, GL, Dismukes, WE: Rifampin treatment of prosthetic valvc endocarditis due to *Staphylococcus epidermidis. Rev. Infect. Dis. (Suppl.) 5*:S543–S548, 1983.
43. Watanakunakorn, C, Guerriero, JC: Interaction between vancomycin and rifampin against *Staphylococcus aureus. Antimicrob. Agents Chemother. 19*:1089–1091, 1981.
44. Zinner, SH, Lagast, H, Klastersky, J: Antistaphylococcal activity of rifampin and other antibiotics. *J. Infect. Dis. 144*:365–371, 1981.
45. Tuazon, CU, Lin, MYC, Sheagren, JN: In vitro activity of rifampicin alone and in combination with nafcillin and vancomycin against pathogenic strains of *Staphyloccus aureus. Antimicrob. Agents Chemother. 13*:759–761, 1978.
46. Peard, MC, Fleck, DG, Garrod, LP, Waterworth, PM: Combined rifampin and erythromycin for bacterial endocarditis. *Br. Med. J. 4*:410–411, 1970.
47. Norden, CW: Experimental chronic staphylococcal osteomyelitis in rabbits: Treatment with rifampin alone and in combination with other antimicrobial agents. *Rev. Infect. Dis. (Suppl.) 5*:S491–S494, 1983.
48. Karchmer, AW, Archer, GL, Dismukes, WE: *Staphylococcus epidermidis* causing prosthetic valve endocarditis: Microbiologic and clinical observations as guides to therapy. *Ann. Intern. Med. 98*:447–455, 1983.
49. Bayer, AS, Lam, K: Vancomycin + rifampin in experimental endocarditis due to methicillin-resistant *Staphylococcus aureus* in vitro-in vivo correlations. Abstr 24th Interscience Conference on Antimicrobial Agents and Chemotherapy, 1984, p. 151, American Society for Microbiology, Washington, D.C.
50. Ricci, J: Discordant results of in-vitro testing for rifampin-cloxacillin synergy against *Staphylococcus aureus*. Abstr 24th Interscience conference on Antimicrobial Agents and Chemotherapy, 1984, p. 170, American Society for Microbiology, Washington, D.C.
51. Vachyanond, P: Staphylococcal CNS infections treated with vancomycin and rifampin. *Arch. Neurol. 41*:637–639, 1984.
52. Norden, CW, Fierer, J, Bryant, RE, et al.: Chronic staphylococcal osteomyelitis: Treatment with regimens containing rifampin. *Rev. Infect. Dis. (Suppl.) 5*:S495–S501, 1983.
53. Kerry, DW, Hamilton-Miller, JMT, Brumfitt, W: Trimethoprim and rifampicin: In vitro activities separately and in combination. *J. Antimicrob. Chemother. 1*:417–427, 1975.
54. Arioli, V, Berti, M, Carniti, G, et al.: Interaction between rifampicin and trimethoprim in vitro and in experimental infections. *J. Antimicrob. Chemother. 3*:87–94, 1977.

55. Greenwood, D, Andrew, J: Rifampicin plus nalidixic acid: A rational combination for the treatment of urinary infection. *J. Antimicrob. Chemother.* *4*:533–538, 1978.
56. Shanson, DC, Leung, T: Susceptibility of *Salmonella typhi* to rifamycins and novobiocin. *J. Antimicrob. Chemother.* *2*:81–86, 1976.
57. Chaudhary, S, Bilinsky, SA, Hennessy, JL, et al.: Penicillin V and rifampin for the treatment of group A streptococcal pharyngitis: A randomized trial of 10 days penicillin vs 10 days penicillin with rifampin during the final 4 days of therapy. *J. Pediatr.* *106*:481–485, 1985.
58. Zuravleff, JJ, Yu, VL, Yee, RB: Ticarcillin-tobramycin-rifampin: in vitro synergy of the triplet combination against *Pseudomonas aeruginosa*. *J. Lab. Clin. Med.* *101*: 896-902, 1983.
59. Yu, V, Peacock, JE, Zuravleff, JJ, et al.: Rifampin therapy for refractory *Pseudomonas aeruginosa* infections. Abstr 24th Interscience Conference on Antimicrobial Agents and Chemotherapy, 1984, p. 308, American Society for Microbiology, Washington, D.C.
60. Beggs, WH, Sarosi, GA, Walker, MI: Synergistic action of amphotericin B and rifampin against *Candida* species. *J. Infect. Dis.* *133*:206–209, 1976.
61. Kobayashi, GS, Zse-Chuen, CC, Schlessinger, D, Medoff, G: Effects of rifamycin derivatives, alone and in combination with amphotericin B, against *Histoplasma capsulatum*. *Antimicrob. Agents Chemother.* *5*:16–18, 1974.
62. Fujita, NK, Edwards, JE, Jr.: Combined in vitro effect of amphotericin B and rifampin on *Cryptococcus neoformans*. *Antimicrob. Agents Chemother.* *19*:196–198, 1981.
63. Rifkind, D, Crowder, ED, Hyland, RN: In vitro inhibition of *Coccidioides immitis* strains with amphotericin B plus rifampin. *Antimicrob. Agents Chemother.* *6*:783–784, 1974.
64. Kitahara, M, Seth, VK, Medoff, G, Kobayashi, GS: Activity of amphotericin B, 5-fluorocytosine, and rifampin against six clinical isolates of *Aspergillus*. *Antimicrob. Agents Chemother.* *9*:915–919, 1976.
65. Kitahara, M, Kobayashi, GS, Medoff, G: Enhanced efficacy of amphotericin B and rifampicin combined in treatment of murine histoplasmosis and blastomycosis. *J. Infect. Dis.* *133*:663–668, 1975.
66. Shalit, I, Guruswamy, A, Welch, DF, Marks, MI: Rifampin enhancement of amphotericin B activity against *Rhizopus*. Abstr Amer Soc Microbiol, 85th Annual Meeting, 1985, p. 368, American Society for Microbiology, Washington, D.C.
67. Hull, PR: Systemic histoplasmosis and oesophageal obstruction due to *Histoplasma* granulomas. *S. Afr. Med. J.* *55*:639–643, 1979.
68. Gontilini, M, Brucker, G, Danis, M, et al.: Dix cas d'histoplasmose: Aspects cliniques, biologiques et thérapeutiques. *Ann. Med. Interne (Paris)* *131*:209–212, 1980.
69. Ribner, B, Keusch, GT, Hanna, BA, Perloff, M: Combination amphotericin B-rifampin therapy for pulmonary aspergillosis in a leukemia patient. *Chest* *70*:681–683, 1976.
70. Arroyo, T, Medoff, G, Kobayashi, GS: Therapy of murine aspergillosis with amphotericin B in combination with rifampin or 5-fluorocytosine. *Antimicrob. Agents Chemother.* *11*:21–25, 1977.
71. Graybill, JR, Ahrens, J: Interaction of rifampin with other antifungal agents in experimental murine candidiasis. *Rev. Infect. Dis. (Suppl.)* *5*:S620–S625, 1983.
72. Huppert, M, Pappagianis, D, Sun, SH, et al.: Effect of amphotericin B and rifampin against *Coccidioides immitis* in vitro and in vivo. *Antimicrob. Agents Chemother.* *9*:406–413, 1976.
73. Winslow, DL, Damme, J, Dieckman, E: Delayed bactericidal activity of β-lactam antibiotics against *Listeria monocytogenes*: Antagonism of chloramphenicol and rifampin. *Antimicrob. Agents Chemother.* *23*:555–558, 1983.

74. Scheld, WM: Evaluation of rifampin and other antibiotics against *Listeria monocytogenes* in vitro and in vivo. *Rev. Infect. Dis. (Suppl.) 5*:S593–S599, 1983.
75. Velo, GP, Vettori, G: Ricerche sull'assorbimento orale e sull eliminazione urinaria della rifampicina. *Gazz. Int. Med. Chir. 73*:2799–2804, 1968.
76. Acocella, G: Clinical pharmacokinetics of rifampicin. *Clin. Pharmacokinet. 3*:108–127, 1978.
77. Siegler, DI, Burley, DM, Bryant, M, et al.: Effect of meals on rifampicin absorption. *Lancet 2*:197–198, 1974.
78. Boman, G, Hanngren, Å, Malmborg, A, et al.: Drug interaction: Decreased serum concentrations of rifampicin when given with P.A.S. *Lancet 1*:800, 1971.
79. Acocella, G: Pharmacokinetics and metabolism or rifampin in humans. *Rev. Infect. Dis. (Suppl.) 5*:S428–S432, 1983.
80. Pawlowska, I, Tniewski, T: Studies of pharmacokinetics of rifampicin in the body of patients with pulmonary tuberculosis. *Arzneimittelforsch. 29*:1906–1911, 1979.
81. Council on Drugs, American Medical Association: Evaluation of a new antituberculous agent. *JAMA 220*:414–415, 1972.
82. McCracken, GH, Ginsburg, CM, Zweighaft, TC, Clahsen, J: Pharmacokinetics of rifampin in infants and children: Relevance to prophylaxis against *Haemophilus influenzae* type B disease. *Pediatrics 66*:17–21, 1980.
83. Nitti, V, Virgilio, R, Particolo, MR, Iuliano, A: Pharmacokinetic study of intravenous rifampicin. *Chemotherapy 23*:1–6, 1977.
84. Jenne, JW, Beggs, WH: Correlation of in vitro and in vivo kinetics with clinical use of isoniazid, ethambutol, and rifampin. *Am. Rev. Respir. Dis. 107*:1013–1021, 1973.
85. Pechere, JC, Tancrede, C: Evolution des concentrations senques et urinaires de la rifampicine au cours des traitements. *Pathol. Biol. 17*:155–158, 1969.
86. Acocella, G, Buniva, G, Flauto, V, Nicolis, FB: Absorption and elimination of the antibiotic rifampicin in newborns and children. In: *Proceedings of the Sixth International Congress of Chemotherapy*, Vol. 2, University of Tokyo Press, 1969, pp. 755--760.
87. Sensi, P, Maggi, N, Furesz, S, Maffii, G: Chemical modifications and biological properties of rifamycins. *Antimicrob. Agents Chemother. 19*:699–714, 1967.
88. Furesz, S: Chemical and biological properties of rifampicin. *Antibiot. Chemother. 16*:316–351, 1970.
89. Bowman, G, Malmborg, AS: Rifampicin in plasma and pleural fluid after single oral doses. *Eur. J. Clin. Pharmacol. 7*:51–58, 1974.
90. Binda, G, Domenichini, E, Gottardi, A, et al.: Rifampicin. A general view. *Arzneimittelforsch. 12a*:1907–1978, 1971.
91. Suter, F, Maserati, R, Concia, E, et al.: Rifampicin in collections of pus—a kinetic study in human abscesses. *J. Antimicrob. Chermother. 13*:43–47, 1984.
92. Grosset, J: The efficacy of short-course chemtherapy for tuberculosis. *Bull. Pan Am. Health Organ. 14*:139–149, 1980.
93. Curci, G, Cava, FD, Vitalo, L: Distribution of rifamycin AMP in blood and cerebospinal fluid. *Minerva Med. 60*:2399–2402, 1969.
94. Sippel, JE, Mikhail, IS, Girgis, NI: Rifampin concentrations in cerebrospinal fluid of patients with tuberculous meningitis. *Am. Rev. Respir. Dis. 109*:579–580, 1974.
95. D'Oliveira, JJG: Cerebrospinal fluid concentrations of rifampin in meningeal tuberculosis. *Am. Rev. Respir. Dis. 106*:432–437, 1972.
96. Lee, EL, Robinson, MJ, Thong, ML, Puthucheary, SD: Rifamycin in neonatal flavobacteria meningitis. *Arch. Dis. Child. 51*:209–213, 1976.
97. Mandell, GL: The antibacterial activity of rifampin: Emphasis on the relation to phagocytes. *Rev. Infect. Dis. (Suppl.) 5*:S463–S467, 1983.
98. Lorber, B: Rifampin in chronic granulomatous disease. *N. Engl. J. Med. 303*:111, 1980.

99. Lyons, RW: Orange contact lenses from rifampin. *N. Engl. J. Med. 300*:372–373, 1979.
100. Capelle, P, Dhumeaux, D, Mora, M, Feldmann, G, Berthelot, P: Effects of rifampicin on liver function in man. *Gut 13*:366–371, 1972.
101. Jeanes, CWL, Jessamine, AG, Eidus, L: Treatment of chronic drug-resistant pulmonary tuberculosis with rifampicin. *Can. Med. Assoc. J. 106*:884–888, 1972.
102. Sharpstone, P: Diseases of the urinary system. Prescribing for patients with renal failure. *Br. Med. J. 2*:36–37, 1977.
103. Bennett, WM, Muther, RS, Parker, RA, et al.: Drug therapy in renal failure: Dosing guidelines for adults. Part I. Antimicrobial agents, analgesics. *Ann. Intern. Med. 93*:62–89, 1980.
104. American Academy of Pediatrics: Meningococcal infections. In: *Report of the Committee on Infectious Diseases*, 19th ed, 1982, pp. 139–141.
105. American Academy of Pediatrics: Revision of recommendation for use of rifampin prophylaxis of contacts of patients with *Haemophilus influenzae* infection. *Pediatrics 74*:301–302, 1984.
106. Simon, HJ, Yin, EJ: Microassay of antimicrobial agents. *Appl. Microbiol. 19*: 573–579, 1970.
107. Weber, A, Opheim, KE, Smith, AL, Wong, K: High-pressure liquid chromatographic quantitation of rifampin and its two major metabolites in urine and serum. *Rev. Infect. Dis. (Suppl.) 5*:S433–S439, 1983.
108. Wardell, WM, McQueen, EG: Urinary excretion of rifampicin and its metabolites as an index of rifampicin blood levels. *N.Z. Med. J. 72*:393–396, 1970.
109. Mouton, RP, Mattie, H, Swart, K, Kreukniet, J, Dewael, J: Blood levels of rifampicin, desacetylrifampicin, and isoniazid during combined therapy. *J. Antimicrob. Chemother. 5*:447–454, 1979.
110. Sirot, J, Lopitaux, R, Cluzel, R, Delisle, JJ, Sauvezie, B: Diffusion de la rifampicine dans l'os non-infecté chez l'homme. *Ann. Microbiol. (Paris) 128B*:229–236, 1977.
111. Newman, R, Doster, BE, Murray, FJ, et al.: Rifampin in initial treatment of pulmonary tuberculosis. *Am. Rev. Respir. Dis. 109*:216–232, 1974.
112. Fox, W, Mitchinson, DA: Short-course chemotherapy for pulmonary tuberculosis. *Am. Rev. Respir. Dis. 111*:325–353, 1975.
113. Wolinsky, E, Gomez, F, Zimpfer, F: Sporotrichoid *Mycobacterium marinum* infection treated with rifampin-ethambutol. *Am. Rev. Respir. Dis. 105*:964–967, 1972.
114. Mandell, F, Wright, PF: Treatment of atypical cervical adenitis with rifampin. *Pediatrics 55*:39–43, 1975.
115. Bullock, WE: Rifampin in the treatment of leprosy. *Rev. Infect. Dis. (Suppl.) 5*: S606–S613, 1983.
116. WHO Study Group: Chemotherapy of leprosy for control programmes. *WHO Tech. Rep. Ser. 675*:7–33, 1982.
117. Cooper, ER, Ellison, RT, Smith, GS et al.: Rifampin-resistant meningococcal disease in a contact patient given prophylactic rifampin. *Pediatrics 108*:93–96, 1986.
118. Glode, MP, Daum, RS, Boies, EG, et al.: Effect of rifampin chemoprophylaxis on carriage eradication and new acquisition of *Haemophilus influenzae* type b in contacts. *Pediatrics 76*:537–542, 1985.
119. Massanari, RM, Donta, ST: The efficacy of rifampin as adjunctive therapy in selected cases of staphylococcal endocarditis. *Chest 73*:371–375, 1978.
120. Sande, MA, Scheld, WM: Combination antibiotic therapy of bacterial endocarditis. *Ann. Intern. Med. 92*:390–395, 1980.
121. George, T, Burch, K, Magilligan, DJ, Jr.: Rifampin in the management of early prosthetic *Staphylococcus epidermidis* endocarditis. *Ann. Thorac. Surg. 29*:74–75, 1980.

122. Farr, B, Mandell, GL: Rifampin. In: *Principles and Practice of Infectious Diseases*, 2nd ed. (GL Mandell, RG Douglas, Jr., and JE Bennett, eds.), John Wiley & Sons, New York, 1985, pp. 216–220.
123. Faville, RJ, Zaske, DE, Kaplan, EL, et al.: *Staphylococcus aureus* endocarditis: Combined therapy with vancomycin and rifampin. *JAMA 240*:1963–1965, 1978.
124. Norden, CW, Shaffer, M: Treatment of experimental chronic osteomyelitis due to *Staphylococcus aureus* with vancomycin and rifampin. *J. Infect. Dis. 147*:352–357, 1983.
125. Desplaces, N, Gutmann, L, Acar, JF: Twice-daily oral therapy for chronic staphylococcal osteomyelitis. Abstr 24th Interscience Conference on Antimicrobial Agents and Chemotherapy, 1984, p. 140, American Society for Microbiology, Washington, D.C.
126. Ring, JC, Cates, KL, Belani, KK, et al.: Rifampin for CSF shunt infections caused by coagulase-negative staphylococci. *J. Pediatr. 93*:317–319, 1979.
127. Wheat, LJ, Kohler, RB, White, AL, White, A: Effect of rifampin on nasal carriers of coagulase-positive staphylococci. *J. Infect. Dis. 144*:127, 1981.
128. Locksket, RNM, Cigeb, NKM, Qyubb, TC, et al.: Multiply antibiotic-resistant *Staphylococcus aureus*: Introduction, transmission, and evolution of nosocomial infection. *Ann. Intern. Med. 97*:317–324, 1982.
129. Tanz, RR, Shulman, ST, Barthel, MJ, et al.: Penicillin plus rifampin eradicates pharyngeal carriage of group A streptococci. *J. Pediatr. 106*:876–880, 1985.
130. Centers for Disease Control: Pneumococcal meningitis caused by chloramphenicol and tetracycline resistant type 23 pneumococcus—Australia. *MMWR 28*:500, 1979.
131. Radetsky, MS, Johansen, TL, Lauer, BA, et al.: Multiply resistant pneumococcus causing meningitis: Its epidemiology within a day-care center. *Lancet 2*:771–773, 1981.
132. Centers for Disease Control: Multiple-antibiotic resistance of pneumococci—South Africa. *MMWR 27*:1, 1977.
133. Llorens-Terol, J, Busquets, RM: Brucellosis treated with rifampicin. *Arch. Dis. Child. 55*:486–488, 1980.
134. Swartz, MN: Clinical aspects of Legionnaire's disease. *Ann. Intern. Med. 90*:492–495, 1979.
135. Fraser, DW, Wachsmuth, IK, Bopp, C, Feeley, JC, Tsai, TF: Antibiotic treatment of guinea-pigs infected with agent of Legionnaire's disease. *Lancet 1*:175–178, 1978.
136. Ezer, G, Soothill, FJ: Intracellular bactericidal effect of rifampin in both normal and chronic granulomatous disease polymorphs. *Arch. Dis. Child. 49*:463–466, 1974.
137. Darougar, S, Viswalingam, M, Treharne, JD, Kinnison, JR, Jones, BR: Treatment of TRIC infection of the eye with rifampicin or chloramphenicol. *Br. J. Ophthalmol. 61*:255–259, 1977.
138. Darougar, S, Jones, BR, Viswalingam, N, et al.: Topical therapy of hyperendemic trachoma with rifampicin, oxytetracycline, or spiramycin eye ointments. *Br. J. Ophthalmol. 64*:37–42, 1980.
139. Ferlauto, JJ, Wells, DH: *Flavobacterium menintosepticum* in the neonatal period. *South. Med. J. 74*:757–759, 1981.
140. Brumfitt, W, Dixson, S, Hamilton-Miller, JMT: Use of rifampin for the treatment of urinary tract infections. *Rev. Infect. Dis. (Suppl.) 5*:S573–S582, 1983.
141. Suter, F, Maserati, R, Carnevale, G, et al.: Management of staphylococcal endocarditis in drug addicts. Combined therapy with oral rifampicin and aminoglycosides. *J. Antimicrob. Chemother. 13(Suppl.)*:57–60, 1984.
142. Clumeck, N, Marcelis, L, Amiri-Lamraski, MH, Gordts, B: Treatment of severe staphylococcal infections with a rifampicin-minocycline association. *J. Antimicrob. Chemother. 13(Suppl.)*:17–22, 1984.

143. Nessi, R, Fowst, G: Clinical use of rifampicin in combination for non-mycobacterial infections: A survey of published evidence. *J. Int. Med. Res.* *7*:179–186, 1979.
144. Naveh, Y, Friedman, A: Rifampicin therapy in Gram-negative bacteraemia in infancy. *Arch. Dis. Child.* *48*:967–969, 1973.
145. Band, JD, Fraser, DW: Adverse effects of two rifampicin dosage regimens for the prevention of meningococcal infection. *Lancet* *1*:101–102, 1984.
146. Grosset, J, Leventis, S: Adverse effects of rifampin. *Rev. Infect. Dis. (Suppl.)* *5*: S440–S446, 1983.
147. Girling, DJ, Hitze, KL: Adverse reactions to rifampicin. *Bull. WHO* *57*:45–49, 1979.
148. Zierski, M: Adverse reactions under intermittent rifampicin regimens. *Chemotherapy* *4*:385–392, 1976.
149. Worlledge, S: Rifampicin-induced antibodies. *Chemotherapy* *4*:273–278, 1976.
150. O'Mahoney, MG, Kar, CW: Relationship between rifampicin-dependent antibody scores, serum rifampicin concentrations and symptoms in patients with adverse reactions to intermittent rifampicin treatment. *Clin. Allergy* *3*:353–362, 1973.
151. Girling, DJ: Adverse reaction to rifampicin in antituberculosis regimens. *J. Antimicrob. Chemother.* *3*:115–132, 1977.
152. Eule, H, Werner, E, Winsel, K, Iwainsky, H: Intermittent chemotherapy of pulmonary tuberculosis using rifampicin and isoniazid for primary treatment: The influence of various factors on the frequency of side-effects. *Tubercle* *55*:81–89, 1974.
153. Lee, CW, Lim, JH, Kang, HJ: Pemphigus foleaceus induced by rifampicin. *Br. J. Dermatol.* *111*:619–622, 1984.
154. Wong, P, Bottorff, MB, Heritage, RW, et al.: Acute rifampin overdose: A pharmacokinetic study and review of the literature. *J. Pediatr.* *104*:781–783, 1984.
155. Boriello, SP, Jones, RH, Phillips, I: Rifampicin-associated pseudomembranous colitis. *Br. Med. J.* *281*:1180–1181, 1980.
156. Moriarty, HJ, Scobie, BA: Pseudomembranous colitis in a patient on rifampicin and ethambutol. *N.Z. Med. J.* *91*:294–295, 1980.
157. O'Connor, RP, Silva, J, Jr., Fekety, R: Rifampicin and antibiotic-associated colitis. *Lancet* *1*:499, 1981.
158. Scheuer, PJ, Summerfield, JA, Lal, S, Sherlock, S: Rifampicin hepatitis. *Lancet* *1*: 421–425, 1974.
159. O'Brien, RJ, Long, MW, Cross, FS, Lyle, MA, Snider, DE, Jr.: Hepatotoxicity from isoniazid and rifampin among children treated for tuberculosis. *Pediatrics* *72*: 491–499, 1983.
160. Rahajoe, NN, Rahajoe, N, Boediman, I, et al.: The treatment of tuberculous meningitis in children with a combination of isoniazid, rifampicin, and streptomycin—preliminary report. *Tubercle* *60*:245–250, 1979.
161. Lal, S, Singhal, SN, Burley, DM, Crossley, G: Effect of rifampicin and isoniazid on liver function. *Br. Med. J.* *1*:148–150, 1972.
162. Ramachandran, P: Chemotherapy of tuberculous meningitis with isoniazid plus rifampicin—interim finding in a trial in children. *Indian J. Tuberc.* *27*:54–58, 1980.
163. Visudhiphan, P, Chiemehanya, S: Evaluation of rifampin in the treatment of tuberculous meningitis in children. *J. Pediatr.* *87*:983–986, 1975.
164. Casteels-Van Daele, M, Igodt-Ameye, L, Corbeel, L, et al.: Hepatotoxicity of rifampicin and isoniazid in children. *J. Pediatr.* *86*:739–741, 1975.
165. Pratt, TH: Rifampicin-induced organic brain syndrome. *JAMA* *241*:2421–2422, 1979.
166. Hatfield, JW: Rifampicin-induced thrombocytopenia. *Postgrad. Med. J.* *56*:59–60, 1980.
167. Lakshminarayan, S, Sahn, SA, Hudson, LD: Massive haemolysis caused by rifampin. *Br. Med. J.* *2*:282–283, 1973.

168. Inman, WH: Study of fatal bone marrow depression with special reference to phenylbutazone and oxyphenbutazone. *Br. Med. J. 1*:1500–1505, 1977.
169. Lee, M, Berger, HW: Eosinophilia caused by rifampin. *Chest 77*:579, 1980.
170. Blajchman, MA, Lowry, RC, Pettit, JE, Stradling, P: Rifampicin-induced immune thrombocytopenia. *Br. Med. J. 3*:24–26, 1970.
171. Graber, CD, Jevaily, J, Galphin, RL, et al.: Light chain proteinuria and humoral immunoincompetence in tuberculous patients treated with rifampin. *Am. Rev. Respir. Dis. 107*:713–717, 1973.
172. Winter, RJD, Banks, RA, Collins, CMP, Hoffbrand, BI: Rifampicin-induced light chain proteinuria and renal failure. *Thorax 39*:952–953, 1984.
173. Chan, WC, O'Mahoney, MG, Yu, DYC, Yu, RYH: Renal failure during intermittent rifampicin therapy. *Tubercle 56*:191–198, 1975.
174. Flynn, CT, Rainford, DJ, Hope, E: Acute renal failure and rifampicin: Danger of unsuspected intermittent dosage. *Br. Med. J. 2*:482, 1974.
175. Davison, AG, Empey, DW: Acute renal failure following reintroduction of rifampicin after a prolonged interval. *Br. J. Dis. Chest 75*:103–104, 1981.
176. Aquinas, M, Allan, WGL, Horsfall, PAL, et al.: Adverse reactions to daily and intermittent rifampicin regimens for pulmonary tuberculosis in Hong Kong. *Br. Med. J. 1*:765–771, 1972.
177. Grassi, GG, Pozzi, E: Effect of rifampicin on delayed hypersensitivity reactions. *J. Infect. Dis. 126*:542–544, 1972.
178. Pogo, BGT: Specific inhibition by rifampicin of transcription in human lymphocytes stimulated by phytohemagglutinin. *J. Cell Biol. 55*:515–519, 1972.
179. Mukerjee, P, Schuldt, S, Kasik, JE: Effect of rifampin on cutaneous hypersensitivity to purified protein derivative in humans. *Antimicrob. Agents Chemother. 4*: 607–611, 1973.
180. Sanders, WE: Rifampin. *Ann. Intern. Med. 85*:82–86, 1976.
181. Rocker, I: Rifampicin in early pregnancy. *Lancet 2*:48, 1977.
182. Steen, JSM, Stainton-Ellis, DM: Rifampicin in pregnancy. *Lancet 2*:604–605, 1977.
183. Brodie, MJ, Boobis, AR, Dollery, CT, et al.: Rifampicin and vitamin D metabolism. *Clin. Pharmacol. Ther. 27*:810–814, 1980.
184. Shah, SC, Sharma, RK, Hemangini, Chitle, AR: Rifampicin induced osteomalacia. *Tubercle 62*:207–209, 1981.
185. Kenwright, S, Levi, AJ: Impairment of hepatic uptake of rifamycin antibiotics and its therapeutic implications. *Lancet 2*:1401–1405, 1973.
186. Fallon, RJ, Lees, AW, Allan, GW, Smith, J, Tyrrell, WF: Probenecid and rifampin serum levels. *Lancet 2*:792–794, 1975.
187. Engelhard, D, Stutman, HR, Marks, MI: Interaction of ketoconazole with rifampin and isoniazid. *N. Engl. J. Med. 311*:1681–1683, 1984.
188. Jesequel, AM, Orlandi, F, Tenconi, LT: Changes of the smooth endoplasmic reticulum induced by rifampicin in human and guinea-pig hepatocytes. *Gut 12*:984–987, 1971.
189. Schoene, B, Fleischmann, RA, Remmer, H: The cytochrome p-450 content and the activities of various microsomal enzymes in human liver. *Proc. Eur. Soc. Stud. Drug Tox. 13*:249–253, 1973.
190. Zilly, W, Breimer, DD, Richter, E: Pharmacokinetic interactions with rifampicin. *Clin. Pharmacokinet. 2*:61–70, 1977.
191. Kyriazopoulou, V, Parparousi, O, Vegenakis, AG: Rifampicin-induced adrenal crisis in Addisonian patients receiving corticosteroid replacement therapy. *J. Clin. Endocrinol. Metab. 59*:1204–1206, 1984.
192. Skolnick, JL, Stoler, BS, Katz, DB, Anderson, WH: Rifampin, oral contraceptives, and pregnancy. *JAMA 236*:1382, 1976.

193. Bussey, HI, Merritt, GJ, Hill, EG: The influence of rifampin on quinidin and digoxin. *Arch. Intern. Med. 144*:1021–1023, 1984.
194. Kreek, MJ, Garfield, JW, Gutjahr, CL: Rifampin-induced methadone withdrawal. *N. Engl. J. Med. 294*:1104–1106, 1976.
195. McAllister, WAC, Thompson, PJ, Al-Habet, SM, Rogers, HJ: Rifampicin reduces effectiveness and bioavailability of prednisolone. *Br. Med. J. 286*:923–925, 1983.
196. Buffington, GA, Dominguez, JH, Piering, WG, et al.: Interaction of rifampin and glucocorticoids. Adverse effect on renal allograft function. *JAMA 236*:1958–1960, 1976.
197. Hendrickse, W, McKiernan, J, Pickup, M, Lowe, J: Rifampicin-induced non-responsiveness to corticosteroid treatment in nephrotic syndrome. *Br. Med. J. 1*: 306, 1979.
198. Baciewicz, AM, Self, TH: Rifampin drug interactions. *Arch. Intern. Med. 144*: 1667–1671, 1984.
199. Bowman, G, Eliasson, K, Odar-Cederlöf, I: Acute cardiac failure during treatment with digitoxin: An interaction with rifampicin. *Br. J. Clin. Pharmacol. 10*:89–90, 1980.
200. Novi, C, Bissoli, F, Simonati, V, et al.: Rifampin and digoxin: Possible drug interaction in a dialysis patient. *JAMA 244*:2521–2522, 1980.
201. Prober, CG: Effect of rifampin on chloramphenicol levels. *N. Engl. J. Med. 312*: 788–789, 1985.
202. Bolt, HM, Kappus, H, Bolt, M: Rifampicin and oral contraception. *Lancet 2*: 1280–1281, 1974.
203. Back, DJ, Breckenridge, AM, Crawford, F, et al.: The effect of rifampicin on norethisterone pharmacokinetics. *Eur.J. Clin. Pharmacol. 15*:193–197, 1979.
204. Rahn, KH, Mooy, J, Böhm, R, Vet, AVD: Reduction of bioavailability of verapamil by rifampin. *N. Engl. J. Med. 312*:920–921, 1985.
205. O'Reilly, A: Interaction of sodium warfarin and rifampin. *Ann. Intern. Med. 81*: 337–340, 1974.
206. Self, TH, Morris, T: Interaction of rifampin and chlorpropamide. *Chest 77*:800–801, 1980.
207. Zilly, W, Breimer, DD, Richter, E: Induction of drug metabolism in man after rifampicin treatment measured by increased hexobarbital and tolbutamide clearance. *Eur. J. Clin. Pharmacol. 9*:219–227, 1975.
208. Cole, AJL, Bate, J, Gyde, OHB: Rifampicin and folate and vitamin B_{12} assays. *Br. Med. J. 2*:53, 1973.

20
Antituberculous Therapy

E. KANTA SUBBARAO AND MELVIN I. MARKS*
University of Oklahoma Health Sciences Center, Oklahoma City, Oklahoma

There have been major changes in the therapy of tuberculosis in the past decade, including new chemotherapeutic agents and short-course and intermittent chemotherapy.

The incidence of tuberculosis in the United States in 1983 was 10.2 cases per 10,000 population, with 1360 cases in children under 15 years of age (1). The diagnosis of tuberculosis may be difficult to establish in children since they may have few symptoms, are less likely to have positive bacterial cultures, and may have extrapulmonary disease. The diagnosis often rests upon a history of exposure to tuberculosis, a positive tuberculin skin test, and abnormal physical, laboratory, and radiological findings (2). If a source case is known, susceptibility data on the isolate of the source case can guide therapy (3). The goals of therapy are to

1. Prevent infection in close contacts
2. Prevent progression of infection to active disease
3. Achieve lifetime control of disease for the patient

Many of the currently used chemotherapeutic agents have been available for several decades. The reader should be aware that much of the pharmacokinetic data were obtained over the years by different methods that have varying sensitivity. Data in the pediatric population are incomplete and in several instances have been derived by extrapolation from the adult experience.

First-line drugs for the treatment of tuberculosis include isoniazid, rifampin, ethambutol, and streptomycin. Rifampin is discussed in a separate chapter (Chapter 19). Tables 1, 2, and 3 summarize bacterial susceptibilities, pharmacokinetics, and adverse effects and toxicities of the first-line antituberculous drugs, isoniazid, ethambutol, and streptomycin.

**Present affiliation*: Miller Children's Hospital/Memorial Medical Center, Long Beach, California

Table 1 Usual Susceptibility of Various Mycobacteria to First-line Drugs

Drug	*M. tuberculosis*	*M. marinum*	*M. avium*	*M. kansasii*
Isoniazid 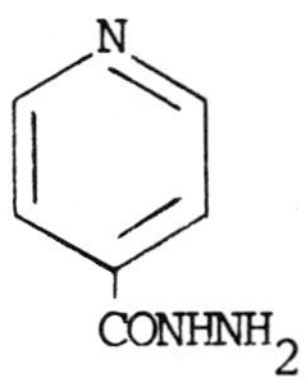	0.2 μg/ml	Resistant	Resistant	5 μg/ml
Ethambutol 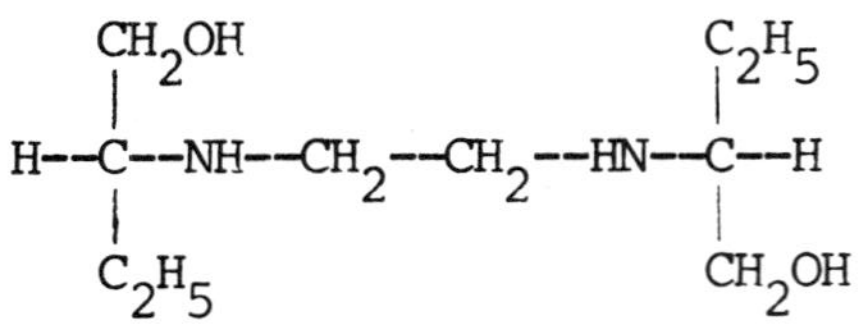	1–2 μg/ml	Variable	Variable	Sensitive
Streptomycin sulfate $(C_{21}H_{39}N_7O_{12})_2 \cdot 3H_2SO_4$.	0.1–10 μg/ml (mainly <2 μg/ml)	Sensitive	Resistant	Sensitive

Table 2 Summary of Pharmacokinetic Data on Isoniazid, Ethambutol, and Streptomycin

Drug	Dosage	Gastro-intestinal absorption	Time to peak serum concentration (hr)	Peak serum concentration (μg/ml)	Serum half-life (min)	Penetration into cerebrospinal fluid	Major metabolites	Major site of metabolism or excretion
Isoniazid	Newborns, 3–5 mg/kg day^{-1}; infants and children, 10–20 mg/kg day^{-1}; adults, 4–5 mg/kg day^{-1}, up to 300 mg/day	+	1–2	Slow acetylators, 19.9 ± 4.3; rapid acetylators, 14.2 ± 5.8	Slow acetylators, 110–>400 (mean, 288); rapid acetylators, 35–110 (mean, 80)	+	Acetylisoniazid; isonicotinic acid; monoacetylhydrazine	Hepatic, renal
Ethambutol	15 mg/kg day^{-1}	+	2–4	3.3–5.6	240 ± 30	+	Unchanged form; aldehyde; butyric acid	Renal
Streptomycin	Children, 20–40 mg/kg; adults, 0.75–1 g/day	–	1–2 after intramuscular dose	40–60	162	+ with meningitis		Renal

Table 3 Toxicities and Adverse Effects of Isoniazid, Ethambutol, and Streptomycin

Drug	Main toxicity	Adverse effects	Comments
Isoniazid	Hepatitis, peripheral neuropathy, acute overdose causes central nervous system symptoms	Fever, skin rash, development of antinuclear antibodies	Hepatitis seen less frequently in children than in adults
Ethambutol	Optic neuritis	Peripheral neuropathy, arthritis, rash	
Streptomycin	Ototoxicity, renal toxicity	Fever, neuromuscular blockade, myocarditis, hepatic necrosis	Hearing loss seen in infants born to mothers treated with streptomycin during pregnancy

I. ISONIAZID

Isoniazid is probably the most important of the antituberculous drugs. It was discovered in 1952 and has a remarkably simple chemical structure, the hydrazine of isonicotinic acid (Figure 1). It is a colorless, odorless, crystalline powder that is soluble in water (4).

A. Mechanism of Action

The mechanism of action of isoniazid is not entirely clear; it was thought to act by selective inhibition of nucleic acid synthesis of mycobacteria (5). There are now data linking the mycobactericidal activity of isoniazid to inhibition of synthesis of mycolic acids (6), which are important constituents of the mycobacterial cell wall.

B. Antimicrobial Activity

Isoniazid is a bactericidal drug with its greatest effect on actively multiplying extracellular organisms in a neutral or slightly alkaline environment (7). Most strains of *Mycobacterium tuberculosis* are susceptible to isoniazid at 0.2 μg/ml, whereas most strains of *Mycobacterium marinum (balnei)* and *Mycobacterium avium* are resistant (even at 5 μg/ml); *Mycobacterium kansasii* is susceptible at a higher concentration than *M. tuberculosis* (8).

Isoniazid resistance patterns in the United States depend upon such factors as prior exposure to antituberculous drugs and, in immigrants, the prevalence of resistance in their country of origin. Problems posed by drug resistance are addressed later in this chapter.

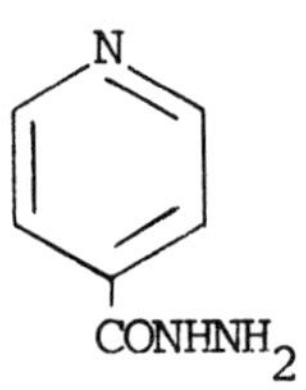

Figure 1 Chemical structure of isoniazid.

C. Clinical Pharmacology

Isoniazid is rapidly and almost completely absorbed from the small intestine. Plasma concentrations peak 1-2 hr after oral administration and fall in about 6 hr (9,10). Absorption is decreased with concomitant ingestion of antacids (11) or food (12). Plasma concentrations after oral administration are lower in rapid compared with slow acetylators (9), e.g., a mean of 19.9 μg/ml at 1 hr following a 15-mg/kg dose in slow acetylators and 14.2 μg/ml in rapid acetylators.

The drug is widely distributed intra- and extracellularly, with concentrations in the cerebrospinal fluid at 1 hr equal to one-fifth of those in plasma (13). Other sites of distribution include pleural fluid, saliva, and feces. Isoniazid crosses the placenta and is excreted in breast milk. Plasma protein binding does not occur to any significant extent. The apparent volume of distribution is 61 ± 11% of body weight or 43 liters in adults. Half-life in slow acetylators ranges from 100 to >400 min (average, 288 min) and in rapid acetylators 35-110 min (average, 80 min) (14). The half-life in children ranges from 96 to 288 min, and plasma concentrations are higher in children than in adults, possibly as a reflection of the higher per kilogram dose (15).

Comparative studies on six U.S. preparations (16) and a sustained-release preparation (17) show no significant differences between the preparations with regard to bioavailability or resultant peak serum concentrations.

The rate of elimination of isoniazid is dependent upon acetylator phenotype, which is determined by two major alleles. Rapid acetylators are homozygotes and acetylate isoniazid five to six times more rapidly than slow acetylators (heterozygotes) (18).

Figure 2 depicts the metabolism of isoniazid. Acetylation is quantitatively the most important pathway. Acetylisoniazid is biotransformed to isonicotinic acid and monoacetylhydrazine. Isonicotinic acid is then conjugated with glycine and excreted by the

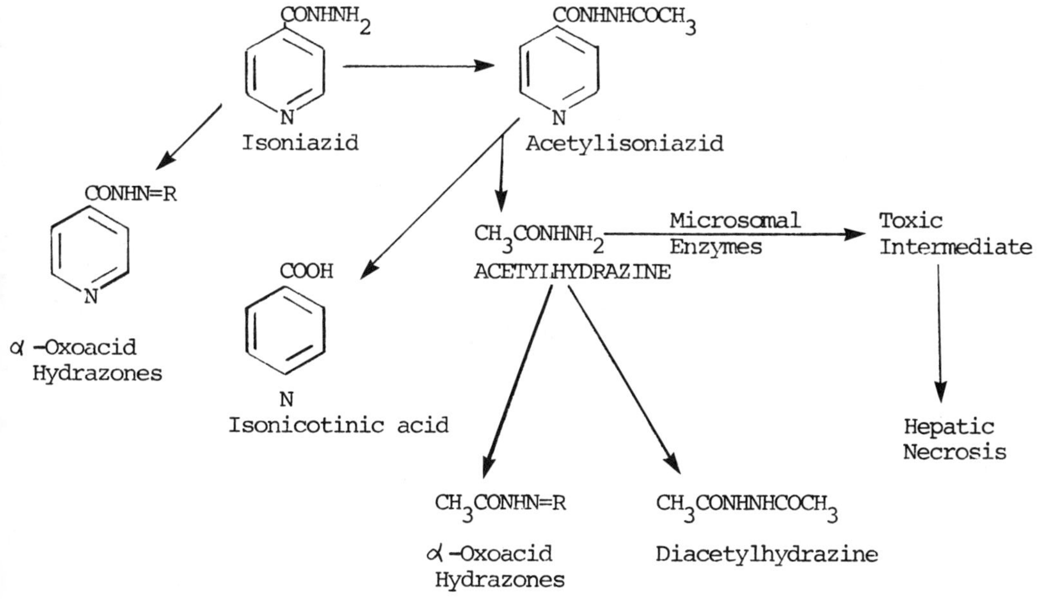

Figure 2 Metabolism of isoniazid.

kidneys. Monoacetylhydrazine is further biotransformed to diacetylhydrazine. Renal clearance of isoniazid and hydrazines is 46 ± 3 ml/min in adults. Renal excretion contributes approximately 27 and 11% to total body clearance in slow and rapid acetylators, respectively.

Metabolites excreted in the urine are reflective of acetylator status in that rapid acetylators excrete 12.4% as isoniazid and 41.2% as acetylisoniazid, whereas slow acetylators excrete 27.1 and 18.47%, respectively (14). Isonicotinic acid accounts for up to 10% urinary excretion in rapid and 30% in slow acetylators (18).

Acetylator status can be identified by several methods. In one, urine is collected 6–8 hr after drug administration and an "inactivation index" (ratio of acetylisoniazid to isoniazid) is calculated (14). Another tests urine or blood 4½ hr after administration of a 10-mg/kg oral dose of sulfamethazine by a modification of Evan's method (19). In the United States, approximately 42% of whites and 59% of blacks are rapid acetylators. There is a predominance of rapid acetylators in the Far East; people of European and African descent are intermediate acetylators. The acetylator phenotype is most important in dosing of isoniazid in intermittent therapy.

The pharmacokinetics of isoniazid are altered in renal failure with a trend toward prolongation of half-life, but there appears to be no direct correlation with the serum creatinine levels (20). Dosage reduction and monitoring of serum concentrations are recommended in adults if the serum creatinine is above 1.2 μg/dl (21).

In liver disease, all patients showed a prolongation of half-life that correlated most closely with serum bilirubin levels.

D. Preparations and Dosage

Isoniazid is available as

1. Isoniazid injection U.S.P. and B.P.
2. Isoniazid syrup 1 g per 100 ml U.S.P.
3. Isoniazid elixir BPC 1973, 50 mg INH per 5 ml
4. Isoniazid tablets U.S.P. and B.P.
5. Combinations with rifampin and ethambutol

E. Recommended Dosage

Newborns: 3–5 mg/kg day^{-1} for the first 2 months of life followed by 5–10 mg/kg day^{-1} (22).
Infants and children: 10–20 mg/kg day^{-1} in single or divided doses up to 300 mg/day.
Older children and adults: 4–5 mg/kg day^{-1} up to 300 mg daily.

Higher doses have been used in intermittent chemotherapy regimens, as will be discussed later in this chapter. Similar doses may be given by the intramuscular or intravenous routes in patients who are unable to take the medication by mouth.

F. Assays

Various methods of assay of activity of isoniazid and its metabolites are available using colorimetry, fluorometry (23), bioassay, radioimmunoassay (24), and high-performance liquid chromatography (HPLC).

G. Toxicity

Toxic effects of isoniazid can be dose dependent and dose independent.

1. Dose-Dependent Toxicities

Peripheral neuropathy occurs most often in chronic alcoholics, slow acetylators, and malnourished patients owing to inhibition of pyridoxal phosphate (vitamin B_6). Complaints include numbness or tingling, and parasthesias accompanied by muscle aches with muscle atrophy and fasciculations may develop. Symptoms reverse with cessation of therapy unless muscle weakness has set in (25). Pyridoxine, 10 mg daily for every 100 mg of isoniazid administered, can prevent the occurrence of this complication in high-risk groups (26). There are no pediatric reports associating isoniazid with these side effects.

Acute overdose with isoniazid causes toxic effects by inhibiting the activity of pyridoxal phosphate in the brain. Seizures occur due to decreased γ-aminobutyric acid concentrations in the brain (27). Patients present with hyperpyrexia, respiratory distress, intractable seizures (28,29), and coma. A severe metabolic acidosis occurs and is thought to be due to lactic acidosis induced by convulsions (30). Serum isoniazid concentrations may range from 8 to 35 μg/ml. The management of acute isoniazid poisoning (31,32) includes attention to supportive measures with administration of pyridoxine (1 g for each 1 g of ingested isoniazid) and diazepam (33) for control of seizures. Isoniazid is dialyzable (28). Chronic overdose was reported in a patient who presented with bizarre behavior and focal seizures (34).

2. Dose-Independent Toxicity

Hepatitis is the most important toxicity of isoniazid and is thought to be due to hydrazine, a product of isoniazid metabolism (35). Mild hepatic injury occurs fairly often and is usually transient despite continuation of therapy (36). Patients at increased risk for hepatotoxicity include the elderly, alcoholics, and patients with a previous history of biliary tract or liver disease (37). The incidence of hepatitis in children is lower than in adults, although there are case reports of fulminant hepatitis in the pediatric population (38,39). The reported incidence of asymptomatic hepatotoxicity in children ranges from 4 to 7.5% (36,40); in adolescents, 10% (41); and in adults, 10-22% (34). In one series in children only 0.8% required discontinuation of therapy (36).

Clinically overt hepatic injury is rare under 20 years of age. There is some correlation with rapid acetylator status, since these patients have an increase in the production of free hydrazine (35).

Controversy exists about the increased incidence of hepatotoxicity with combined use of isoniazid and rifampin. In a retrospective study of 874 children, of whom 430 received isoniazid and rifampin concurrently, there were 16 reports of hepatitis with only 2 in children receiving isoniazid alone (42). The overall hepatotoxic reaction rates were 3.2% for patients receiving rifampin and 0.5% for those receiving isoniazid. Biopsy findings are not helpful in differentiating isoniazid-induced disease from other possible causes of hepatitis. Cessation of therapy is followed by the resolution of signs and symptoms in all patients within 1 year. Fatalities are rare in children. Since the extent of hepatic injury induced by isoniazid encompasses a spectrum, with the majority of cases mild and transient, biochemical tests of liver function should be obtained only when indicated by clinical symptomatology.

Fever (43) is a common symptom following use of isoniazid and may appear with the first dose and disappear with cessation of therapy with isoniazid.

Skin rashes, including exfoliative dermatitis (44), morbilliform rashes, acne (45), and pellagra responsive to nicotinamide therapy (46), have been reported.

Neutropenia and a Coombs-positive hemolytic anemia (47) have been reported. Isoniazid has also been known to unmask a pyridoxine-dependent behavior disorder (48).

A delayed hypersensitivity type of reaction (49) has been reported, as have allergic reactions to isoniazid (50).

In adults, isoniazid therapy induced the formation of antinuclear antibodies in 22.4% of patients (51). Lupuslike syndromes have also been described (52,53).

Combined use of isoniazid and ethambutol may result in bilateral optic neuropathy (54).

Glycosuria has been reported following isoniazid administration (55).

Follow-up studies on patients who were exposed to isoniazid in utero show no increase in childhood cancers (56). Isoniazid was embryotoxic in mice (56), but studies in humans show no significant differences from control populations in birth weights, sex ratios, birth rates, or incidence of anomalies (57).

H. Drug Interactions (Table 4)

1. With rifampin, a toxic hepatitis may develop that differs from the hepatotoxicity induced by isoniazid alone (9) in that the peak incidence is higher and occurs earlier with the combination.
2. Diphenylhydantoin: phenytoin toxicity occurs in patients receiving both drugs, especially in slow acetylators (9,58), due to a noncompetitive inhibition resulting in accumulation of unmetabolized phenytoin. Phenytoin dosage in such patients must be reduced.
3. Warfarin: interaction with isoniazid results in increased activity of warfarin (59).
4. Carbamezapine: isoniazid results in a prompt decrease (approximately 45%) in hepatic clearance of carbamezapine, presumably by inhibition of microsomal metabolism of the drug (60).

Table 4 Interactions of Isoniazid with Other Drugs

During	Result of interaction	Comment	Reference
Rifampin	Toxic hepatitis		9
Diphenylhydantoin (phenytoin)	Accumulation of unmetabolized phenytoin due to a noncompetitive inhibition	Dosage of phenytoin must be reduced	9, 58
Warfarin	Increased activity of warfarin		59
Carbamezapine	Decrease in hepatic clearance of carbamezapine due to inhibition of microsomal metabolism		61
Levodopa	Due to a monoamine oxidase deficiency		62
Prednisolone	Decrease in isoniazid concentration due to enhanced renal clearance		61

5. Prednisolone causes a significant decrease in the concentration of isoniazid by enhanced renal clearance (61).
6. Levodopa interactions occur due to a monoamine oxidase deficiency (62).
7. Histamine poisoning following tuna fish (63) or skipjack ingestion (64) owing to isoniazid's activity as a potent diamine oxidase inhibitor.
8. Ingestion of cheese may induce reactions including hypertensive crises due to elevated monoamines (65).

II. ETHAMBUTOL

Ethambutol is rarely used in children under 5 years of age because of difficulty in monitoring for ocular toxicity. Ethambutol is the dextrorotatory isomer of 2,2′-ethylene diimino-di-1-butanol dihydrochloride (see Figure 3). The levo isomer has no significant activity against mycobacteria (66). Ethambutol is a white, odorless crystalline compound that is highly soluble in water (67).

A. Mechanism of Action

The mechanism of action is not entirely known but is thought to be due to a disturbance in nucleic acid synthesis (66). Ethambutol rapidly enters cells by diffusion, but its effect is seen only in rapidly proliferating cells (68) in which, after an initial delay, multiplication is arrested.

Although traditionally classed as a bacteriostatic drug, there is recent evidence to suggest that ethambutol has a bactericidal effect on intracellular bacilli infecting macrophages (69).

B. Antimicrobial Activity

Of 170 strains of *M. tuberculosis*, 24% were inhibited by less than 1 μg/ml and 76% by less than 5 μg/ml (the majority were inhibited by 1-2 μg/ml). Similar minimum inhibitory concentrations (MIC) were obtained against *Mycobacterium bovis* and the photochromogens, but susceptibility of the scotochromogens and nonchromogens was variable (70). Resistance develops when ethambutol is used alone.

C. Clinical Pharmacology

Ethambutol is rapidly but incompletely absorbed from the gastrointestinal tract (71), and serum concentrations are proportional to the dosage and enhanced by administration with food (72). Accumulation up to 10% occurs with continued administration of the

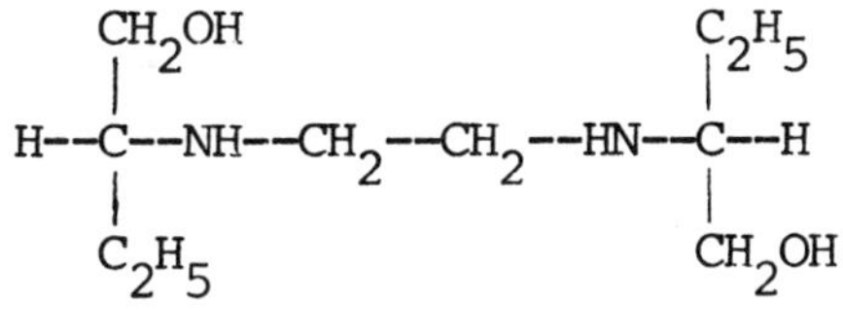

Figure 3 Chemical structure of ethambutol.

drug (73). Peak plasma concentrations after oral administration occur within 2-4 hr; e.g., concentrations measured by gas-liquid chromatography following a 25-mg/kg oral dose are 3.3-5.6 mg/ml; peak serum concentrations after an intravenous dose of 15 mg/kg are 11.6-15.4 μg/kg. Ethambutol is rapidly distributed into most tissues, including red blood cells. In animals, an affinity for lung tissue and pulmonary macrophages has been demonstrated (74,75). Ethambutol crosses the blood-brain barrier in meningitis (76,77), and cerebrospinal fluid concentrations of 1 μg/ml are detected in 30% (78) to 60% (79) of patients, although concentrations are dependent upon the dosage administered, time of assay, and inflammation of the meninges (79). The amount of ethambutol bound to plasma proteins is 20-30%.

Figure 4 depicts the metabolism of ethambutol. By conversion to aldehyde and butyric acid forms (Figure 4), 8-15% of administered ethambutol is metabolized. Of an oral dose or an intravenous dose of 25 mg/kg, 54-67 and 79%, respectively, are excreted unchanged in the urine (74,80). Over 144 hr, 67-74% of the drug is excreted in the urine and 12-19% is excreted in the feces. Half-life following an oral dose is 4.1 ± 0.5 hr. Renal clearance is 428.2 ± 59.3 ml/min.

In patients undergoing hemodialysis, ethambutol exhibits a markedly reduced half-life; recovery from dialysis fluid accounts only for a small portion of the administered dose (81).

D. Preparations and Dosage

Ethambutol is available commercially in oral form only as ethambutol syrup, 500 mg/ml, ethambutol tablets and capsules, Myambutol (Lederle, UK), as 100- and 400-mg tablets, and in combination with isoniazid.

The recommended dosage is 15 mg/kg day^{-1} in a single dose in children and adults.

E. Toxicity

1. Dose-Dependent Toxicity

The most important toxicity of ethambutol is optic neuritis, which may be unilateral or bilateral. The incidence of ocular toxicity with a 15 mg/kg day^{-1} dose ranges from 1 to 5% (81,82). There are two types of involvement: (1) central involvement of papillomacular fibers from macular ganglion cells presenting with diminished acuity, central scotoma, and loss of green color vision; and (2) periaxial involvement of fibers presenting with a defect in peripheral isopters, with little or no loss of acuity and normal green color sense. Recovery occurs after cessation of therapy, and recovery time is related to the severity of the defect (71). The exact mechanism of ocular toxicity is not known, but it is likely that

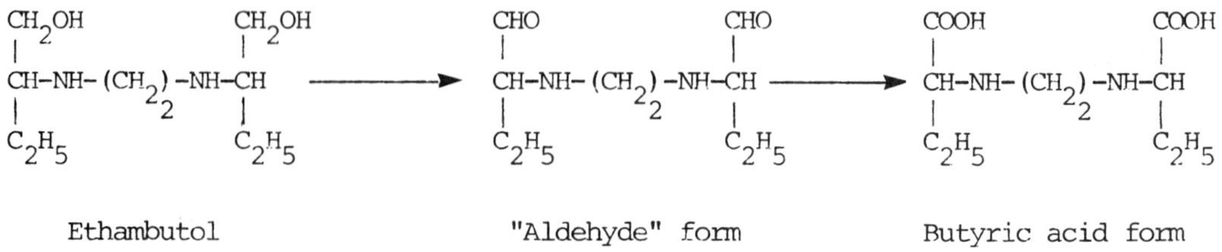

Figure 4 Metabolism of ethambutol.

multiple attacks of retrobulbar neuritis will result in more permanent damage than a single attack (82).

2. Dose-Independent Toxicity

Peripheral neuropathy has been described in some susceptible patients (83-85). Ethambutol can cause gouty arthritis (86,87) due to hyperuricemia by decreasing the renal clearance of uric acid (88,89). An erythematous generalized maculopapular rash (90) and toxic epidermolysis (91) have also been described. Toxic interstitial nephritis (92) may develop with use of ethambutol, but gastrointestinal intolerance is uncommon.

III. STREPTOMYCIN

This aminoglycoside antibiotic is a white hygroscopic powder, freely soluble in water isolated from *Streptomyces griseus*. Its bactericidal activity against *M. tuberculosis* was noted in the 1940s, and it became a major component of antituberculous therapy regimens. Owing to its toxicity and the need for parenteral administration, streptomycin is used less often now, particularly in children, and is generally reserved for drug-resistant cases. Dihydrostreptomycin is more stable than streptomycin but can cause sudden irreversible deafness; hence it is no longer in use.

A. Mechanism of Action

The mechanism of action of streptomycin is through inhibition of protein synthesis at the 30S ribosomal subunit (93).

B. Antimicrobial Activity

Streptomycin is bactericidal against extracellular tubercle bacilli (7). The MIC against *M. tuberculosis* range from 0.1 to 10 μg/ml, with the majority inhibited by 2 μg/ml. *M. marinum* and *M. kansasii* are susceptible in vitro; while most *M. avium* (8) are resistant to streptomycin.

C. Clinical Pharmacology

Streptomycin is poorly absorbed after oral administration, but following intramuscular injection, it passes rapidly into the blood, reaching a peak about 1 hr later. The volume of distribution is approximately 30% of body weight. Peak plasma concentrations following the injection of 0.25-1 g are 40-60 μg/ml. Serum half-life is 2.7 hr, and in premature infants it is 10.7 hr. It is loosely bound to plasma proteins. The drug penetrates poorly into cerebrospinal fluid, although inflammation of the meninges permits greater diffusion of the drug. It also diffuses into saliva, milk, ocular fluid, and pleural fluid and crosses the placental barrier. The majority of the drug is excreted in the urine by glomerular filtration (94,95).

D. Preparations and Dosage

Streptomycin is available as a streptomycin sulfate injection, and the dosage is 20-40 mg/kg day^{-1} in children and 1 g/day in adults. In premature infants, this dosage is modified to 5 mg/kg every 12 hr for the first week of life, and in newborns 10-20 mg/kg day^{-1} is recommended (94).

E. Toxicity

1. Dose-Dependent Toxicities

Most important is eighth nerve damage, which first manifests as vertigo or nystagmus and may be detected quite early by audiometry (96). The incidence of ototoxicity is reduced by limiting the total administered dose to 20–30 g in adults. A dose-dependent neuromuscular blockade has been reported with the use of streptomycin (94).

2. Dose-Independent Toxicities

These include hypersensitivity reactions, febrile reactions, myocarditis, hepatic necrosis (94), and an immune hemolytic anemia (97). The use of streptomycin during pregnancy has resulted in hearing loss in offspring (98).

IV. SECOND-LINE DRUGS

The second-line drugs used in tuberculous therapy are described in this section. Table 5 lists their dosages and adverse effects.

A. Pyrazinamide

Pyrazinamide was first shown to be effective in tuberculosis in 1952. The potential for hepatotoxicity and lack of adequate information on the use in children limits pyrazinamide to a "second-line" status. The mechanism of action is not known, but pyrazinamide appears to act well in an acidic medium (4) and is bactericidal against intracellular mycobacteria (7).

Pyrazinamide is absorbed from the gastrointestinal tract extremely rapidly and completely (99). Peak concentrations occur at 2 hr and are proportionate to dosage over the range of 0.5–5 g. The serum half-life is 4–10 hr (mean, 6.1 hr). The drug is rapidly distributed through the body water and is present in cerebrospinal fluid at concentrations equal to serum concentrations (100). It is metabolized in the liver, and its most important metabolite is pyrazinoic acid (101). Unchanged drug (4%) and pyrazinoic acid (30%) are excreted in the urine.

The adult dose is 20–35 mg/kg to a maximum of 3 g daily. The daily dose in children is 20 mg/kg and should be given in three to four divided doses.

The toxicity of pyrazinamide is mainly hepatic, producing elevated transaminase values in 10% of patients (102,103). Another important side effect is hyperuricemia (104), which results in arthralgia.

In combination with other antituberculous drugs, pyrazinamide plays an important role in the first 2 months of therapy, owing to killing of intracellular bacilli.

B. Ethionamide

Ethionamide, a thioamide derivative of ethylisonicotinic acid, was synthesized in 1956 (105). Experience with use of ethionamide in children is limited. Its action is bacteriostatic, with MIC of 0.6–1.2 μg/ml against *M. tuberculosis*. MIC against *M. balnei* (*avium*) and the scotochromogens range from 20 to 40 μg/ml; the susceptibility pattern of photochromogens resembles that of *M. tuberculosis*.

Ethionamide is rapidly absorbed from the gastrointestinal tract. A dose of 500 mg orally in adults results in serum concentrations of 12, 6, and 3 μg/ml at 3, 6, and 9 hr,

Table 5 Summary of Doses and Toxicities of the Second-line Antituberculous Drugs

Drug	Daily dosage	Major toxicities	Other adverse effects
Pyrazinamide	Children, 20 mg/kg; adults, 20–35 mg/kg	Hepatitis, hyperuricemia, arthralgia	
Ethionamide	Children, 12–15 mg/kg; adults, 0.5–1 g	Gastrointestinal intolerance	Hepatitis; central nervous system symptoms, e.g., somnolence, depression, acute psychotoxicity; goitrous hypothyroidism
Para-Aminosalicylic acid	Children, 200 mg/kg; adults, 9–12 g	Gastrointestinal intolerance	Hepatotoxicity, neutropenia, thrombocytopenia
Capreomycin	Children, 20 mg/kg; adults, 1 g	Ototoxicity, renal toxicity, electrolyte abnormalities	Hematologic and hepatic toxicity, rash, neuromuscular blockade
Cycloserine	Children, 5–15 mg/kg; adults, 0.5–1 g	Somnolence, hyperreflexia, mental confusion, convulsions	

respectively (106). However, absorption may be inconsistent (105). The drug is widely distributed in the tissues, including cerebrospinal fluid, where peak levels occur 3 hr following a dose (107). Ethionamide is extensively metabolized (108), and $<1\%$ is excreted unchanged in the urine. The biologic half-life is 2-4 hr. Ethionamide is available as tablets (U.S.P. and B.P.). The dosage in children is 12-15 mg/kg day^{-1} to a maximum of 750 mg/day and in adults is 0.5-1 g daily in divided doses (4). The drug is not well tolerated, with only 43% of patients tolerating 500 mg orally (109).

Toxicities include gastrointestinal intolerance in up to 80% of patients. Hepatitis occurs occasionally, and central nervous system (CNS) toxicities, including headaches, are seen in 77% (110). Somnolence, depression, and acute psychotic reactions have been reported (111,112). Other adverse effects include rash, pruritus, gynecomastia, menorrhagia, and impotence. Goitrous hypothyroidism (113,114) occurs due to the inhibition of organification in thyroid tissues; complete resolution of the hypothyroidism is seen with discontinuation of therapy. If therapy must be continued, replacement thyroid hormone may be required. Use in combination with pyrazinamide may result in an increased incidence of hepatotoxicity (115). Ethionamide is teratogenic in animals (116).

C. Para-Amino-Salicylic Acid (PAS)

The use of PAS has declined in recent years, primarily owing to its minimal antibacterial activity, the bulky oral formulation, and gastrointestinal side effects. PAS is a bacteriostatic drug, and its main role in the past was to delay emergence of resistance to isoniazid (117). Its action resulted from inhibition of the folic acid metabolic pathway (118). It is rapidly absorbed following oral administration and is extensively bound to protein. The main metabolic pathway is by acetylation in the liver, and up to 80% is excreted in the urine. The half-life is reported as 0.8-1.9 hr. The recommended dosage in children is 200 mg/kg day^{-1} and in adults is 9-12 g/day. The most commonly reported adverse effect of PAS is gastrointestinal irritation. Others include hepatotoxicity, neutropenia, and thrombocytopenia (119,120).

D. Cycloserine

Cycloserine was discovered in 1954 in cultures of *Streptomyces orchidaceus* and *Streptomyces garyphalus* (121). It is structurally similar to D-alanine. The mechanism of action is thought to be by inhibition of early formation of microbial cell walls. It acts in vitro as a weak mycobacteriostatic agent, and there is controversy about its bactericidal activity in vivo (118). Its activity against *M. tuberculosis* in vitro results in complete inhibition of growth at 10-20 μg/ml. It is active against bacilli resistant to the first-line drugs. Resistance develops to cycloserine when used as a single agent. Cycloserine is completely and rapidly absorbed from the gastrointestinal tract, with peak blood concentrations at 3-4 hr. There is a tendency for the drug to accumulate in the first 3 days of therapy.

The drug is widely distributed in body tissues and fluids including cerebrospinal fluid. The major route of excretion is renal, with 64% of the administered drug excreted in the urine within 72 hr.

Cycloserine is available in the form of capsules, which may deteriorate in tropical climates (122). The recommended dose in children is 5-15 mg/kg day^{-1} and in adults is 500 mg to 1 g/day. Dosage must be adjusted in renal failure. The toxicity of cycloserine is mainly neurological, with somnolence, hyperreflexia, mental confusion, and convulsions.

The use of divided doses limited to 250 mg may reduce the risk of convulsions. The use of cycloserine in combination with isoniazid is often effective.

E. Capreomycin

Capreomycin is a polypeptide antibiotic isolated from *Streptomyces capreolus* and was first made available in 1961 (122). It is related to viomycin. Capreomycin is bacteriostatic against *M. tuberculosis*; however, its mechanism of action is unknown. Cross-resistance occurs among viomycin, neomycin, and kanamycin (123). The drug is not absorbed after oral administration. Peak serum concentrations obtained after 1 g of capreomycin administered intramuscularly are 20–30 μg/ml in adults (124). Data in children are not available. There is no accumulation of the drug with continued use. Of the administered drug, 52% is excreted in the urine within 12 hr. The recommended dose in adults is 1 million units (equivalent to 1 g) daily to a maximum of 20,000 units/kg or 20 mg/kg day^{-1}. Dosage adjustments should be made in patients with renal failure.

Toxicities resemble those of streptomycin (renal toxicity and ototoxicity). The renal effects are reversible with discontinuation of therapy. Serum electrolyte abnormalities include hypokalemia, hypomagnesemia, hypocalcemia, and hyperchloremic alkalosis (125), probably as a result of a drug-induced hyperaldosteronism. Other side effects include eosinophilia, leukocytosis, bleeding diathesis, arthropathy, liver enzyme elevations (126), urticaria, maculopapular rash, and neuromuscular blockade following intravenous use (124).

F. Ansamycin

The new agent, ansamycin, is a spiropiperidyl rifamycin that has improved activity against *M. avium-intracellulare*. The use of ansamycin so far has been restricted to patients with the acquired immunodeficiency syndrome, with life-threatening disease due to *M. avium-intracellulare* (127).

Kanamycin and viomycin are rarely used in the present-day therapy of tuberculosis.

V. PREVENTION OF INFECTION (CHEMOPROPHYLAXIS)

Tuberculosis occurs as a result of a silent infection that may remain clinically inapparent for years. Once infected, the risk of reactivation persists for life. There are some groups that are clearly at an increased risk (Table 6). Children are considered at high risk because the tuberculin conversion rate among children exposed to active disease in a household may reach 25% and because they have an increased risk of development of more serious forms of disease, e.g., miliary tuberculosis.

Isoniazid prophylaxis reduces the incidence of active disease during the year of therapy by 70–80%, and protection persists in up to 50% of subjects over a 20-year period (128). The level of protection provided by isoniazid was best in compliant patients and in patients who received 52 weeks of therapy (129). In individual patient groups, the risks and benefits of isoniazid prophylaxis must be weighed carefully. In a 30-year follow-up study, 1882 children were enrolled and followed for a mean of 6.5 years (130). Only 8 patients developed active tuberculosis—a morbidity rate of 4.2 per 1000. There were 316 patients under 4 years of age, none of whom developed disease. The incidence of isoniazid toxicity, chiefly hepatotoxicity, is more of a concern in adults. The reader is referred to the section on isoniazid in this chapter for details.

Table 6 Indications for Isoniazid Prophylaxis

Tuberculin-positive asymptomatic contacts of newly discovered cases
Tuberculin-negative children in close contact with patients with active infection
Newly infected asymptomatic persons with a tuberculin conversion within 2 years
Immunocompromised hosts
Hematologic or reticuloendothelial malignancy
Systemic steroids for a prolonged period of time
Silicosis
Chronic renal insufficiency
Diabetes mellitus, especially if poorly controlled
Nutritional deficiency and weight $\leqslant$ 15% of ideal body weight
Heroin addicts

The dosage of isoniazid employed in prophylaxis is 10 mg/kg day^{-1}, to a maximum of 300 mg/day in children and 300 mg/day in adults to be administered for 1 year. A 9-month regimen should be effective but has not been evaluated (131).

In patients in whom compliance is a problem, twice weekly supervised administration of 15 mg/kg for 1 year is recommended.

A. Special Situations in Prophylaxis

1. Isoniazid Resistance

Prophylaxis has not been well studied in patients infected with isoniazid-resistant strains. In those at very high risk, e.g., immunocompromised hosts, rifampin at 10 mg/kg up to 600 mg/day may be given in addition to isoniazid (128) until susceptibility data from the source case become available.

2. Tuberculin-negative contacts

In children with a history of close contact with tuberculosis patients, the tuberculin reaction soon after exposure may be negative. In such patients, isoniazid prophylaxis should be initiated and the tuberculin reaction should be rechecked 3 months later. If still negative and the contact is broken or effectively treated, therapy may be discontinued. If the reaction is positive, however, therapy should be continued for 1 year (128).

3. Children Born to Mothers with Tuberculosis

These patients are at risk of acquiring the infection during or following delivery. If the mother is asymptomatic (i.e., skin test positive only), observation of the child, in conjunction with PPD skin tests, at 3 and 12 months is adequate. If the mother has inactive pulmonary disease or is receiving antituberculous chemotherapy, isoniazid should be administered to the infant at 10 mg/kg for 3–4 months. PPD reactions must be followed at 4 and 6 months. In mothers with active or disseminated disease, infants should be treated with 10 mg/kg isoniazid and followed with PPD skin tests at 4, 6, and 12 months.

When noncompliance is anticipated and in populations of high endemicity for tuberculosis, an alternative to the use of isoniazid (or adjunctive with isoniazid) is

Table 7 Contraindications to Isoniazid Chemoprophylaxis

Active tuberculosis
History of previous adequate therapy for tuberculosis
INH allergy
Active liver disease
Defer (if possible) therapy in pregnant women
INH resistance

vaccination of the infants with BCG and isolation of the infant from the mother until effective protection is demonstrated by asymptomatic tuberculin conversion in the infant. This may take 6–8 weeks to achieve, and such lengthy separation may have emotional consequences upon the mother and the infant (132).

Contraindications to isoniazid chemoprophylaxis are listed in Table 7 (133).

VI. TREATMENT OF TUBERCULOSIS

The aim of therapy of tuberculosis is to achieve control of the disease for the lifetime of the patient. Effective therapy first became possible with the discovery of chemotherapeutic agents with activity against mycobacteria. Combinations of these agents were found to be effective in arresting the disease, preventing relapses, and reducing the likelihood of development of bacterial resistance.

In recent years, several factors have contributed to a change in the approach to management of tuberculosis:

1. The discovery of rifampin, a potent bactericidal drug that is very effective in combination with isoniazid
2. The demonstration in field trials of the efficacy of ambulatory treatment with well-tolerated, orally administered drugs (134)
3. Studies that indicate that the risk to household contacts from sputum-positive index cases decreases with the initiation of chemotherapy (135)
4. The finding that two bactericidal drugs used in combination could cure tuberculosis in experimental animals in a much shorter period of time than was previously recognized (7)
5. The recognition that intermittent or "pulse" administration (e.g., twice weekly) of the drugs was as effective as daily therapy if "pulse therapy" was utilized following an initial phase of daily doses
6. The concept that there are distinct populations of tubercle bacilli in disease states against which therapy can be targeted: extracellular actively multiplying organisms (susceptible to isoniazid, rifampin, and streptomycin), a population of organisms with spurts of metabolic activity (susceptible to the action of rifampin), a population of bacilli within macrophages (susceptible to pyrazinamide), and a dormant population (which is difficult to eradicate with drugs) (7)

Table 8 Guidelines for Short-course Chemotherapy (American Thoracic Society and Centers for Disease Control)

Initial phase (2–8 weeks)
Isoniazid, 10 mg/kg day^{-1} up to 300 mg daily
plus
Rifampin, 10–20 mg/kg day^{-1} up to 600 mg daily
Continuation phase (for 9 months or 6 months from first negative sputum culture)
Isoniazid plus rifampin in doses mentioned above
or
Twice weekly isoniazid, 15 mg/kg, plus rifampin, 600 mg

The current approach to uncomplicated pulmonary tuberculosis is to treat patients in an ambulatory situation with a combination of drugs aimed specifically at the subpopulations of bacilli, with daily or intermittent administration for 9 months. There are obvious advantages to such short-course chemotherapy, including rapid conversion to negative culture, fewer treatment failures, fewer relapses, and no additional toxic effects. Trials of short-course chemotherapy include an extensive, well-controlled trial by the British Thoracic and Tuberculosis Association (BTTA) (136,137), the Singapore trial by the British Medical Research Council (138), and the experience in the United States in Arkansas (139). Based on these studies, the American Thoracic Society and Centers for Disease Control have published guidelines for short-course chemotherapy (140), which are summarized in Table 8. Briefly, an initial phase of 2–8 weeks of isoniazid at 10 mg/kg day^{-1} up to 300 mg daily with rifampin, 10–20 mg/kg day^{-1} up to 600 mg daily, is followed by a continuation phase of daily self-administration of both drugs in the same dose or supervised twice weekly administration of isoniazid at 15 mg/kg and rifampin at 600 mg for 9 months or longer (i.e., 6 months from the first negative sputum culture). There is evidence that addition of a third drug in the initial phase offers no advantage (141).

The recommendations for short-course chemotherapy in children were made by extrapolation from the adult experience (142). There are limited published data on short-course chemotherapy in children (143); however, in one series of 50 patients, excellent results were obtained (144).

Contraindications to short-course chemotherapy are outlined in Table 9 (140). There are several reports in the literature of regimens employing durations of 6 months or less (145,146); however, there are not yet enough data to support their use in children.

Table 9 Contraindications to Short-course Antituberculous Chemotherapy

Extrapulmonary tuberculosis
Drug-resistant tuberculosis
Patients with complicating medical conditions, e.g., silicosis, diabetes, immunocompromised states
Patients with active liver disease
Persistent or progressive infection

A. Extrapulmonary Tuberculosis

1. CNS Tuberculosis and Tubercular Meningitis

Successful treatment requires the use of bactericidal drugs that achieve adequate concentrations in the cerebrospinal fluid. Three-drug combinations are used initially (147, 148): isoniazid plus rifampin plus streptomycin. Ethambutol is used instead of streptomycin in children over 5 years of age. Pyrazinamide is added if drug-resistant strains are suspected. The recommended minimal duration of treatment is 18 months. Appropriate changes should be made in the regimen based upon susceptibility tests when available. The role of steroids in tuberculous meningitis is not clear. There is evidence that use of low-dose (1 mg/kg) steroids for the initial 30 days is beneficial in reducing intracranial pressure (149,150).

Hydrocephalus may develop during the course of the disease and may be treated with serial ventricular needle aspirations and acetazolamide (151) or by placement of a ventriculoperitoneal shunt.

Tuberculomas and tuberculous brain abscesses should be treated with combination chemotherapy; surgery may occasionally be required as well (152).

2. Miliary Tuberculosis

This form of disease is due to hematogenous dissemination. Therapy should be initiated with three drugs, including both isoniazid and rifampin (the third being streptomycin or ethambutol) and should be continued for 2 years (148).

3. Tuberculous Lymphadenopathy

Unlike localized disease due to atypical organisms, chemotherapy is the mainstay of therapy, with surgery added only if spontaneous drainage is imminent (148).

4. Skeletal Tuberculosis

Treatment with antituberculosis drugs for 18–24 months is indicated. Surgery, though important, has a limited role. It may be indicated if there is progression of disease despite therapy or if the location so demands, e.g., spinal cord compression or a paravertebral abscess (153).

5. Renal Tuberculosis

Renal tuberculosis is best treated with chemotherapy including isoniazid, rifampin, and ethambutol. Despite reports of short-course chemotherapy (154,155), we recommend the conventional 18 months of therapy in view of reports of persistence of viable bacilli detected in nephrectomy specimens after 6–8 months of therapy (156). Surgery may be indicated, e.g., nephrectomy in localized disease or reconstructive procedures for correction of strictures.

6. Congenital Tuberculosis

Intrauterine infection occurs rarely. Therapy includes isoniazid at 10-15 mg/kg day^{-1}, rifampin at 15 mg/kg day^{-1}, and streptomycin at 20 mg/kg day^{-1} for 3 months, followed by continuation of isoniazid and rifampin for 18 months (148,157).

7. Other Sites

Other possible sites of involvement include the abdomen, pericardium, skin, and eyes (158), in all of which combined therapy is indicated for 18 months. Topical steroids may be indicated in ocular disease.

The role of systemic steroids in the treatment of tuberculosis has not been evaluated in a well-controlled fashion. Steroids are often used early in the course of miliary tuberculosis, extensive pulmonary disease, and tuberculous meningitis. It is not known whether the use of steroids alters the prognosis, but it may contribute to a general feeling of well-being and an improved appetite.

Therapy of tuberculosis in pregnancy deserves mention (159). The risks of therapy in pregnant women with infection but no active disease probably outweigh the benefits of prophylaxis and can be deferred till the postpartum period. However, active disease should be treated, and the recommended drugs include isoniazid and ethambutol.

B. Adjuncts to Drug Therapy in Tuberculosis

The control and treatment of tuberculosis should involve a public health organization. In fact, the choice of chemotherapeutic regimens must take into account several local factors, e.g., geographic, social, cultural, and economic considerations (160). Continued surveillance of the patient and contacts is vitally important in control of disease in a population. Compliance monitoring can be done by urine tests, pill counting, and written instructions to the patients. Follow-up bacteriology and x-rays should be obtained every 2 or 3 months until improvement is seen.

VII. DRUG-RESISTANT TUBERCULOSIS

Resistance of mycobacteria to drugs may be primary or secondary. Primary drug resistance is seen in patients with no history of previous exposure to the drugs. It is seen in up to 6.9% of cases surveyed. There is a highly significant inverse relationship with age. Primary drug resistance is seen in 14% of patients 0–10 years of age and 3.6% of patients 90–99 years of age. Resistance to isoniazid is seen in 4%, streptomycin 3.8%, and ethionamide 1.1%. All others occur at <1% (161). There is a great variation in the geographic distribution of resistant organisms, and the local susceptibility patterns must be kept in mind during the selection of drugs for therapy. Table 10 provides a list of patients in whom drug susceptibility testing of the initial isolate is indicated. Primary drug resistance to more than one agent is rare and is estimated to occur at a rate of 1×10^{-11} to 1×10^{-12} (162).

Acquired drug resistance is seen in patients who have previously been treated for tuberculosis. It occurs more rapidly when a drug is used alone or in combination with a

Table 10 Indications for Drug Susceptibility Testing in Isolates from Patients with Tuberculosis

Populations known to have a high prevalence of drug resistance, e.g., Asians, Hispanics
Patients who have been treated for tuberculosis in the past
Patients who fail to become culture negative by month 4 of therapy
Persons who have been exposed to drug-resistant tuberculosis

drug of low efficacy and also in patients who are noncompliant. The management of drug-resistant disease is difficult. Drug susceptibility data are not available for a few weeks. Also, second-line drugs are not as well tolerated. Initial therapy should include at least two bactericidal drugs—one of which should be rifampin, since resistance to rifampin and ethambutol is not common (163). In patients with relapses, it is wise to add at least two drugs to which the patient has had no prior exposure. Therapy should be continued for the conventional 18-24 months. The regimen should be altered appropriately when drug susceptibility data become available (164,165) or when toxicity mandates.

VIII. ATYPICAL MYCOBACTERIAL INFECTIONS

Atypical mycobacteria are widely distributed in the environment, and children are constantly exposed to them. The extent of disease depends upon host factors.

A. Localized Disease

The most common manifestation of atypical mycobacterial disease in children is cervical lymphadenopathy (166), usually associated with few if any systemic symptoms. Management is surgical (167), with total excision of the node, abscess tract, and any involved skin. Cure rates of 92% have been described with surgery alone. Antituberculous drugs are indicated only in the rare patient in whom total surgical excision is not possible. Incision and drainage alone result in unacceptably low cure rates and the frequent development of draining fistulas.

B. Disseminated Disease

This is rare in children but may occur in immunocompromised patients. The commonest organism is *M. avium-intracellulare*, which demonstrates multiple drug resistance in vitro. There are no controlled studies evaluating combination regimens, but the generally accepted practice has been to use five or six drugs for a year (if tolerated), the most commonly employed agents being rifampin, ethambutol, isoniazid, ethionamide, cycloserine, and streptomycin. This is followed by the use of rifampin, ethambutol, and clofazimine for the second year (127).

Current research of tuberculosis therapy centers around new medications and shortened regimens. A recent report of in vitro activity of ciprofloxacin (168) against mycobacteria is one such example.

REFERENCES

1. Centers for Disease Control: Tuberculosis. *MMWR* Annual Summary, 62–64, 1983.
2. Inselman, LS: Tuberculosis in children: Update on diagnosis and therapy. *J. Respir. Dis. 4*:11–25, 1983.
3. Steiner, P, Rao, M, Mitchell, M, Steiner, M: Primary drug-resistant tuberculosis in children. *Am. J. Dis. Child. 139*:780–782, 1985.
4. Reynolds, JEF (ed.): Tuberculostatics and tuberculocides. In: *Martindale : The Extra Pharmacopeia*, 28th ed., Pharmaceutical Press, London, 1982, pp. 1564–1585.
5. Gangadharam, PRJ, Harold, FM, Schaefer, WB: Selective inhibition of nucleic acid synthesis in *Mycobacterium tuberculosis* by isoniazid. *Nature 198*:712–714, 1963.
6. Takayama, K, Wang, L, David, HL: Effect of isoniazid on the in vivo mycolic acid synthesis, cell growth, and viability of *Mycobacterium tuberculosis. Antimicrob. Agents Chemother. 2*:29–35, 1972.

7. Dutt, AK, Stead, WW: Present chemotherapy for tuberculosis. *J. Infect. Dis. 146*: 698–704, 1982.
8. Van Scoy, RE: Antituberculosis agents. Isoniazid, rifampin, streptomycin, ethambutol. *Mayo Clin. Proc. 52*:694–700, 1977.
9. Weber, WW, Hein, DW: Clinical pharmacokinetics of isoniazid. *Clin. Pharmacokinet. 4*:401–422, 1979.
10. Mount, FW, Anastasiades, AA, Schnack, GA: Control study of biologically active isoniazid in serum of children with primary tuberculosis. *Am. Rev. Respir. Dis. 83*: 173–183, 1961.
11. Hurwitz, A, Schlozman, DL: Effects of antacids on gastrointestinal absorption of isoniazid in rat and man. *Am. Rev. Respir. Dis. 109*:41–47, 1974.
12. Melander, A, Danielson, K, Hanson, A, Jansson, L, Rerup, C, Schersten, B, Thulin, T, Wahlin, E: Reduction of isoniazid bioavailability in normal men by concomitant intake of food. *Acta Med. Scand. 200*:93–97, 1976.
13. Des Prez, R, Boone, IU: Metabolism of C^{14}-isoniazid in humans. *Am. Rev. Respir. Dis. 84*:42–51, 1961.
14. Eidus, L, Ling, GM, Harnanansingh, AMT: Isoniazid excretion in fast and slow inactivators and its practical aspect for phenotyping. *Arzneimittelforsch. 21*:1696–1699, 1971.
15. Olson, WA, Pruitt, AW, Dayton, PG: Plasma concentrations of isoniazid in children with tuberculous infections. *Pediatrics 67*:876–878, 1981.
16. Gelber, R, Jacobsen, P, Levy, L: A study of the availability of six commercial formulations of isoniazid. *Clin. Pharmacol. Ther. 10*:841–848, 1969.
17. Jalsenjak, I, Nixon, JR, Senjkovic, R, Stivic, I: Sustained-release dosage forms of microencapsulated isoniazid. *J. Pharm. Pharmacol. 32*:678–680, 1980.
18. Ellard, GA, Gammon, PT: Pharmacokinetics of isoniazid metabolism in man. *J. Pharm. Biopharm. 4*:83–113, 1976.
19. Weber, WW, Brenner, W: A filter paper method for determining isoniazid acetylator phenotype. *Am. J. Hum. Genet. 26*:467–473, 1974.
20. Gold, CH, Buchanan, N, Tringham, V, Viljoen, M, Strickwold, B, Moodley, GP: Isoniazid pharmacokinetics in patients in chronic renal failure. *Clin. Nephrol. 6*: 365–369, 1976.
21. Bowersox, DW, Winterbauer, RH, Stewart, GL, Orme, B, Barron, E: Isoniazid dosage in patients with renal failure. *N. Engl. J. Med. 289*:84–87, 1973.
22. Peonides, A, Katz, G: Prophylactic isoniazid dosage in newborn infants. *Arch. Dis. Child. 52*:165, 1977.
23. Olson, WA, Dayton, PG, Israili, ZH, Pruitt, AW: Spectrophotofluorometric assay for isoniazid and acetyl isoniazid in plasma adapted to pediatric studies. *Clin. Chem. 23*: 745–748, 1977.
24. Schwenk, R, Kelly, K, Tse, KS, Sehon, AH: A radioimmunoassay for isoniazid. *Clin. Chem. 21*:1059–1062, 1975.
25. Goldman, AL, Braman, SS: Isoniazid: A review with emphasis on adverse effects. *Chest 62*:71–77, 1972.
26. Honeycutt, WM, Huldin, DH: Reactions to isoniazid. *Arch. Dermatol. 88*:126–130, 1963.
27. Miller, J, Robinson, A, Percy, AK: Acute isoniazid poisoning in childhood. *Am. J. Dis. Child. 134*:290–292, 1980.
28. Terman, DS, Teitelbaum, DT: Isoniazid self-poisoning. *Neurology (N.Y.) 20*:299–304, 1970.
29. Cameron, WM: Isoniazid overdose. *Can. Med. Assoc. J. 118*:1413–1415, 1978.
30. Chin, L, Sievers, ML, Herrier, RN, Picchioni, AL: Convulsions as the etiology of lactic acidosis in acute isoniazid toxicity in dogs. *Toxicol. Appl. Pharmacol. 49*: 377–384, 1979.

31. Brown, CV: Acute isoniazid poisoning. *Am. Rev. Respir. Dis. 105*:206–216, 1972.
32. Yarbrough, BE, Wood, JP: Isoniazid overdose treated with high-dose pyridoxine. *Ann. Emerg. Med. 12*:303–305, 1983.
33. Sievers, ML, Herrier, RN, Chin, L, Picchioni, AL: Treatment of isoniazid overdose. *JAMA 247*:583–584, 1982.
34. Rubin, DH, Carbone, J, Fong, B, Borowitz, D, Leven, R, Grossman, M: Chronic isoniazid poisoning. *Clin. Pediatr. 22*:518–519, 1983.
35. Mitchell, JR, Zimmerman, HJ, Ishak, KG, Thorgeirsson, UP, Timbrell, JA, Snodgrass, WR, Nelson, SD: Isoniazid liver injury: Clinical spectrum, pathology, and probable pathogenesis. *Ann. Intern. Med. 84*:181–192, 1976.
36. Spyridis, P, Sinaniotis, C, Papadea, I, Oreopoulos, L, Hadjiyiannis, S, Papadatos, C: Isoniazid liver injury during chemoprophylaxis in children. *Arch. Dis. Child. 54*: 65–67, 1979.
37. Gronhagen-Riska, C, Hellstrom, PE, Froseth, B: Predisposing factors in hepatitis induced by isoniazid-rifampin treatment of tuberculosis. *Am. Rev. Respir. Dis. 118*: 461–466, 1978.
38. Bistritzer, T, Barzilay, Z, Jonas, A: Isoniazid-rifampin-induced fulminant liver disease in an infant. *J. Pediatr. 97*:480–482, 1980.
39. Vanderhoof, JA, Ament, ME: Fatal hepatic necrosis due to isoniazid chemoprophylaxis in a 15-year-old girl. *J. Pediatr. 88*:867–868, 1976.
40. Stein, MT, Liang, D: Clinical hepatotoxicity of isoniazid in children. *Pediatrics 64*: 499–505, 1979.
41. Litt, IF, Cohen, MI, McNamara, H: Isoniazid hepatitis in adolescents. *J. Pediatr. 89*:133–135, 1976.
42. O'Brien, RJ, Long, MW, Cross, FS, Lyle, MA, Snider, DE, Jr.: Hepatotoxicity from isoniazid and rifampin among children treated for tuberculosis. *Pediatrics 72*:491–499, 1983.
43. Dasta, JF, Prior, JA: Isoniazid-induced fever. *Chest 75*:196–197, 1979.
44. Rosin, MA, King, LE, Jr.: Isoniazid-induced exfoliative dermatitis. *South. Med. J. 75*:81, 1982.
45. Cohen, LK, George, W, Smith, R: Isoniazid-induced acne and pellagra. *Arch. Dermatol. 109*:377–381, 1974.
46. Thomas, RHM, Payne, CMER, Black, MM: Isoniazid-induced pellagra. *Br. Med. J. 283*:287–288, 1981.
47. Robinson, MG, Foadi, M: Hemolytic anemia with positive Coombs' test. *JAMA 208*: 656–658, 1969.
48. Brenner, A, Wapnir, RA: Pyridoxine-dependent behavioral disorder unmasked by isoniazid. *Am. J. Dis. Child. 132*:773–776, 1978.
49. Rudoy, R, Stuemky, J, Poley, JR: Isoniazid administration and liver injury. *Am. J. Dis. Child. 125*:733–736, 1973.
50. Periman, P, Venkataramani, TK: Acute arthritis induced by isoniazid. *Ann. Intern. Med. 83*:667–668, 1975.
51. Rothfield, NF, Bierer, WF, Garfield, JW: Isoniazid induction of antinuclear antibodies. *Ann. Intern. Med. 88*:650–652, 1978.
52. Zingale, SB, Minzer, L, Rosenberg, B, Lee, SL: Drug-induced lupus-like syndrome. *Arch. Intern. Med. 112*:63–66, 1963.
53. Alarcon-Segovia, D: Drug-induced lupus syndromes. *Mayo Clin. Proc. 44*:664–681, 1963.
54. Karmon, G, Savir, H, Zevin, D, Levi, J: Bilateral optic neuropathy due to combined ethambutol and isoniazid treatment. *Ann. Ophthalmol. 11*:1013–1017, 1979.
55. Dickson, I: Glycosuria and diabetes mellitus following I.N.A.H. therapy. *Med. J. Aust. 1*:325–326, 1962.

56. Hammond, EC, Selikoff, IJ, Robitzek, EH: Isoniazid therapy in relation to later occurrence of cancer in adults and in infants. *Br. Med. J. 2*:792–795, 1967.
57. Ludford, J, Doster, B, Woolpert, SF: Effect of isoniazid on reproduction. *Am. Rev. Respir. Dis. 108*:1170–1174, 1973.
58. Kutt, H, Brennan, R, Dehejia, H, Verebely, K: Diphenylhydantoin intoxication. *Am. Rev. Respir. Dis. 101*:377–384, 1970.
59. Rosenthal, AR, Self, TH, Baker, ED, Linden, RA: Interaction of isoniazid and warfarin. *JAMA 238*:2177, 1977.
60. Wright, JM, Stokes, EF, Sweeney, VP: Isoniazid-induced carbamazepine toxicity and vice versa. *N. Engl. J. Med. 307*:1325–1327, 1982.
61. Sarma, GR, Kailasam, S, Nair, NGK, Narayana, ASL, Tripathy, SP: Effect of prednisolone and rifampin on isoniazid metabolism in slow and rapid inactivators of isoniazid. *Antimicrob. Agents Chemother. 18*:661–666, 1980.
62. Morgan, JP: Isoniazid and levodopa. *Ann. Intern. Med. 92*:434, 1980.
63. Uragoda, CG: Histamine poisoning in tuberculous patients after ingestion of tuna fish. *Am. Rev. Respir. Dis. 121*:157–159, 1980.
64. Senanayake, N, Vyravanathan, S, Kanagasuriyam, S: Cerebrovascular accident after a "skipjack" reaction in a patient taking isoniazid. *Br. Med. J. 2*:1127–1128, 1978.
65. Lejonc, JL, Gusmini, D, Brochard, P: Isoniazid and reaction to cheese. *Ann. Intern. Med. 91*:793, 1979.
66. Forbes, M, Peets, EA, Kuck, NA: Effect of ethambutol on mycobacteria. *Ann. N.Y. Acad. Sci. 135*:726–731, 1966.
67. Leading article: Ethambutol. *Tubercle 47*:292–295, 1966.
68. Forbes, M, Kuck, NA, Peets, EA: Mode of action of ethambutol. *J. Bacteriol. 84*: 1099–1103, 1962.
69. Crowle, AJ, Sbarbaro, JA, Judson, FN, May, MH: The effect of ethambutol on tubercle bacilli within cultured human macrophages. *Am. Rev. Respir. Dis. 132*: 742–745, 1985.
70. Kearlson, AG: The in vitro activity of ethambutol (dextro-2,2′-[ethylenediimino]-1-butanol) against tubercle bacilli and other microorganisms. *Am. Rev. Respir. Dis. 84*:905–906, 1961.
71. Place, VA, Peets, EA, Buyske, DA, Little, RR: Metabolic and special studies of ethambutol in normal volunteers and tuberculous patients. *Ann. N.Y. Acad. Sci. 135*:775–795, 1966.
72. Place, VA, Thomas, JP: Clinical pharmacology of ethambutol. *Am. Rev. Respir. Dis. 87*:901–904, 1963.
73. Lee, CS, Gambertoglio, JG, Brater, DC, Benet, LZ: Kinetics of oral ethambutol in the normal subject. *Clin. Pharmacol. Ther. 22*:615–621, 1977.
74. Liss, RH, Letourneau, RJ, Schepis, JP: Distribution of ethambutol in primate tissues and cells. *Am. Rev. Respir. Dis. 123*:529–532, 1981.
75. Kelly, RG, Kaleita, E, Eisner, HJ: Tissue distribution of [^{14}C]ethambutol in mice. *Am. Rev. Respir. Dis. 123*:689–690, 1981.
76. Pilheu, JA, Maglio, F, Cetrangolo, R, Pleus, AD: Concentrations of ethambutol in the cerebrospinal fluid after oral administration. *Tubercle 52*:117–122, 1971.
77. Place, VA, Pyle, MM, de la Huerga, J: Ethambutol in tuberculous meningitis. *Am. Rev. Respir. Dis. 99*:783–785, 1969.
78. Gundert-Remy, U, Klett, M, Weber, E: Concentration of ethambutol in cerebrospinal fluid in man as a function of the non-protein-bound drug fraction in serum. *Eur. J. Clin. Pharmacol. 6*:133–136, 1973.
79. Bobrowitz, ID: Ethambutol in tuberculous meningitis. *Chest 61*:629–632, 1972.
80. Lee, CS, Marbury, TC, Benet, LZ: Clearance calculations in hemodialysis: Application to blood, plasma, and dialysate measurements for ethambutol. *J. Pharm. Biopharm. 8*:69–81, 1980.

81. Barron, GJ, Tepper, L, Iovine, G: Ocular toxicity from ethambutol. *Am. J. Ophthalmol. 77*:256–260, 1974.
82. Leibold, JE: The ocular toxicity of ethambutol and its relation to dose. *Ann. N.Y. Acad. Sci. 135*:904–909, 1966.
83. Nair, VS, LeBrun, M, Kass, I: Peripheral neuropathy associated with ethambutol. *Chest 77*:98–100, 1980.
84. Aelony, Y, Locks, MO: Peripheral neuropathy associated with ethambutol. *Chest 78*:898, 1980.
85. Tugwell, P, James, SL: Peripheral neuropathy with ethambutol. *Postgrad. Med. J. 48*:667–670, 1972.
86. Khanna, BK: Acute gouty arthritis following ethambutol therapy. *Br. J. Dis. Chest 74*:409–410, 1980.
87. Self, TH, Fountain, FF, Taylor, WJ, Jr., Sutliff, WD: Acute gouty arthritis associated with the use of ethambutol. *Chest 71*:561–562, 1977.
88. Postlethwaite, AE, Kelley, WN: Studies on the mechanism of ethambutol-induced hyperuricemia. *Arthritis Rheum. 15*:403–409, 1972.
89. Postlethwaite, AE, Bartel, AG, Kelley, WN: Hyperuricemia due to ethambutol. *N. Engl. J. Med. 286*:761–762, 1972.
90. Pasricha, JS, Kanwar, AJ: Skin eruption caused by ethambutol. *Arch. Dermatol. 113*:1122–1123, 1977.
91. Pegram, PS, Jr., Mountz, JD, O'Bar, PR: Ethambutol-induced toxic epidermal necrolysis. *Arch. Intern. Med. 141*:1677–1678, 1981.
92. Collier, J, Joekes, AM, Philalithis, PE, Thompson, FD: Two cases of ethambutol nephrotoxicity. *Br. Med. J. 2*:1105–1106, 1976.
93. Davis, BD: Streptomycin resistance and the study of ribosomal structure and function. *N. Engl. J. Med. 283*:1405–1406, 1970.
94. Simon, HJ: Streptomycin, kanamycin, neomycin and paromomycin. *Pediatr. Clin. North Am. 15*:73–83, 1968.
95. Robson, JM, Sullivan, FM: Antituberculosis drugs. *Pharmacol. Rev. 15*:169–223, 1963.
96. Ballantyne, J: Iatrogenic deafness. *J. Laryngol. Otol. 84*:967–1000, 1970.
97. Letona, JM-L, Barbolla, L, Frieyro, E, Bouza, E, Gilsanz, F, Fernandez, MN: Immune haemolytic anaemia and renal failure induced by streptomycin. *Br. J. Haematol. 35*:561–571, 1977.
98. Robinson, GC, Cambon, KG: Hearing loss in infants of tuberculous mothers treated with streptomycin during pregnancy. *N. Engl. J. Med. 271*:949–951, 1964.
99. Ellard, GA: Absorption, metabolism and excretion of pyrazinamide in man. *Tubercle 50*:144–158, 1969.
100. Forgan-Smith, R, Ellard, GA, Newton, D, Mitchison, DA: Pyrazinamide and other drugs in tuberculous meningitis. *Lancet 2*:374, 1973.
101. Roboz, J, Suzuki, R, Yu, TA-F: Mass fragmentographic determination of pyrazinamide and its metabolites in serum and urine. *J. Chromatogr. 147*:337–347, 1978.
102. Danan, G, Pessayre, D, Larrey, D, Benhamou, JP: Pyrazinamide fulminant hepatitis: An old hepatotoxin strikes again. *Lancet 2*:1056–1057, 1981.
103. Pretet, S, Liard, R, Perdrizet, S: Pyrazinamide, a major antituberculosis drug. *Lancet 1*:399, 1982.
104. Horsfall, PAL, Plummer, J, Allan, WGL, Girling, DJ, Nunn, AJ, Fox, W: Double blind controlled comparison of aspirin, allopurinol and placebo in the management of arthralgia during pyrazinamide administration. *Tubercle 60*:13–24, 1979.
105. Weinstein, HJ, Hallett, WY, Sarauw, AS: The absorption and toxicity of ethionamide. *Am. Rev. Respir. Dis. 86*:576–578, 1962.
106. Rist, N, Grumbach, F, Libermann, D: Experiments on the antituberculous activity of alpha-ethylthioisonicotinamide. *Am. Rev. Tuber. Pulmon. Dis. 79*:1–5, 1959.

107. Hughes, IE, Oxon, BM, Smith, H, Kane, PO: Ethionamide: Its passage into the cerebrospinal fluid in man. *Lancet 1*:616–617, 1962.
108. Johnston, JP, Kane, PO, Kibby, MR: The metabolism of ethionamide and its sulphoxide. *J. Pharm. Pharmacol. 19*:1–9, 1967.
109. Gupta, DK: Acceptability of thioamides. I. Ethionamide. *J. Postgrad. Med. 23*: 175–180, 1977.
110. Fox, W, Robinson, DK, Tall, R: A study of acute intolerance to ethionamide, including a comparison with prothionamide, and of the influence of a vitamin b-complex additive in prophylaxis. *Tubercle 50*:125–143, 1969.
111. Narang, RK: Acute psychotic reaction probably caused by ethionamide. *Tubercle 53*:137–138, 1972.
112. Lansdown, FS, Beran, M, Litwak, T: Psychotoxic reaction during ethionamide therapy. *Am. Rev. Respir. Dis. 95*:1053–1055, 1967.
113. Drucker, D, Eggo, MC, Salit, IE, Burrow, GN: Ethionamide-induced goitrous hypothyroidism. *Ann. Intern. Med. 100*:837–839, 1984.
114. Moulding, T, Fraser, R: Hypothyroidism related to ethionamide. *Am. Rev. Respir. Dis. 101*:90–94, 1970.
115. Schless, JM, Allison, RF, Inglis, RM, White, EF, Topperman, S: The use of ethionamide in combined drug regimens in the re-treatment of isoniazid-resistant pulmonary tuberculosis. *Am. Rev. Respir. Dis. 91*:728–737, 1965.
116. Anon: Safety of antimicrobial drugs in pregnancy. *Med. Lett. 27*:93–95, 1985.
117. Sattler, A: The present status of PAS in tuberculosis therapy. *Am. Rev. Respir. Dis. 85*:927–928, 1962.
118. Yoshikawa, TT, Fujita, NK: Antituberculous drugs. *Med. Clin. North Am. 66*: 209–219, 1982.
119. Eisner, EV, Kasper, K: Immune thrombocytopenia due to a metabolite of para-aminosalicylic acid. *Am. J. Med. 53*:790–796, 1972.
120. Feigin, RD, Zarkowsky, HF, Shearer, W, Anderson, DC: Thrombocytopenia following administration of paraaminosalicylic acid. *J. Pediatr. 83*:502–503, 1973.
121. Storey, PB, McLean, RL: A current appraisal of cycloserine. *Antibiot. Med. Clin. Ther. 4*:223–232, 1957.
122. Rao, KVN, Eidus, L, Evans, C, Kailasam, S, Radhakrishna, S, Somasundaram, PR, Stott, H, Subbammal, S, Tripathy, SP: Deterioration of cycloserine in the tropics. *Bull. WHO 39*:781–789, 1968.
123. Tsukamura, M: Cross-resistance relationships between capreomycin, kanamycin, and viomycin resistances in tubercle bacilli from patients. *Am. Rev. Respir. Dis. 99*:780–782, 1969.
124. Editorial: Capreomycin-evaluation of a new antituberculous agent. *JAMA 223*: 179–180, 1973.
125. Holmes, AM, Hesling, CM, Wilson, TM: Capreomycin-induced serum electrolyte abnormalities. *Thorax 25*:608–611, 1970.
126. Danilov, G: Capreomycin regimen in the treatment of tuberculosis. *Mod. Med. Can. 28*:131–135, 1973.
127. Iseman, MD, Corpe, RF, O'Brien, RJ, Rosenzwieg, DY, Wolinsky, E: Disease due to *Mycobacterium avium-intracellulare. Chest 87*:139S–149S, 1985.
128. Koch-Weser, D, Barrett-Connor, EL, Comstock, GW, Grzybowski, S, Smith, DW: Preventive treatment of tuberculosis. *Chest 87*:128S–134S, 1985.
129. International Union Against Tuberculosis Committee on Prophylaxis: Efficacy of various durations of isoniazid preventive therapy for tuberculosis: Five years of follow-up in the IUAT trial. *Bull. WHO 60*:555–564, 1982.
130. Hsu, KHK: Isoniazid in the prevention and treatment of tuberculosis. *JAMA 229*: 528–533, 1974.

131. Jacobs, RF, Abernathy, RS: The treatment of tuberculosis in children. *Pediatr. Infect. Dis. 4*:513–517, 1985.
132. Hughes, WT: Tuberculosis today. *Pediatr. Infect. Dis. 2(Suppl.)*:S37–S39, 1983.
133. Noble, J: Isoniazid prophylaxis re-examined. *N. Engl. J. Med. 285*:687–689, 1974.
134. Pilheu, JA: Ambulatory treatment of pulmonary tuberculosis with ethambutol-isoniazid. *Chest 58*:497–500, 1970.
135. Gunnels, JJ, Bates, JH, Swindoll, H: Infectivity of sputum-positive tuberculous patients on chemotherapy. *Am. Rev. Respir. Dis. 109*:323–330, 1974.
136. Angel, JH: BTA short-course chemotherapy studies. *Chest 80*:722–724, 1981.
137. Somner, AR: Short-course chemotherapy in pulmonary tuberculosis. A controlled trial by the British Thoracic Association. *Lancet 1*:1182–1183, 1980.
138. Singapore Tuberculosis Service/British Medical Research Council: Controlled trial of intermittent regimens of rifampicin plus isoniazid for pulmonary tuberculosis in Singapore. *Lancet 2*:1105–1109, 1975.
139. Dutt, AK, Jones, L, Stead, WW: Short-course chemotherapy for tuberculosis with largely twice-weekly isoniazid-rifampin. *Chest 75*:441–447, 1979.
140. Iseman, MD, Albert, R, Locks, M, Raleigh, J, Sutton, F, Farer, LS: Guidelines for short-course tuberculosis chemotherapy. *Am. Rev. Respir. Dis. 121*:611–614, 1980.
141. Stead, WW, Good, WE: Contribution of a third drug to various two-drug regimens in the treatment of tuberculosis. *Am. Rev. Respir. Dis. 121*:463 (abstract), 1980.
142. Smith, MHD: What about short course and intermittent chemotherapy for tuberculosis in children? *Pediatr. Infect. Dis. 1*:298–303, 1982.
143. Addington, WW, Albert, RK, Bass, JB, Jr., Catlin, BJ, Loudon, RG, Seggerson, J, Slutkin, G: Standard therapy for tuberculosis 1985. *Chest 87*:117S–127S, 1985.
144. Abernathy, RS, Dutt, AK, Stead, WW, Moers, DJ: Short-course chemotherapy for tuberculosis in children. *Pediatrics 72*:801–806, 1983.
145. Mehrotra, ML, Gautam, KD, Chaube, CK: Shortest possible acceptable effective chemotherapy in ambulatory patients with pulmonary tuberculosis. Part II. Results during the 24 months after the end of chemotherapy. *Am. Rev. Respir. Dis. 129*:1016–1017, 1984.
146. Snider, DE, Graczyk, J, Bek, E, Rogowski, J: Supervised six-months treatment of newly diagnosed pulmonary tuberculosis using isoniazid, rifampin, and pyrazinamide with and without streptomycin. *Am. Rev. Respir. Dis. 130*:1091–1094, 1984.
147. Rahajoe, NN, Rahajoe, N, Boediman, I, Said, M, Lazuardi, S: The treatment of tuberculous meningitis in children with a combination of isoniazid, rifampicin and streptomycin–preliminary report. *Tubercle 60*:245–250, 1979.
148. Lorin, MI, Hsu, KHK, Jacob, SC: Treatment of tuberculosis in children. *Pediatr. Clin. North Am. 30*:333–348, 1983.
149. Escobar, JA, Belsey, MA, Duenas, A, Medina, P: Mortality from tuberculous meningitis reduced by steroid therapy. *Pediatrics 56*:1050–1055, 1975.
150. O'Toole, RD, Thornton, GF, Mukherjee, MK, Nath, RL: Dexamethasone in tuberculous meningitis. *Ann. Intern. Med. 70*:39–48, 1969.
151. Visudhiphan, P, Chiemchanya, S: Hydrocephalus in tuberculous meningitis in children: Treatment with acetazolamide and repeated lumbar puncture. *J. Pediatr. 95*:657–660, 1979.
152. Wouters, EFM, Hupperts, RMM, Vreeling, FW, Greve, LH, Janevski, B, Willebrand, D, Berfelo, WF: Successful treatment of tuberculous brain abscess. *J. Neurol. 232*: 118–119, 1985.
153. Davidson, PT, Horowitz, I: Skeletal tuberculosis. *Am. J. Med. 48*:77–84, 1970.
154. Gow, JG: Genitourinary tuberculosis: A 7-year review. *Br. J. Urol. 51*:239–244, 1979.

155. Gow, JG, Barbosa, S: Genitourinary tuberculosis. A study of 1117 cases over a period of 34 years. *Br. J. Urol. 56*:449–455, 1984.
156. Mallo, N, Dalet, F, Villavicencio, H: Treatment of renal tuberculosis. *Eur. Urol. 4*:269–273, 1978.
157. Hageman, J, Shulman, S, Schreiber, M, Luck, S, Yogev, R: Congenital tuberculosis: Critical reappraisal of clinical findings and diagnostic procedures. *Pediatrics 66*:980–984, 1980.
158. Dinning, WJ, Marston, S: Cutaneous and ocular tuberculosis: A review. *J. R. Soc. Med. 78*:576–581, 1985.
159. Scheinhorn, DJ, Angelillo, VA: Antituberculous therapy in pregnancy. *West. J. Med. 127*:195–198, 1977.
160. Fox, W: Whither short-course chemotherapy? *Br. J. Dis. Chest 75*:331–357, 1981.
161. Centers for Disease Control: Primary resistance to antituberculosis drugs—United States. *MMWR 32*:521–523, 1983.
162. Mitchell, RS: Control of tuberculosis. *N. Engl. J. Med. 276*:842–848, 1967.
163. Jeanes, CWL, Jessamine, AG, Eidus, L: Treatment of chronic drug-resistant pulmonary tuberculosis with rifampin and ethambutol. *Can. Med. Assoc. J. 106*: 884–888, 1972.
164. Dutt, AK, Stead, WW: Managing—and preventing—drug resistant tuberculosis. *J. Respir. Dis. 1*:12–18, 1980.
165. Glassroth, J, Robins, AG, Snider, DE, Jr.: Tuberculosis in the 1980s. *N. Engl. J. Med. 302*:1441–1450, 1980.
166. Rivron, MJ, Hughes, EA, Sibert, JR, Jenkins, PA: Cervical lymphadenitis in childhood due to mycobacteria of the Fortuitum group. *Arch. Dis. Child. 54*:312–313, 1979.
167. Schaad, UB, Votteler, TP, McCracken, GH, Jr., Nelson, JD: Management of atypical mycobacterial lymphadenitis in childhood: A review based on 380 cases. *J. Pediatr. 95*:356–360, 1979.
168. Marinis, E, Legakis, NJ: In-vitro activity of ciprofloxacin against clinical isolates of mycobacteria resistant to antimycobacterial drugs. *J. Antimicrob. Chemother. 16*: 527–530, 1985.

21

DNA-Gyrase Inhibitors: Nalidixic Acid, Quinolones, and Novobiocin

MICHAEL J. MUSZYNSKI,* JOHN C. CHRISTENSON, AND RONALD K. SCRIBNER
University of Oklahoma Health Sciences Center, Oklahoma City, Oklahoma

Nalidixic acid and novobiocin are the oldest representatives of two classes of DNA-gyrase inhibiting antimicrobials, which are now known to act on different subunits of the enzyme. Nalidixic acid and related quinolones affect the DNA-gyrase A subunit; novobiocin and coumermycins act on the B subunit.

Nalidixic acid was synthesized in 1962 along with a number of naphthyridine-carboxylic acids after similar chloroquine synthesis derivatives were found to exhibit antibacterial activity. It was marketed the following year for the therapy of urinary tract infections due to gram-negative bacteria (1,2). Nalidixic acid became the prototype for the early cinnoline, pyridopyrimidine, and quinolone antibiotics that soon followed. During the past 6–8 years, interest has refocused on the quinolone class of antimicrobials and many new agents have been developed to provide a greater potency, broader antimicrobial spectrum, and improved tissue penetration while maintaining the advantage of oral bioavailability (3).

Novobiocin was discovered in 1955 as an extracellular product of *Streptomyces niveus* and *Streptomyces spheroides* (4). Analogs of novobiocin, such as coumermycin, are the subjects of new research into agents effective against methicillin-resistant staphylococci (5).

Our understanding of the DNA-gyrase inhibitors, especially the newer quinolones, is still evolving. Basic chemistry, human pharmacokinetic, and clinical efficacy data for the newer agents are not extensive, but they are rapidly expanding.

I. CHEMISTRY

A. A-Subunit Inhibitors

This group of antimicrobials can be divided into two classes based on their heterocyclic ring structure: the naphthyridines (Figure 1A) and the quinolones (Figure 1D). Nalidixic

**Present affiliation*: Orlando Regional Medical Center, Orlando, Florida

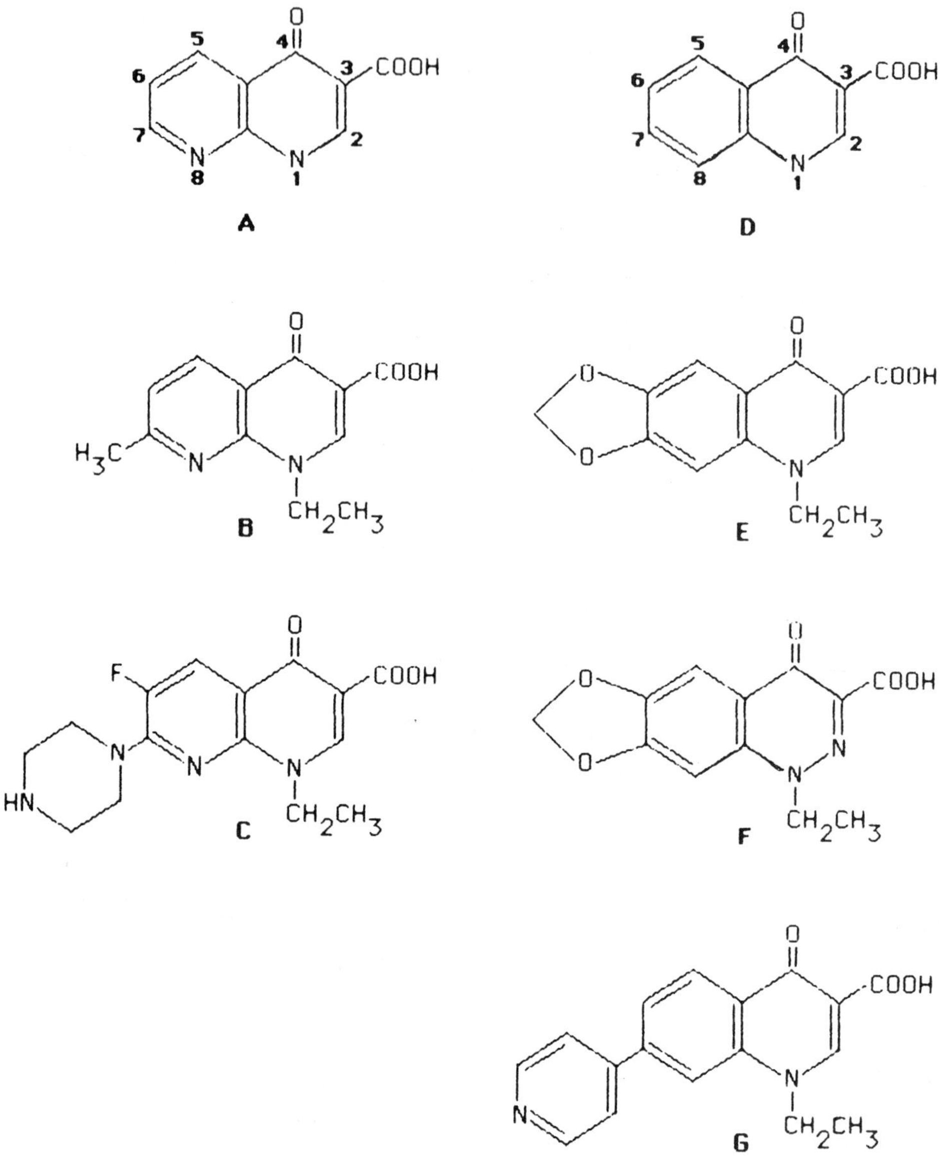

Figure 1 Structures of the naphthyridines and older quinolones: (A) naphthyridine antibiotic parent structure, (B) nalidixic acid, (C) enoxacin, (D) 4-quinolone, (E) oxolinic acid, (F) cinoxacin, (G) rosoxacin.

acid (Figure 1B) is the oldest naphthyridine antimicrobial, and enoxacin (Figure 1C) is the newest member of this class. Oxolinic acid (Figure 1E), introduced in 1967 as an analog of nalidixic acid, is considered the prototypic quinolone antimicrobial. Although there has been temptation to further classify quinolones into "generations" as has been done with the cephalosporins, it would probably be best to avoid such terminology and group the quinolones according to functionally important modifications on the ring structure (6).

Structure-activity relationships of the A-subunit inhibitors have recently been reviewed (6). Modifications at each of the ring structure sites (Figure 1A and D) have been evaluated for effects on pharmacokinetic properties, antimicrobial potency, and antimicrobial spectrum. The presence of a 2-carbon fragment, or its spatial equivalent, at position 1 is important to antimicrobial activity. The naphthyridines and most of the quinolones have an ethyl group at this position, but ciprofloxacin has a 3-carbon ring at position 1 (Figures 1 and 2). Recently, two quinolones with a 4-fluorophenol group substitution at position 1 were found to be active against a variety of gram-negative and gram-positive bacteria and comparable in antimicrobial activity to ethyl-substituted quinolones (7,8). This substitution did not appear to offer major advantages over the 2-carbon chain; however, that good antibacterial activity was preserved is rationale to evaluate other substitutions at position 1.

Modifications at postion 2 have not been particularly advantageous and have not been extensively studied. Cinoxacin (Figure 1F) differs from oxolinic acid (Figure 1E) only by a nitrogen atom in position 2, which enhances gastrointestinal absorption but at a cost of lower in vitro antibacterial activity.

The carboxylic acid group at position 3 and the ketone moiety at position 4 of the basic naphthyridine and quinolone structures are essential for DNA-gyrase inhibition. Other substitutions at either of these positions will abolish anti-DNA-gyrase activity.

Modifications at position 5 have not resulted in significant changes in antibacterial activity. A small advantage in absorption and tissue penetration may be achieved with an NH_2 modification at this position.

The newest quinolone antibiotics are characterized by alterations at positions 6, 7, and 8. One of the most important advances in quinolone chemistry was the chance addition of a fluorine atom to position 6. This resulted in greatly enhanced in vitro activity against gram-negative bacilli and cocci and improved activity against gram-positive cocci (3). Substitutions of various organic moieties or other halogens have not improved antibacterial activity. These fluoroquinolones (Figure 2) will also achieve excellent antibacterial concentrations at many different body sites. This has not been the case for nalidixic acid or the early quinolones, of which acceptable concentrations have occurred only in urine. Accordingly, the older agents have been limited to the therapy of urinary tract infections (9).

All newer quinolones (Figure 2) and the fluorinated naphthyridine, enoxacin (Figure 1C), have an aromatic side chain at position 7. In general, derivatives bisubstituted at positions 6 and 7 are more potent than agents monosubstituted at either position (10). Rosoxacin (Figure 1G) was the first monosubstituted quinolone available for clinical study with an aromatic substitution at position 7. The incidence of central nervous system (CNS) side effects seemed to be increased by this substitution, a problem that has been greatly reduced by bisubstitution and using a piperazine ring at position 7 (6). The 6-fluoro-7-piperazino-4-quinolone compounds have antimicrobial activity superior to compounds with other position 7 modifications (10).

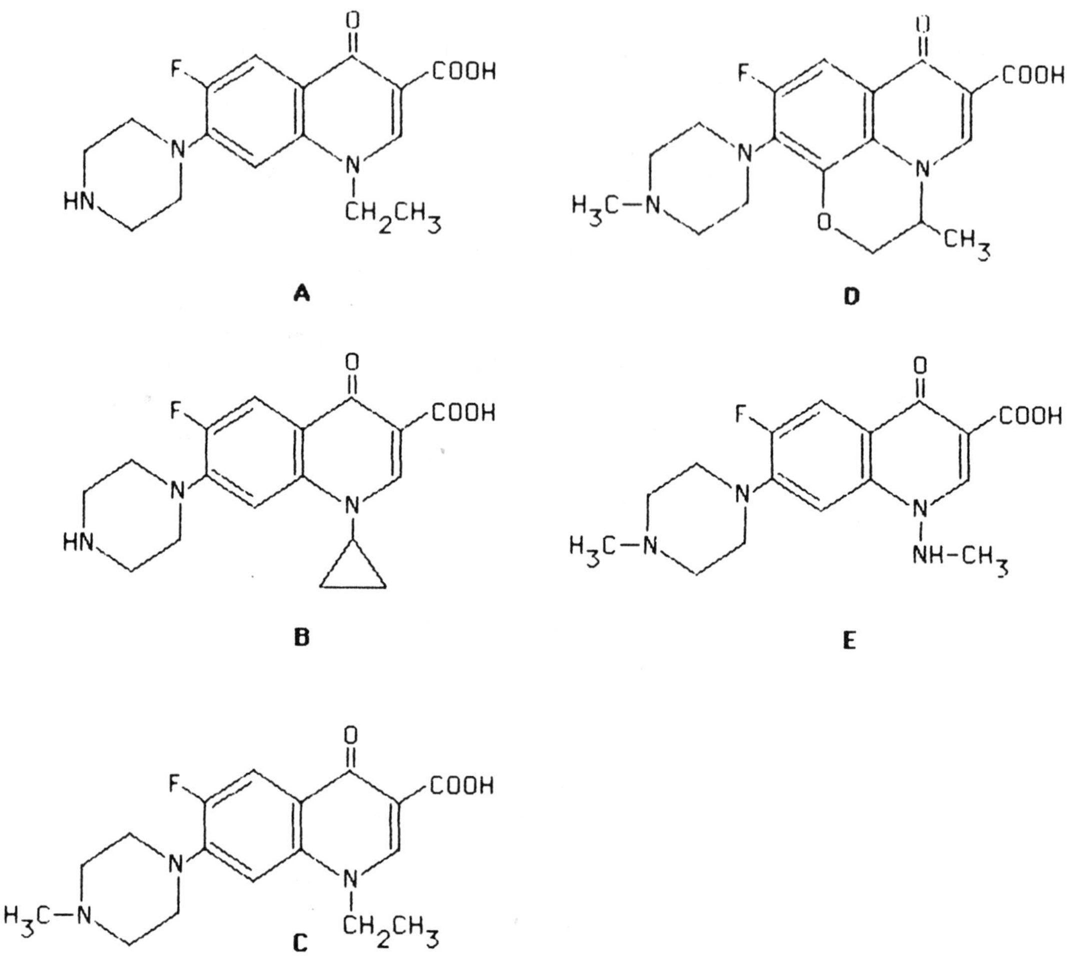

Figure 2 Structures of the fluoroquinolones: (A) norfloxacin, (B) ciprofloxacin, (C) pefloxacin, (D) ofloxacin, (E) amifloxacin.

The basic nitrogen in the piperazine ring is necessary for the most efficient delivery of the compound to the active site of DNA-gyrase (6). The mechanism of transport is not known. More recent examples of modification of the piperazine ring are pefloxacin and amifloxacin (Figures 2C, E). A methyl group on the piperazine ring of these agents was shown to enhance bioavailability even further (3), and membrane permeability mutants of *Escherichia coli* (*nal* B mutants) were shown to be most susceptible to the more bioavailable quinolones (1).

Modification of position 7 with a fluorine atom has created a new class of bifluorinated compounds more active against gram-positive organisms than other quinolones (11).

Substitutions at position 8, of which ofloxacin (Figure 2D) is the main example, produce increased activity against anaerobic and gram-positive bacteria.

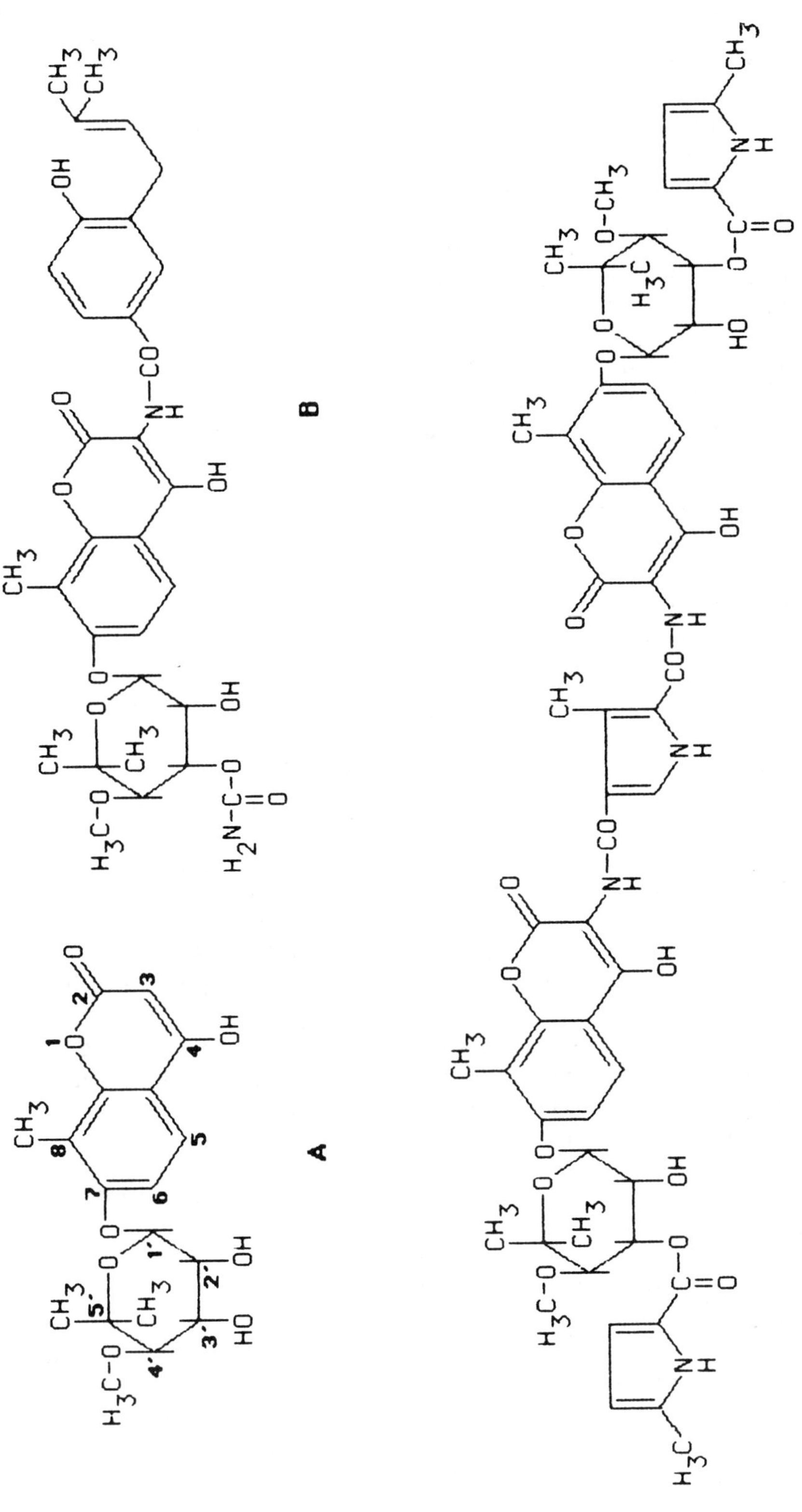

Figure 3 Structures of DNA-gyrase B-subunit inhibitors: (A) 4-hydroxy-8-methylcoumarin-noviose sugar core, (B) novobiocin, (C) coumermycin A1.

B. B-Subunit Inhibitors

Inhibitors of the DNA-gyrase B subunit have a common 4-hydroxy-8-methylcoumarin core glycosidally attached at position 7 to a noviose sugar (Figure 3A). Novobiocin (Figure 3B) has a benzoic acid moiety substituted at position 3 and an amide group at the 3′ position of the noviose sugar. Both the noviose sugar and its 3′ substitution are necessary for DNA-gyrase inhibition and antibacterial activity. The coumarin core alone has no effect on DNA-gyrase (12).

Modifications at position 3 significantly alter antibacterial activity. The larger the substituted moiety, the greater is the antibacterial effect, but without significant variations in DNA-gyrase inhibition (12). Compounds with large carboxyl substitutions at position 3 may penetrate the bacterial cell more efficiently.

The coumermycins are structurally similar to novobiocin, with a 5-methylpyrrole instead of an amide group at the 3′-noviose position. Coumermycin A1, the most active of these compounds, is a symmetrical molecule with a duplication of the coumarin-noviose-5-methylpyrrole structure on either side of a central 2,4-dicarboxamido-3-methylpyrrole (Figure 3C). Coumermycin A1 is a more potent DNA-gyrase inhibitor than novobiocin, possibly due to this bifunctional structure (12).

II. MECHANISMS OF ACTION

The circular chromosomal DNA of prokaryotic cells exists in a supercoiled form. This energetic state is essential for the processes of DNA repair, replication, transcription, transposition, and recombination (13). The amount of DNA supercoiling, or topological state of the DNA, is controlled by a balance of activities within a class of enzymes termed the DNA topoisomerases. Two types of DNA topoisomerases have been described; type I acts through transient single-strand breaks in the DNA, and type II involves double-strand breaks. DNA-gyrase is a type II topoisomarase with a number of recently described functions, including ATP-dependent negative supercoiling of DNA, relaxation of supercoiled DNA in the absence of ATP, hydrolysis of ATP in the presence of DNA, catenation and decatenation of duplex DNA, and double-stranded breakage of DNA in the presence of sodium dodecyl sulfate, proteinase K, and oxolinic acid (13). DNA gyrase mediates the energy-requiring process of superhelical twisting accomplished by passage of a DNA duplex through a double-strand break in the DNA, followed by resealing of the strands.

DNA-gyrase is a tetramer of proteins, consisting of two 100–105 kilodalton A subunits encoded by the *gyr*A gene and two 90–95 kilodalton B subunits encoded by the *gyr*B gene. The naphthyridine and quinolone antimicrobials interact with the A subunit (13). High-level nalidixic acid mutants at the *gyr*A locus are cross-resistant to the newer quinolones (14,15).

The exact mechanism of action of the quinolones is not definitely known (3), but the actual target may be the DNA itself rather than DNA-gyrase (16). Necessary interactions between enzyme and DNA may then be prevented. Nalidixic acid and quinolones probably produce an aberrant covalent linkage between DNA breaks and the DNA-gyrase enzyme (1), thus A-subunit inhibitors may in effect prevent the DNA resealing process.

The complete picture is undoubtably more complex. Inhibitors of protein synthesis, such as rifampin and chloramphenicol, will antagonize the bactericidal action of nalidixic acid and the quinolones, but not their bacteriostatic properties (1,13,17,18). This suggests that protein is necessary for bacterial killing. Ciprofloxacin and ofloxacin are not as susceptible as other quinolones to this effect. The existence of at least two bactericidal mechanisms for ciprofloxacin and ofloxacin, one of which cannot be abolished by rifampin, would explain this phenomenon (1).

Concentrations of A-subunit inhibitor in excess of the most bactericidal concentration result in inhibition of protein synthesis (1,18,19). At this point the agents become bacteriostatic. Smith suggested that this paradox may be due to "an extreme deficiency of negative supercoiling," which would result in decreased RNA synthesis and a deficiency of the protein essential for bacterial killing (1).

The target for novobiocin and coumermycins is the B subunit of DNA-gyrase, which mediates the ATPase, or energy coupling reaction, required for DNA supercoiling (13, 20). These agents appear to block the binding of ATP to the subunit.

III. ANTIMICROBIAL ACTIVITY AND RESISTANCE

Recent interest in the quinolone derivatives has resulted in a plethora of published reports on the activity of norfloxacin (21,22), enoxacin (23,24), ofloxacin (25,26), ciprofloxacin (27,28), pefloxacin (29), and amifloxacin (30,31). A compilation of minimum inhibitory concentrations (MIC) of four new quinolones, cinoxacin, and nalidixic acid against bacteria isolated from pediatric patients is shown in Table 1. The activities of pefloxacin and amifloxacin are similar to those of enoxacin and norfloxacin against *Pseudomonas aeruginosa, Hemophilus influenzae*, and Enterobacteriaceae. Pefloxacin appears similar to ofloxacin in its activity against *Staphylococcus aureus* (32).

All the newer quinolones are highly active against *H. influenzae, Neisseria gonorrhoeae*, and *Neisseria meningitidis*. Additionally, excellent activity is seen against organisms causing gastrointestinal infections, including pathogenic Enterobacteriaceae, *Aeromonas* spp., and *Campylobacter jejuni*.

Activity of the quinolones against anaerobes is much less dramatic. Ofloxacin and ciprofloxacin have the highest activity, with MIC_{90} (concentration required to inhibit 90% of isolates) values of 4–8 μg/ml for *Bacteroides* spp., *Clostridium* spp., and anaerobic gram-positive cocci (26,32–35). Whether these concentrations of drug are attainable at sites of infection is questionable. Enoxacin, pefloxacin, amifloxacin, and norfloxacin have even less activity and probably no clinical utility against these organisms (32,36).

In vitro activity of fluoroquinolones, especially ciprofloxacin, against mycobacteria has been investigated by various authors (37–39). Ciprofloxacin is inhibitory to *Mycobacterium tuberculosis* and *Mycobacterium fortuitum* (MIC_{90} = 1.56 μg/ml), intermediately inhibitory to *Mycobacterium xenopi, Mycobacterium marinum (balnei)* (MIC_{90} = 3.12 μg/ml), and *Mycobacterium kansasii* (MIC_{90} = 6.25 μg/ml), but not inhibitory to most strains of *Mycobacterium avium-intracellulare* and *Mycobacterium chelonae* (MIC_{90} = 12.5 μg/ml) (38). Ofloxacin may have useful activity against *M. tuberculosis* (MIC_{90} = 1 μg/ml) but not against *M. avium-intracellulare* (MIC_{90} = 16 μg/ml) (39). Additionally, these agents appear to be mycobactericidal at concentrations close to the inhibitory concentrations.

Ciprofloxacin and ofloxacin appear to have useful activity against *Chlamydia trachomatis* (MIC_{90} = 1–4 μg/ml) and *Ureaplasma urealyticum* (MIC_{90} = 4–8 μg/ml); enoxacin may be effective against some strains (40–44). Ofloxacin has reasonable activity against *Mycoplasma pneumoniae* (MIC_{90} = 1.56 μg/ml) but is less active against *Mycoplasma hominis* (MIC_{90} = 8 μg/ml) (44,45).

Ciprofloxacin was effective in suppressing chicken embryo mortality at a concentration of 1 μg/g in eggs infected with *Rickettsia conorii*. Using the same strain in a Vero cell plaque assay, 0.25 μg/ml was inhibitory and 0.5 μg/ml was rickettsiacidal (46).

Table 1 Comparative In Vitro Activities of Quinolone Antimicrobials Against Pediatric Bacterial Isolates

Bacterium	Antimicrobial agent	MIC (μg/ml)		
		50%	90%	Range
Pseudomonas aeruginosa	Ciprofloxacin	0.12	1	≤0.015-8
	Norfloxacin	1	2	0.25-4
	Enoxacin	1	2	≤0.06-4
	Ofloxacin	2	4	0.12-16
P. aeruginosa (tobramycin resistant)	Ciprofloxacin	0.5	1	≤0.12-4
	Norfloxacin	2	4	0.25-16
	Enoxacin	2	4	1-8
	Ofloxacin	4	8	0.12-8
P. cepacia	Ciprofloxacin	8	16	0.12-16
	Norfloxacin	16	>16	1->16
	Enoxacin	16	>16	2->16
	Ofloxacin	16	>16	1->16
P. maltophilia	Ciprofloxacin	1	4	0.12-8
	Norfloxacin	8	16	2->16
	Enoxacin	2	4	1-8
	Ofloxacin	16	>16	4->16
Pseudomonas spp.	Ciprofloxacin	0.06	0.5	≤0.015-0.5
	Norfloxacin	0.5	4	0.06-4
	Enoxacin	≤0.12	0.5	≤0.12-1
	Ofloxacin	0.5	8	≤0.12-16
Escherichia coli	Nalidixic acid	4	4	2-16
	Cinoxacin	2	4	1-4
	Ciprofloxacin	0.25	≤0.015	≤0.015
	Norfloxacin	0.03	0.06	≤0.015-0.06
	Enoxacin	0.12	0.25	≤0.06-1
	Ofloxacin	0.03	0.06	≤0.015-0.06
Serratia spp.	Nalidixic acid	2	4	1-64
	Cinoxacin	4	16	2-64
	Ciprofloxacin	0.03	0.12	≤0.015-0.5
	Norfloxacin	0.12	1	0.03-2
	Enoxacin	0.25	0.25	≤0.06-8
	Ofloxacin	0.06	0.25	≤0.015-2
Shigella spp.	Nalidixic acid	4	4	2-16
	Ciprofloxacin	≤0.015	≤0.015	≤0.015-0.12
	Norfloxacin	≤0.015	0.03	≤0.015-1
	Enoxacin	0.12	0.25	≤0.06-0.5
	Ofloxacin	0.03	0.06	≤0.015-0.25
Salmonella spp.	Nalidixic acid	4	8	2-64
	Ciprofloxacin	≤0.015	≤0.015	≤0.015-0.12
	Norfloxacin	0.06	0.12	≤0.015-0.5
	Enoxacin	0.12	0.25	≤0.12-0.25
	Ofloxacin	0.06	0.06	0.06-0.12
Yersinia enterocolitica	Nalidixic acid	2	2	1-32
	Ciprofloxacin	≤0.015	≤0.015	≤0.015-0.03

Table 1 (Continued)

Bacterium	Antimicrobial agent	MIC (μg/ml) 50%	90%	Range
	Norfloxacin	0.03	0.03	≤0.015–0.03
	Enoxacin	≤0.12	≤0.12	≤0.12
	Ofloxacin	0.06	0.06	≤0.03–0.25
Aeromonas spp.	Ciprofloxacin	≤0.008	≤0.008	≤0.008–0.015
	Enoxacin	≤0.008	≤0.03	≤0.008–0.06
	Ofloxacin	≤0.008	≤0.015	≤0.008–0.06
Other Enterobacteriaceae[a]	Ciprofloxacin	≤0.015	0.06	≤0.015–1
	Norfloxacin	0.06	0.25	≤0.015–8
	Enoxacin	0.25	0.5	≤0.06–1
	Ofloxacin	0.06	0.12	≤0.015–2
Staphylococcus aureus	Ciprofloxacin	0.12	0.12	0.12–0.5
	Norfloxacin	0.5	1	0.12–2
	Enoxacin	0.5	1	0.5–2
	Ofloxacin	0.12	0.25	0.06–0.25
Methicillin-resistant *S. aureus*	Ciprofloxacin	0.12	0.25	0.06–0.25
	Norfloxacin	0.5	1	0.5–1
	Enoxacin	0.5	1	0.25–1
	Ofloxacin	0.12	0.25	0.03–0.25
Staphylococcus spp. (coagulase negative)	Ciprofloxacin	0.12	0.25	≤0.015–1
	Norfloxacin	0.5	2	0.03–4
	Enoxacin	0.5	2	0.25–8
	Ofloxacin	0.06	1	≤0.06–16
Enterococci	Ciprofloxacin	1	2	0.5–4
	Norfloxacin	4	8	2–>32
	Enoxacin	8	16	4–16
	Ofloxacin	2	2	1–4
Streptococcus pneumoniae	Ciprofloxacin	2	4	1–4
	Norfloxacin	4	8	2–16
	Enoxacin	8	16	4–16
	Ofloxacin	2	2	1–4
S. agalactiae (Group B)	Ciprofloxacin	0.5	2	0.5–1
	Norfloxacin	4	4	2–8
	Enoxacin	2	2	2–4
	Ofloxacin	1	2	1–2
S. pyogenes (Group A)	Ciprofloxacin	0.5	1	0.25–1
	Norfloxacin	1	2	0.25–2
	Enoxacin	4	>8	2–>8
	Ofloxacin	1	2	0.5–2
Hemophilus influenzae[b]	Ciprofloxacin	0.15	0.015	≤0.004–0.03
	Norfloxacin	0.03	0.03	≤0.015–0.06
	Enoxacin	0.06	0.06	0.03–0.12
	Ofloxacin	0.03	0.06	≤0.015–0.06
Neisseria meningitidis	Ciprofloxacin	0.008	0.008	≤0.001–0.008
	Norfloxacin	0.015	0.015	≤0.001–0.015

Table 1 (Continued)

Bacterium	Antimicrobial agent	MIC (μg/ml) 50%	90%	Range
	Enoxacin	0.015	0.015	⩽0.001–0.015
	Ofloxacin	0.008	0.008	⩽0.001–0.008
N. gonorrhoeae[c]	Nalidixic acid	1	1	0.5–2
	Ciprofloxacin	0.002	0.008	⩽0.001–0.008
	Norfloxacin	0.002	0.008	⩽0.001–0.03
	Enoxacin	0.015	0.015	0.015–0.06
	Ofloxacin	0.002	0.004	⩽0.001–0.03
Gardnerella vaginalis	Nalidixic acid	128	>256	64–>256
	Ciprofloxacin	0.5	8	0.5–8
	Norfloxacin	2	8	0.5–8
	Enoxacin	2	8	1–16
	Ofloxacin	1	4	0.5–8
Campylobacter jejuni	Nalidixic acid	8	8	2–16
	Ciprofloxacin	0.12	0.25	0.06–0.5
	Norfloxacin	0.25	0.25	0.12–0.5
	Enoxacin	0.06	0.12	0.06–0.25
	Ofloxacin	0.25	0.25	0.12–0.5

[a]Includes *Enterobacter* spp., *Citrobacter* spp., *Proteus mirabilis, Proteus vulgaris, Morganella morganii, Providencia* spp., and *Klebsiella* spp.
[b]Includes β-lactamase producing strains and chloramphenicol acetyltransferase producing strains.
[c]Includes penicillinase-producing strains.
Source: Data were compiled from References 23, 25, 27, 29, 56, and 59.

CI-934 is the first biflourinated quinolone developed specifically for gram-positive antibacterial activity. In vitro results indicate good activity against *Staphylococcus* spp. (MIC_{90} = 0.2 μg/ml), *Streptococcus* spp. (MIC_{90} = 0.4 μg/ml), and some activity against enterococci (MIC_{90} = 3.1 μg/ml) (11). Unfortunately, activity against gram-negative bacteria is greatly reduced compared with other fluoroquinolones.

Although reports of combinations of quinolones with other antimicrobials are sparse, a pattern is beginning to emerge. Against gram-negative rods, particularly *P. aeruginosa*, quinolone-aminoglycoside combinations appear indifferent. Quinolone-β-lactam combinations have shown significant synergy (up to 56% for ciprofloxacin-azlocillin) against the same organisms (47–49). Against *S. aureus*, combinations of enoxacin and either dicloxacillin, cephalexin, cefaclor, or rifampin were indifferent (50). Particularly intriguing is the synergy seen against *S. aureus* when ofloxacin, norfloxacin, or enoxacin (DNA-gyrase A-subunit inhibitors) are combined with coumermycin, a DNA-gyrase B-subunit inhibitor (5). Antagonism appears to be extremely rare, except with rifampin and chloramphenicol, as previously discussed.

The in vitro activity of fluoroquinolones against aerobic bacteria is affected little by inoculum size, medium composition, or presence of serum (2,23,25,27); however, certain quinolones lose some activity when the medium pH is less than 5 and lose even more activity when the medium is urine (23–25,27).

The mechanisms of resistance to nalidixic acid and quinolone antimicrobials are not well understood, but it has been fairly well established that resistance is not plasmid mediated (51). In fact, quinolones have been shown to eliminate various resistance plasmids from bacteria (52,53). Resistance to newer quinolones will develop in a gradual stepwise manner when bacteria are transferred serially through increasing concentrations of these agents (54,55). Single-step, high-level resistance mutants are recovered at very low frequencies. The mutation frequency for bacteria exposed to enoxacin ranges from 1 in 2.8×10^9 colony-forming units for *P. aeruginosa* to less than 1 in 10^{11} colony-forming units for *Salmonella* sp. (54).

Nalidixic acid and cinoxacin are useful only against aerobic gram-negative organisms other than *Pseudomonas*. Oxolinic acid is several times more active against these bacteria and has moderate activity against *Staphylococcus* spp. (56). The usefulness of the newer compounds will depend on patient pharmacokinetics. Serum concentration and tissue penetration data available at present (see below) suggest that most gram-negative aerobes will be susceptible to the newer quinolones, as will most strains of *S. aureus*. Ciprofloxacin and ofloxacin may also have clinically useful activity against certain strains of streptococci and anaerobes.

Novobiocin is active against *S. aureus* and *Streptococcus pneumoniae* and has some activity against other gram-positive bacteria and some strains of *Proteus* (57). Coumermycin has considerable activity against certain Enterobacteriaceae and many gram-positive bacteria (5). Of recent interest is the excellent activity against methicillin-resistant staphylococci. The MIC_{90} of coumermycin A1 for methicillin-resistant *S. aureus* and methicillin-resistant *Staphylococcus epidermidis* is 0.05 μg/ml or less (5,58).

IV. CLINICAL PHARMACOLOGY

A. Nalidixic Acid

Most pharmacokinetic studies of nalidixic acid have been with oral preparations, and pharmacokinetic parameters are summarized in Table 2 (60-62). Of an orally administered dose, 96% is rapidly absorbed through the gastrointestinal tract. Studies done by Barbeau and Belanger demonstrated an increase in the area under the curve concentrations (AUC) and elimination half-lives in elderly volunteers (327.7 ± 44.2 μg/ml hr^{-1} and 11.5 ± 2.8 hr, respectively) compared with younger volunteers, suggesting diminishing clearance with advancing age (60).

Nalidixic acid is oxidized in the liver to a biologically active metabolite, 7-hydroxynalidixic acid, which reaches a peak serum concentration 1 hr after the dose (61). The estimated rate of metabolism is 32%. Of the absorbed parent compound, 56% is conjugated with glucuronide and less than 4% is recovered unchanged in the feces. The 7-hydroxynalidixic acid is further metabolized in the kidney to an inactive compound, 7-carboxynalidixic acid, which is eliminated in the urine. This renal metabolite is undetectable in serum (62). Of the 7-hydroxynalidixic acid, 4% is then eliminated as a glucuronide-conjugated form. Between 72 and 101% of the administered oral dose of nalidixic acid (mean, 81%) will be recovered in urine within 24 hr, and alkalinization of the urine will increase excretion of the biologically active forms. Concentrations of nalidixic acid in renal parenchyma are much higher than concomitant serum concentrations (63).

Tablets of 250, 500, and 1000 mg or a 250 mg in 5 ml suspension are available. A citrated formulation is available in the United Kingdom (64). The recommended dosage

Table 2 Pharmacokinetics of Older DNA-gyrase Inhibitors[a]

	Nalidixic acid	Oxolinic acid	Cinoxacin
Dose	1.0 g	750 mg twice a day	500 mg
C_{max} (μg/ml)	15–30	2.1–3.6[d]	16.1 ± 1.5
t_{max} (hr)	2–4	2–6	1–2
AUC 0→∞ (μg/ml hr^{-1})	156.3 ± 26.0[b]	—	—
$t_{½\,\beta}$ (hr)	2.7 ± 0.7[b]	6–7	1.20–0.25
V_d (liter/kg)	0.47 ± 0.11	—	0.20–0.25
Protein binding (%)	89–91	77–81	68–73
Urine recovery 0–24 hr (%)	81[c]	50[d]	48–54
References	60–62	67, 148	72, 74, 75

[a]Data expressed as range, mean ± SD, or percentage.
[b]Data from young adult volunteers.
[c]Only 20% is biologically active.
[d]Data from multiple dosing schedule. Single 750-mg dose: C_{max} = 0.81 μg/ml; and urine recovery in first 8 hr is 0.55%.

of the antibiotic without citrate for adults is 4 g daily divided in four equal doses at 6-hr intervals. A dose of 50 mg/kg day^{-1} divided in four equal doses has been recommended for children over 3 months of age (65).

Nalidixic acid is not indicated in patients with a creatinine clearance below 20 ml/min. For adults with creatinine clearances of 20–50 ml/min and 50–80 ml/min, respectively (66), 1 g twice a day and 1 g three times a day are recommended.

B. Oxolinic Acid

Oxolinic acid has also been studied as an oral agent for the treatment of urinary tract infections (67) (see also Reference 148). Single-dose pharmacokinetics in healthy volunteers demonstrate a mean peak concentration of 1.4 μg/ml 3 hr after a 750-mg oral dose (67). During multiple dosing, peak serum concentrations tended to be at least four to five times higher (Table 2). The elimination half-life has been estimated between 6 and 7 hr. The urine recovery of oxolinic acid at steady state is less than that for nalidixic acid (67); however, a greater percentage of the oxolinic acid elimination products have antimicrobial activity. Urine concentrations in children 24 hr after a dose have ranged from 5.0 to 10.2% of the total administered dose (68), and amounts as high as 20% have been recovered in feces.

In a study of adult patients with chronic urinary tract infections and impaired renal function, a 750-mg oral dose achieved a peak serum concentration of 6.1 μg/ml 2 hr later (69). Since drug accumulation does not occur in patients with impaired renal function, no dosage adjustment is required (70).

The main metabolite of oxolinic acid is a glucuronide compound, which is biologically inactive (71). The recommended dosage for adults was 750 mg twice daily. For children a daily dose of 15-20 mg/kg day^{-1} divided in two equal doses was recommended (69).

C. Cinoxacin

Mean peak serum concentrations of 7.1, 15.5, and 20.9 μg/ml have been achieved after oral doses of 250, 500, and 1000 mg of cinoxacin (72). Food decreased serum concentrations of cinoxacin by approximately 30%. During multiple oral doses of 250 mg every 6 hr, 500 mg every 6 hr, and 1000 mg every 12 hr, peak serum concentrations ranged between 3 and 10, 13 and 21, and 18 and 28 μg/ml, respectively. Over 90% of these doses were absorbed.

Of an orally administered dose, 60% is recovered in the urine as unchanged drug (72). High pressure anion exchange chromatography has identified seven to nine urinary metabolites (73). Of an administered dose, 33% is conjugated to glucuronide; other metabolites include a glucuronidase, a sulfatase-hydrolyzable conjugate, and an acid-hydrolyzable conjugate.

Peak serum concentrations in patients with impaired renal function (creatinine clearance below 30 mg/ml) are approximately twice as high as in normal individuals (74). The elimination half-life is increased from 1.1 to 12.1 hr in such patients, but bioavailability is not affected by renal function (75). Alkalinization of the urine will enhance the renal excretion of cinoxacin but may reduce its antibacterial activity (76). Probenecid has been shown to interfere with the tubular excretion of cinoxacin (77).

Burt and co-workers have evaluated the tissue penetration of cinoxacin (78). A single 500-mg oral dose achieved mean concentrations of 70.1 μg/g in kidney, 12.6 μg/g in muscle, and 4.7 μg/g in adipose tissue with a concomitant serum concentration of 11.7 μg/ml. A 500-mg twice daily oral dose achieved a 2.3 μg/g mean prostatic tissue concentration with a concomitant mean serum concentration of 8.1 μg/ml. Cinoxacin is supplied as 250- or 500-mg pulvules. The recommended dosage for adults is 500 mg twice daily (65). In patients with severe renal impairment (creatinine clearance < 20 ml/min), a single 250-mg daily dose has been suggested (66). Reduced doses of 250 mg three times a day for patients with a creatinine clearance of 50–80 ml/min and 250 mg two times a day for those with a clearance of 20–50 ml/min were also recommended.

D. Ciprofloxacin

Ciprofloxacin is rapidly absorbed following oral administration, achieving peak serum concentrations of approximately 3.0 μg/ml 1.25 hr after a 500-mg dose (79). Table 3 summarizes pharmacokinetic data for ciprofloxacin and the newer quinolones. The C_{max}, t_{max} and bioavailability values for ciprofloxacin are similar for tablet and solution preparations (80). Relative bioavailability varies between 74 and 79%, and serum concentrations are directly proportional to the administered dose (81,82). For example, oral doses of 250, 500, and 750 mg resulted in serum concentrations of 1.35–1.42, 2.60–2.89, and 3.41–4.21 μg/ml, respectively (81). The administration of ciprofloxacin with meals interferes with drug absorption and delays C_{max} (83).

Pharmacokinetic studies using an intravenous preparation demonstrated a rapid decrease in serum concentration from 2.1 μg/ml at 5 min to 0.56 μg/ml at 30 min, which suggests rapid distribution in the tissues (84). Mean volume of distribution was 177 liters.

Extravascular concentration in blister fluid (which mimics a mild inflammatory reaction) surpasses antibactericidal concentrations of many pathogens (Tables 1 and 3). Ciprofloxacin can also significantly accumulate in tissues. For example, prostate and seminal vesicle tissue have been shown to have concentrations 125–618% higher than the serum (85), tonsils 150% higher (86), and lung tissue 300–900% higher (87). High con-

Table 3 Pharmacokinetics of Newer DNA-gyrase Inhibitors[a]

	Ciprofloxacin, 500 mg PO	Norfloxacin, 400 mg PO	Enoxacin, 600 mg PO	Ofloxacin, 600 mg PO
Serum				
C_{max} (μg/ml)	2.3 ± 0.7	1.45 ± 0.09	3.7 ± 0.5	5.2–22.2
t_{max} (hr)	1.25 ± 0.5	1–2.0	0.75–3.0	0.5–1.0
$t_{½β}$ (hr)	3.9 ± 0.8	2.8–5.9	6.2 ± 1.1	7.1 ± 1.1
AUC 0→∞ (μg/ml hr^{-1})	9.9 ± 2.43	6.26 ± 2.03	28.8 ± 4.9	57.5 ± 11.3
Bioavailability (%)	71.7 ± 13.2	50	70	90
Protein binding (%)	20	14	–	6
Volume distribution (L)	145–218	25–35[b]	1.5–4.9 liters/kg	123.6 ± 6.5
Blister fluid				
C_{max} (μg/ml)	1.4 ± 0.36	1.01 ± 0.27	3.0 ± 0.5	5.2 ± 0.9
t_{max} (hr)	2.6 ± 0.97	2.3 ± 0.37	3.3 ± 1.2	5.3 ± 0.8
$t_{½β}$ (hr)	5.6 ± 2.4	3.5 ± 0.79	7.2 ± 2.5	6.75–11.0
AUC ∞ (μg/ml hr^{-1})	11.6 ± 4.1	5.74 ± 1.60	32.8 ± 7.1	71.8 ± 13.2
Urine recovery				
0–24 hr (%)	30.6 ± 9.8	30	61.2	72.9
References	79, 80, 84	100, 149, 150	109–111	116, 118, 119

[a]Data expressed as range, mean ± SD, or mean percentage.
[b]Extrapolated from animal studies.

centrations can also be achieved in bone, cartilage (88), uterus, and oviducts (89,90). Concentrations in bronchial secretions have been 30–79% less than concomitant serum concentrations (91). In normal volunteers, salivary concentrations vary widely between 30 and 45% of serum concentrations (81). Studies done by Shalit and associates demonstrated that ciprofloxacin peritoneal fluid concentrations were approximately 60% of the serum value after a 750-mg single oral dose (92). Studies done in cystic fibrosis patients showed an adequate gastrointestinal absorption achieving C_{max} and AUC comparable to normal individuals (93–95). Pancreatic enzyme supplementation did not significantly alter these results.

In a study of patients with end-stage renal disease, serum concentrations were slightly higher and t_{max} values were slightly longer compared with normal volunteers (C_{max} 1.7 vs. 1.5 μg/ml; t_{max} 1.7 vs. 1.0 hr) (96). Also, the renal patients had a larger AUC (mean, 14.3 μg/ml hr^{-1}) and prolonged elimination half-life (mean, 8.7 hr).

At least four metabolites of ciprofloxacin, designated M1, M2, M3, and M4, have been identified and are similar to those of the other quinolones (see below). The proportion of metabolites (especially M1 and M2) to the total amount of drug excreted in the urine increased from 29.7% after an intravenous dose to 42.7% after an oral dose, suggesting a first pass effect in the liver (97,98). The M3 and M4 metabolites have in vitro antimicrobial activity comparable to that of norfloxacin (99).

E. Norfloxacin

The pharmacokinetics for a 400-mg oral dose of norfloxacin are summarized in Table 3. Bioavailability appears to be approximately 70% (100). Serum concentrations and AUC are similar to ciprofloxacin and increase proportionally with increasing dose. Swanson and associates demonstrated that these increases were linear unless the dose was higher than 800 mg (101). Decreased absorption or variations in elimination or distribution may explain this nonlinear phenomenon.

The exact volume of distribution of norfloxacin in humans is not known, owing to the lack of an intravenous preparation. Data extrapolated from animal studies suggest a volume of distribution of 25-35 liters (102).

Active renal tubular secretion of norfloxacin is suggested by the high rate of renal clearance (mean, 285 ml/min), and probenecid interferes with elimination (103). A total of six urinary metabolites have been described, each with a modification of the piperazine ring (104). The oxo form (M1) and the ethylenediamine form (M2) are the two major metabolites, found in urine as 20% and 4% of the administered parent compound. Neither compound is detectable in serum. The other four metabolites account for less than 1% of the administered dose, and 30% of an oral dose is recovered in urine unchanged.

The elimination half-life and AUC are elevated in patients with impaired renal function and are not altered by hemodialysis (105-107). The dose should be reduced by one-half in those patients with creatinine clearance below 20 ml/min (102). Although the liver metabolizes norfloxacin, patients with hepatic dysfunction have pharmacokinetic parameters similar to those in healthy volunteers (105).

Oral administration of norfloxacin has resulted in antibacterially appropriate concentrations in prostatic tissue and biliary secretions (108). Concentrations in inflammatory tissues are comparable to those of ciprofloxacin. Norfloxacin has also been detected in breast milk and neonatal cord blood (100).

F. Enoxacin

In normal volunteers, an oral dose of 600 mg achieved a peak serum concentration range of 2.9-4.3 μg/ml (Table 3). Enoxacin is absorbed more slowly than either ciprofloxacin or norfloxacin; however, higher enoxacin concentrations can be achieved in inflamed tissues. The elimination half-life of enoxacin is longer when compared with ciprofloxacin and norfloxacin (109,110), which may allow for a once daily dosing schedule for certain infections. Enoxacin's large apparent volume of distribution is similar to that of other quinolones (111).

The four metabolites of enoxacin identified by high-pressure liquid chromatography vary by oxo, amino, formyl, or acetyl alterations in the piperazine ring (109). The oxo form is the major metabolite and accounts for 15% of the enoxacin recovered in urine (109). Urine recovery within the first 48 hr is approximately 70% of the total dose as assessed by microbiologic assay, and about 60% by high-pressure liquid chromatography (HPLC) (111).

Enoxacin penetrates well into extravascular fluid (Table 3). The cerebrospinal fluid-plasma AUC ratio in animals with uninfected meninges after a 12.5-mg/kg intravenous dose was 0.33 and doubled in the presence of inflamed meninges (112). In humans with chronic bronchitis, a sputum penetration of 90% of peak serum enoxacin concentration has been demonstrated (113). Sputum-serum AUC ratios were 1.0 or slightly above.

Rannikko and Malmborg reported mean prostatic tissue concentrations of 4.1 μg/g, with a concomitant mean serum concentration of 2.4 μg/ml (114). Concentrations in the biliary tract are also higher than serum concentrations (115).

G. Ofloxacin

The pharmacokinetics of ofloxacin in normal volunteers given a 600-mg oral dose are summarized in Table 3 (116). As with the other quinolones, peak serum concentrations and AUC tend to be directly proportional to the administered dose. Blister penetration is approximately 125% of serum, based on AUC data. Human lung tissue-plasma ratios were approximately 3.5 for normal lungs and 4.0 for inflamed lung tissue, based on peak plasma concentrations (117). A concentration of 4.4 μg/ml may be detected in saliva after a 600-mg dose.

Approximately 90% of an ofloxacin dose is excreted unchanged in urine (118). Less than 5% can be found as metabolites in the urine, mainly as desmethylofloxacin and ofloxacin *N*-oxide. As with other quinolones, active renal tubular excretion is the major mechanism of elimination (119). Patients with impaired renal function have prolonged elimination half-lives inversely proportional to renal function (120,121).

H. Pefloxacin

In humans, peak serum concentration of pefloxacin is achieved between 1 and 3 hr after administration. The C_{max} is similar to that of enoxacin, but the elimination half-life of pefloxacin is significantly greater than that of the other quinolones.

In a study of oral pefloxacin in healthy adult volunteers, a 400-mg dose resulted in a mean C_{max} of 3.84 μg/ml by HPLC and 3.77 μg/ml by microbiologic assay (122). Mean elimination half-lifes were 8.6 and 10.1 hr by the same respective methods, indicative of different elimination rates for microbiologically active metabolites. The major metabolites described for pefloxacin are pefloxacin glucuronide, pefloxacin *N*-oxide, and norfloxacin (produced by demethylation of pefloxacin in the liter). Of a pefloxacin dose, 26% appears to be eliminated in the urine as a N-oxide compound, which like the glucuronide form has little antibacterial activity. A total of 20% has been recovered as norfloxacin and 8.7% as pefloxacin, both with excellent antibacterial activity (123). Protein binding has been estimated to be between 20 and 30% (124) and apparent volume of distribution between 1.7 and 2.6 liters/kg (124,125).

Animal studies have demonstrated good tissue penetration for pefloxacin (122,124). In humans, cerebrospinal fluid concentrations at 1, 6, and 24 hr after a 1-hr, 400-mg intravenous infusion were 0.84 ± 0.60, 2.76 ± 0.45, and 0.76 ± 0.33 μg/ml, respectively (126). In a study by Wolf and associates, good cerebrospinal concentrations were achieved with oral or intravenously administered pefloxacin (127).

Multiple dosing of 400 mg twice daily achieved bone concentrations between 2 and 9 μg/g (128). Studies have demonstrated good penetration into sputum (129) and heart valve tissue (130). Pharmacokinetic studies performed in cystic fibrosis patients failed to demonstrate any significant differences compared to healthy patients (131).

I. Other Quinolones

Human pharmacokinetics of amifloxacin and the older quinolone, rosoxacin, have not been studied in detail. Data on the metabolism and disposition of amifloxacin in animals have been published recently (132,133).

Rosoxacin has been studied as a possible therapeutic alternative in the treatment of gonorrhea, and preliminary animal pharmacokinetic data are available (134).

J. Novobiocin

Both oral and parenteral formulations of novobiocin have been evaluated. Toxicity associated with the parenteral form led to the development of novobiocin as an oral agent (135). Oral novobiocin is better absorbed in a fasting state, achieving a peak serum concentration 2 hr after dose (136). The t_{max} for novobiocin given after meals is around 4–5 hr. In an early clinical study, a dose of 20–30 mg/kg achieved a C_{max} of 3.2–25.6 μg/ml; 40–60 mg/kg resulted in a 6.4–100 μg/ml peak concentration after multiple dosing (137).

Studies of novobiocin tissue penetration have demonstrated no detectable drug in pleural or ascitic fluid after a 500-mg single oral dose despite concomitant serum concentrations greater than 50 μg/ml; however, significant concentrations were achieved after multiple dosing (137). Novobiocin does not cross the blood-brain barrier (138,139).

Novobiocin is 90% protein bound and has a mean elimination half-life of 8 hr (136). The major site of elimination is through the biliary tract, and its use in patients with hepatobiliary disease is not recommended. Only 3% of an oral dose of novobiocin is recovered in urine in a 24-hr period.

Novobiocin is currently supplied as tablets and suspension and at one time in combination with tetracycline hydrochloride (65). The recommended adult dose is 250–500 mg orally every 6 hr. For children, 30 mg/kg daily divided in three equal doses at 8-hr intervals has been suggested. Doses as high as 100 mg/kg have been used in serious infections (140).

K. Coumermycin A1

Little has been published on the pharmacokinetics of coumermycin antibiotics in humans. Kaplan demonstrated in four healthy adult volunteers that a single oral dose of 50 mg coumermycin A1 achieved a peak serum concentration of approximately 1.0 μg/ml 2.5–5.0 hr after the dose and a 100-mg oral dose resulted in a mean peak of 2.0 μg/ml (141). Approximately 14–28% of the administered dose was absorbed by the gastrointestinal tract. The elimination half-life varied from 14.8 to 46.3 hr.

V. DRUG ASSAYS

Microbiologic assays for the DNA-gyrase inhibitors are well standardized and have been utilized for a variety of biologic fluids, being easy to perform and relatively inexpensive. Major disadvantages of these methods include the need to stock bacterial reference strains (e.g., American Type Culture Collection strains of *Klebsiella pneumoniae* and *E. coli*) (142), a 24- to 48-hr waiting period for results, and the subjective nature of reading zones of bacterial inhibition. The sensitivity of the microbiological assay is as good as HPLC for the active compounds (143).

A colorimetric assay for novobiocin was developed in the late 1950s, but it lacked sensitivity, especially for serum samples, and was unreliable for concentrations less than 5.0 μg/ml (144).

Spectrofluorometry has been used for many years for the determination of body fluid and tissue concentrations of nalidixic acid, oxolinic acid, cinoxacin (72,74), pefloxacin (122), and many of the other quinolones, requiring sample volumes of approximately 0.5 ml. This method will detect only the parent compound of these drugs;

however for nalidixic acid, it detects the parent compound and the main metabolite, 7-hydroxynalidixic acid (60). The lower limits of sensitivity are 0.1 μg/ml for serum and 1.0 μg/ml for urine.

The majority of the metabolism and disposition data of DNA-gyrase inhibitors is derived from HPLC methods. HPLC is rapid, sensitive, and able to detect parent compounds and multiple metabolites (145–147). For example, the method for pefloxacin has a sensitivity threshold of 0.1 μg/ml for plasma and cerebrospinal fluid. The lower limit of sensitivity for ciprofloxacin using similar methods is 0.006 μg/ml. The amount of specimen required varies from as small as 0.3–0.5 ml for serum to 10 ml for urine (148). HPCL systems for the quinolones have recently been modified to reduce interference encountered in biologic fluids. Reversed-phase columns for ciprofloxacin and norfloxacin HPLC systems have improved metabolite detection (38).

VI. THERAPEUTIC INDICATIONS

Nalidixic acid, oxolinic acid, cinoxacin, and norfloxacin are the only A-subunit inhibitors that have been marketed. The newer quinolones are currently available on an investigational basis only. Nalidixic acid has been extensively evaluated in the therapy of urinary tract infections (6) and less well investigated for bacillary diarrheal disease (151) and selective decontamination of the gastrointestinal tract (152). The emergence of resistant organisms during therapy and problems with side effects have led practitioners to prefer other agents (e.g., sulfonamides and β-lactams). Some authors have argued that the higher doses of nalidixic acid (4 g/day for adults) will limit the emergence of resistance (153). Despite these concerns, nalidixic acid is considered an effective agent for the treatment of lower urinary tract infection (151,154–158) in both adults and children and a reasonable alternative for upper tract infection (6,154).

In comparative studies, oxolinic acid appeared to be as effective as nalidixic acid in treating urinary tract infections (9,159,160) in both children and adults; however, the emergence of resistance was a problem (160). Because of its narrow therapeutic-toxic ratio, oxolinic acid therapy is rarely indicated in any age group (6).

Cinoxacin has been shown to be as effective as nalidixic acid or trimethoprim-sulfamethoxazole for uncomplicated acute urinary tract infections due to susceptible organisms (161). Prospective studies in adults have demonstrated a clinical efficacy at least equal to that of amoxicillin or nitrofurantoin. Single-dose studies or clinical trials in patients with pyelonephritis have not been performed. The prophylactic efficacy of cinoxacin is questionable, as two studies have demonstrated protection from recurrent urinary tract infection but a follow-up study showed no difference in recurrence between cinoxacin and placebo groups (161). The early emergence of resistant bacteria is a problem with cinoxacin, but the incidence appears to be less than with nalidixic acid. Studies of cinoxacin in the pediatric population are lacking, since its use in prepubertal patients has not been recommended (161).

The list of clinical indications for the newer quinolones is evolving, as early clinical studies are just now being reported. Unfortunately, toxicity to cartilagenous tissue may limit their usefulness in prepubescent patients.

Randomized, comparative studies have demonstrated the efficacy of the newer quinolone, norfloxacin, in the treatment of uncomplicated urinary tract infections (162–169). Its efficacy in pyelonephritis and complicated infections is less certain. In two of the studies, patients with probable upper tract involvement were successfully treated

(164,168). Another study suggested that norfloxacin was superior to amoxicillin in elderly patients with complicated infections (166). A similar success rate in complicated infections has been reported in an open evaluation of ciprofloxacin (170). In clinical trials in which norfloxacin susceptibilities were prospectively followed, resistance associated with therapeutic failure occurred in 1% of cases (171). Quinolones may be useful in difficult to treat urinary infections, such as those due to *P. aeruginosa*; however, more study is needed (172).

Norfloxacin is also efficacious in the therapy of uncomplicated urethritis due to β-lactamase negative and positive *N. gonorrhoeae* (173). Enoxacin has similarly been shown to be effective in patients with gonococcal urethritis or cervicitis (174). In vitro studies suggest the potential use of several newer quinolones against other genital pathogens (42-44), such as genital *Mycoplasma* (45), *C. trachomatis* (40,175), and possibly *U. urealyticum* (175).

Clinical applications that have been less well investigated include gastrointestinal, skin and soft tissue, bone and joint, and respiratory tract infections. Early reports of quinolones in the treatment of shigellosis, typhoid fever, and the *Salmonella typhi* carrier state have been promising (176,177). As with nalidixic acid, quinolones may also prove to be useful for the selective decontamination of the bowel (178).

Quinolones may add a new dimension to the therapy of pulmonary infections secondary to *Legionella* (179), mycoplasma (45), and mycobacteria (37-39). Rapid emergence of resistance will limit their use for *P. aeruginosa* infections, especially in cystic fibrosis patients (180-183). The efficacy shown in experimental models of osteomyelitis (184) and endocarditis, which included methicillin-resistant *S. aureus* (185), have been encouraging. Because of their broad spectrum of activity, quinolones have potential for the treatment of mixed soft tissue infections or systemic infections in immunocompromised hosts. The topical therapy of burn wounds with silver-quinolone preparations is yet another potential application (186).

The broad spectrum of in vitro antimicrobial activity, oral bioavailability, long elimination half-lives, excellent tissue penetration, and high achievable concentrations in bile and urine form the basis for the great therapeutic potential of the quinolones. It remains to be seen whether this encouraging preliminary data will translate into in vivo efficacy in human infections other than those of the urinary tract.

Novobiocin is rarely used today. Its relatively high incidence of side effects (4), the emergence of novobiocin-resistant strains, and the availability of many other safe and effective antistaphylococcal antibiotic alternatives have made routine therapy with novobiocin impractical. Originally seen as a promising agent for the therapy of serious gram-positive bacterial infections, there are currently no indications for the clinical use of novobiocin.

Coumermycin remains an investigational agent. An in vitro study has identified coumermycin as a potential prophylactic antibacterial when incorporated into acrylic orthopedic cement (187).

VII. TOXICITY

Toxicity and adverse reactions reported with nalidixic acid, cinoxacin, and oxolinic acid are similar and vary mainly in incidence. Gastrointestinal side effects, such as abdominal pain, nausea, vomiting, and diarrhea, are more common with nalidixic acid and cinoxacin, occurring in 13-16% of patients (188). Central nervous system reactions can occur with any of the three but are more frequently associated with oxolinic acid, especially in elderly patients (61). As many as 10-12% of patients treated with nalidixic acid or cinoxacin may complain of headache, dizziness, drowsiness, or visual disturbances (188). More serious central nervous system reactions, including convulsions and psychosis, have been reported (189). Nalidixic acid may actually lower the seizure threshold, since most seizures attributed to this drug have been in patients with underlying convulsive disorders. Acute increases in intracranial pressure, associated with headache and vomiting, papilledema, electroencephalographic abnormalities, and focal neurological signs, have also been reported (190). Many of these cases involved infants; the oldest patient reported was 16 years of age. The pathophysiologic basis is unknown, and no predictors of occurrence have been identified. The central nervous system effects of these agents tend to be self-limited and resolve after prompt discontinuation of therapy. These drugs should not be used in patients under 3 months of age or in patients with neurological disorders. The marketed DNA-gyrase inhibitors should be used with caution in children.

Rashes have occurred in patients receiving nalidixic acid, cinoxacin, or oxolinic acid, including photosensitivity reactions. Nalidixic acid appears to be the most potent photosensitizer (191). Patients receiving these antibiotics and the related newer quinolones should be warned to avoid excessive exposure to sunlight.

Nalidixic acid can precipitate hemolysis in patients with glucose-6-phosphate dehydrogenase deficiency (192). Other blood dyscrasias, cholestatic jaundice, and elevated renal function tests have been reported but are unusual.

The most serious side effect concerning the pediatric patient is an arthropathy, which has been occasionally reported with nalidixic acid (193) and demonstrated in prepubescent laboratory animals treated with the newer quinolones. Joint and tendon involvement in adults has also been reported (172). The future of the newer quinolones in pediatric infectious disease depends on whether cartilage toxicities are confirmed in humans. Until then, these agents should be avoided in individuals whose skeletal development is incomplete (172).

Other toxicities of the newer quinolones are similar to those of nalidixic acid and may be less frequent. In the clinical trials of norfloxacin, side effects have rarely been severe enough to require the cessation of therapy.

The incidence of untoward effects due to novobiocin has been reported as high as 20% (4). Novobiocin is a potent sensitizing compound causing skin rashes in 10-15% of patients taking the drug for longer than 5 days (194). Gastrointestinal side effects are also quite common but usually not severe enough to prevent patients from taking the drug. Novobiocin can raise serum bilirubin levels of newborn infants either by displacement of bilirubin from albumin or inhibition of glucuronyltransferase (4).

VIII. CONTRAINDICATIONS

The use of nalidixic acid or the quinolones is contraindicated in patients with known seizure disorders. Nalidixic acid should not be used in patients under 3 months of age. The quinolones are contraindicated in prepubescent patients until the concern of cartilage toxicity is resolved. Novobiocin has been contraindicated in neonates. Safety in pregnancy or while breast feeding has not been established for any of the DNA-gyrase inhibitors.

IX. DRUG INTERACTIONS

As previously mentioned, the antibacterial activity of the DNA-gyrase inhibitors acting at the A subunit are antagonized by antibiotics that inhibit protein synthesis. Combinations with rifampin or chloramphenicol should be avoided, although in vivo correlates have not been well described. Desplaces and co-workers reported that 6 of 6 patients with chronic staphylococcal osteitis were cured with the combination of pefloxacin and rifampin, compared with 13 of 16 patients treated with pefloxacin alone (195). The prevention of pefloxacin resistance by rifampin in vivo may have been more important to clinical outcome than antibiotic antagonism demonstrable in vitro. Nitrofurantoin can also interfere with the action of nalidixic and oxolinic acids (196).

Enoxacin has been shown to interfere with theophylline metabolism, often leading to theophylline toxicity in patients taking both drugs (113,197). Patients placed on pefloxacin (198) or ofloxacin (199) while receiving a theophylline preparation did not appear to have this problem. Whether this phenomenon is peculiar to enoxacin is not yet known.

Since nalidixic acid and the quinolones may be epileptigenic, the concomitant use of central nervous stimulants should be avoided.

Novobiocin, a coumarin derivative, may add to the activity of the coumarin-type anticoagulants. Nalidixic acid may displace oral anticoagulants from binding sites on albumin. Nalidixic acid can also produce false-positive urine glucose reactions when using Benedict's solution, but not with the glucose oxidose method (192).

REFERENCES

1. Smith, JT: Awakening the slumbering potential of the 4-quinolone antibacterials. *Pharm. J. 233*:299–305, 1984.
2. Lesher, GY, Froelich, EJ, Gruett, MD, Bailey, JH, Brundage, RP: 1,8-Naphthyridine derivatives. A new class of chemotherapeutic agents. *J. Med. Pharm. Chem. 5*:1063–1065, 1962.
3. Wolfson, JS, Hooper, DC: The fluoroquinolones: Structures, mechanisms of action and resistance, and spectra of activity in vitro. *Antimicrob. Agents Chemother. 28*:581–586, 1985.
4. Riley, HD: Vancomycin and novobiocin. *Med. Clin. North Am. 54*:1277–1289, 1970.
5. Neu, HC, Chin, N-X, Labthavikul, P: Antimicrobial activity of coumermycin alone and in combination with other antibiotics. *Antimicrob. Agents Chemother. 25*: 687–689, 1984.
6. Schentag, JJ, Domagala, JM: Structure-activity relationships with the quinolone antibiotics. *Res. Clin. Forums* 7:9–15, 1985.
7. Stamm, JM, Hanson, CW, Chu, DTW, Bailer, R, Vojtko, C, Fernandes, PB: In vitro evaluation of A-56619 (Difloxacin) and A-56620: New aryl-fluoroquinolones. *Antimicrob. Agents Chemother. 29*:193–200, 1986.
8. Smith, BR, LeFrock, JL, Donato, JB, Joseph, WS, Weber, SJ: In vitro activity of A-56619 and A-56620, two new aryl-fluoroquinolone antimicrobial agents. *Antimicrob. Agents Chemother. 29*:355–358, 1986.
9. Albrecht, R: Development of antibiotic agents of the nalidixic acid type. *Prog. Drug Res. 21*:9–104, 1977.
10. Koga, H, Itoh, A, Murayama, S, Suzue, S, Irikura, T: Structure-activity relationships of antibacterial 6,7- and 7,8-disubstituted 1-alkyl-1,4-dihydro-4-oxoquinoline-3-carboxylic acids. *J. Med. Chem. 23*:1358–1363, 1980.

11. Cohen, MA, Griffin, TJ, Bien, PA, Heifetz, CL, Domagala, JM: In vitro activity of CI-934, a quinolone carboxylic acid active against gram-positive and -negative bacteria. *Antimicrob. Agents Chemother. 28*:766–772, 1985.
12. Hooper, DC, Wolfson, JS, McHugh, GL, Winters, MB, Swartz, MN: Effects of novobiocin, coumermycin A1, clorobiocin, and their analogs on *Escherichia coli* DNA gyrase and bacterial growth. *Antimicrob. Agents Chemother. 22*:662–671, 1982.
13. Gellert, M: DNA topoisomerases. *Annu. Rev. Biochem. 50*:879–910, 1981.
14. Crumplin, GC, Kenwright, M, Hirst, T: Investigations into the mechanism of action of the antibacterial agent norfloxacin. *J. Antimicrob. Chemother. 13(Suppl. B)*:9–23, 1984.
15. Traub, WH: Incomplete cross-resistance of nalidixic acid and pipemidic acid-resistant variants of *Serratia marcescens* against ciprofloxacin, enoxacin, and norfloxacin. *Chemotherapy 31*:34–39, 1985.
16. Shen, LL, Pernet, AG: Mechanism of inhibition of DNA gyrase by analogues of nalidixic acid: The target of the drug is DNA. *Proc. Natl. Acad. Sci. USA 82*:307–311, 1985.
17. Deitz, WH, Cook, TM, Goss, WA: Mechanism of action of nalidixic acid on *Escherichia coli*. III. Conditions required for lethality. *J. Bacteriol. 91*:768–773, 1966.
18. Crumplin, GC, Smith, JT: Nalidixic acid: An antibacterial paradox. *Antimicrob. Agents Chemother. 8*:251–261, 1975.
19. Stevens, PJE: Bactericidal effect against *Escherichia coli* of nalidixic acid and four structurally related compounds. *J. Antimicrob. Chemother. 6*:535–542, 1980.
20. Sugino, A, Higgins, NP, Brown, PO, Peebles, CL, Cozzarelli, NR: Energy coupling in DNA gyrase and the mechanism of action of novobiocin. *Proc. Natl. Acad. Sci. USA 75*:4838–4842, 1978.
21. Norrby, SR, Jonsson, M: Antibacterial activity of norfloxacin. *Antimicrob. Agents Chemother. 23*:15–18, 1983.
22. Khan, MY, Gruninger, RP, Nelson, SM, Klicker, RE: Comparative in vitro activity of norfloxacin (MK-0366) and ten other oral antimicrobial agents against urinary bacterial isolates. *Antimicrob. Agents Chemother. 21*:848–851, 1982.
23. Chartrand, SA, Scribner, RK, Weber, AH, Welch, DF, Marks, MI: In vitro activity of CI-919 (AT-2266), an oral antipseudomonal compound. *Antimicrob. Agents Chemother. 23*:658–663, 1983.
24. Chin, N-X, Neu, HC: In vitro activity of enoxacin, a quinolone carboxylic acid, compared with those of norfloxacin, new β-lactams, aminoglycosides, and trimethoprim. *Antimicrob. Agents Chemother. 24*:754–763, 1983.
25. Scribner, RK, Weber, A, Marks, MI: In vitro activity of ofloxacin against bacterial isolates from pediatric patients. In: *Ofloxacin DL-8280*; Selected Proceedings from the 24th Interscience Conference on Antimicrobial Agents and Chemotherapy, Excerpta Medica, Tokyo, 1985, pp. 14–21.
26. Sato, K, Matsuura, Y, Inoue, M, Une, T, Osada, Y, Ogawa, H, Mitsuhashi, S: In vitro and in vivo activity of DL-8280, a new oxazine derivative. *Antimicrob. Agents Chemother. 22*:548–553, 1982.
27. Weber, AH, Scribner, RK, Marks, MI: In vitro activity of ciprofloxacin against pediatric pathogens. *Chemotherapy 31*:456–465, 1985.
28. Eliopoulos, GM, Gardella, A, Moellering, RC: In vitro activity of ciprofloxacin, a new carboxyquinoline antimicrobial agent. *Antimicrob. Agents Chemother. 25*:331–335, 1984.
29. Clarke, AM, Zemcov, SJV, Campbell, ME: In vitro activity of pefloxacin compared to enoxacin, norfloxacin, gentamicin and new β-lactams. *J. Antimicrob. Chemother. 15*:39–44, 1985.
30. Pohlod, DJ, Saravolatz, LD: In vitro susceptibilities of 393 recent clinical isolates to

WIN 49375, cefotaxime, tobramycin, and piperacillin. *Antimicrob. Agents Chemother. 25*:377–379, 1984.
31. Cornett, JB, Wagner, RB, Dobson, RA, Wentland, MP, Bailey, DM: In vitro and in vivo antibacterial activities of the fluoroquinolone WIN 49375 (amifloxacin). *Antimicrob. Agents Chemother. 27*:4–10, 1985.
32. Van Caekenberghe, DL, Pattyn, SR: In vitro activity of ciprofloxacin compared with those of other new fluorinated piperazinyl-substituted quinoline derivatives. *Antimicrob. Agents Chemother. 25*:518–521, 1984.
33. Chin, N-X, Neu, HC: Ciprofloxacin, a quinolone carboxylic acid compound active against aerobic and anaerobic bacteria. *Antimicrob. Agents Chemother. 25*:319–326, 1984.
34. Prabhala, RH, Rao, B, Marshall, R, Bansal, MB, Thadepalli, H: In vitro susceptibility of anaerobic bacteria to ciprofloxacin (Bay 09867). *Antimicrob. Agents Chemother. 26*:785–786, 1984.
35. Wise, R, Andrews, JM, Edwards, LJ: In vitro activity of Bay 09867, a new quinoline derivative, compared with those of other antimicrobial agents. *Antimicrob. Agents Chemother. 23*:559–564, 1983.
36. King, A, Shannon, K, Phillips, I: The in vitro activities of enoxacin and ofloxacin compared with that of ciprofloxacin. *J. Antimicrob. Chemother. 15*:551–558, 1985.
37. Gay, JD, DeYoung, DR, Roberts, GD: In vitro activities of norfloxacin and ciprofloxacin against *Mycobacterium tuberculosis, M. avium* complex, *M. chelonei, M. fortuitum*, and *M. kansasii. Antimicrob. Agents Chemother. 26*:94–96, 1984.
38. Collins, CH, Uttley, HC: In vitro susceptibility of mycobacteria to ciprofloxacin. *J. Antimicrob. Chemother. 16*:575–580, 1985.
39. Fenlon, CH, Cynamon, MH: Comparative in vitro activities of ciprofloxacin and other 4-quinolones against *Mycobacterium tuberculosis* and *Mycobacterium intracellulare. Antimicrob. Agents Chemother. 29*:386–388, 1986.
40. Heessen, FWA, Muytjens, HL: In vitro activities of ciprofloxacin, norfloxacin, pipemidic acid, cinoxacin, and nalidixic acid against *Chlamydia trachomatis. Antimicrob. Agents Chemother. 25*:123–124, 1984.
41. Heppleston, C, Richmond, S, Bailey, J: Antichlamydial activity of quinolone carboxylic acids. *J. Antimicrob. Chemother. 15*:645–647, 1985.
42. Rettig, PJ, Scribner, RK, Rollerson, WJ, Welch, DF, Marks, MI: In vitro activity of CI-919 and norfloxacin against sexually transmitted pathogens. Abstracts of the 23rd Interscience Conference on Antimicrobial Agents and Chemotherapy, Las Vegas, abstract 696, October 1983.
43. Rettig, PJ, Rollerson, WJ, Scribner, RK, Marks, MI: In vitro activity of ofloxacin and other quinolones against sexually transmitted pathogens. Program and Abstracts of the 24th Interscience Conference on Antimicrobial Agents and Chemotherapy, Washington, D.C., abstract 986, October 1984.
44. Rettig, PJ, Haddad, PA, Scribner, RK, Marks, MI: Susceptibility of cervicovaginal pathogens to newer fluoroquinolones. Program and Abstracts of the 25th Interscience Conference on Antimicrobial Agents and Chemotherapy, Minneapolis, abstract 576, September 1985.
45. Osada, Y, Ogawa, H: Antimycoplasmal activity of ofloxacin (DL-8280). *Antimicrob. Agents Chemother. 23*:509–511, 1983.
46. Raoult, D, Roussellier, P, Galicher, V, Perez, R, Tamalet, J: In vitro susceptibility of *Rickettsia conorii* to ciprofloxacin as determined by suppressing lethality in chicken embryos and by plaque assay. *Antimicrob. Agents Chemother. 29*:424–425, 1986.
47. Haller, I: Comprehensive evaluation of ciprofloxacin-aminoglycoside combinations against *Enterobacteriaceae* and *Pseudomonas aeruginosa* strains. *Antimicrob. Agents Chemother. 28*:663–666, 1985.

48. Moody, JA, Peterson, LR, Gerding, DN: In vitro activity of ciprofloxacin combined with azlocillin. *Antimicrob. Agents Chemother. 28*:849–850, 1985.
49. Muszynski, MJ, Scribner, RK, Marks, MI: In vitro activity of ciprofloxacin, in combination with other antimicrobials, against *Pseudomonas aeruginosa* isolates from patients with cystic fibrosis. Abstracts of the 85th Annual Meeting of the American Society for Microbiology, Las Vegas, abstract A19, March 1985.
50. Chartrand, SA, Scribner, RK, Marks, MI, Welch, DF: Oral antibiotic effective against *Pseudomonas aeruginosa*. Abstracts of the 22nd Annual Meeting of the Cystic Fibrosis Club, San Francisco, May 1981, p. 45.
51. Burman, LG: Apparent absence of transferrable resistance to nalidixic acid in pathogenic gram-negative bacteria. *J. Antimicrob. Chemother. 3*:509–516, 1977.
52. Hooper, DC, Wolfson, JS, McHugh, GL, Swartz, MD, Tung, C, Swartz, MN: Elimination of plasmid pMG110 from *Escherichia coli* by novobiocin and other inhibitors of DNA gyrase. *Antimicrob. Agents Chemother. 25*:586–590, 1984.
53. Weisser, J, Wiedemann, B: Elimination of plasmids by new 4-Quinolones. *Antimicrob. Agents Chemother. 28*:700–702, 1985.
54. Scribner, RK, Welch, DF, Marks, MI: Low frequency of bacterial resistance to enoxacin in vitro and in experimental pneumonia. *J. Antimicrob. Chemother. 16*: 597–603, 1985.
55. Barry, AL, Jones, RN: Cross-resistance among cinoxacin, ciprofloxacin, DJ-6783, enoxacin, nalidixic acid, norfloxacin, and oxolinic acid after in vitro selection of resistant populations. *Antimicrob. Agents Chemother. 25*:775–777, 1984.
56. Barry, AL, Jones, RN, Thornsberry, C, Ayers, LW, Gerlach, EH, Sommers, HM: Antibacterial activities of ciprofloxacin, norfloxacin, oxolinic acid, cinoxacin, and nalidixic acid. *Antimicrob. Agents Chemother. 25*:633–637, 1984.
57. Weinstein, L: Antibiotics. IV. Miscellaneous antimicrobial, antifungal, and antiviral agents. In: *The Pharmacological Basis of Therapeutics* (LS Goodman and A Gilman, eds.), Macmillan, New York, 1970, pp. 1269–1370.
58. Aldridge, KE, Janney, A, Sanders, CV: Comparison of the activities of coumermycin, ciprofloxacin, teicoplanin, and other non-β-lactam antibiotics against clinical isolates of methicillin-resistant *Staphylococcus aureus* from various geographical locations. *Antimicrob. Agents Chemother. 28*:634–638, 1985.
59. San Joaquin, VH, Scribner, RK, Pickett, DA, Welch, DF: Antimicrobial susceptibility of *Aeromonas* species isolated from patients with diarrhea. *Antimicrob. Agents Chemother. 30*:794–795, 1986.
60. Barbeau, G, Belanger, PM: Pharmacokinetics of nalidixic acid in old and young volunteers. *J. Clin. Pharmacol. 22*:490–496, 1982.
61. McChesney, EW, Froelich, EJ, Lesher, GY, Crain, AVR, Rosi, D: Absorption, excretion, and metabolism of a new antibacterial agent, nalidixic acid. *Toxicol. Appl. Pharmacol. 6*:292–309, 1964.
62. Ferry, N, Cuisinaud, G, Pozet, N, Zech, PY, Sassard, J: Nalidixic acid kinetics after single and repeated oral doses. *Clin. Pharmacol. Ther. 29*:695–698, 1981.
63. Jameson, RM: Tissue concentration of nalidixic acid in chronic pyelonephritis. *Br. Med. J. 2*:621–622, 1965.
64. Dulake, C, Adam, G, Allenby, F, Anderson, AR, Clark-Jones, A, Cure, SMF: A new citrated formulation of nalidixic acid (Mictral U.K.) for the treatment of acute cystitis. *J. Int. Med. Res. 9*:177–180, 1981.
65. Wade A, Reynolds JEF (eds.): *Martindale. The Extra Pharmacopeia*. The Pharmaceutical Press, London, 1982, pp. 1049–1053.
66. Cameron, DW, Ronald, AR: The older DNA-gyrase inhibitors. *Res. Clin. Forums 7*: 81–87, 1985.
67. Mannisto, PT: Pharmacokinetics of nalidixinic acid and oxolinic acid in healthy women. *Clin. Pharmacol. Ther. 19*:37–46, 1975.

68. Shapera, RM, Matsen, JM: Oxolinic acid therapy for urinary tract infections in children. *Am. J. Dis. Child. 131*:34–37, 1977.
69. Madsen, PO, Rhodes, PR: Oxolinic acid, a new chemotherapeutic agent in the treatment of urinary tract infection. *J. Urol. 105*:870–872, 1971.
70. Guyer, BM: Drug profile: Prodoxol (oxolinic acid). *J. Int. Med. Res. 2*:458–460, 1974.
71. Dicarlo, FJ, Crew, MC, Melgar, MD, Roemer, S, Ringel, SM, Haynes, LJ, Wilson, M: Oxolinic acid metabolism by man. *Arch. Int. Pharmacodyn. 174*:413–427, 1968.
72. Black, HR, Israel, KS, Wolen, RL, Brier, GL, Obermeyer, BD, Ziege, EA, Wolny, JD: Pharmacology of cinoxacin in humans. *Antimicrob. Agents Chemother. 15*:165–170, 1979.
73. Wolen, RL, Obermeyer, BD, Ziege, EA, Black, HL: Metabolic fate of cinoxacin (1-ethyl-1,4-dihydro-4-oxo[1,3]dioxolo-[4,5-g] cinnoline-3-carboxylic acid) in man. *Clin. Pharmacol. Ther. 19*:119, 1976.
74. Ohkawa, M, Sugata, T, Sawaki, M, Okasho, A, Kuroda, K, Yamada, H: Pharmacokinetics of cinoxacin in normal volunteers and patients with impaired renal function. *J. Antimicrob. Chemother. 8*:447–451, 1981.
75. Maigaard, S, Frimodt-Moller, N, Welling, PG, Madsen, PO: Cinoxacin: Pharmacokinetics and tolerance in patients with normal and impaired renal function. *Antimicrob. Agents Chemother. 16*:411–416, 1979.
76. Barbhaiya, RH, Gerber, AU, Craig, WA, Welling, PG: Influence of urinary pH on the pharmacokinetics of cinoxacin in humans and on antibacterial activity in vitro. *Antimicrob. Agents Chemother. 21*:472–480, 1982.
77. Rodriquez, N, Madsen, PO, Welling, PG: Influence of probenecid on serum levels and urinary excretion of cinoxacin. *Antimicrob. Agents Chemother. 15*:465–469, 1979.
78. Burt, RAP, Morgan, T, Payne, JP, Bonner, RM: Cinoxacin concentrations in plasma, urine, and prostatic tissue after oral administration to man. *Br. J. Urol. 49*:147–152, 1977.
79. Crump, B, Wise, R, Dent, J: Pharmacokinetics and tissue penetration of ciprofloxacin. *Antimicrob. Agents Chemother. 24*:784–786, 1983.
80. Davis, RL, Koup, JR, Williams-Warren, J, Weber, A, Smith, AL: Pharmacokinetics of three oral formulations of ciprofloxacin. *Antimicrob. Agents Chemother. 28*:74–77, 1985.
81. Gonzalez, MA, Uribe, F, Moisen, SD, Fuster, AP, Selen, A, Welling, PG, Painter, B: Multiple-dose pharmacokinetics and safety of ciprofloxacin in normal volunteers. *Antimicrob. Agents Chemother. 26*:741–744, 1984.
82. Hoffler, H, Dalhoff, A, Gau, W, Beermann, D, Michl, A: Dose- and sex-independent disposition of ciprofloxacin. *Eur. J. Clin. Microbiol. 3*:363–366, 1984.
83. Ledergerber, B, Bettex, J-D, Joos, B, Flepp, M, Luthy, R: Effect of standard breakfast on drug absorption and multiple-dose pharmacokinetics of ciprofloxacin. *Antimicrob. Agents Chemother. 27*:350–352, 1985.
84. Wise, R, Lockley, RM, Webberly, M, Dent, J: Pharmacokinetics of intravenously administered ciprofloxacin. *Antimicrob. Agents Chemother. 26*:208–210, 1984.
85. Boerema, JBJ, Debruyne, FMJ, Dalhoff, A: Intraprostatic concentrations of ciprofloxacin after intravenous administration. *Lancet 2*:695–696, 1984.
86. Falser, N, Dalhoff, A, Weuta, H: Ciprofloxacin concentrations in tonsils following single and repeated administration. Abstract of the 14th International Congress of Chemotherapy, Kyoto, Japan, abstract P-37-86, June 1985.
87. Schlenkhoff, D, Mayer, M, Dalhoff, A: Penetration of ciprofloxacin into human lung-tissue following a single intravenous administration. Abstract of the 14th International Congress of Chemotherapy, Kyoto, Japan, abstract S-40-11, June 1985.
88. Braun, R, Durig, M, Harder, F: Penetration of ciprofloxacin into bone tissues. Ab-

stract of the 14th International Congress of Chemotherapy, Kyoto, Japan, abstract P-37-85, June 1985.
89. Pavic, N, Frankhauser-Mauri, C, Weuta, H: Pharmacokinetics of ciprofloxacin in uterine and tubal tissue after single and repeated application. Abstracts of the 14th International Congress of Chemotherapy, Kyoto, Japan, abstract P-37-87, June 1985.
90. Goormans, E, Dalhoff, A, Kazzaz, B, Branolte, J: Penetration of ciprofloxacin into gynecological tissues following oral and intravenous administration. *Chemotherapy 32*:7–17, 1986.
91. Bergogne-Berezin, E, Berthelot, G, Even, P, Stern, M, Reynaud, P: Penetration of ciprofloxacin into bronchial secretions. *Eur. J. Clin. Microbiol. 5*:197–200, 1986.
92. Shalit, I, Greenwood, RB, Marks, MI, Pederson, JA, Frederick, DL: Pharmacokinetics of single-dose oral ciprofloxacin in patients undergoing chronic ambulatory peritoneal dialysis. *Antimicrob. Agents Chemother. 30*:152–156, 1986.
93. Bender, SW, Dalhoff, A, Shah, PM, Strehl, R, Posselt, H-G: Ciprofloxacin pharmacokinetics in patients with cystic fibrosis. *Infection 14*:17–21, 1986.
94. Blumer, JL, Stern, RC, Myers, CM, Klinger, JD, Reed, MD: Pharmacokinetics and pharmacodynamics of ciprofloxacin in cystic fibrosis. Abstracts of the 14th International Congress of Chemotherapy, Kyoto, Japan, abstract S-40-14, June 1985.
95. Goldfarb, J, Wormser, GP, Inchiosa, MA, Guideri, G, Diaz, M, Gandhi, R, Goltzman, C, Mascia, AV: Single-dose pharmacokinetics of oral ciprofloxacin in patients with cystic fibrosis. *J. Clin. Pharmacol. 26*:222–226, 1986.
96. Boelaert, J, Valcke, Y, Schurgers, M, Daneels, R, Rosseneu, M, Rosseel, MT, Bogaert, MG: The pharmacokinetics of ciprofloxacin in patients with impaired renal function. *J. Antimicrob. Chemother. 16*:87–93, 1985.
97. Hoffken, G, Lode, H, Prinzing, C, Borner, K, Koeppe, P: Pharmacokinetics of ciprofloxacin after oral and parenteral administration. *Antimicrob. Agents Chemother. 27*:375–379, 1985.
98. Brogard, J-M, Jehl, F, Monteil, H, Adloff, M, Blickle, J-F, Levy, P: Comparison of high-pressure liquid chromatography and microbial assay for the determination of biliary elimination of ciprofloxacin in humans. *Antimicrob. Agents Chemother. 28*: 311–314, 1985.
99. Zeiler, H-J, Petersen, U, Gau, W: Antibacterial activity of the metabolites of ciprofloxacin identified in human urine. Program and Abstracts of the 24th Interscience Conference on Antimicrobial Agents and Chemotherapy, Washington, D.C., abstract 983, October 1984.
100. Holmes, B, Brogden, RN, Richards, DM: Norfloxacin: A review of its antibacterial activity, pharmacokinetic properties and therapeutic use. *Drugs 30*:482–513, 1985.
101. Swanson, BN, Boppana, VK, Vlasses, PH, Rotmensch, HH, Ferguson, RK: Norfloxacin disposition after sequentially increasing oral doses. *Antimicrob. Agents Chemother. 23*:284–288, 1983.
102. Fillastre, JP, Hannedouche, T, Leroy, A, Humbert, G: Pharmacokinetics of norfloxacin in renal failure. *J. Antimicrob. Chemother. 14*:439, 1984.
103. Shimada, J, Yamaji, T, Ueda, Y, Uchida, H, Kusajima, H, Irikura, T: Mechanism of renal excretion of AM-715, a new quinolonecarboxylic acid derivative, in rabbits, dogs, and humans. *Antimicrob. Agents Chemother. 23*:1–7, 1983.
104. Wise, R: Norfloxacin—a review of pharmacology and tissue penetration. *J. Antimicrob. Chemother. 13(Suppl. B)*:59–64, 1984.
105. Eandi, M, Viano, I, Di Nola, F, Leone, L, Genazzani, E: Pharmacokinetics of norfloxacin in healthy volunteers and patients with renal and hepatic damage. *Eur. J. Clin. Microbiol. 2*:253–259, 1983.
106. Arrigo, G, Cavaliere, G, D'Amico, G, Passarella, E, Brocali, G: Pharmacokinetics of norfloxacin in chronic renal failure. *J. Clin. Pharmacol. Ther. Toxicol. 23*:491–496, 1985.

107. Hughes, PJ, Webb, DB, Asscher, AW: Pharmacokinetics of norfloxacin (MK 366) in patients with impaired kidney function—some preliminary results. *J. Antimicrob. Chemother. 13(Suppl. B)*:55–57, 1984.
108. Bologna, M, Vaggi, L, Forchett, CM, Martin, E: Bactericidal intraprostatic concentrations of norfloxacin. *Lancet 2*:280, 1983.
109. Wise, R, Lockley, R, Dent, J, Webberly, M: Pharmacokinetics and tissue penetration of enoxacin. *Antimicrob. Agents Chemother. 26*:17–19, 1984.
110. Wise, R, Lockley, R, Webberly, M, Adhami, ZN: The pharmacokinetics and tissue penetration of enoxacin and norfloxacin. *J. Antimicrob. Chemother. 14(Suppl. C)*: 75–81, 1984.
111. Wolf, R, Eberl, R, Dunky, A, Mertz, N, Chang, T, Goulet, JR, Latts, J: The clinical pharmacokinetics and tolerance of enoxacin in healthy volunteers. *J. Antimicrob. Chemother. 14(Suppl. C)*:63–69, 1984.
112. Tho, TV, Armengaud, A, Davet, B: Diffusion of enoxacin into the cerebrospinal fluid in dogs with healthy meninges and with experimental meningitis. *J. Antimicrob. Chemother. 14(Suppl. C)*:57–62, 1984.
113. Davies, BI, Maesen, FPV, Teengs, JP: Serum and sputum concentrations of enoxacin after single oral dosing in a clinical and bacteriological study. *J. Antimicrob. Chemother. 14(Suppl. C)*:83–89, 1984.
114. Rannikko, S, Malmborg, AS: Enoxacin concentration in human prostatic tissue after oral administration. *J. Antimicrob. Chemother. 17*:123, 1986.
115. Flowerdew, A, Walker, E, Karran, SJ: Evaluation of the biliary pharmacokinetics of oral enoxacin, a new quinolone antibiotic. Abstracts of the 14th International Congress of Chemotherapy, Kyoto, Japan, abstract S-42-13, June 1985.
116. Lockley, MR, Wise, R, Dent, J: The pharmacokinetics and tissue penetration of ofloxacin. *J. Antimicrob. Chemother. 14*:647–652, 1984.
117. Couraud, L, Fourtillan, JB, Saux, MC, Bryskier, A, Vincent, DU, Laurier, M: Diffusion of ofloxacin in human lung tissue. *Infection 14*(Suppl. B):S65–S66, 1986.
118. Humbert, G, Borsa, F, Couet, W, Fourtillan, JB, du Laurier, MV, Bryskier, A: Pharmacokinetics of ofloxacin in young healthy subjects. Abstracts of the 14th International Congress of Chemotherapy, Kyoto, Japan, abstract S-41-3, June 1985.
119. Nomura, H, Tsumura, M, Tachizawa, H, Kamiya, A, Okumura, K, Hori, R: Quantitative investigation on renal handling of ofloxacin in man. Abstracts of the 14th International Congress of Chemotherapy, Kyoto, Japan, abstract WS-9-7, June 1985.
120. Washida, H, Tsugaya, M, Hirao, N, Sakagami, H, Iwase, Y, Fujimoto, T: Absorption and excretion of ofloxacin in patients with impaired renal function. Abstracts of the 14th International Congress of Chemotherapy, Kyoto, Japan, abstract P-36-57, June 1985.
121. Nakano, H, Nihira, H, Kamiya, A, Hori, R: Influence of renal impairment on multiple-dose pharmacokinetics of ofloxacin. Program and Abstracts of the 24th Interscience Conference on Antimicrobial Agents and Chemotherapy. Washington, D.C., abstract 773, October 1984.
122. Montay, G, Goueffon, Y, Roquet, F: Absorption, distribution, metabolic fate, and elimination of pefloxacin mesylate in mice, rats, dogs, monkeys, and humans. *Antimicrob. Agents Chemother. 25*:463–472, 1984.
123. Sorgel, F, Bruning, I, Stephan, U, Lang, E: The pharmacokinetics of pefloxacin and its metabolites in healthy volunteers. 14th International Congress of Chemotherapy, Kyoto, Japan, abstract S-41-9, June 1985.
124. Contrepois, A, Daldoss, C, Pangon, B, Garaud, J-J, Kecir, M, Sarrazin, C, Vallois, J-M, Carbon, C: Pefloxacin in rabbits: Protein binding, extravascular diffusion, urinary excretion and bactericidal effect in experimental endocarditis. *J. Antimicrob. Chemother. 14*:51–57, 1984.

125. Barre, J, Houin, G, Tillement, JP: Dose-dependent pharmacokinetic study of pefloxacin, a new antibacterial agent, in humans. *J. Pharm. Sci. 73*:1379–1382, 1984.
126. Dow, J, Chazal, J, Frydman, AM, Janny, P, Woehrle, R, Djebbar, F, Gaillot, J: Transfer kinetics of pefloxacin into cerebro-spinal fluid after one hour I.V. infusion of 400 mg in man. *J. Antimicrob. Chemother. 17*(Suppl. B):81–87, 1986.
127. Wolff, M, Regnier, B, Daldoss, C, Nkam, M, Vachon, F: Penetration of pefloxacin into cerebrospinal fluid of patients with meningitis. *Antimicrob. Agents Chemother. 26*:289–291, 1984.
128. Dellamonica, P, Bernard, E, Etesse, H, Garraffo, R: The diffusion of pefloxacin into bone and the treatment of osteomyelitis. *J. Antimicrob. Chemother. 17* (Suppl. B):93–102, 1986.
129. Zimmermann, I, Schmidt, EW, Ritzerfeld, W, Ulmer, WT: Pefloxacin concentrations in sputum and blood in patients with chronic obstructive bronchitis. Abstracts of the 14th International Congress of Chemotherapy, Kyoto, Japan, abstract P-35-50, June 1985.
130. Brion, N, Lessana, A, Mosset, F, Lefevre, JJ, Montay, G: Penetration of pefloxacin in human heart valves. *J. Antimicrob. Chemother. 17*(Suppl. B):89–92, 1986.
131. Sorgel, F, Stephan, U, Bruning, I, Wiesemann, HG, Dominick, H-C, Heidbohmer, A: The pharmacokinetics of pefloxacin in patients with cystic fibrosis and healthy volunteers. Abstracts of the 14th International Congress of Chemotherapy, Kyoto, Japan, abstract S-41-10, June 1985.
132. Johnson, JA, Benziger, DP: Metabolism and disposition of amifloxacin in laboratory animals. *Antimicrob. Agents Chemother. 27*:774–781, 1985.
133. McCoy, LF, Crawmer, BP, Benziger, DP: Analysis of amifloxacin in plasma and urine by high-pressure liquid chromatography and intravenous pharmacokinetics in rhesus monkeys. *Antimicrob. Agents Chemother. 27*:769–773, 1985.
134. Kullberg, MP, Koss, R, O'Neil, S, Edelson, J: High-performance liquid chromatographic analysis of rosoxacin and its N-oxide metabolite in plasma and urine. *J. Chromatogr. 173*:155–163, 1979.
135. Larson, EJ, Connor, ND, Swoap, OF, Runnels, RA, Prestrud, MC, Eble, TE, Freyburger, WA, Veldkamp, W, Taylor, RM: Novobiocin, a new antibiotic. VI. Toxicology. *Antibiot. Chemother. 6*:226–230, 1956.
136. Taylor, RM, Miller, WL, Van der Brook, MJ: Streptonivicin, a new antibiotic. V. Absorption, distribution, and excretion. *Antibiot. Chemother. 6*:162–170, 1956.
137. Simon, HJ, McCune, RM, Dineen, PAP, Rogers, DE: Studies on novobiocin, a new antimicrobial agent. *Antibiot. Med. 2*:205–218, 1956.
138. Bayne, GM, Strickland, SC, Gylfe, JM, Boger, WP: Novobiocin: A study of plasma and spinal fluid concentrations in man. *Antibiot. Med. 2*:166–172, 1956.
139. Lin, F-K, Coriell, LL: Novobiocin, a laboratory and clinical evaluation. *Antibiot. Med. 2*:268–276, 1956.
140. Finland, M, Nichols, RL: Novobiocin. *Curr. Ther. 179*:84–92, 1957.
141. Kaplan, SA: Pharmacokinetic profile of coumermycin A1. *J. Pharm. Sci. 59*:309–313, 1970.
142. Joos, B, Ledergerber, B, Flepp, M, Bettex, J-D, Luthy, R, Siegenthaler, W: Comparison of high-pressure liquid chromatography and bioassay for determination of ciprofloxacin in serum and urine. *Antimicrob. Agents Chemother. 27*:353–356, 1985.
143. Jehl, F, Gallion, C, Debs, J, Brogard, JM, Monteil, H, Minck, R: High-performance liquid chromatographic method for determination of ciprofloxacin in biological fluids. *J. Chromatogr. 339*:347–357, 1985.

144. Boxer, GE, Shonk, CE: A colorimetric determination of novobiocin in serum or plasma. *Antibiot. Chemother. 6*:589–597, 1956.
145. Boppana, VK, Swanson, BN: Determination of norfloxacin, a new nalidixic acid analog, in human serum and urine by high-performance liquid chromatography. *Antimicrob. Agents Chemother. 21*:808–810, 1982.
146. Cuisinaud, G, Ferry, N, Seccia, M, Bernard, N, Sassard, J: Determination of nalidixic acid and its two major metabolites in human plasma and urine by reversed-phase high-performance liquid chromatography. *J. Chromatogr. 181*:399–406, 1980.
147. Weber, A, Chaffin, D, Smith, A, Opheim, KE: Quantitation of ciprofloxacin in body fluids by high-pressure liquid chromatography. *Antimicrob. Agents Chemother. 27*:531–534, 1985.
148. Montay, G, Blain, Y, Roquet, F, Le Hir, A: High-performance liquid chromatography of pefloxacin and its main active metabolites in biological fluids. *J. Chromatogr. 272*:359–365, 1983.
149. Albrecht, R: Development of antibacterial agents of the nalidixic acid type. *Prog. Drug Res. 21*:9–104, 1977.
150. Adhami, ZN, Wise, R, Weston, D, Crump, B: The pharmacokinetics and tissue penetration of norfloxacin. *J. Antimicrob. Chemother. 13*:87–92, 1984.
151. Haltalin, KC, Nelson, JD, Kusmiesz, HT: Comparative efficacy of nalidixic acid and ampicillin for severe shigellosis. *Arch. Dis. Child. 48*:305–312, 1973.
152. Wade, JC, de Jongh, CA, Newman, KA, Crowley, J, Wiernik, PH, Schimff, SC: Selective antimicrobial modulation as prophylaxis against infection during granulocytopenia: Trimethoprim-sulfamethoxazole vs. nalidixic acid. *J. Infect. Dis. 147*: 624–634, 1983.
153. Stamey, TA, Bragonje, J: Resistance to nalidixic acid. *JAMA 236*:1857–1860, 1976.
154. Preiksaitis, JK, Thompson, L, Harding, GKM, Marrie, TH, Hoban, S, Ronald, AR: A comparison of efficacy of nalidixic acid and cephalexin in bacteriuric women and their effect on fecal and periurethral carriage of enterobacteriaceae. *J. Infect. Dis. 143*:603–608, 1981.
155. Ahlmen, J, Sigurdsson, J, Wohrm, A, Calmenius, C, Merck, C, Bucht, H: Effect of a three-day course of nalidixic acid in the frequency-dysuria syndrome with significant bacteriuria in women. *Scand. J. Infect. Dis. 15*:71–74, 1983.
156. Winwick, JG, Savage, SJ: A comparison of a 3-day course of mictral with a 7-day course of ampicillin in the treatment of urinary tract infection. *J. Int. Med. Res. 9*: 58–61, 1981.
157. Ronald, AR, Turck, M, Petersdorf, RG: A critical evaluation of nalidixic acid in urinary tract infections. *N. Engl. J. Med. 275*:1081–1089, 1966.
158. Kneebone, GM: A clinical appraisal of nalidixic acid in urinary tract infection in childhood. *Med. J. Aust. 2*:947–949, 1965.
159. Sabbour, MS, El Bokl, MA, Osman, LM: Experiences on the efficacy and safety of nalidixic acid, oxolinic acid, cinoxacin and norfloxacin in the treatment of urinary tract infections (UTI). *Infection 12*:377–380, 1984.
160. Clark, H, Brown, NK, Wallace, JF, Turck, M: Emergence of resistant organisms as a function of dose in oxolinic acid therapy. *Am. J. Med. Sci. 261*:145–148, 1971.
161. Sisca, TS, Heel, RC, Romankiewicz, JA: Cinoxacin. A review of its pharmacological properties and therapeutic efficacy in the treatment of urinary tract infections. *Drugs 25*:544–569, 1983.
162. Gimarellou, H, Tsaragarahis, J, Petrikkos, G, Daikos, GK: Norfloxacin versus co-trimoxazole in the treatment of lower urinary tract infections. *Eur. J. Clin. Microbiol. 2*:266–269, 1983.

163. Goldstein, EJC, Alpert, ML, Ginsberg, BP: Norfloxacin versus trimethoprim-sulfamethoxazole in the therapy of uncomplicated, community-acquired urinary tract infections. *Antimicrob. Agents Chemother. 27*:422–423, 1985.
164. Guerra, JG, Falconi, E, Palomino, JC, Benavente, L, Antunez de Mayolo, E: Clinical evaluation of norfloxacin versus cotrimoxazole in urinary tract infections. *Eur. J. Clin. Microbiol. 2*:260–265, 1983.
165. Haase, DA, Harding, GKM, Thomson, MJ, Kennedy, JK, Urias, BA, Ronald, AR: Comparative trial of norfloxacin and trimethoprim-sulfamethoxazole in the treatment of women with localized, acute, symptomatic urinary tract infections and antimicrobial effect on periurethral and fecal microflora. *Antimicrob. Agents Chemother. 26*:481–484, 1984.
166. Leigh, DA, Smith, EC, Marriner, J: Comparative study using norfloxacin and amoxycillin in the treatment of complicated urinary tract infections in geriatric patients. *J. Antimicrob. Chemother. 13(Suppl. B)*:79–83, 1984.
167. Reeves, DS, Lacey, RW, Mummery, RV, Mahendra, M, Bint, AJ, Newsom, SWB: Treatment of acute urinary infection by norfloxacin or nalidixic acid/citrate: A multi-centre comparative study. *J. Antimicrob. Chemother. 13(Suppl. B)*:99–105.
168. Sabbaj, J, Hoagland, VL, Shih, WJ: Multiclinic comparative study of norfloxacin and trimethoprim-sulfamethoxazole for treatment of urinary tract infections. *Antimicrob. Agents Chemother. 27*:297–301, 1984.
169. Watt, B, Chait, I, Kelsey, MC, Newsom, SWB, Newsom, RA, Smith, J, Toase, PD, Deaney, NB, Round, EM, Vogel, R, Currie, WJC: Norfloxacin versus cotrimoxazole in the treatment of uncomplicated urinary tract infections—a multi-centre trial. *J. Antimicrob. Chemother. 13(Suppl. B)*:89–94, 1984.
170. Boerema, J, Boll, B, Muytjens, H, Branolte, J: Efficacy and safety of ciprofloxacin (Bay 09867) in the treatment of patients with complicated urinary tract infections. *J. Antimicrob. Chemother. 16*:211–217, 1985.
171. Hooper, DC, Wolfson, JS: The fluoroquinolones: Pharmacology, clinical uses, and toxicities in humans. *Antimicrob. Agents Chemother. 28*:716–721, 1985.
172. Van Poppel, H, Wegge, M, Dammekens, H, Chysky, V: Oral treatment of *Pseudomonas*-induced urinary tract infections with ciprofloxacin. *Chemotherapy 32*:83–87, 1986.
173. Crider, SR, Colby, SD, Miller, LK, Harrison, WO, Kerbs, SBJ, Berg, SW: Treatment of penicillin-resistant *Neisseria gonorrhoeae* with oral norfloxacin. *N. Engl. J. Med. 311*:137–140, 1984.
174. Notowicz, A, Stotz, E, Van Klingeren, B: A double blind study comparing two doses of enoxacin for the treatment of uncomplicated urogenital gonorrhoea. *J. Antimicrob. Chemother. 14(Suppl. C)*:91–94, 1984.
175. Aznar, J, Caballero, MC, Lozano, MC, de Miguel, C, Palomares, JC, Perea, EJ: Activities of new quinoline derivatives against genital pathogens. *Antimicrob. Agents Chemother. 27*:76–78, 1985.
176. Ramirez, CA, Bran, JL, Mejia, CR, Garcia, JF: Open, prospective study of the clinical efficacy of ciprofloxacin. *Antimicrob. Agents Chemother. 28*:128–132, 1985.
177. Hudson, SJ, Ingham, HR, Snow, MH: Treatment of *Salmonella typhi* carrier state with ciprofloxacin. *Lancet 1*:1047, 1985.
178. De Vries-Hospers, HG, Welling, GW, Van der Waaij, D: Norfloxacin for selective decontamination: A study in human volunteers. *Prog. Clin. Biol. Res. 181*:259–262, 1985.
179. Saito, A, Sawatari, K, Fukuda, Y, Nagasawa, M, Koga, H, Tomonaga, A, Nakazato, H, Fujita, K, Shigeno, Y, Suzuyama, Y, Yamaguchi, K, Izumikawa, K, Hara, K:

Susceptibility of *Legionella pneumophila* to ofloxacin in vitro and in experimental *Legionella* pneumonia in guinea pigs. *Antimicrob. Agents Chemother. 28*:15–20, 1985.

180. Miller, MG, Ghoneim, AT, Littlewood, JM: Use of enoxacin in a patient with cystic fibrosis. *Lancet 1*:646, 1985.
181. Eron, LJ, Harvey, L, Hixon, DL, Poretz, DM: Ciprofloxacin therapy of infections caused by *Pseudomonas aeruginosa* and other resistant bacteria. *Antimicrob. Agents Chemother. 27*:308–310, 1985.
182. Chapman, ST, Speller, DCE, Reeves, DS: Resistance to ciprofloxacin. *Lancet 2*: 39, 1985.
183. Scully, BE, Neu, HC, Parry, MF, Mandell, W: Oral ciprofloxacin therapy of infections due to *Pseudomonas aeruginosa. Lancet 1*:819–822, 1986.
184. Norden, CW, Shinners, E: Ciprofloxacin as therapy for experimental osteomyelitis caused by *Pseudomonas aeruginosa. J. Infect. Dis. 151*:291–294, 1985.
185. Sullam, PM, Tauber, MG, Hackbarth, CJ, Chambers, HF, Scott, KG, Sande, MA: Pefloxacin therapy for experimental endocarditis caused by methicillin-susceptible or methicillin-resistant strains of *Staphylococcus aureus. Antimicrob. Agents Chemother. 27*:685–687, 1985.
186. Modak, S, Stanford, J, Friedlaender, J, Fox, P, Fox, CL, Jr.: Control of burn wound infections by pefloxacin and its silver derivative. *Burns 10*:170–178, 1984.
187. Beeching, NJ, Thomas, MG, Roberts, S, Lang, SDR: Comparative in-vitro activity of antibiotics incorporated in acrylic bone cement. *J. Antimicrob. Chemother. 17*: 173–184, 1986.
188. Burt, RAP: Review of adverse reactions associated with cinoxacin and other drugs used to treat urinary tract infections. *Urology 23*:101–107, 1984.
189. Poe, TE, Marion, GS, Jackson, DS: Seizures due to nalidixic acid therapy. *South. Med. J. 77*:539–540, 1984.
190. Gedroyc, W, Shorvon, SD: Acute intracranial hypertension and nalidixic acid therapy. *Neurology (N.Y.) 32*:212–215, 1982.
191. Moore, DE, Hemmens, VJ, Yip, H: Photosensitization by drugs: Nalidixic and oxolinic acids. *Photochem. Photobiol. 39*:57–61, 1984.
192. Andriole, VT: Urinary tract agents: Quinolones, nitrofurantoin, and methenamine. In: *Principles and Practice of Infectious Diseases* (GL Mandell, RG Douglas Jr., and JE Bennett, eds.), John Wiley and Sons, New York, 1985, pp. 244–253.
193. Bailey, RR, Natale, R, Linton, AL: Nalidixic acid arthralgia. *Can. Med. Assoc. J. 107*:604–607, 1972.
194. Welch, H, Lewis, CN, Putnam, LE, Randall, WA: A study of the sensitizing potential of novobiocin. *Antibiot. Med. 3*:27–32, 1956.
195. Desplaces, N, Gutmann, L, Acar, JF: Twice-daily oral therapy for chronic staphylococcal osteitis (CSO) with a new quinolone pefloxacin (PEF) alone or in combination with rifampin (RIF). Program and Abstracts of the 24th Interscience Conference on Antimicrobial Agents and Chemotherapy, abstract 279, 1984.
196. Westwood, GPC, Hooper, WL: Antagonism of oxolinic acid by nitrofurantoin. *Lancet 1*:460, 1975.
197. Wijnands, WJA, van Herwaarden, CLA, Vree, TB: Enoxacin raises plasma theophylline concentrations. *Lancet 2*:108–109, 1984.
198. Maesen, FPV, Teengs, JP, Baur, C, Davies, BI: Quinolones and raised plasma concentrations of theophylline. *Lancet 2*:530, 1984.
199. Fourtillan, JB, Granier, J, Saint-Salvi, B, Salmon, J, Surjus, A, Tremblay, D, Vincent Du Laurier, M, Beck, S: Pharmacokinetics of ofloxacin and theophylline alone and in combination. *Infection 14(Suppl. 1)*:S67–S69, 1986.

22
Nitrofurans

WAYNE M. SULLENDER
Stanford University School of Medicine, Stanford, California

The nitrofurans in common human use in the United States are nitrofurantoin, nitrofurazone, and furazolidone. Nifurtimox is available through the Centers for Disease Control.

I. HISTORY

The first nitrofurans were synthesized in the 1930s, and the antimicrobial activities of these compounds were described during World War II (1). Since that time, over 3500 nitrofurans have been synthesized. In addition to their use in clinical medicine, they have been used as additives to the food of humans and animals and as disinfectants (2).

II. CHEMISTRY

The nitrofurans are yellow crystalline photosensitive compounds that are only slightly soluble in water (2). They are one of a group of nitroheterocylic compounds composed of a heterocyclic 5-membered ring bound to a primary nitro group (3). The structure of nitrofurantoin, 1-[(5-nitrofurfurylidene)amino] hydantoin, is shown in Figure 1. Furazolidone, nitrofurazone, and nifurtimox result from the substitution of different nitro groups attached to the heterocyclic ring.

A structural aspect that appears to be important for antibacterial activity is the nitrofuran binding via a vinyl group to a nitrogen group. The presence of the 5-nitro group on the furan ring is associated with antimicrobial, mutagenic, and oncogenic activity (4).

III. MECHANISMS OF ACTION

The precise mechanisms of action are not defined. Metabolic activity requires reduction of the nitro group. Resultant intermediate forms are important for antimicorbial, mutagenic, and carcinogenic activity (5). The nitrofurans inhibit the synthesis of DNA, RNA,

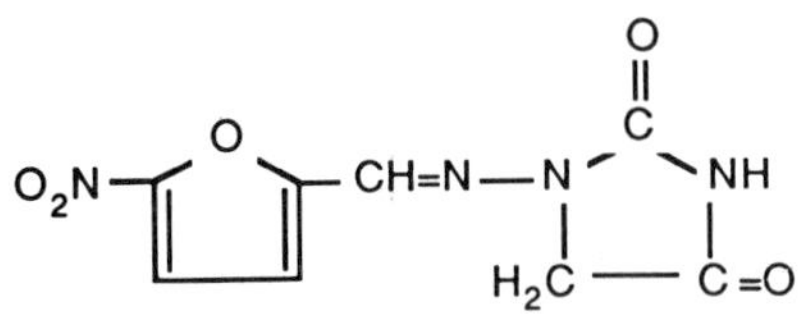

Figure 1 Chemical structure of nitrofurantoin.

and some proteins. They also damage bacterial DNA (6,7). The production of activated oxygen species may partially account for the therapeutic effect of nitrofurtimox against trypanosoma cruzi (7).

IV. ANTIMICROBIAL ACTIVITY AND RESISTANCE

The nitrofurans have a broad spectrum of antibacterial activity. The range of minimum inhibitory concentrations (MIC) of nitrofurantoin and nitrofurazone against a variety of gram-positive and gram negative organisms is shown in Table 1. In general, organisms with an MIC of $\leqslant 32$ μg/ml are considered susceptible. Disk diffusion susceptibility tests utilize a disk containing 300 μg nitrofurantoin, with a zone diameter of $\geqslant 17$ mm defined as susceptible. The approximate MIC correlation is $\leqslant 25$ μg/ml (10). The susceptibility patterns of common clinical isolates are shown in Table 2.

The in vitro activity of furazolidone against a variety of enteric pathogens has recently been assessed. The bacterial agents associated with diarrhea are generally susceptible (Table 3), as is the protozoa *Giardia lamblia* (2,11,12).

Bacterial resistance can be induced to the nitrofurans in vitro. However, changes in patterns of resistance have been negligible during years of use. The most common cause

Table 1 Antibacterial Activity of Nitrofurantoin and Nitrofurazone

	MIC (μg/ml)	
Organisms	Nitrofurantoin	Nitrofurazone
Staphylococcus aureus	0.5–30	6–12
Streptococcus pyogenes	0.05–13	6–50
S. viridans	8	25
S. faecalis	4–125	25–100
Neisseria gonorrhoeae	0.3–10	0.1–10
Escherichia coli	0.4–512	3–12
Proteus spp.	7.5–>300	40–100
Klebsiella, Enterobacter spp.	25–>200	10–100
Salmonella spp.	5–100	3–100
Shigella spp.	3–100	3–25
Pseudomonas aeruginosa	>200	>200
Serratia marcescens	$\leqslant$50–>300	50–100

Source: Compiled from References 2, 8, and 9.

Table 2 Nitrofurantoin Susceptibility

Organisms	% Susceptible[a]
Gram-negative	
Escherichia coli	96
Citrobacter freundii	88
Enterobacter cloacae	64
E. aerogenes	56
Klebsiella pneumoniae	61
Acinetobacter sp.	12–19
Morganella morganii	15
Proteus mirabilis	11
P. vulgaris	16
Providencia rettgeri	12
Serratia marcescens	11
Pseudomonas aeruginosa	1
Gram-positive	
Staphylococcus aureus	97
S. epidermidis	96
Streptococcus faecalis	94
Streptococcus, β-hemolytic (non-group A)	97
Streptococcus viridans	92

[a]Results of susceptibility tests on organisms isolated from patients in 252 hospitals in the United States, 1983. Testing done by disk diffusion using Kirby-Bauer technique.
Source: Based on data from Atkinson (9).

Table 3 Antibacterial Activity of Furazolidone

Organism	Furazolidone MIC (μg/ml)
Enterotoxigenic *Escherichia coli*	⩽0.5–4
Salmonella spp.	⩽0.5–2
Shigella spp.	⩽0.5–2
Vibrio cholerae	3
Yersinia enterocolitica	16–128
Campylobacter jejuni	⩽0.5
Aeromonas hydrophila	⩽0.5–1
Plesiomonas shigelloides	⩽0.5
Vibrio parahaemolyticus	⩽0.5–1

Source: Compiled from References 2 and 11.

of bacterial resistance is a deficiency in cellular nitrofuran reductase activity following chromosomal mutations. Weak plasmid-mediated resistance has been described but is thought to occur uncommonly (5).

V. CLINICAL PHARMACOLOGY

A. Absorption

Nitrofurantoin is well absorbed after oral administration. Most of this absorption occurs in the small intestine, with little gastric absorption. Even though well absorbed, with 90% average absolute availability, plasma concentrations are low, usually less than 1 μg/ml (2). Maximum serum nitrofurantoin concentrations of 0.4 μg/ml are attained approximately 2 hr after a 50-mg dose administered orally to fasting adults (13).

The macrocrystalline nitrofurantoin preparation is absorbed at a slower rate than the microcrystalline form (14). Absorption of all available nitrofurantoin preparations is enhanced by the presence of food (15). There are no published reports on blood concentrations of nitrofurantoin in children. An intravenous preparation was available in the past, and intramuscular forms have been used in kinetics studies. Even with increased intravenous doses, therapeutic plasma concentrations are not attained (3). A trial of rectal administration using suppositories in children showed inadequate absorption, with peak urine concentrations of 9.2 μg/ml and only 0.52% of the administered rectal dose recovered in the urine in 12 hr (16).

Furazolidone administered orally results in little absorption (2). Pharmacokinetic studies in children are not available. Nitrofurazone is used primarily as a topical agent. In a study in human volunteers, 1.13% of the total cutaneous daily dose of nitrofurazone was recovered in the urine (2). Nitrofurazone and nifurtimox are well absorbed by the oral route, but only low plasma concentrations are attained (17).

B. Distribution

Between 60 and 90% of nitrofurantoin is bound to plasma proteins (13,18). After oral administration of nitrofurantoin, cerebrospinal fluid, aqueous humor, and prostatic fluid concentrations are less than those of blood; concentrations attained in the thoracic lymphatic systems are similar to those attained in blood, and the drug is concentrated in the bile and urine. Using ^{14}C-labeled drug, radioactivity can be demonstrated in most tissues of the body. Minute amounts can be found in the liver and kidney after intravenously administered nitrofurantoin (2). The diffusion of nitrofurantoin into the interstitial tissue of the renal medulla has been shown to occur, and the concentration in renal medullary lymphatics may exceed that of serum (19). The drug crosses the placenta and may be found in breast milk (20). After intravenous infusion, the V_{dss} is 40.3 liters (SD = 8.5 liters) in adult males (13).

C. Metabolism

Inactivation of nitrofurantoin appears to take place in a variety of body tissues, with about two-thirds of the drug rapidly metabolized (21). The liver may play a major role in inactivation of nitrofurantoin (3,19,21).

Table 4 Nitrofurantoin Urinary Excretion in Children After Oral Suspension Administration[a]

Time (hr)	Urine concentration (μg/ml) ($\bar{\chi}$ ± SE) Age 2–14 months (n = 7)	3–11 years (n = 5)
3	118 ± 33	125 ± 37
6	45 ± 12	152 ± 46
9	21 ± 4	116 ± 31
12	24 ± 11	204 ± 83
Amount excreted in urine in 12 hr as % total dose	25.07 ± 5.7%	44.32 ± 16.07%

[a]Nitrofurantoin suspension administered at a 3.5 mg/kg dose orally.
Source: From References 27 and 28.

D. Elimination

Nitrofurantoin is excreted in the urine by glomerular filtration, with a small amount undergoing tubular secretion and reabsorption. One-third of an orally administered dose appears unchanged in the urine (3). The concentration of the drug in the urine is linearly related to creatinine clearance. At a creatinine clearance rate less than 60 ml/min, concentrations may be inadequate to inhibit common urinary tract pathogens (22).

The elimination $t_{1/2}$ for adults is commonly described as 20 min, although a more recent study defined it as 58.1 ± 15 min (3,13). Plasma clearance is 0.69 ± 0.06; renal is 0.32 ± 0.09 liters/min. In fasting adults, after an oral dose of 50 mg nitrofurantoin, urinary T_{max} is 105 ± 64 min and C_{max} 132 ± 116 μg/ml. The duration of urine concentrations in excess of 32 μg/ml is 90 ± 54 min (13).

A total of seven studies of nitrofurantoin urinary excretion in children have been published (16,23–28). Tables 4 and 5 depict results published by Wierzba et al. in Poland

Table 5 Nitrofurantoin Urinary Excretion in Children after Oral Administration (see also Table 4)

Population studied (number, age)	Form of drug	Dose	Peak urine concentration	% Drug excreted in urine	Reference
n = 32, 6–15 years	Syrup	100 mg		22.3% in 4 hr	26
n = 17, 4 weeks to 11 months	Drops	5 mg/kg	66 μg/ml	26.4% in 6 hr	
n = 5, <1 year	Perles	5 mg/kg	65 μg/ml	30.3% in 6 hr	25
n = 6, 1–4 years	Not specified	5 mg/kg day^{-1}	Peak at 3–4 hr	36.6% in 24 hr	
				27.2% in 24 hr	24

in 1982 and 1984 (27,28). Older children (3-11 years), compared with younger children (2-14 months), had higher and more sustained nitrofurantoin urinary concentrations, with a greater percentage of total drug recovered in the urine in 12 hr in the older age group. The three other studies in children receiving various nitrofurantoin preparations orally are summarized in Table 5.

VI. PREPARATIONS

Nitrofurantoin: Suspension, 25 mg in 5 ml; 50- and 100-mg tablets; macrocrystals, 25-, 50-, and 100-mg capsules. Dosage, 5-7 mg/kg day^{-1} every 6 hr PO for 7-10 days [acute urinary tract infection (UTI)] or 1-2 mg/kg day^{-1} every 1-2 days PO (chronic dose for recurrent UTI). Adults, 200-400 mg/day for 7-10 days every 6 hr PO (acute UTI) or 50-100 mg/day PO (chronic dose for recurrent UTI).

Furazolidone: Suspension, 50 mg in 15 ml, 100-mg tablets. Dosage, 5-9 mg/kg day^{-1} every 6 hr for 7-10 days. Adults, 100 mg four times a day PO for 10 days.

Nitrofurazone: Topical preparations, as 0.2% nitrofurazone in polyethylene glycols or in a water-miscible base.

VII. DRUG ASSAYS

The techniques used have included spectrophotometric, polarographic, electrochemical, biologic, and high-performance liquid chromatographic (HPLC) methods. The nitromethane-thiamine method has been preferred (14). HPLC has been shown to be sensitive and accurate for the determination of nitrofurantoin concentrations in urine and plasma (29).

VIII. THERAPEUTIC INDICATIONS

Nitrofurantoin is not indicated as a first-line agent for the therapy of uncomplicated urinary tract infections in children (30-32).

Nitrofurantoin has been used effectively for the treatment of acute urinary tract infections and for prophylaxis of recurrent urinary tract infections. Because it does not achieve therapeutic concentrations in serum or most tissues, it should not be used for patients who may have bacteremia; in fact, it has been suggested that it be used only in lower tract or chronic recurrent urinary tract infections (3,33).

Furazolidone may be used for the therapy of intestinal infections, and its chief role in the United States currently is in the therapy of giardiasis. An efficacy of about 80% is reported, compared with over 90% with quinacrine and metronidazole (34). The broad range of enteric organisms susceptible to furazolidone might indicate a role for its use in bacterial diarrheal disease, but its clinical efficacy is not established (11,33,35). Experience in China has suggested efficacy in the therapy of peptic ulcer disease, with the authors postulating a possible mechanism being its activity against gastric campylobacterlike organisms (36).

Nitrofurazone is useful in the topical therapy of burn patients and prophylactically in skin graft recipients (37). Nifurtimox is available through the Centers for Disease Control for the therapy of trypanosomiasis (17).

IX. TOXICITY

The severity and increasing incidence of side effects of nitrofurantoin, in addition to its documented mutagenesis and possible risk of carcinogenesis, should preclude its use unless alternative drugs are unavailable (30-32). In several countries it has been removed from the market (32).

Gastrointestinal side effects, usually nausea and vomiting, are the most frequent toxicities of nitrofurantoin. They are dose and concentration related and occur after oral or intravenous administration of the drug (30). The macrocrystalline preparation causes fewer intestinal side effects, possibly owing to its slower absorption. The microcrystalline, in contrast to the macrocrystalline form, causes minor symptoms in 38 vs. 17%. These symptoms are of sufficient severity to cause discontinuation of therapy in 16% of those receiving microcrystalline nitrofurantoin and 4.3% of patients administered the macrocrystalline drug (30,38). Symptoms may be decreased by ingestion of the drug with food or beverage or by lowering the dose.

Polyneuropathy may also occur, typically in patients with impaired renal function. It has been described in children (30). A decrease in motor nerve conduction time may occur even in normal individuals treated with nitrofurantoin. In most cases, complete or partial improvement occurs after discontinuing nitrofurantoin, but death may occur if therapy continues (3,30). Individuals should be advised to report any early signs of neuritis.

Pulmonary toxicities may also occur. In Sweden, in the period 1966-1976, nitrofurantoins were implicated in 10-12% of all reported adverse drug reactions, more than any other single drug. Of these, 48% were pulmonary reactions, usually of an acute nature (39). Of these patients, three-quarters required hospitalization. The median age at onset was 62 years, with women predominating (40). Children were rarely involved (40,41). An acute reaction is typically seen after 1-2 weeks of therapy and appears to be a hypersensitivity reaction. Chronic fibrosing pulmonary reactions are less common and may represent a toxic reaction due to active oxygen radicals generated during nitrofurantoin metabolism. This is analagous to the lung injury of paraquat, a lung-toxic herbicide (42).

Allergic reactions involving the skin comprise up to 42% of the adverse reactions reported for nitrofurantoin (39). Hepatotoxicity is not common, but the development of chronic active hepatitis, occasionally ending fatally, has been described. Hemolysis in individuals with glucose-6-phosphate dehydrogenase deficiency and other erythrocytic enzyme deficiencies has been reported. Nitrofurantoin may impart a brown color to the urine. Sperm counts as well as sperm mobility may be reduced (30). One case of brown staining of the teeth in a child has been reported, thought to be due to direct contact with the suspension (3). Patients with glutathione synthetase deficiency may be at an increased risk of nitrofurantoin toxicity (43).

The nitrofurans are as a class mutagenic, and many are known to induce cancer in experimental animals. Carcinogenesis has not been shown for nitrofurantoin, although evaluation has been limited. Mutagenesis in bacterial systems has been shown, and high doses of nitrofurantoin induce DNA damage in rat livers and possibly in human fibroblast cultures (44,45). No association between human birth defects and nitrofurantoin has been shown, but a study with pregnant mice administered high doses of nitrofurantoin and nitrofurazone revealed a low frequency of anomalies in newborn mice (46).

The toxicities of furazolidone are similar to those of nitrofurantoin, with gastrointestinal, hepatic, neuropathic, dermatologic, and hematologic effects described (30).

These systemic effects occur even though it is poorly absorbed. Brown discoloration of the urine may occur. Furazolidone has a monamine oxidase inhibitory effect, possibly mediated by its metabolites. It may interact with drugs that inhibit monamine oxidase, indirect acting sympathomimetic amines, amphetamines, and tyramine-containing foods (30,47).

Nitrofurazone appears to cause relatively few systemic effects, although limited absorption does occur. Topical reactions, such as irritation and sensitization, have been described in a small number of treated patients. Polyethylene glycol is used as a carrier in some preparations and may be toxic in patients with impaired renal function (37). Nitrofurazone and furazolidone are mutagenic and carcinogenic in animals (7,48).

Nitrofurantoin may interfere with tests for glucose using reducing reagents, causing falsely positive tests for glucose in the urine or artifactual elevations in blood glucose concentrations. Creatinine concentrations may also be minimally elevated (30).

X. CONTRAINDICATIONS

Nitrofurans should not be used in infants, particularly premature and young infants, owing to their unknown capacity for metabolism and elimination of these compounds (31,33).

Any degree of renal impairment precludes the use of nitrofurantoin because of the risk of accumulation of drug with resultant toxicities, especially neurotoxicity. Also, with impaired renal function adequate concentrations of drug are not found in the urine.

Pre-existing conditions that might be exacerbated by a toxic nitrofurantoin reaction are contraindications to its use, such as polyneuropathy, allergic pneumonitis, lung fibrosis, hemolytic anemia, or hepatitis.

Urinary tract infections that might be associated with bacteremia or tissue invasion, or any systemic infections, are contraindications to the use of nitrofurantoin (31).

XI. DRUG INTERACTIONS

Nitrofurantoin inhibits the antibacterial effect of nalidixic acid, and the efficacy of estrogen is decreased (30). Disulfiramlike reactions may be seen when nitrofurantoin or furazolidone is taken in combination with alcohol (3,30). Probenicid blocks the secretion of nitrofurantoin (49). Furazolidone also has a monamine oxidase inhibitory effect and may interact with various drugs and tyramine-containing foods, as described in Section IX.

REFERENCES

1. Bryan, GT: Occurrence, production, and uses of nitrofurans. In: *Carcinogenesis–A Comprehensive Survey*, Vol. 4, *Nitrofurans: Chemistry, Metabolism, Mutagenesis, and Carcinogenesis* (GT Bryan, ed.), Raven Press, New York, 1978, pp. 1–11.
2. Chamberlain, RE: Chemotherapeutic properties of prominent nitrofurans. *J. Antimicrob. Chemother.* 2:325–336, 1976.
3. Kucers, A, Bennett, NM, eds.: *The Use of Antibiotics*, 3rd ed., J. B. Lippincott, Philadelphia, 1979, pp. 749–760.
4. Ichikawa, M: Chemistry of nitrofurans. In: *Carcinogenesis–A Comprehensive Survey*, Vol. 4, *Nitrofurans: Chemistry, Metabolism, Mutagenesis, and Carcinogenesis* (GT Bryan, ed.), Raven Press, New York, 1978, pp. 13–57.

5. Rabin, HR, Lockerby, DL: Resistance to nitrofurans and nitroimidazoles. In: *Antimicrobial Drug Resistance* (LE Bryan, ed.), Academic Press, Orlando, Florida, 1984, pp. 317–343.
6. McCalla, DR: Mutagenicity of nitrofuran derivatives: Review. *Environ. Mutagen. 5*: 745–765, 1983.
7. McCalla, DR: Nitrofurans. In: *Antibiotics*, Vol. 5, Part 1, *Mechanism of Action of Antibacterial Agents* (FE Hahn, ed.), Springer-Verlag, Berlin, 1979, pp. 176–213.
8. Garrod, LP, Lambert, HP, O'Grady, F, eds.: *Antibiotic and Chemotherapy*, 5th ed. Churchill Livingstone, Edinburgh, 1981, pp. 44–49.
9. Atkinson, BA: Species incidence and trends of susceptibility to antibiotics in the United States and other countries: MIC and MBC. In: *Antibiotics in Laboratory Medicine*, 2nd ed. (V Lorian, ed.), Williams and Wilkins, Baltimore, 1986, pp. 995–1162.
10. Acar, JF, Goldstein, FW: Disk susceptibility test. In: *Antibiotics in Laboratory Medicine*, 2nd ed. (V Lorian, ed.), Williams and Wilkins, Baltimore, 1986, pp. 27–63.
11. Carlson, JR, Thornton, SA, DuPont, HL, West, AH, Mathewson, JJ: Comparative in vitro activities of ten antimicrobial agents against bacterial enteropathogens. *Antimicrob. Agents Chemother. 24*:509–513, 1983.
12. Boreham, PFL, Phillips, RE, Shepherd, RW: The sensitivity of *Giardia intestinalis* to drugs in vitro. *J. Antimicrob. Chemother. 14*:449–461, 1984.
13. Hoener, B, Patterson, SE: Nitrofurantoin disposition. *Clin. Pharmacol. Ther. 29*: 808–816, 1981.
14. Conklin, JD: The pharmacokinetics of nitrofurantoin and its related bioavailability. *Antibiot. Chemother. 25*:233–252, 1978.
15. Rosenberg, HA, Bates, TR: The influence of food on nitrofurantoin bioavailability. *Clin. Pharmacol. Ther. 20*:227–232, 1976.
16. Voemel, W, Kienitz, M, Sauer, W. Untersuchungen zur rectalen Resorption von Nitrofurantoin. *Arzneimittelforsch. 19*:333–336, 1969.
17. James, DM, Gilles, HM: *Human Antiparasitic Drugs: Pharmacology and Usage*, John Wiley and Sons, Chichester, England, 1985, p. 77.
18. Mannsto, PT, Lamminsivu, U: Nitrofurantoin is highly bound to plasma protein. (letter). *J. Antimicrob. Chemother. 9*:327–328, 1982.
19. Andriole, VT: Urinary tract agents: Quinolones, nitrofurantoin, and methenamine. In: *Anti-infective Therapy* (GL Mandell, RG Douglas, Jr., and JE Bennett, eds.), John Wiley and Sons, New York, 1985, pp. 263–267.
20. Norris, SN, Mandell, GI: Tables of antimicrobial agent pharmacology. In: *Anti-infective Therapy* (GL Mandell, RG Douglas, Jr., and JE Bennett, eds.), John Wiley and Sons, New York, 1985, pp. 484–485.
21. Conklin, JD: The pharmacokinetics of nitrofurantoin and its related bioavailability. *Antibiot. Chemother. 25*:233–252, 1978.
22. Sachs, J, Geer, T, Noell, P, Kunin, C: Effect of renal function on urinary recovery of orally administered nitrofurantoin. *N. Engl. J. Med. 278*:1032–1035, 1968.
23. Lippman, RW, Wrobel, CJ, Rees, R, Hoyt, R. A theory concerning recurrence of urinary infection: Prolonged administration of nitrofurantoin for prevention. *J. Urol. 80*:77–81, 1958.
24. Guedeke, R, Kollman, W, Schirrmeister, J. Endogene kreatin clearance und Furadantinausscheidung bei Kindersn. In: *Proceedings of the III International Congress of Chemotherapy*, Stuttgart, Germany, July 22–27, 1963, Vol. 1 (HP Kuemmerle, ed.), Georg Thieme Verlag, Stuttgart, 1964, pp. 581–585.
25. Voemel, W, Kienitz, M, Krueger, D, Betzien, G. Experimentelle und klinische Untersuchungen zur Anwendung von Furadantintropfen in der Kinderheilkunde. *Med. Welt 18*:1453–1458, 1967.

26. Prumersk, Zastrow, J, Depersdorff, J: Der Einfluss von Vitamin B_6 aud die Nifurantinausscheidung bei Kindern. *Dtsch. Gesundheitswesen 29*:1258–1259, 1974.
27. Wierzba, K, Wankowicz, B, Rogoyski, A, Prokopczyk, J, Piekarczyk, A, Kaminska, E, Bozkowa, K: Experimental and clinical pharmacokinetics of nitrofurantoin in the early period of life. *Padiatr. Padol. 17*:293–299, 1982.
28. Wierzba, K, Wancowicz, B, Prokopczyk, J, Piekarczyk, A: Badania nad farmakokintyka lekow w ustoroju rozwijajacyn sie. *Pediatr. Pol. 59*(II):955–963, 1984.
29. Aufrere, MB, Hoener, B, Vore, ME: High performance liquid-chromatographic assay for nitrofurantoin in plasma and urine. *Clin. Chem. 23*:2207–2217, 1977.
30. Dukes, MNG (ed.): *Meyler's Side Effects of Drugs*, Elsevier, Amsterdam, 1984, pp. 549–569.
31. Enzensberger, R, Stille, W: Die Stellung des Nitrofurantoins heute. *Dtsch. Med. Wochensch. 26*(108):1330–1333, 1983.
32. Eichenwald, HF: Antimicrobial therapy in infants and children: Update 1976–1985. Part II. *J. Pediatr. 107*:337–345, 1985.
33. Eichenwald, HF, McCracken, GH, Jr, Metz, H, Stroder, J: The nitrofurans. In: *Practical Pediatric Therapy* (HF Eichenwald and J Stroder, eds.), VCH Publishers, Deerfield Beach, Florida, 1985, pp. 803–804.
34. Turner, JA: Giardiasis and infections with *Dientamoeba fragilis. Pediatr. Clin. North Am. 32*:865–880, 1985.
35. DuPont, HL, Ericsson, CD, Galindo, E, Wood, LV, Morgan, D, Bitsura, JAM, Mendiola, JG: Furazolidone versus ampicillin in the treatment of traveler's diarrhea. *Antimicrob. Agents Chemother. 26*:160–163, 1984.
36. Zheng, ZT, Wang, ZY, Chu, YX, Li, YN, Li, QF, Lin, SR, Xu, ZM: Double-blind short-term trial of furazolidone in peptic ulcer (letter). *Lancet 8436*:1048–1049, 1985.
37. Hooper, G, Covarrubias, J: Clinical use and efficacy of furacin: A historical perspective. *J. Int. Med. Res. 11*:289–293, 1983.
38. Kalowski, S, Rudford, N, Kincaid-Smith, P: Crystalline and macrocrystalline nitrofurantoin in the treatment of urinary-tract infection. *N. Engl. J. Med. 290*:385–387, 1974.
39. Holmberg, L, Boman, G, Bottiger, LE, Eriksson, B, Spross, R, Wessling, A: Adverse reactions to nitrofurantoin. *Am. J. Med. 69*:733–738, 1980.
40. Holmberg, L, Boman, G: Pulmonary reactions to nitrofurantoin. *Eur. J. Respir. Dis. 62*:180–189, 1981.
41. Rantala, H, Kirvela, O, Anttolainen, I: Nitrofurantoin lung in a child (letter). *Lancet 8145*:799–800, 1979.
42. Bus, JS, Gibson, JE: Role of activated oxygen in chemical toxicity. In: *Drug Metabolism and Drug Toxicity* (JR Mitchell and MG Horning, eds.), Raven Press, New York, 1984, pp. 21–32.
43. Spielberg, SP, Gordon, GB: Nitrofurantoin cytotoxicity. *J. Clin. Invest. 67*:37–41, 1981.
44. Russo, P, Pala, M, Nicolo, G, Santi, L, Panodi, S: DNA damage in liver of rats treated with nitrofurantoin. *Mutat. Res. 105*:377–382, 1982.
45. Hirsch-Kauffman, M, Herrlich, P, Schweiger, M: Nitrofurantoin damages of DNA of human cells. *Klin. Wochenschr. 56*:405–407, 1978.
46. Schardein, JR: *Chemically Induced Birth Defects*, Marcel Dekker, New York, 1985, pp. 379, 384.
47. Craft, JC: Giardia and giardiasis in childhood. *Pediatr. Infect. Dis. 1*:196–211, 1982.
48. World Health Organization International Agency for Research on Cancer. Monographs on the Evaluation of the Carcinogenic Risk of Chemicals to Humans. Some Food Additives, Feed Additives, and Naturally Occurring Substances. IARC Working Group on the Evaluation of Carcinogenic Risk of Chemicals to Humans which met in Lyon, 19–26 October, 1982.
49. Buzard, JA, Bender, RC, Nohle, EG, Humphrey, DT, Paul, MF: Renal tubular transport of nitrofurantoin. *Am. J. Physiol. 202*:1136–1138, 1962.

23
Methenamine

PAMELA S. DIAZ
Stanford University School of Medicine, Stanford, California

The compound methenamine (hexamethylene tetramine, hexamethyleneamine) was first described by Butlerow in 1860 (1), but it was not until 1894 that Nicolaier reported on its antibacterial properties (2). In 1924 De Eds' list of reported usages included typhoid fever, pneumonia, nephritis, septicemia, typhus, tuberculosis, prostatitis, bronchitis, and malaria (3). Usage was narrowed once studies were completed demonstrating that formaldehyde (the active compound of methenamine) was only found in gastric washings and in the urine. Currently, methenamine is used solely as a urinary tract antiseptic.

I. CHEMISTRY

Methenamine is a synthetic cyclic hydrocarbon that forms an odorless crystal or white crystalline powder that is freely soluble in water or in alcohol (4). Its free structure is represented in Figure 1. In accordance with the equation,

$$4H^+ + (CH_2)_6N_4 + 6H_2O \rightleftharpoons 4NH_4^+ + 6HCHO$$

hexamethyleneamine + water ⇌ ammonia + formaldehyde

one molecule of methenamine will yield six molecules of formaldehyde upon complete hydrolysis.

There are two major derivatives of this structure in clinical usage. The first is methenamine mandelate, which is composed of 48% methenamine and 52% mandelic acid; the second is methenamine hippurate, a combination of 44% methenamine and 56% hippuric acid (4). Both moieties, mandelic acid and hippuric acid, were added to enhance the hydrolysis of methenamine to formaldehyde (the active compound) by providing a more acidic environment.

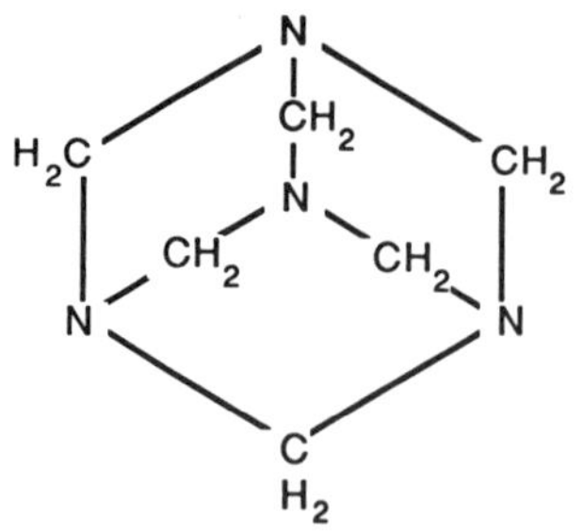

Figure 1 Methenamine.

II. MECHANISMS OF ACTION

Methenamine itself has no antibacterial action. All antibacterial activity is dependent upon the liberation of formaldehyde from methenamine in an acid medium. Formaldehyde is a nonspecific antibacterial agent, and once generated, it is equally bactericidal in an acid or alkaline medium (5). The antibacterial action of formaldehyde is related to its ability to precipitate proteins—hence its nonspecificity.

III. ANTIMICROBIAL ACTIVITY AND RESISTANCE

Virtually all organisms, including gram positive, gram negative, and fungi, are sensitive to formaldehyde. Waterworth determined that almost all bacteria are susceptible to free formaldehyde at about the same concentration (6). Jackson and Stamey have shown that a formaldehyde concentration of 20 μg/ml was bacteriostatic for all bacteria tested after 6 hr incubation and bactericidal after 24 hr (7). Two independent publications demonstrated inhibition of bacterial growth in all urine samples tested if they contained 18-25 μg/ml or greater of formaldehyde (8,9). Resistance has not been shown to develop, even with prolonged therapy (8,10,11). In addition, Duca and Scudi observed no resistance to methenamine with organisms that had in vitro induction of resistance to sulfathiazole or streptomycin (10,11). Methenamine, however, is less effective against urea-splitting organisms owing to the high pH that they render.

IV. CLINICAL PHARMACOLOGY

A. Absorption and Bioavailability

Methenamine is rapidly absorbed from the gastrointestinal tract (12-14). Although 70-90% of an oral dose is absorbed, the remaining 10-30% is hydrolyzed in the gastrointestinal tract to formaldehyde and excreted in the stool. Little if any of this hydrolyzed formaldehyde is absorbed from the gastrointestinal tract into the bloodstream. Klinge et al. studied 10 volunteers who ranged in age from 21 to 42 years (14). They were given 1 g methenamine hippurate twice daily. Data at steady state was comparable to that after one dose. Maximum serum concentration (C_{max}) at steady state was 35.2 mg/liter, and C_{min} was 4.3 mg/liter. The time to attain peak concentration (T_{max}) was approximately 1 hr.

B. Distribution

There are no data regarding the binding of methenamine to proteins.

Methenamine is widely distributed. Klinge et al. showed that the average volume of distribution V_d is approximately 0.56 liter/kg, which is close to total body water (14). Methenamine has been found in virtually every compartment of the body, including CSF, synovial tissue, pericardium, both aqueous and vitreous humors of the eye, saliva, middle ear and nasal sinuses, tears, bronchi, bile, lochia, and in breast milk (15,16).

Despite this wide distribution, only gastric juice and urine are capable of releasing formaldehyde (15). The drug, in particular, appears to be inactive in plasma with little or no release of formaldehyde. This is probably secondary to the plasma pH and methenamine pK_a of 4.8 (12,17).

C. Excretion and Metabolism

Methenamine is eliminated by the kidneys. The clearance from blood is considerably less than the glomerular filtration rate (18). Methenamine appears in the urine in small quantities within 30 min of dosage, and approximately 90% of a dose will be excreted within 24 hr (19). The reported $t_{1/2}$ of methenamine has ranged between 2 and 6 hr, depending upon the preparation used and the assay for determination (14,20,21). If the drug is administered as methenamine mandelate or methenamine hippurate, the mandelic or hippuric acid is rapidly excreted in the urine unchanged and there does not appear to be any tubular reabsorption (19).

Once in the urine, methenamine must be hydrolyzed to formaldehyde to generate any antibacterial action. Although there is debate on particular aspects, it is clear from the cumulative data that certain properties are important in attaining therapeutic concentrations of methenamine and for the hydrolysis of methenamine to formaldehyde. These include the pH of the urine, the time allowed for hydrolysis, and the volume of urine in the bladder at the time of hydrolysis (9,12,13,22).

Several investigators have demonstrated the necessity of an acid pH to produce formaldehyde (3,5,8,9,15,16). The exact pH that is optimal is debated, although most investigators agree that the pH needs to be less than 6.0 for necessary amounts of formaldehyde to be generated. However, despite apparently optimal urine pH levels, only small amounts of formaldehyde are found. Of methenamine, 2-20% is converted to formaldehyde in optimally acid urine (13,19). The time to reach the maximal concentration of formaldehyde generated has ranged from 30 min to 3 hr (4,7,9,19).

Along with urinary pH, the time allowed for hydrolysis to occur is also important (9,22). Musher and Griffith have shown that if the urine flow rate increases from 31 to 58 ml/hr, the concentration of formaldehyde drops 60%, from 60 to 25 μg/ml (22).

The third factor is the volume of urine in the bladder at the time of hydrolysis. The greater the volume of urine, the more dilute the formaldehyde becomes, thus decreasing its overall concentration. Also, urine that is produced by diuresis is more alkaline and therefore inhibits the hydrolysis of methenamine (8,17).

D. Preparation, Dosages, Regimens, and Routes of Administration

Methenamine is only available in oral formulation. The three derivatives most often used are methenamine, methenamine mandelate, and methenamine hippurate. Frequently, these preparations are enteric coated. The percentage of hydrolysis in the gastrointestinal tract is reduced, but the rate of absorption is decreased with enteric coating (4). Peak concentrations are then obtained in 3-8 hr.

Optimal dosages have not been established for children; however, recommended dosages have been as follows (23):

Methenamine mandelate: 50-75 mg/kg day^{-1} divided four times daily
Methenamine hippurate: 25-50 mg/kg day^{-1} divided twice daily

V. DRUG ASSAY

The measurement of methenamine is without value since it has no antibacterial activity. A variety of assays have been used to measure formaldehyde. Originally, the Tanenbaum-Bricker method was widely used for measuring formaldehyde concentrations (24). This assay has inherent problems. The Tanenbaum-Bricker method converts 20-30% of residual methenamine to formaldehyde owing to its own acidity. More recently, the Riker method, or a modification by Jackson and Stamey, which converts less than 1% of residual methenamine to formaldehyde, has been used.

Generally, all assays for determining concentrations of formaldehyde have limitations. They must be performed on fresh urine in order to minimize spontaneous hydrolysis of methenamine to formaldehyde. However, even fresh urine has been shown to release formaldehyde despite storage at −20°C (8).

VI. THERAPEUTIC INDICATIONS

Methenamine has been evaluated for usage in the treatment of acute and chronic urinary tract infections. It has also been evaluated for the prophylaxis of urinary tract infections in patients with indwelling urinary catheters or in patients with recurrent urinary tract infections.

It has no place in the therapy of an acute urinary tract infection, and there is conflicting evidence in its usefulness in treating chronic bacteriuria. Methenamine is ineffective in the prophylaxis of patients with indwelling catheters (25).

The most effective use of methenamine is as prophylaxis against recurrent episodes of urinary tract infections. The three pediatric studies supporting this indication are summarized in Table 1 (26-28). All three studies found methenamine to effectively decrease urinary tract infection rates with little overall toxicity.

VII. TOXICITY

Methenamine is generally well tolerated. The list of toxic gastrointestinal side effects include nausea, vomiting and diarrhea, cramps, and anorexia. Renal toxicity has been reported, with urgency, dysuria, albuminuria, hematuria, bladder irritation, and painful micturition observed. Rarely, crystalluria has been reported in patients with decreased urinary flow rates (29). One patient had generalized edema, urticaria, and dyspnea (30). Other hypersensitivity reactions have occurred, and two elderly patients on prolonged therapy developed lipoid pneumonitis (31). There has been no evidence of bone marrow depression or liver damage, although one study described transient elevations of SGOT and SGPT (32).

Table 1 Comparative Experience of Methenamine Usage in Pediatric Patients

	Holland and West	Elo et al.	Petersen
Number of patients	20	91	20
Sex	All female	3 Males, 88 females	All female
Age	1 and $\frac{2}{12}$ to 12 and $\frac{6}{12}$ years	6 months to 15 years	5–12 years
Daily dosage	Methenamine mandelate, 2 g/m^2	Methenamine hippurate: 250 mg, <6 years; 500 mg, 6–12 years; 1 g, >12 years	Methenamine hippurate, 0.5 g
Length of therapy	2.25 years (9 months to 4 years)	3 months	12 months
Study design	Compared infection rate in patients prior to therapy and during therapy	Compared methenamine to nitrofurantoin and sulfisoxazole for prophylaxis of recurrent infections	Compared infection rate in patients prior to therapy, during therapy, and post-therapy
Results	Infection rate decreased from 1 in 2.6 months to 1 in 15 months	Methenamine recurrence rate least when used as prophylaxis after adequate therapy	Infection rate per patient-years down from 3.1 to 0.7; postprophylaxis, rate increased to 1.4 over a 12-month period

Reported toxicity in the pediatric population is limited to the three publications concerned with the use of methenamine for urinary tract infection prophylaxis and one example of an 8-g overdosage in a 2½ year old (33). This patient had severe lower urinary tract irritative symptoms and gross hematuria with azotemia. Toxicity reported in the other three publications was limited to headache, local irritation, dysuria, and possibly hematuria (26–28). These three papers combined have an overall toxicity frequency of 3.8%.

Although methenamine has been used since the late 1800s, it has not been studied longitudinally in terms of its carcinogenicity. As yet, there are no human data, but concerns have been raised regarding animal data results (34–36). The potential for development of gastric, bladder, or urinary tract carcinoma is at this time unknown. Considering the length of therapy in many patients, this may be an important issue.

VIII. CONTRAINDICATIONS

Methenamine is not recommended for patients with renal failure or severe degrees of renal impairment (4,19,30,37). If acidifying agents are added, the additional acid load may be dangerous in uremia (29,37). However, patients with mild renal impairment can tolerate the drug and it may still be used in decreased dosages (12,29).

Methenamine is contraindicated in hepatic insufficiency because of the ammonia released when it is hydrolyzed to formaldehyde (4,29). It should be avoided in patients with gout, as urate crystals may precipitate in the urine (30,37).

Although no relationship has been found between methenamine and increased teratogenicity, during pregnancy it should be used with caution and only when clearly indicated (38,39).

Patients with allergies to methenamine or dyes should avoid these preparations. Hiprex (one form of methenamine hippurate) contains the dye tartrazine (FD&C yellow no. 5) and may cause allergic reactions. These reactions may occur more frequently in patients sensitive to aspirin (4).

IX. DRUG INTERACTIONS

One drug interaction has been reported. Formaldehyde and sulfamethizole form an insoluble precipitate in acid urine and therefore should not be used together (40). Several interactions with clinical test determinations have also been documented. Formaldehyde interferes with the fluorometric procedures for determining urinary catecholamine and vanillylmandelic acid, causing erroneously high results (41). It also causes falsely low urine estriol concentration and false elevations of 17-hydroxycorticosteroid concentrations with the Porter-Silber method (42,43). Falsely depressed 5-hydroxyindoleacetic acid concentrations (5-HIAA) are also seen (44). Methenamine mandelate also results in a positive screening test for keto acids and interferes with amino acid determinations (45).

REFERENCES

1. Butlerow, A: Ueber ein neues Methylenderivat. *Liebig Ann. Chem. 115*:322, 1860.
2. Nicolaier, A: Ueber die therapeutische Verwendung des Hexamethylentetramin. *Zentralb. Med. Wissensch. 32*:897, 1894.
3. De Eds, F: Fate of hexamethylenamin in the body and its bearing on systemic antisepsis. *Arch. Intern. Med. 34*:511–528, 1924.

4. G. K. McEvoy (ed.), Urinary anti-infectives; Methenamine. In: *Drug Information 86*, American Society of Hospital Pharmacists, Bethesda, Maryland, 1986, pp. 364–365.
5. Shohl, AT: Hexamethylenamine: Its quantitative factors in therapy. *J. Urol. 4*: 419–437, 1920.
6. Waterworth, PM: A misapplication of the sensitivity test: Mandelamine discs. *J. Med. Lab. Technol. 14*:163, 1962.
7. Jackson, J, Stamey, T: The Riker method for determining formaldehyde in the presence of methenamine. *Invest. Urol. 9*(2):124–129, 1971.
8. Miller, H, Phillips, E: Antibacterial correlates of urine drug levels of hexamethylenetetramine and formaldehyde. *Invest. Urol. 8*(1):21–33, 1970.
9. Musher, D, Griffith, D: Generation of formaldehyde from methenamine: Effect of pH and concentration, and antibacterial effect. *Antimicrob. Agents Chemother. 6*(6):708–711, 1974.
10. Duca, C, Scudi, J: Some antibacterial properties of mandelamine. *Proc. Soc. Exp. Biol. Med. 66*:123–126, 1947.
11. Scudi, J, Duca, C: Some antibacterial properties of mandelamine (methenamine mandelate). *J. Urol. 61*(2):459–467, 1949.
12. Knight, V, Draper, J, et al.: Methenamine mandelate: Antimicrobial activity, absorption and excretion. *Antibiot. Chemother. II*(12):615–635, 1952.
13. Gandelman, AL: Methenamine mandelate: Antimicrobial activity in urine and correlation with formaldehyde levels. *J. Urol. 97*:533–536, 1967.
14. Klinge, E, et al.: Pharmacokinetics of methenamine in healthy volunteers. *J. Antimicrob. Chemother. 9*:209–216, 1982.
15. Hanzlick, P, Collins, RJ: Hexamethylenamin: The liberation of formaldehyde and the antiseptic efficiency under different chemical and biological conditions. *Arch. Intern. Med. 12*:578–612, 1913.
16. Levy, LH, Strauss, A: A clinical and bacteriological study of hexamethylenamin as a urinary antiseptic. *Arch. Intern. Med. 14*:730–742, 1914.
17. Stamey, TA: General and specific principles of therapy. In: *Urinary Infections*, Williams and Wilkins, Baltimore, 1972, pp. 264–269.
18. Scudi, J, Reinhard, J: Absorption and distribution, and renal excretion of mandelamine. *J. Lab. Clin. Med. 33*:1304–1310, 1948.
19. Kucers, A, Bennett, N: Methenamine mandelate and methenamine hippurate. In: *The Use of Antibiotics* (N Bennett, ed.), William Heinemann Medical Books, London, 1979, pp. 792–795.
20. Allgren, LG, Persson, B, Sorbo, B: Biological fate of methenamine in man. *Acta Obstet. Gynecol. Scand. 58*:287–293, 1979.
21. Jackson, EA, McLeod, DC: Pharmacokinetics and dosing of antimicrobial agents in renal impairment, Part II. *Am. J. Hosp. Pharm. 31*:137–148, 1974.
22. Musher, D, Griffith, D, Richie, Y: The generation of formaldehyde from methenamine—effect of urinary flow and residual volume. *Invest. Urol. 13*(5):380–382, 1976.
23. Nelson, JD: Antimicrobial drugs with dosage forms and usual dosages. In: *1985 Pocketbook of Pediatric Antimicrobial Therapy*, 6th ed. (TM Tracy and C Eckart, eds.), Williams and Wilkins, Baltimore, 1985, p. 70.
24. Tanenbaum, M, Bricker, C: Microdeterminations of free formaldehyde. *Anal. Chem. 23*:354–357, 1951.
25. Vainrub, B, Musher, D: Lack of effect of methenamine in suppression of, or prophylaxis against, chronic urinary infection. *Antimicrob. Agents Chemother. 12*(5): 625–629, 1977.
26. Holland, N, West, C: Prevention of recurrent urinary tract infections in girls. *Am. J. Dis. Child. 105*:560–567, 1963.

27. Elo, J, Sarna, S, Ahava, K, Lepo, A: Methenamine hippurate in urinary tract infections in children: Prophylaxis, treatment and side effects. *J. Antimicrob. Chemother. 4*:355–365, 1978.
28. Petersen, S: Long-term prophylaxis with methenamine hippurate in girls with recurrent urinary tract infections. *Acta Paediatr. Scand. 67*:597–599, 1978.
29. Mandell, GL, Sande, MA: Agents for urinary tract infections; methenamine. In: *The Pharmacological Basis of Therapeutics* (AG Gilman, LS Goodman, et al., eds.), Macmillan, New York, 1985, pp. 1108–1109.
30. Freeman, R, et al.: Prevention of recurrent bacteriuria with continuous chemotherapy. U.S. Public Health Service Cooperative Study. *Ann. Intern. Med. 69*(4): 655–672, 1968.
31. Timmerman, RJ, Schroer, JA: Lipoid pneumonia caused by methenamine mandelate suspension. *JAMA 225*:1524–1525, September, 1973.
32. Gibson, GR: A clinical appraisal of methenamine hippurate in urinary tract infection. *Med. J. Aust. 24*:167–170, January 1970.
33. Ross, R, Jr., Conway, G: Hemorrhagic cystitis following accidental overdose of methenamine mandelate. *Am. J. Dis. Child. 119*:86–87, 1970.
34. Ashby, J, Leferre, P: Formaldehyde generators: Relationship between stability, lipophilicity and carcinogenic potency. *Carcinogenesis 3*(11):1273–1276, 1982.
35. Ariens, EJ, et al.: Beware of formaldehyde in disguise. *Eur. J. Clin. Pharmacol. 23*: 373–375, 1982.
36. Moller, JO: Cancer risk from formaldehyde. *Lancet 2*:480–481, 1980.
37. Freeman, RB, et al.: Long-term therapy for chronic bacteriuria in men. U.S. Public Health Service Cooperative Study. *Ann. Intern. Med. 83*(2):133–147, 1975.
38. Heinonen, OP, Slone, D, Shapiro, S: Evaluation of drugs in relation to malformations which may originate during early or late embryogenesis, *Birth Defects and Drugs In Pregnancy*, Publishing Sciences Group, Littleton, Mass., 1977, pp. 434–436.
39. Schardein, JL: Antimicrobial Agents. In: *Chemically Induced Birth Defects*, (FJ DiCarlo, FW Oehme, eds.), Marcel Dekker, New York, 1985, pp. 381 and 384.
40. Lipton, JH: Incompatability between sulfamethiazole and methenamine mandelate. *N. Engl. J. Med. 268*:92–93, January 1963.
41. Klotz, MO, Richter, H, Meuffels, M: Interference by formaldehyde-forming drugs in the determination of urinary catecholamines. *Clin. Chem. 10*:372–373, April 1964.
42. Carlstrom, K, Lunell, NO: Interference of antiseptics containing hexamethylene tetraamine (Hiprex) with the estimation of urinary oestriol excretion during pregnancy. *Acta Obstet. Gynecol. Scand. 54*:387–388, 1975.
43. Braverman, LE, Reinstein, H, Loayza, H, et al.: Formaldehyde-forming drugs and urinary 17-hydroxycorticosteroids. *Clin. Chem. 14*:374–377, April 1968.
44. Shils, ME: Interference by formaldehyde drugs in the quantitative determination of urinary hydroxyindoleacetic acid. *Clin. Chem. 13*:397–405, May 1967.
45. Roesel, R, et al.: Interference by methenamine mandelate in screening for organic and amino acid disorders. *Clin. Chim. Acta 100*:55–58, 1980.

24
Antiseptics

E. LEE FORD-JONES
The Hospital for Sick Children, Toronto, Ontario, Canada

Antiseptics are relatively insoluble chemicals that are applied to living tissue to destroy microorganisms or limit their growth (1,2). There is very little information about the use of antiseptics in children, and unless otherwise stated the following information has been obtained from studies in adults.

I. GENERAL PRINCIPLES

There are a few situations in which antiseptics are of proven value. In general, their greatest use is in prophylaxis, on healthy skin and mucous membranes. It is essential to differentiate between the antiseptic as an antimicrobial agent (efficacy) and the usefulness of the antiseptic in actual practice (effectiveness).

A. Factors Influencing Efficacy

The differences in response of microorganisms to chemical and physical agents vary widely, bacterial endospores being most resistant, followed by tubercle bacilli, fungal spores, small or nonlipid viruses, vegetative fungi, medium-sized or lipid viruses, and vegetative bacterial cells. Among the vegetative bacteria, which have the highest lipid content, the gram-negative organisms are the most resistant. The rate of germicidal action approximates first-order kinetics, varying with the concentration, temperature, pH, and vehicle of application (3).

B. Factors Influencing Effectiveness

Antiseptics are applied locally because of toxicity that would make systemic administration unacceptable. The properties listed in Table 1 are desirable for antiseptics. In order for an antiseptic to be effective in use, it is vital that certain conditions be met. These are listed in Table 2. It is particularly important that the contact time be adequate. For example, the time necessary for a 50% reduction in bacterial count on the skin of the hands and arms is about 0.6 min for 70% ethanol and 7 min for 1:1000 benzalkonium

Table 1 Desirable Properties of Antiseptics

Broad spectrum of germicidal activity
Germicidal rather than germistatic
Low degree and incidence of resistance
Retention of potency in presence of inflammatory exudates and body fluids, dilutions
Rapid and sustained action
Low surface tension for ease of application, dispersibility
Pleasant esthetic qualities (odor, color, lack of staining)
Inexpensive
For application to intact skin, lipid solubility
High therapeutic index (no local damage, impairment of healing, systemic assumption with taking)

Source: Adapted from Reference 3.

Table 2 Factors Influencing Effectiveness of an Antiseptic in Use

Diffusion, penetration, binding
Mechanical cleaning–good physical cleaning must precede; organic material may protect bacteria from penetration by the agent or directly inactivate certain agents
Inactivating contact materials, e.g., benzalkonium chloride and cotton fibers
Use–dilution
Contamination
Contact time

Source: Adapted from Reference 3.

Table 3 Acute and Chronic Adverse Effects of Antiseptics

Interference with healing and tissue repair
Systemic side effects resulting from drug absorption
Acute local effects (erythema, edema, formation of nodules or pustules, necrosis
Chronic local effects (sensitization, carcinogenesis)
Poisoning
Suppression of normal flora
Emergence of resistant pathogens
Interference with action of other topically applied drugs
Staining of skin

chloride. The promotional literature frequently neglects this vitally important point (3). The concentration must be considered since the rate of action is not necessarily directly proportional to the concentration.

Potential toxic effects may be acute or chronic, local or systemic, and are listed in Table 3. Of particular importance in preterm infants is the high permeability of the skin to drugs. Infants of 32 weeks' gestation or less show marked drug absorption and high skin water losses, effects not present after 2 weeks of age or in infants of 37 weeks' gestation or more (4).

Contamination of many antiseptics, including chlorhexidine, iodophors, alcohol, hexachlorophene, and benzalkonium chloride, has been described, leading to pseudobacteremia as well as local and systemic infections.

II. EVALUATION OF ANTIMICROBIAL ACTIVITY

Many different methods are currently used to evaluate antimicrobial activity. In general, these methods are not well standardized and few comparative studies have been performed (2,3,5,6). There are some good controlled studies of surgical (7) and urinary tract antiseptics. Testing methods should be reliable (reproducible) and valid (accurately measure the outcome of importance). There is no satisfactory standard method for in vitro kinetic study of the virucidal activity of antiseptics (8,9).

To determine the efficacy of an antiseptic, a variety of tests are recommended by the U.S. Food and Drug Administration (FDA) as outlined in Table 4 (1,9). Testing is required for both the individual antimicrobial ingredient and the finished formulation.

Table 4 In Vivo Methods for Evaluating Topical Antimicrobial Agents on Human Skin

Test	Purpose	Method
Occlusion test	Measure ability to prevent expansion of resident microflora, i.e., bacteriostatic effect	Impermeable dressing applied to forearm and measurements made at 24 and 48 hr
Expanded flora test	Measure ability to suppress dense proliferating population of microorganisms, i.e., bactericidal effect	Prior application of impermeable occlusive dressing followed by application of agent with measurements between 10 min and 48 hr
Persistent test	Measures ability of agent to establish a reservoir in the horny layer	Repeated application over 4 days followed 24 hr later by application of occlusive dressing
Ecological shift test	Determines major alteration in cutaneous ecology	Quantitative cultures following three 48-hr applications of agent and occlusive dressing
Serum activation test	Determine if the presence of serum proteins interferes with antimicrobial activity	Generate wound through inoculation with 50! ammonium hydroxide and bacteria; apply agent and occlusive dressing for 24 hr

Source: From References 1 and 9.

The importance of counteracting the activity of the antiseptic through the use of an appropriate neutralizer cannot be overemphasized (10).

Although much of the emphasis has been on in vitro testing, it is now recognized that the determination of effectiveness through adequate clinical trials is necessary. Such studies are expensive and time consuming to carry out in North America because of the relative rarity of infections.

A. Microbiology

The microbial flora of the skin can be classified as transient or resident (11,12). Transient flora are easily acquired by touching contaminated surfaces. These organisms are not firmly attached and can be removed by careful cleansing. Transient pathogens may be recovered from hospital personnel in large numbers (13). Up to 10^7 *Staphylococcus aureus* and gram-negative bacteria have been recovered from the hands of nurses through patient care or laboratory specimen contact (13,14). Although 99% of gram-negative organisms die within 2 min of application, 10^5 bacteria may remain on the fingers for up to 90 min (15). Resident flora, however, are more permanent constituents of the skin, and these are firmly attached and multiply there. Resident bacteria generally includes *Staphylococcus epidermidis* and *Propionobacterium* species and occasionally pathogenic gram-negative organisms. Regardless of the agent used, vigorous mechanical cleaning is necessary.

B. Principles of Prophylactic Skin Degerming

Tests usually involve sampling of the hands of a number of subjects and counting the number of organisms before and after application of antiseptics (15-20). Bacterial counts are obtained by rinsing hands in a bowl or plastic bag containing broth and the appropriate neutralizer. Alternatively, the fingertips may be sampled by rubbing them on bacteriologic media in a petri dish. Degerming efficacy is stated as a percentage reduction of microorganisms following treatment compared with a control group. Biopsy is probably the most sensitive technique (11,21), and other methods continue to be evaluated (22-24). Extrapolation of efficacy measured as reduction in bacterial concentration to the actual effectiveness of an agent in preventing infection is extremely difficult.

Immediate action refers to the reduction of the natural skin flora measured immediately after completion of a given washing procedure and must be assessed separately for transient and resident flora. The results of studies to determine the impact of a 2-min wash on resident flora, which are more difficult to remove than transient flora, are shown in Table 5. It can be seen that at best only an 80-90% reduction in flora can be achieved with a single wash. Maki et al. (25) studied a 15-sec wash in personnel naturally acquiring gram-negative organisms through patient contact. He showed significant reductions of organisms followed chlorhexidine washes but not soap with alcoholic rinse or povidone-iodine washes.

Cumulative effect refers to the kill achieved after several applications over a period of time. The cumulative effect of regular use improves the performance of almost any hand disinfectant (Table 5).

Persistent action of the agent over time is primarily important for surgical scrubs and preoperative skin preparations. To measure such an effect, organisms in glove fluid or washings are counted. The gloved hand method has been remarkably reliable (15). Less commonly, inocula of *S. aureus* or *Escherichia coli* may be introduced into the skin at

Table 5 Immediate and Cumulative Action of Antibacterial Hand Washes Against Resident Skin Flora

Hand wash preparation	Concentration active agent	% Reductions		References
		Single wash, immediate	Repeated washes, cumulative	
Chlorhexidine	4% w/v	86.7 X 3.0	99.2 X 0.2	Lowbury and Lilly
		88.1 X 2.4	98.2 X 1.6	Ayliffe et al.
		74	77	Jarvis et al.
		92.1	98.0	Askgaard
		89.1		Ojajärvi
			98.8	Rosenberg et al.
Povidone-iodine	7.5% w/v	68.0 X 6.8	97.7 X 0.7	Lowbury and Lilly
		87	85	Jarvis et al.
		42.0		Ojajärvi
Hexachlorophene	3% w/v	51.1 X 4.8	98.4 X 0.8	Lowbury and Lilly
	2% w/v	58.2	96.3	Askgaard
	3% w/v	41.3		Ojajärvi
Bar soap	Unmedicated	3.3 X 8.3	25.9 X 5.1	Lowbury and Lilly
		23.3	20.4	Askgaard
		14.6 X 2.8	30.5 X 17.3	Ayliffe et al.
		-22.2		Ojajärvi

Source: Reproduced with permission of J.F. Gardner, K.G. Gray and Lea & Febiger, Philadelphia (26).

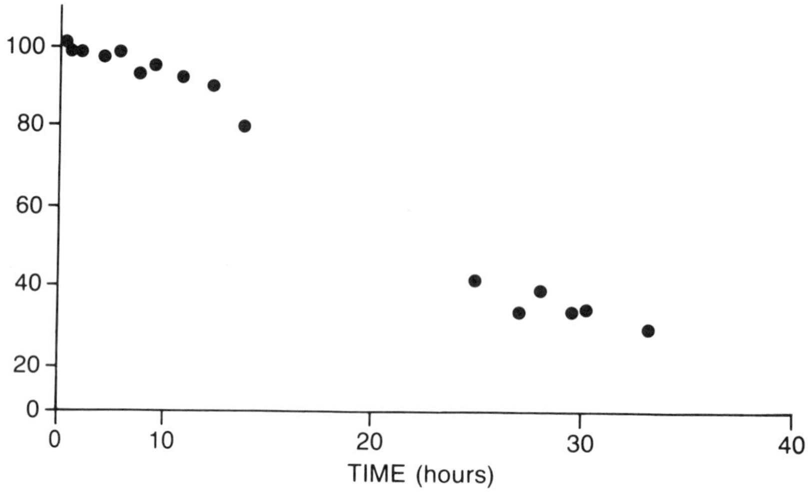

Figure 1 Chlorhexidine curve. Reproduced with permission of NDA Hibiclens, ICI United States Inc., and Lea and Febiger (26).

various times after application of the antiseptic. Chlorhexidine and hexachlorophene have a persistent effect when measured by finger streak sampling methods, but povidone-iodine, which is water soluble, and alcohol do not. Persistence, as demonstrated by inoculation of bacterium on the skin after chlorhexidine or alcohol treatment, has been demonstrated 1 hr after chlorhexidine but not alcohol application. Using radiolabeled chlorhexidine, persistence of 90% for 5 hr and 26% for 29 hr has been demonstrated, as shown in Figure 1 (26).

In the *rebound effect*, ordinary scrubbing with hexachlorophene may be followed during succeeding days of nonuse by temporary excessive regeneration of the cutaneous flora of the hands and arms (27).

III. IN VIVO TESTING OF SKIN DEGERMING

Modern studies of disinfection of artifically contaminated skin have given very contradictory results. For example, "soap and water" was reported to be superior to chlorhexidine detergent in water if, initially, the contaminating bacteria are merely dried passively on the skin. However, if the bacterial suspension is rubbed into the skin before drying the position is completely reversed. Presumably the more firmly attached bacteria are no longer adequately removed by soap, water, and gentle hand rubbing. When skin biopsy is used to evaluate skin antiseptics, the following reductions in counts are obtained (21):

Iodine in ethanol, 96%
Iodophor (PVP-1), 89%
Chlorhexidine in ethanol, 88%

Table 6 Testing the Safety and Efficacy of Antiseptics

Antimicrobial activity (e.g., MIC, Kelsey-Sykes procedure, emergence of resistance)
Episomatic test for skin and mucosa tolerance (e.g., primary irritation, potential allergy, photosensitivity, effect on wound healing and skin pigmentation, effect of total skin flora, accumulation)
Pharmacological tests (e.g., degree of absorption through intact and abraded skin and mucus membranes following single and multiple exposure, inhalation studies for aerosols)
Toxicological tests (e.g., LD_{50}, target organs, tissue distribution, metabolic rates, and rate and route of excretion; teratogenic, mutagenic, and reproductive effects)
Pharmaceutical application and in-use tests

Source: From Weuffer, W, and Kramar, A: Definition, Prophylactic Value and Toxic Hazard in the Use of Antiseptics. *J. Hyg. Epidemiol. Microbiol. Immunol. 1*:104, 1980.

60% Isopropanol, 83%
70% Ethanol, 83%
Chlorhexidine (aqueous), 82%
Benzalkonium chloride (aqueous), 39%
Thiomersal (aqueous), 37% (35)

Additional in vivo tests are listed in Table 6. Detailed descriptions of evaluation of the health care personnel hand wash, preoperative preparation of the patient, and surgical hand scrub may be found elsewhere (2,28). A comparative summary of the effects of these agents is found in Table 7. The iodophors and chlorhexidine gluconate are active against a greater bacterial spectrum and retain their action for a prolonged period of time. Alcohol should not be included as a final rinse since it will remove the resident germicidal barrier.

Table 7 Comparison of Common Antiseptic Agents

Agent	Alcohol	Chlorhexidine	Hexachlorophene	Iodine-Iodophor
Spectrum of bacterial activity	Gram-positive and gram-negative	Gram-positive and most gram-negative	Gram-positive	Gram-positive and gram-negative
Immediate effect	Good	Good	Poor	Good
Persistent effect	Poor	Good	Good	Poor
Cumulative effect	Good	Good	Good	Good
Rebound effect	–	–	Yes	–
Active in the presence of blood, pus, soap	No	Yes	No	No
Toxicity in infants	Burns with pooling		Vacuolar myelinopathy in babies < 1500 g	Biochemical hypothyroidism in babies < 37 weeks

Table 8 Cellular Targets for Nonantibiotic Antibacterial Drugs[a]

	Acid	Acridine dyes	Alcohols	Chlorhexidine	Copper II salts	Formaldehyde	Hexachlorophene	Hydrogen peroxide
Cell wall	+	+	+			+		
Cytoplasmic membrane	+							
Action membrane potentials			+				+	
Action on membrane enzymes								
Electron transport chain							+	
Adenosine triphosphatase				+	+			
Enzymes with thiol groups	+	+		+		+	+	+
Action on membrane permeability		+	+,++	+	+			
Cytoplasm								
General coagulation		+++	+++	+++	+++	+++	+++	
Ribosomes		+						+
Nucleic acids		+						
Thiol groups	+	+		+	+	+		+
Amino groups	+			+		++,+	+	
Highly reactive compounds				+				

[a]Crosses indicating activity, which appear in several columns for a given compound, demonstrate the multiple actions for the compound concerned. This activity is nearly always concentration dependent, and the number of crosses indicates the order of concentration at which the effect is elicited; i.e., +, elicited at low concentrations; +++, elicited at high concentrations. When a cross appears in only one target column, this is the only known site of action of the drug.

Source: Modified from A. D. Russell, W. B. Hugo, and G. A. J. Ayliffe, Disinfection mechanisms. In: *Principles and Practice of Disinfection, Preservation and Sterilisation*, with permission, Blackwell Scientific Publications, Boston, p. 159, 1982.

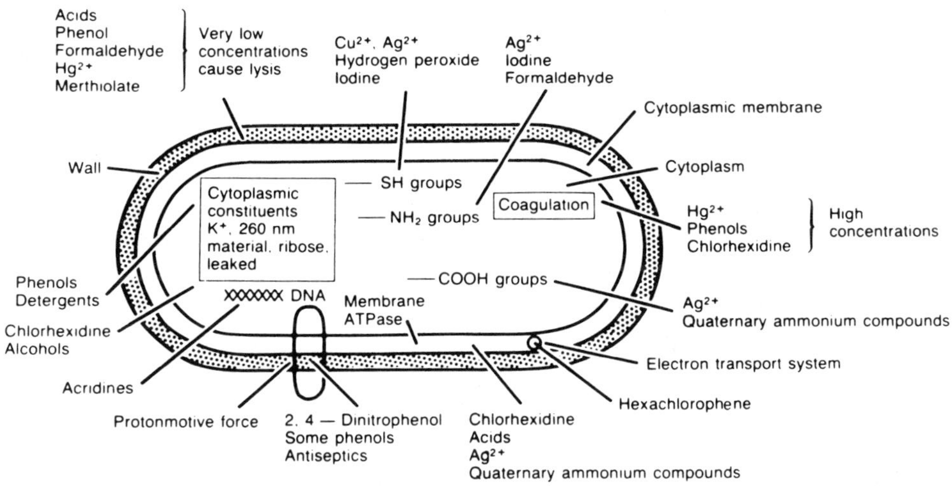

Figure 2 Main sites of action for antiseptics. Modified from A. D. Russell, W. B. Hugo, and G. A. J. Ayliffe, Disinfection Mechanisms, *Principles and Practice of Disinfection, Preservation and Sterilisation*, with permission, Blackwell Scientific Publications, Boston, p. 158, 1982.

IV. SITES OF ACTIONS

It is difficult to define the exact mechanism of action of each agent since more than one cell constituent may be affected and the differentiation of primary and secondary effects are difficult to determine. Information about the cellular targets has been obtained in the same way as for other antimicrobial agents. These are outlined in Figure 2 and Table 8.

V. ANTISEPTIC RESISTANCE

Resistance may be intrinsic and related to inherent qualities of the bacteria, virus, or spore forms. Bacteria generally acquire resistance to antiseptics much less readily than to antibiotics, but there is also evidence to suggest that plasmids may be responsible for acquired resistance of gram-positive and gram-negative bacteria to antiseptics, disinfectants, and preservatives. Plasmid-mediated resistance to Hg^{2+}, organomercury, hexachlorophene, and silver has been described (29). Resistance may be linked to plasmids that specify resistance to antibiotics.

VI. SPECIFIC AGENTS

The use of acids as antiseptics is primarily of historical interest. Readers are referred to several reviews on this topic (1,3,30).

A. Alcohols

1. Benzyl Alcohol

Benzyl alcohol is commonly used as a preservative in multidose injectable pharmaceuticals, including physiologic saline or water. It has been associated with a fatal toxic syndrome in premature infants, but generally only when used to flush intravenous catheters (31). Benzyl alcohol is normally oxidized rapidly to benzoic acid, conjugated with glycose in the liver, and excreted as hippuric acid. In premature infants this enzyme may not be developed and benzoic acid may accumulate, leading to metabolic acidosis (31,32).

2. Isopropyl and Ethyl Alcohol

a. Chemistry. The germicidal activity of aliphatic alcohols increases with increase in their molecular weight and lipid solubility up to tertiary alcohols in which micelle formation limits the availability of free alcohol (3).

b. Mechanism of Action. It is most likely that alcohol exerts its antibacterial effect by denaturing proteins. Protein is denatured more readily in the presence of water, explaining why absolute ethyl alcohol is less effective than combinations with water. There is some evidence that it also exerts a bacteriostatic effect through the inhibition of the production of metabolites for rapid cell division. In addition it may inhibit enzymes necessary for spore germination or affect microorganisms by direct lysis (3).

c. Antimicrobial Activity and Resistance. Unlike ethyl alcohol, the bactericidal action of isopropyl alcohol increases with concentration. Common nonsporing bacteria in a moist state are destroyed within 5 min by any strength of alcohol above 40%, whereas organisms in a dry state require concentrations of 60–70%. Bacterial spores are not killed even after 24 hr of exposure, although their growth may be temporarily inhibited. Other miscellaneous microbes, such as tubercle bacilli, are also resistant (21), whereas the effect on fungi and viruses is variable. The application of 70% ethanol as a single wipe, which is then allowed to evaporate, can be expected to reduce bacterial counts by only 75% or less. Alcohol produces sublethal changes to some bacteria, possibly by increasing their vulnerability to a second antiseptic, and it is therefore sometimes combined with chlorhexidine. Ethyl alcohol also appears to increase the germicidal activity of chlorhexidine, iodine, iodophors, and hexachlorophene.

Isopropyl alcohol in concentrations above 70% is slightly more germicidal than ethyl alcohol; 35% isopropanol readily destroys the lipid membrane of respiratory syncytial virus (RSV) within 60 sec (32), but its effect on other viruses is variable or unknown.

Its wide spectrum of activity, low toxicity, and rare hypersensitivity have made it a popular agent, and the lack of systemic absorption is of particular importance in neonates. It is colorless (unless coloring is desirable) and therefore does not impair visualization of vessels, and it is inexpensive. The flammable, volatile nature of alcohol as well as the stinging effect on puncture sites have been considered drawbacks to more widespread use. Ethanol is less irritating and drying and has a less offensive smell than isopropanol. A disadvantage of alcohol is its failure to exert any persistent effect.

d. Interactions. Alcohol may inactivate benzylpenicillin (33).

e. Preparation and Dosage. For routine use, 70% by weight is recommended because it is less expensive than stronger solutions, it spreads evenly, wets efficiently, dries slowly, and is almost completely innocuous.

f. Therapeutic Indications. These include (1) skin preparation when other agents are contraindicated or as part of a two-phase antiseptic procedure (e.g., alcohol-chlorhexidine in premature infants (34); (2) application after routine iodine or iodophor degerming to improve visualization of the area; (3) venipuncture in a nonimmunocompromised host undergoing phlebotomy other than a blood culture; and (4) skin preparation in a patient with allergy to other agents. A contact time of 2 min is required. Its role in hand degerming requires further study, although European data are encouraging (35-38).

g. Assay. Gas chromatography can be used for quantitative and qualitative alcohol determinations.

h. Absorption. Absorption of alcohol has not been reported during routine clinical use. Acute ethanol intoxication (blood alcohol concentrations of 295 mg per 100 ml) has occurred in a preterm infant of 1800 g following local application of alcohol-soaked compresses on the legs as a treatment for puncture hematomas (39). Skin cleansing of the umbilicus and lumbar puncture site with methylated spirits in a 27-week 985-g baby resulted in a blood ethanol concentration of 259 mg per 100 ml and a methanol concentration of 26 mg per 100 ml (40).

Ethanol should not be applied to open wounds, where it forms a coagulum under which bacteria may thrive. Alcohol may also remove bactericidal substances from the skin, leaving the skin with decreased bactericidal activity.

i. Adverse Effects. Isopropanol causes vasodilation, so that puncture sites may bleed. Eczematous reactions or an uncomfortable feeling of dryness has been reported during use of isopropyl alcohol as it defats the skin when used repeatedly, particularly in concentrated solution and large volumes. This may be avoided by using 0.5 ml or less. Toxicity has been reported as a result of use in premature infants of very low birth weight in whom isopropyl alcohol was used for electrocardiogram (ECG) lead contact and as preparation of the umbilical stump. Second- and third-degree burns resulted possibly as a result of local hypoperfusion (39,40-43).

Mouthwashes contain up to 26.9% ethanol, and their accessibility and attractiveness to children continue to result in numerous poisonings—422 in an 18-month period according to the U.S. National Poison Center (39,44-46).

Bacterial spores have occasionally been recovered from various concentrations of alcohol.

j. Contraindications. Prompt drying of the skin of small premature infants after antisepsis to avoid pooling of the agent is advisable. Because alcohol coagulates wound fluids, it is not recommended for use on wounds. There is little evidence to support the notion that blood specimens drawn for alcohol levels are contaminated by the use of an alcohol pad.

B. Biguanides

1. Chemistry

The formula for chlorhexidine is shown in Figure 3.

2. Mechanism of Action

One of the most important attributes of chlorhexidine is its strong affinity for skin, to which it is adsorbed and where it persists for several hours, as shown in Figure 1. Chlorhexidine causes a leakage of organic and inorganic cell constituents through its effect on the semipermeable cell membrane at low concentrations. At higher concentrations cyto-

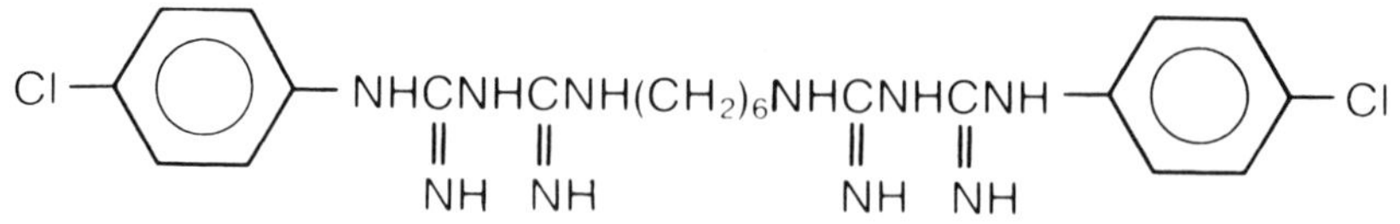

Figure 3 Structure of chlorhexidine.

plasmic constituents are precipitated and leakage is not great (26). Chlorhexidine uptake on the bacterial surface is dependent on the availability of negatively charged groups on the bacterial surface that are favored by a neutral or alkaline alcohol pH.

3. Antimicrobial Activity

It is bactericidal to vegetative forms of bacteria at concentrations of 100 μg/ml and above while exerting bacteriostatic effects to 1 μg/ml or even lower. Most gram-positive bacteria are inhibited by concentrations of 10 μg/ml; gram-negative bacteria require 50 μg/ml. The lowest recommended concentration is 200 μg/ml. It is not virucidal and the minimum inhibitory concentrations (MIC) of chlorhexidine gluconate for *Aspergillus* and *Nocardia* species are high (3,26). Chlorhexidine detergent rapidly destroys respiratory syncytical virus; however, the virucidal component is primarily the detergent base, not the chlorhexidine (32).

4. Resistance

Despite long-term use, most organisms appear to retain their sensitivity to chlorhexidine. Chlorhexidine-resistant *Pseudomonas* species have been described. This resistance is postulated to result from a reduced content of lipopolysaccharide and hence decreased adsorption by the cell wall. Resistance of *Pesudomonas aeruginosa* to chlorhexidine may be more common than that to antibiotics. Methicillin- and gentamicin-resistant strains of *S. aureus* may also be relatively resistant to chlorhexidine (47), although not to the high concentrations of chlorhexidine used in clinical practice. Chlorhexidine-resistant strains also show multiple antibiotic resistance (48). Although repeated use in a nursery setting has not resulted in selection of gram-negative bacteria, adults using chlorhexidine for 6 months had significantly more gram-negative bacilli in their axillae and groins than controls.

5. Interactions

The bactericidal action is not adversely affected by the presence of blood or serum protein (49). There is some evidence of synergy with neomycin, gentamicin (50), sulfadiazine (51), and polymycins (52) against some bacterial strains.

6. Preparation and Dosage

A variety of formulations containing chlorhexidine are available for use on skin and mucosal surfaces (Table 9). Other preparations containing chlorhexidine acetate and diphosphanilate are available.

7. Therapeutic Indications

a. Skin Preparation. Because of the high permeability of neonatal skin to antiseptics and the frequency with which coagulase-negative staphylococci have emerged as

Table 9 Examples of Chlorhexidine Formulations Available in North America and Europe

Formulation	Trade name	Therapeutic indication(s)
Detergent chlorhexidine (4%, 2%)	Hibiclens, Hibiscrub	Surgical hand scrub; patient preoperative showering, bathing, skin preparation; health care personnel handwashing; wound cleansing
Alcoholic (70%); chlorhexidine (0.5%) with skin emollient	Hibistat, Hibisol	Germicidal, hand rinse, skin preparation
Chlorhexidine (1%) mouth rinses and gels	Corsodyl, Hibitane, Dental Gel	Oral surgery
Chlorhexidine (0.5%) imprefracted gauze	Bactigras	Superficial wound care

pathogens, cleansing with 70% isopropyl alcohol followed by a 60-sec application of chlorhexidine (0.5% in 70% ethanol) has been studied (34) and shown to be ineffective. This is possibly because of the high density of coagulase-negative staphylococci on the skin of many infants who are maintained in incubators and have increased skin hydration (11). Two-phase antisepsis may facilitate penetration of chlorhexidine deeper into the epidermis, and alcohol may increase vulnerability to a second antiseptic by causing sub-lethal damage to some bacteria.

b. Hand Washing. Chlorhexidine, 4%, is an appropriate agent for a 15-sec routine hand wash and a 2-min surgical wash. Chlorhexidine, 2%, may be equally effective (53). Chlorhexidine, 0.5%, in 70% isopropyl alcohol is appropriate as a hand cleaner when running water is not available, but only if the hands are physically clean (54).

c. Preoperative Bathing and Skin Preparation. Washes or showers with chlorhexidine will reduce bacterial counts at the operative site and wound infection, particularly if used repeatedly. A preliminary study of a 0.5% chlorhexidine gluconate spray as a preoperative preparation is encouraging (55). Chlorhexidine gloconate, 4%, may have short-term advantages over an iodophor for the skin preparation of hemodialysis patients because of the longer duration of action (56).

d. Neonatal Washing. Chlorhexidine gluconate appears to be the most promising agent for routine neonatal skin care in the event of a neonatal staphylococcal epidemic since the withdrawal of hexachlorophene-containing products (57) and the emergence of staphylococcal colonization and infection (58-61). It has been recommended for neonatal bathing as a 4% (3), 0.4%, or 0.04% solution (58-62), but absorption has not been studied adequately. In a pilot study of 51 full-term neonates undergoing various wash regimens with 0.4% chlorhexidine gluconate, no chlorhexidine was detected in the blood of any treated infant using a gas-liquid chromatographic method with a sensitivity limit of 0.1 μg/ml (57). Chlorhexidine, 0.04%, may be less effective than hexachlorophene (63). A 14-month trial of 0.04% chlorhexidine in 3500 babies showed clinical tolerance, but microbiologic effects and blood concentrations were not studied (58).

e. Other Uses. Chlorhexidine applied to umbilical cords also appears to be more effective than ethanol in decreasing groups B and G streptococci colonization (64).

Chlorhexidine 4% w/v has been approved for use in the cleansing of wounds as it is nontoxic and does not delay wound healing. A nasal cream has been used for staphylococcal carriers (65,66). Creams containing 0.02% w/v chlorhexidine with silver sulfadiazine may be effective topical burn therapy, particularly in the perineum, where *Pseudomonas* colonization is common. In studies of burn wounds in rats, chlorhexidine diphosphanilate was found to be equivalent to silver sulfadiazine (67). No evidence of cross-resistance with sulfonamide-resistant strains of gram-negative organisms was found. Chlorhexidine, 1%, in natural or gel forms, is the most important dental antiseptic in current use (3,68). It is a useful supragingival dental plaque inhibitor, provided it is used only for brief periods to avoid tooth staining. The taste may be bitter. It has also been used for denture stomatitis and aphthous ulcers and improving postoperative healing rates of periodontal wounds (26). Chlorhexidine gluconate and acetate have been used for irrigation of the bladder, disinfection of the meatus, and bladder installation; however, its efficacy in preventing infection has not yet been established (69,70). Lavage with aqueous solutions of chlorhexidine may be effective in controlling peritoneal sepsis, but it does precipitate in chloride ion so that it is not recommended for dilution in saline and hence not recommended for ambulatory dialysis.

8. Assays

Low concentrations of chlorhexidine may be measured colorimetrically by a reaction with alkaline sodium hypobromite; samples containing larger amounts may be measured by dissolving evaporated residue in glacial acetic acid and potentiometrically titrating against perchloric acid using a glass electrode. Radioactive and gas-liquid chromatography with electron capture (sensitivity limit, 0.1 μg/ml) methods may also be used (26).

9. Absorption

Systemic absorption has not been documented in studies of adult volunteers using contact times of 3 hr or repeated use over three 5-day weeks. The absorption of chlorhexidine in neonatal cord care is unlikely in term infants (71) but may occur in preterm infants treated with 1% solution of chlorhexidine in ethanol (72).

10. Adverse Reactions

In four adults accidentally given the agent by vein, no adverse effects were documented (3). Skin irritation and sensitization has not been documented, apart from minor dryness when a rigorous scrubbing schedule is followed. Contact dermatitis and photosensitivity may occur in 8% of patients. Chlorhexidine, particularly if used in combination with detergents and alcohol, causes sensory neural hearing loss when in contact with the middle ear. Constant use of a chlorhexidine-containing mouthwash can cause gingival bleeding and staining of the teeth (73). Chlorhexidine interacts with tetrabromophenol, the pH indicator included in dipsticks for proteinuria. False-positive dipstick readings for protein may be obtained in urine contaminated by the antiseptics (74).

11. Contamination

Flavobacterium meningosepticum, P. aeruginosa, P. picketti, and *P. cepacia* contamination of dilute aqueous chlorhexidine has been described (75-80).

C. Dyes

1. Antimicrobial Activity and Mechanism of Action

Triphenylmethane dyes are basic and include crystal violet, brilliant green, and malachite green. They are extremely active against gram-positive species, and efficacy is greater at pH 7 than at pH 5. They have a prolonged antibacterial effect after a single application (81,82). However, they do not prevent gram-negative multiplication and unless used daily they are not effective against group B streptococci as well (82–87).

2. Acceptability and Toxicity

Triple dyes are not widely used because they stain the patient, clothing, and bedding, as well as the hands of the people manufacturing and administering it, and there are other acceptable modes of therapy. Crystal violet has been associated with necrotic skin reactions in babies, and sensitization to brilliant green has been reported (88,89). Daily alcohol application to a cord stump originally treated with triple dye may promote prolonged adherence of the cord, although this is controversial (90).

3. Therapeutic Use

Their use has been recommended in therapy of tinea capitis, trench mouth, tinea pedis, moniliasis, and trichomoniasis. They have a dramatic impact on *S. aureus* colonization of the cord and nose of neonates, decreasing levels of colonization more than any other currently available agent (91–96).

D. Iodine and Iodine Compounds

1. Chemistry

Iodine has been used as an antiseptic for years, but its chemistry is poorly understood. One hypothesis is that the concentration of "free" iodine (the elemental iodine in solution) is responsible for the observed antimicrobial activity (3,91,92). The solubility of iodine in water at pH 7.5 is 0.15%, but it is more soluble in 70% ethanol. To increase iodine content, NaI is included.

A carrier of high molecular weight like pyrrolidone nitrogen of polyvinyl pyrrolidone (PVP) increases the solubility of iodine as micellar aggregates and provides a sustained release reservoir of iodine. These compounds are known as iodophors. These aqueous solutions contain the same particles as do the pure iodine solutions, but none can equal the germicidal activity of iodine. These surface-active carriers improve wetting properties and interaction with organic soil and fat. The percentage of iodine complexed with a carrier (iodophor) is not constant at all concentrations but decreases with dilution so that there is more free iodine in a dilute solution (91). In 10% povidone-iodine (which contains 1% "available iodine"), the free iodine concentration is only 0.001%. In a 10-fold dilution (0.1% povidone-iodine), the content of free iodine rises because of dissociation of the complex (3). The paradoxical increase in bacterial killing at lower concentrations of PVP is shown in Figure 4. Considerable variability is seen between strains (93).

2. Mechanism of Action (94,95)

Iodine penetrates the cell wall of microorganisms rapidly and is assumed to

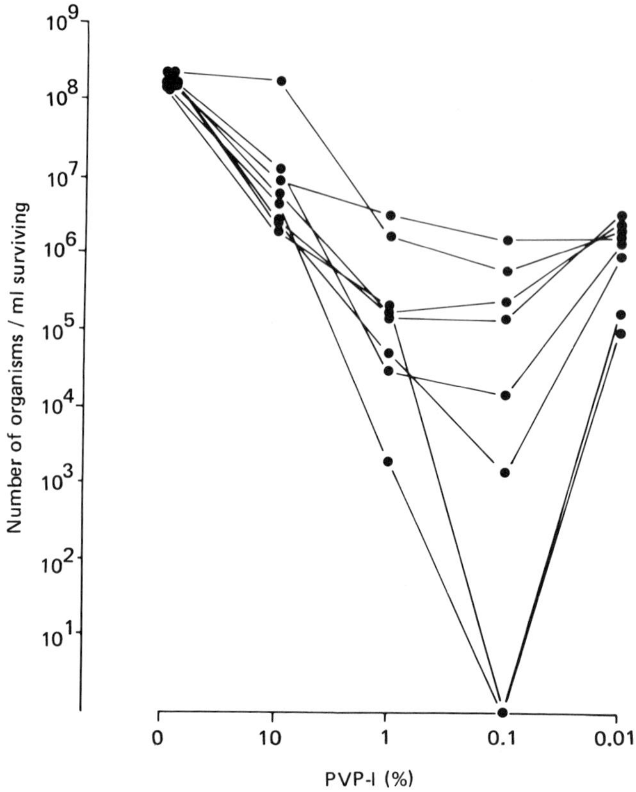

Figure 4 Killing of staphylococci is paradoxically increased at lower concentrations of PVP-I, but considerable variability is observed between strains. From (93), with permission.

1. Block positions of hydrogen bonding in amino acids and nucleotides
2. Oxidize the S-H group of cysteine to prevent formation of S-S bridges in the synthesis of protein
3. React with phenolic OH group of tyrosine
4. React with carbon bond of unsaturated fatty acids leading to a change in physical properties of the lipids and membrane immobilization (3,96)

3. Antimicrobial Activity and Resistance

Iodine and complex iodophors are the only antiseptics to act reliably against bacterial spores as well as vegetative microorganisms. Iodine kills bacteria, enteric viruses, rhinovirus (97), protozoan cysts, mycobacteria, spores of bacilli, clostridia, fungi, and *Trichomonas*. Various amounts of iodine are required, and test conditions have varied considerably with respect to pH, temperature, concentration and type of iodine, exposure time, amount, and time of dissolved organic and inorganic substances. Ethanol enhances germicidal activity and a 1% solution will kill 90% of the bacteria on the skin in 90 sec; 5% will kill 90% of the bacteria within 60 sec.

Povidone-iodine is bacteriostatic at 640 μg/ml and bactericidal at 960 μg/ml against *S. aureus*, whereas *Mycobacterium tuberculosis* is resistant (3). A standard surgical scrub with 10% povidone-iodine decreases the cutaneous bacterial population by about 85%, leaving a higher residual population than do 1% iodine or 4% chlorhexidine. Within hours the population returns to normal and the agent is therefore less effective than chlorhexidine. Repeated applications are not required, but since these agents are water soluble no protective film is left once rinsed off the skin.

4. Resistance

Some gram-negative bacteria can acquire extraordinary resistance to free iodine in the concentration of approximately 1–2 ppm free iodine. It may be that true bacterial resistance of PVP-I does not occur and that the observed phenomenon of incomplete killing is primarily determined by exposure time (97).

5. Interaction

Iodine may inactivate benylpenicillins (33).

6. Preparation and Dosage

a. Iodine. Iodine is available in 2% and 5% (Lugol's) solutions and tincture of alcohol. Generally aqueous solutions are preferred because they are less irritating. These contain iodine and potassium or sodium iodide in water, ethyl alcohol, and glycerol (96).

b. Iodophors. Iodophors consisting of iodine bound to povidone iodine are available in aerosols, surgical detergent scrubs, ointments, solutions, shampoos, douches, pads, and vaginal gels. The scrub differs from the solution in that it contains detergent.

Povidone-iodine, the best known iodophor, contains 10% bound iodine and 1% available iodine. Iodophors are available in a variety of forms, such as 10% applicator solutions, 2% scrubs, aerosol sprays, foams and vaginal gels, ointments, powders, mouthwashes, perineal washes, and surgical gels (97). A new iodine preparation with low available iodine content (0.01%) has been patented (98) for use as a germicidal hand wash although its efficacy is not yet established (53). A 5% povidone-iodine solution is expected to show more rapid liberation of iodine (99).

7. Therapeutic Indications

Iodine solutions, used chiefly for skin disinfection, are probably superior to any other agent for its immediate effect (3,96). Iodophors are widely used for preoperative preparations of the skin (100), surgical disinfection of hands, and disinfection prior to transfusions and infusions (101). Iodophors are one of three antiseptics recommended by the American Centers for Disease Control (102).

In adults, povidone-iodine is used for disinfection of the eye, skin (103), mucous membranes, surgical wounds, and burns (104–106), as well as for pleuritis, peritonitis (107,108), wound infections, and cutaneous candidiasis. In these latter conditions its efficacy is questionable (109–111). Its use in children should be discouraged because of the questionable efficacy and potential toxicity following absorption. None of these studies emphasize the removal of blood, pus, or organic material from the wounds and cavities, although it is well known that they bind iodine and decrease the iodine content and antibacterial effect (109–112). There is strong evidence that addition of antibacterial substances to urinary drainage bags is not effective (113,114); however, recent reports have suggested that the incidence of bacteriuria is reduced in patients in whom povidone-iodine is added to the drainage bag (115). The use of povidone ointment at peripheral intravenous sites has been associated with lower rates of *Candida* species colonization, but *S. aureus* colonization of the catheters continued to occur (116).

More properly controlled prospective studies are needed to establish the true prophylactic value of these agents compared with others (117,118). Even accepting the consensus that preoperative scrubbing and rinsing of the hands of health personnel with iodophors decreases the incidence of nosocomial infections, the effects of povidone-iodine on skin flora are not as marked as with 1% iodine tincture or 0.5% chlorhexidine (3) and the duration of action is much less than with chlorhexidine. The common belief that disinfection of the skin, mouth, or wounds with povidone-iodine protects against postoperative infections does not seem to be supported by a number of recent studies (2,27,119-121).

For topical antiseptics prior to venipuncture, a 0.5% solution of iodine in water or in 70% alcohol (tincture of iodine) may be used. After application, the iodine should dry for 30 sec and then be washed off with 70% alcohol to reduce the chance of burns. Iodophors may be substituted but ideally should not be washed off after application because their germicidal action may be augmented by the sustained release of free iodine. Alcohol, 70%, is an acceptable disinfectant if the patient is sensitive to iodine. There is no difference in bacterial counts between a 10-min two-brush scrub with povidone-iodine and a 5-min brush or sponge scrub using the same antibacterial solutions (96, 117,118).

8. Pharmacokinetics

Blood concentrations of iodine are directly related to the concentration used, the frequency of applications, and the status of renal function, as the kidneys are the main route of iodine excretion (109). Concern has arisen with regard to thyroid function because of the local application of iodine-containing agents on intact skin in children (122,123), to wounds (124-128) or burns (124-129), and to intact neonatal skin (129-134) or the mother's vaginal mucosa (129-137). Significant vaginal absorption of PVP-I has occurred after a single 2-min application in which the serum iodine concentration remained elevated for at least an hour. Absorbed iodine is bound to plasma proteins and secreted by the kidney.

9. Wound Healing

The effect of single applications of 70% isopropyl alcohol and 10% povidone-iodine solution on partial-thickness wounds in rabbits inoculated with *S. aureus* has been evaluated, and only very limited efficacy in superficial wounds has been demonstrated. A 1% solution shows no significant difference in leukocyte migration, fibroblastic activity, and wound cellularity compared with control wounds irrigated with normal saline (110), whereas inhibition of this activity occurs at 5 and 10% concentrations. Povidone-iodine did not affect the healing rate of superficial wounds uninoculated with bacteria.

10. Toxicity

Most adverse reports have followed topical application of 70% tincture of iodine and include fever, headache, delirium, coma, coryza, shock, cyanosis, vomiting and diarrhea, rashes range from localized hemorrhagic eruption to generalized urticaria, erythema, and exfoliative dermatitis (39,43,138-141). Contact dermatitis (142) and allergy or cross-sensitivity to iodine (3) have been described in as many as 12% of users. Iodophors produce less pain, staining, and irritation than tincture of iodine.

Iodides easily cross the placenta from mother to fetus and may produce profound effects on fetal thyroid function (129-137). It has also been demonstrated that the extensive topical application of an iodine antiseptic (Betadine) to premature infants appears to produce a reversible transient hypothyroidism state most marked in infants under 32 weeks' gestation (129-134). These investigators have theorized that there is an enhanced sensitivity and vulnerability to the induction of transient neonatal hypothyroidism in premature infants. In addition, metabolic acidosis, inhibition of lymphocyte blastogenesis, neutropenia, and possible renal effects have also been reported with high concentrations (140).

Some forms of iodophor may be associated with lower rates of absorption than others, hence there may be toxicity.

Iodine-containing solutions can cause a positive haem (Hemoccult) reaction even if present in only small amounts (143,144). Betadine solution has produced a positive test without developer at dilutions from 1:100 to 1:10,000, although a developer was needed to produce a positive test at full strength or 1:10 dilution and with Lugol's solution.

Aspiration pneumonia has followed preparation of the oral cavity with povidone-iodine when the endotracheal tube was not sufficiently inflated (145). Fatalities have resulted from oral ingestion when 30-50 ml of iodine tincture have been taken (3).

11. Contraindications

PVP-I should be avoided in patients with known iodine hypersensitivity since there is enough free iodine available to cause allergic contact dermatitis.

It should be used only with great caution in intravaginal antisepsis for pregnant women and not routinely in infants $<$ 37 weeks of age.

12. Contamination

Pseudomonas cepacia was recovered from blood cultures of 52 patients in four hospitals in New York City over a 7-month period in 1980 (146). Epidemiologic investigations indicated that this was a pseudobacteremia in which *P. cepacia* entered blood culture tubes from povidone-iodine left on the skin prior to venipuncture. The source was believed to be the water deionization treatment system, which introduced high concentration of bacteria of 10^5-10^7 ml^{-1} that could survive for long periods in 10% povidone-iodine solution containing 1% available iodine. Innate bacterial resistance to iodine or protection of bacteria from iodine by slime or organic materials has been proposed as mechanisms of survival of the bacteria.

E. Halogens: Chlorine-Containing Solutions

Chlorine has been used since 1915, when Dakin introduced 0.45-0.50% sodium hypochlorite for wound antisepsis during World War I.

1. Chemistry

Both free and undisassociated hypochloric acid are germicidal, although free chlorine is more active than combined chlorine.

2. Antimicrobial Activity and Resistance

At pH7, most bacteria are killed by 0.10-0.25 ppm (parts per million) within 15-30 sec. Among the vegetative bacteria, *E. coli* is generally more resistant to chlorine than others. Fungi, protozoa, and viruses also appear to be sensitive (3,147).

3. Therapeutic Indications

Although hypochlorite is inactivated by organic material, it has been used for wound infections. This compound has been shown to dissolve necrotic tissue and to delay clotting (3). It has been used in peritoneal dialysis systems. It is unstable and must be prepared fresh. Sodium hypochlorite solutions, 0.1-1.25%, have been used in controlling athlete's foot infections. Sodium hypochloride may be added to hydrotherapy water to kill organisms on the burn surface. At a water concentration of 850 μg/ml, a one to two log arithmic decrease of bacteria in burn wound surface may be achieved. Because of its instability, hypochlorite has to be prepared fresh before every use.

F. Oxidizing Agents

1. Hydrogen Peroxide

Hydrogen peroxide is able to change the microbial environment by producing a powerful oxidant, the hydroxyl free radical. However, its use as an antiseptic has generally been abandoned as it is unstable in solution and is rapidly decomposed by tissue catalase.

2. Benzoyl Peroxide

The efficacy of benzoyl peroxide in the treatment of acne is generally recognized. It effectively suppresses both aerobes and *Propionobacterium acnes*, presumably by breakdown to benzoic acid and nascent oxygen, resulting in a fall of porphyrin and free fatty acid levels.

G. Phenols

1. Hexachlorophene

a. Chemistry. Phenols have a wide spectrum of activity depending on para substitutions of an alkyl chain up to six carbon atoms in length, halogenation, and nitration. The formula for hexachlorophene (HCP) is shown in Figure 5.

b. Mechanism of Action. Low concentrations of hexachlorophene interrupt the bacterial electron transport chain and inhibit membrane-bound enzymes; higher concentrations rupture bacterial membranes (121).

c. Antimicrobial Activity and Resistance. Hexachlorophene has good gram-positive activity but is generally bacteriostatic rather than bactericidal against gram-negative organisms. A 3% solution will kill *S. aureus* within 15-30 sec, but 24 hr or more are needed for some gram-negative bacteria.

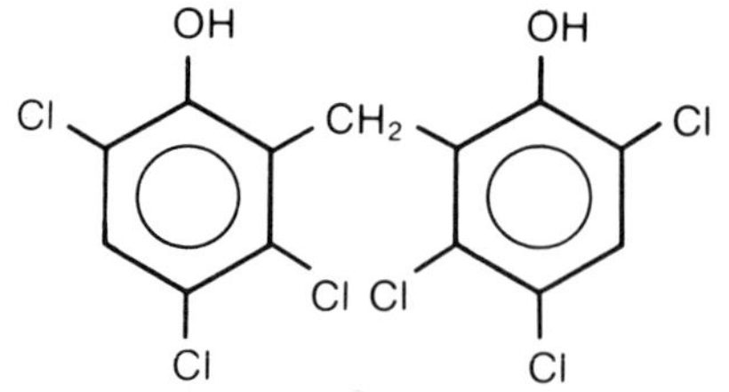

Figure 5 Structure of hexachlorophene.

Ordinary scrubbing followed by days of nonuse result in temporary excessive regeneration of resident bacteria (rebound affect). Its use in nursery population results in the emergence of gram-negative resistant organisms within 1 week (3).

The presence of blood or serum proteins has been shown to adversely affect the bactericidal activity of hexachlorophene, but it does not lose its activity in the presence of soap.

d. Preparation and Dosage. It is available as a 3% cleansing emulsion and as 0.75 and 0.33% liquid soap and 0.5% powder, depending on federal regulations.

e. Assay. A gas-liquid chromatography method modified by Ferry and McQuin appears to be a sensitive and reproducible for measuring plasma concentrations of hexachlorophene (3).

f. Pharmacokinetics. Normal Skin. Animal studies involving both rats and newborn rhesus monkeys show absorption and consequently neurotoxicity similar to that occurring in humans. Hexachlorophene has been detected in the serum of individuals scrubbing hands and forearms with for 10 min, five times a day, 6 days a week for a total of 58 days. Resulting concentrations of 0.05-0.07 μg/ml were not associate with signs of toxicity (148).

Of five adult patients with third-degree burns undergoing daily or more frequent bathing with 3% hexachlorophene, three developed neurological signs associated with hexachlorophene concentrations between 71.0 and 180.4 μmol/liter. The remaining two patients had no clinical findings, although serum concentrations were 82.9 and 537 μmol/liter (149,150).

Full-term Infants: Hexachlorophene concentrations ranging from 0.022 to 1.58 μmol/liter with a mean of 0.266 μmol/liter have been reported in blood specimens taken from 50 newborn infants undergoing routine daily bathing with a 3% hexachlorophene emulsion. No clinical toxicity was noted (149).

Premature Infants: In a report of 10 premature infants who were given total body hexachlorophene baths for 13-82 days, the highest blood concentration (3.88 μmol/liter occurred in a premature infant weighing 822 g at birth. None of the infants had neurological signs, and in follow-up of 33 such infants there were no neurological or developmental abnormalities at 6 months of age.

g. Therapeutic Use. Neonatal (149-152): In 1973, drug-regulating authorities in the United States, Canada, and the United Kingdom introduced regulations to restrict preparations containing hexachlorophene in concentrations greater than 0.75%. In retrospective human studies, there has been no convincing evidence that bathing full-term infants who have intact skin with hexachlorophene is hazardous.

Effectiveness has been demonstrated in several centers. Plueckhahn has shown in a trial between 1960 and 1963 that 3% hexachlorophene was the agent responsible for a decrease in infant staphylococcal sepsis in the maternity wing. In 1965, Simon showed that the routine use of hexachlorophene for skin care of infants was highly effective even in an overcrowded Central American maternity hospital. Similar decreases have been reported in England, where 0.33% hexachlorophene powder has been used in infant skin care since 1957. The use of 0.75% hexachlorophene emulsion has been associated with increased staphylococcal disease, suggesting it is less effective than a 3% emulsion.

The 0.33 or 0.5% hexachlorophene talcum powder or 3% hexachlorophene emulsion may be appropriate and effective antistaphylococcal preparations for use in the skin care of normal newborn infants in maternity hospital.

Preoperative Bathing: Hexachlorophene is particularly useful in elective surgery, where the operative site can be washed with hexachlorophene three or four times per day for several days preoperatively, although chlorhexidine may now be a better choice. It is particularly useful in such areas as the hands, feet, face, and ears, which are difficult to disinfect by ordinary methods, as well as mucous membranes (anus, vagina, and external genitalia).

h. Adverse Effects. In September 1972, a list of adverse reactions with hexachlorophene compiled for the FDA included 13 infant deaths associated with topical use; 9 in burn victims; 2 neonates with congenital icthyosis; a 4-year-old boy who received pHisohex enemas on alternate days for 1 month in the treatment of megacolon; and a 7-month-old premature infant with a rash (149).

i. Reproduction (153,154). A 15% malformation rate (major and minor malformations combined) among the infants of exposed nurse-mothers and a 3.4% rate among offspring of unexposed nurse-mothers has been reported. Although this retrospective cohort study reveals an odds ratio of 4.4, it is not clear if the assiduousness of case finding was equivalent in both groups.

j. Neurotoxicity (149,150,155–160). In a postmortem survey of 20 of 97 low-birth-weight (less than 1750 g) newborn infants who had received limited skin disinfection with 3% HCP emulsion, Anderson et al. found 4 cases who had developed spongiform myelinopathy (HCP concentration in the cerebrum between 6 and 281 ng/g). Another 9 of these 20 infants had detectable amounts of HCP in the brain (HCP between 3 and 40 ng/g) but no myelinopathy.

Plueckhahn observed 63 infants with spongy vacuolization of the central nervous system (CNS) at autopsy between 1959 and 1969, of whom 57 had undergone routine antiseptic skin care (3 or more washings) with a 3% emulsion. All 57 infants weighed 2000 g or less at birth. Such vacuolization did not occur in infants weighing more than 2000 g at birth. Mature human myelin is apparently not affected. This vacuolization in premature infants is probably a manifestation of simple transient edema due to physical interaction of hexachlorophene with the hydrophobic lipid droplets that precede myelination in the CNS of the fetus. This vacuolation appears to be reversible when induced experimentally in infant monkeys (149).

In 1972, an epidemic of unexplained neurological illness in which 204 children became ill and 36 died occurred in four areas of France (161). Affected children presented with erythematous, edematous, ulcerative skin lesions mainly in the diaper area, irritability, drowsiness, vomiting, anorexia, and diarrhea. In more severe cases, convulsions developed followed by weakness, lethargy, and coma. A total of 12 victims had typical vacuolization of the white matter at autopsy. The body powder contained 6.3% hexachlorophene, a white powder similar in appearance to talc.

k. Cutaneous. The application of high concentrations of hexachlorophene may result in erythema and ulceration of normal skin surfaces. *Contamination* with gram-negative organisms, including *E. coli, Klebsiella* sp., and *P. aeruginosa*, has been reported (3).

l. Contraindications. It would appear unwise to use 3% HCP emulsion on the skin of infants weighing under 1750 g during at least the first 2 weeks of life. Its use should be avoided in patients with exfoliative skin disorders.

2. Other Phenols

Chlorophene (*O*-benzyl-*p*-chlorophenol) is bactericidal to gram-positive and gram-negative bacteria and is virucidal to lipid-containing viruses. It is an ingredient of vestal LPH (3).

Hexyl resorcinol is used at a concentration of 1:1000 in pharyngeal antiseptics.

Para-tertiary amylphenol is bactericidal for most gram-positive and gram-negative bacteria, excluding *P. aeruginosa*, and is a component of vestal LPH (3).

Thymol is included in a variety of ointments lotions for acne, analgesia, and cough drops. Its concentration in mouthwashes may be too low to be effective (3).

Triclosan [(2,4-didrchlorophenoxy]-5-chlorophenol, has broad-spectrum activity except against *P. aeruginosa*. A 0.5% tincture has been studied for hand washing (3,162).

H. Silver

1. Chemistry

Inorganic silver salts are highly germicidal in solution (3,163).

2. Mechanism of Action

Silver complexes with electron donor groups containing sulfur, oxygen, or nitrogen, including the bases contained in DNA. Denaturation of protein and disruption of the cell membrane with formation of blobs results in death of the organism. Silver-protein complexes formed under high concentrations of silver ions are applied to tissue and provide a reservoir for the sustained release of silver ions.

3. Antimicrobial Activity

Silver, 1%, effectively kills gram-positive and gram-negative bacteria and fungi. Silver nitrate appears to effectively kill gram-negative and gram-positive bacteria depending on the concentration and time during which the compound is allowed to act. The antibacterial activity of silver sulfadiazine is outlined in Table 10 (163).

Silver sulfadiazine is less soluble than silver nitrate, so that very little protein and chloride ion are precipitated, avoiding problem of hyponatremia, hypochlorema, and adherent eschars. Clinical data confirm the ease with which the concentrations necessary to kill bacteria are achieved in topical preparations.

4. Resistance

There is increasing incidence of silver- and/or sulfadiazine-resistant organisms in hospital. Resistance is plasmid mediated and may include tolerance to other sulfa drugs, heavy metals, and β-lactam antibiotics as well. A burn unit strain of *Salmonella typhinurium* that was resistant to silver nitrate, mercuric chloride, and antibiotics transferred resistance to *E. coli* in vitro. A burn unit strain of *P. aeruginosa* resistant to silver nitrate and gentamicin regained its sensitivity to silver nitrate on subculture, but gentamicin resistance persisted, showing that the two resistances may not be genetically linked.

Sulfadiazine-resistant stains may be silver nitrate sensitive. A center using sulfadiazine widely found sulfadiazine-resistant gram-negative *Klebsiella* that could transfer resistance.

5. Preparation and Dosage

Silver sulfadiazine, 1–3%, is internationally recognized as a prophylactic agent in burn wounds and other dermal conditions. Cerium nitrate silver sulfadiazine is also used.

Table 10 Susceptibility to Silver Sulfadiazine of Bacterial Species

Species	Strain identification no.	MIC[a] (μg silver sulfadiazine per ml)
Providencia	1505	12.5
Proteus rettgeri	1157	6.25
	1689	1.56
P. vulgaris	1677	1.56
Pseudomonas fluorescens	1477	6.25
	1618	<0.78
	1604	6.25
Streptococcus pyogenes	1686	12.5
	3264A	3.13
	3264B	1.56
	1693	12.5
Corynebacterium diphtheriae	1685	12.5
Clostridium perfringens	1687	100
	1694	100
Serratia	1101	6.25
	1254	3.13
Escherichia coli	RTF	3.13
	1200	25
	1334	6.25
Pseudomonas aeruginosa	1186	1.56
P. multiphilia	1422	<0.78
	1610	25
Klebsiella	1415	50
Enterobacter	1249	1.56
	1521	1.56
Proteus mirabilis	1231	1.56
Herellea	1642	6.25
Staphylococcus aureus	1212	50
	1436	25
S. epidermidis	1202	25
Enterococcus (group D streptococcus)	1561	50

[a]Minimal inhibitory concentrations were determined by twofold dilutions in trypticase soy broth.
Source: From HS Carr, TJ Wlodkowski, HS Rosenkranz, Silver sulfadiazine: In vitro antibacterial activity. *Antimicrob. Agents Chemother. 4*:585–587, 1973, with permission.

Continuous application of 0.25 or 0.50% of aqueous silver nitrate to gauze dressings for myelomeningocele sac antiseptics have effectively prevented infection. An ideal bandage for use in promoting healing of skin is one that closes the wound to prevent bacterial contamination, has an antibacterial effect itself, reduces fluid and protein losses, maintains adequate electrolyte balance at the wound surface, and, if possible, stimulates healing while reducing pain. Recently, the addition of silver ion to pigskin xenografts has been shown to result in timed release of silver ions at the wound surface. The effect is immediate and lasts for the 10 days, during which the graft remains adherent. Efficacy has been demonstrated in more rapid re-epithelialization (6.8 vs. 14.2 days) using silver sulfadiazine during therapy of the indolent ulcers of Hansen's disease (164).

6. Therapeutic Use

All these agents are of value prophylactically to prevent burn wound colonization and sepsis until the wound heals as in the case of the partial-thickness injury or until the wound is debrided or excised and grafted. Silver sulfadiazine is administered as a 1% cream in the prophylactic treatment of burns. Increases in wound healing have been noted with silver sulfadiazine compared with neomycin, polysporin, and bacitracin (165).

Water-soluble silver nitrate is used in 10% strength for mouth rinses, as 0.5% (w/w) strength for application to second- and third-degree burns, as 1% for the prevention of ophthalmia neonatorum, as 2% for the same purpose added with 0.85% sodium chloride, and at 2% or less for other eye uses and bladder irrigation.

Toughened silver nitrate as a moistened pencil is used primary for the cauterization of wounds and removal of granulomatous tissue and warts.

Silver acetate is used in creams eye, lotions, and drops.

Silver citrate is dusted on wounds and delicate membranes.

Silver lactate is used at dilutions of 1:100 and 1:2500 antiseptic and astringent.

Silver picrate has been used in glycerine suppositories. Silver 2,2′-methyl-bis is used topically as a 1% solution, cream, or emulsion for burns, varicose ulcers, and pressure sores.

7. Toxicity

As a sulfa, silver sulfadiazine may accordingly cause allergic reactions. It occasionally causes reversible neutropenia in children. Leukopenia may be potentiated if cimetidine is also used. Silver nitrate in a concentration of over 1% and exposure beyond a minute or two can lead to cauterization of the cornea. Silver nitrate, 1%, is associated with the development of conjunctivitis. Repeated use of sulfadiazine on wounds can result in sodium and chloride depletion, hyperosmolarity, argyrism, and methemoglobulinemia through bacterial reduction to nitrate (165). Although the electrolyte disturbance can easily be corrected, the bluish discoloration of the skin mucosa and viscera are virtually permanent (39).

REFERENCES

1. Food and Drug Administration: 1978. OTC Topical Antimicrobial Products. Tentative Final Monograph (21 CFR Part 33), *Federal Register* January 6, *43*(4):1210–1249.
2. Bruch, MK: Methods of testing antiseptics: Antimicrobials used topically in humans. In: *Disinfection Sterilization and Preservation*, 3rd ed. (SS Block, ed.) Lea and Febiger, Philadelphia, 1983, pp. 946–963.

3. Harvey, SC: Antiseptics and disinfectants. In: *The Pharmacological Basis of Therapeutics*, 7th ed. (LS Goodman, AG Gilman, TW Rall, and F Murad, eds.), Macmillan, New York, 1985, pp. 959–979.
4. Harpin, VA, Rutter, N: Barrier properties of the newborn infant's skin. *J. Pediatr. 102*:419–425, 1983.
5. Hall, R, Denton, G, Bucknall, RA: Use and evaluation of antiseptics for the treatment of intact and broken skin (wounds) in hospital. In: *Disinfectants: Their Use and Evaluation of Effectiveness*, Academic Press, New York, 1981, pp. 109–121.
6. Leyden, JJ, Stewart, R, Kligman, AM: Updated in vivo methods for evaluating topical antimicrobial agents on human skin. *J. Invest. Dermatol. 72*:165–170, 1979.
7. Berry, AR, Watt, B, Goldacre, MJ, Thomson, JW, McNair, TJ: A comparison of the use of povidone-iodine and chlorhexidine in the prophylaxis of postoperative wound infection. *J. Hosp. Infect. 3*:55–63, 1982.
8. Boudouma, M, Enjalbert, L, Didier, J: A simple method for the evaluation of antiseptic and disinfectant virucidal activity. *J. Virol. Methods 9*:271–276, 1984.
9. Chen, JHS, Koski, TA: Methods of testing virucides. In: *Disinfection, Sterilization and Preservation*, 3rd ed. (SS Block, ed.), Lea and Febiger, Philadelphia, 1983, pp. 981–997.
10. MacKinnon, IH: The use of inactivators in the evaluation of disinfectants. *J. Hyg. (Camb.) 73*:189–195, 1974.
11. Selwyn, S, Ellis, H: Skin bacteria and skin disinfection reconsidered. *Br. Med. J. 1*:136–140, 1972.
12. Lilly, HA, Lowbury, EJL, Wilkins, MD: Limits to progressive reduction of resident skin bacteria by disinfection. *J. Clin. Pathol. 32*:382–385, 1979.
13. Ayliffe, GAG, Babb, JR, Quoraishi, AH: A test for "hygienic" hand disinfection. *J. Clin. Pathol. 31*:923–929, 1978.
14. Greene, VW: Hospital sterilization practices. In: CRC Handbook Series in Clinical Laboratory Science, Section E; *Clinical Microbiology* (D Seligson, ed.), CRC Press Inc., Cleveland, Ohio, 1977, pp. 415–444.
15. Filho, PPG, Stumpf, M, Cardoso, CL: Survival of gram-negative and gram-positive bacteria artificially applied on the hands. *J. Clin. Microbiol. 21*:652–653, 1985.
16. Larson, E: Handwashing and skin physiologic and bacteriologic aspects. *Infection Control 6*:14–23, 1985.
17. Larson, E: Current handwashing issues. *Infection Control 5*:15–17, 1984.
18. Reybrouck, G: Role of the hands in the spread of nosocomial infections. 1. *J. Hosp. Infect. 4*:103–110, 1983.
19. Rotter, ML: Hygienic hand disinfection. *Infection Control 5*:18–22, 1984.
20. Reber, H: Rationale and testing of degerming procedures. *Infection Control 5*: 28–31, 1984.
21. Selwyn, S: Evaluating skin disinfectants in vivo by excision biopsy and other methods. *J. Hosp. Infect. 6 (Suppl. A)*:37–43, 1985.
22. Hartmann, AA: A comparison of the effect of povidone-iodine and 60% *n*-propanol on the resident flora using a new test method. *J. Hosp. Infect. 6 (Suppl. A)*:73–80, 1985.
23. Gundermann, KO, Christiansen, B, Holler, C: New methods for determining preoperative and postoperative skin disinfection. *J. Hosp. Infect. 6 (Suppl. A)*:51–57, 1985.
24. Newsom, SWB, Matthews, J: Studies on the use of povidone-iodine with the "hygienic hand disinfection" test. *J. Hosp. Infect. 6 (Suppl. A)*:45–50, 1985.
25. Maki, DG, Zilz, MA, Alvarado, CJ: Evaluation of antibacterial efficacy of four agents for handwashing. Current chemotherapy and infectious disease. Proc 11th Int Cong Chem 11: 1979, p. 1089.

26. Gardner, JF, Gray, KG: Chlorhexidine. In: *Disinfection, Sterilization and Preservation*, 3rd ed. (SS Block, ed.), Lea and Febiger, Philadelphia, 1983, pp. 251-270.
27. Altemeier, WA: Surgical antiseptics. In: *Disinfection, Sterilization and Preservation*, 3rd ed. (SS Block, ed.), Lea and Febiger, Philadelphia, 1983, pp. 493–504.
28. MacKintosh, CA, Hoffman, PN: An extended model for transfer of micro-organisms via the hands: Differences between organisms and the effect of alcohol disinfection. *J. Hyg.* *92*:345–355, 1984.
29. Russell, AD: The role of plasmids in bacterial resistance to antiseptics, disinfectants and preservations. *J. Hosp. Infect.* *6*:9–19, 1985.
30. Kevorkian, CG, Merrit, JL, Ilstrup, DM: Methenamine mandelate with acidification: An effective urinary antiseptic in patients with neurogenic bladder. *Mayo Clin. Proc.* *59*:523–529, 1984.
31. Gershanik, J, Boecler, B, Ensley, H, McCloskey, S, George, W: The gasping syndrome and benzyl alcohol poisoning. *N. Engl. J. Med.* *307*:1384–1388, 1982.
32. Platt, J, Bucknall, RA: The disinfection of respiratory syncytial virus by isopropanol and a chlorhexidine-detergent handwash. *J. Hosp. Infect.* *6*:89–94, 1985.
33. Schwartz, MA, Buckwalter, FH: Pharmaceutics of penicillin. *J. Pharm. Sci.* *51*: 1119–1128, 1962.
34. Champagne, S, Fussell, S, Scheifele, D: Evaluation of skin antisepsis prior to blood culture in neonates. *Infection Control* *5*:489–491, 1984.
35. Lilly, HA, Lowbury, EJL, Wilkins, MD, Zaggy, A: Delayed antimicrobial effects of skin disinfection by alcohol. *J. Hyg. (Lond.)* *82*:497–500, 1979.
36. Meers, PD, Yeo, GA: Shedding of bacteria and skin squames after handwashing. *J. Hyg. (Lond.)* *81*:99–105, 1978.
37. Nystrom, B: The merits of alcohol as a skin degerming agent. *Infection Control* *6*: 4, 1985.
38. Gruer, LD, Babb, JR, Davies, JG, Ayliffe, GAJ, Adu, D, Michael, J: Disinfection of hands and tubing of CAPD patients. *J. Hosp. Infect.* *5*:305–312, 1984.
39. Reybrouck, G: Antiseptic drugs and disinfectants. In: *Side Effects of Drugs*, Annual 6 (MNG Dukes and J Elis, eds.), Excerpta Medica, Princeton, 1982, pp. 236-239.
40. Harpin, V, Rutter, N: Percutaneous alcohol absorption and skin necrosis in a preterm infant. *Arch. Dis. Child.* *57*:477–479, 1982.
41. Weintraub, Z, Iancu, TC: Isopropyl alcohol burns. *Pediatrics* *69*:506, 1982.
42. Schick, JB, Milstein, JM: Burn hazard of isopropyl alcohol in the neonate. *Pediatrics* *68*:587–588, 1981.
43. Reybrouck, G: Antiseptic drugs and disinfectants. In: *Side Effects of Drugs*, Annual 7 (MNG Dukes and J. Elis, eds.), Excerpta Medica, Princeton, 1983, pp. 265–270.
45. Varma, BK, et al.: Mouthwash-induced hypoglycemia. *Am. J. Dis. Child.* *132*: 930–931, 1978.
46. Weller-Fahy, ER, Berger, LR, Troutman, WG: Mouthwash: A source of acute ethanol intoxication. *Pediatrics* *66*:302–305, 1980.
47. Brumfitt, W, Dixson, S, Hamilton-Miller, JRT: Resistance to antiseptics in methicillin and gentamicin resistant *Staphylococcus aureus*. *Lancet*, June 22:1442–1443, 1985.
48. Nakahara, H, Kozukue, H: Isolation of chlorhexidine-resistant *Pseudomonas aeruginosa* from clinical lesions. *J. Clin. Microbiol.* *15*:166–168, 1982.
49. Lowbury, EJL, Lilly, HA: The effect of blood on disinfection of surgeons' hands. *Br. J. Surg.* *61*:19–21, 1974.
50. Barnham, M, Kerby, J: Antibacterial activity of combinations of chlorhexidine with neomycin and gentamicin. *J. Hosp. Infect.* *1*:77, 1980.
51. Quesnel, LB, Al-Najjar, AR, and Buddhävudhikrai, P: Synergism between chlorhexidine and sulfadiazine. *J. App. Bacteriol.* *45*:397–405, 1978.

52. Al-Najjar, AR, Quesnel, LB: Synergism between chlorhexidine and polymycins against *Pseudomonas aeruginosa. J. Appl. Bacteriol. 47*:469–476, 1979.
53. Stiles, ME, Sheena, AZ: Efficacy of low-concentration iodophors for germicidal hand washing. *J. Hyg. (Lond.) 94*:269–277, 1985.
54. Schwab, K: The use of germicidal hand rinse. *Infection Control 4*:73, 1983.
55. Brown, TT, Ehrlich, CE, Stehman, FB, Golichowski, AM, Madura, JA, Eitzen, HE: A clinical evaluation of chlorhexidine gluconate spray as compared with iodophor scrub for preoperative skin preparation. *Surg. Gynecol. Obstet. 158*:363–366, 1984.
56. Goldblum, SE, Ulrich, JA, Goldman, RS, Reed, WP, Avasthi, PS: Comparison of 4% chlorhexidine gluconate in a detergent base (Hibiclens) and povidone-iodine (Betadine) for the skin preparation of hemodialysis patients and personnel. *Am. J. Kidney Dis. II*:548–552, 1983.
57. O'Neill, J, Hosmer, M, Challop, R, Driscoll, J, Speck, W, Sprunt, K: Percutaneous absorption potential of chlorhexidine in neonates. *Curr. Ther. Res. 31*:485, 1985.
58. Maloney, MH: Chlorhexidine. Hexachlorophene substitute in the nursery. *Nursing Times*, Vol. 71, ICNA Suppl., Contact 3:21, September 11, 1975.
59. Scopes, JS, Eykyn, S, Phillips, I: Staphylococcal infection in the newborn. *Lancet*, December 7:1392, 1974.
60. Tuke, W: Hibiscrub in the control of staphylococcal infection in neonates. *Nursing Times*, Vol. 71, ICNA Suppl., Contact 3:20, September 11, 1975.
61. Lowbury, EJL, Lilly, HA: Use of 4% chlorhexidine detergent solution (Hibiscrub) and other methods of skin disinfection. *Br. Med. J. 1*:510–515, 1973.
62. Seeberg, S, Brinkhoff, B: Epidemiology and control of staphylococcal pyoderma among newborn infants: Evaluation of a method for routine cord care with 4 per cent chlorhexidine-detergent solution. *J. Hosp. Infect. 5*:121–136, 1984.
63. Fares, E, Selwyn, S, Sethra, T: Chlorhexidine detergent and other alterations to hexachlorophene for use in maternity nurseries. *J. Clin. Pathol. 30*:785–786, 1977.
64. Bygdeman, S, Hambraeus, A, Henningsson, A, Nystrom, B, Skoglund, C, Tunell, R: Influence of ethanol with and without chlorhexidine on the bacterial colonization of the umbilicus of newborn infants. *Infection Control 5*:275–278, 1984.
65. Williams, JD, Waltho, CA, Ayliffe, GAJ, Lowbury, EJL: Trials of five antibacterial creams in the control of nasal carriage of *Staphylococcus aureus. Lancet*, August 19: 390–395, 1967.
66. Bryan, CS, Wilson, RS, Meade, P, Sill, LG: Topical antibiotic ointments for staphyloccal nasal carriers: Survey of current practices and comparison of bacitracin and vancomycin ointments. *Infection Control 1*:153–156, 1980.
67. McManus, AT, Denton, CL, Mason, AD, Jr.: Topical chlorhexidine diphosphanilate (WP-973) in burn wound sepsis. *Arch. Surg. 119*:206–211, 1984.
68. Fine, PD: A clinical trial to compare the effect of two antiseptic mouthwashes on gingival inflammation. *J. Hosp. Infect. 6 (Suppl. A)*:189–193, 1985.
69. Noy, MF, Smith, CA, Watterson, LL: The use of chlorhexidine in catheter bags. *J. Hosp. Infect. 3*:365–367, 1982.
70. Gillespie, WA, Simpson, RA, Jones, JE, Nashef, L, Teasdale, C, Speller, DCE: Does the addition of disinfectant to urine drainage bags prevent infection in catheterised patients? *Lancet*, May 7:1037–1039, 1983.
71. Alder, VG, Burman, D, Simpson, RA, Fysh, J, Gillespie, WA: Comparison of hexachlorophene and chlorhexidine powders in prevention of neonatal infection. *Arch. Dis. Child. 55*:277–280, 1980.
72. Aggett, PJ, Cooper, LLV, Ellis, SH, McAinsh, J: Percutaneous absorption of chlorhexidine in neonatal cord care. *Arch. Dis. Child. 56*:878–882, 1981.
73. Ainamo, J, Asikainen, S, Paloheimo, L: Gingival bleeding after chlorhexidine mouth rinses. *J. Clin. Periodontol. 9*:337–345, 1982.

74. Rudensky, B: False-positive test for protein using dipsticks: Contamination with chlorhexidine antiseptic. *JAMA 246*:1089, 1981.
76. Rosenberg, A, Alatary, SD: Chlorhexidine and contaminants. *Ann. Intern. Med. 84*: 752, 1976.
77. Coyle-Gilchrist, MM, Crewe, P, Roberts, G: *Flavobacterium meningosepticum* in the hospital environment. *J. Clin. Pathol. 29*:824–826, 1976.
78. Anyiwo, CE, Coker, AO, Daniel, SO: *Pseudomonas aeruginosa* in postoperative wounds from chlorhexidine solutions. *J. Hosp. Infect. 3*:189–191, 1982.
79. Kahan, A, Philippon, A, Weber, S, DeGeorges, M: Is chlorhexidine an essential drug? *Lancet*, September 29:759–760, 1984.
81. Czarlinsky, DK, Hall, RT, Barnes, WG, et al.: Staphylococcal colonization in a newborn nursery, 1971–1976. *Am. J. Epidemiol. 109*:218–225, 1979.
82. Speck, WT, Driscoll, JM, Polin, RA, et al.: Staphylococcal and streptococcal colonization of the newborn infant: Effect of antiseptic cord care. *Am. J. Dis. Child. 131*: 1005–1008, 1977.
83. Speck, WT, Driscoll, JM, O'Neil, J, Rosenkranz, HS: Effect of antiseptic cord care on bacterial colonization in the newborn infant. *Chemotherapy 26*:372–376, 1980.
84. Buffenmyer, CL, McDonald, HM: Changing pattern of neonatal colonization with triple-dye crod prophylaxis. *Am. J. Infect. Control 8*:41, 1980.
85. Andrich, MP, Golden, SM: Umbilical cord care. A study of bacitracin ointment vs. triple dye. *Clin. Pediatr. 23*:342–344, 1984.
86. Barrett, FF, Mason, EO, Jr., Fleming, D: The effect of three cord-care regimens on bacterial colonization of normal newborn infants. *J. Pediatr. 94*:796–800, 1979.
87. Wald, ER, Snyder, MJ, Gutberlet, RL: Group B β hemolytic streptococcal colonization. *Am. J. Dis. Child. 131*:178–180, 1977.
88. Bielicky, T, Novak, M: Contact-group sensitization to triphenyl methane dyes: Gentian violet, brilliant green and malachite green. *Arch. Dermatol. 100*:540–543, 1969.
89. Bjornberg, A, Mobacken, H: Necrotic skin caused by 1% gentian violet and brilliant green. *Acta Derm. Venereol. (Stockh.) 52*:55–60, 1972.
90. Schuman, AJ, Oscol, BA: The effect of isopropyl alcohol and triple dye on umbilical cord separation time. *Milit. Med. 150*:49–50, 1985.
91. Berkelman, RL, Holland, BW, Anderson, RL: Increased bactericidal activity of dilute preparations of povidone-iodine solutions. *J. Clin. Microbiol. 15*:635–639, 1982.
92. Favero, MS: Iodine—champagne in a tin cup. *Infection Control 3*:30–32, 1982.
93. Gocke, DJ, Ponticas, S, Pollack, W: In vitro studies of the killing of clinical isolates by povidone-iodine solutions. *J. Hosp. Infect. 6 (Suppl. A)*:59–66, 1985.
94. Rackur, H: New aspects of mechanism of action of povidone-iodine. *J. Hosp. Infect. 6 (Suppl. A)*:13–23, 1985.
95. Gottardi, W: The influence of the chemical behaviour of iodine on the germicidal action of disinfectant solutions containing iodine. *J. Hosp. Infect. 6 (Suppl. A)*:1–11, 1985.
96. Gottardi, W: Iodine and iodine compounds. In: *Disinfection, Sterilization and Preservation*, 3rd ed. (SS Block, ed.), Lea and Febiger, Philadelphia, 1983, pp. 183–196.
97. Hendley, JO, Mika, LA, Gwaltey, JM: Evaluation of virucidal compounds for inactivation of rhinovirus on hands. *Antimicrob. Agents Chemother. 14*:690–694, 1978.
98. U.S. Patent: Germicidal iodine compositions with enhanced iodine stability. U.S. Patent No. 4271149, June 2, 1981.
99. Pollack, W, Iny, O: A physico-chemical study of PVP-I solutions leading to the reformulation of "Betadine" preparations (5% PVP-I). *J. Hosp. Infect. 6 (Suppl. A)*: 25–32, 1985.

100. Georgiade, G, Riefkohl, R, Georgiade, N, Georgiade, R, Wildman, MF: Efficacy of povidone-iodine in pre-operative skin preparation. *J. Hosp. Infect. 6 (Suppl. A)*: 67–71, 1985.
101. Maki, DG, Goldmann, DA, Rhame, FS: Infection control in intravenous therapy. *Ann. Intern. Med. 79*:867–887, 1973.
102. Simmons, BP: CDC guidelines for the prevention and control of nosocomial infections. Guideline for prevention of surgical wound infections. *Am. J. Infect. Control 11*:133–143, 1983.
103. Apt, L, Isenberg, SJ, Yoshimori, R: Antimicrobial preparation of the eye for surgery. *J. Hosp. Infect. 6 (Suppl. A)*:163–172, 1985.
104. Zellner, PR, Bugyi, S: Povidone-iodine in the treatment of burn patients. *J. Hosp. Infect. 6 (Suppl. A)*:139–146, 1985.
105. Bickerstaff, KI, Regnard, C: Prophylactic povidone-iodine spray in accidental wounds. *J. R. Coll. Surg. Edinb. 29*:234–236, 1984.
106. de Kock, M: Topical burn therapy comparing povidone-iodine ointment or cream plus aserbine, and povidone-iodine cream. *J. Hosp. Infect. 6 (Suppl. A)*:127–132, 1985.
107. Sindelar, WF, Brower, ST, Merkel, AB, Takesue, EI: Randomised trial of intraperitoneal irrigation with low molecular weight povidone-iodine solution to reduce intra-abdominal infectious complications. *J. Hosp. Infect. 6 (Suppl. A)*:103–114, 1985.
108. Vallance, S, Waldron, R: Antiseptic vs. saline lavage in purulent and faecal peritonitis. *J. Hosp. Infect. 6 (Suppl. A)*:87–91, 1985.
109. Zamora, JL: Povidone-iodine and wound infection. *Surgery 95*:121–122, 1984.
110. Viljanto, J: Disinfection of surgical wounds without inhibition of normal wound healing. *Arch. Surg. 115*:253–256, 1980.
111. Rodeheaver, G, Bellamy, W, Kody, M, Spatafora, G, Fitton, L, Leyden, K, Edlich, R: Bactericidal activity and toxicity of iodine-containing solutions in wounds. *Arch. Surg. 117*:181–186, 1982.
112. Lacey, RW: Antibacterial activity of povidone-iodine against non-sporing bacteria. *J. Appl. Bacteriol. 46*:443–449, 1979.
113. Kunin, CM: The drainage bag additive saga. *Infection Control 6*:261–262, 1985.
114. Cass, AS, Ireland, GW: Antibacterial perineal washing for prevention of recurrent urinary tract infections. *Urology XXV*:492–494, 1985.
115. van den Broek, PJ, Daha, THJ, Mouton, RP: Bladder irrigation with povidone-iodine in prevention of urinary-tract infections associated with intermittent urethral catheterisation. *Lancet*, March 9:563–565, 1985.
116. Maki, DG, Band, JD: A comparative study of polyantibiotic and iodophor ointments in prevention of vascular catheter-related infection. *Am. J. Med. 70*:739–744, 1981.
117. Galle, PC: Reassessment of the surgical scrub. *Surg. Gynecol. Obstet. 147*:215–218, 1978.
118. Dineen, D: An evaluation of the duration of the surgical scrub. *Surg. Gynecol. Obstet. 129*:1181–1184, 1969.
119. Davies, J, Babb, JR, Ayliffe, GAJ, Wilkins, MD: Disinfection of the skin of the abdomen. *Br. J. Surg. 65*:855–858, 1978.
120. Elek, SD, Conen, PE: The virulence of *Staphylococcus pyogenes* for man. A study of the problems of wound infection. *Br. J. Exp. Pathol. 38*:573–586, 1957.
121. Special problems in hospital antisepsis. In: *Principles and Practice of Disinfection, Preservation and Sterilization* (AD Russell, WB Hugo, and GAJ Ayliffe, eds.), Blackwell Scientific, Boston, 1982, pp. 262–284.
122. Block, SH: Thyroid function abnormalities from the use of topical Betadine solution on intact skin of children. *Cutis 26*:88–89, 1980.

123. Lyen, KR, Finegold, D, Orsini, R, Herd, JE, Parks, JS: Transient thyroid suppression associated with topically applied povidone-iodine. *Am. J. Dis. Child. 136*: 369–370, 1982.
124. Arnonoff, GR, Friedman, SJ, Doedens, DJ, Lavelle, KJ: Increased serum iodide concentration from iodine absorption through wounds treated topically with povidone-iodine. *Am. J. Med. Sci. 279*:173–177, 1980.
125. Rogers, DM, Blouin, GS, O'Leary, JP: Povidone-iodine wound irrigation and wound sepsis. *Surg. Gynecol. Obstet. 157*:426–430, 1983.
126. deJong, TE, Vierhout, RJ, van Vroonhoven, TJ: Povidone-iodine irrigation of the subcutaneous tissue to prevent surgical wound infections. *Surg. Gynecol. Obstet. 155*:221–224, 1982.
127. Lewis, DA, Leaper, DJ, Speller, DCE: Prevention of bacterial colonization of wounds at operation: Comparison of iodine-impregnated ("Ioban") drapes with conventional methods. *J. Hosp. Infect. 5*:431–437, 1984.
128. Lavelle, KJ, Doedens, DJ, Kleit, SA, Forney, RB: Iodine absorption in burn patients treated topically with povidone-iodine. *Clin. Pharmacol. Ther. 17*:355–362, 1975.
129. Quagliana, JM: Effect of topical povidone-iodine (Betadine) on serum protein-bound iodine. *J. Clin. Endocrinol. 23*:395–397, 1963.
130. Clemens, P, Plettner, C, Gruttner, R: Use of povidone-iodine for intravaginal and periumbilical antisepsis. *J. Pediatr. 106*:348, 1985.
131. l'Allemand, D, Gruters, A, Heideman, P, Schurnbrand, P: Iodine-induced alterations of thyroid function in newborn infants after prenatal and perinatal exposure to povidone-iodine. *J. Pediatr. 102*:935–937, 1983.
132. Bachrach, LK, Burrow, GN, Gare, DJ: Maternal-fetal absorption of povidone-iodine. *J. Pediatr. 104*:158–159, 1984.
133. Theodoropoulos, T, Braverman, LE, Vagenakis, AG: Iodide-induced hypothyroidism: A potential hazard during perinatal life. *Science 205*:502–503, 1979.
134. Chabrelle, JP, Rossier, A: Goitre and hypothyroidism in the newborn after cutaneous absorption of iodine. *Arch. Dis. Child. 53*:495–498, 1978.
135. Galina, MP, Avnet, ML, Einhorn, A: Iodides during pregnancy: An apparent cause of neonatal death. *N. Engl. J. Med. 267*:1124–1127, 1962.
136. Vorrherr, H, Vorherr, UF, Mehta, P, Ulrich, JA, Messer, RH: Vaginal absorption of povidone-iodine. *JAMA 244*:2628–2629, 1980.
137. Jacobson, JM, Hankins, GV, Young, RL, Hauth, JC: Changes in thyroid function and serum iodine levels after prepartum use of a povidone-iodine vaginal lubricant. *J. Reprod. Med. 29*:98–100, 1984.
138. Reybrouck, G: Antiseptic and disinfectants. In: *Side Effects of Drugs*, Annual 8 (MNG Dukes and J Elis, eds.), Elsevier, New York, 1984, pp. 243–247.
139. Goodman, LJ, Kaplan, RL, Landau, W, Jung, E, Barrett, JE, Levin, S, Harris, AA: A urine preservative system to maintain bacterial counts. A laboratory and clinical evaluation. *Clin. Pediatr. 24*:383–386, 1985.
140. Ninnemann, JL: Suppressor cell induction by povidone-iodine: In vitro demonstration of a consequence of clinical burn treatment with Betadine. *J. Immunol. 126*:1905–1908, 1981.
141. Marks, JG, Jr.: Allergic contact dermatitis to povidone-iodine. *J. Am. Acad. Dermatol. 6*:473–475, 1982.
143. Bar-Or, D, Mark, JA: False-positive haem detection due to povidone-iodine. *Lancet* September 12:589, 1981.
144. Orchard, JL, Lawson, R: False-positive hemoccult reaction caused by Betadine. *N. Engl. J. Med. 311*:199, 1983 (letter).
145. Howe, DJ: Aspiration pneumonia from povidone-iodine (Betadine): Report of case. *J. Oral Surg. 39*:224, 1981.

146. Berkelman, RL, Lewin, S, Allen, JR, Anderson, RL, Budnick, LD, Shapiro, S, Friedman, SM, Nicholas, P, Holzman, RS, Haley, RW: Pseudobacteremia attributed to contamination of povidone-iodine with *Pseudomonas cepacia*. *Ann. Intern. Med. 95*:32–36, 1981.
147. Dychdala, GR: Chlorine and chlorine compounds. In: *Disinfection, Sterilization and Preservation*, 3rd ed. (SS Block, ed.), Lea and Febiger, Philadelphia, 1983, p. 157.
148. Butcher, HR, Ballinger, WF, Gravens, DL, Dewar, NE, Ledlie, EF, Barthel, WF: Hexachlorophene concentrations in the blood of operating room personnel. *Arch. Surg. 107*:70–74, 1973.
149. Plueckhahn, VD, Ballard, BA, Banks, JM, Collins, RB, Flett, PR: Hexachlorophene preparations in infant antiseptic skin care: Benefits, risks and the future. *Med. J. Aust. 2*:555–560, 1978.
150. Plueckhahn, VD, Banks, J: Hexachlorophene toxicity, the newborn child and the staphylococcus. *Med. J. Aust. 1*:897–903, 1972.
151. Committee on Fetus and Newborn: Skin care of newborns. *Pediatrics 54*:682–683, 1974.
152. Evans, ZA, Rendtorff, RC, Robinson, H, Rosenberg, EW: Ecological influence of hexachlorophene on skin bacteria. *J. Invest. Dermatol. 60*:207–214, 1973.
153. Janerich, DT: Environmental causes of birth defects: The hexachlorophene issue. *JAMA 241*:830–831, 1979.
154. Check, W: New study shows hexachlorophene is teratogenic in humans. *JAMA 240*:513–514, 1978.
155. Cooperman, EM: Hexachlorophene in the nursery. *Can. Med. Assoc. J. 117*:205–206, 1977.
156. Powell, H, Swarner, O, Gluck, L, Lampert, P: Hexachlorophene myelinopathy in premature infants. *J. Pediatr. 82*:976–981, 1973.
157. Kimbrough, RD, Gaines, TB: Hexachlorophene effects on the rat brain. *Arch. Environ. Health 23*:114–118, 1971.
158. Shuman, RM, Leech, RW, Alvord, EC: Neurotoxicity of hexachlorophene in the human. 1. A clinicopathologic study of 248 children. *Pediatrics 54*:689–695, 1974.
159. Gowdy, JM, Ulsamer, AG: Hexachlorophene lesions in newborn infants. *Am. J. Dis. Child. 130*:247–250, 1976.
160. Anderson, JM, Cockburn, F, Forfar, J, Harkness, RA, Kelly, RW, Kilshaw, B: Neonatal spongioform myelinopathy after restricted application of hexachlorophane skin disinfectant. *J. Clin. Pathol. 34*:25–29, 1981.
161. Martin-Bouyer, G, Toga, M, Lebreton, R, Stolley, PD, Lockhart, J: Outbreak of accidental hexachlorophene poisoning in France. *Lancet* January 9:91–95, 1982.
162. Bartzokas, CA, Gibson, MF, Graham, R, Pinder, DC: A comparison of triclosan and chlorhexidine preparations with 60 percent isopropyl alcohol for hygienic hand disinfection. *J. Hosp. Infect. 4*:245–255, 1983.
163. Grier, N: Silver and its compounds. In: *Disinfection, Sterilization and Preservation*, 3rd ed. (SS Block, ed.), Lea and Febiger, Philadelphia, 1983, pp. 375–389.
164. Ersek, RA, Lorio, J: The most indolent ulcers of the skin treated with porcine xenografts and silver ions. *Surg. Gynecol. Obstet. 158*:431–436, 1984.
165. Kulick, MI, Lewis, NS, Bansal, V, Warpeha, R: Hyperosmolality in the burn patient: Analysis of an osmolal discrepancy. *J. Trauma 20*:223–228, 1980.

Part IV
Antifungal Drugs

25
Amphotericin B

ALLAN S. LAU
The Hospital for Sick Children, Toronto, Ontario, Canada

Amphotericin A and B are the two antibiotics produced by *Streptomyces nodosus*, an actinomycete isolated from soil from Templadora on the Orinoco River. The separation and purification of amphotericin B (from that of amphotericin A) for clinical use was accomplished by Vandeputte et al. in 1956 (1). Since then, amphotericin B has remained the drug of choice for the treatment of many systemic fungal infections (2,3). It continues to have potent fungistatic and fungicidal properties against most pathogenic fungal species, only a few of which have developed resistance.

I. CHEMISTRY

Amphotericin B is a polyene antibiotic (4). The polyene antibiotics comprise a complex group of some 200 compounds, produced by various *Streptomyces* species, of which only amphotericin B is sufficiently well tolerated to allow its systemic use in humans. Chemically, polyenes are characterized by a large macrolide ring of carbon atoms, closed by the formation of an internal lactone or ester bond. They differ in the number of carbon atoms, hydroxyl residues, conjugated double bonds (5-7). Amphotericin B is a heptaene macrolide with a mycosamine linked by a glycosidic bond to the hydroxyl group on carbon-19 in the macrolactone ring (Figure 1). All seven double bonds are in the trans conformation (4). These conjugated bonds form the hydrophobic part of the molecule, and the hydroxyl groups and the sugar moiety form the hydrophilic part. This structural arrangement confers an amphiphilic property that is undoubtedly important in the interaction of the drug with biologic membranes.

Amphotericin B also contains a primary amino group and a free carboxyl group. The drug is amphoteric—hence its name—capable of behaving as a base and an acid simultaneously. It is insoluble in water and unstable at extremes of pH. The antifungal activity of the drug is maximum between pH 6.0 and 7.5; activity decreases at low pH (8).

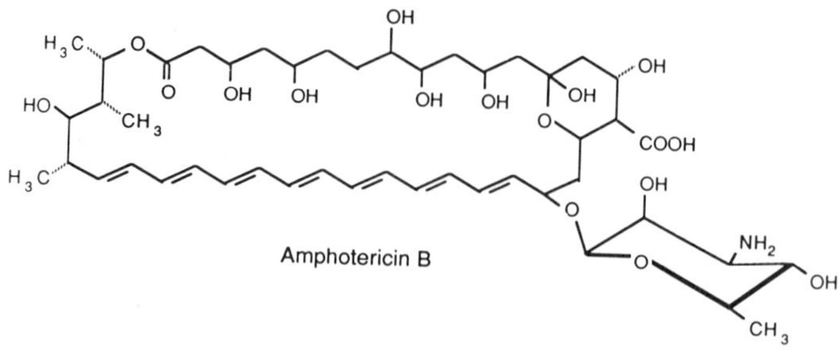

Figure 1 Molecular structure of amphotericin B, showing common structural features of polyenes with a macrolide ring consisting of conjugated double bonds and hydroxyl groups. (From References 4–7.)

II. MECHANISM OF ACTION

Soon after the purification of amphotericin B, several investigators independently demonstrated that polyene antibiotics promote leakage of intracellular K^+ and other cellular constituents of eukaryotic cells (9–11). Further studies indicated that the anticellular action of amphotericin B is due to an interaction of the drug with sterol in the cell membrane. This is supported by the fact that the presence of sterol in natural or artificial membranes renders them sensitive to amphotericin B action (5,6,11,12). In addition, the presence of free sterol into the culture medium antagonizes the anticellular effects of amphotericin B, as demonstrated in studies on *Saccharomyces cerevisiae* and *Candida albicans* (13). Prokaryotic organisms, containing no sterols in their cell membranes, are resistant to amphotericin B action (14).

Recent studies have investigated the mechanisms of action of amphotericin B at a molecular level, using artificial membrane preparations, such as multilamellar or small sonicated unilamellar vesicles. The interaction between the membrane models and amphotericin B were studied by various kinds of spectroscopic methods, including electronic absorption, electronic paramagnetic resonance, and nuclear magnetic resonance (13,15,16). These in vitro experiments support the hypothesis that incorporation of the polyene into the membrane results in the production of aqueous pores consisting of an annulus of amphotericin B and ergosterol (12,17,18). It has been suggested that the hydroxyl region of the polyene faces the interior of this hypothetical pore, thus creating an aqueous channel for the transfer of ions. Further evidence of amphotericin B-sterol interaction was derived from Scatchard analysis of the binding of amphotericin B to lecithin-sterol membranes monitored by electronic absorption; a single complex of 1:1 stoichiometry was observed (19). This polyene-sterol interaction is reversible both in vitro (18) and in vivo (20), and the fungal inhibitory effect would appear to result from the loss of K^+ ion and other intracellular constituents. Indeed, the fungistatic effect of amphotericin B on *C. albicans* can be abolished by the concomitant addition of K^+ and Mg^{2+} to the culture medium (21). In this case, the antibiotic interacts with the plasma membrane but the intracellular concentration of K^+ and Mg^{2+} remains constant.

Despite its growth inhibitory effect, this polyene-induced leakage of intracellular molecules, following reversible binding of amphotericin B to cell surface sterols, may not be the sole mechanism of the lethal action of amphotericin B (22). Studies by Kotler-

Brajiburg et al. indicated that the lethal action of amphotericin B is associated with an irreversible energy-dependent binding of the antibiotic to fungal cell membranes (23). Biochemical events following this irreversible binding and subsequent processes leading to target cell death remain to be investigated. To complicate the matter further, it has been shown that amphotericin B is capable of inducing permeability changes to K^+ and glucose in sterol-free membrane models, although to a lesser extent than in the presence of sterol (24,25).

Both fungal and mammalian cells contain sterols, ergosterol in fungi and cholesterol in mammals (Figure 2). The anticellular effects of amphotericin B are more inhibited by the simultaneous addition of free ergosterol than cholesterol in the culture medium (26). Also, a lower concentration of amphotericin B can be used to induce K^+ leakage from ergosterol-containing membranes than from cholesterol-containing membranes (27). The binding of amphotericin B to sterol is a relatively specific process, with a 10-fold higher affinity for ergosterol than for cholesterol. The basis for this preferred binding of amphotericin B to ergosterol is not fully understood. It is thought that the double bond at carbon-7 in ring B of the ergosterol molecule is responsible for this interaction (28). Other polyenes, such as filipin, also exhibit specific binding to sterol derivatives. However, it shows higher avidity for cholesterol than for ergosterol. Consequently, this polyene product elicits more anticellular effects and damage to the host cells than to the fungal cells (26). This increase in host cell toxicitics limits its use clinically for systemic mycosis.

In addition to its direct antifungal effects, amphotericin B appears to have immunoregulatory properties. Recent studies indicate that, at low concentrations, amphotericin B has paradoxical stimulatory effects on cell proliferation, including that of fungal and mammalian cells in culture. In vitro experiments showed that the polyene is capable of polyclonal B-cell activation of murine lymphocytes (29,30), activation of murine macrophages for phagocytosis, and tumor cell killing (31,32). In animal studies, humoral immunostimulation by amphotericin B was consistently observed with augmented IgM and IgG responses (33). The drug can also potentiate cell-mediated immunity and delayed hypersensitivity (34,35). It has been postulated that a selective toxic effect on suppressor T cell by amphotericin B could account for the immunopotentiating properties observed (36). Another interesting immunomodulatory effect of the drug is its antineoplastic property on advanced syngenic leukemia in AKR mice (37). This antitumor action has

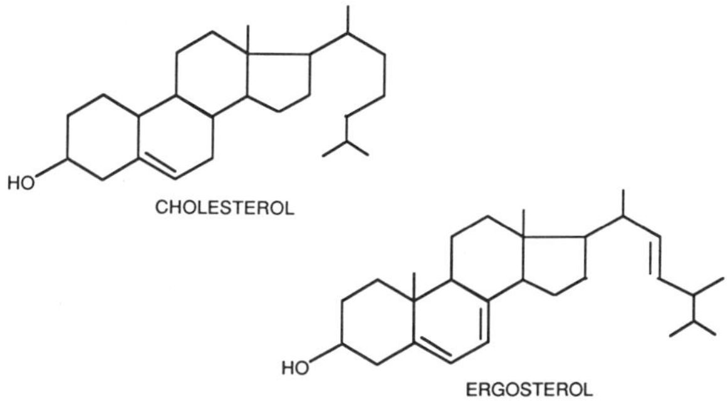

Figure 2 Chemical structures of cholesterol and ergosterol, candidates for specific binding on the plasma membrane with amphotericin B.

been demonstrated to be immune mediated. However, under different experimental conditions, a paradoxical immunosuppressive effect of amphotericin was observed (38,39). These immunomodulatory effects may have clinical importance, particularly in the immunocompromised host with disseminated systemic fungal infections.

In summary, both in vitro and in vivo studies indicate that the pharmacological basis of therapeutic effects of amphotericin B on fungal infections is very complex. The drug has a direct effect on fungal cells mediated by specific binding to the cell surface ergosterol. In addition, this polyene antibiotic modulates the immunologic responses of the host.

III. SPECTRUM OF ANTIFUNGAL ACTIVITY

Amphotericin B is active against many species of fungi, including dermatophytes (*Epidermophyton, Microsporum*, and *Trichophyton*), dimorphic fungi (*Blastomyces dermatitidis, Coccidioides immitis, Paracoccidioides brasiliensis*, and *Histoplasma capsulatum*) molds (*Aspergillus* and *Penicillum*), and yeasts (*Candida* species and *Cryptococcus neoformans*). Minimal inhibitory concentrations (MIC) of amphotericin B for these pathogenic fungi are presented in Table 1 (40). The MIC obtained from different laboratories vary considerably. Such factors as inoculum size, temperature and duration of incubation, and composition of culture medium contribute to the variations of MIC observed. In general, the MIC of these pathogenic fungi range from 0.04 to 0.8 μg/ml. The drug is either fungistatic or fungicidal, depending on the sensitivity of individual fungal species and the concentration of the antibiotic used in the experiment. In addition to its antifungal activities, amphotericin B is toxic to such protozoa as *Entamoeba, Leishmania, Naeglaria*, and *Trypanosoma* (7).

A variety of antimicrobial agents has been studied in combination with amphotericin B. Flucytosine is perhaps the most extensively investigated in this regard. Early studies demonstrated that flucytosine reduced the minimal inhibitory concentration of amphotericin B against *Candida* and cryptococcal species in vitro (41). The combination of these drugs also favorably improves the outcome, than using either drug alone, in the treatment of experimental infections caused by *Candida* and *Cryptococcus* (42-44). In humans, improved outcome has also been demonstrated in the treatment of cryptococcal and

Table 1 Minimal Inhibitory Concentration of Amphotericin B Against Pathogenic Fungi

Organism	MIC (μg/ml)
Blastomyces dermatidis	0.05–0.5
Coccidioides immitis	0.2–0.8
Histoplasma capsulatum	0.4–1.0
Aspergillus sp.	0.14–>8.0
Candida sp.	0.09–1.0
Cryptococcus neoformans	0.2–1.0
Mucor sp.	0.1–>40
Sporotrichum schenkii	0.07–13
Toruloposis glabrata	0.1–0.4

Source: Adapted from Chemel and Louria, Reference 40.

candidal meningitis (45,46). The mechanism of this synergistic interaction remains to be investigated. However, it has been hypothesized that the selective binding of amphotericin B to ergosterol induces increases in the permeability of the fungal membranes, thereby allowing better penetration of flucytosine to exert its anticellular effects. The demonstrable synergistic effects appear to be fungal species specific, as the combination shows no synergism against *H. capsulatum, B. dermatitidis*, or *C. immitis*.

Some combinations of antifungals have demonstrated antagonism in vitro. For example, both miconazole and ketoconazole appear to decrease the effectiveness of the antifungal action of amphotericin B (47,48). The mechanism of this antagonism has been attributed to their inhibition of ergosterol synthesis, with consequent reduction in binding of amphotericin B to the target cells (47).

Enhancement of the antifungal activity of amphotericin B has also been demonstrated when it has been used concurrently with rifampin or monocycline (49-53). For instance, rifampin, which has no antifungal activity by itself, reduces the concentration of amphotericin B required to inhibit the growth of *Aspergillus, Candida,* or *Histoplasma* in vitro (49-51). Similar synergistic effects of the combination against *H. capsulatum* and *B. dermatitidis* infections have been demonstrated in mice (52). Likewise, minocycline enhances the activity of amphotericin B on *Candida* and *Cryptococcus* species (53). These observed synergistic effects are not always consistent (54). Currently, there are no clinical studies supporting the use of these combinations.

The occurrence of amphotericin-resistant mutants of *C. albicans* has been reported sporadically in immunocompromised hosts (55,56) but has not yet posed a serious problem clinically. Most of the in vitro studies on fungal resistance have been conducted with mutagen-treated cultures or serial subcultures of strains of *C. albicans* or *C. immitis* in increasing concentrations of amphotericin. Resistant mutants of *C. albicans* have an altered colonial morphology, slower rate of growth, and decreased virulence for animals. Interestingly, amphotericin B resistance in these strains appears to be associated with an alteration in the sterol composition of the fungal membrane, resulting from a block in ergosterol biosynthesis (55,57,58).

IV. PHARMACOKINETICS

Although amphotericin B has been used as the principal systemically administered antifungal agent for more than two decades, pharmacological studies are scarce. Most of the studies were done in adults, with little or no data on the disposition of the drug in children (59-61). Amphotericin B is poorly absorbed from the gastrointestinal tract. Oral intake of 3 g of the antibiotic produces plasma concentrations of approximately 0.1 μg/ml. Intravenous administration of the drug is therefore required to attain therapeutic concentrations. Following a daily dose of 0.4-0.6 mg/kg, the serum peak concentrations range from 0.5 to 2 μg/ml. The average steady-state concentration of the drug in plasma approaches 0.5 μg/ml (59).

During intravenous therapy, the drug molecule segregates from the colloidal admixture of amphotericin-desoxycholate, the formulation used to enhance colloidal dispersion of the insoluble antibiotic for intravenous administration (62). More than 95% of the drug subsequently binds to serum proteins (63), principally to cholesterol moieties carried on β-lipoproteins (64). More than 90% of the drug leaves the circulation promptly and possibly is bound to cholesterol-containing cytoplasmic membranes. Amphotericin B is stored in the liver, muscles, and other organs and returns into the circulation slowly (60).

Atkinson and Bennett (60) postulated a three-compartment model for the distribution behavior of amphotericin B in adults: the drug is introduced into a central intravascular compartment and rapidly distributed into two peripheral extravascular compartments, of which one is fast and the other slow to equilibrate. About two-thirds of the administered drug is located in the latter compartment when steady state is achieved. Initially, the drug is rapidly eliminated, with a half-life of 24 hr. In the second elimination phase, the half-life of amphotericin B was computed to be approximately 15 days, reflecting slow release of the drug from a peripheral compartment of high storage capacity. In adults this slow-equilibrating compartment possesses a volume of 220 liters compared with 30 liters of the other two compartments. The total distribution volume is very large (4 liters/kg), indicating high storage capacity. This model is in accord with previous pharmacological studies of the drug (61).

Atkinson and Bennet also attempted to calculate the time taken to reach steady state utilizing two different dose regimens (60). With the first regimen, amphotericin B was given at 1 mg on the first day and 5, 10, and 15 mg on the subsequent 3 days, respectively. The serum concentrations required for antifungal activity (0.3-0.5 μg/ml) were reached only on day 4 and were maintained for 10 hr. In contrast, with the second regimen (25 mg on days 1 and 2; 30 mg on days 3 and 4), the desired serum concentrations were achieved on day 2 and maintained thereafter. The results of this study constitute the pharmacological basis for recommending an initial dose of at least 0.3 mg/kg of amphotericin B for severely ill patients with disseminated mycosis rather than a test done of 1 mg/kg.

Renal excretion of amphotericin B is very slow, and only 3% of a dose is excreted in active form (59,65). Pre-existing renal or hepatic failure has no effect on the plasma concentrations of the drug. Even in anephric patients, there is no accumulation of the drug (66). Biliary excretion accounts for less than 20% of the drug dose (65). Following cessation of intravenous therapy, the drug can be detected in urine for at least 8 weeks. Hemodialysis does not alter blood concentrations of the drug (63).

Concentrations of amphotericin B in body fluids are lower than that of serum, as shown in Table 2 (67). In the pleura, peritoneum, and synovium, approximately 50% of the serum concentrations are achieved. The drug readily crosses the placenta barrier. There is little penetration into the cerebrospinal fluid even in the presence of inflamma-

Table 2 Concentrations of Amphotericin B in Body Fluids

Source	Body fluid (μg/ml)	Serum (μg/ml)
Pleura	0.66	1.02
Peritoneum	0.22-0.32	0.4-1.7
Joint synovium	0.29	0.78
Cerbrospinal fluid	0.05	1-2.12
Vitreous humor	0.05-0.17	0.3-1.0
Bronchial secretion	0-0.16	1.36
Cord blood	0.37	1.26
Amniotic fluid	0.16	1.26

Source: Adapted from Polak, Reference 67.

tion. Likewise, concentrations in vitreous humor, bronchial secretion, and amniotic fluid are very low (67).

Until recently there have been no detailed studies concerning the clinical pharmacology of amphotericin B in neonates or infants. Consequently, guidelines for the use of this drug in these age groups were extrapolated from those of the adult studies. In a recent study, Baley et al. studied the pharmacokinetics of the drug in 13 preterm infants treated for fungal infection at 22 ± 16 days of life (68). Amphotericin dose was serially increased in most infants from 0.1 to 0.5 mg/kg·day, given intravenously over 4-6 hr. Three infants received 0.8 mg/kg day^{-1}. Of 5 patients studied during the first dose, only 2 who received 0.8 mg/kg had detectable concentrations. Although 9 neonates had elimination of amphotericin between doses, 4 showed a plateau resulting in drug accumulation. Steady-state pharmacokinetic parameters were $T_{1/2}$ of 25.5 ± 25.5 hr; V_d 4.7 ± 6.1 liters/kg; and clearance 26.3 ± 20 ml/min 1.73 m^2.

Concentrations in cerebrospinal fluids corresponded to 40-90% of plasma levels. The authors concluded that in order to achieve therapeutic concentrations, the initial dose should be at least 0.5 mg/kg day^{-1}. The dose interval should be at least 24 hr, and serum concentrations should be monitored to avoid drug accumulation (68). Cherry et al. (69) reported concentrations of amphotericin B in serum and cerebrospinal fluid (CSF) of a 4 1/2-year-old child receiving 1.2 mg/kg intravenously on alternate days. The serum trough concentration 44 hr after administration of the drug was 0.48 μg/ml. The concentration simultaneously attained in the CSF was 0.24 μg/ml. In a recent report, random determination of serum amphotericin concentrations yielded a range of 0.29-0.43 μg/ml in a 3-year-old child, whereas the concentrations in a neonate ranged from 2.3 to 5.0 μg/ml (70). Both patients were treated with 0.5 mg/kg day^{-1} of amphotericin B.

V. PREPARATIONS, ROUTES OF ADMINISTRATION, AND DOSAGE

The commercially available preparation of amphotericin B for parenteral use is marketed in 50-mg vials that also contain 41 mg desoxycholate (to effect a colloidal dispersion of the insoluble antibiotic) and 25.2 mg sodium phosphate buffer. Less than 1% of the preparation is amphotericin A and other impurities. The contents of the vial should be reconstituted in 10 ml sterile water and administered intravenously in 5% dextrose in water to make a final concentration of no more than 0.1 mg/ml. Solutions of other electrolytes, preservatives, or acidic pH buffers should not be added, as they cause precipitation of the colloid (71). The infusion bottle does not require light shielding (72). The drug decomposes slowly in solution, but the effect is negligible under usual conditions of intravenous administration over 4-6 hr. Even without aggregation, the colloidal solution is partially retained by a 0.22-μm pore filter (73); therefore hyperalimentation lines should use 0.45-μm pore filters. Fever and chills in response to intravenous administration of the drug may be alleviated by the addition of 0.7 mg/kg of hydrocortisone hemisuccinate in some patients. Meperidine may also be effective in this regard (74). Heparin (1 U/ml) is customarily added to the infusion, although there is no proof that this decreases thrombophlebitis.

There is no consensus on the most effective dosage and schedule for the administration of amphotericin B. In adults, therapy is commonly begun with a small test dose of 1 mg, given intravenously over 20-30 min. Subsequent to the test dose, vital signs are monitored closely. A patient with a rapidly progressive infection, with good cardiopulmonary status and a mild reaction to the test dose, can be given immediately 0.3

mg/kg of amphotericin B over a period of 2-6 hr. If the patient is chronically debilitated with cardiopulmonary impairment or has a severe reaction to the test dose, a smaller second dose, such as 5 or 10 mg, should be used. This may then be increased by 5-10 mg to a final daily dose of 0.5-0.7 mg/kg over a period of 5-7 days (2,3,13). Therapy for indolent mycosis may also be initiated slowly to avoid undesirable side effects. In children, we usually start with 0.25 mg/kg and increase the amount by 0.25 mg/kg daily until the full daily maintenance dose of 1 mg/kg is achieved.

Daily maintenance doses of 1.5 mg/kg have been used and recommended. However, such regimens have no proven therapeutic advantages and often cause renal toxicity. Others have suggested that daily doses of 0.3-0.5 mg/kg may be adequate for the treatment of most mycoses, provided that the serum concentration of amphotericin B can be measured. Amphotericin B may be administered on alternate days by doubling the recommended daily dose without affecting therapeutic efficacy (3). In adults the individual dose given should not exceed 70 mg in the alternate-day schedule, even if the daily dose is more than 35 mg. Doses above 70 mg have no proven additional efficacy but are often associated with toxicity. Apart from its convenience and more ambulation for the patient, this alternate-day regimen does not reduce the incidence of nephrotoxicity but may increase the occurrence of febrile reactions. Likewise, the individual dose given in children should not exceed 1.0 mg/kg every other day.

VI. DRUG ASSAYS

Concentrations of amphotericin B in biologic fluids have been measured by bioassays (59). Recently, newer techniques, including rubidium 86 release (75), radiometric respirometry (76), and high-pressure liquid chromatography (77), have been described. The latter is the most promising method to follow the pharmacological behavior of the drug in patients. It is an accurate, reproducible, and relatively simple procedure for the measurement of the drug. A further advantage of this method is that it only requires 50 μl serum for the assay and is therefore particularly useful for pediatric patients.

VII. THERAPEUTIC USES

Amphotericin B is the drug of choice for most systemic fungal infections, including aspergillosis, blastomycosis, candidiasis, coccidioidomycosis, cryptococcosis, histoplasmosis, mucormycosis, paracoccidioidomycosis, and extracutaneous sporotrichosis (2,3,13). The duration of therapy with amphotericin B varies with the nature, severity, progression of the fungal infection, and development of drug toxicities. These untoward effects may necessitate temporary cessation of therapy or a reduction in the dose of intravenous infusion. There are no good objective data on the appropriate length and total dose of therapy for most systemic mycoses. In general, adult patients are treated with a total dose of 1.5-2.0 g of amphotericin B over a period of 6-12 weeks. In the pediatric population, this can be extrapolated as 20-30 mg/kg for the total dose of treatment. A low-dose regimen has been recommended for certain types of candidal infections, including infections limited to the skin, esophagus, or urinary tract (8,78). In this protocol, an adult patient receives a total dose of 100-200 mg (0.3 mg/kg day^{-1} in a pediatric patient) of amphotericin B over 7-10 days.

In addition to intravenous administration, local instillation of amphotericin B may be utilized in certain types of fungal infection. Sporotrichosis or coccidioidomycosis of joints may benefit from intra-articular injections of 5-15 mg of the drug, depending on joint size (79). This route should be used only when it is necessary to deliver a high dose of the drug to a confined site; the safety of this route of administration is not established. Bladder irrigations with amphotericin B, 50 μg/ml, in distilled water have been used in candidal cystitis (80). Corneal irrigations with 1 mg/ml are beneficial but irritating in corneal keratomycosis. Indeed, Hill et al. reported therapeutic success in direct instillation of 40 μg amphotericin B into the anterior chamber of the eye in an infant with endophthalmitis due to *Candida* (81).

In children with coccidioidal or candidal meningitis, intravenous therapy should be accompanied by intrathecal administration of amphotericin B. The drug can be injected into the lumbar or cisternal space, or it may be directly injected into the ventricles by means of an Ommaya reservoir (82,83). In older, cooperative children, amphotericin B can be injected in the lumbar area and the patient placed into the Trendelenburg position to enhance distribution. Cisternal injection is subsequently used, because of the higher incidence of arachnoiditis associated with the lumbar route. In young children, intraventricular therapy using an Ommaya device is preferred. After a test dose of 0.025 mg, the amount is progressively increased until a maintenance dose of 0.1-0.5 mg is achieved. At that time, therapy can be given every other day, alternating with intravenous administration. However, in infants, the initial intrathecal dose should be 0.01 mg, gradually increased over a period of 7 days to 0.1 mg given every other day (84). In the case of coccidioidal meningitis, the duration of CSF treatment usually exceeds that of intravenous therapy and may extend for years until CSF cultures are negative for at least 1 year (82). Unavoidable side effects of ventricular injection include nausea, vomiting, fever and chills, headaches, and occasionally paralysis of lower extremities, disturbances of bladder and bowel functions, seizures, and coma (85). The addition of 5-15 mg hydrocortisone to the injection mixture may alleviate some side effects.

With advances in cancer chemotherapy and improved survival of immunocompromised patients, the judicial use of amphotericin B has become increasingly important. This subject of empirical therapy with the antifungal agent in these delibitated hosts with fever and unidentified infections has been extensively reviewed (86,87). In summary, patients presenting with prolonged neutropenia and refractory fever despite broad-spectrum antibiotics are at high risk of developing systemic fungal infections. These patients should be empirically treated with intravenous amphotericin B. Such therapy should be continued throughout the neutropenic period. If definitive or presumptive evidence for systemic mycosis exists, a full course of therapy should be completed. Otherwise, amphotericin B should be discontinued once the neutropenia has resolved. In addition, prophylactic oral amphotericin B has been examined in patients with acute leukemia (88). The drug at a dose of 250 mg given four times a day orally was effective in reducing the incidence of systemic candidiasis.

There are anecdotal reports of the therapeutic efficacy of different antifungal combinations in the treatment of infections caused by *Aspergillus* (89), *Candida* (90), or *Cryptococcus* (91). Among them, the combination of flucytosine and amphotericin B is the most promising because of the ability of flucytosine to permit lower doses of amphotericin B used and the ability of the latter to prevent drug resistance against the former. A prospective randomized trial has investigated the use of the combination in the management of adults with cryptococcal meningitis (45). In this study, amphotericin B was given at 0.4 mg/kg day^{-1} for 10 weeks when used alone or at 0.3 mg/kg day^{-1} for 6 weeks in combination with 150 mg/kg day^{-1} of flucytosine. Among the 51 patients with cryptococcal meningitis who were randomized for treatment, the combination cured or improved more patients, produced fewer relapses, and resulted in more rapid sterilization of the cerebrospinal fluid. Nephrotoxicity was significantly less with the combination, although side effects of flucytosine, including neutropenia, thrombocytopenia, and diarrhea, occurred frequently. In fact, combination regimens with amphotericin B doses in excess of 0.3 mg/kg day^{-1} or 0.6 mg/kg every other day cause sufficient azotemia to make concurrent administration of flucytosine difficult. With these high doses, the amphotericin B-sparing function of flucytosine is abolished.

In a retrospective review, the therapeutic efficacy of combined therapy with amphotericin B and flucytosine for candidal meningitis was observed in children (46). In this study, 11 of the 17 patients examined were 12 months of age or younger; 7 of them were neonates. Although 2 of the premature neonates died, all others improved with the combination therapy. Interestingly, three *Candida* isolates from these infants were resistant to flucytosine, with MIC of more than 50 μg/ml; one of these was also resistant to amphotericin B, with MIC of 625 μg/ml. However, all patients on the combination therapy were cured and recovered with no major impairment (46).

In summary, the clinical experience to date indicates that combination therapy of amphotericin B and flucytosine provides effective treatment for patients with cryptococcal or candidal meningitis. Such therapeutic regimens may allow a lower daily dose of amphotericin B, thereby alleviating the toxicity of amphotericin B during the prolonged course of therapy. Combination therapy also allows avoidance of intrathecal administration of amphotericin B.

VIII. DERIVATIVES OF AMPHOTERICIN B

Attempts to improve the therapeutic-toxicity ratio of amphotericin B led to the synthesis of several derivatives. Among them, amphotericin B methyl ester is an ester derivative that retains antifungal activity (92). In vivo studies on animals demonstrated that the derivative has less nephrotoxicity than the parent compound (93,94). Unfortunately, recent clinical trials have reported severe leukoencephalopathy in patients receiving this drug (95). Consequently, further studies have been suspended.

Lopez-Berestein et al. have developed a technique of liposomal encapsulation of amphotericin B. They have reported a decrease in toxicity and enhancement in efficacy in experimental candidiasis in mice (96,97). A preliminary clinical trial of the liposomal-encapsulated amphotericin B revealed favorable clinical responses in 67% of the patients with cancer treated for systemic fungal infections (98).

IX. TOXICITIES

The toxicity of amphotericin B in humans is significant and can be categorized into acute and chronic effects. The acute toxicities during the course of therapy include fever, chills, nausea, vomiting, flushing, generalized pain, headache, and, less frequently, seizures, hypotonia, and transient mild bone marrow suppression with leukopenia, anemia, or thrombocytopenia. In adults, 50% of the initial intravenous injections of the drug are associated with chills and 20% with vomiting and high temperature up to 40°C. With the progression of therapy, patients usually become tolerant to these side effects. These can be ameliorated with premedications, such as meperidine, phenothiazines, antihistamines, and hydrocortisone (2,3,8,13). In both adults and children, thrombophlebitis at the infusion site is common. Convulsions and cardiac arrhythmias, although rare, may occur, especially during rapid infusion of amphotericin B with concentrations exceeding 0.1 mg/ml. Amphotericin B frequently induces a normochromic, normocytic anemia associated with very low concentrations of erythropoietin (99). Occasionally, leukopenia and thrombocytopenia may occur (100). These hematologic disturbances are transient and subside after cessation of the drug therapy. Lethal pulmonary reaction with the combined use of amphotericin B and leukocyte transfusions have been reported (101). Simultaneous administration of the drug with leukocytes should be avoided.

Renal dysfunction is the most important toxic effect of amphotericin B. In 93% of adult patients, the glomerular filtration rate falls about 40% immediately following initiation of therapy (102). It usually stabilizes at 20-60% of the normal filtration rate throughout the treatment course. This is associated with elevations of blood urea and creatinine and with hypokalemia. If renal function further deteriorates, the drug should be discontinued for a few days to allow the serum creatinine level to fall below 3.5 mg per 100 ml. This is necessary to help keep nausea and vomiting from causing excessive discomfort, dehydration, and cachexia. Following improvement of renal functions, the previously administered dose can be reinstituted for the completion of therapy. In most patients, renal functions return to normal months after cessation of amphotericin B treatment. However, some patients after receiving 4 g or more of the drug sustain as much as 50% reduction in glomerular filtration rate for an extended period of time (102,103). The degree of renal damage appears to correlate with the total dose of amphotericin B received and is believed to result from drug-induced renal vasoconstriction as well as from the direct toxicity of amphotericin B on renal tubules (104). Other renal abnormalities include distal renal tubular acidosis, cylindruria, and impaired urinary concentrating ability (105-107). Hypokalemia due to urinary potassium loss may be profound and requires vigorous replacement therapy. Although concomitant administration of mannitol or sodium bicarbonate prevents nephrotoxicity in animals (108,109), human studies with mannitol have not documented a protective effect (110).

There are few data on the toxicity of amphotericin B in infants and children. Cherry et al. reviewed the literature on children aged between 2 months and 12 years who received amphotericin B for 2 weeks or more (69). They found a similar incidence of nephrotoxicity compared to that of adults when the doses received by the pediatric patients were corrected to dosage per 1.73 m. Of 19 children whose renal functions were studied during therapy, 12 had abnormalities: 7 with only proteinuria and 5 with elevated blood urea, proteinuria, and cylinduria. Also, of 13 children whose renal functions were assessed 3 months after cessation of therapy, only 3 had a slight to moderate degree of nephrotoxicity. In another retrospective study, Wilson et al. reviewed the course of amphotericin B therapy in 20 children with cancer (111). They found azotemia (BUN $>$ 20 mg/dl) in 96%, and hypokalemia ($K^+ < 3$ mEq/liter) in 46% of treatment courses. The incidence of transient proteinuria and hematuria were found in 15 and 10% of patients, respectively.

In the intensive care setting, the incidence of nephrotoxicity in neonates receiving amphotericin B appears to be highly variable. In two studies including neonates with birth weights less than 1500 g, the drug has been well tolerated (112,113). Nephrotoxicities documented were mild and usually resolved after cessation of the antifungal therapy (112). In contrast, Baley et al. reported profound nephrotoxicity, including severe oliguria or anuria, rises in urea and creatinine, and severe hypokalemia during amphotericin therapy of neonates with a mean birth weight of 788 g (114).

The effect of amphotericin B on the fetus has not been extensively investigated. Several pregnant patients have received the drug systemically without fetal damage (115). Nevertheless, the safety of the drug in pregnancy is not clearly established.

Monitoring of amphotericin B toxicity is absolutely necessary during the course of antifungal therapy. Laboratory studies include hemograms and urinalysis, as well as determinations of serum potassium, magnesium, urea nitrogen, and creatinine. These tests should be obtained as a baseline before treatment and twice a week during therapy. If evidence of increasing toxicity appears, the dose may have to be adjusted.

REFERENCES

1. Vandeputte, J, Wachtel, JL, Stiller, ET: Amphotericin A and B, antifungal antibiotics produced by a streptomyces II. The isolation and properties of the crystalline amphotericins. In: *Antibiotics Annals*, Medical Encyclopedia, Inc., New York, 1956, pp. 587–591.
2. Bennett, JE: Antifungal agents. In: *Principle and Practice of Infectious Diseases* (GL Mandell, RG Douglas, JE Bennett, eds.), Wiley Medical Books, New York, 1984, pp. 263–266.
3. Drugs for the treatment of systemic fungal infection. *Med. Lett. 26*:36–38, 1984.
4. Mechlinski, W, Schaffner, CB, Ganis, P, Avitabile, G: Structure and absolute configuration of the polyene macrolide antibiotic amphotericin B. *Tetrahedron Lett. 44*:3873-3876, 1970.
5. Hamilton-Miller, JMT: Chemistry and biology of the polyene macrolide antibiotics. *Bacteriol. Rev. 37*:166–196, 1973.
6. Norman, AW, Spielvogel, AM, Wong, RG: Polyene antibiotic-sterol interaction. In: *Advances in Lipid Research*, Vol. 14 (R Paoletti and D Kritchecski, eds.), Academic Press, New York, 1976, pp. 127–170.
7. Kobayashi, GS, Medoff, G: Antifungal agents: Recent development. *Annu. Rev. Microbiol. 31*:291, 1977.
8. Sande, MA, Mandell, GL: Antifungal agents: Amphotericin B. In: *The Pharmacologic Basis of Therapeutics* (LS Goodman and A Gilman, eds.), Macmillan, New York, 1985, pp. 1219–1239.
9. Kinsky, SC: Alteration in permeability of *Neurospora crassa* due to polyene antibiotic. *J. Bacteriol. 82*:889–897, 1961.
10. Marini, F, Aynow, P, Lampen, JO: The effect of monovalent cations on the inhibition of yeast metabolism by nystatin. *J. Gen. Microbiol. 24*:51–62, 1961.
11. Hamilton-Miller, JMJ: Fungal sterols and the mode of action of the polyene antibiotics. *Adv. Appl. Microbiol. 17*:109–134, 1974.
12. Kerridge, D: The polyene macrolide antibiotics. *Postgrad. Med. J. 55*:653–656, 1979.
13. Medoff, G, Brajtburg, Kobayashi, GS: Antifungal agents useful in therapy of systemic fungal infections. *Annu. Rev. Pharmacol. Toxicol. 23*:303–330, 1983.
14. Lampen, JO: Interference by polyene antibiotics with specific membrane functions. *Symp. Soc. Gen. Microbiol. 16*:111, 1966.
15. Chen, WC, Bittman, R: Kinetics of association of amphotericin B with vesicles. *Biochemistry 16*:4145–4149, 1977.
16. Brown, JM, Sidebottom, PJ: Theproton magnetic resonance spectrum of amphotericin B. *Tetrahedron 37*:1421–1428, 1981.
17. De Kruijff, B, Demel, RA: Polyene antibiotic-sterol interactions in membranes of *Acholeplasma laidlawii* cells and lecithin liposomes. III. Molecular structures of polyene antibiotic-cholesterol complexes. *Biochim. Biophys. Acta 339*:57–70, 1974.

18. Holz, RW: The effects of the polyene antibiotics nystatin and amphotericin B on thin lipid membranes. *Ann. N.Y. Acad. Sci. 235*:469, 1974.
19. Readio, JD, Bittman, R: Equilibrium binding of amphotericin B and its methyl ester and borate complex to sterols. *Biochim. Biophys. Acta 685*:219–224, 1982.
20. Kerridge, D, Koh, TY, Johnson, AM: The interaction of amphotericin B methyl ester with protoplasts of *Candida albicans. J. Gen. Microbiol. 96*:117–123, 1976.
21. Kerridge, D, Koh, TY, et al.: The production and properties of protoplasts from the dimorphic yeast *Candida albicans*. In: *Microbial and Plant Protoplast* (JF Peberdy, AH Rose, et al., eds.), Academic Press, New York, 1976, p. 230.
22. Chen, CC, Chou, DL, Feingold, DS: Dissociation between ion permeability and the lethal action of polyene antibiotics on *Candida albicans. Antimicrob. Agents Chemother. 13*:914–918, 1978.
23. Kotler-Brajiburg, J, Medoff, G, et al.: Characterization of the binding of amphotericin B to *Saccharomyces cerevisiae* and relationship to the antifungal effects. *Antimicrob. Agents Chemother. 6*:770–776, 1974.
24. Hsu Chen, CC, Feingold, DS: Polyene antibiotic action on lecithin liposomes: Effect of cholesterol and fatty acyl chains. *Biochem. Biophys. Res. Commun. 51*: 972–978, 1973.
25. Archer, DB: Effect of the lipid composition of *Mycoplasma mycoides* subspecies Capri and phosphatidylcholine vesicles upon the action of polyene antibiotics. *Biochim. Biophys. Acta 436*:68–76, 1976.
26. Kotler-Brajtburg, J, Price, HD, Medoff, G, et al.: Molecular basis for the selective toxicity of amphotericin B for yeast and filipin for animal cells. *Antimicrob. Agents Chemother. 5*:377–382, 1974.
27. Teerlink, T, DeKruijff, B, Demel, RA: The action of pimaricin etruscomycin and amphotericin B on liposomes with varying sterol content. *Biochim. Biophys. Acta 599*:484–492, 1980.
28. Feigin, AM, Belousova, I, Yakhimovich, IM: Role of the number and position of double bonds in the four ring sterol nucleus in reaction with polyene antibiotics. *Biofizika 24*:330–331, 1979.
29. Hammarström, L, Smith, E: Mitogenic properties of polyene antibiotics for murine B cells. *Scand. J. Immunol. 5*:37–43, 1976.
30. Hammarström, L, Smith, E: In vitro activating properties of polyene antibiotics for murine lymphocytes. *Acta Pathol. Microbiol. Scand.* [*C*] *85*:277–283, 1977.
31. Lin, HS, Medoff, G, Kobayashi, GS: Effect of amphotericin B on macrophages and their precursors cells. *Antimicrob. Agents Chemother. 11*:154–160, 1977.
32. Chapman, HA, Hibbs, JB: Modulation of macrophage tumoricidal capability by polyene antibiotics: Support for membrane lipid as a regulatory determinant of macrophage function. *Proc. Natl. Acad. Sci. USA 75*:4349–4353, 1978.
33. Little, JR, Blanke, TJ, Valeriote, F, Medoff, G: Immunoadjuvant and antitumor properties of amphotericin B. In: *Immune Modulation and Control of Neoplasia by Adjuvant Therapy* (MA Chirigos, ed.), Raven Press, New York, 1978, pp. 381–387.
34. Shirley, SF, Little, JR: Immunopotentiating effects of amphotericin B. I. Enhanced contact sensitivity in mice. *J. Immunol. 123*:2878–2882, 1979.
35. Shirley, SF, Little, JR: Immunopotentiating effects of amphotericin B. II. Enhanced in vitro responses of murine lymphocytes. *J. Immunol. 123*:2883–2889, 1979.
36. Stobo, JD, Paul, S, Van Scoy, RE, Hermans, PE: Suppressor thymus-derived lymphocytes in fungal infection. *J. Clin. Invest. 57*:319–328, 1976.
37. Medoff, G, Valeriote, F, Lynch, RG, et al.: Synergistic effect of amphotericin B and ,3-Bis(2-chlorethyl)-1-nitrosourea (BCNU) against a syngenic transplantable AKR leukemia. *Cancer Res. 34*:974–978, 1974.

38. Ferrante, A, Rowan-Kelley, B, Thong, YH: Suppression of immunological responses in mice by treatment with amphotericin B. *Clin. Exp. Immunol. 38*:70–76, 1979.
39. Thomas, MZ, Medoff, G, Kobayashi, GS: Changes in murine resistance to *Listeria monocytogenes* infection induced by amphotericin B. *J. Infect. Dis. 127*:373–377, 1973.
40. Chemel, H, Louria, DB: Antifungal antibiotics: Mechanism of action, resistance, susceptibility, testing, and assays of activity in biological fluids. In: *Antibiotics in Laboratory Medicine* (V Lorian, ed.), Williams and Wilkins, Baltimore, 1980, pp. 170–192.
41. Medoff, G, Comfort, M, Kobayashi, GS: Synergistic action of amphotericin B and 5-fluorocytosine against yeast-like organisms. *Proc. Soc. Exp. Biol. Med. 138*:571–574, 1971.
42. Block, ER, Bennett, JE: The combined effect of 5-fluorocytosine and amphotericin B in the therapy of murine cryptococcosis. *Proc. Soc. Exp. Biol. Med. 142*:476–480, 1973.
43. Titsworth, E, Grunberg, E: Chemotherapeutic activity of 5-fluorocytosine and amphotericin B against *Candida albicans* in mice. *Antimicrob. Agents Chemother. 4*:306–308, 1973.
44. Sande, MA, Bowan, CR, Calderone, RA: Experimental *C. albicans* endocarditis. Characterization of the disease and response to therapy. *Infect. Immun. 17*:140–147, 1977.
45. Bennett, JE, et al.: A collaborative study: Amphotericin B-flucytosine in cryptococcal meningitis. *N. Engl. J. Med. 308*:126–131, 1979.
46. Smego, RA, Perfect, JR, Durack, DT: Combined therapy with amphotericin B and 5-flurocytosine for *Candida* meningitis. *Rev. Infect. Dis. 6*:791–801, 1984.
47. Cosgrove, RF, Beezer, AE, Miles, RJ: In vitro studies of amphotericin B in combination with the imidazole antifungal compounds clotrimazole and miconazole. *J. Infect. Dis. 138*:681–685, 1978.
48. Iwen, PC, Miller, NG, McFadden, HW, Jr.: Treatment of murine pulmonary cryptococcosis with ketoconazole and amphotericin B. *J. Infect. Dis. 149*:650, 1984.
49. Edwards, JE, Morrison, J, Henderson, DK, et al.: Combined effects of amphotericin B and rifampin on *Candida* species. *Antimicrob. Agents Chemother. 17*:484–487, 1980.
50. Kitahara, M, Seth, UK, Medoff, G, et al.: Activity of amphotericin B, 5-fluorocytosine and rifampin against six clinical isolates of *Asperigillus. Antimicrob. Agents Chemother. 9*:915–919, 1976.
51. Kobayashi, GS, Medoff, G, Schleissinger, D, et al.: Amphotericin B potentiation of rifampin as an antifungal agent against the yeast phase of *Histoplasma* capsulation. *Science 177*:709–710, 1972.
52. Kitahara, M, Kobayashi, GS, Medoff, G: Enhanced efficacy of amphotericin B and rifampicin combined in treatment of murine histoplasmosis and blastomycosis. *J. Infect. Dis. 133*:663–668, 1976.
53. Lew, M, Beckett, KM, Levin, MJ: Combined activity of minocycline and amphotericin B in vitro against medically important yeasts. *Antimicrob. Agents Chemother. 14*:465–469, 1978.
54. Ernst, JD, Rusnah, M, Sande, MA: Combination antifungal chemotherapy for experimental disseminated candidiasis: Lack of correlation between in vitro and in vivo observations with amphotericin B and rifampin. *Rev. Infect. Dis. 5 (Suppl. 3)*: S626–S630, 1983.
55. Woods, RA, Bard, M, Jackson, IE, Drutz, DJ: Resistance to polyene antibiotics and correlated sterol changes in two isolates of *Candida tropicalis* from a patient with an amphotericin B resistant funguria. *J. Infect. Dis. 129*:53–58, 1974.

56. Dick, JD, Merz, WG, Saral, R: Incidence of polyene-resistant yeasts recovered from clinical specimens. *Antimicrob. Agents Chemother. 18*:158–163, 1980.
57. Hamilton-Miller, JMT: Sterols from polyene-resistant mutants of *Candida albicans. J. Gen. Microbiol. 73*:201–203, 1972.
58. Pierce, AM, Pierce, JR, Unrau A, Oehlschlager, AC: Lipid composition and polyene resistance of *Candida albicans* mutants. *Can. J. Biochem.* 56–135, 1978.
59. Bindschadler, DD, Bennett, JE: A pharmacologic guide to the clinical use of amphotericin B. *J. Infect. Dis. 20*:427–436, 1969.
60. Atkinson, AJ, Bennett, JE: Amphotericin B pharmacokinetics in humans. *Antimicrob. Agents Chemother. 13*:271–276, 1978.
61. Fields, BTH, Bates, JH, Abernathy, RS: Amphotericin B serum concentrations during therapy. *Appl. Microbiol. 19*:955–959, 1970.
62. Jagdis, FA, Mongi, N, Lawrence, RM, et al.: Distribution of radio labelled amphotericin B methyl ester and amphotericin B in non-human primates. In: Sixteen Interscience Conf. Antimicrob Agents Chemother. (abstract). 1976, p. 305, Washington, D.C.
63. Block, ER, Bennett, JE, Liveti, LG, et al.: Flucytosine and amphotericin B: Hemodialysis effect on the plasma concentration and clearance. *Ann. Intern. Med. 80*: 613–617, 1974.
64. Bennett, JE: Amphotericin B binding to serum betalipoprotein. In: *Recent Advances in Medical and Veterinary Mycology* (Iwata, ed.), University of Tokyo Press, 1977, pp. 107–109.
65. Craven, PC, Ludden, TM, Drutz, DJ: Excretion pathways of amphotericin B. *J. Infect. Dis. 140*:329–340, 1979.
66. Felman, HA, Hamilton, JD, Gutman, RA: Amphotericin therapy in an anephric patient. *Antimicrob. Agents Chemother. 4*:402–405, 1973.
67. Polak, A: Pharmacokinetics of amphotericin B and flucytosine. *Postgrad. Med. J. 55*:667–670, 1979.
68. Baley, J, Meyers, C, Kliegman, R, et al.: Pharmacokinetics of amphotericin B and 5 fluorocytosine in neonates. *Pediatr. Res. 20*:201A, 1986.
69. Cherry, JD, Lloyd, CA, Quity, JF, Laskowski, LF: Amphotericin B therapy in children: A review of the literature and a case report. *J. Pediatr. 75*:1063–1069, 1969.
70. Oh, SE, Conley, SB, Pickering, LK: Fungal peritonitis in children undergoing peritoneal dialysis. *Pediatr. Infect. Dis. 4*:62–66, 1985.
71. Jurgens, RW, Jr., DeLuca, PP, Papadimitriou,: Compatibility of amphotericin B with certain large volume parenterals. *Am. J. Hosp. Pharm. 38*:377–378, 1981.
72. Block, ER, Bennett, JE: Stability of amphotericin B in the infusion bottle. *Antimicrob. Agents Chemother. 4*:648–649, 1973.
73. Tipple, M, Shadomy, S, Espinel-Ingrolf, A: Availability of active amphotericin B after filtration through membrane filters. *Am. Rev. Respir. Dis. 115*:879–881, 1977.
74. Burks, LC, Aisner, J, Fortner, CL, Wiernik, PH: Meperidine for the treatment of shaking chills and fever. *Arch. Intern. Med. 140*:483–484, 1980.
75. Cosgrove, RF, Fairbrother, JE: Bioassay method for polyene antibiotics based on the measurement of rubidium efflux from rubidium-loaded yeast cells. *Antimicrob. Agents Chemother. 11*:31–33, 1977.
76. Merz, WG, Fay, D, Thumar, B, et al.: Susceptibility testing of filamentous fungi to amphotericin B by a rapid radiometric method. *J. Clin. Microbiol. 19*:54–56, 1984.
77. Golas, CL, Prober, CG, MacLeod, SM, et al.: Measurement of amphotericin B in serum or plasma by high-performance liquid chromatography. *J. Chromatogr. 278*: 387–395, 1983.
78. Medoff, G, Dismukes, WE, Meade, RH, et al.: A new therapeutic approach to *Candida* infections: A preliminary report. *Arch. Intern. Med. 130*:241–245, 1972.

79. Serstock, DS, Zinneman, HH: Pulmonary and articular sporotrichosis: Report of two cases. *JAMA 233*:1291–1293, 1975.
80. Wise, GJ, Wainstein, S, Goldberg, P, et al.: *Candida* cystitis: Management by continuous bladder irrigation with amphotericin B. *JAMA 224*:1636–1637, 1973.
81. Hill, HR, Mitchell, TG, Matsen, JM, et al.: Recovery from disseminated candidiasis in a premature infant. *Pediatrics 53*:748–752, 1974.
82. Zealear, DS, Winn, WA: The neurosurgical approach in the treatment of coccidioidal meningitis: Report of ten cases. In: *Coccidioidomycosis* (L Ajello, ed.), University of Arizona Press, Tuscon, 1967, pp. 43–53.
83. Pasner, JB: Reservoirs for intraventricular chemotherapy (editorial). *N. Engl. J. Med. 288*:212, 1973.
84. Klein, JD, Yamauchi, T, Horlick, SP: Neonatal candidiasis, meningitis and arthritis: Observations and a review of the literature. *J. Pediatr. 81*:31–34, 1972.
85. Carnevale, NT, Galgiani, JN, Stevens, DA, et al.: Amphotericin B-induced myelopathy. *Arch. Intern. Med. 140*:1189–1192, 1980.
86. Pizzo, PA, Robichaud, KJ, Gill, FA, et al.: Empiric antibiotic and antifungal therapy for cancer patients with prolonged fever and granulocytopenia. *Am. J. Med. 72*: 101–111, 1982.
87. Holleran, WM, Wilburn, JR, De Gregorio, MW: Empiric amphothericin B therapy in patients with acute leukemia. *Rev. Infect. Dis. 7*:619–624, 1985.
88. Guiot, HFL, Van der Meer, JWM, Van Furth, R: Selective antimicrobial modulation of human microbial flora: Infection prevention in patients with decreased host defence mechanisms by selective elimination of potentially pathogenic bacteria. *J. Infect. Dis. 143*:644–654, 1981.
89. Codish, SD, Tobias, JS, Hannigan, M: Combined amphotericin B-flucytosine therapy in *Aspergillus* pneumonia. *JAMA 241*:2418–2419, 1979.
90. Chesny, PJ, Teets, KC, Mulvihill, JJ: Successful treatment of *Candida* meningitis with amphotericin B and 5-flurocytosine in combination. *J. Pediatr. 89*:1017–1019, 1976.
91. Jimbow, T, Tejima, Y, Ikemoto, H: Comparison between 5-fluorocytosine, amphotericin B and the combination administration of these agents in the therapeutic effectiveness for cryptococcal meningitis. *Chemotherapy 24*:374–379, 1978.
92. Huston, AC, Hoeprich, PD: Comparative susceptibility of four kinds of pathogenic fungi to amphotericin B and amphotericin B methyl ester. *Antimicrob. Agents Chemother. 13*:905–909, 1978.
93. Lawrence, RM, Hoeprich, PD: Comparison of amphotericin B and amphotericin B methyl ester: Efficacy in murine coccidioidomycosis and toxicity. *J. Infect. Dis. 133*:168–174, 1976.
94. Jagdis, FA, Hoeprich, PD, Lawrence, RM, et al.: Comparative pharmacology of amphotericin B and amphotericin B methyl ester in the non-human primate. *Macaca mulatta. Antimicrob. Agents Chemother. 12*:582–585, 1977.
95. Ellis, WG, Sobel, RA, Nielsen, SL: Leukoencephalopathy in patients treated with amphotericin B methyl ester. *J. Infect. Dis. 146*:125–137, 1982.
96. Lopez-Berestein, G, Mehta, R, Hopfer, RL, et al.: Treatment and prophylaxis of disseminated infection due to *Candida albicans* in mice with liposome-encapsulated amphotericin B. *J. Infect. Dis. 147*:939–945, 1983.
97. Lopez-Berestein, G, Hopfer, R, Mehta, R, et al.: Prophylaxis of *Candida albicans* infections in neutropenic mice with liposome-encapsulated amphotericin B. *Antimicrob. Agents Chemother. 25*:366–367, 1984.
98. Lopez-Berestein, G, Fainstein, V, Hopfer, R, et al.: Liposomal amphotericin B for the treatment of systemic fungal infections in patients with cancer: A preliminary study. *J. Infect. Dis. 151*:704–710, 1985.

99. MacGregor, RR, Bennett, JE, Ersley, AJ: Erythropoietin concentration in amphotericin B-induced anemia. *Antimicrob. Agents Chemother. 14*:270–273, 1978.
100. Chan, CSP, Tuazon, CU, Lessin, LS: Amphotericin B-induced thrombocytopenia. *Ann. Intern. Med. 96*:332–333, 1982.
101. Wright, DG, Robichand, KF, Pizzo, PA, et al.: Lethal pulmonary reactions associated with the combined use of amphotericin B and leukocyte transfusions. *N. Engl. J. Med. 304*:1185–1189, 1981.
102. Butler, WT, Bennett, JE, Alling, AW, et al.: Nephrotoxicity of amphotericin B: Early and late effects in 81 patients. *Ann. Intern. Med. 61*:175–187, 1964.
103. Maddux, MS, Barriere, SL: A review of complications of amphotericin B therapy: Recommendations for prevention and management. *Drug Intell. Clin. Pharm. 14*: 177–181, 1980.
104. McCurdy, DK, Frederic, M, Elington, JR: Renal tubular acidosis due to amphotericin B. *N. Engl. J. Med. 278*:124–130, 1968.
105. Burgess, JL, Birchall, R: Nephrotoxicity of amphotericin B, with emphasis on changes in tubular function. *Am. J. Med. 53*:77–84, 1972.
106. Jose, PA, Eisner, GM, Hollerman, CE, et al.: Acute renal effects of amphotericin B. *Proc. Soc. Exp. Biol. Med. 137*:224–228, 1971.
107. Finn, JT, Cohen, LH, Steinmetz, PR: Acidifying defect induced by amphotericin B. Comparison of bicarbonate and hydrogen ion permeabilities. *Kidney Int. 11*: 261–266, 1977.
108. Hellebusch, AA, Salama, F, Eadle, E: The use of mannitol to reduce the nephrotoxicity of amphotericin. *Surg. Gynecol. Obstet. 134*:241–245, 1972.
109. Gouge, TH, Andriole, VT: An experimental model of amphotericin B nephrotoxicity with renal tubular acidosis. *J. Lab. Clin. Med. 78*:713–724, 1971.
110. Bullock, WE, Luke, RG, Nutall, CE, et al.: Can mannitol reduce amphotericin B nephrotoxicity? *Antimicrob. Agents Chemother. 10*:555–563, 1976.
111. Wilson, R, Feldman, S: Toxicity of amphotericin B in children with cancer. *Am. J. Dis. Child. 133*:731–734, 1979.
112. Faix, RG: Systemic *Candida* infections in infants in intensive care nurseries: High incidence of central nervous system involvement. *J. Pediatr. 105*:616–622, 1984.
113. Johnson, DE, Thompson, TR, Green, TP, et al.: Systemic candidiasis in very low birth weight infants (<1500 grams). *Pediatrics 73*:138–143, 1984.
114. Baley, JE, Kliegman, RM, Fanaroff, AA: Disseminated fungal infections in very low birth weight infants: Therapeutic toxicity. *Pediatrics 73*:153–157, 1984.
115. Neiberg, AD, Mavromatis, F, Dyke, J, et al.: *Blastomyces* dermatitidis treated during pregnancy. Report of a case. *Am. J. Obstet. Gynecol. 128*:911–912, 1977.

26
Imidazole Antifungals: Miconazole and Ketoconazole

ALAN M. SUGAR
University Hospital of the Boston University Medical Center, Boston, Massachusetts

I. CHEMISTRY

The imidazole compounds possess a wide range of biologic activities, including antibacterial (1,2), antiparasitic (3–5), and antiviral (6), as well as antifungal (7) effects. Synthesis of imidazole derivatives has been achieved by adding various side chains to the 5-membered imidazole nucleus (see Figure 1).

The two common features of antifungal imidazoles required for biologic activity are (1) an unsubstituted imidazole ring and (2) a covalent linkage between the nitrogen in the imidazole ring and the carbon side chain (8). Modifications of the groups attached to the carbon that are found to the imidazole ring affect pharmacological properties more so than antifungal activity.

With the exception of the hydrochloride salt of ketoconazole, the imidazole antifungals are poorly soluble in water. These drugs act as weak bases and have a net positive charge by virtue of being protonated at physiologic pH. These properties have ramifications for the use of the drugs in clinical practice.

A. Miconazole

Miconazole, (1- [2-(2,4-dichlorophenyl)-2-[2,4-dichlorophenyl)methoxy] ethyl)-1H-imidazole), ($C_{18}H_{14}Cl_4N_2O \cdot HNO_3$, molecular weight = 479.16), was synthesized in 1968 by the chemists working in the laboratories of Janssen Pharmaceutica. The compound is a white crystalline powder that is only minimally soluble in water. It is available for intravenous use as a clear, colorless to slightly yellow solution, with a pH of 3.5–5.7. Each milliliter of this solution contains 10 mg miconazole, 0.115 ml polyethylene glycol 40, 1.0 mg lactic acid U.S.P., 0.5 mg methylparaben U.S.P., and 0.05 mg propylparaben U.S.P. in water

B. Ketoconazole

Ketoconazole, *cis*-1-acetyl-4-[4-[[2-(2,4-dichlorophenyl)-2-(1H-imidazol-1-ylmethyl)-1,3-dioxolan-4-yl] methoxy] phenyl] piperazine, ($C_{26}H_{28}Cl_2N_4O_4 \cdot 2HCl$, molecular weight =

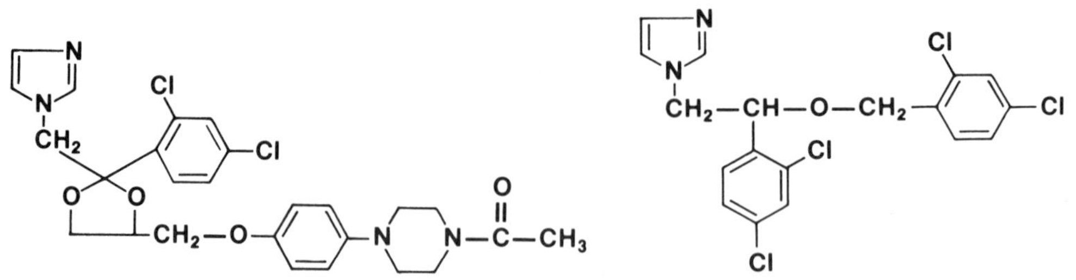

Figure 1 Structure of ketoconazole and miconazole.

531.44) and was also synthesized by scientists at Janssen Pharmaceutica in 1976. Ketoconazole is a white to slightly beige powder. Unlike miconazole, it is well absorbed orally and thus represents the first "broad-spectrum" antifungal drug that can be swallowed.

II. MECHANISM OF ACTION

Imidazoles inhibit fungal synthesis of membrane sterols, resulting in disorganization of the fungal cell membrane (9–11). However, additional effects are thought to be important in explaining their antifungal activity.

In contrast to mammalian cells, which contain cholesterol as the primary membrane sterol, the primary sterol of the fungal cell membrane is ergosterol. This basic difference in fungal and mammalian cell composition probably explains the selective antifungal action of these agents. The imidazoles appear to inhibit 14α-demethylation of lanosterol, the main precursor to ergosterol (12). The accumulation of these ergosterol precursors causes changes in membrane permeability with subsequent failure of the cell to grow or loss of cell viability.

There are several problems with this as the sole explanation for the antifungal effects of these drugs. Changes in cell permeability can be demonstrated using concentrations of the drugs well below those needed to affect growth and viability of the fungus (8). These effects also occur within seconds of the drug coming into contact with the fungus. In addition, gram-positive bacteria (organisms not containing ergosterol in their cell membranes) are inhibited by imidazoles in concentrations similar to those used in experiments with fungi. Thus inhibition of ergosterol synthesis may be important in explaining some of the effects of the imidazoles, but other activities need to be considered.

Other effects of ketoconazole of uncertain clinical significance have been described. For example, ketoconazole inhibits hyphae formation in *Candida albicans* (7). Although controversial, the formation of hyphae and pseudohypae maybe an important correlate of virulence in *C. albicans* (13).

Ketoconazole also seems to act synergistically with host phagocytes to eradicate *C. albicans* (14,15). Interactions of imidazoles with microsomal enzymes (16) and inhibition of triglyceride and fatty acid synthesis (17) are among some of the other potentially relevant effects of these drugs. Ketoconazole has been shown to inhibit the activity of a mitochondrial NADH oxidase in *C. albicans* at clinically achievable concentrations, effectively inhibiting respiration of the yeast (18). Furthermore, ketoconazole has been shown to inhibit cytochrome c oxidase, a component of the distal portion of the mitochondrial respiratory chain (19). The relevance of these various activities to antifungal action is unclear at present. For a more complete discussion of the factors concerning the mechanisms of action of the imidazoles, the reader is referred to the review by Beggs et al. (8).

III. ACTIVITY AND RESISTANCE

Before reviewing the in vitro antifungal activity of miconazole and ketoconazole, it is important to stress that procedures for testing antifungal drugs in the laboratory are not standardized. Even though results are often reported as minimum inhibitory concentrations (MIC) or minimum fungicidal concentrations (MFC), these values do not necessarily parallel determinations of antibacterial activity. This caveat is particularly pertinent when evaluating the imidazoles. There are many variables that influence MIC and MFC values of the imidazoles: composition and pH of the medium (20-22), presence of serum in the medium (1), size of the inoculum (23), and morphological form of the fungus tested (22). Furthermore, the results of in vitro susceptibility testing may not accurately reflect the performance of the drug in animal models of infection or in the clinical situation. Discordance between in vitro susceptibility results and in vivo response to the therapy with the drug are common. The appropriate standardized methods for conducting and interpreting in vitro susceptibility tests have not yet been described. With these reservations in mind, the accumulated data can be reviewed.

The imidazoles are broad-spectrum agents, active against most of the fungi that cause human disease. Notable in the context of pediatric diseases is the susceptibility of almost all strains of *C. albicans*. However, many non-*albicans Candida* have proved to be resistant to the imidazoles when tested in vitro. The agents of dermatophytosis are uniformly susceptible to both miconazole and ketoconazole. Although individual strains of different fungi may vary in their in vitro susceptibility to any of the imidazoles, the only groups of fungi that consistently appear to be resistant in the laboratory, in animal models of infection, and in patients are *Aspergillus* species and the *Zygomycetes*, the agents of mucormycosis. These latter organisms typically have MIC > 10 μg/ml. In contrast, both *Paracoccidioides brasiliensis* and *Pseudallescheria boydii* are exquistely susceptible to both miconazole and ketoconazole, with MIC < 0.1 μg/ml (24). Detailed summaries of the MIC have been published (25).

Activity against both gram-positive bacteria (2), *Plasmodium falciparum* (3), and *Leishmania* (4,5) has been reported, but has yet to be shown to have clinical importance.

IV. CLINICAL PHARMACOLOGY

As the route of administration and pharmacokinetics of miconazole and ketoconazole differ, the drugs will be considered separately.

A. Miconazole

Early studies established that miconazole was absorbed after oral administration but that serum concentrations following oral doses were low. Approximately 30% of the total ingested dose appeared in the serum. As is the case with clotrimazole, a potent inducer of hepatic microsomal enzymes and thus of its own degradation, miconazole was found to be similarly rapidly degraded, presumably in the liver, after oral administration (26). Thus, further attention was directed to studying the behavior of miconazole in the body following intravenous dosing.

Following a 1-g intravenous dose of miconazole in a study involving four normal human volunteers, peak concentrations obtained 15 min following infusion were 6 μg/ml (range, 2-9 μg/ml) (27). After 4 hr the mean plasma concentrations were below 1 μg/ml. Little miconazole is found in the urine (14% recovered in the urine after 6 days). The pharmacokinetics of miconazole has been best fitted to a three-compartment model (28), with a central compartment equilibrating with the fast and slow compartments. The fast compartment represents biodegradation or excretion in the feces; tissue stores represent the slow compartment. The terminal half-life of miconazole is about 24 hr and is not influenced by the presence of renal failure or the use of hemodialysis (28). Patients with impaired renal function have similar plasma concentrations of miconazole, as do those with normal renal function (27). Thus the dose of miconazole need not be altered in the presence of renal failure or when hemodialysis is instituted. About 90% of the drug is protein bound, primarily to serum albumin. Miconazole is widely distributed throughout the body with a volume of distribution V_d approximating 1500 liters in adults. The drug exhibits good penetration into infected joints and vitreous humor. However, significant cerebrospinal fluid (CSF) concentrations are not attained following intravenous administration of miconazole, and very little miconazole is found in the sputum (29). Elimination of miconazole is primarily due to biodegradation and excretion in the feces.

Several pediatric patients have received miconazole and have had serum concentrations reported. Sung et al. treated two infants (30). A 38-day-old male received 6 mg/kg miconazole by intravenous infusion. The serum miconazole concentration was 0.65 μg/ml at 2 hr and 0.18 μg/ml at 6 hr postinfusion. Similarly, after receiving 4 mg/ml, 0.71 and 0.23 μg/ml were detected 1 and 4 hr postinfusion, respectively. The second infant was a 709-g premature male who received 3.8 mg/kg of miconazole, with 2- and 6-hr serum concentrations of 0.53 and 0.19 μg/ml, respectively. At a dose of 6.9 μg/ml, 1.26 and 0.27 μg/ml were detected at these same time points.

Fisher et al. (31) reported on the therapy of a 9-year-old boy who received 10 mg/kg miconazole intravenously. At both 0.5 and 8 hr, <0.5 μg/ml of the drug was detectable in the serum. Other reports of the use of miconazole in children do not comment on the serum concentrations in those patients (32-36). In a review of miconazole, Heel et al. (29) recommend using 20-40 mg/kg day^{-1} in children, with a single dose not to exceed 15 mg/kg.

In addition to the intravenous use of miconazole, this drug can be injected directly into the central nervous system. Intrathecal, intracisternal, and intraventicular administration of miconazole results in detectable CSF concentrations for up to 72 hr. Most of the experience with this mode of therapy has been in patients with coccidioidal meningitis (37).

Miconazole is available for intravenous infusion. The exact doses prescribed are based on the severity and type of fungal infection being treated. Up to 3600 mg/day in three divided doses has been given in the treatment of coccidioidomycosis. In adults with candidiasis, 600-1800 mg/day is recommended, depending on the severity of the infection. Children should receive 20-40 mg/kg day^{-1} in three doses, not to exceed 15 mg/kg for any one dose. The maximal daily dose used in treatment of coccidiodymycosis is 3600 mg.

B. Ketoconazole

Because there are only a limited number of rather small studies upon which to draw conclusions about the pharmacokinetic behavior of ketoconazole, the studies will be reviewed in some detail. This will provide the reader with an opportunity to recognize the limitations of the available information.

In normal volunteers, single doses from 200 to 800 mg of ketoconazole were given and serum concentrations were determined by bioassay or high-performance liquid chromatography (HPLC) (38–41). From these studies it is clear that wide variations in serum concentrations, even in these normal volunteers, occur. Mean peak serum concentrations of ketoconazole following different doses are shown in Table 1.

Studies in normal subjects have provided conflicting results concerning the effect of food on the absorption of ketoconazole. Mannisto et al. (39), using an HPLC method for measuring serum ketoconazole concentrations, studied 10 normal subjects after they received 200 mg ketoconazole while fasting, after a standardized meal, or with 300 ml orange juice. The peak serum concentrations decreased from 4 μg/ml when the drug was taken on an empty stomach to 2 μg/ml following the meal. The orange juice had no appreciable effect on the absorption of ketoconazole in these volunteers. In contrast, Daneshmend et al. (40) studied eight healthy adults following single oral doses of 200, 400, 600, and 800 mg ketoconazole. They found that the absorption of ketoconazole and peak serum concentrations were not altered by the food, even though the standard meal was similar to that used in the study performed by Mannisto et al. These results were similar to those of Brass et al. (41), who found no effect of food on absorption of ketoconazole in seven patients. Whether the method of determination of ketoconazole serum concentrations by HPLC (41) or bioassay (39) can explain these discrepancies has not yet been addressed. Because of the small sample sizes of these studies and the large variations in serum ketoconazole concentrations, the effect of food on absorption of ketoconazole may be masked. Until more data are available, the drug should probably not be administered concomitantly with food.

The half-life of ketoconazole has also been noted to vary over a wide range. In normal volunteers, the half-life has generally ranged from 1 to 2 hr. The $t_{1/2}$ increases with increasing doses: from $t_{1/2} = 1.4$ hr with 200 mg to $t_{1/2} = 3.8$ hr with 800 mg.

There is evidence that the administration of ketoconazole with food may prolong the elimination $T_{1/2}$ and increase the area under the concentration-time curve (AUC) of the drug (42). Similar phenomena have been described with other drugs (e.g., propranolol), and it may be explained by a food-induced decrease in the first-pass (presystemic) clearance of the drug in the liver.

Similarly, there is evidence that multiple doses of ketoconazole may produce the same effect (42). Possible explanations, such as improved absorption, nonlinear elimination, saturable first-pass metabolism, or a change of distribution volume, have been put forward but not yet proven.

Table 1 Approximate Peak Serum Concentrations of Ketoconazole

Dose (mg)	Serum concentration (μg/ml)	Time of peak (hr)
200	4	1–3
400	8–10	1–3
600	15	4–6
800	20	4–6

Children with a variety of fungal infections have been treated with ketoconazole, and several authors have reported the serum concentrations attained. Bardare et al. (43) treated 26 children with invasive candidal infections. Ages ranged from 5 months to 14 years. Some of the patients received the drug as suspension (details of the preparation of this formulation were not given; ketoconazole suspension is not yet available for clinical use), whereas others received the drug in tablets. Serum concentrations of only 0.5 μg/ml were detected in 2 patients who received 3 mg/kg of suspension. However, when the dose was increased to 10 mg/kg, the peak concentration rose to 2 μg/ml. When ketoconazole was given in tablet form, doses of approximately 5 and 9 mg/kg day^{-1} resulted in peak serum concentrations of 3.5 and 6 μg/ml, respectively. The authors concluded that 3 mg/kg three times daily with either formulation was not sufficient to maintain adequate serum concentrations, whereas doses $\geqslant$ 8 mg/kg day^{-1} resulted in appropriate concentrations.

In another study of ketoconazole suspension, Ginsburg et al. (44) administered either tablets crushed in applesauce or a suspension prepared by Janssen Pharmaceutica (FDA approval for this formulation has been applied for) to 12 children with oral candidiasis and superficial dermatophytoses. The ages of the patients were not stated. Each patient received each preparation on two separate occasions, 5-7 days apart. Doses were 5 mg/kg with either preparation, and serum concentrations were determined by HPLC. The commercially prepared suspension provided higher peak serum concentrations at earlier time points. The mean concentration attained 1 hr after administration was 4.4 μg/ml, whereas the mean concentration attained 2 hr after the crushed tablets were administered was 2.6 μg/ml. It is interesting to note that peak concentrations ranged from 0.3 to 8.8 μg/ml after the suspension and 0.4-6.5 μg/ml after the crushed tablets, once again stressing the wide individual variations seen with oral ketoconazole.

An important characteristic of all the studies that have been reviewed here is that very small numbers of normal subjects or patients were studied. In contrast, the multicenter cooperative studies (45-47) sponsored by the National Institutes of Health-National Institute of Allergy and Infectious Diseases-Mycoses Study Group (NIH-NIAID-MSG) involve considerably more patients, and thus, results obtained from these trials are more definitive.

The patients in the initial NIH-NIAID-MSG studies had a variety of mycoses, including coccidioidomycosis, histoplasmosis, sporotrichosis, blastomysosis, and cryptococcosis (45,46). The doses of ketoconazole ranged from 200 to 600 mg/day. A 3-year-old boy received 100 mg/day. As noted in the other studies of ketoconazole pharmacokinetics, large inter- and intrapatient variations were detected. Mean peak (1-3 hr postdose) serum ketoconazole concentrations with 400- and 600-mg doses were 6.0 and 6.3 μg/ml, respectively. Of some concern was the observation that 11 of 97 (11%) samples had undetectable serum concentrations and an additional 13 (13%) contained less than 1 μg/ml. Approximately 30% of the samples contained > 4 μg/ml ketoconazole. There was no correlation between serum ketoconazole concentrations and clinical response. The elimination half-life of ketoconazole remained unchanged with increasing doses, ranging from 3 to 5 hr. Poor response of the fungal infection in patients who are taking ketoconazole may be attributed to poor absorption of the drug.

Absorption of ketoconazole in bone marrow transplant patients is markedly impaired, and the usual 200- or 400-mg/day dose results in extremely low concentrations (48,49). In particular, Hann et al. (48) found that serum ketoconazole concentrations fell precipitously from the third week of therapy until the end of therapy at 5 weeks. Whereas non-bone marrow transplant patients maintained a peak serum concentration of 3-5 μg/ml throughout the study, the bone marrow transplant recipients demonstrated a mean of 0.6 μg/ml 2 hr after a dose at week 3 and < 0.3 μg/ml 2 hr after a dose at weeks 4 and 5. This effect was thought to be due to the extensive mucosal damage experienced by these patients. An increase in clinically evident fungal infections in bone marrow transplant recipients was also observed during this period of impaired ketoconazole absorption. Finally, Hann et al. comment on the similarity of the pharmacokinetic data obtained from the adults and seven children who participated in this study.

Vu Van et al. (49) studied seven bone marrow transplant recipients and found that absorption of ketoconazole was delayed in these patients, peak serum concentrations often occurring 4-6 hr after the administration of a dose. Graft-versus-host disease did not seem to alter the absorption of ketoconazole. The apparent decrease in serum ketoconazole concentrations found by Hann et al. (48) might be explained by their failure to obtain sera at times beyond 2 hr after a dose, but both studies confirm that the absorption of ketoconazole is highly variable. This may explain in part the failure to respond to therapy. Patients with malignancies who are being treated with cytotoxic chemotherapy also demonstrate alterations in absorption of ketoconazole (50). In fact, 200 mg ketoconazole administered every 6 hr was required to maintain steady-state peak serum ketoconazole concentrations of approximately 3 μg/ml (50). There was an increase in the area under concentration-time curve from days 1 and 8 of therapy in patients receiving the drug every 6 hr, whereas this phenomenon was minimal when ketoconazole was administered every 12 hr. These investigators confirmed that very little active ketoconazole is excreted in the urine (<1% of administered dose).

Ketoconazole has been found to be widely distributed throughout the body. Following a single dose of 200 mg, the drug has been found in low but detectable concentrations in urine, saliva, sebum, cerumen, and skin (51-53). Approximately 90% of ketoconazole in the serum is protein bound. Ketoconazole is metabolized by oxidation, *o*-dealkylation, and aromatic hydroxylation. These metabolites, which are devoid of antifungal activity, are ultimately excreted from the body in the feces (54).

Reports concerning the penetration of ketoconazole into the cerebrospinal fluid are conflicting. Craven et al. (55) treated six patients with high doses of ketoconazole (800 or 1200 mg/day) with or without the use of amphotericin B. Peak ventricular CSF ketoconazole concentrations of 0.2 μg/ml were detected at 2 and 4 hr after an 800-mg dose. The corresponding mean peak serum concentration in these patients was 11.5 ± 4.0 μg/ml. Lumbar CSF concentrations at 4 and 8 hr were 0.3 and 0.24 μg/ml, respectively, both higher than those seen in the ventricular CSF at those times. No detectable ketoconazole was seen in either CSF compartment at 24 hr following the dose. After a 1200-mg dose, peak serum concentrations increased to about 16 μg/ml. Lumbar fluid ketoconazole concentrations again exceeded those in the ventricular fluid, with lumbar CSF concentrations at 4 hr ranging from 0.27 to 1.65 μg/ml. The penetration of ketoconazole into lumbar CSF was calculated to be 5.4 ± 2.6%, with penetration into the ventricular CSF 1.9 ± 0.8%.

In contrast to these results, we have recently analyzed the data from a third NIH-NIAID-MSG study in patients with coccidioidal meningitis who were treated with doses of ketoconazole ranging from 800 to 2000 mg/day (47). Of 23 CSF samples analyzed, only 5 obtained from four patients had CSF ketoconazole concentrations >1 μg/ml (see Table 2). There was no clear relationship between actual dose administered and subsequent CSF ketoconazole concentration. Those CSF samples containing >1 μg/ml of

Table 2 Lumbar Cerebrospinal Fluid Ketoconazole Concentrations

Dose (mg/day)	[Ketoconazole] (μg/ml) hours postdose			
	1–3	4–6	7–9	10–23
800	0.203	0.299	0.264	0.620
1200	0.175	0.554	0.358	0.563
1600	0.527	0.613	NA[a]	1.200
2000	0.257	0.460	0.817	0.078

[a]Not available.

ketoconazole were obtained at daily doses of 1600 mg (two samples), 1800 mg (one sample), and 2000 mg (two samples) at 1-4 hr following ingestion of the drug. Because of the very wide fluctuations in serum ketoconazole concentrations seen in this study, no definite statement about the degree of ketoconazole penetration into the CSF could be made. It was a general impression that some patients did remarkably well while on ketoconazole alone, supporting similar findings by Craven et al. (55). This is interesting when comparing the low CSF ketoconazole concentrations obtained with the usual minimal inhibitory concentration (MIC) of ketoconazole to *Coccidioides immitis*, about 1 μg/ml (56). Perhaps the degree of penetration of ketoconazole into the CSF is not the critical determinant of successful therapy of coccidioidal meningitis. Further studies to investigate this notion are warranted.

In the coccidioidal meningitis study, there were 5 children who were treated with ketoconazole. Their ages ranged from 1.5 to 8.5 years, and doses of ketoconazole were either 200 or 400 mg/day. CSF ketoconazole concentrations ranged from undetectable to 0.5 μg/ml. Peak serum concentrations in this small number of patients were comparable with those seen in the adult patients.

Ketoconazole is currently available only in tablet form containing 200 mg per tablet. An application for approval of suspension of this formulation is pending in the United States. Currently recommended doses of ketoconazole are 200-400 mg/day in a single administration. Higher doses have been used in certain instances, but the proper dose for any of the indications is not established.

In children, a dose equal to or greater than 8 mg/kg day^{-1} was associated with adequate serum concentrations of ketoconazole (43). In summary, ketoconazole is absorbed to a much greater extent than miconazole following oral administration and does not appear to induce the hepatic microsomal enzymes that increase its own metabolism, as does miconazole. However, ketoconazole exhibits a marked propensity for intra- and interpatient variability of serum concentrations. Thus, in critically ill patients who require immediate antifungal therapy, a parenteral agent, especially amphotericin B, should be used. If serum concentrations of ketoconazole can be readily obtained, ketoconazole may be considered for initial therapy in these patients. This would be a desirable option in the patient who cannot tolerate amphotericin B.

These studies were performed using one of the several available bioassays (57-60) or HPLC techniques (61-64). None of these assays have been widely applied as the standard assay for use in either research or in the performance of clinical studies. Even so, modifications of the bioassay are still being made in an attempt to make them more easily adaptable to the clinical situation should the need arise (65). Some of the variability in the reported serum concentrations of these drugs may be explained by the differences in methodology.

V. CLINICAL INDICATIONS

Miconazole is approved in the United States for use in patients with coccidioidomycosis, candidiasis (including chronic mucocutaneous candidiasis), cryptococcosis, and paracoccidioidomycosis. Ketoconazole is approved for the treatment of coccidioidomycosis, histoplasmosis, paracoccidioidomycosis, chronic mucocutaneous candidiasis, oral candidiasis, candiduria, and chromomycosis. In the absence of comparative trials of different antifungal agents and with the proliferation of in vitro susceptibility data and in vivo experience with various animal models of fungal disease, there is a tendency to extrapolate this information to the therapy of human mycoses. However, this temptation should be resisted in most instances until enough experience is gained using the imidazoles in the treatment of these infections (66). Because of the rarity of many fungal diseases, it is unlikely that comparative trials can be performed. For those more common mycoses, such as candidiasis, the present dilemma for the physician is making correct and timely diagnoses. It is impossible to conduct studies designed to evaluate differing therapies if the diagnosis of the infection is doubtful. Thus, we have a situation in which clinical decisions are made on the basis of empirical recommendations (67), which often differ depending upon the source of the information. Furthermore, the effect of reporting bias in influencing the number of reports of successfully treated patients as opposed to treatment failures is hard to judge, and therefore, the literature provides little basis on which to make a thoughtful decision concerning the efficacy of these antifungal drugs. Most physicians will agree, however, that the seriously ill patient infected by most fungal pathogens should be treated with amphotericin B, as it is a much more reliable agent to use.

The disease whose management has most clearly benefited from the introduction of ketoconazole is chronic mucocutaneous candidiasis (68,69,70). Patients who are treated with ketoconazole usually show a dramatic resolution of their lesions, and if therapy is continued for several months, even the nail lesions resolve. Unfortunately, perhaps because the immunologic defects in these patients persist despite treatment (71), recurrences are common after therapy is discontinued.

Therefore, attempts to control the disease includes chronic daily or every 2-3 day suppressive therapy with ketoconazole. Although ketoconazole seems to be nontoxic to patients treated with long-term ketoconazole in these studies, the isolation of ketoconazole-resistant *C. albicans* has been reported (72). The role of intermittent exposure of the fungus to the antifungal agent in the selection of resistant organisms is not yet known.

Most patients with systemic candidiasis are seriously ill and thus require parenteral therapy. Because of the extensive clinical experience with amphotericin B, most physicians elect to use this drug rather than miconazole or ketoconazole for these patients. However, anecdotal reports suggest that certain patients may fare well with either of the imidazoles (73). Much more experience with the imidazoles is needed to place this information in proper perspective.

In patients with paracoccidioidomycosis and pseudallescheriosis, both exceedingly rare diseases in children, an imidazole is preferred over amphotericin B because of the demonstrated clinical efficacy (74,74). Because ketoconazole is administered orally, it is the logical choice for the prolonged periods of time required for adequate therapy of these mycoses.

Miconazole has proved to be useful in selected cases of coccidioidomycosis (76). When intrathecal therapy is required in patients with coccidioidal meningitis and amphotericin B can no longer be tolerated, miconazole has been reported to be an acceptable alternative in doses ranging from 20 mg twice a day to 20 mg every other day (37).

Early experience with miconazole made it clear that intravenous courses of up to 7 months were still complicated by relapses in about one-third of patients (24). Fortunately, as has been demonstrated by recently completed trials conducted by the NIH-NIAID-MSG, ketoconazole has proved to be effective in patients involving skin and soft tissues, bones and joints, and chronic infections of the lung.* The response to ketoconazole did not seem to be dose dependent, but patients often showed gratifying responses to this therapy. However, relapses were frequent even after more than 6 months of therapy. It appears that prolonged therapy with ketoconazole (more than 1 year) is probably necessary; however, the exact duration of therapy to achieve a cure is not known. In addition, ketoconazole appeared to be well tolerated even when taken for several years.

Experts generally agree that the treatment of choice for cryptococcal meningitis should include amphotericin B and flucytosine (77). As is true for other fungal infections, reports of successes and failures using either miconazole or ketoconazole have appeared in the literature. Animal studies (78,79) and anecdotal clinical reports (80) notwithstanding, the use of imidazoles in the treatment of systemic cryptococcosis must still be regarded as experimental.

VI. TOXICITY

A. Miconazole

It was originally hoped that miconazole would replace amphotericin B because it was significantly less toxic and had a broad spectrum of activity. However, it soon was realized that miconazole displayed several important adverse effects as well as no demonstrable advantage over amphotericin B in most clinical situations. Table 3 lists the side effects

Table 3 Adverse Effects Associated with Miconazole

Hyponatremia	Pruritus	Diarrhea
Phlebitis	Hyperlipidemia[a]	Acute toxic psychosis
Anemia	Hyperesthesia	Anaphylaxis
Nausea	Euphoria	Cardiorespiratory arrest[b]

[a]Due to the cremophor carrier.
[b]May be due to the rate of infusion and concentration of the drug. See text for details.

*Galgiani, J. N., et al.: Ketoconazole treatment of coccidioidomycosis. II. 400 vs 800 mg/day with provision for ascending dose. Results in bone/joint and soft tissue disease. Abstracts of the Twenty-fourth Interscience Conference on Antimicrobial Agents and Chemotherapy. No. 1102, 1984; Graybill, J. R., et al.: Ketoconazole treatment of coccidioidomycosis: 400 vs 800 mg/day, with provision for ascending dose. I. Clinical characteristics and results in chronic pulmonary disease. Abstracts of the Twenty-fourth Interscience Conference on Antimicrobial Agents and Chemotherapy. No. 1103, 1984.

attributed to miconazole. The most common side effects include pruritus, (often without a rash), nausea, vomiting, diarrhea, skin rash, and fever and chills. In past, phlebitis was a common problem; this has resolved to a large extent following the introduction of a new buffered formulation of miconazole. The absence of renal or hepatic toxicity is notable. The precise frequency of the various side effects is difficult to determine, as various series report reaction rates between 1 and 50%.

Perhaps the most disturbing of all of the side effects of miconazole are the anaphylactic reactions (81) and cardiorespiratory arrests (82). Obviously, patients who have demonstrated hypersensitivity to imidazole derivatives should not be given miconazole or ketoconazole. Cardiac and/or respiratory arrest independent of an anaphylactic reaction can be seen, especially if infusion rates are shorter than 1 hr and if the volume of diluent containing miconazole is less than 200 ml. Fainstein and Bodey (82) therefore recommended that infusions should be given over more than 60 min and in a volume of greater than 200 ml. Precise recommendations for these parameters in small infants and children are not available, but as dilute a solution as possible over at least 60 min should be given in those patients who require therapy with miconazole.

B. Ketoconazole

When the early studies with ketoconazole were conducted using doses of less than 400 mg/day, this drug appeared to be relatively free of serious adverse effects. Adverse reactions noted included nausea, vomiting, or anorexia and skin rash. Other less frequently noted side effects include photophobia, paresthesias, thrombocytopenia, amenorrhea, and abnormalities of liver function tests (see Table 4).

Once doses in excess of 400 mg/day were prescribed, the frequency of the more common side effects, such as gastrointestinal upset, increased to almost 50% of patients (47) and certain endocrinologic disturbances were observed. The gastrointestinal reactions

Table 4 Adverse Effects Associated with Ketoconazole

Nausea
Vomiting
Anorexia
Gynecomastia
Oligospermia (azospermia)
Menorrhagia or metrorrhagia
Hepatitis
Alopecia
Pruritus
Rash
Photophobia
Paresthesias
Thrombocytopenia
Suppression of testosterone synthesis
Suppression of adrenal steroidogenesis[a]

[a]Of uncertain clinical significance.

and endocrine effects appear to be dose related: 18% of patients taking 400 mg/day vs. 42–50% taking 800–1600 mg/day develop nausea and/or vomiting. Only 4 and 13% of men on 400 or 800 mg/day, respectively, developed gynecomastia, compared with approximately 30% of these patients taking 1200–200 mg/day (47).

The first indication that ketoconazole could affect the endocrine system was the development of gynecomastia in some male patients (83). Studies of the mechanism of this effect revealed that ketoconazole inhibits testicular testosterone synthesis by blocking C_{17-20} lyase, a cytochrome P_{450}-mediated hydroxylation step (84,85). C_{17-20} lyase is one of two enzymes that mediate the conversion of 17α-hydroxyprogesterone to androstenedione. Such a block in this metabolic sequence causes an accumulation of 17α-hydroxyprogesterone and a decrease in androstenedione and testosterone. These results have been verified in vitro (86). Ketoconazole was also found to displace sex steroids from serum binding globulins (87), and the ratio of free estradiol to free testosterone was noted to be increased (88), possibly representing the mechanism for the gynecomastia. The inhibitory effects of ketoconazole on testosterone serum concentrations decrease as the concentration of ketoconazole in the serum decreases. Therefore, maintenance of high serum concentrations of ketoconazole by giving several doses of the drug per day may have a more profound inhibitory effect on serum testosterone concentrations and block the escape from this effect that occurs when ketoconazole is administered as a single daily dose (89). The implications of these effects are important when the use of ketoconazole is considered in the pubescent patient, particularly in boys. It is likely that the normal onset of puberty will be delayed if testosterone synthesis is suppressed. However, as long as the serum ketoconazole concentrations drop to low levels for some part of the day, testosterone synthesis should continue.

Ketoconazole may also cause suppression of cortisol synthesis by the adrenal cortex. Both in vitro and in vivo effects have been noted (90,91). The mechanism seems to involve cytochrome P_{450}-dependent enzymes, similar to the effects on testosterone synthesis (92). In general this effect is of no clinical significance, although a recent report suggests that symptoms of adrenal insufficiency can occur (93). Adrenal steroidogenesis is inhibited in a dose-dependent manner, similar to the inhibition of testosterone synthesis.

The antihormonal effects of ketoconazole have been used to the therapeutic benefit of some patients. For example, multiple daily dosing has been used successfully in treating patients with prostate cancer (94), and in three boys (aged 3.3–3.9 years) with precocious puberty a subsequent decrease in serum testosterone concentrations was observed following the institution of ketoconazole (95). Not unexpectedly, during the first week of ketoconazole therapy, the boys exhibited a blunted adrenal response to synthetic adrenocorticotropic hormone (ACTH). However, by 1 month of continuous ketoconazole therapy, adrenal reserve returned to normal. Furthermore, normal diurnal cortisol rhythm was preserved. These results are encouraging in that patients who are maintained on ketoconazole for prolonged courses of therapy for fungal infections should not encounter problems of adrenal insufficiency, especially if the ketoconazole is taken only once daily.

As more patients were treated with ketoconazole, an idiosyncratic hepatitis was recognized as one of the more serious adverse reactions. The reactions do not appear to be dose related (96). In a comprehensive review, Lewis et al. (96) analyzed 33 cases of hepatitis thought to be caused by ketoconazole. Of the 33 patients, 21 were women 40 years of age or older. The mean duration of therapy before the onset of liver dysfunction was 49 days, with a range of 11–168 days. These investigators calculated that the incidence of ketoconazole-induced hepatitis was 1 in 15,000 exposed individuals. In that series, 2 children were reported. The first, a 17-year-old male with chronic mucocutaneous candidiasis, received 200 mg ketoconazole every day or every other day. He developed elevated transaminases on day 135 of ketoconazole treatment and fully recovered from the hepatitis. The second child was a 5-year-old boy with chronic mucocutaneous candidiasis. He developed marked transaminase elevations after receiving 100 mg/day of ketoconazole for 166 days. Ketoconazole was discontinued, and this patient receovered within 6 weeks.

Because of the variable length of time until onset of hepatic dysfunction, Lewis et al. recommend that biochemical tests of liver function be monitored every 2 weeks for the first 2 months and then every 1 or 2 months for the duration of ketoconazole therapy (96). Any unexplained gastrointestinal symptoms should be evaluated with the appropriate tests of liver function. If liver dysfunction is present, ketoconazole should be discontinued. When ketoconazole is discontinued at the onset of hepatitis, the outcome is good. Patients who have had allergic reactions to imidazole compounds should not receive either of these antifungals.

VII. DRUG INTERACTIONS

A. Miconazole

Probably because of the relatively infrequent use of miconazole in large numbers of patients, there have been few reports of drug interactions. Deresinski et al. (97) have noted that the anticoagulant effect of Coumadin (warfarin) may be potentiated by miconazole. In vitro antagonism between miconazole and amphotericin B has been noted. This effect is presumably due to the alterations in the fungal cell membrane induced by miconazole, which results in a decrease in membrane ergosterol, the target sterol to which amphotericin B binds.

B. Ketoconazole

Several clinically important interactions between ketoconazole and other drugs have been reported. Since ketoconazole requires gastric acidity for the dissolution of the tablets and subsequent absorption of active drug (98,99), any drug that decreases acid secretion in the stomach will decrease ketoconazole serum concentrations. Antacids and histamine H_2-receptor blockers, such as cimetidine and ranitidine, have markedly decreased absorption of ketoconazole.

An interaction between rifampin or isoniazid and ketoconazole has been documented in a 2-year-old child with tuberculosis (100). The authors suggested that the decrease in ketoconazole serum concentrations could be explained on the basis of increased metabolism of the antifungal drug, but no data were provided to support this hypothesis. A further finding in that study was that the concurrent administration of ketoconazole and rifampin appeared to markedly impair the absorption of rifampin: an approximately 60% decrease in rifampin concentrations was observed. Administration of the two drugs 12 hr apart had no effect on rifampin serum concentrations.

Ketoconazole has been found to elevate serum concentrations of cyclosporin (101–104). The mechanism of this effect is not established but may involve the inhibition of cyclosporin metabolism. A result of this interaction is an increase in incidence of nephrotoxicity attributed to cyclosporin.

Interactions between amphotericin B and imidazoles have been evaluated. Because polyene antifungals, like amphotericin B, bind to membrane ergosterol and depend on this for their activity, imidazoles have been found to antagonize the effects of amphotericin B. This presumably is the result of inhibition of ergosterol synthesis by the imidazole. Schaffner and Frick (105) demonstrated in an animal model of disseminated aspergillosis that initial treatment of infected mice with ketoconazole, followed by amphotericin B, seriously compromised their survival when compared with mice that did not receive initial therapy with ketoconazole. Unfortunately, this effect extends to *C. albicans*, at least in vitro (106). The ramifications for patient care and the use of prophylactic antifungals in the immunocompromised patient are not clear. The preliminary evidence, however, is worrisome and should serve to discourage the widespread use of imidazoles for questionable indications.

REFERENCES

1. Van Cutsem, JM, Thienpont, D: Miconazole, a broad-spectrum antimycotic agent with antibacterial activity. *Chemotherapy 17*:392–404, 1972.
2. Sud, IJ, Feingold, DS: Action of antifungal imidazoles on *Staphylococcus aureus. Antimicrob. Agents Chemother. 22*:470–474, 1982.
3. Pfaller, MA, Krogstad, OJ: Imidazole and polyene activity against chloroquine-resistant *Plasmodium falciparum. J. Infect. Dis. 144*:372–375, 1981.
4. Berman, JD: Activity of imidazoles against *Leishmania tropica* in human macrophage cultures. *Am. J. Trop. Med. Hyg. 30*:566–569, 1981.
5. McCabe, RE, Remington, JS, Araujo, FG: Ketoconazole inhibition of intracellular multiplication of *Trypanasoma cruzi* and protection of mice against lethal infection with the organism. *J. Infect. Dis. 150*:594–601, 1984.
6. Pottage, J, Kessler, H, Goodrich, J, Hurley, T, Levin, S: Antiviral effects of ketoconazole. *Clin. Res. 31*:736A, 1983.
7. Borgers, M: Mechanism of action of antifungal drugs, with special reference to the imidazole derivatives. *Rev. Infect. Dis. 2*:520–534, 1980.
8. Beggs, WH, Andrews, FA, Sarosi, GA: Action of imidazole-containing antifungal drugs. *Life Sci. 28*:111–118, 1981.
9. Borgers, M, Van den Bossche, H, De Brabander, M: The mechanism of action of the new antimycotic ketoconazole. *Am. J. Med. 74*(1B):2–8, 1983.
10. Pye, GW, Marriott, MS: Inhibition of sterol C14 demethylation by imidazole-containing antifungals. *Sabouraudia 20*:325–329, 1982.
11. Heeres, J, Van den Bossche, H: Antifungal chemotherapy. In: *Annual Reports in Medicinal Chemistry* (LM Werbel, ed.), Academic Press, New York, 1980, pp. 139–148.
12. Sud, IJ, Feingold, DS: Heterogeneity of action mechanisms among antimycotic imidazoles. *Antimicrob. Agents Chemother. 20*:71–74, 1981.
13. Stanley, VC, Hurley, R: The growth of *Candida* species in cultures of mouse peritoneal macrophages. *J. Pathol. 97*:357–366, 1969.
14. De Brabander, M, Aerts, F, Van Cutsem, J, Van den Bossche, H, Borgers, M: The activity of ketoconazole in mixed cultures of leukocytes and *Candida albicans. Sabouraudia 18*:197–210, 1980.
15. Cutler, JE, Poor, AH: Effect of mouse phagocytes on *Candida albicans* in in vivo chambers. *Infect. Immun. 31*:1110–1116, 1981.
16. Niemegeers, CJE, Levron, JCL, Awouters, F, Janssen, PAJ: Inhibition and induction of microsomal enzymes in the rat. A comparative study of four antimycotics: Miconazole, econazole, clotrimazole, and ketoconazole. *Arch. Intern. Pharmacodyn. Ther. 251*:26–38, 1981.

17. Van den Bossche, H, Willemsens, G, Cools, W, Lauwers, WFJ, Lejeune, L: Biochemical effects of miconazole on fungi. Inhibition of ergosterol biosynthesis in *Candida albicans. Chem. Biol. Interact. 21*:59–78, 1978.
18. Uno, J, Shigematsu, ML, Arai, T: Primary site of action of ketoconazole on *Candida albicans. Antimicrob. Agents Chemother. 21*:912–918, 1982.
19. Shigematsu, ML, Uno, J, Arai, T: Effect of ketoconazole on isolated mitochondria from *Candida albicans. Antimicrob. Agents Chemother. 21*:919–914, 1982.
20. Beggs, WH: Influence of pH on ketoconazole activity against *Candida parapsilosis* and *Candida albicans. Res. Commun. Chem. Pathol. Pharmacol. 37*:495–498, 1982.
21. Minagawa, H, Kitaura, K, Nakamizo, N: Effects of pH on the activity of ketoconazole against *Candida albicans. Antimicrob. Agents Chemother. 23*:105–107, 1983.
22. Odds, FC: Laboratory evaluation of antifungal agents: A comparative study of five imidazole derivatives of clinical importance. *J. Antimicrob. Chemother. 6*:749–761, 1980.
23. Galgiani, JN, Stevens, DA: Antimicrobial susceptibility testing of yeasts: A turbidometric technique independent of inoculum size. *Antimicrob. Agents Chemother. 10*: 721–726, 1976.
24. Stevens, DA: Miconazole in the treatment of systemic fungal infections. *Am. Rev. Respir. Dis. 116*:801–806, 1977.
25. Drutz, DJ: Newer antifungal agents and their use, including an update on amphotericin B and flucytosine. In: *Current Clinical Topics in Infectious Diseases* (JS Remington and MN Swartz, eds.), McGraw-Hill, New York, 1982, pp. 97–135.
26. Plempel, M: Pharmacokinetics of imidazole antimycotics. *Postgrad. Med. J. 55*: 662–666, 1979.
27. Boelaert, J, Daneels, R, Van Landuyt, H, Symoens, J: Miconazole plasma levels in healthy subjects and in patients with impaired renal function. *Chemotherapy 6*:165–169, 1976.
28. Lewi, PJ, Boelaert, J, Daneels, R, De Meyere, R, Van Landuyt, H, Heykants, JJP, Symoens, J, Wynants, J: Pharmacokinetic profile of intravenous miconazole in man. Comparison of normal subjects and patients with renal insufficiency. *Eur. J. Clin. Pharmacol. 10*:49–54, 1976.
29. Heel, RC, Brogden, RN, Pakes, GE, Speight, TN, Avery, GS: Miconazole: A preliminary review of its therapeutic efficacy in systemic fungal infections. *Drugs 19*: 7–30, 1980.
30. Sung, JP, Rajani, K, Chopra, DR, Grendahl, JG, Haws, EB: Miconazole therapy for systemic candidiasis in a conjoined (siamese) twin and a premature newborn. *Am. J. Surg. 138*:688–691, 1979.
31. Fisher, JF, Duma, RJ, Markowitz, SM, Shadomy, S, Espinel-Ingroff, A, Chew, WH: Therapeutic failures with miconazole. *Antimicrob. Agents Chemother. 13*:965–968, 1978.
32. Evers, KG, Knoop, UF: Miconazole treatment of *Candida* sepsis in aminophenazone induced agranulocytosis. *Acta Paediatr. Belg. 31*:151–153, 1978.
33. Wade, TR, Jones, HE, Chanda, JJ: Intravenous miconazole therapy of mycotic infections. *Arch. Intern. Med. 139*:784–786, 1979.
34. Clarke, M, Davies, DP, Odds, F, Mitchell, C: Neonatal systemic candidiasis treated with miconazole. *Br. Med. J. 2*:354, 1980.
35. de Mol, P, Laureys, W, Dorchy, H: Neonatal meningitis due to *Candida albicans*, associated with osteomyelitis; failure to respond to miconazole. *J. Infection 5*: 195–197, 1982.
36. McDougall, PN, Fleming, PJ, Speller, DCE, Daish, P, Speidel, BD: Neonatal systemic candidiasis: A failure to respond to intravenous miconazole in two neonates. *Arch. Dis. Child. 57*:884–886, 1982.

37. Deresinski, SC, Lilly, RB, Levine, HB, Galgiani, JN, Stevens, DA: Treatment of fungal meningitis. *Arch. Intern. Med. 137*:1180–1185, 1977.
38. Daneshmend, TK, Warnock, DW, Ene, MD, Johnson, EM, Potten, MR, Richardson, MD, Williamson, PJ: Influence of food on the pharmacokinetics of ketoconazole. *Antimicrob. Agents Chemother. 25*:1–3, 1984.
39. Mannisto, PT, Mantyla, R, Nykanen, S, Lamminsivu, U, Ottoila, P: Impairing effect of food on ketoconazole absorption. *Antimicrob. Agents Chemother. 21*:730–733, 1982.
40. Daneshmend, TK, Warnock, DW, Turner, A, Roberts, CJC: Pharmacokinetics of ketoconazole in normal subjects. *J. Antimicrob. Chemother. 8*:299–304, 1981.
41. Brass, C, Galgiani, JN, Blaschke, TF, Defelice, R, O'Reilly, RA, Stevens, DA: Disposition of ketoconazole, an oral antifungal, in humans. *Antimicrob. Agents Chemother. 21*:151–158, 1982.
42. Daneshmend, TK, Warnock, DW, Ene, MD, Johnson, EM, Parker, G, Richardson, MD, Roberts, CJC: Multiple dose pharmacokinetics of ketoconazole and their effects on antipyrine kinetics in man. *J. Antimicrob. Chemother. 12*:185–188, 1983.
43. Bardare, M, Tortorano, AM, Pietrogrande, MC, Viviani, MA: Pharmacokinetics of ketoconazole and treatment evaluation in candidal infections. *Arch. Dis. Child. 59*: 1068–1071, 1984.
44. Ginsburg, CM, McCraken, GH, Jr., Olsen, K: Pharmacology of ketoconazole suspension in infants and children. *Antimicrob. Agents Chemother. 23*:787–789, 1983.
45. Dismukes, WE, Stamm, AM, Graybill, JR, et al.: Treatment of systemic mycoses with ketoconazole: Emphasis on toxicity and clinical response in 52 patients. *Ann. Intern. Med. 98*:13–20, 1983.
46. Shadomy, S, Espinel-Ingroff, A, Tartaglione, TA, Dismukes, WE, the NIAID Mycoses Study Group: Treatment of systemic mycoses with ketoconazole: Studies of ketoconazole serum levels. *Mykosen 29*:195–209, 1986.
47. Sugar, AM, Stevens, DA, Galgiani, JN, Graybill, JR, Dismukes, WE, Cloud, G, the NIAID Mycoses Study Group: Pharmacokinetics and toxicity of high dose ketoconazole: Results of multicenter randomized trials in disseminated coccidioidomycosis. In preparation.
48. Hann, IM, Prentice, HG, Keaney, M, Corringham, R, Blacklock, HA, Fox, J, Gascoigne, E, Van Cutsem, J: The pharmacokinetics of ketoconazole in severely immunocompromised patients. *J. Antimicrob. Chemother. 10*:489–496, 1982.
49. Vu Van, H, Piens, MA, Archimbaud, E, Monier, MF, Guyotat, D, Mojon, M, Fiere, D: Serum levels of ketoconazole in bone marrow transplanted patients. *Nouv. Rev. Fr. Hematol. 25*:241–244, 1983.
50. Maksymiuk, AW, Levine, HB, Bodey, GP: Pharmacokinetics of ketoconazole in patients with neoplastic diseases. *Antimicrob. Agents Chemother. 22*:43–46, 1982.
51. Heel, RC: Pharmacokinetic properties. In: *Ketoconazole in the Management of Fungal Disease* (HB Levine, ed.), ADIS Press, Balgowlah, Australia, 1982, pp. 67–73.
52. Schafer-Korting, M, Korting, HC, Dorn, M, Mutschler, E: Ketoconazole concentrations in human skin blister fluid and plasma. *Int. J. Clin. Pharmacol. Ther. Toxicol. 22*:371–374, 1984.
53. Harris, R, Jones, HE, Artis, WM: Orally administered ketoconazole: Route of delivery to the stratum corneum. *Antimicrob. Agents Chemother. 24*:876–882, 1983.
54. Medoff, G, Kobayashi, GS: Strategies in the treatment of systemic fungal infections. *N. Engl. J. Med. 302*:145–155, 1980.
55. Craven, PC, Graybill, JR, Jorgensen, JH, Dismukes, WE, Levine, BE: High-dose ketoconazole for treatment of fungal infections of the central nervous system. *Ann. Intern. Med. 98*:160–167, 1983.
56. Brass, C, Galgiani, JN, Campbell, SC, Stevens, DA: Therapy of disseminated or pulmonary coccidioidomycosis with ketoconazole. *Rev. Infect. Dis. 2*:665–660, 1980.

57. Levine, HB, Cobb, JM: Oral therapy for experimental coccidioidomycosis with R41,400 (ketoconazole), a new imidazole. *Am. Rev. Respir. Dis. 118*:715–721, 1978.
58. Harvey, RP, Isenberg, RA, Stevens, DA: Molecular modifications of imidazole compounds: Studies of activity and synergy in vitro and of pharmacology and therapy of blastomycosis in a mouse model. *Rev. Infect. Dis. 2*:559–569, 1980.
59. Clayton, YM, Wingfiled, HJ: Bioassay of ketoconazole in human serum. *Clin. Res. Rev. 1*:189–193, 1981.
60. Jorgensen, JH, Alexander, GA, Graybill, JR, Drutz, DJ: Sensitive bioassay for ketoconazole in serum and cerebrospinal fluid. *Antimicrob. Agents Chemother. 20*:59–62, 1981.
61. Swezey, SF, Giacomini, KM, Abang, A, Brass, C, Stevens, DA, Blaschke, TF: Measurement of ketoconazole, a new antifungal agent, by high-performance liquid chromatography. *J. Chromatogr. 227*:510–515, 1982.
62. Pascucci, VL, Bennett, J, Narang, PK, Chatterji, DC: Quantitation of ketoconazole in biological fluids using high-performance liquid chromatography. *J. Pharm. Sci. 72*:1467–1469, 1983.
63. Alton, KB: Determination of the antifungal agent, ketoconazole in human plasma by high-performance liquid chromatography. *J. Chromatogr. 221*:337–344, 1980.
64. Andrews, FA, Peterson, LR, Beggs, WH, Crankshaw, D, Sarosi, GA: Liquid chromatographic assay of ketoconazole. *Antimicrob. Agents Chemother. 19*:110–113, 1981.
65. Bodet, CA, III, Jorgensen, JH, Drutz, DJ: Simplified bioassay method for measurement of flucytosine or ketoconazole. *J. Clin. Microbiol. 22*:157–160, 1985.
66. Bennett, JE, Remington, JS: Miconazole in cryptococcosis and systemic candidiasis: A word of caution. *Ann. Intern. Med. 94*:708–709, 1981.
67. Sugar, AM: The polyene macrolide antifungal drugs. In: *The Antimicrobial Agent*, Annual 2 (PK Peterson, J Verhoef, Eds.), Elsevier, Amsterdam, pp. 228–237, 1987.
68. Petersen, EA, Alling, DW, Kirkpatrick, CH: Treatment of chronic mucocutaneous candidiasis with ketoconazole. A controlled clinical trial. *Ann. Intern. Med. 93*: 791–795, 1980.
69. Rosenblatt, HM, Byrne, W, Ament, ME, Graybill, J, Stiehm, ER: Successful treatment of chronic mucocutaneous candidiasis with ketoconazole. *J. Pediatr. 97*: 657–660, 1980.
70. Fanconi, S, Seger, R, Joller, P, Issler, C, Schar, G: Intermittent ketoconazole therapy of chronic mucocutaneous candidiasis in childhood. *Eur. J. Pediatr. 139*: 176–180, 1980.
71. Hughes, WT, Bartley, DL, Patterson, GG, Tufenkeji, H: Ketoconazole and candidiasis: A controlled study. *J. Infect. Dis. 147*:1060–1063, 1983.
72. Horsburgh, CR, Kirkpatrick, CH: Long-term therapy of chronic mucocutaneous candidiasis with ketoconazole: Experience with twenty-one patients. *Am. J. Med. 74*(1B):23–29, 1983.
73. Tudehope, DI, Rigby, B: Neonatal systemic candidiasis treated with miconazole and ketoconazole. *Med. J. Aust. 1*:480–481, 1983.
74. Lutwick, LI, Rytel, MW, Yanez, JP, Galgiani, JN, Stevens, DA: Deep infections from *Petriellidium boydii* treated with miconazole. *JAMA 241*:272–273, 1979.
75. Galgiani, JN, Stevens, DA, Graybill, JR, Stevens, DL, Tillinghast, AJ, Levine, HB: *Pseudallescheria boydii* infections treated with ketoconazole. Clinical evaluations of seven patients and in vitro susceptibility results. *Chest 86*:219–224, 1984.
76. Stevens, DA: Miconazole in the treatment of coccidioidomycosis. *Drugs 26*:347–354, 1983.
77. Bennett, JE, Dismukes, WE, Duma, RJ, et al.: A comparison of amphotericin B alone and combined with flucytosine in the treatment of cryptococcal meningitis. *N. Engl. J. Med. 301*:126–131, 1979.

78. Graybill, JR, Kaster, SR, Drutz, DJ: Comparative activities of Bay n7133, ICI 153,066, and ketoconazole in murine cryptococcosis. *Antimicrob. Agents Chemother. 24*:829–834, 1983.
79. Iwen, PC, Miller, NG, McFadden, HW, Jr.: Treatment of murine pulmonary cryptococcosis with ketoconazole and amphotericin B. *J. Infect. Dis. 149*:650, 1984.
80. Weinstein, L, Jacoby, I: Successful treatment of cerebral cryptococcoma and meningitis with miconazole. *Ann. Intern. Med. 93*:569–571, 1980.
81. Van Dijke, CPH, Veerman, FR, Haverkamp, HCH: Anaphylactic reactions to ketoconazole. *Br. Med. J. 287*:1673, 1983.
82. Fainstein, V, Bodey, GP: Cardiorespiratory toxicity due to miconazole. *Ann. Intern. Med. 93*:432–433, 1980.
83. Defilice, R, Johnson, DG, Galgiani, JN: Gynecomastia with ketoconazole. *Antimicrob. Agents Chemother. 19*:1073–1074, 1981.
84. Pont, A, Williams, PL, Azhar, S, Reitz, RE, Bochra, C, Smith, ER, Stevens, DA: Ketoconazole blocks testosterone synthesis. *Arch. Intern. Med. 142*:2137–2140, 1982.
85. Santen, RJ, Van den Bossche, H, Symoens, J, Brugmans, J, De Coster, R: Site of action of low dose ketoconazole on androgen biosynthesis in men. *J. Clin. Endocrinol. Metab. 57*:732–736, 1983.
86. Sikka, SC, Swerdloff, RS, Rajfer, J: In vitro inhibition of testosterone biosynthesis by ketoconazole. *Endocrinology 116*:1920–1925, 1985.
87. Grosso, DS, Boyden, TW, Parmenter, RW, Johnson, DG, Stevens, DA, Galgiani, JN: Ketoconazole inhibition of testicular secretion of testosterone and displacement of steroid hormones from serum transport proteins. *Antimicrob. Agents Chemother. 23*:207–212, 1983.
88. Pont, A, Goldman, ES, Sugar, AM, Siiteri, PK, Stevens, DA: Ketoconazole causes an increased estradiol to testosterone ratio: Probable explanation for gynecomastia. *Arch. Intern. Med. 145*:1429–1431, 1985.
89. Pont, A, Graybill, JR, Craven, PC, Galgiani, JN, Dismukes, WE, Reitz, RE, Stevens, DA: High-dose ketoconazole therapy and adrenal and testicular function in humans. *Arch. Intern. Med. 144*:2150–2153, 1984.
90. Kowal, J: The effect of ketoconazole on steroidogenesis in cultured mouse adrenal cortex tumor cells. *Endocrinology 112*:1541–1543, 1983.
91. Pont, A, Williams, PL, Loose, DS, Feldman, D, Reitz, RE, Bochra, C, Stevens, DA: Ketoconazole blocks adrenal steroid synthesis. *Ann. Intern. Med. 97*:370–372, 1982.
92. Loose, DS, Kan, PB, Hirst, MA, Marcus, RA, Feldman, D: Ketoconazole blocks adrenal steroidogenesis by inhibiting cytochrome P_{450}-dependent enzymes. *J. Clin. Invest. 71*:1495–1599, 1983.
93. Tucker, WS, Snell, BB, Island, DP, Gregg, CR: Reversible adrenal insufficiency induced by ketoconazole. *Arch. Intern. Med. 253*:2413–2414, 1985.
94. Trachtenberg, J, Halpern, N, Pont, A: Ketoconazole: A novel and rapid treatment for advanced prostatic cancer. *J. Urol. 130*:152–153, 1983.
95. Holland, FJ, Fishman, L, Bailey, JD, Fazekas, ATA: Ketoconazole in the management of precocious puberty not responsive to LHRH-analogue therapy. *N. Engl. J. Med. 312*:1023–1028, 1985.
96. Lewis, JH, Zimmerman, HJ, Benson, GD, Ishak, KG: Hepatic injury associated with ketoconazole therapy. Analysis of 33 cases. *Gastroenterology 86*:503–513, 1984.
97. Deresinski, SC, Galgiani, JN, Stevens, DA: Miconazole treatment. *112*:1541–1543, 1983.
98. Van Der Meer, JW, Keuning, JJ, Scheijgrond, HW, Heykants, J, Van Cutsem, J, Brugmans, J: The influence of gastric acidity on the bio-availability of ketoconazole. *J. Antimicrob. Chemother. 6*:552–554, 1980.

99. Carlson, JA, Mann, HJ, Canafax, DM: Effect of pH on disintegration and dissolution of ketoconazole tablets. *Am. J. Hosp. Pharm. 40*:1334–1336, 1983.
100. Englehard, D, Stutman, HR, Marks, MI: Interaction of ketoconazole with rifampin and isoniazid. *N. Engl. J. Med. 311*:1681–1683, 1984.
101. Ferguson, RM, Sutherland, DER, Simmons, RL, Najarian, JS: Ketoconazole, cyclosporin metabolism, and renal transplantation. *Lancet 2*:882–883, 1982.
102. Dieperink, H, Moeller, J: Ketoconazole and cyclospirin. *Lancet 2*:1217, 1982.
103. Daneshemnd, TK: Ketoconazole-cyclosporin interaction. *Lancet 2*:1342–1343, 1982.
104. Cunningham, C, Burke, MD, Whiting, PH, Simpson, JG, Wheatley, DN: Ketoconazole, cyclosporin, and the kidney. *Lancet 2*:1464, 1982.
105. Schaffner, A, Frick, PG: The effect of ketoconazole on amphotericin B in a model of disseminated aspergillosis. *J. Infect. Dis. 151*:902–910, 1985.
106. Sud, IJ, Feingold, DS: Effect of ketoconazole on the fungicidal action of amphotericin B in *Candida albicans. Infect. Immun. 23*:185–187, 1983.

27
5-Fluorocytosine

CHARLES G. PROBER
Stanford University School of Medicine, Stanford, California

5-Fluorocytosine (5-FC) is a fluorinated pyrimidine. It was synthesized in 1957 during a search for antileukemia drugs. Although it was not found to be effective for the therapy of leukemia, in 1964 it was found to effectively treat candidemia in mice (1). Its effectiveness as an antifungal agent in humans was first reported in 1967 (2). It was released in the United States in 1972 (3).

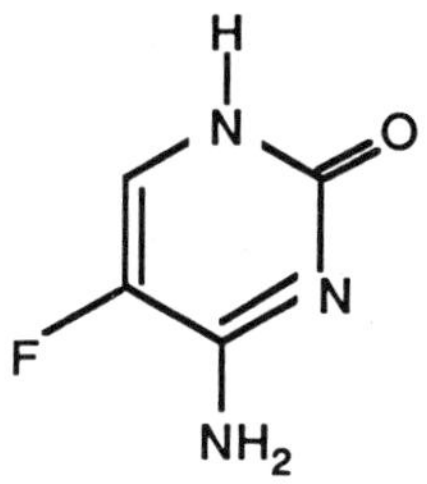

5-Fluorocytosine

I. MODE OF ACTION AND SPECTRUM OF ACTIVITY

5-FC is an antifungal agent without inherent antibacterial activity. It enters fungal cells under the action of permeases and is then deaminated in sensitive fungi by cytosine deaminase to 5-fluorouracil (5-FU). 5-FU acts as an inactive pyrimidine substitute leading to the production of nonfunctioning RNA with consequent alteration in protein synthesis (4–6). It has also been suggested that further conversion to fluorodeoxyuridine monophosphate results in the inhibition of thymidylate synthetase activity and hence DNA synthesis (5–7).

Fungi that are usually inhibited by attainable serum concentrations of 5-FC include most strains of *Cryptococcus neoformans*, many *Candida, Torulopsis, Phialophora, Sporotrichum*, Chromomycosis, and some isolates of *Aspergillus*, including *Aspergillus fumigatus*, *Aspergillus flavus*, and *Aspergillus niger* (4). In one study, which utilized disk diffusion sensitivity testing of 216 pathogenic and commensal yeasts, 95% of 78 *C. neoformans*, 96% of 27 *Torulopsis*, 85% of 53 non-*albicans Candida* species, and 77% of 58 species of *C. albicans* were inhibited by <16 μg/ml of 5-FC (8). A more recent study demonstrated that only 57% of 137 *C. albicans* clinical isolates were completely susceptible to <50 μg/ml of 5-FC (8a). Of the isolates, 51% were partially resistant in that there was sparse slow growth on medium containing 50 μg/ml of 5-FC. Interestingly, these partially resistant isolates gave rise to variants that were highly resistant. This observation may explain the tendency of resistance to readily develop if 5-FC is used alone. When measured by agar dilution, the minimal inhibitory concentrations (MIC) for sensitive cryptococci and *Candida* are generally <5 μg (5,9) and most *Torulopsis glabrata* are <25.6 μg (10). Several in vitro assessments of the activity of 5-FC against yeasts have consistently noted marked differences between the MIC and minimal bactericidal concentrations (MBC) for most strains, exemplifying the fungistatic nature of this compound (9,11,12). Synergistic interactions against *Candida* and cryptococci have been noted when 5-FC has been combined with amphotericin B (13–18), polymyxin B, or an imidazole (17–20).

Both primary resistance of fungi to 5-FC and the development of resistance during therapy are important factors that limit the use of this drug. Fungi that often display primary resistance to 5-FC include *Histoplasma, Blastomyces, Aspergillus* species, most dermatophytes, and from 3 to 53% of *Candida* strains (4,6,8,8a). Resistance emerging during serial passage in vitro or during treatment occurs with *Candida, Cryptococcus*, and *Torulopsis* isolates (4,5). This resistance often develops as a single-step mutation, resulting from the loss of cytosine deaminase activity (21). Other mechanisms of resistance that have been described include loss of permease (22) or uridine monophosphate pyrophosphorylase activity (23) and alteration of uridine monophosphate kinase, an enzyme essential to fungal growth (24). The overproduction of pyrimidines also has been implicated as a mechanism of resistance development in response to 5-FC treatment (22,23). Although the rate of induction of resistance in vitro has been shown not to be influenced by the concentration of 5-FC (23), it has been observed that the emergence of resistance in vivo is more likely to occur at lower (100 mg/kg day^{-1}) rather than at higher (150 mg/kg day^{-1}) doses of 5-FC (25).

II. PHARMACOKINETICS

Concentrations of 5-FC may be measured by a variety of assays, which include bioassay (26), fluorimetric assay (27), and high-performance liquid chromatography (HPLC) performed on a reversed-phase column (28) or on a cation-exchange column (29). The HPLC systems perform more favorably as they are more rapid, simple, sensitive, and specific when compared with microbiologic assays (28). A novel approach to estimating 5-FC concentrations was recently described by Noble et al. (30). This involved measuring the serum creatinine concentration by the Jaffe reaction (31) and also by the Kodak Ektachem system. As the Kodak system also detects 5-FC, the difference between these two values approximated the serum concentration of 5-FC. The correlation coefficient comparing these calculated concentrations with bioassay values was 0.982.

The absorption of 5-FC from the gastrointestinal tract is rapid and complete (4). When serum concentrations have been compared after oral and intravenous administration, the calculated bioavailability in normal subjects has ranged from 76 to 89% (32).

Bioavailability is reduced to 40–76% in patients with end-stage renal failure (33). The rate but not extent of absorption has been shown to be decreased with encapsulation, food, and antacids (32). Absorption is also delayed up to 10 hr in patients with impaired renal function (34).

In adults, peak serum concentrations (C_{max}) are usually attained 1–2 hr after an oral dose (4) and are in the range of 16–56 μg/ml after a dose of 25 mg/kg (9,25,35) and 23–86 μg/ml after 37.5 mg/kg (25). The large deviations in serum concentrations after oral doses are indicative of marked interpatient variation (25,32). The only data derived from the treatment of children revealed peak serum concentrations greater than 20 μg/ml in eight children after a unit dose of 25 mg/kg (36).

The volume of distribution V_d of 5-FC ranges from 400 to 700 ml/kg, approximating the value of total body water (19,32,34). The protein binding of 5-FC in vitro is minimal (2.9–4%) and is not affected by drug concentration (37). It is assumed that, because of the low molecular weight and sparse protein binding, 5-FC distributes widely. Data derived from rats sacrificed 6 hr after a dose revealed concentrations more than 50% of serum concentrations in liver, kidney, spleen, heart, lung, brain, fat, and muscle (38). Similarly, data from dogs also demonstrated excellent distribution of 5-FC into intrabronchial secretions, with concentrations 76% of simultaneous serum concentrations (39). Although there are only limited data on the distribution of 5-FC in humans, it has been found to attain therapeutic concentrations in saliva, peritoneal fluid, joint fluid, and cerebrospinal fluid (CSF) in treated patients (5). Data on the concentrations attained in CSF are the most extensive and indicate concentrations in excess of 75% of serum concentrations (9,33,40).

Although less than 4% of administered 5-FC is metabolized (41,42), studies in two patients and two volunteers given 2 g 5-FC demonstrated sustained concentrations of 5-FU > 100 ng/ml measured by a sensitive gas chromatographic-mass spectrometric assay (41). In addition, 20 of 41 serum samples from seven patients treated with 5-FC and amphotericin B were found to contain concentrations of 5-FU > 1000 ng/ml (41). These concentrations of 5-FU are comparable to those attained in patients with cancer receiving 12–15 mg/kg of 5-FU. It is probable that the hematologic toxicities of 5-FC are related to this metabolism to 5-FU.

Of administered 5-FC, 85–95% is excreted unchanged in the urine in the first 24 hr after a dose (4,28,43). Elimination is by filtration without significant secretion or reabsorption (43). The amount of 5-FC excreted in the stool ranges from 0.5 to 10.8% (38). The plasma clearance of 5-FC approximates creatinine clearance (37), and urine concentrations of the drug exceed serum concentrations by at least 20-fold (33,36).

The elimination half-life of 5-FC in the presence of normal renal function ranges from 3.3 to 8 hr (4,32,37,43). The half-life of 5-FC has been noted to be slightly prolonged in neonates (44) and in the presence of compromised renal function (5,33,37,45, 46). The degree of prolongation of the half-life is roughly proportional to the degree of serum creatinine elevation (32,37). Amphotericin B-induced renal dysfunction has been found to increase 5-FC concentrations by 14–142% (40).

Hemodialysis results in effective 5-FC clearance (32,33,37,46). Clearance has been found to increase as flow through the dialyzer increases (33). Peritoneal dialysis also effectively removes 5-FC (33). A supplementary dose of 5-FC is therefore recommended after dialysis, if dialysis is carried out every 48–72 hr (37).

The clearance of 5-FC does not seem to be altered in the presence of hepatic dysfunction, although published human data are limited to one patient recovering from postnecrotic cirrhosis (35). Kinetics of 5-FC was also unaltered among 10 New Zealand rabbits before and after hepatic insult caused by the administration of carbon tetrachloride (35).

III. TOXICITY

5-Fluorocytosine is a relatively safe antifungal agent. Side effects are usually mild, and when they occur, they only rarely necessitate discontinuation of therapy. Gastrointestinal intolerance occurs in approximately 6% of patients (47). In severe cases, mucosal necrosis and intestinal perforation have been described (48,49). Abnormal liver function tests occur in about 5–10% of patients in a dose-related fashion (4,47). These patients are usually asymptomatic, and this effect appears to be reversible (4). It has been suggested that liver function be monitored weekly during the administration of 5-FC.

Leukopenia and/or thrombocytopenia occur in 5–30% of patients (47,50,51). This is especially likely to occur in subjects with renal dysfunction or in those also receiving amphotericin B. It has also been noted with an especially high frequency among adults with the acquired immunodeficiency syndrome (51). This toxic reaction is usually dose and serum concentration related, occurring when concentrations exceed 100–125 μg/ml for prolonged periods (33,50,52). However, these high serum concentrations are not universally associated with hematosuppression. In one study, concentrations $>$ 100 μg/ml were noted among 5 of 14 patients, none of whom had leukopenia or thrombocytopenia (50). These toxic reactions are the most common reasons for discontinuing 5-FC, and they usually become manifest 10–26 days into a course of treatment (50). Death resulting from neutropenia-induced sepsis has been described (52,53). There is evidence to suggest that the myelosuppressive effects of 5-FC result from its in vivo conversion to 5-FU (41). The erythroid cell line, at least in vitro, is more resistant to the effects of 5-FC and the suppression of mammalian cell lines in vitro is completely reversed by uracil (54).

Uncommon side effects of 5-FC include rashes, headache, and hallucinations (4).

Other than the delayed absorption of 5-FC by coadministration of aluminum or magnesium hydroxide (33) and the delayed excretion resulting from the coadministration of amphotericin B, drug interactions with 5-FC have not been described as an important problem.

IV. CLINICAL USES

The clinical uses of 5-FC are limited. It has been used alone in the treatment of non-life-threatening urinary tract infections caused by sensitive strains of *Candida* (55) and in treating the chronic skin infection, chromomycosis (56). Because of the tendency of fungi to develop resistance to 5-FC when it is used alone, it is generally administered in combination with amphotericin B. Its best established application in this regard is in the treatment of meningitis caused by *C. neoformans*. In the study that best supports this use, 50 patients were randomized to receive amphotericin B alone for 10 weeks or amphotericin B in combination with 5-FC for 6 weeks (50). The combination therapy cured or improved more patients, had fewer failures or relapses, more rapidly sterilized the CSF, and caused less nephrotoxicity. Other, less well supported clinical circumstances in which 5-FC is often prescribed in combination with amphotericin B include the treatment of endocarditis caused by *Candida* (3), ophthalmitis caused by *Candida* (57), pulmonary infections caused by cryptococci (58), and a variety of infections caused by

T. glabrata, A. fumigatus, and *Sporotrichum schenckii* (58). This combination is also recommended for the treatment of neonatal candidiasis, especially in light of the fact that central nervous system involvement is quite common in this population of patients (59).

V. DOSE RECOMMENDATIONS

The usual recommended dose of 5-FC in patients with normal renal function is 100-200 mg/kg day^{-1} divided into four doses (4,5). Dose adjustment is necessary in those with compromised renal function. The duration of treatment is dependent upon the severity of infection and clinical response and is usually in the range of 6–10 weeks. The drug is supplied in 250- and 500-mg capsules and in a 1% intravenous formulation.

REFERENCES

1. Grunberg, E, Titsworth, E, Bennett, M: Chemotherapeutic activity of 5-fluorocytosine. *Antimicrob. Agents Chemother. 3*:566–568, 1963.
2. Grunberg, E, Prince, HN, Utz, JP: Observations on the activity of two newer antifungal agents saramycetin and 5-fluorocytosine. Int Congr Chemother., 5th, Vienna, 1967, pp. 69–76.
3. Utz, JP: Flucytosine. *N. Engl. J. Med. 286*:777–778, 1972.
4. Ashe, WD, Jr., Van Reken, DE: 5-fluorocytosine: A brief review. *Clin. Pediatr. 16*: 364–366, 1977.
5. Bennett, JE: Flucytosine. *Ann. Intern. Med. 86*:319–322, 1977.
6. Koldin, MH, Medoff, G: Antifungal chemotherapy. *Pediatr. Clin. North Am. 30*:49–61, 1983.
7. Diaso, RB, Bennett, JE, Meyers, CE: mode of action of 5-fluorocytosine. *Biochem. Pharmacol. 27*:703–707, 1978.
8. Utz, CJ, Shadomy, S: Antifungal activity of 5-fluorocytosine as measured by disc diffusion susceptibility testing. *J. Infect. Dis. 135*:970–974, 1977.

8a. Defever, KS, Whelan, WL, Rogers, AL, Beneke, ES, Veselenak, JM, Soll, DR: *Candida albicans* resistance to 5-fluorocytosine: Frequency of partially resistant strains among clinical isolates. *Antimicrob. Agents Chemother. 22*:810–815, 1982.

9. Shadomy, S: In vitro studies with 5-fluorocytosine. *Appl. Microbiol. 17*:871–877, 1969.
10. Schonebeck, J, Ansehn, S: 5-fluorocytosine resistance in *Candida* species and *Torulopsis glabrata. Sabouraudia 11*:10–20, 1973.
11. Shadomy, S, Kirchofdf, CF, Ingroff, AE: In vitro activity of 5-fluorocytosine against *Candida* and *Torulopsis* species. *Antimicrob. Agents Chemother. 3*:9–14, 1973.
12. Speller, DCE, Davies, MG: Sensitivity of yeasts to 5-fluorocytosine. *J. Med. Microbiol. 6*:315–321, 1973.
13. Rabinovich, S, Shaw, BD, Bryant, T, Donta, ST: Effect of 5-fluorocytosine and amphotericin B on *Candida albicans* infection in mice. *J. Infect. Dis. 130*:28–31, 1974.
14. Pollak, A, Scholer, HJ: Combination of amphotericin B and 5-fluorocytosine. In: *Chemotherapy*, Vol. 6, (JD Williams, and AM Geddes, eds.), Plenum Press, New York, 1976, pp. 137–142.
15. Medoff, G, Comfort, M, Kobayashi, GS: Synergistic action of amphotericin B and 5-fluorocytosine against yeast-like organisms. *Proc. Soc. Exp. Biol. Med. 138u*:571–574, 1971.
16. Kwan, CN, Medoff, G, Kobayashi, GS, Schlessinger, D, Raskas, HJ: Potentiation of the antifungal effects of antibiotics by amphotericin B. *Antimicrob. Agents Chemother. 2*:61–65, 1972.

17. Block, ER, Bennett, JE: The combined effect of 5-fluorocytosine and amphotericin B in the therapy of murine cryptococcosis. *Proc. Soc. Exp. Biol. Med. 142*:476–480, 1973.
18. Titsworth, E, Grunberg, E: Chemotherapeutic activity of 5-fluorocytosine and amphotericin B against *Candida albicans* in mice. *Antimicrob. Agents Chemother. 4*: 306–308, 1973.
19. Dupont, B, Drouhet, E: In vitro synergy and antagonism of anti-fungal agents against yeast-like fungi. *Postgrad. Med. J. 55*:683–686, 1979.
20. Beggs, WE, Sarosi, GA: Combined activity of ketoconazole and 5-fluorocytosine on potentially pathogenic yeasts. *Antimicrob. Agents Chemother. 21*:355–357, 1982.
21. Hoeprich, PD, Ingraham, JL, Kleker, E, Winship, MJ: Development of resistance to 5-fluorocytosine in *Candida parapsilosis* during therapy. *J. Infect. Dis. 130*:112–118, 1974.
22. Jund, R. Lacroute, F: Genetic and physiological resistance to 5-fluoropyrimidines in *Saccharomyces cerevisiae. J. Bacteriol. 102*:607–615, 1970.
23. Normark, S, Schonebeck, J: In vitro studies of 5-fluorocytosine resistance in *Candida albicans* and *Torulopsis glabrata. Antimicrob. Agents Chemother. 2*:114–121, 1972.
24. Ingraham, JL, Naeuhard, J: Cold-sensitive mutants of *Salmonella typhimurium* defective in uridine monophosphate kinase (pyr H). *J. Biol. Chem. 247*:6259–6265, 1972.
25. Shadomy, S: Further in vitro studies with 5-fluorocytosine. *Infect. Immun. 2*:484–488, 1970.
26. Kaspar, RL, Drutz, DJ: Rapid, simple bioassay for 5-fluorocytosine in the presence of amphotericin B. *Antimicrob. Agents Chemother. 7*:462–465, 1975.
27. Wade, D, Sudlow, G: Fluorometric measurement of 5-fluorocytosine in biological fluids. *J. Pharm. Sci. 62*:828–829, 1973.
28. Bury, RW, Mashford, ML, Miles, HM: Assay of flucytosine (5-fluorocytosine) in human plasma by high-pressure liquid chromatography. *Antimicrob. Agents Chemother. 16*:529–532, 1979.
29. Diasio, RB, Wilburn, ME, Shadomy, S, Espinel-Ingroff, A: Rapid determination of serum 5-fluorocytosine levels by high-performance liquid chromatography. *Antimicrob. Agents Chemother. 13*:500–504, 1978.
30. Noble, MA, Harper, B, Grant, AG, Bernstein, M: Rapid determination of 5-fluorocytosine levels in blood. *J. Clin. Microbiol. 20*:996–997, 1984.
31. Jaffe, M: Ueber den Niederschlag welchen Pikrinsaeure in normalem Harn erzeuget und ueber eine neue Reaktion des Kreatinins. *Z. Phys. Chem. 10*:391–400, 1886.
32. Cutler, RE, Blair, AD, Kelly, MR: Flucytosine kinetics in subjects with normal and impaired renal function. *Clin. Pharmacol. Ther. 24*:333–342, 1978.
33. Daneshmed, TK, Warnock, DW: Clinical pharmacokinetics of systemic antifungal drugs. *Clin. Pharmacokinet. 8*:17–42, 1983.
34. Dawborn, JK, Page, MD, Schiavone, DJ: Use of 5-fluorocytosine in patients with impaired renal function. *Br. Med. J. 4*:382–384, 1973.
35. Block, ER: Effect of hepatic insufficiency on 5-fluorocytosine concentrations in serum. *Antimicrob. Agents Chemother. 3*:141–142, 1973.
36. Holt, RJ, Newman, RL: The antimycotic activity of 5-fluorocytosine. *J. Clin. Pathol. 26*:167–174, 1973.
37. Block, ER, Bennett, JE, Livoti, LG, Klein, WJ, MacGregor, RR, Henderson, L: Flucytosine and amphotericin B: Hemodialysis effects on the plasma concentration and clearance, studies in man. *Ann. Intern. Med. 80*:613–617, 1974.
38. Koechlin, BA, Rubio, F, Palmer, S, Gabriel, T, Duschinsky, R: The metabolism of 5-fluorocytosine-2(^{14})C and of cytosine-(^{14})C in the rat and the disposition of 5-fluorocytosine-2(^{14})C in man. *Biochem. Pharmacol. 15*:435–446, 1966.

39. Pennington, JE, Block, ER, Reynolds, HY: 5-fluorocytosine and amphotericin B in bronchial secretions. *Antimicrob. Agents Chemother. 6*:324–326, 1974.
40. Block, ER, Bennett, JE: Pharmacological studies with 5-fluorocytosine. *Antimicrob. Agents Chemother. 1*:476–482, 1972.
41. Diasio, RB, Lakings, DE, Bennett, JE: Evidence for conversion of 5-fluorocytosine to 5-fluorouracil in humans: Possible factor in 5-fluorocytosine clinical toxicity. *Antimicrob. Agents Chemother. 14*:903–908, 1978.
42. Polak, A, Eschenhof, E, Fernex, M, Scholer, HJ: Metabolic studies with 5-fluorocytosine-6(^{14})C in mouse, rat, rabbit, dog, and man. *Chemotherapy 22*:137–153, 1976.
43. Wade, DN, Sudlow, G: The kinetics of 5-fluorocytosine elimination in man. *Aust. N.Z. J. Med. 2*:153–158, 1972.
44. Drouhet, E, Borderon, JC, Borderon, E, Boulard, P: Evolution des concentrations serique de 5-fluorocytosine chez les prematures. *Bull. Soc. Fr. Mycol. Med. 3*:37–40, 1974.
45. Schonebeck, J, Polak, A, Fernex, M, Scholar, HJ: Pharmacokinetic studies on the oral antimyotic agent 5-fluorocytosine in individuals with normal and impaired kidney function. *Chemotherapy 18*:321–336, 1973.
46. Drouhet, E, Babinet, P, Chapusot, JP, Kleinknecht, D: 5-Fluorocytosine in the treatment of candidiasis with acute renal insufficiency. *Biomedicine 19*:408–414, 1973.
47. Fernex, M: Klinische Erfahrung mit 5-fluorocytosin in der Behandlung von systemischen Mykosen. 11 Wissensch Tag deutschspr Myokol Ges, Basel, 1974.
48. Harder, EJ, Hermans, PE: Treatment of fungal infections with flucytosine. *Arch. Intern. Med. 135*:231–237, 1975.
49. Utz, JP: Current and future chemotherapy of central nervous system fungal infections. *Adv. Neurol. 6*:127–132, 1974.
50. Bennett, JE, Dismukes, WE, Duma, RJ, Medoff, G, Sande, MA, Gallis, H, Leonard, J, Fields, BT, Bradshaw, M, Haywood, H, McGee, ZA, Cate, TR, Cobbs, CG, Warner, JF, Alling, DW: A comparison of amphotericin B alone and combined with flucytosine in the treatment of cryptococcal meningitis. *N. Engl. J. Med. 301*:126–131, 1979.
51. Kovacs, JA, Kovacs, AA, Polis, M, Wright, WC, Gill, VJ, Tuazon, CV, Gelmann, EP, Lane, HC, Longfield, R, Overturf, G, Macher, AM, Fauci, AS, Parrillo, JE, Bennett, JE, Masur, H: Cryptococcosis with the acquired immunodeficiency syndrome. *Ann. Intern. Med. 103*:533–538, 1985.
52. Kaufman, CA, Frame, PT: Bone marrow toxicity associated with 5-fluorocytosine therapy. *Antimicrob. Agents Chemother. 11*:244–247, 1977.
53. Meyer, R, Axelrod, JL: Fatal aplastic anemia resulting from flucytosine. *JAMA 228*: 1573, 1974.
54. Koeffler, HP, Golde, DW: 5-fluorocytosine inhibition of hematopoiesis in vitro and reversal of inhibition by uracil. *J. Infect. Dis. 139*:438–443, 1979.
55. Schonebeck, J, Steen, L, Tarnvik, A: 5-Fluorocytosine treatment of *Candida* infections of the urinary tract and other sites. *Scand. J. Urol. Nephrol. 6*:37–43, 1972.
56. Mauceri, AA, Cullen, SI, Vandevelde, AG, Johnson, JE: Flucytosine. An effective oral treatment for chromomycosis. *Arch. Dermatol. 109*:873–876, 1974.
57. Robertson, DM, Riley, FC, Hermans, PE: Endogenous *Candida* oculomycosis: Report of two patients treated with flucytosine. *Arch. Ophthalmol. 91*:33–38, 1974.
58. Herman, PE, Keys, TF: Antifungal agents used for dee-seated mycotic infections. *Mayo Clin. Proc. 58*:223–231, 1983.
59. Johnson, DE, Thompson, TR, Green, TP, Ferrieri, P: Systemic candidiasis in very low-birth-weight infants ($\leqslant$1500 grams). *Pediatrics 73*:138–143, 1984.

Part V
Antiviral Agents

28

Vidarabine Therapy of Herpesvirus Infections in Childhood

RICHARD J. WHITLEY
University of Alabama at Birmingham, Birmingham, Alabama

The pyrimidine analog 5-iodo-2′-deoxyuridine (idoxuridine, IDU) was the first drug developed for the treatment of viral infections. Studies performed in the early 1960s showed that this drug was useful for the treatment of herpes simplex keratoconjunctivitis. Although the licensure of idoxuridine began an era of testing of antiviral drugs, it was not until the development of vidarabine in the early 1970s that interest in the feasibility of parenteral antiviral therapy began to develop. Early developments with vidarabine and, subsequently, acyclovir have established antiviral chemotherapy's role in the physician's armamentarium. Advances in the therapy of viral infections were once only the basis of discussion among clinical and biomedical investigators; however, these advances have now been applied by the practicing physician to the management of human viral diseases. Most of these advances have been achieved in the treatment of adult viral infections. However, the past few years have recognized the established use of antiviral drugs in the treatment of severe and life-threatening diseases of childhood. The development of specific and selective inhibitors of viral replication is especially important in the treatment of herpesvirus infections.

The ability of drugs to distinguish enzymes responsible for viral replication from those enzymes necessary for cell replication has led to the development of compounds with low toxicity and broader clinical applicability. Controlled studies utilizing appropriate biostatistical designs have identified viral infections amenable to therapy. During the conduct of controlled studies, the natural history and pathogenesis of many herpesvirus infections has been elucidated and the need for prompt diagnosis of these infections further reiterated. This last point, the need for rapid and specific viral diagnosis, warrants further emphasis. If further advances in the treatment of human herpesvirus infections are to be achieved, particularly for diseases in which clinical manifestations are vague and nonspecific, such as herpes simplex encephalitis, rapid diagnostic procedures must be available at the time of clinical presentation of illness in order for the appropriate deployment of an antiviral drug. This chapter will focus on the developments of vidarabine, a drug that has provided a foundation for the development of newer and more specific antiviral compounds with enhanced therapeutic activity. Studies performed with vidarabine have provided a model for the development and evaluation of other antiviral drugs for clinical pharmacology as well as the determination of therapeutic activity.

I. HISTORY

Vidarabine, 9-β-D-arabinofuranosyl adenine or adenine arabinoside, was synthesized in the early 1960s as a potential anticancer agent (1,2). The compound was found to have antiviral activity against herpes simplex and vaccinia virus in cell culture by the French investigators led by De Rudder and colleagues (3). At approximately the same time, investigators at Parke Davis and Company, Ann Arbor, Michigan, and Southern Research Institute, Birmingham, Alabama, found similar significant antiviral activity of an antibiotic concentrate derived from the fermentation of *Streptomyces antibioticus*. It was not until several years later, however, in 1967, that this concentrate was identified as vidarabine, a compound that could be prepared inexpensively by fermentation or isolated along with several other arabinosyl nucleosides from the Caribbean sponge *Cryptotithia crypta* (4–6). Detailed reviews of these compounds appeared within the first decade of their discovery (7,8).

II. ACTIVITY AND MECHANISM OF ACTION

Following the initial in vitro reports of Privat de Garilhe and De Rudder of vidarabine's activity against herpes simplex (3), Miller and colleagues demonstrated that other DNA viruses, particularly varicella zoster virus and cytomegalovirus, were also sensitive to this compound when studied in other cell systems (5). These observations prompted comparisons with the then existing antiviral compounds idoxuridine and cytosine arabinoside (9,10). The findings of a variety of investigators were similar; namely, vidarabine was the most potent antiviral identified at this time, followed in order by idoxuridine and cytosine arabinoside. Investigators at Southern Research Institute proposed that the therapeutic index of vidarabine was better than the other two compounds because of decreased cellular toxicity within an efficacious dose range (6).

The tissue culture observations, not only of vidarabine but also of cytosine arabinoside and idoxuridine, led to investigations of the mechanism of action of these compounds. Unfortunately, even in 1986, our knowledge of the mechanism of action of vidarabine is not nearly as complete as that of other antiviral agents, such as acyclovir, currently under investigation (11).

Vidarabine is phosphorylated, as are other nucleoside analogs, to its triphosphate derivative. Cohen has summarized the mechanism of action of vidarabine (12). In spite of deamination to arabinosyl hypoxanthine, the parent compound is transported into cells, where phosphorylation to the mono-, di-, and triphosphate derivatives occurs. The triphosphate derivative, then, acts as a competitive inhibitor of herpes simplex virus DNA polymerase (13,14). In addition, vidarabine is incorporated into the growing DNA molecule (15,16). Furthermore, it appears as though the triphosphate derivative of vidarabine suppresses virally induced DNA polymerase slightly more than cellular DNA polymerases; however, it has been difficult to confirm these observations (15). Thus, the essential mechanism of action of vidarabine, although not precisely defined, appears similar to that of idoxuridine (17,18). Like idoxuridine, vidarabine is a first-generation antiviral compound, being a nonselective inhibitor of both host cell and viral replication. There is a potential for cellular toxicity that appears to be dose related. This latter effect is to be expected because of the lack of selective inhibition of virally induced enzymes.

III. PHARMACOLOGY

Studies of the pharmacokinetics, safety, and potential clinical usefulness of vidarabine have been summarized (19,20). It should be emphasized that most studies assessing the pharmacology of antiviral drugs have been performed in adults with only limited studies in children. Vidarabine is no exception. The studies of vidarabine can be summarized according to the following. First, human beings and higher animal species (such as simians), when given vidarabine, deaminate the parent compound to arabinosyl hypoxanthine, a derivative that has antiviral activity although significantly less than that of the parent compound. In contrast, lower animal forms oxidize vidarabine to xanthine, which is freely excreted in the urine. This latter observation implies the need for caution when interpreting experimental data generated from animal species that oxidize rather than deaminate this drug. Second, as indicated from radioactive tracer studies, the plasma half-life of vidarabine is approximately 4 hr. However, when re-evaluated by high-pressure liquid chromatography (HPLC), these patterns of clearance of radioactivity indicated a shorter half-life. These studies were performed principally in adults; thus, age variation may not have been identified. Third, additional radioactive tracer studies have demonstrated the accumulation of active drug and metabolites within erythrocytes for 5-7 days after dosing with persistence for as long as 3 weeks. These observations have been extended to terminal leukemic patients whose tissues were examined several weeks after dosing for the presence of active compound. The highest drug concentrations were found in kidney, liver, and spleen; somewhat lower concentrations were obtained from skeletal muscle and, importantly, brain. Fourth, during and as long as 10 days after therapy, vidarabine and its metabolites were found in the cerebrospinal fluid at approximately one-half the concentration of the corresponding plasma levels. Fifth, multidose pharmacokinetic studies in humans have demonstrated that the primary extracellular metabolite was arabinosyl hypoxanthine. During a constant infusion, arabinosyl hypoxanthine concentrations peak at the termination of a period of a 12-hr infusion, resulting in concentrations of 4–8 μg/ml. Vidarabine was present but only at barely detectible concentrations of approximately 0.2 μg/ml, the lower limit of detection. These data imply no extracellular accumulation of vidarabine and its immediate conversion to the hypoxanthine derivative. Even at present, there are no data regarding intracellular drug accumulation following multidose administration. Finally, vidarabine is cleared from the body by the kidney with nearly 60% of the dosage appearing in the urine as arabinosyl hypoxanthine over the first 24 hr after administration. Consequently, the dose should be reduced to avoid toxicity in cases of renal insufficiency. All these data provided the foundation for expanded field trials in humans.

During the conduct of these studies there was virtually no evidence of toxicity that would contradict the availability of this compound for controlled clinical investigations.

Limited studies of the pharmacology of vidarabine have been performed in children and neonates. When comparing plasma concentrations generated from pharmacokinetics studies in adults, apparent findings in newborns would indicate that higher dosages of medication are required to achieve similar plasma concentrations of arabinosyl hypoxanthine and vidarabine (21,22). Such studies have important implications for therapy of the newborn, particularly with neonatal herpes simplex virus infection.

IV. CLINICAL CONTROLLED TRIALS

Vidarabine was the first of the parenterally administered antiviral drugs for which unequivocal efficacy was demonstrated. Following the assessment of the clinical pharmacology of vidarabine, a series of uncontrolled studies defined therapeutic regimens, established both safety and tolerance, and identified targeted diseases and viruses for evaluation in controlled trials. The uncontrolled studies will not be considered further but can be reviewed (23-31). The controlled studies will be reviewed, indicating the value of vidarabine and the pitfalls encountered in the evaluation of antiviral compounds.

A. Herpes Simplex Encephalitis

One of the first advances in therapy of any viral infection, and the first for parenteral antiviral therapy, was the demonstration that vidarabine treatment decreased the mortality of biopsy-proven herpes simplex encephalitis. Through the National Institute of Allergy and Infectious Diseases (NIAID) Collaborative Antiviral Study Group, vidarabine therapy of biopsy-proven disease in a double-blind, placebo-controlled study decreased mortality from 70% in placebo recipients to 28% at 1 month and 40% at 6 months after the initiation of treatment in drug recipients (32). Because of small numbers of patients in the original controlled trial, a follow-up investigation of biopsy-proven disease was performed to verify mortality and define long-term morbidity. In this study, vidarabine administered at a dosage of 15 mg/kg day^{-1} by continuous infusion over 12 hr at a concentration of 0.5 mg/mg resulted in a mortality of 40% overall (33). Both age and level of consciousness at the time of institution of treatment influenced outcome in biopsy-proven disease. Outcome was significantly better for patients less than 30 years of age who were lethargic or semicomatose compared with those individuals who were comatose. For individuals over 30 years of age outcome was poorer overall. The data indicate that successful treatment can be achieved more readily in the younger patient and certainly in patients with a higher level of consciousness. These data provided the basis for the licensure of vidarabine for the treatment of herpes simplex virus infections of the central nervous system.

Prompt institution of antiviral therapy is mandatory. Once a brain biopsy has been performed, antiviral therapy is administered to patients with suspect herpes simplex encephalitis. If the brain biopsy is positive in tissue culture for herpes simplex virus, then treatment is continued for a full 14 days. On the other hand, if the biopsy is negative, therapy is usually discontinued at the end of 5 days of treatment.

Obvious problems in the assessment of patients with focal encephalitis is the method of diagnosis and the time that has elapsed prior to therapeutic intervention (34,35).

Recently, two double-blind comparative trials have evaluated vidarabine and acyclovir for the management of herpes simplex encephalitis (35,36). In these studies, it has been learned that acyclovir administered at dosages of 10 mg/kg every 8 hr over the period of 10 days is superior to vidarabine for treatment of this disease entity. As shown in Figure 1, the overall mortality in children and adults with acyclovir therapy 13 months after the onset of disease is 29%. Nearly 40% of acyclovir-treated patients return to normal function following this disease. As was recognized in the original studies with vidarabine, age and, in this circumstance, Glasgow coma score were predictive of long-term outcome. As shown in Figure 2, younger patients who had a Glasgow coma score in excess of 6 were more likely to return to normal function than individuals whose Glasgow coma score was less or equal to 6. The score of 6 is equated to a level of consciousness of coma. Glasgow coma scores in excess equate with levels of consciousness of semicoma and lethargy. For children, the early institution of acyclovir therapy can lead to a near 90% return to normal function. Significant adverse clinical and laboratory effects were

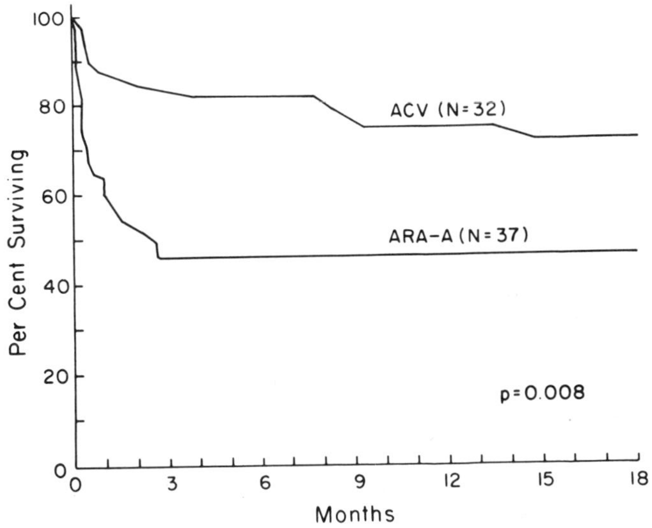

Figure 1 Comparison of survival in patients with biopsy-proven herpes simplex encephalitis treated with vidarabine (ARA-A) or acyclovir (ACV); P = 0.008. *Source*: *N. Engl. J. Med. 314*:144–149, 1986, with permission.

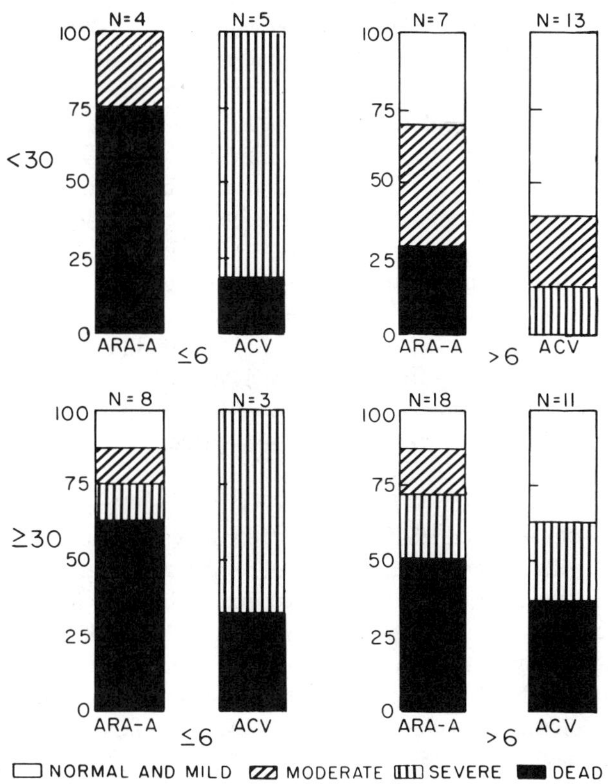

Figure 2 Morbidity after vidarabine (ARA-A) or acyclovir (ACV) treatment of biopsy-proven herpes simplex encephalitis, according to age (<30 vs. ⩾30) and the Glasgow coma score (⩽6 vs. >6). The scale at left side of each column indicates percentages (0–100). *Source*: *N. Engl. J. Med. 314*:144–149, with permission.

not encountered in these studies with either medication. These data indicate that acyclovir is the treatment of choice for herpes simplex encephalitis. The data from the NIAID Collaborative Antiviral Study Group were similar to those derived from a collaborative group of Swedish investigators utilizing different diagnostic criteria (36).

B. Neonatal Herpes Simplex Virus Infection

Following the demonstration that vidarabine was useful for the treatment of herpes simplex encephalitis, the efficacy of vidarabine for neonatal herpes simplex virus (HSV) infections was shown (37,38).

Because knowledge of the extent of disease with or without therapy is of prognostic value for long-term outcome, a disease classification scheme for neonatal HSV infection has been generated. Classification is essential for evaluating therapeutic outcome. Babies are classified as having either disseminated or localized disease. Disseminated infection involves multiple organs with or without involvement of the central nervous system (CNS). Localized infection can be subdivided into two categories. Disease can remain localized to the CNS without involvement of other organs. Finally, disease can remain localized to the skin, eyes, or mouth (SEM) without involvement of other sites. Historically, babies with CNS or disseminated disease have accounted for approximately 85% of children with neonatal herpes simplex virus infection (39,40). In the absence of therapy, mortality for these babies is in excess of 80% and less than 10% of babies develop normally. In contrast, babies with disease localized to the SEM have no mortality, but without therapy, 20-30% will develop long-term neurological impairment.

Over the past several years, the clinical presentation of neonatal herpes simplex virus infection has changed. Now, only approximately 50% of children have CNS or disseminated neonatal herpes simplex virus infection at presentation and the remainder will have involvement of the SEM (41). This can be attributed in large part to earlier recognition of babies with neonatal herpes simplex virus infection and the introduction of safe and efficacious antiviral therapy that has prevented disease progression.

Vidarabine at dosages of 15 and 30 mg/kg day^{-1} has been shown to decrease mortality in babies with CNS and disseminated disease from 70 to 40% overall, as shown in Figure 3 (37). Furthermore, following recovery from infection, nearly 30% of babies with such severe forms of infection develop normally. Babies treated for SEM involvement have no mortality, and only approximately 10% will develop neurological impairment.

Dosages of 15 and 30 mg/kg day^{-1} administered for 10 days lead to no difference in the overall mortality or morbidity from neonatal HSV infection (38); however, the higher dosage of vidarabine was associated with a decreased frequency of progressive disease. Specifically, in the absence of therapy it has been recognized that 70% of babies with SEM involvement will progress to either CNS or disseminated infection (37,39). When vidarabine is administered at 15 mg/kg day^{-1}, the frequency of progression can be decreased to 24%; at a dosage of 30 mg/kg day^{-1}, the frequency of progression is decreased to 2% (41). Thus, the recommended dosage for vidarabine therapy of neonatal herpes simplex virus infections is 30 mg/kg day^{-1}.

C. Ocular Infections

Herpes simplex infections of the eye are amenable to antiviral therapy. These infections are the most common viral cause of blindness in developed societies. Herpes simplex

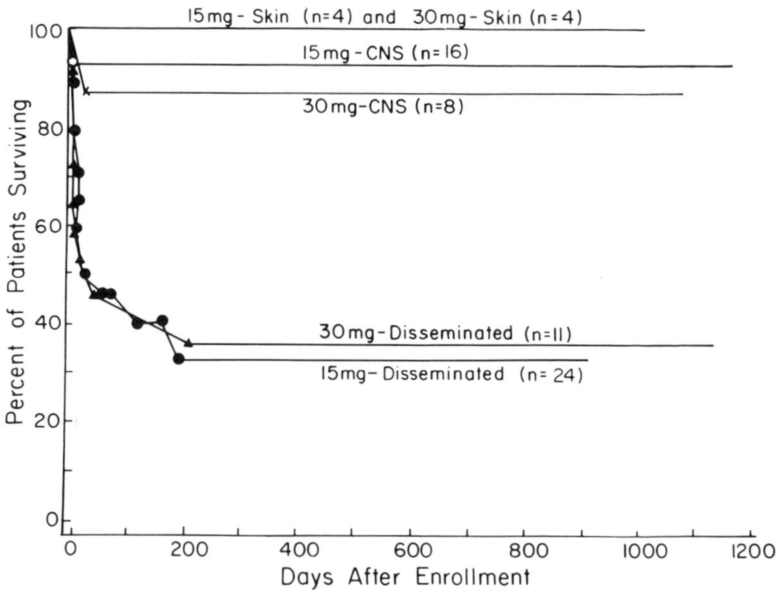

Figure 3 Survival of newborns with herpes simplex virus according to disease classification and dose of vidarabine. *Source*: *Pediatrics 72*:779–785, 1983, with permission.

keratoconjunctivitis is characterized by tearing, photophobia, discharge, and characteristic dendritic lesions. In the absence of therapy, these lesions can progress to geographic ulcers of the cornea. As has been well documented for other mucocutaneous herpes simplex infections, recurrences are common.

Idoxuridine, trifluorothymidine (TFT), and vidarabine ophthalmic have all been shown to be effective in the treatment of these ocular infections. For practical purposes, the child presumed to have herpes simplex virus infection of the eye should be followed most carefully by an ophthalmalogist.

D. Mucocutaneous Herpes Simplex Virus Infection

Mucocutaneous herpes simplex virus infections include those of the oropharynx, either primary herpes gingivostomatitis or recurrent herpes labialis, genitalia, or skin. Significant advances have been achieved in the management of genital herpes simplex virus infections with acyclovir (42–44), but no data indicate efficacy for vidarabine therapy of these clinical conditions.

Herpes simplex virus infections in the immunocompromised host are significantly more debilitating than those encountered in the normal individual. In contrast to the usual circumstance of asymptomatic primary infection in the normal child, infection in the immunocompromised host can be associated with significant morbidity. Mucositis with associated herpes simplex infection can lead to anorexia, severe pain, and decreased caloric intake, as well as facial scarring. Such clinical presentations are particularly common in patients undergoing bone marrow transplantation or on induction chemotherapy for acute lymphoblastic leukemia. In such circumstances, the administration of vidarabine has not been of established clinical value. A controlled trial utilizing a crossover study design demonstrated accelerated defervescence and loss of pain; however, there was no clinical benefit for healing (45).

E. Varicella Zoster Virus Infections

Chickenpox in the child with malignancy, especially acute lymphoblastic leukemia, has been associated with a 30% incidence of visceral complications, particularly pneumonitis (46,47). Mortality overall can be as high as 15-20% in the absence of antiviral therapy. The natural history of disease in these patients is characterized by a prolonged period of vesicle formation associated with, most likely, prolonged viremia. Approximately 50% of patients will continue to form new lesions for at least 1 week. Herpes zoster of childhood, on the other hand, is most frequently encountered following induction therapy for Hodgkin's disease or other solid tumors appearing during the teenage years. In the absence of antiviral therapy, nearly 50% of patients with Hodgkin's disease will progress to cutaneous dissemination (25% of all immunocompromised patients) and nearly half of the patients who develop cutaneous dissemination will develop evidence of visceral complications, including hepatitis, pneumonitis, and meningoencephalitis (48-50). Mortality from these complications has been reported to be 5-8% overall. The associated morbidity and mortality of varicella zoster virus infections in the immunocompromised host has made these infections targets for both prophylactic and therapeutic intervention.

Antiviral therapy with vidarabine was first shown to be efficacious for herpes zoster virus infections in the mid-1970s (51) and, subsequently, for chickenpox (47,49).

Studies of herpes zoster in the immunocompromised host have demonstrated that treatment with vidarabine will beneficially influence the outcome of these infections. Specifically, vidarabine therapy, administered at a dosage of 10 mg/kg day^{-1} for a period of 5 days, is associated with accelerated cessation of new lesion formation and decreased time to total pustulation and scabbing. In addition, the frequency of cutaneous dissemination and visceral complications is significantly decreased in treated compared with placebo recipients. Finally, both acute neuritis and postherpetic neuralgia are decreased more readily in those patients receiving drug than their counterpart placebo recipients. This latter issue is less of a problem in the management of herpes zoster in pediatric patients compared with that in the elderly. A similar series of studies has been performed with acyclovir in somewhat different patient populations (52). These studies have demonstrated that, although acyclovir has little effect on the events of cutaneous healing, it does prevent progressive disease and significantly decreases the appearance of visceral complications. Recently, it has been learned that vidarabine was inferior to acyclovir for the therapy of localized zoster in a significantly sicker patient population, namely, bone marrow transplant recipients. Cutaneous dissemination and accelerated healing were clinically more apparent in the acyclovir recipients (53).

Chickenpox is also amenable to antiviral therapy. Both vidarabine and acyclovir successfully decreased the appearance of visceral complications and death associated with chickenpox in the immunocompromised host (47,54). From a therapeutic standpoint, it is reasonable to seek hospitalization of the high-risk child, namely, the organ transplant recipient or the cancer patient, especially those on induction chemotherapy, for administration of intravenous antiviral therapy. Either medication will lead to a satisfactory outcome from a therapeutic standpoint, predicated on published data.

V. TOXICITY

Adverse effects of vidarabine are relatively few. Thus, the therapeutic index for this drug appears satisfactory for its utilization in high-risk patients. Vidarabine recipients may experience nausea, vomiting, and diarrhea more frequently than with acyclovir. In addition, rash, weakness, and thrombophlebitis at the site of infusion have been described. Central nervous system untoward effects, including dizziness, ataxia, tremor, hallucinations, and psychoses, are associated with doses above 20 mg/kg day^{-1}. Mutogenicity and carcinogenicity associated with the drug have been suggested.

ACKNOWLEDGMENTS

Studies reported by the author were initiated under and supported by a contract (NO1-A1-62554) with the Development and Application Branch of the National Institute of Allergy and Infectious Diseases and by grants from the National Center Institute (CA-13148), the General Clinical Research Centers Programs (RR-032) of the National Institutes of Health, and the State of Alabama.

REFERENCES

1. Lee, W, Benietz, A, Goodman, L, Baker, BR: *J. Am. Chem. Soc. 82*:2648, 1960.
2. Resit, EJ, Benitez, A, Goodman, L, et al.: *J. Org. Chem. 27*:3274, 1962.
3. De Rudder, J, Andreeff, F, Privat de Garilhe, M: Action inhibitrice de la 9-beta-D-xylofuranosyl-adenine sur la multiplication du virus de l'herpes en culture cellulaire. *C.R. Acad. Sci. (Paris) 264*:677–680, 1967.
4. Dixon, GJ, Sidwell, RW, Miller, FA, et al.: Antiviral activity of 9-β-D-arabirofuranosyladenine. I. Activity against intracerebral vaccinia virus infections in mice. *Antimicrob. Agents Chemother.* 172–179, 1968.
5. Miller, FA, Dixon, GJ, Ehrlich, J, et al.: Antiviral activity of 9-β-D-arabinofuranosyladenine. I. Cell culture studies. Proceedings 8th Interscience Conference on Antimicrobial Agents in Chemotherapy, pp. 136–147, 1968.
6. Schardein, JL, Sidwell, RW: Antiviral activity of 9-β-D-arabinofuranosyladenine. III. Reduction in evidence of encephalitis in treated herpes-simplex-infected hamsters. Proceedings 8th Interscience Conference on Antimicrobial Agents in Chemotherapy, pp. 155–160, 1968.
7. Suhadolnik, RJ: Nucleoside antibiotics. VI. Biosynthesis of the pyrrolopyrimidine nucleoside antibiotic toyocamycin by *Streptomyces rimosus. Nucleoside Antibiotics*, John Wiley and Sons, New York, 1970.
8. Cohen, SS: Virus-induced synthesis of enzymes. *Prog. Nucl. Acid Res. Mol. Biol. 5*:238–248, 1966.
9. Buthala, DA: Cell culture studies on antiviral agents. I. Action of cytosine arabinoside and some comparisons with 5-iodo-2-deoxyuridine. *Proc. Soc. Exp. Biol. Med. 115*:69–77, 1964.
10. Fiala, M, Chow, AW, Miyasaki, K: Susceptibility of herpesviruses to three nucleoside analogues and their combinations and enhancement of the antiviral effect of acid pH. *J. Infect. Dis. 129*:82–85, 1974.
11. Schaeffer, HJ, Beauchamp, L, de Miranda, P, Elion, GB, Baver, DJ, Collins, P: 9-(2-Hydroxyethoxymethyl)guanine activity against viruses of the herpes group. *Nature 272*:583–585, 1978.
12. Cohen SS: The mechanisms of lethal action of arabinosyl cytosine (ara-C) and arabinosyl adenine (ara-A). *Cancer 40*:509–18, 1977.

13. Furth, JJ, Cohen, SS: Inhibition of mammalian DNA polymerase by the 5′-triphosphate of 9-beta-D-arabinofuranosyladenine. *Cancer Res. 28*:2061–2067, 1968.
14. York, JL, LePage, GA: A proposed mechanism for the action of 9-β-D-arabinofuranosyladenine as an inhibitor of the growth of some ascites cells. *Can. J. Biochem. 44*:19, 1966.
15. Schwartz, PM, Shipman, C, Drach, JC: Antiviral activity of arabinosyladenine and arabinosylhyoxanthine in herpes simplex virus-infected KB cells: Selective inhibition of viral deoxyribonucleic acid synthesis in the presence of an adenosine deaminase inhibitor. *Antimicrob. Agents Chemother. 10*:64–74, 1976.
16. Plunkett, W, Lapi, L, Ortiz, PJ, et al.: Penetration of mouse fibroblasts by the 5′-phosphate of 9-beta-D-arabinofuranosyladenine and incorporation of the nucleotide into DNA. *Proc. Natl. Acad. Sci. USA 71*:73–77, 1974.
17. Prussoff, WH, Bakhle, YS: Cellular and antiviral effects of halogenated deoxyribonucleosides. *Ann. N.Y. Acad. Sci. 130*:135–150, 1965.
18. Kaplan, AS, Ben-Porat, T, Kamiya, T: Mechanism of inhibition of cellular DNA synthesis by pseudorabies virus. Incorporation of 5-bromodeoxyuridine and 5-iododeoxyuridine into viral DNA and its effect on the infective process. *Ann. N.Y. Acad. Sci. 130*:22–29, 226–239, 1965.
19. Whitley, RJ, Chien, LT, Buchanan, RA, Alford, CA: *Perspectives in Virology*, Academic Press, New York, 1975, pp. 315–336.
20. Glazko, AJ, Chang, T, Drach, JC, Mourer, DR, Borondy, PE, Schneider, H, Croskey, L, Maschewske, E: Species differences in the metabolic disposition of adenine arabinoside. *Adenine Arabinoside: An Antiviral Agent* (D Pavon-Langston, RA Buchanan, and CA Alford, Jr., Eds.), Raven Press, 1975, pp. 111–133.
21. Bryson, Y, Connor, JD, Hebblewaite, D: Pharmacology and efficacy of ARA-A in neonates. 19th Interscience Conference on Antimicrobial Agents and Chemotherapy, Abstract 974, Boston, 1979.
22. Shope, TC, Kauffman, RE, Bowman, D, Marcus, EL: Pharmacokinetics of vidarabine in the treatment of infants and children due to herpes viruses. *J. Infect. Dis. 148*: 721–725, 1983.
23. Ch'ien, LT, Dismukes, WD, Whitley, RJ, Buchanan, RA, Alford, CA, Cannon, NJ: Effect of adenine arabinoside on severe herpesvirus hominis infections in man. *J. Infect. Dis. 128*:658–663, 1973.
24. Luby, JP, Jones, SR, Johnson, MT, Mikulec, D: Sensitivities of herpes simplex virus types 1 and 2 and varicella-zoster virus to adenine arabinoside and hypoxanthine arabinoside. *Adenine Arabinoside: An Antiviral Agent* (D Pavon-Langston, RA Buchanan, and CA Alford, Jr., Eds.), Raven Press, 1975, pp. 171–175.
25. Johnson, MT, Luby, JP, Buchanan, RA: Treatment of varicella-zoster virus infections with adenine arabinoside. *J. Infect. Dis. 131*:225–229, 1975.
26. Luby, JP, Johnson, MT, Buchanan, RA, Chien, L, Whitley, RJ, Alford, CA: Adenine arabinoside therapy of varicella-zoster virus infections. Summary of phase II studies. *Adenine Arabinoside: An Antiviral Agent* (D Pavon-Langston, RA Buchanan, and CA Alford, Jr., Eds.), Raven Press, 1975, pp. 237–246.
27. Ch'ien, LT, Whitley, RJ, Nahmias, A, Lewin, E, Bellanti, J, Linnemann, CC, Frenkel, LD, Buchanan, RA, Alford, CA: Antiviral chemotherapy and neonatal herpes simplex virus infection: A pilot study—experience with adenine arabinoside. *Pediatrics 55*:678–685, 1975.
28. Abel, R, Kaufman, HE, Sugar, J: Effect of intravenous adenine arabinoside on herpes simplex keratouveitis in humans. *Adenine Arabinoside: An Antiviral Agent* (D Pavon-Langston, RA Buchanan, and CA Alford, Jr., Eds.), Raven Press, 1975, pp. 393–400.

29. Baublis, JV, Whitley, RJ, Chien, LT, Alford, CA: Treatment of CMV infection in infants and adults. *Adenine Arabinoside: An Antiviral Agent* (D Pavon-Langston, RA Buchanan, and CA Alford, Jr., Eds.), Raven Press, 1975, pp. 247–260.
30. Ch'ien, LT, Whitley, RJ, Alford, CA, et al.: Adenine arabinoside for therapy of herpes zoster in immunosuppressed patients: Preliminary results of a collaborative study. *J. Infect. Dis. 133(Suppl. A)*:184–191, 1976.
31. Rytel, MW, Kaufman, M: Clinical efficacy of adenine arabinoside in therapy of cytomegalovirus infections in renal allograft recipients. *J. Infect. Dis. 133*:202–205, 1976.
32. Whitley, RJ, Soong, SJ, Hirsch, MD, Karchmer, AW, Dolin, R, Galasso, G, Dunnick, JK, Alford, CA, Jr., the NIAID Collaborative Antiviral Study Group: Herpes simplex encephalitis: Vidarabine therapy and diagnostic problems. *N. Engl. J. Med. 304*: 313–318, 1981.
33. Whitley, RJ, Soong, SJ, Dolin, R, Galasso, GJ, Chien, LT, Alford, CA, the Collaborative Study Group: Adenine arabinoside therapy of biopsyproved herpes simplex encephalitis. *N. Engl. J. Med. 297*:289–294, 1977.
34. Nahmias, AJ, Whitley, RJ, Visintine, AN, Takei, Y, Alford, CA, the NIAID Collaborative Antiviral Study Group: Herpes simplex virus encephalitis: Laboratory evaluations and their diagnostic significance. *J. Infect. Dis. 145*:829–836, 1982.
35. Skoldenberg, B, Forsgren, M, Alestig, K, et al.: Acydovin versus vidarabine in herpes simplex encephalitis. *Lancet 2*:707–711, 1984.
36. Whitley, RJ, Alford, CA, Jr., Hirsch, MS, Schooley, RT, Luby, JP, Aoki, FY, Hanley, D, Nahmias, AJ, Soong, AJ, the NIAID Collaborative Antiviral Study Group: Vidarabine versus acydoviz therapy in herpes simplex encephalitis. *N. Engl. J. Med. 314*: 144–149, 1986.
37. Whitley, RJ, Nahmias, AJ, Soong, SJ, Galasso, GG, Fleming, CL, Alford, CA, Jr., the NIAID Collaborative Antiviral Study Group with special assistance from J Connor, Y Bryson, C Linnemann: Vidarabine therapy of neonatal herpes simplex virus infections. *Pediatrics 66*:495–501, 1980.
38. Whitley, RJ, Yeager, A, Kartus, P, Bryson, Y, Connor, JD, Nahmias, AJ, Soong, SJ, the NIAID Collaborative Antiviral Study Group: Neonatal herpes simplex infection: Follow-up evaluation of vidarabine therapy. *Pediatrics 72*:778–785, 1983.
39. Nahmias, JD, Keyserling, H, Whitley, RJ: *Herpesviruses and Virus Chemotherapy: Pharmacological and Clinical Approaches*. Excerpta Medica, Amsterdam, 1985, pp. 145–149.
40. Whitley, RJ, Hutto, C: Neonatal herpes simplex virus infections. *Pediatr. Rev. 7*: 119–126, 1985.
41. Whitley, RJ, Hutto, C, Corey, L, Arvin, A, Nahmias, AJ, Alford, CA, Jr., Soong, SJ, the NIAID Collaborative Antiviral Study Group: Changing presentation of neonatal herpes simplex virus (HSV) infections, Abstract, 20th Interscience Conference on Antimicrobial Agents and Chemotherapy, Minneapolis, 1985.
42. Corey, L, Nahmias, AJ, Guinan, ME, et al.: A trial of topical acyclovir in genital herpes simplex virus infections. *N. Engl. J. Med. 306*:1313–1319, 1982.
43. Bryson, YJ, Dillon, M, Lovett, M, et al.: Treatment of first episodes of genital herpes simplex virus infection with oral acyclovir. A randomized double-blind controlled trial in normal subjects. *N. Engl. J. Med. 308*:916–921, 1983.
44. Corey, L, Adamo, HG, Brown, ZA, et al.: Genital herpes simplex virus infections: Clinical manifestations, course and complications. *Ann. Intern. Med. 98*:958–972, 1983.
45. Gnann, JW, Whitley, RJ: Current status of antiviral therapy, *IM-Internal Medicine for the Specialist 4*:49, 1983.

46. Feldman, S, Hughes, WT, Daniel CB: Varialla in children with cancer: Seventy seven cases. *Pediatrics 56*:388–397, 1975.
47. Whitley, RJ, Hilty, M, Haynes, R, Bryson, Y, Connor, JD, Soong, SJ, Alford, CA, Jr., NIAID Collaborative Antiviral Study Group: Vidarabine therapy of varicella in immunosuppressed patients. *J. Pediatr. 101*:125–131, 1982.
48. Dolin, R, Reichman, RC, Mazur, MW, et al.: NIH Conference. Herpes zoster-varicella infections in immuno-suppressed patients. *Ann. Intern. Med. 89*:375–388, 1978.
49. Whitley, RJ, Chien, LT, Dolin, R, Galasso, GJ, Alford, CA, Jr., the Collaborative Antiviral Study Group: Adenine arabinoside therapy of herpes zoster in the immunosuppressed. *N. Engl. J. Med. 294*:1193–1199, 1976.
50. Whitley, RJ, Soong, SJ, Dolin, R, Betts, R, Linnemann, C, Jr., Alford, CA, Jr., the NIAID Collaborative Antiviral Study Group: Early vidarabine therapy to control the complications of herpes zoster in immunosuppressed patients. *N. Engl. J. Med. 307*: 971–975, 1982.
51. Gluckman, E, Lotsberg, J, Devergie, A, et al.: Oral acyclovir prophylactic treatment of herpes simplex infection after bone marrow transplantation. *J. Antimicrob. Chemother. 12*:161–167, 1982.
52. Balfour, HH, Jr., Bean, B, Laskin, OL, et al.: Acyclovir halts progression of herpes zoster in immunocompromised patients. *N. Engl. J. Med. 308*:1448–1453, 1983.
53. Shepp, DM, Dandliker, PS, Meyers, JD: Treatment of varicella-zoster virus infections in severely immunocompromised patients. A randomized comparison of acyclovir and vidarabine. *N. Engl. J. Med. 314*:208–212, 1986.
54. Prober, CG, Kirk, LE, Keeney, RE: Acycloviz therapy of chickenpox in immunosuppressed children: A collaborative study. *J. Pediatr. 101*:622–625, 1982.

29
Acyclovir

PAUL S. LIETMAN
Johns Hopkins University School of Medicine, Baltimore, Maryland

Acyclovir is an effective and relatively nontoxic antiherpesvirus agent that has rapidly achieved the status of a standard in antiviral chemotherapy. Its discovery followed the initial synthesis of structural analogs of adenosine in an attempt to create inhibitors of adenosine deaminase (1) as potential immunosuppressants. One such adenosine analog, which might be called acycloadenosine since it lacks the 2′ and 3′ carbon atoms of the cyclic ribose ring, was found to have some, albeit minimal, activity in an in vitro screening test against the herpes simplex virus in cultured cells. A rational search for more potent agents related to "acycloadenosine" led to the discovery that the analogous derivative of guanosine, initially called acycloguanosine and now known as acyclovir, was an extremely potent antiherpes agent. In an elegant series of studies, the mechanism of antiviral action and the rationale for selective toxicity to viral replication as contrasted to host cell function was elucidated during the preclinical phase of drug development (2,3). After the acquisition of evidence for effectiveness in animal models of herpes simplex infections and after preclinical toxicology studies had established the likelihood of minimal toxicity, a series of carefully conducted human investigations efficiently defined the pharmacokinetics of acyclovir in humans, the lack of appreciable human toxicity, and the clinical effectiveness in the treatment of established herpes simplex infections in both immunocompromised and immunocompetent patients, as well as the effectiveness in preventing the recrudescence of herpes simplex infections. Additional and continuing clinical studies have extended and refined the therapeutic place of acyclovir in additional herpes infections in humans.

The lessons learned in the efficient establishment of the clinical place of acyclovir through well-designed prospective, controlled, randomized, and blinded clinical trials should serve as a model for the clinical development of future antiviral agents.

I. CHEMISTRY

Acyclovir may be viewed as an acyclic derivative of guanosine (or deoxyguanosine), lacking the 2′ and 3′ carbon atoms of the cyclic ribose ring.

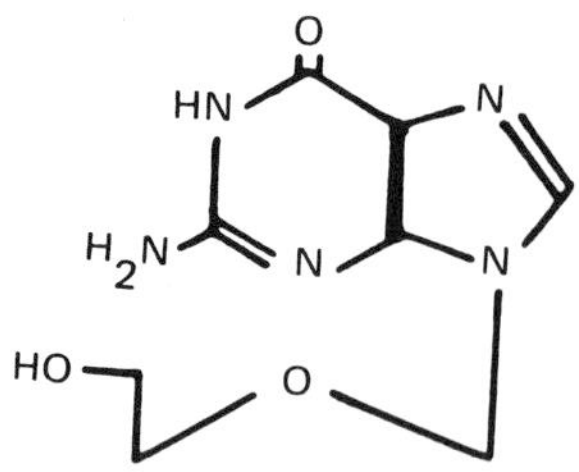

Acyclovir

The critical features of the molecule are its resemblance to deoxyguanosine and its lack of the 2′ and 3′ carbon atoms of the cyclic ribose ring. The resemblance to deoxyguanosine is important in order to serve as a substrate for the viral deoxynucleoside kinase that initiates activation of the drug (see below) and in order for the fully activated drug, as acyclovir triphosphate, to serve as an inhibitor of the viral DNA polymerase that uses deoxyguanosine triphosphate as one of its substrates. The lack of the 2′ and 3′ carbon atoms of the cyclic ribose ring is important since the addition of an acyclovir molecule to a growing viral DNA chain is chain terminating as a consequence of its inability to accept another nucleoside that would normally be added to the hydroxyl group on the 3′ carbon of deoxyguanosine.

Numerous derivatives of acyclovir that retain these two critical features have been synthesized, and some of these may be developed in the future as antiviral agents or as prodrugs that are converted to acyclovir in vivo.

II. MECHANISM OF ACTION

Acyclovir inhibits herpesvirus replication and is selectively toxic to viral DNA synthesis, in contrast to host cell DNA synthesis, as a result of the differential selectivity of each of two enzymologic reactions involving the deoxynucleoside kinases and DNA polymerases (2,3).

Acyclovir is converted to acyclovir monophosphate in herpes-infected cells, but not in uninfected cells, as a result of the ability of the herpes-induced deoxynucleoside kinase (commonly called the herpes thymidine kinase) to utilize acyclovir as a substrate and the inability of any kinase in the uninfected cell to utilize acyclovir effectively as a substrate. Consequently, acyclovir monophosphate is formed only in herpes-infected cells. Selectivity at this step of initial phosphorylation also explains the spectrum of activity of acyclovir. Acyclovir is active only if the infecting virus provides the requisite information necessary for the host cell to synthesize a new deoxynucleoside kinase that can act upon acyclovir as a substrate. It appears that most viruses outside the herpes family do not supply the necessary information, and even within the herpes family, the cytomegalovirus does not and the Epstein-Barr (EB) virus probably does not supply the necessary information (4). Thus, within the herpes family, only herpes simplex viruses (HSV) I and II and varicella zoster viruses (VZV) produce the appropriate deoxynucleoside kinases in infected cells. Mutants of these viruses have been described that are unable to induce the necessary enzyme, thus leading to acyclovir resistance (see below).

Acyclovir monophosphate is further phosphorylated to acyclovir diphosphate by a cellular guanosine monophosphate kinase (5), and the resultant acyclovir diphosphate is in turn phosphorylated to acyclovir triphosphate by other cellular enzymes. The phosphorylated derivatives of acyclovir that are formed in infected cells accumulate to high concentrations, possibly in part because of the charged nature of the added phosphate groups (2,3).

The second site of selectivity is the DNA polymerase (6-9). The herpesviruses also contain information for a new DNA polymerase, and it also differs from the host cells' own DNA polymerases in such a way that the herpes DNA polymerase is preferentially inhibited by acyclovir triphosphate as compared with the host cell enzymes.

Thus acyclovir exerts its antiviral effect as a result of its activation to acyclovir triphosphate in a multistep process that is pivotally dependent on an initial phosphorylation by a herpes deoxynucleoside kinase, its accumulation as acyclovir triphosphate only in infected cells, and the ability of acyclovir triphosphate to inhibit preferentially the herpes DNA polymerase and terminate the growth of nascent herpes DNA chains. The impressive selectivity of its effect results from the inability of uninfected host cells to phosphorylate the drug and, therefore, the inability of uninfected host cells to accumulate acyclovir triphosphate, and also from the relative insensitivity of the host cell DNA polymerases to acyclovir triphosphate.

III. ANTIVIRAL ACTIVITY AND RESISTANCE

Quantification of the in vitro antiviral activity of and resistance to acyclovir is not yet standardized or validated in terms of clinical relevance. The uncertainties that currently exist are due to several factors. First, the currently used method of in vitro quantification involves the incubation of infected cells with known and constant drug concentrations over a period of time followed by measuring the antiviral effect. The assessment of antiviral effect may be by quantification of the number of virus particles released into the medium either as measured by the number of DNA molecules released or by the cytopathologic effects of the released infectious viral units. Second, the relationship between the observed effects and the drug concentrations can be expressed as the concentration that causes a 50% inhibition of viral replication (ID_{50}), a 99% inhibition (the ID_{99}), or any other predetermined degree of inhibition. Third, the complexities are enormously amplified by the fact that the activity observed will vary depending on both the host cell line chosen and the concentrations of several constituents of the growth medium used for cell culture, especially the essential nucleosides (10). Finally, the validation of any in vitro measure of antiviral activity must ultimately rest on the proven clinical applicability of the values measured. To date there is only enough information to allow very rough correlations between in vitro data and in vivo success or failure. Nevertheless, some broad conclusions appear to be of some value at the present time, and surely new information will be forthcoming that will expand our knowledge.

In general, herpes simplex viruses, both type I and type II, are inhibited 50% (ID_{50}) by acyclovir concentrations of less than 2 μg/ml (<0.89 μM) when tested in Vero cells using a dye-uptake assay to quantify viral cytopathologic effects (see Table 1) (11,12). Other methods of quantifying the ID_{50} of various virus strains appear to produce lower ID_{50}, but the virtue of the dye-uptake assay is in its use in over a thousand clinical isolates in a uniform manner. It is generally accepted that herpes simplex type I is somewhat more sensitive to acyclovir than type II, but the overlap is considerable and the differences appear to be small and clinically meaningless. Published data are far less extensive for the varicella zoster virus, Epstein-Barr virus, or cytomegalovirus (CMV), and

Table 1 In Vitro Sensitivities of Herpesviruses to Acyclovir

Virus	Plaque reduction assays[a] (μg/ml)	Dye-uptake assay[b]
HSV I	0.004–0.4	95% <2 μg/ml
HSV II	0.01–1.45	95% <2 μg/ml
VZV	0.36–1.4	
EB	1.5–25	
CMV	2.25–50	

[a]Adapted from a compilation by Collins (12).
[b]From Dekker et al. (11).

the assays used have been more diverse. In general, however, the varicella zoster virus is inhibited 50% (ID_{50}) by less than 2 μg/ml using methods that are generally productive of lower ID_{50} than the dye-uptake method (11,12). The Epstein-Barr virus appears to require from 2-25 μg/ml, and the cytomegalovirus usually requires more than 25 μg/ml for 50% inhibition (11,12).

Since 95% of clinical isolates of herpes simplex virus are inhibited 50% by less than 2 μg/ml, the level of 2 μg/ml has been suggested as a cutoff point to define herpes simplex virus resistance to acyclovir, assuming the dye-uptake method is used (11). Using this criterion, the incidence of "resistance" to acyclovir has been rather uncommon to date. Nevertheless, resistance can occur both in clinical isolates and in laboratory settings.

The biochemical mechanisms that have been associated with in vitro resistance include an altered herpes deoxynucleoside kinase that is less efficient in phosphorylating acyclovir, an absence of this enzyme entirely, and an altered herpes DNA polymerase that is less susceptible to inhibition by acyclovir triphosphate (11,13).

The clinical relevance of resistant herpes simplex viruses remains somewhat uncertain. It does appear that increasing resistance can occur during acyclovir therapy, although this acquisition of resistance seems to be uncommon to date. It also appears that, even though resistance may occur during therapy, subsequent recrudescence in the same patient usually, if not always, is caused by the original sensitive strain that has persisted in the latent state in ganglia (14).

IV. CLINICAL PHARMACOLOGY

A. Absorption and Bioavailability

Acyclovir is absorbed to only a limited extent after oral administration. The oral bioavailability appears to vary from about 15% at oral doses of 100 mg to about 5% at oral doses of 600 mg in adults (15). It can probably be assumed that children, outside the newborn period, absorb acyclovir similarly. No data exist with respect to oral absorption in the newborn. After an oral dose of acyclovir, peak plasma levels are achieved at about 2 hr (16). The peak plasma levels achieved at steady state, after repeated oral dosing every 4 hr, range from about 0.5 μg/ml after 200 mg per dose to about 1.3 μg/ml after 600 mg per dose in adults (16). Although relatively low, these peak levels are well above the ID_{50} of most strains of HSV and even many strains of VZV. Furthermore, clinical evidence attests to the effectiveness of oral acyclovir in several clinical situations (see below).

Topical acyclovir is minimally absorbed into the systemic circulation. Direct absorption (at least a small extent) into the surface cells does seem to occur since evidence exists to substantiate the effectiveness of topical acyclovir in several clinical situations (see below) and since acyclovir must be internalized to be effective. The extent of local intracellular absorption remains controversial and may differ between two existing topical formulations, one available in the United States and the other marketed in the United Kingdom and Europe.

Intravenous acyclovir is, of course, completely absorbed. Intramuscular acyclovir is not available.

B. Protein Binding

Acyclovir is bound to plasma proteins to an extent of only about 15% (17). Although no published studies address the issue of bilirubin displacement in the newborn, it would seem unlikely that this would represent a clinical problem.

C. Distribution

Acyclovir distributes well into most tissues, including the brain, where cerebrospinal fluid (CSF) levels in humans of about 50% of plasma levels (18) suggest the probability of even higher brain tissue levels. Again, the proven efficacy of acyclovir in herpes encephalitis (see below) attests to the achievement of at least effective brain tissue levels. Heart, lung, and liver appear to attain levels similar to those in the plasma, and kidney levels considerably exceed plasma levels (19). Acyclovir enters saliva, vaginal secretions, and zoster vesicular fluid quite well (16). Acyclovir, as expected, crosses the placenta, although the extent and rate have not been defined (20). Although breast milk levels have not been reported, acyclovir would be expected to enter breast milk. However, the concentrations are likely to be low, considering the volume of milk usually ingested and the low oral bioavailability of acyclovir, and insufficient to produce either therapeutic levels or toxicity in the nursing infant.

The volume of distribution at steady state in children is about 70% of body weight in adults (18) and somewhat greater in newborns when expressed as a percentage of weight (as opposed to somewhat less when expressed as liters/1.73 m^2) (21).

D. Elimination

Acyclovir is metabolized to only a small extent (<15%) in adults with normal renal function (17).

Acyclovir is excreted nearly quantitatively into the urine as unchanged drug, with very little appearing in the feces (17). The mechanism of renal elimination involves predominantly glomerular filtration, with some contribution by active renal tubular secretion (22). Consequently, one would expect that the newborn, whose glomerular filtration rate (GFR) and tubular secretory capacity are both "immature," would eliminate acyclovir more slowly than the adult, and this is borne out by the very limited studies in newborns (Table 2). In newborns, the plasma clearance of acyclovir is about 100 ml/min/1.73 m^2, as contrasted with an adult plasma clearance of about 300 ml/min/1.73 m^2, and the half-life of the β phase is about 4 hr in newborns as compared with a $T_{1/2}\beta$ of about 2.5 hr in adults (18,21).

Acyclovir elimination is decreased in patients with renal glomerular (and possibly in those with renal tubular) dysfunction. Adult dosing regimens have been proposed for

Table 2 Elimination of Acyclovir

	Vd_{ss} (liters/1.73 m^2)	Cl_{tot} (ml/min/1.73 m^{-2})	$T_{1/2}\beta$ (hr)
Neonates	27.5 ± 7.0	109 ± 39	3.78 ± 1.21
Children	44.7 ± 15.4	335 ± 109	2.52 ± 1.04
Adults	49.7 ± 14.5	327 ± 80	2.48 ± 0.64

patients with all degrees of glomerular dysfunction (18,23), and the same principles also apply in children.

E. Preparations, Dosages, Regimens, and Routes

Acyclovir is available in topical, oral, and intravenous formulations.

Topical acyclovir is available in the United States as an ointment containing 5% (50 mg/g) acyclovir in a propylene glycol base. In the United Kingdom, topical acyclovir is marketed as a 5% cream (an aqueous preparation in propylene glycol). The dosing regimen involves the application of sufficient ointment (or cream) to cover the lesions every 3 hr, six times a day. The usual duration of treatment for genital herpes is 7 days.

Oral acyclovir is available in capsules, each containing 200 mg acyclovir. The recommended adult oral dosing regimen is 200 mg every 4 hr while awake, that is, five doses per day, for 10 days for the treatment of initial genital herpes. For the chronic suppressive therapy of recurrent genital herpes, 200 mg three times (or up to five times) a day for up to 6 months is approved. For the intermittent therapy of recurrent genital herpes, 200 mg five times a day for 5 days is recommended.

The relatively higher ID_{50} for VZV would seem to explain the lack of effectiveness of the usual HSV dosing regimens for zoster. Higher doses, in the range of 800 mg five times a day, may be of value (24) but are as yet unproven and not approved by the FDA.

V. DRUG ASSAYS

Acyclovir can be accurately and sensitively measured in plasma (as well as urine, saliva, secretions, CSF, vesicle fluid, and tissues) by radioimmunoassay (25,26). The assay can be performed on 100 μl plasma, with a lower limit of detection of 0.5 pmol/100 μl and a coefficient of variation of 4.5-9.6%. It is also possible to measure acyclovir by high-pressure liquid chromatography but the method is far more time consuming and cumbersome (25,27).

It should be noted that, at the present time, the relationship between plasma acyclovir levels and either effectiveness or toxicity is not established. Therefore, the routine therapeutic monitoring of acyclovir plasma levels is unnecessary.

VI. THERAPEUTIC INDICATIONS

Acyclovir is of proven value in a rather large number of diverse clinical herpetic infections.

For initial genital herpes, oral acyclovir is the most convenient method of treatment but topical acyclovir is also of proven value. Intravenous acyclovir is also of proven value but is usually inconvenient.

Unfortunately, there are no data addressing the efficacy of acyclovir for initial labial herpes, a disease producing significant gingivostomatitis in children.

For the treatment of recurrent genital herpes, oral acyclovir is again most convenient, although intravenous therapy is also of proven value. Topical acyclovir appears to have a marginal effect with respect to clinical symptomatology.

For recurrent labial herpes, no formulation of acyclovir is approved in the United States, although the cream that is available in the United Kingdom appears to provide some clinical benefit (28).

For the treatment of herpes simplex infections in immunosuppressed patients, intravenous acyclovir is of proven value (29). Topical acyclovir is also of value and may have a place in non-life-threatening situations (30). Oral acyclovir is also of value but frequently difficult for the sick immunosuppressed patient to take.

For the suppression of or prophylaxis against recrudescence of herpes simplex in the immunosuppressed patient, either intravenous (31,32) or oral (33-37) acyclovir is of proven value.

For the suppression of or prophylaxis against recrudescence of genital herpes in non-immunosuppressed patients, oral acyclovir is of proven value (38-40).

For herpes simplex encephalitis, intravenous acyclovir is of proven value and is superior to the only alternative, that is, vidarabine (41,42).

For neonatal herpes, acyclovir is of proven value (43). A very well designed study comparing acyclovir with vidarabine in neonatal herpes has not detected a clinically significant difference. The dosage of intravenous acyclovir is 10 mg/kg per dose every 8 hr in that study.

For the treatment of varicella zoster infections in immunocompromised patients, intravenous acyclovir is of proven value, especially in preventing visceral and cutaneous dissemination (44).

For the treatment of zoster in adults, intravenous acyclovir is of some value, although no effect on the worrisome postherpetic neuralgia was seen (45).

No studies have addressed the value of acyclovir in chicken pox in otherwise healthy children.

Several generalizations appear to be applicable to the therapeutic use of acyclovir in herpetic infections. First, it is advantageous to initiate treatment as early as possible in order to maximize the value of treatment. This is most dramatically demonstrated in herpes encephalitis but is applicable elsewhere as well. This is logical since the drug is quite effective in stopping viral replication but probably can do nothing to save cells already producing virus. Second, the drug should stop viral replication quite promptly but clinical healing will not be immediate and the results of therapy, in terms of clinically apparent resolution, may be rather slow. Third, the most obvious clinical results will be seen in severe illnesses, whereas more short-lived and less serious illnesses yield more subtle or more marginal clinical benefit.

VII. TOXICITY

Acyclovir is remarkably nontoxic, at least to date. No life-threatening side effects have been attributed to the drug, and only rarely have even moderately severe side effects been associated with (but not necessarily caused by) acyclovir. Rarely, seizures and other central nervous system effects have been reported concurrently with acyclovir administration in adults, almost always in severely ill patients who are also receiving a multiplicity of other drugs. Nevertheless, the report of seizures occurring concurrently with acyclovir in an otherwise healthy person with herpes zoster suggests that a causal relationship may in fact exist (46).

Transient renal glomerular dysfunction, manifest as a decrement in GFR or an increment in serum creatinine has been reported, usually following rapid intravenous administration (47). This is rarely seen following the recommended infusion times of 1 hr.

Local irritation at the site of intravenous extravasation can clearly occur. This is primarily attributable to the high pH of the intravenous formulation, which is necessary to keep acyclovir in solution.

Each of these side effects has occurred primarily or exclusively after intravenous administration. After oral administration, only nonspecific gastrointestinal symptoms that are mild and reversible have been reported. After topical administration, only mild local irritation has occasionally been reported.

Acyclovir has not been teratogenic in mice, rats, or rabbits to date, and there is no evidence for teratogenicity in humans. However, very few pregnant women have received the drug during the period of organogenesis. No fetal effects have been described after administration of acyclovir later in pregnancy in animals or in humans.

Acyclovir does not appear to be carcinogenic in animals.

In vitro mutagenicity testing has been extensive, and the results seem to show little evidence for a significant mutagenic effect although a clastogenic effect has been demonstrated in Chinese hamsters and in two mammalian systems (human lymphocytes and mouse lymphoma cells in vitro) acyclovir was mutagenic and produced chromosomal damage at concentrations at least 25 times the plasma levels achieved in humans (48).

VIII. CONTRAINDICATIONS

There are no known contraindications to acyclovir.

IX. DRUG INTERACTIONS

The only drug-drug interaction that has been demonstrated with acyclovir is the interaction with probenecid, an inhibitor of renal organic acid secretion, which leads to a modest (30%) prolongation of the half-life of acyclovir (22). The effect of acyclovir on the pharmacokinetics of other drugs that are secreted by the organic acid secretory mechanism has not been investigated.

REFERENCES

1. Schaeffer, HJ, Gurwara, S, Vince, R, and Bittner, S: *J. Med. Chem. 14*:367, 1971.
2. Elion, GB, Furman, PA, Fyfe, JA, de Miranda, P, Beauchamp, L, and Schaeffer, HJ: *Proc. Natl. Acad. Sci. USA 74*:5716, 1977.
3. Schaeffer, HJ, Beauchamp, L, de Miranda, P, Elion, GB, Bauer, DJ, and Collins, P: *Nature 272*:583, 1978.
4. Pagano, JS, and Datta, AK: *Am. J. Med. 73*(Suppl.):18, 1982.
5. Miller, WH, and Miller, RL: *J. Biol. Chem. 255*:7204, 1980.
6. Furman, PA, St. Clair, MH, Fyfe, JA, Rideout, JL, Keller, PM, and Elion, GB: *J. Virol. 32*:72, 1979.
7. St. Clair, MH, Furman, PA, Lubbers, CM, and Elion, GB: *Antimicrob. Agents Chemother. 18*:741, 1980.

8. Derse, D, Cheng, Y-C, Furman, PA, St. Clair, MH, and Elion, GB: *J. Biol. Chem. 256*:11447, 1981.
9. Furman, PA, St. Clair, MH, and Spector, T: *J. Biol. Chem. 259*:9575, 1984.
10. Elion, GB: In *Antiviral Chemotherapy: New Directions for Clinical Application and Research* (J Mills and L Corey, eds.), Elsevier, New York, 1986, p. 118.
11. Dekker, C, Ellis, MN, McLaren, C, Hunter, G, Rogers, J, and Barry, DW: *J. Antimicrob. Chemother. 12*(Suppl. B):137, 1983.
12. Collins, P: *J. Antimicrob. Chemother. 12*(Suppl. B):19, 1983.
13. Field, HJ: *J. Antimicrob. Chemother. 12*(Suppl. B):129, 1983.
14. Straus, SE, Rooney, JF, Sever, JL, Seidlin, M, Nusinoff-Lehrman, S, and Cremer, K: *Ann. Intern. Med. 103*:404, 1985.
15. Brigden, D, Fowle, A, and Rosling, A: In *Developments in Antiviral Therapy* (P Collier and M Oxford, eds.), Academic Press, New York, 1980, p. 53.
16. Laskin, O: *Clin. Pharmacokinet. 8*:187, 1983.
17. de Miranda, P, Good, SS, Laskin, OL, Krasny, HC, Connors, JD, and Lietman, PS: *Clin. Pharmacot. Ther. 30*:662, 1981.
18. Blum, MR, Liao, SHT, and de Miranda, P: *Am. J. Med. 73*(Suppl. 2):186, 1982.
19. Wade, JC, Hintz, M, McGuffin, RW, Springmeyer, SC, Connor, JD, and Meyers, JD: *Am. J. Med. 73*(Suppl.):249, 1982.
20. Greffe, BS, Dooley, SL, Deddish, RB, and Krasny, HC: *J. Pediatr. 108*:1020, 1986.
21. Hintz, M, Connor, JD, Spector, SA, Blum, MR, Keeney, RE, and Yeager, AS: *Am. J. Med. 73*(Suppl.):210, 1982.
22. Laskin, OL, de Miranda, P, King, DH, Page, DA, Longsstreth, JA, Rocco, L, and Lietman, PS: *Antimicrob. Agents Chemother. 21*:804, 1982.
23. Laskin, OL, Longstreth, JA, Whelton, A, Rocco, L, Lietman, PS, Krasny, HC, and Keeney, RE: *Clin. Pharmacol. Ther. 31*:594, 1982.
24. McKendrick, MW, McGill, JI, Bell, AM, Hickmott, E, and Burke, C: *Lancet 2*:925, 1984.
25. Quinn, RP, de Miranda, R, Gerald, L, and Good, SS: *Anal. Biochem. 98*:319, 1979.
26. Skubitz, KM, Quinn, RP, and Lietman, PS: *Antimicrob. Agents Chemother. 21*: 352, 1982.
27. Land, G, and Bye, A: *J. Chromatogr. 224*:51, 1981.
28. Fiddian, AP, Yeo, JM, Stubbings, R, and Dean, D: *Br. Med. J. 286*:1699, 1983.
29. Meyers, JD, Wade, JC, Mitchell, CD, Saral, R, Leitman, PS, Durack, DT, Levin, MJ, Segreti, AC, and Balfour, HH, Jr.: *Am. J. Med. 73*(Suppl.):22, 1982.
30. Whitley, R, Barton, N, Collins, E, Whelchel, J, and Diethelm, AG: *Am. J. Med. 73* (Suppl.):236, 1982.
31. Saral, R, Burns, WH, Laskin, OL, Santos, GW, and Lietman, PS: *N. Engl. J. Med. 305*:63, 1981.
32. Saral, R, Ambinder, RF, Burns, WH, Angelopulos, CM, Griffin, DE, Burke, PJ, and Lietman, PS: *Ann. Intern. Med. 99*:773, 1983.
33. Gluckman, E, Lotsberg, J, Devergie, A, Zhao, XM, Melo, R, Gomez-Morales, M, Nebout, T, Mazeron, MC, and Perol, Y: *Lancet 2*:706, 1983.
34. Wade, JC, Newton, B, Flournoy, N, and Meyers, JD: *Ann. Intern. Med. 100*:823, 1984.
35. Anderson, H, Scarffe, JH, Sutton, RNP, Hickmott, E, Brigden, D, and Burke, C: *Br. J. Cancer 50*:45, 1984.
36. Pettersson, E, Hovi, T, Ahonen, J, Fiddian, AP, Salmela, K, Hockerstedt, K, Eklund, B, von Willebrand, E., and Hayry, P: *Transplantation 39*:279, 1985.
37. Seale, L, Jones, CJ, Kathpalia, S, Jackson, GG, Mozes, M, Maddux, MS, and Packham, D: *JAMA 254*:3435, 1985.
38. Strauss, SE, Takiff, HE, Seidlin, M, Bachrach, S, Lininger, L, DiGiovanna, JJ, Western, KA, Smith, HA, Nusinoff, S, Lehrman, Creagh-Kirk, T, and Alling, DW: *N. Engl. J. Med. 310*:1545, 1984.

39. Douglas, JM, Critchlow, C, Benedetti, J, Mertz, GJ, Connor, JD, Hintz, MA, Gahnlander, A, Remington, M, Winter, C, and Corey, L: *N. Engl. J. Med. 310*:1551, 1984.
40. Mindel, A, Weller, IVD, Faherty, A, Sutherland, S, Hindley, D, Fiddian, AP, and Adler, MW: *Lancet 2*:57, 1984.
41. Skoldenberg, B, Forsgren, M, Alestig, K, Bergstrom, T, Burman, L, Dahlqvist, E, Forkman, A, Fryden, A, Lovgren, K, Norlin, K, Norrby, R, Olding-Stenkvist, E, Stiernstedt, G, Uhnoo, I, and de Vahl, K: *Lancet 2*:707, 1984.
42. Whitley, RJ, Alford, CA, Hirsch, MS, Schooley, RT, Luby, JP, Aoki, FY, Hanley, D, Nahmias, AJ, Soong, PDS-J, and the NIAID Collaborative Group: *N. Engl. J. Med. 314*:144, 1986.
43. Whitley, RJ, and the NIAID Collaborative Antiviral Study Group: *J. Antimicrob. Chemother. 12*(Suppl. B):105, 1983.
44. Balfour, HH, Bean, B, Laskin, OL, Ambinder, RJ, Meyers, JD, Wade, JC, Zaia, JA, Aeppli, D, Kirk, LE, Segreti, AC, and Keeney, RE: *N. Engl. J. Med. 308*:1448, 1983.
45. Peterslund, NA, Seyer-Hansen, K, Ipsen, J, Esmann, V, Schonheyder, H, and Juhl, H: *Lancet 2*:827, 1981.
46. Cohen, SMZ, Minkove, JA, Zebley, JW, III, and Mulholland, JH: *Ann. Intern. Med. 100*:920, 1984.
47. Fiddian, AF, Brigden, D, Yeo, JM, and Hickmott, EA: *Antiviral Res. 4*:99, 1984.
48. Clive, D, Turner, NT, Hozier, J, Batson, AG, and Tucker, WE, Jr.: *Fund. Appl. Toxicol. 3*:587, 1983.

30
Ribavirin

CHARLES G. PROBER
Stanford University School of Medicine, Stanford, California

Ribavirin was first synthesized in 1970 as part of a major program to search for a compound with broad antiviral activity (1). The rationale for the synthesis of a compound of this type was to develop an agent with the potential to affect enzymatic processes common to all viruses, such as viral-induced nucleic acid and protein synthesis. Much work has been done with ribavirin since its original synthesis. This work includes defining its in vitro spectrum of activity, assessing its efficacy in a variety of animal models, expanding its formulations (most recently to include an aerosolized form), and exploring its efficacy in the therapy of infections caused by an expanding number of human viruses, ranging from respiratory viruses to the recently discovered human immunodeficiency virus (HIV). Although the aerosolized formulation of this drug has been licensed, the ultimate place of each form of this agent in our antiviral armamentarium has yet to be completely defined.

I. MODE OF ACTION AND SPECTRUM OF ACTIVITY

Ribavirin has a molecular weight of 244 daltons, a ribose moiety, and a triazole ring. Its observed antiviral activity appears to be directly related to its structural resemblance to natural nucleosides; x-ray crystallography shows that it most closely resembles guanosine (2). Ribavirin is phosphorylated intracellularly to its 5′-phosphate derivatives by cellular enzymes; the major metabolite responsible for antiviral activity is the triphosphate (3).

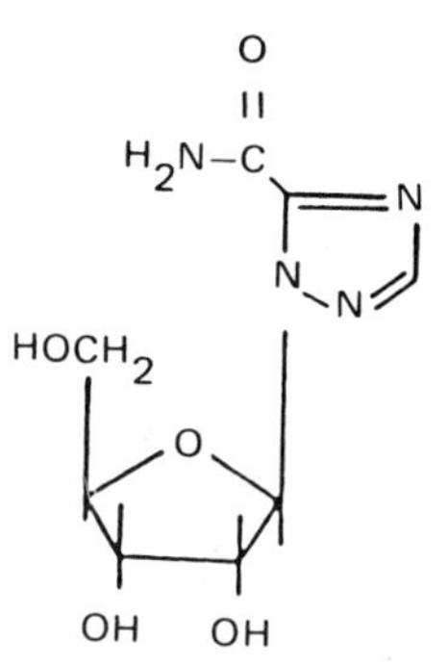

Ribavirin

The precise mechanisms of antiviral activity of ribavirin have been studied most extensively for the influenza viruses (4-6). Ribavirin's virustatic effects may be exerted through at least three mechanisms: a decrease in the intracellular nucleoside pool presumed to be due to competitive inhibition of inosimic acid (IMP) dehydrogenase and two virus-specific actions. These actions are inhibition of 5′-cap formation of mRNA and inhibition of the function of virus-coded RNA polymerases necessary to initiate and elongate viral mRNA. This potential for viral inhibition at more than one site, it is hoped, will reduce the eventual development of resistance to ribavirin.

Ribavirin has a broad range of antiviral activity on both DNA and RNA viruses (2, 7-10). It is virostatic. Its reported activity varies appreciably according to the cell line used in the assay, the concentration of virus inoculum used to infect the cells, and the specific viral strain (10). Viruses that are reportedly inhibited by attainable concentrations of ribavirin include influenza A and B, respiratory syncytial virus, parainfluenza viruses 1 and 3, some adenoviruses, rubeola, herpes simplex types 1 and 2, cytomegalovirus, hepatitis A, bunyaviruses, togaviruses, and arenaviruses, including Lassa fever virus (11). The ranges of reported inhibitory concentrations for these viruses are broad. Susceptible DNA viruses are generally inhibited by concentrations of ribavirin approximately ranging from 1 to 32 μg/ml; herpes simplex viruses are inhibited by concentrations at the lower end of the range and adenoviruses inhibited by concentrations at the higher end. The RNA viruses are usually more sensitive to ribavirin; the range of inhibitory concentrations for susceptible isolates being approximately 0.0032-10 μg/ml. It has also been shown in cultures of human adult T lymphocytes to suppress the replication of the retrovirus responsible for causing the acquired immunodeficiency syndrome (12). The lowest effective in vitro dose was in the range of 7.5-12.5 μg/ml.

II. PHARMACOKINETICS

There are only limited data on the disposition of ribavirin in humans. Most of the available data have been summarized by Connor et al. (13), including kinetics after oral, intravenous, and aerosol administration. Most of the data after oral and intravenous administration have been derived from studies conducted in adults, whereas most of the data after aerosol administration have been derived from studies conducted in children.

A group of four adults being treated for Lassa fever in Sierra Leone had plasma concentrations in the range of 0.4-1.3 μg/ml 2½ hr after an oral dose of 5 mg/kg of ribavirin. In the same patient population, the range of maximum plasma concentrations attained was 13--21 μg/ml in 11 individuals receiving 7.5 mg/kg and 23-25 μg/ml in eight individuals after an intravenous dose of 15 mg/kg of ribavirin.

Aerosol administration of ribavirin has been accomplished by means of a Collison generator adapted to deliver a continuous flow of small particles (mass medium diameter of 1.4 μm) for extended periods (14). Using a ribavirin concentration of 20 mg/ml in the reservoir of the delivery system and a constant flow rate of nebulized aerosol, it has been estimated that 0.82 mg/kg hr^{-1} of drug is deposited upon the respiratory membrane (15). This estimate assumes that 70% of the inhaled drug is delivered to the respiratory epithelium. The actual dose delivered per hour varies and is dependant on the patient's ventilation and lung pathology.

Plasma concentrations of ribavirin have been measured after aerosol administration to several nonintubated children. Plasma concentrations have tended to increase as the duration of aerosolization has increased. The mean concentration of ribavirin at the end of 2.5 hr of aerosolization was 0.19 μg/ml, whereas it was 0.28 μg/ml after 5.0 hr and 1.10 μg/ml after 8 hr of aerosolization (13). Mean plasma concentrations attained in three nonintubated children treated at Children's Hospital in Boston with 20 hr/day of aerosolized ribavirin were 0.68, 2.03, and 2.38 μg/ml, respectively (K McIntosh, unpublished data, Reference 13). Accumulation of ribavirin after successive doses was not noted when the duration of aerosolization was 2.5-5.0 hr, but it was noted when the duration was 8 hr. After the longer duration, plasma concentrations increased from 0.88 μg/ml after the first dose to 1.53 μg/ml after the third dose. We have measured ribavirin concentrations in two intubated children who were receiving 16 hr/day of aerosolized drug. The maximum plasma concentrations observed were 1.13 and 1.60 μg/ml, respectively. In two similar children studied by McIntosh, plasma concentrations ranged from 2.0 to 26.75 μg/ml (K McIntosh, unpublished data, Reference 13). Concentrations of ribavirin in the respiratory secretions collected from intubated children at the end of a 8 to 20-hr cycle of aerosolization have ranged from 250 to 1925 μg/ml (13).

Although the metabolism and tissue distribution of ribavirin have been studied extensively in rats, there are only limited data in nonhuman primates and humans (16,17). After oral or intravenous administration of radiolabeled ribavirin to monkeys, less than 1% of the drug is found in the lungs; 45-60% is excreted in the urine within 3 days (16, 17). In humans, the majority of ribavirin is excreted undegraded or as 1,2,4-triazole-carboxamide. The major excretory route is the kidneys. The approximate plasma half-life of ribavirin is 9 hr, and its half-life in tracheal secretions is 1-2 hr (13). Ribavirin is concentrated and retained in erythrocytes (3). In an analysis of 20 simultaneously obtained plasma and erythrocyte samples, we have found concentrations of ribavirin to be 29- to 306-fold higher within erythrocytes. Absolute concentrations within the erythrocytes ranged from 13.5 to 91.5 μg/ml. The erythrocytic half-life of ribavirin has been estimated to be 40 days (16).

III. TOXICITY

Ribavirin appears to be a very safe antiviral agent. Its only consistent adverse effect reported to date is a dose-dependent transient anemia (18). In monkeys, this effect has been attributed to more rapid extravascular clearing of erythrocytes and suppression of release of mature erythrocytes from the bone marrow (3). Oral or intravenous administration of ribavirin to patients with Lassa fever has been associated with hemolysis and anemia (19). This anemia was reversible and always followed by a brisk erythrocytosis. It has not been observed in children who have received aerosolized ribavirin. Early investigations of the effectiveness of oral ribavirin administered to adults to prevent or treat influenza infections also showed transient elevations of serum bilirubin (20-22). However, this side effect has not been observed in subsequent clinical trials.

Ribavirin administered by aerosolization occasionally has been associated with bronchospasm, but it has been difficult to determine whether this is due to the infecting respiratory virus or to the treatment. When the U.S. Food and Drug Administration (FDA) released ribavirin for aerosolization in late 1985, they required that a package insert statement be made warning against the use of this agent in intubated, ventilated patients. The reason for this warning was the observation that ribavirin can precipitate within the ventilator apparatus, including the endotracheal tube, resulting in increased positive end expiratory pressure and increased positive inspiratory pressure. Accumulation of fluid in tubing has also been noted. We, however, have reported on the safe administration of the drug during mechanical ventilation of 15 young children with respiratory syncytial virus (RSV) infection (23). During the ribavirin aerosol treatments, evidence of precipitation and excessive condensation in ventilator tubing was monitored hourly, and filters and valves were changed routinely every 1-4 hr. In addition, a heated wire was used in the tubing to reduce aerosol condensation. The effect of ribavirin on the young and developing lung is unknown, and long-term evaluation is needed (11).

Because ribavirin has been found to be teratogenic and/or embryolethal in multiple animal species, it is contraindicated in pregnant women. It is also recommended that pregnant female health care personnel avoid inadvertent exposure to the aerosol.

IV. CLINICAL USES

In North America, only the aerosolized formulation of ribavirin is licensed. It has been found to be effective in the treatment of lower respiratory tract infections caused by influenza A (24-26), influenza B (15,26), and RSV (27-30). Isolated case reports have also suggested that aerosolized ribavirin may be effective in the treatment of severe respiratory virus infections caused by RSV and parainfluenza in immunodeficient children (31,32). In contradistinction to the favorable results reported with aerosolized ribavirin, ribavirin administered by the oral route has not been of consistent benefit in the therapy of respiratory virus infections (21,22,23).

The decision to prescribe ribavirin therapy in an individual patient is difficult. Although the drug has demonstrable efficacy as noted above, it requires prolonged inhalation (12-20 hr/day) and is expensive. It would seem reasonable to use ribavirin in patients severely ill with lower respiratory tract disease caused by RSV or influenza and in those at particular high risk of a poor outcome (e.g., children with chronic lung disease or congenital heart disease). It may even be reasonable to prescribe therapy for any patient ill enough to be admitted to the hospital with an infection caused by one of these agents; this, however, is not yet established.

Oral or intravenous ribavirin is clearly effective at reducing the mortality rate in patients with Lassa fever (19). Maximum effectiveness was noted if treatment was initiated within the first 6 days after the onset of fever, but even if treatment was initiated later, mortality was significantly reduced. The authors thus concluded that ribavirin should be used at any point in the illness as well as for postexposure prophylaxis. Animal studies also suggest a role for ribavirin in the treatment of other arenavirus infections. For example, the prolonged survival of animals infected with either Junin virus, the agent of Argentine hemorrhagic fever, or with Machupo virus, the agent of Bolivian hemorrhagic fever, has been demonstrated (34). However, a fatal encephalitis subsequently ensues in these animals.

V. DOSAGE AND ADMINISTRATION

Ribavirin is available only for aerosolized use in North America. It is supplied as a sterile, lyophilized powder that does not contain any preservatives. Upon reconstitution, it has a pH of 5.0-6.9 and is colorless, odorless, and tasteless. The aerosol is delivered by a small particle aerosol generator (SPAG-2). The aerosol may be delivered into an infant oxygen hood, a face mask, or an oxygen tent. With due caution, as outlined above, it may also be administered in ventilated patients through the endotracheal tube. The recommended drug concentration is 20 mg/ml as the starting solution in the drug reservoir of the SPAG unit. The daily duration of aerosolization should be 12-18 hr, and treatment should be given for 3-7 days, with the actual duration depending upon clinical response.

REFERENCES

1. Witkowski, JT, Robins, RK, Sidwell, RW, Simon, LN: Design, synthesis, and broad spectrum antiviral activity of 1-β-D-ribofuranosyl-1,2,4-triazole-3-carboxamide and related nucleosides. *J. Med. Chem. 15*:1150-1154, 1972.
2. Prusiner, P, Sundaralingam, M: A new class of synthetic nucleoside analogues with broad-spectrum antiviral properties. *Nature* [*New Biol.*] *244*:116-118, 1973.
3. Canonico, PG, Kende, M, Huggins, JW: The toxicology and pharmacology of ribavirin in experimental animals. In: *Clinical Applications of Ribavirin* (RA Smith, V Knight, and JAD Smith, eds.), Academic Press, New York, 1984, pp. 65-77.
4. Wray, SK, Gilbert, BE, Noall, MW, Knight, V: Mode of action of ribavirin: Effect of nucleoside pool alterations on influenza virus ribonucleoprotein synthesis. *Antiviral Res. 5*:29-37, 1985.
5. Wray, SK, Gilbert, BE, Knight, V: Effect of ribavirin triphosphate on primer generation and elongation during influenza virus transcription in vitro. *Antiviral Res. 5*: 39-48, 1985.
6. Smith, RA: Background and mechanisms of action of ribavirin. In: *Clinical Applications of Ribavirin* (RA Smith, V Knight, and JAD Smith, eds.), Academic Press, New York, 1984, pp. 1-18.
7. Crumpacker, CS: Overview of ribavirin treatment of infection caused by RNA viruses. In: *Clinical Applications of Ribavirin* (RA Smith, V Knight, and JAD Smith, eds.), Academic Press, New York, 1984, pp. 33-37.
8. Kirsi, JJ, North, JA, McKernan, PA, Murray, BK, Canonico, PG, Huggins, JW, Srivastava, PC, Robins, RK: Broad-spectrum antiviral activity of 2-β-D-ribofuranosylselenazole-4-carboxide, a new antiviral agent. *Antimicrob. Agents Chemother. 24*:353-361, 1983.
9. Sidwell, RW, Huffman, JH, Khare, GP, Allen, LB, Witkowski, JT, Robins, RK: Broad-spectrum antiviral activity of virazole: 1-β-D-ribofuranosyl-1,2,4-triazole-3-carboxamide. *Science 177*:705-706, 1972.
10. Sidwell, RW: In vitro and in vivo inhibition of DNA viruses by ribavirin. In: *Clinical Applications of Ribavirin* (RA Smith, V Knight, and JAD Smith, eds.), Academic Press, New York, 1984, pp. 19-32.
11. Hall, CB: Ribavirin: Beginning the blitz on respiratory viruses? *Pediatr. Infect. Dis. 4*:668-671, 1985.
12. McCormick, JB, Mitchell, SW, Getchell, JP, Hicks, DR: Ribavirin suppresses replication of lymphadenopathy-associated virus in cultures of human adult T lymphocytes. *Lancet 2*:1367-1369, 1984.
13. Connor, JD, Hintz, M, Van Dyke, R, McCormick, JB, and McIntosh, K: Ribavirin pharmacokinetics in children and adults during therapeutic trials. In: *Clinical Applications of Ribavirin* (RA Smith, V Knight, and JAD Smith, eds.), Academic Press, New York, 1984, pp. 107-123.
14. Wilson, SZ, Knight, V, Moore, R, Larson, EW: Amantadine small-particle aerosol: Generation and delivery to man. *Proc. Soc. Exp. Biol. Med. 161*:350-354, 1979.
15. McClung, HW, Knight, V, Gilbert, BE, Wilson, SZ, Quarles, JM, Divine, GW: Ribavirin aerosol treatment of influenza B virus infection. *JAMA 249*:2671-2674, 1983.
16. Catlin, DH, Smith, RA, Samuels, AI: ^{14}C-ribavirin: Distribution and pharmacokinetic studies in rats, baboons, and man. In: *Ribavirin: A broad Spectrum Antiviral Agent* (RA Smith, and W Kirkpatrick, eds.), Academic Press, New York, 1980, pp. 83-98.

17. Ferrara, EA, Oishi, JS, Wannemacher, RW, Jr., Stephen, EL: Plasma disappearance, urine excretion, and tissue distribution of ribavirin in rats and Rhesus monkeys. *Antimicrob. Agents Chemother. 19*:1042–1049, 1981.
18. Shulman, NR: Assessement of hematologic effects of ribavirin in humans. In: *Clinical Applications of Ribavirin* (RA Smith, V Knight, and JAD Smith, eds.), Academic Press, New York, 1984, pp. 79–92.
19. McCormick, JB, King, IJ, Webb, PA, Scribner, CL, Craven, RB, Johnson, KM, Elliot, LH, Belmont-Williams, R: Lassa fever: Effective therapy with ribavirin. *N. Engl. J. Med. 314*:20–26, 1986.
20. Cohen, A, Togo, Y, Khakoo, R, Waldman, R, Sigel, M: Comparative clinical and laboratory evaluation of the prophylactic capacity of ribavirin, amantadine hydrochloride, and placebo in induced human influenza type A. *J. Infect. Dis. 133*(Suppl. A):114–120, 1976.
21. Magnussen, CR, Douglas, RG, Jr., Betts, RF, Roth, FK, Meager, MP: Double-blind evaluation of oral ribavirin (Virazole) in experimental influenza A virus infection in volunteers. *Antimicrob. Agents Chemother. 12*:498–502, 1977.
22. Smith, CB, Charette, RP, Fox, JP, Conney, MK, Hall, CB: Lack of effect of oral ribavirin in naturally occurring influenza A virus (H1N1) infection. *J. Infect. Dis. 141*:548–554, 1980.
23. Wilson, CM, Arvin, AM, Frankel, LR, Smith, DW, Prober, CG: The safe administration of aerosolized ribavirin during mechanical ventilation of young children with respiratory syncytial virus (RSV) infection. Abstract 372, Twenty-sixth Interscience Conference on Antimicrobial Agents and Chemotherapy, American Society for Microbiology, 1986.
24. Knight, V, Wilson, SZ, Quarles, JM, Greggs, SE, McClung, HW, Waters, BK, Cameron, RW, Zerwas, JM, Couch, RB: Ribavirin small-particle aerosol treatment of influenza. *Lancet 1*:945–949, 1981.
25. Wilson, SZ, Gilbert, BE, Quarles, JM, Knight, V, McClung, HW, Moore, RV, Couch, RB: Treatment of influenza A (H1N1) virus infection with ribavirin aerosol. *Antimicrob. Agents Chemother. 26*:200–203, 1984.
26. Gilbert, BE, Wilson, SZ, Knight, V, Couch, RB, Quarles, JM, Dure, L, Hayes, N, Willis, G: Ribavirin small-particle aerosol treatment of infections caused by influenza virus strains A/Victoria/7/83 (H1N1) and B/Texas/1/84. *Antimicrob. Agents Chemother. 27*:309–313.
27. Taber, LH, Knight, V, Gilbert, BE, McClung, HW, Wilson, SZ, Norton, HJ, Thurson, JM, Gordon, WH, Atmar, RL, Schlaudt, R: Ribavirin aerosol treatment of bronchiolitis associated with respiratory syncytial virus infection in infants. *Pediatrics 72*: 613–618, 1983.
28. Hall, CB, Walsh, EE, Hruska, JF, Betts, RF, Hall, WJ: Ribavirin treatment of experimental respiratory syncytial viral infection. A controlled double-blind study in young adults. *JAMA 249*:2666, 1983.
29. Hall, CB, McBride, JT, Walsh, EE, Bell, DM, Gala, CL, Hildreth, S, Ten Eyck, LG, Hall, WJ: Aerosolized ribavirin treatment of infants with respiratory syncytial viral infection: A randomized double-blind study. *N. Engl. J. Med. 308*:1443–1447, 1983.
30. Hall, CB, McBride, JT, Gala, CL, Hildreth, SW, Schnabel, KC: Ribavirin treatment of respiratory syncytial viral infection in infants with underlying cardiopulmonary disease. *JAMA 254*:3047–3051, 1985.
31. McIntosh, K, Kurachek, SC, Cairns, LM, Burns, JC, Goodspeed, B: Treatment of respiratory viral infection in an immunodeficient infant with ribavirin aerosol. *Am. J. Dis. Child. 138*:305–308, 1984.

32. Gelfand, EW, McCurdy, B, Rao, CP, Middleton, PJ: Ribavirin treatment of viral pneumonitis in severe combined immunodeficiency disease. *Lancet 2*:732–733, 1983.
33. Salido-Rengall, F, Nasser-Quinones, H, Briseno-Garcia, B: Clinical evaluation of 1-beta-D-ribafuranosyl-1,2,4-triazole-3-carboxamide (ribavirin) in a double blind study during an outbreak of influenza. *Ann. N.Y. Acad. Sci. 284*:272–277, 1977.
34. Huggins, JW, Jahrling, P, Kende, M, Canonica, PG: Efficacy of ribavirin against virulent RNA virus infections. In: *Clinical Applications of Ribavirin* (RA Smith, V Knight, and JAD Smith, eds.), Academic Press, New York, 1984, pp. 49–63.

31
Interferon

ANN M. ARVIN
Stanford University School of Medicine, Stanford, California

> The contagion of the measles, if it be taken a sufficient time before inoculation, so that the eruption may commence before the variolous fever comes on, stops the progress of the smallpox in the inoculated wound, and delays it until the measles-fever has finished its career.
>
> Erasmus Darwin, M.D., F.R.S., in *Zoonomia or, The Laws of Organic Life*, Second American Edition, Vol. II, 1803, p. 208

This description of the inhibition of vaccinia virus replication in patients with measles probably represents the first description of the effect of interferon in vivo. Modern investigation of interferons begins with the observation by Isaacs and Lindemann of the efficacy of interferon in protecting cells against viral infection in vitro (1).

Interferons (IFN) are a group of glycoproteins that are synthesized by mammalian cells upon induction with viruses, double-stranded ribonucleic acids (RNA), and other compounds (2,3). These proteins have been evaluated as antiviral substances because of the observation that viral replication was inhibited in vitro if tissue culture cells were exposed to interferon prior to challenge with virus. In addition to their antiviral effects, interferons alter mammalian cell growth and differentiation and regulate the host immune response. The cell growth and immunoregulatory effects have led to the assessment of interferons as antitumor agents (4) and for treatment of diseases that may have an immunologic component in their pathogenesis, e.g., multiple sclerosis (5).

The interferons are now classified as α-IFN, β-IFN and γ-IFN. α-IFN is identified primarily as a product of leukocytes, especially mononuclear cells; β-IFN is synthesized by fibroblasts and epithelial cells. Lymphoblastoid cells are another source of IFN that is predominantly α-IFN but also contains some β-IFN. γ-IFN is produced by T lymphocytes and is recognized for its immunoregulatory effects, such as the induction of virus-specific T-lymphocyte cytotoxicity. α-IFN and β-IFN bind to cell surface receptors that differ from those involved in the attachment of γ-IFN. α-IFN and β-IFN show a considerable degree of homology between their respective nucleotide and amino acid sequences. γ-IFN shows little overall biochemical relationship to α- and β-IFN but does contain a few amino acid sequences that are quite similar. Differences in receptor specificity and other molecular differences may provide a basis for the antiviral synergy between α-IFN or β-IFN and γ-IFN that has been observed in vitro. The IFNs characteristically exhibit a high degree of species specificity that requires the use of human IFN for the treatment of human disease.

The assessment of IFN efficacy for the treatment of human viral infections and of malignant diseases was limited by the difficulty of large-scale preparation of human IFN before the development of recombinant DNA technology (6). The production of all three types of IFN has now been accomplished using these methods. Most clinical trials of IFN have been carried out using human leukocyte α-IFN (7). This material contained 10^5–10^6 international units IFN per milligram protein, which is less than 1% pure IFN (6). The clinical efficacy of pure recombinant α-IFN has been very similar to that of the crude leukocyte α-IFN preparation, e.g., as therapy for herpes zoster in immunocompromised patients. That the recombinant IFNs are not glycosylated does not appear to reduce their biologic activity. The double-stranded RNA inducers of IFN are polyinosinic:polycytidylic acid (poly IC) and poly IC-poly L-lysine (poly ICLC). Interferon inducers have been administered to achieve in vivo IFN production by the host (8–10). Poly ICLC may prove to be more effective for human administration because it is degraded less rapidly than poly IC.

I. MECHANISM OF ACTION

The mechanisms by which the IFNs inhibit viral replication are incompletely understood. The induction of the antiviral state requires new cellular RNA and protein synthesis. Interference with viral uncoating, transcription of viral mRNA, viral protein synthesis, and the assembly of whole virions have been demonstrated (2,3). As antiviral agents, the IFNs have the advantage of a broad spectrum of activity against RNA as well as DNA viruses. The IFNs in combination with acyclovir have demonstrated an additive or synergistic effect in vitro against herpes simplex, varicella zoster, and cytomegalovirus (11–14). Adenine arabinoside did not interfere with the inhibition of herpes simplex by α-IFN, but its antiviral effect was not enhanced (15). The direct antiviral activity of the IFNs may also be enhanced in vivo by their immunomodulating effects.

Most assays for the detection of IFN activity are bioassays that demonstrate the protection of a cell monolayer against infection with a challenge virus. The original plaque reduction assay was done using serial dilutions of the sample to be tested, which were incubated on human fibroblast cells for 24 hr, following which the monolayers were rinsed and incubated with an inoculum of vesicular stomatitis virus (16). An agar overlay was added, the plates were incubated for 24 hr, and the plaques were counted after staining with neutral red. Other challenge viruses and other cell lines have also been used, and the bioassay method has been adapted to microtiter plates. IFN units determined by bioassay are expressed as units per milliliter relative to a reference standard (Research Resources Branch, Antiviral Substances Program, National Institute of Allergy and Infectious Diseases). The type of IFN detected is demonstrated by neutralization of the IFN activity with reference antisera to α-, β-, or γ-IFN. γ-IFN can be measured with a radioimmunoassay method - Interferon-Gamma RIA, Centocor Inc., Malvern, Pennsylvania (17).

II. PHARMACOLOGY

A. Route of Administration

The IFNs have been administered by intramuscular injection in most clinical trials. Intravenous administration is usually avoided because of rapid removal from serum and because of the complication of hypotension in a few instances. Topical application of IFN to the nasal mucosa has been used for the prevention and treatment of respiratory viral infections. Herpes keratitis has been treated topically with an ophthalmic preparation of IFN. A few patients have been treated with intralesional injections of IFN for warts, injections into a tumor mass, e.g., medulloblastoma, or direct instillation into the cerebrospinal fluid. The topical and intralesional routes of administration do not produce detectable serum concentrations of IFN. Poly IC and poly ICLC can be administered by intramuscular or intravenous injection.

B. Pharmacokinetics

The mechanism for the metabolism of the IFNs is not certain. Catabolism of IFN proteins by the liver is probably the primary metabolic pathway for their removal. Renal clearance occurs, but there is evidence for tubular reabsorption. IFN activity was not detectable in the urine of patients receiving leukocyte α-IFN. The interferon inducers are hydrolyzed by ribonucleases in serum and tissues.

Most adult trials with leukocyte α-IFN have been carried out using doses of $3-10 \times 10^6$ units per dose as a once or twice daily injection (18-26). The range of serum IFN concentrations in these patients has been approximately 100-1000 units/ml. IFN at these doses is cleared from the serum in 6-24 hr. Equivalent serum concentrations of α-IFN can be maintained throughout a 24-hr period by continuous intravenous infusion. The IFNs do not cross the blood-brain barrier in that cerebrospinal fluid (CSF) titers are undetectable in patients who have high serum concentrations.

Mean peak serum concentrations of IFN after the intravenous administration of poly ICLC at doses of 0.5-27.0 mg/m^2 range from 15 to 10,000 U/ml and occur at 8 hr after intravenous injection. IFN is detectable in the cerebrospinal fluid after poly ICLC administration at concentrations related to the poly ICLC dose and ranging up to 1000 U/ml (11).

Data concerning the pharmacokinetics of the IFNs and IFN inducers in children is limited (18,27-29). Immunocompromised children treated with leukocyte α-IFN for varicella at doses of $1.75-3.5 \times 10^5$ U/kg day^{-1} had serum concentrations ranging from 40 to 200 U/ml. Infants given the same material for rubella infections at doses of 5×10^5 to 7×10^5 U/kg day^{-1} had serum concentrations of 40-279 U/ml. One infant treated with the higher dose had a serum concentration of 3000 U/ml. Infants with cytomegalovirus infections given lower doses, i.e., 1.7×10^5 to 5×10^5, had serum concentrations of 22-460 U/ml, with most values below 100 U/ml.

The pharmacokinetics of γ-IFN, using recombinant γ-IFN, is under investigation.

C. Toxicity

The major toxicities of IFN therapy include the "flulike" symptoms of fever, malaise and fatigue, and leukopenia. The side effects of IFN are dose related. The toxic effects seen with pure recombinant α_2-IFN have been the same as those observed with the administration of the crude material (30,31). Of healthy subjects given recombinant α_2-IFN for genital herpes simplex virus (HSV), 38% had clinical side effects at 3×10^6 U per dose compared with 15% of placebo recipients. A transient, mild leukopenia was noted in 28% of IFN recipients at 3×10^6 U per dose and in 55% of participants who received 5×10^6 U per dose. Of the participants who received the higher dose of IFN, 20% also had transient thrombocytopenia. Among immunocompromised patients given leukocyte α-IFN, there was a tendency for IFN recipients to have lower leukocyte counts but the decrease did not require the discontinuation of therapy. The study of IFN efficacy against cytomegalovirus infection in bone marrow transplant recipients demonstrated that doses $\leqslant 1.6 \times 10^5$ U/kg day^{-1} did not reduce the leukocyte count significantly in this severely immunocompromised population. Thrombocytopenia has also occurred with leukocyte α-IFN but is less common than leukopenia. Poly ICLC induces side effects that include fever, nausea, leukopenia, thrombocytopenia, and others also observed with α-IFN therapy (8–10). Combination therapy with IFN and vidarabine or IFN and acyclovir appears to have the potential to cause significant neurological toxicity. Patients given exceptionally high doses of α-IFN alone, whether leukocyte or recombinant preparations, may also develop neurological symptoms (31,32). Confusional states were reported in 8 of 11 patients given these preparations at doses of 100×10^6 U/m^2 by continuous intravenous infusion to maintain serum concentrations from 432–2500 U/m^2 (33). Most of these patients had significant electroencephalographic (EEG) abnormalities and also had elevated liver enzymes. Infants treated with IFN have had febrile reactions, transient increases in SGOT, and reduced weight gain (28,29). Hair loss has occurred with prolonged courses of treatment given to patients with hepatitis B or laryngeal papillomatosis (34). All the toxicities observed with IFN administration have resolved when the drug was discontinued. Topical intranasal application of α-IFN was associated with minor nasal bleeding and small punctate bleeding points in the nasal mucosa. Douglas et al. reported such toxicity among 41 of 345 IFN recipients compared to 11 of 330 placebo recipients ($p = 0.00002$) (35). When Hayden et al. evaluated patients who were given repeated courses of nasal α_2-IFN, no decrease in tolerance of the preparation was noted (36).

III. CLINICAL EFFICACY OF IFN FOR VIRAL INFECTIONS

A. Herpesviruses

Leukocyte α-IFN was effective for the treatment of primary and recurrent varicella zoster virus (VZV) infections in immunocompromised patients in prospective, randomized, placebo-controlled trials. Of 44 patients with varicella, 23 received IFN (27). The initial dose was $0.4\text{–}2.5 \times 10^5$ U/kg day^{-1}. In the second phase, patients received 3.5×10^5 U/kg day^{-1} for 2 days and 1.75×10^5 U/kg day^{-1} for 3 days. The IFN recipients had a decrease in the number of days of new lesion formation compared with the placebo recipients. Of subjects in the second phase of the study, 92% had no new lesions for 24 hr by day 6 compared with 45% of placebo recipients ($p < 0.025$). Of 21 placebo recipients, 3 died of progressive varicella; 2 of 23 IFN recipients died late after the onset of varicella (2–3 weeks). None of the survivors who received IFN developed life-threatening dissemination compared with 3 of 18 placebo recipients (see Table 1).

Leukocyte α-IFN was evaluated by Merigan et al. for the treatment of herpes zoster in adult patients with malignancy (18). The dose in the initial phase of the study was

Table 1

Infection	IFN preparation	Patient population	Indication	Clinical efficacy, antiviral effect
Varicella	Leukocyte	Immunocompromized	Treatment	Yes
Herpes zoster	Leukocyte and α_2-IFN	Immunocompromized	Treatment	Yes
Herpes labialis	Leukocyte	Normal	Prophylaxis	Yes
	Leukocyte and α_2-IFN	Immunocompromized	Prophylaxis	Yes
Herpes genitalis	α_2-IFN	Normal	Treatment	No
Congenital cytomegalovirus	Leukocyte	Infant	Treatment	No
Cytomegalovirus pneumonia	Leukocyte	Immunocompromized	Prophylaxis	No
	Leukocyte	Immunocompromized	Treatment	No
Cytomegalovirus retinitis	Leukocyte	Immunocompromized	Treatment	No
	Leukocyte	Immunocompromized	Treatment	No
Rhinovirus upper respiratory infection	α_2-IFN	Normal	Prophylaxis	Yes
Laryngeal papillomatosis	Leukocyte	Normal	Treatment	Yes
Condyloma acuminatum	Leukocyte	Normal	Treatment	Yes
Hepatitis B	Leukocyte and fibroblast	Normal	Treatment	Only a few patients

4.2×10^4 U/kg day^{-1}, the dose in the second phase was 1.7×10^5 U/kg day^{-1}, and the highest dose was 5.1×10^5 U/kg day^{-1}. Given for an average of 8 days, the highest dose of IFN decreased the progression of herpes zoster in the primary dermatome and reduced the number of days of continued progression of the local infection. Cutaneous dissemination did not occur in the patients receiving the highest dose regimen, but approximately one-third of placebo recipients in each phase of the trial developed lesions outside the primary dermatome. Although there were no fatal complications, 6 of 45 placebo recipients developed serious dissemination compared with 1 of 45 IFN recipients. These complications included encephalitis and postherpetic paresis. Postherpetic neuralgia was also significantly reduced with the two higher dose regimens. Severe pain occurred in 8 of 29 placebo vs. 2 of 29 IFN recipients.

Most recently, recombinant α-IFN has been used for the treatment of herpes zoster in adults with malignancy (30). Two dosage schedules, 3.6×10^7 U/kg day^{-1} for 7 days and 6.8×10^7 U/kg day^{-1} for 7 days, were used. The higher dose regimen was dropped because of significant adverse effects. The 3.6×10^7 U/kg dosage reduced cutaneous dissemination in this patient population. Of 24 interferon recipients, 3 developed cutaneous lesions outside the primary dermatome compared with 12 of 23 placebo recipients.

Preliminary data suggest potential efficacy of IFN for treatment of primary herpes simplex 1 or 2 (HSV) infections (37). Pazin et al. demonstrated that leukocyte α-IFN prophylaxis decreased the reactivation of HSV-1 after trigeminal root decompression (20). Patients were enrolled in a placebo-controlled trial 1 day before surgery and received 7×10^4 U/kg day^{-1} of IFN for 5 days. Herpetic lesions were significantly reduced among IFN recipients (26%) compared with placebo recipients (56%). Viral isolation from the oropharynx occurred in only 42% of IFN recipients vs. 83% of placebo recipients.

The efficacy of leukocyte α-IFN for HSV prophylaxis among renal transplant recipients was examined by Cheeseman et al. (22). The IFN dose was 3×10^6 U per dose for 15 doses over the first 6 weeks after transplant. This patient population was highly immunocompromised, particularly the subgroup receiving antithymocyte globulin. HSV excretion in the oropharynx and the development of HSV lesions was not diminished by IFN prophylaxis.

In a recent study, recombinant α-IFN was evaluated for the treatment of genital HSV (31). Most of these infections were probably HSV-2. The patient population was composed of healthy subjects with genital HSV who typically experienced a prodrome prior to the eruption of lesions. The subjects were treated at <24 hr after the onset of prodromal symptoms. The dosage schedule was 3×10^6 U/day for 2 days or 5×10^6 U/day for 2 days. The frequency and the time to develop herpetic lesions and the duration of lesions was not reduced by comparison with a placebo control group.

The efficacy of leukocyte α-IFN in patients with cytomegalovirus (CMV) infection has been examined in several clinical trials. IFN therapy in a study of infants who were excreting CMV in the urine as a result of congenital CMV infection was associated with a transient decrease in the titer of CMV in urine, but shedding was not eliminated during any of five treatment courses (28).

The efficacy of human leukocyte IFN as prophylaxis against CMV infection in renal transplant recipients was evaluated in a study of IFN administered for 6 weeks beginning on the day of transplantation (22). Recurrent urinary CMV excretion began earlier among placebo recipients than IFN recipients. CMV viremia was significantly reduced by IFN therapy in patients not receiving antithymocyte globulin. In a further study, Hirsch et al.

found that leukocyte α-IFN given at a dose of 3×10^6 U three times a week for 6 weeks and then twice a week for 8 weeks after renal transplant produced a marked reduction of CMV syndromes compared with placebo (1 of 20 IFN vs. 7 of 22 placebo patients, p = 0.03) (23). Opportunistic infections occurred only in the placebo group, which suggests a reduction in CMV-related immunosuppression.

Leukocyte α-IFN was not effective for the treatment of established CMV pneumonia in bone marrow transplant recipients when given alone (2×10^4 and 6×10^5 U/kg day^{-1}) or in combination with acyclovir (24,38).

Leukocyte α-IFN has also been tested against another form of established CMV infection, CMV retinitis (25). A group of four patients with severe immunosuppression, which was caused by acquired immunodeficiency syndrome in three cases, received IFN at doses from 5 to 36×10^6 U/day for 19-62 days. There was no significant effect upon viral excretion, and the clinical infection progressed during the course of therapy.

A group of seven patients with acquired immunodeficiency syndrome were treated with recombinant γ-IFN at doses of 2×10^6 U/m^2 or 20×10^6 U/m^2 five times a week for 3–14 weeks with no effect upon excretion of CMV (39).

B. Respiratory Viruses

Intranasal IFN has been evaluated for the prophylaxis and treatment of respiratory viral infections caused by rhinoviruses, coronavirus, and influenza A virus (35,36). Volunteers who were experimentally infected with rhinovirus had less severe clinical symptoms and a reduction in the amount of virus replication when given 14×10^6 U per dose of human leukocyte IFN from 2 days before until 2 days after inoculation with the virus. Recombinant α_2-IFN was effective in preventing rhinovirus infections among family contacts of naturally infected individuals. Douglas et al. found that users of intranasal α_2-IFN spray at a dosage of 5×10^6 U per dose applied to the nasal mucosa daily for 7 days had 86% fewer clinical illnesses and 76% fewer days of respiratory symptoms compared with placebo recipients (35). Hayden et al. also proved the efficacy of intranasal α_2-IFN in reducing rhinovirus transmission in the family setting (36). Illness caused by rhinovirus occurred in 2 of 27 IFN recipients compared with 12 of 34 placebo recipients ($p = 0.02$; efficacy = 79%). No beneficial effect was observed for influenza A and parainfluenza virus infections at this dosage.

C. Papillomaviruses

Initial clinical trials of IFN therapy for papillomavirus infections have indicated some therapeutic efficacy (40,41). Leukocyte α-IFN has been administered systemically to treat juvenile laryngeal papillomatosis. Although treatment did not eliminate the need for surgical intervention in this disease, IFN recipients required surgery less frequently. Intramuscular lymphoblastoid IFN has been given to patients with condylomata acuminata with regression of symptoms. Intralesional injection of condylomata acuminata and verucca plantaris with recombinant α_2-IFN and β-IFN was also associated with regression of these forms of papillomavirus infection.

D. Hepatitis B Virus

Leukocyte α-IFN and fibroblast IFN have been evaluated for antiviral activity against chronic hepatitis B infection (42,43). Patients treated with IFN had three patterns of response, including a permanent elimination of hepatitis B surface antigen from serum and from liver cells (type I), a fall in hepatitis B surface antigen titer in serum but persistence in liver cells (type II), and no change in hepatitis B surface antigen in serum or liver cells (type III). However, the majority of patients with chronic hepatitis B infection did not show eradication of the chronic infection. Combination therapy with IFN and vidarabine failed to increase the numbers of patients with a type I clinical response and was associated with more toxicity. Fibroblast β-IFN has also been evaluated in patients with chronic hepatitis B with similar results. Chronic hepatitis B infection is the target of new clinical trials designed to examine the potential in vivo synergy of β- and γ-IFN (44).

REFERENCES

1. Isaacs, A, Lindemann, J: Virus interference. I. The interferon. *Proc. R. Soc. Lond.* [*Biol.*] *147*:258–267, 1957.
2. Stewart, WE, II: *The Interferon System*, Springer-Verlag, Berlin, 1979.
3. Friedman, RM: *interferons, A Primer*, Academic Press, New York, 1981.
4. Merigan, TC, Sikora, K, Breeden, JH, Levy, R, Rosenberg, SA: Preliminary observations on the effects of human leukocyte interferon in non-Hodgkin's lymphoma. *N. Engl. J. Med. 299*:1449–1453, 1978.
5. Knobler, RL, Panitch, HS, Braheny, SL, Sipe, JC, Rice, GPA, Huddlestone, JR, Francis, GS, Hooper, CJ, Kamin-Lewis, RM, Johnson, KP, Oldstone, MBA, Merigan, TC: Systemic alpha-interferon therapy of multiple sclerosis. *Neurology 34*:1273–1279, 1984.
6. Pestka, S, Maeda, S, McCandliss, R, Levy, WR, Familletti, PC, Sloma, A, Hobbs, DS: Human interferons: Purification of the proteins and their expression in bacteria. In: *The Clinical Potential of Interferons* (R Kono and J Vilcek, eds.), University of Tokyo Press, Tokyo, 1982, pp. 369–380.
7. Cantell, K, Hirvonen, S: Large scale production of human leukocyte interferon containing 10^8 units per ml. *J. Gen. Virol. 39*:541–543, 1978.
8. Guggenheim, MA, Baron, S: Clinical studies of an interferon inducer, polyriboinosinic-polyribocytidylic acid [Poly(1)-Poly(C)] in children. *J. Infect. Dis. 136*:50–58, 1977.
9. Levy, H, Riley, F, Levine, A, Salazar, A, Engle, WK, Durie, B, Leventhal, B, Whiznant, J, Lampkin, B, Krown, S: Preliminary clinical studies with poly (ICLC). In: *The Clinical Potential of Interferons* (R Kono and J Vilcek, eds.), University of Tokyo Press, Tokyo, 1982, pp. 111–125.
10. Levine, AS, Sivulich, M, Wiernick, PH, Levy, HB: Initial clinical trials in cancer patients of poly (ICLC)—a highly effective interferon inducer. *Cancer Res. 39*:1645–1652, 1979.
11. Levin, MJ, Leary, PL: Inhibition of human herpes virus by combination of acyclovir and human leukocyte interferon. *Infect. Immun. 32*:995–999, 1981.
12. Stanwick, TL, Schinazi, RF, Campbell, DF, Nahmias, AJ: Combined antiviral effect of interferon and acyclovir on herpes simplex virus types 1 and 2. *Antimicrob. Agents Chemother. 19*:672–677, 1981.
13. Hammer, SM, Kaplan, JL, Lowe, BR, Hirsch, MS: Alpha interferon and acyclovir treatment of herpes simplex virus in lymphoid cell cultures. *Antimicrob. Agents Chemother. 21*:634–640, 1982.
14. Smith, CA, Wigdahl, B, Rapp, F: Synergistic antiviral activity of acyclovir and interferon on human cytomegalovirus. *Antimicrob. Agents Chemother. 24*:325–332, 1983.
15. Bryson, YJ, Kronenberg, LH: Combined antiviral effects of interferon, adeninine arabinoside, hypoxanthine arabinoside and adenine monophosphate in human fibroblast cultures. *Antimicrob. Agents Chemother. 11*:299–306, 1977.

16. Merigan, TC: A plaque inhibition assay for human interferon employing human neonate skin fibroblast monolayers and bovine vesicular stomatitis virus. In: *In Vitro Methods in Cell-mediated Immunity* (BR Bloom and PR Glade, eds.), Academic Press, New York, 1971, pp. 489–499.
17. Chang, T, et al.: Use of monoclonal antibodies as sensitive and specific probes for biologically active human gamma interferon. *Proc. Natl. Acad. Sci. USA 81*:5219–5221, 1984.
18. Merigan, TC, Rand, KH, Pollard, RB, Abdallah, PS, Jordan, GW, Fried, RP: Human leukocyte interferon for the treatment of herpes zoster in patients with cancer. *N. Engl. J. Med. 298*:891–897, 1978.
19. Merigan, TC, Gallagher, JG, Pollard, RB, Arvin, AM: Short course interferon therapy in treatment of herpes zoster in cancer patients. *Antimicrob. Agents Chemother. 19*: 193–195, 1980.
20. Pazin, GJ, Armstrong, JA, Lam, MT, Tarr, GC, Janetta, PJ, Ho, M: Prevention of reactivated herpes simplex infection by human leukocyte interferon after operation on the trigeminal root. *N. Engl. J. Med. 301*:225–230, 1979.
21. Haverkos, HW, Pazin, GJ, Armstrong, AJ, Ho, M: Follow-up of interferon treatment of herpes simplex. *N. Engl. J. Med. 303*:699–700, 1980.
22. Cheeseman, SH, Rubin, RH, Stewart, JA, et al.: Controlled clinical trial of prophylactic human leukocyte interferon in renal transplantation: Effects on cytomegalovirus and herpes simplex virus infections. *N. Engl. J. Med. 300*:1345–1349, 1979.
23. Hirsch, MS, Schooley, RT, Cosimi, AB, et al.: Effects of interferon-alpha on cytomegalovirus reactivation syndrome in renal transplant recipients. *N. Engl. J. Med. 308*:1489–1493, 1983.
24. Myers, JD, McGuffin, RW, Neiman, PE, Singer, JW, Thomas, ED: Toxicity and efficacy of human leukocyte interferon for treatment of cytomegalovirus pneumonia after marrow transplantation. *J. Infect. Dis. 141*:555–562, 1980.
25. Chou, SW, Dylewski, JS, Gaynon, MW, Egbert, PR, Merigan, TC: Alpha-interferon administration in cytomegalovirus retinitis. *Antimicrob. Agents Chemother. 25*:25–28, 1984.
26. Cheeseman, SH, Henle, W, Rubin, RH, et al.: Epstein-Barr virus infection in renal transplant recipients: Effects of antithymocyte globulin and interferon. *Ann. Intern. Med. 93*:39, 1980.
27. Arvin, AM, Kushner, JH, Feldman, S, Baehner, RL, Hammond, D, Merigan, TC: Human leukocyte interferon for the treatment of varicella in children with cancer. *N. Engl. J. Med. 306*:761–765, 1982.
28. Arvin, AM, Yeager, AS, Merigan, TC: Effect of leukocyte interferon on urinary excretion of cytomegalovirus by infants. *J. Infect. Dis. 133s*:A205–210, 1976.
29. Arvin, AM, Merigan, TC, Schmidt, N: Interferon administration to infants with congenital rubella. *Antimicrob. Agents Chemother. 21*:259–261, 1982.
30. Winston, D, Eron, L, Ho, M, Pazin, G, Kessler, H, Sartino, G, Gallagher, J, Ho, W, Champlin, R, Bernhardt, L, Bigley, J, Nadler, P: Treatment of herpes zoster in immunocompromised cancer patients with recombinant leukocyte A interferon (abstract). In: *The 1985 TNO-ISIR Meeting on the Interferon System*, October 1985.
31. Radolf, J, Wofsy, C, Niland, N, Lovett, M, Dillon, M, Fall, H, Hauer, L, Bigley, J, Rosenbaum, D, Gordin, F, Nadler, P, Mills, J, Bryson, Y: Recombinant leukocyte interferon A treatment during prodromal symptoms of recurrent herpes genitalis (abstract). In: *The 1985 TNO-ISIR Meeting on the Interferon System*, October 1985.
32. Scott, GM, Secher, DS, Flowers, D, Bate, J, Cantell, K, Tyrell, DAJ: Toxicity of interferon. *Br. Med. J. 282*:2345–2353, 1981.
33. Rohatiner, AZS, Prior, PF, Burton, AC, Smith, AT, Balkwill, FR, Lister, TA: Central nervous system toxicity of interferon. *Br. J. Cancer 47*:419–422, 1983.

34. Ingimarsson, S, Cantell, K, Strander, H: Side effects of long-term treatment with human leukocyte interferon. *J. Infect. Dis. 140*:560–563, 1979.
35. Douglas, RM, Moore, BW, Miles, HB, Davies, LM, Graham, NMH, Ryan, P, Worswick, DA, Albrecht, JK: Prophylactic efficacy of intranasal alpha$_2$-interferon against rhinovirus infections in the family setting. *N. Engl. J. Med. 314*:65–70, 1986.
36. Hayden, FG, Albrecht, JK, Kaiser, DL, Gwaltney, JM: Prevention of natural colds by contact prophylaxis with intranasal alpha$_2$-interferon. *N. Engl. J. Med. 314*: 71–75, 1986.
37. Ho, M, et al.: In: *Proceedings of New Directions in Antiviral Chemotherapy Symposium* (J Mills, ed.), in press, 1986.
38. Wade, JC, McGuffin, RW, Springmeyer, SC, Newton, B, Singer, JW, Myers, JD: Treatment of cytomegaloviral pneumonia with high-dose acyclovir and human leukocyte interferon. *J. Infect. Dis. 148*:557–562, 1983.
39. Drew, WL, Conant, M, Volberding, P: In: *Proceedings of the New Directions in Antiviral Chemotherapy Symposium* (J Mills, ed.), in press, 1986.
40. Reichman, RC: Use of interferons for papillomavirus infections. In: *Proceedings of the New Directions in Antiviral Chemotherapy Symposium* (J Mills, ed.), in press, 1986.
41. Oriel, JD: Human papillomaviruses. In: *Proceedings of the New Directions in Antiviral Chemotherapy Symposium* (J Mills, ed.), in press, 1986.
42. Greenberg, HB, Pollard, RB, Lutwick, LI, Gregory, PB, Robinson, WS, Merigan, TC: Effect of human leukocyte interferon in hepatitis B virus infection in patients with chronic active hepatitis. *N. Engl. J. Med. 295*:517–522, 1976.
43. Desmyter, J, Ray, MB, Degrotte, J, Bradburne, AF, Desnet, VJ, Edy, VG, Billiau, A, Desomer, P, Mortelmans, J: Administration of human fibroblast interferon in chronic hepatitis B infection. *Lancet 2*:645–647, 1976.
44. Fleischmann, WR, Georgiades, JA, Osborne, LC, Johnson, HM: Potentiation of interferon activity by mixed preparations of fibroblast and immune interferon. *Infect. Immun. 26*:248–253, 1979.

Part VI
Antiparasitic Drugs

32
Antimalarial Drugs

JOSE ANTONIO JESUS BODINO AND EDUARDO L. LOPEZ
Children's Hospital of Buenos Aires, Buenos Aires, Argentina

The global potential for transmission of malarial infections has risen again over the past 15 years. Many of the attempts at eradication launched all over the world 30 years ago met with failure, mainly due to the development of resistance to insecticides, e.g., dichlorodiphenyltrichloroethane (DDT), and to antimalarial drugs, especially chloroquine resistance by *Plasmodium falciparum*. Although most temperate regions continue to be largely free of malaria, prevalence of the disease in other areas has increased markedly and the potential for transmission is approaching its original level (1).

Other factors also account for this. Undue reliance on highly encouraging initial results led to the premature discontinuance or weakening of malaria control campaigns involving the combined use of chemotherapy and insecticides. This in turn has caused the disease to upsurge drastically after a few years, as reported in Sri Lanka, India, and Pakistan (2).

The worldwide phenomenon of increased migration has been determinant in the resurgence of malaria. The new cases reported in developed countries are for the most part imported, for example, service personnel or refugees coming from such malarious regions as Vietnam and Indonesia. However, the possibility of locally acquired mosquito-transmitted infection cannot be ruled out, since very brief exposures have been shown to suffice for inoculation. Some such cases have occurred in France, Switzerland (2), and the United States (3).

To deal with still another barrier to malaria control, i.e., resistance to DDT, different insecticides have been tried. Some are petroleum derivatives, and their high cost makes extensive spraying with these products almost impracticable. In other cases the peculiar habits of vectors prevent the effective use of insecticides.

Notwithstanding these setbacks, a number of more or less recent advances provide some basis for optimism. The in vitro cultivation of *P. falciparum* (4) has proven fundamental for the development of new chemotherapeutic compounds. A promising line of investigation aims at interfering with the process of attachment to and penetration of erythrocytes by merozoites, on the grounds that the most compromising effects of malaria on humans are those brought about during the asexual intraerythrocytic phase of

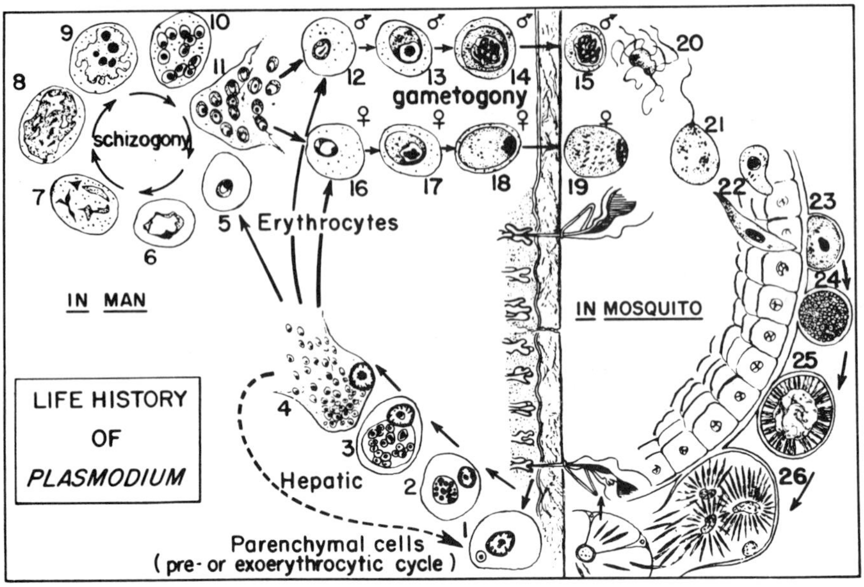

Figure 1 Life cycle of *Plasmodium*. From Wilcox, *Manual for the Microscopical Diagnosis of Malaria in Man*. National Institute of Health, U.S.P.H.S., Bulletin 180.

plasmodia (Figure 1). Another major achievement expected to contribute to the development of vaccines is the isolation of antigens from parasites in different stages of maturation (5).

Thus the skills and imagination of multidisciplinary research teams are confronted with the challenge to improve methods of malaria vector control, to develop new effective and safe antimalarial drugs, and to advance research projects eventually leading to the creation of antimalarial vaccines.

I. CLASSIFICATION

Antimalarial compounds may be classified according to the parasitic stage on which they exert their primary action. The functions an antimalarial agent is expected to fulfill either alone or in combination with others, can be roughly outlined as follows.

Causal prophylaxis prevents liver stages, i.e., sporozoites (and hypnozoites in *Plasmodium vivax* and *Plasmodium ovale*), from developing into pre-erythrocytic schizonts.

Suppressive treatment involves the administration of small doses of drugs capable of destroying erythrocytic parasites, to prevent clinical symptoms and/or parasitemia.

Suppressive cure, in the presence of *P. falciparum* and *P. malariae*, can be obtained by continuing suppressive treatment for about 6 weeks after leaving an endemic area, to ensure interruption of parasite development into the erythrocytic stage.

Clinical cure is achieved by giving higher doses of the same type of drugs as for suppressive treatment, to eliminate the largest number of parasites present in a clinical attack.

Radical cure, which for *P. falciparum* and *P. malariae* infections can be equated to suppressive cure, in the presence of *P. ovale* and *P. vivax*, on the other hand, also necessitates the use of agents that can eliminate the dormant liver forms.

Table 1 Classification of Blood Schizontocides

Main site of action	Compound	Chemical class
Para-aminobenzoic acid incorporation (PABA blockers)[a]	Dapsone	Sulfone
	Sulfadoxine	Sulfonamide
	Sulfalene	Sulfonamide
Folate metabolism (dihydrofolate reductase inhibitors)	Proguanil[b]	Biguanide
	Pyrimethamine	Pyrimidine
Hemoglobin digestion products	Chloroquine	4-Aminoquinoline
	Amodiaquine	4-Aminoquinoline (and Mannich base)
	Quinine	Aminoalcohol
	Mefloquine	Aminoalcohol
	Halofantrine	Aminoalcohol
Protein metabolism (?)	Artemisine (qinghaosu)	Sesquiterpene lactone
	Artesunate (hemisuccinyl derivative of qinghaosu)	Sesquiterpene ester
Protein synthesis (?)	Tetracyclines	Naphthacene derivatives

[a]Little, if any, action on *P. vivax*.
[b]Through its active metabolite, cycloguanil.

A. Blood Schizotocides

These compounds act upon the asexual intraerythrocytic stages of human plasmodia and may be classified as shown in Table 1 (6). Drugs belonging to this group aim to interrupt schizogony and terminate clinical attacks. Antimalarials that are effective against asexual erythrocytic stages may have no gametocytocidal properties and may be ineffective against exoerythrocytic stages. A patient may be free of schizogonic parasites yet still be infectious owing to the persistence of gametocytes in the circulating blood or may still relapse owing to reinfection of the bloodstream from the tissue.

B. Tissue Schizontocides

These compounds may be divided in two groups. Primary tissue schizontocides are used for causal prophylaxis. They act upon primary tissue forms that lodge in the liver prior to initiating the erythrocytic stage of infection. Hypnozoitocides are used to prevent relapses and affect the dormant liver forms or hypnozoites, now believed to be responsible for the production of true relapses in *P. vivax* infections (7) and possibly also in *P. ovale* infections. Currently available drugs belonging to these two groups are listed in Table 2 (6).

C. Gametocytocides

These compounds destroy the sexual erythrocytic forms of plasmodia and prevent the transmission of malaria to mosquitoes.

D. Sporontocides

These drugs ablate the transmission of malaria by preventing or inhibiting the formation of oocysts and sporozoites in infected mosquitoes. Primaquine and chloroguanide are the major antimalarials with this type of action.

Another approach to the classification of antimalarial agents advanced by James and Gilles (8) has gained general acceptance. By dividing the principal antimalarial compounds into four "arbitrary" groups, as shown on Table 3, it avoids the pitfalls encountered in classifying in terms of specific antimalarial activity, because of the varied other effects that some drugs exert.

Table 2 Classification of Tissue Schizontocides

Stage affected	Site of action	Compound	Chemical class
PE[a] schizont	Mitochondria	Primaquine[b]	8-Aminoquinoline
PE schizont	Folate metabolism (?)	Proguanil	Biguanide
PE schizont	Folate metabolism (?)	Pyrimethamine	Pyrimidine
PE schizont	PABA incorporation[c]	Sulfadoxine	Sulfonamide
Hypnozoite	Unknown	Primaquine[b]	8-Aminoquinoline

[a]Pre-erythrocytic.
[b]Possibly through an active metabolite.
[c]Not confirmed in any human species of *Plasmodia.*

Table 3 Main Antimalarial Drugs

Drug	Chemical classification	Dynamic classification
Quinine	4-Quinolinemethanol	Rapidly acting blood schizontocides
Mefloquine	4-Quinolinemethanol	
Chloroquine	4-Aminoquinoline	
Amodiaquine	4-Aminoquinoline	
Qinghaosu	Sesquiterpene lactone	
Sulfadoxine	Sulfonamide	Antifolates type I
Sulfalene	Sulfonamide	
Dapsone	Sulfone	
Proguanil	Biguanide	Antifolates type II
Chlorproguanil	Biguanide	
Pyrimethamine	2,4-Diaminopyrimidine	
Primaquine	8-Aminoquinoline	Tissue schizontocide

References

1. Bruce-Chwatt, IJ: Man against malaria: Conquest or defeat. *Trans. R. Soc. Trop. Med. Hyg. 73*:605–617, 1979.
2. Wyler, DJ: Malaria resurgence, resistance and research (first of two parts). *N. Engl. J. Med. 308*:875–878, 1983.
3. Randall, G, Seidel, JS: Malaria. *Pediatr. Clin. North Am. 32*:893–916, 1985.
4. Trager, W, Jensen, JB: Human malaria parasites in continuous culture. *Science 193*: 673–675, 1976.
5. Wyler, DJ: Malaria resurgence, resistance and research (second of two parts). *N. Engl. J. Med. 308*:934–940, 1983.
6. World Health Organization: Drug resistance in human pathogenic plasmodia. In: *Advances in Malaria Chemotherapy*, Technical Report Series 711, World Health Organization, Geneva, 1984, pp. 10–60.
7. Krotoski, WA, et al.: Demonstration of hypnozoites in sporozoite-transmitted *Plasmodium vivax* infection. *Am. J. Trop. Med. Hyg. 31*:1291–1293, 1982.
8. James, DN, Gilles, HM: Malaria. In: *Human Antiparasitic Drugs: Pharmacology and Usage* (DM James and HM Gilles, eds.), John Wiley, Chichester, 1985, pp. 120–164.

II. CHLOROQUINE AND ITS CONGENERS

Chloroquine was the first of the 4-aminoquinolines to be synthesized and tested for antimalarial activity. During World War II, an extensive cooperative program of antimalarial research was implemented in the United States. Chloroquine was among the many 4-aminoquinolines investigated. The pharmacokinetics of this drug were described in 1946 and 1948 (1-3). By the end of World War II, it came to light that as early as 1934 the Germans had synthesized and studied chloroquine under the name of Resochin. It is still the most widely used member of the 4-aminoquinoline group, an effective schizontocide having also some gametocytocidal power. Its spectrum of activity is very similar to that of quinine, and its effects are more rapid.

A. Chemistry

Chloroquine has the following structural formula:

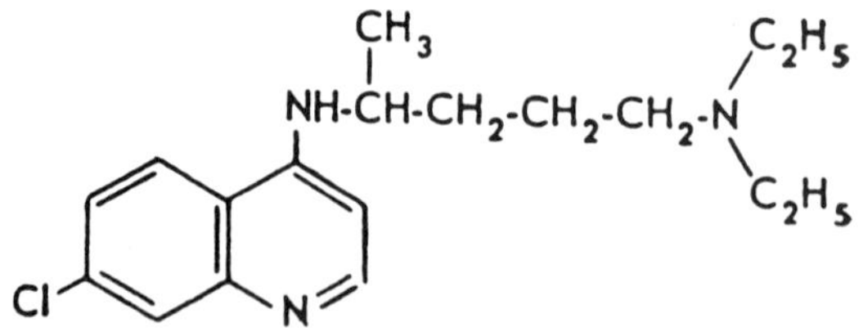

It is a white, bitter powder that forms stable solutions in water. It is available as a diphosphate.

Chloroquine bears close resemblance to quinacrine, featuring the same alkyl side chain. It differs from quinacrine in that it has a quinoline instead of an acridine nucleus. It lacks the methoxy moiety. Pamaquine and pentaquine, earlier 8-aminoquinoline antimalarials, differ from chloroquine in the position of the alkyl side chain. Chloroquine also has a chlorine instead of a methoxy nuclear substituent. There are dextrorotatory, levorotatory, and racemic forms of chloroquine, which are indistinguishable in potency tests in duck malaria. The dextrorotatory isomer seems to be less toxic in mammals than the levorotatory isomer. The 4-aminoquinolines having a chlorine atom in position 7 of the quinoline show marked antimalarial activity in both avian and human malaria. Activity is reduced with methyl substitution in position 3 of the quinoline and completely nullified with an additional substitution in position 8.

A more in-depth analysis of these mechanisms is presented by Berliner and co-workers (2) and Coatney and co-workers (4).

Amodiaquine is a congener of chloroquine featuring the following structural formula:

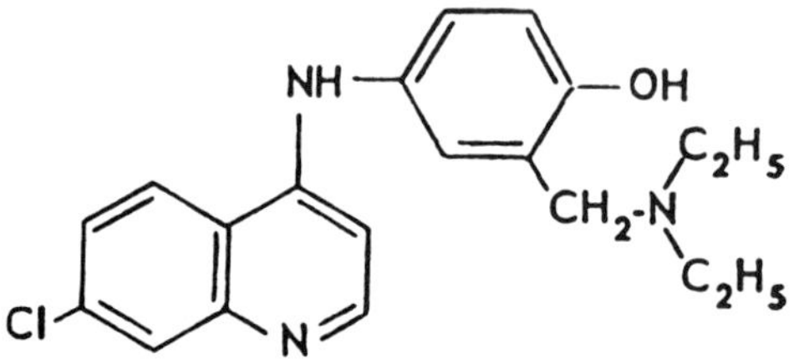

It has been used as an alternative drug when severe hypersensitivity reactions to chloroquine arose. Early in vitro and in vivo studies suggested amodiaquine to be more effective than chloroquine, particularly against certain strains of *P. falciparum* with decreased sensitivity to chloroquine. In addition, recent clinical studies in Kenya (5,6) again seem to support the notion that the degree of efficacy of amodiaquine is higher than that of chloroquine. Also, preliminary results based on a sensitive high-performance liquid chromatographic (HPLC) assay technique suggest that amodiaquine patterns of disposition may differ from those of chloroquine (7). More conclusive data are awaited.

Hydroxychloroquine is considered essentially equivalent to chloroquine, the difference being that one of the N-ethyl substituents of chloroquine is β-hydroxylated. Hydroxychloroquine has proven effective against normally sensitive parasites.

B. Mechanisms of Action

Chloroquine is a rapidly acting blood schizontocide whose primary mechanism of action has not yet been elucidated. It is clear that it affects hemoglobin digestion by parasites, but the molecular processes involved continue to be controversial. Hematin (ferriprotoporphyrin IX) (8), a transient breakdown product of hemoglobin within the parasites, causes plasmodial and host membranes to disrupt. It has been hypothesized that parasites synthesize a "segregating protein" that aggregates with hematin to form the innocuous pigment hemozoin. It has also been maintained that an even more hemolytic complex resulting from chloroquine binding to hematin kills the plasmodia by disrupting parasite-host membranes (9). The first change observed in parasites exposed to chloroquine is a rapid aggregation of all the existing hemozoin granules into a large clump (8), but the binding of the drug to hematin remains to be demonstrated.

It has been shown that chloroquine and quinine can inhibit macromolecular synthesis in malaria parasites. The effect on DNA is markedly greater than on RNA and protein synthesis. As this appears to be a first indicator of the site and mechanism of their antimalarial action, further studies on isolated nucleic acids have been conducted, including the binding interactions of these drugs with DNA. Chloroquine forms a complex with DNA by intercalation, i.e., the drug molecule inserts itself between base pairs of double-stranded DNA. Intercalation is common to all rapidly acting blood schizontocides, except mefloquine (10). This drug does not bind to DNA despite close structural and biologic similarities with the other members of the group. Hence, intercalation is not a prerequisite for this type of antimalarial action.

C. Antimalarial Activity and Resistance

Chloroquine exerts no activity against the exoerythrocytic tissue stages of plasmodia. It is highly effective against the asexual erythrocytic phase of *P. vivax* and *P. falciparum*, as well as against gametocytes of *P. vivax*. It is more effective than quinine in suppressing vivax malaria.

In the acute malaria attack, chloroquine rapidly controls clinical symptoms and parasitemia. Patients become completely afebrile within 24–48 hr after administration of therapeutic doses; thick smears of peripheral blood are generally negative for parasites by 48–72 hr. Except for certain strains in Central and South America, Southeast Asia, Africa and India, it completely cures falciparum malaria (Table 4). Chloroquine, like quinine, does not prevent relapses of vivax malaria but substantially lengthens the interval between relapses.

The in vitro susceptibility to chloroquine of some strains of *P. falciparum* has been studied more extensively than susceptibility to other antimalarials. These studies made it possible to relate parasite sensitivity in vitro to the response of nonimmune individuals treated with chloroquine (11).

Complete inhibition of schizont formation at chloroquine concentrations of 1.0 or 1.1 μmol/liter (320 μg/liter of blood) indicates infection with chloroquine-sensitive parasites. Maturation to schizonts at concentrations up to 1.5 or 2.0 μmol/liter (480–640 μg/liter of blood) has been defined as the RI level of resistance, at concentrations up to 2.4 or 3.0 μmol/liter (800–960 μ/liter of blood) as the RII level of resistance, and above 4 μmol/liter (1200 μg/liter of blood) as the RIII level of resistance in nonimmune individuals (see Figure 1) (11).

Table 4 Areas with Reported Chloroquine-Resistant *Plasmodium falciparum*

Africa[a]	Asia
Angola	Burma
Burundi	China (Hainan Island and southern provinces)
Central African Republic	Indonesia[b]
Comoros	Kampuchea[a]
Gabon	Laos[c]
Kenya	Malaysia
Madagascar	Philippines (Luzon, Basilan, Mindoro, Palawan and Mindanao Islands; Sulu Archipelago)
Malawi	Thailand
Mozambique	Vietnam
Namibia	Oceania[a]
Rwanda	Papua New Guinea
Sudan (northern provinces)	Solomon Islands
Tanzania	Vanuatu
Uganda	Indian subcontinent[a]
Zaire (northeastern)	Bangladesh (north and east)
Zambia (northeastern)	India
South America	Pakistan (Rawalpindi)
Bolivia	
Brazil[d]	
Colombia	
Ecuador[e]	
French Guiana	
Guyana	
Panama (east of the Canal zone, including San Blas Islands)	
Peru (northern provinces)	
Surinam	
Venezuela	

[a]Malaria risk exists in most urban areas.
[b]Malaria risk exists in urban areas of Timor and Kalimantan provinces. Irian Jaya should be considered in Oceania.
[c]Malaria risk exists in all urban areas except Vientiane.
[d]Malaria risk exists in urban areas of interior Amazon river region.
[e]Malaria risk exists in urban areas of Esmeraldas, Manabi, El Oro, and Guayas provinces including city of Guayaquil. Malaria risk in urban areas is limited to the above indications.
Source: From Reference 9.

D. Clinical Pharmacology

The first communications on the pharmacokinetics of chloroquine were published in the 1940s (1-3). Further studies appeared in the 1960s (12,13). New techniques, more sensitive and more specific, have been used over the last 5 years that have allowed determinations of the drug and its metabolites in body fluids and tissues (14,15).

Recent studies in healthy volunteers and children with malaria demonstrate that chloroquine is rapidly and almost completely absorbed from the gastrointestinal tract. Less than 10% of the administered dose is found in the stools.

In one study (16), 300 mg chloroquine base were given in the form of tablets or solution to healthy male adults weighing between 65 and 91 kg. Peak plasma concentrations

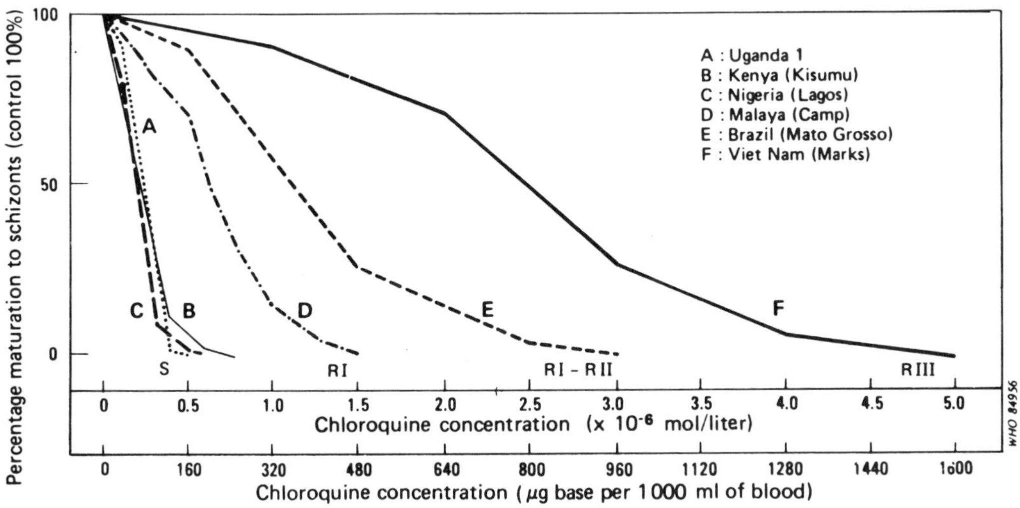

Figure 2 Chloroquine sensitivity of *P. falciparum* in vitro and in vivo. (From Reference 11. Reproduction authorized by the World Health Organization.)

of 73 ± 12 μg/liter were reached in 1-6 hr (mean, 3 hr). Mean bioavailability was 78% after intravenous administration and 89% after oral administration. Children with malaria received 10 mg chloroquine per kilogram body weight in the form of tablets (17). Peak plasma concentrations of 250 ± 30 μg/liter were reached in 2 hr. The absorption half-life was 0.56 hr. Plasma concentrations of chloroquine obtained 30 min after the administration of an oral dose of 10 mg/kilogram are usually well above the therapeutic level for sensitive *P. falciparum* (17,18).

Slow intravenous infusion of 300 mg chloroquine given to healthy adults over a period of about 25 min results in peak plasma concentrations 10 times higher than those attained after an oral dose (16). In developing countries, chloroquine is often taken without prescription as the first-line home remedy in the presumptive treatment of fevers. Walker and co-workers (18) found that approximately 50% of children diagnosed as having malaria in a teaching hospital in Nigeria had measurable plasma chloroquine concentrations before treatment was initiated. If chloroquine is given intravenously to such patients, the plasma concentrations attained may be high enough to produce severe and even fatal cardiotoxicity.

No recent studies have been performed to investigate intramuscular absorption of chloroquine in the human. In the rabbit, 10 mg/kg IM resulted in plasma concentrations twice as high as those attained after a comparable dose taken orally (19).

There is no need to administer chloroquine parenterally because the drug is almost completely absorbed following oral administration. If the patient is unable to take it by mouth, quinine may be given intravenously (quinine dihydrochloride, 10 mg/kg body weight in physiological saline solution at 10 ml/kg body weight, administered by intravenous infusion over 2-4 hr every 8-12 hr until the patient is able to take oral medication (20).

Chloroquine is approximately 50% bound to plasma proteins (21,22). The percentage binding to human serum albumin is less than the percentage binding to plasma

(21). The nonalbumin proteins to which chloroquine is bound have been shown to include α_1-acid glycoprotein (22). Aspirin does not affect chloroquine-protein binding when both are given during the treatment of acute malaria.

After absorption, chloroquine is distributed throughout the body. Early studies showed that the drug accumulated in the tissues; the concentrations recorded for the spleen, kidney, lungs, heart, and liver are 300–500 times higher than those in plasma (2, 12,23). Brain and spinal cord contain only 10–30 times the concentration in plasma. The drug has affinity to melanin-containing tissue of the skin and eye (24,25).

Chloroquine has an exceptionally large apparent volume of distribution, 116–285 liter/kg (mean, 204 liter/kg) (16). Frisk-Holmberg and co-workers, using a high-performance liquid chromatographic method, estimated the volume of distribution for plasma chloroquine to be 1000 liter/kg (26). This degree of tissue sequestration affects drug bioavailability in the central compartments, but this can be compensated for by administering a loading dose three times the subsequent dose on the first day of treatment.

The concentration of chloroquine in red blood cells has always been of interest to investigators. Early studies (27,28) showed that the erythrocyte-plasma chloroquine concentration ratio was approximately 100 in mice infected with *Plasmodium berghei* and only 10 in noninfected mice. Mice infected with chloroquine-resistant parasites had a lower ratio than those infected with sensitive strains. Similar studies have been performed in children with acute malaria (17). The erythrocyte concentration of chloroquine was higher than the plasma concentration during a sampling period of 7 days. At a stage of high parasitemia the ratio was 21, falling to a value of about 5.3 after 4 days, when parasitemia had completely disappeared. Hence there is a preferential concentration of chloroquine in human red blood cells that is further enhanced when red blood cells are infected with malaria parasites. A value of 4.8 for the unparasitized erythrocyte-plasma chloroquine concentration ratio was calculated in Swedish volunteers (16). This value is similar to that found in African children (17).

Leukocytes and thrombocytes concentrate even more than erythrocytes (29). Because of elution of chloroquine into the serum during clotting, serum concentrations are usually higher than those in plasma.

Peak concentrations of chloroquine in erythrocytes and in plasma have been observed to occur at the same time (16,17). In contrast, peak concentrations in different organs (lungs, heart, liver, and kidney) were reached at different times, and these values differed from those in plasma and red blood cells (24,25).

A loading dose is essential to achieve and maintain effective plasma concentrations because of the avidity of tissues for chloroquine. When the drug is discontinued after 2 weeks of daily administration, plasma concentration and urinary excretion decrease, with a half-life of 6–7 days for the next 4 weeks; then urinary excretion half-life increases to about 17 days. Small amounts may be found in the urine for several years (30). Daily oral dosage of 300 μg chloroquine base result in a steady-state concentration in plasma of about 125 μg/liter. Peak concentration of the drug in plasma varies between 150 and 250 μg/liter with a weekly dose of 0.5 g. Just prior to the succeeding dose, the range is between 20 and 40 μg/liter. This compares to the therapeutic concentration of about 30 μg/liter for drug-sensitive *P. falciparum* and 15 μg/liter for *P. vivax*. After single or weekly doses, the half-life of the drug in plasma is about 3 days (30).

Chloroquine is 7-chloro-4-(4′-diethylamino-1′-methylbutylamino)quinoline. By side-chain de-ethylation, it successively metabolizes in the liver, first to desethyl, and then to bidesethylchloroquine, which is a primary amine. This compound can be deaminated to form an alcohol (the 4′-hydroxy compound), which is oxidized to the 4′-carboxylic acid derivative. Successive dealkylation of the side chain ultimately produces the compound 7-chloro-4-aminoquinoline (23,31). The main metabolite varies in the different species. In humans it is desethylchloroquine (13,16,32).

After intravenous administration of 300 mg chloroquine, the desethylchloroquine concentration in plasma was approximately 20–35% that of chloroquine (16). After oral administration of the same amount of drug, the peak plasma concentration of the metabolite was 10–20 μg/liter, and the time to reach peak concentrations was approximately the same as for the parent compound. Concentrations of chloroquine and desethylchloroquine in plasma of children receiving a dose of 10 mg/kg of chloroquine were measured by Walker and co-workers (18). Desethylchloroquine was detected in the plasma after 30 min and reached a peak concentration within 2–12 hr (the same as for the parent compound). The concentration of the metabolite remained at a value of 25–40% that of chloroquine, which was 250 μg/liter, after the peak concentration had been reached. Desethylchloroquine also has the same profile of distribution and tissue binding as chloroquine (32).

There may be individual variations in the pattern of distribution of chloroquine and its desethyl metabolite. Adverse reactions to chloroquine may be related to these variations. A study was performed by Olatunde on two groups of African subjects, those who itched after receiving chloroquine and those who did not (33). Plasma concentrations were found to be similar in both groups, but the skin from subjects prone to chloroquine-induced pruritus contained higher concentrations of chloroquine and lower concentrations of the metabolite than the skin from the other subjects.

Desethylchloroquine is active against chloroquine-sensitive plasmodia (34).

Chloroquine is slowly eliminated from the body. After a single dose of 300 mg, the drug and its metabolite can be detected in the plasma for up to 52 days (16). The decline of the plasma concentrations with time after a single dose is polyexponential, suggesting a multicompartmental distribution. After peak concentrations have been reached, drug concentrations in erythrocytes and in plasma show a parallel decline, indicating that an equilibrium is soon established and subsequently maintained between these two media (16,17). Tissues, instead, behave as separate compartments, with slower elimination rate constants than plasma. Their decline phase of the log concentration-time curves diverges from that of the plasma curve with time (24,25).

Determination of the real half-life of a drug depends on the identification of the true terminal log linear elimination phase. The continuous redistribution of chloroquine from large tissue stores to plasma practically prevents the exact determination of its half-life. Estimates of the plasma half-life of chloroquine will therefore vary according to the duration of the sampling. The longer the sampling period is, the greater the number of exponential functions of the log concentration-time curve obtained, the flatter the terminal slope, and the longer the half-life. Grossly different values for the plasma half-life of chloroquine have been reported by different authors over the years, e.g., 2.5 days (1), 7–14 days (16), and 1–2 months (26). These differences may be explained by the different duration of the respective samplings.

The kinetics of chloroquine have been said to be dose dependent, on the basis of a study in which three different doses (250, 500, and 1000 mg) of the drug were given and three significantly different half-lives (3.1, 42.9, and 312 hr, respectively) were obtained (35). Examination of this report reveals that sampling lasted for only 50 hr after the 500-mg dose and for 1176 hr after the 1000-mg dose (36). Different exponential functions of the concentration-time curves were analyzed; obviously, this procedure was bound to result in different half-lives. Recent studies have failed to confirm that chloroquine kinetics are dose dependent (16,37).

The total plasma clearance of chloroquine has been estimated in 355-950 ml/min (mean, 722 ml/min) (16). Other authors (26), however, using a highly sensitive assay method, report a total plasma clearance of 1.6 ml/min kg^{-1}.

Renal clearance accounts for 51% of the total clearance; it has been found to be 260–765 ml/min (mean, 412 ml/min). Since the value for renal clearance exceeds that of glomerular filtration, the drug is probably excreted by both glomerular filtration and tubular secretion. The kidney is the main route of elimination of chloroquine; the drug has been detected in the urine for 119 days after a dose of 300 mg. In the first 24 hr (13), 10% was excreted. Subsequent urinary excretion decreases exponentially, with a computed total quinoline urinary recovery between 50 and 60% of the administered dose. Chloroquine is predominantly excreted unchanged. Desethylchloroquine accounts for less than 25% of the excreted drug. Another 10% appears in the feces.

E. Preparation, Dosage, Regimens, and Routes of Administration

Chloroquine phosphate (Aralen) is supplied in 250-mg and 500-mg tablets. Approximately 60% of the diphosphate represents the base. Chloroquine hydrochloride is available for parenteral injection in 5-ml vials containing 50 mg/ml, equivalent to 40 mg/ml base. The liquid preparation Nivaquine (sulfate) is available outside the United States.

The base equivalence of chloroquine is as follows:

167 mg diphosphate = 100 mg base
136 mg sulfate = 100 mg base

The adult prophylactic dose is 300 mg base (500 mg salt) once weekly, beginning 1-2 weeks prior to, during, and continuing for 6 weeks after exposure in a malarious area.

The pediatric prophylactic dose is 5 mg base (8.3 mg salt) per kilogram once weekly up to a maximum of 300 mg base, 500 mg salt, beginning 1-2 weeks prior to, during, and continuing for 6 weeks after exposure in a malarious area.

The adult therapeutic regimen is as follows:

Dose 1, 600 mg at once
Dose 2, 300 mg 6 hr after dose 1
Dose 3, 300 mg 18 hr after dose 2
Dose 4, 300 mg 24 hr after dose 3

The pediatric therapeutic regimen is as follows:

Dose 1, 10 mg base (16.6 mg salt) per kilogram initially (maximum 600 mg base)
Dose 2, 5 mg base (8.3 mg salt) per kilogram 6 hr after dose 1
Dose 3, 5 mg base (8.3 mg salt) per kilogram 18 hr after dose 2
Dose 4, 5 mg base (8.3 mg salt) per kilogram 24 hr after dose 3
(doses 2-4 maximum 300 mg base)

These regimens are indicated for all plasmodia, except chloroquine-resistant *P. falciparum.*

Chloroquine hydrochloride (Aralen hydrochloride, 5-ml vials equaling 200 mg base; i.e., 1 ml = 40 mg base) should be used only if parenteral administration is required for the treatment of severe *P. falciparum* infection until the patient is able to take oral medication. The dosage is 5 mg base IM per kilogram initially, and subsequently at 6-hr intervals until oral medication can be taken. Chloroquine hydrochloride is not recommended because of its potential toxicity, e.g., hypotension and circulatory collapse (17,38).

Hydrochloroquine sulfate (Plaquenil) is available in 200-mg tablets, each equaling 155 mg base; 400 mg hydrochloroquine sulfate is equivalent to 500 mg chloroquine phosphate. It may be used as an alternative agent for malaria prophylaxis at a dosage of 5 mg base (6.8 mg salt) once weekly, 1-2 weeks prior to, during, and for 6 weeks after exposure in a malarious region.

Amodiaquine, a congener of chloroquine, may also be given as an alternative agent for malaria prophylaxis, although proprietary preparations are available only in certain countries. Basoquin, amodiaquine base, is presented as a suspension containing 150 mg in each 5 ml, and as 150 mg tablets. Camoquin, amodiaquine hydrochloride, is presented as a pediatric suspension containing 50 mg base in each 5 ml and as tablets containing either 200 or 600 mg base (130 mg dihydrochloride dehydrate = 100 mg base).

The adult prophylactic dosage of amodiaquine is 400 mg base (520 mg salt) once weekly, beginning 1-2 weeks prior to exposure and continuing for 6 weeks after leaving a malarious area.

The pediatric prophylactic dosage is 7 mg base (9 mg salt) per kilogram once weekly, 1-2 weeks prior to, during, and for 6 weeks after exposure in a malarious area.

F. Drug Assays

Chloroquine monitoring has been done by gas chromatographic techniques (39). Gas chromatography-mass spectrometry and spectrodensitometry have proven adequate for pharmacokinetic studies. However, the most sensitive method for this purpose is high-performance liquid chromatography with ultraviolet or fluorescence detection (40). A technique has recently been devised to determine chloroquine and monodesethylchloroquine levels in blood using HPLC with fluorescence detection to analyze 0.1-ml samples taken by fingerprick and preserved on filter paper (41).

G. Therapeutic Indications

Chloroquine is mainly used for clinical or suppressive cure of malaria. It acts on the asexual erythrocytic stages of malaria parasites to interrupt erythrocytic schizogony and terminate clinical attacks.

It is also used to treat extraintestinal amebiasis and has anti-inflammatory effects as well.

The drug has been occasionally employed in the treatment of rheumatoid arthritis and more frequently for diskoid lupus erythematosus; its efficacy in the latter condition is controversial (42).

Chloroquine has been utilized successfully to treat porphyria cutanea tarda, solar urticaria, and polymorphous light eruptions (43).

H. Toxicity

The drug is well tolerated by patients receiving the recommended prophylactic dose regimens but may induce untoward effects at the dosages needed to treat clinical attacks.

These effects, for the most part minor and reversible, include gastrointestinal upset, pruritus, mild transient headache, and blurred vision. Only rarely is it necessary to discontinue drug administration because of intolerance. A small proportion of individuals, however, show a high degree of intolerance. All symptoms readily disappear when the drug is withheld. Chloroquine may cause discoloration of nail beds and mucous membranes.

Toxicity is dose dependent. Toxic effects are seen following chronic administration involving greater doses than those needed to control malaria. Large doses given to healthy volunteers occasionally caused visual symptoms, bleaching of the hair, T-wave abnormalities in the electrocardiogram (ECG), headache, and weight loss. The observed toxic effects caused no incapacity and were reversible upon withdrawal of the drug (1).

High daily doses of chloroquine, e.g., 200 mg or over, given for long-term treatment of diseases other than malaria (lupus) can result, once the cumulative dose exceeds 100 g base, in irreversible retinopathy, probably related to deposition of the drug in melanin-rich tissues (44). In contrast to the permanent retinopathy, crystalline deposition in the cornea and lens disappears after discontinuance of the drug. Chloroquine-induced retinopathies have occurred frequently in patients receiving high doses of the drug for the treatment of collagen diseases, but a small number of cases of retinopathy has also been reported in individuals who have taken chloroquine for malaria prophylaxis at weekly doses of 600 mg or daily doses of 100 mg for prolonged periods. This toxic effect can be avoided if the dose does not exceed 200 mg (42,45). Good and Shader (46) report neuropsychiatric disturbances associated with overdosage of chloroquine.

No definite evidence has been found yet of fetal abnormalities due to chloroquine administration during pregnancy.

I. Contraindications

Chloroquine should be used with caution in the presence of hepatic disease, owing to the high concentrations it reaches in the liver tissue. It may be contraindicated in severe gastrointestinal, neurological, or blood disorders. If such disorders occur in the course of therapy, chloroquine administration should be withheld.

Periodical ophthalmologic examination is recommended in long-term treatments (46).

J. Drug Interactions

The concomitant use of chloroquine with gold or phenylbutazone should be avoided because all three agents tend to produce dermatitis. Chloroquine given at the recommended prophylactic dosage has been shown to be associated with lower mean titers of neutralizing antibody after intradermal administration of human diploid cell rabies vaccine (47). Further investigation is needed to establish the immunosuppressive effects of chloroquine associated with different vaccine antigens and to identify its mechanism of action on the immune response.

References

1. Alving, AS, Eichelberger, L, Craige, B, Jr., Jones, R, Jr., Whorton, CM, Pullman, TN: Studies on the chronic toxicity of chloroquine (SN-7618). *J. Clin. Invest. 27*:60–65, 1948.
2. Berliner, RW, Earle, DP, Jr., Taggart, JV, Zybrod, CG, Welch, WJ, Conan, NJ, Bauman, E, Scudder, ST, Shannon, JA: Studies on the chemotherapy of the human

malarias. VI. The physiological disposition, antimalarial activity, and toxicity of several derivatives of 4-aminoquinolines. *J. Clin. Invest. 27*:98–107, 1948.
3. Most, H, et al.: Chloroquine for acute attacks of vivax malaria. *JAMA 131*:963–967, 1946.
4. Coatney, GR, Cooper, WC, Eddy, NB, Greenberg, J: *Survey of Antimalarial Agents: Chemotherapy of* Plasmodium gallinaceum *Infections; Toxicity; Correlation of Structure and Action*, Public Health Service Monograph 9, U.S. Government Printing Office, Washington, D.C., 1953.
5. Spencer, HC, Oloo, AJ, Watkins, WM, Sixmith, DG, Churchill, FC, Koech, DI: Amodiaquine is more effective than chloroquine against *Plasmodium falciparum* malaria on Kenya coast. *Lancet 1*:956–957, 1984.
6. Watkins, WM, Sixmith, DG, Spencer, HC, Boriga, DA, Karluki, DM, Kipingor, T, Koech, DK: Effectiveness of amodiaquine as treatment for chloroquine-resistant *Plasmodium falciparum* infections in Kenya. *Lancet 1*:357–359, 1984.
7. White, NJ: Clinical pharmacokinetics of antimalarial drugs. *Clin. Pharmacokinet. 10*: 187–215, 1985.
8. Chou, AC, Chevli, R, Fitch, CD: Ferriprotoporphyrin IX fulfills the criteria for identification as the chloroquine receptor of malaria parasites. *Biochemistry 19*: 1543–1549, 1980.
9. Fitch, CD: Mode of action of antimalarial drugs. In: *Malaria and the Red Cell*, CIBA Foundation Symposium 94, Pitman, London, 1983, pp. 222–232.
10. Davidson, MW, Griggs, BG, Jr., Boykin, DW, Wilson, WD: Molecular structural effects involved in the interaction of quinoline methanolamines with DNA. Implications for antimalarial action. *J. Med. Chem. 20*:1117–1122, 1977.
11. World Health Organization: Drug resistance in human pathogenic plasmodia. In: *Advances in Malaria Chemotherapy*, Technical Report Series 711, World Health Organization, Geneva, 1984, pp. 10–60.
12. McChesney, EW, McAuliff, JP: Laboratory studies of the 4-aminoquinoline antimalarials. I. Some biochemical characteristics of chloroquine, hydroxychloroquine and SN-7718. *Antibiot. Chemother. 11*:800–810, 1961.
13. McChesney, EW, et al.: Metabolism of chloroquine-3-^{14}C in the rhesus monkey. *Biochem. Pharmacol. 16*:2444–2447, 1967.
14. Adelusi, SA, Salako, LA: Improved fluorimetric assay of chloroquine in biological samples. *J. Pharm. Pharmacol. 32*:711–712, 1980.
15. Alvan, G, Ekman, L, Lindstrom, P: Determination of chloroquine and its desethyl metabolite in plasma, red blood cells and urine by liquid chromatography. *J. Chromatogr. 229*:241–247, 1982.
16. Gustafsson, LL, Walker, O, Alvan, G, Beerman, B, Estevez, F, Gleisner, L, Lindstrom, B, Sjoqvist, F: The disposition of chloroquine in man after single intravenous and oral doses. *Br. J. Clin. Pharmacol. 15*:471–479, 1983.
17. Adelusi, SA, Dawodu, AH, Salako, LA: Kinetics of the uptake and elimination of chloroquine in children with malaria. *Br. J. Clin. Pharmacol. 14*:483–487, 1982.
18. Walker, O, Dawodu, AH, Adeyokunnu, AA, Salako, LA, Alvan, G: Plasma chloroquine and desethylchloroquine concentrations in children during and after chloroquine treatment for malaria. *Br. J. Clin. Pharmacol. 16*:701–706, 1983.
19. Salako, LA, Adelusi, SA: Plasma, whole blood and red blood cell kinetics of chloroquine after oral and parenteral administration in rabbits. *Arch. Int. Pharmacodyn. Ther. 261*:4–15, 1983.
20. World Health Organization: Use of antimalarial drugs. In: *Advances in Malaria Chemotherapy*, Technical Report Series 711, World Health Organization, Geneva, 1984, pp. 60–90.
21. Adelusi, SA, Salako, LA: Protein binding of chloroquine in the presence of aspirin. *Br. J. Clin. Pharmacol. 13*:451–452, 1982.

22. Walker, O, Birkett, DJ, Alvan, G, Gustafsson, LL, Sjoqvist, F: Characterization of chloroquine plasma protein binding in man. *Br. J. Clin. Pharmacol. 15*:365–377, 1983.
23. McChesney, EW, Conway, WD, Banks, WF, Rogers, JE, Shekosky, JM: Studies of the metabolism of some compounds of the 4-amino-7-chloroquine series. *J. Pharmacol. Exp. Ther. 151*:482–493, 1966.
24. Adelusi, SA, Salako, LA: Tissue and blood concentrations of chloroquine following chronic administration in the rat. *J. Pharm. Pharmacol. 34*:733–735, 1982.
25. Adelusi, SA, Salako, LA: Kinetics of the distribution and elimination of chloroquine in the rat. *Gen. Pharmacol. 13*:433–437, 1982.
26. Frisk-Holmberg, M, Bergquist, Y, Termone, E, Domeij-Nyberg, B: The single dose kinetics of chloroquine and its major metabolite desethyl-chloroquine in healthy subjects. *Eur. J. Clin. Pharmacol. 26*:521–530, 1984.
27. Macomber, PB, et al.: Chloroquine: Physiological basis of drug resistance in *Plasmodium berghei. Science 152*:1374–1375, 1966.
28. Warhurst, DC, Hockley, DJ: Mode of action of chloroquine on *Plasmodium berghei* and *P. cynomolgi. Nature 214*:935–936, 1967.
29. Bergqvist, Y, Domeij-Nyberg, B: Distribution of chloroquine and its metabolite desethyl-chloroquine in human blood cells and its implication for the quantitative determination of these compounds in serum and plasma. *J. Chromatogr. 272*:137–148, 1983.
30. Webster, LT, Jr.: Drugs used in the chemotherapy of protozoal infections. Malaria. In: *The Pharmacological Basis of Therapeutics*, 7th ed., (A Goodman, LS Goodman, TW Rall, and F Murad, eds.), Macmillan, New York, 1985, pp. 1029–1048.
31. Kuroda, K: Detection and distribution of chloroquine metabolites in human tissues. *J. Pharmacol. Exp. Ther. 137*:156–161, 1962.
32. Fletcher, KA, et al.: Studies on the metabolism of chloroquine in rhesus monkeys and human subjects. *Trans. R. Soc. Trop. Med. Hyg. 69*:6, 1975.
33. Olatunde, IA: Chloroquine concentrations in the skin of rabbits and man. *Br. J. Pharmacol. 43*:335–340, 1971.
34. Aderounmu, AF, Fleckestein, L: Pharmacokinetics of chloroquine diphosphate in the dog. *J. Pharmacol. Exp. Ther. 226*:633–639, 1983.
35. Frisk-Holmberg, M, Bergqvist, Y, Domeij-Nyberg, B, Hellstrom, L, Jansson, F: Chloroquine serum concentrations and side effects: Evidence of dose-dependent kinetics. *Clin. Pharmacol. Ther. 25*:345–350, 1979.
36. World Health Organization: Recent progress in chemotherapeutic research. In: *Advances in Malaria Chemotherapy*, Technical Report Series 711, World Health Organization, Geneva, 1984, pp. 91–156.
37. Aderounmu, AF, Lindstrom, B: Are chloroquine kinetics really dose-dependent? *Abstracts, 2nd World Conference on Clinical Pharmacology and Therapeutics*, Washington, D.C., 1983, p. 82.
38. Darlow, B, Vrbova, H, Stace, J: Acute malaria in children from Mandang: Endemicity, clinical presentation and treatment. *Papua New Guinea Med. J. 224*:85–95, 1981.
39. Berqvist, Y, Eckerbom, S: Simultaneous determination of chloroquine and its desethyl metabolite in human plasma by gas chromatography. *J. Chromatogr. 226*: 91–97, 1981.
40. Bergqvist, Y, Frisk-Holmberg, M: Sensitive method for the determination of chloroquine and its metabolite desethylchloroquine in human plasma and urine by high-performance liquid chromatography. *J. Chromatogr. 221*:119–127, 1980.
41. Patchen, LC, Mount, DL, Schwartz, IK, Churchill, FC: Analysis of filter-paper-absorbed finger-prick blood samples for chloroquine and its major metabolite using

high-performance liquid chromatography with fluorescence detection. *J. Chromatogr. 278*:81–89, 1983.
42. Dubois, EL: Antimalarials in the management of discoid and systemic lupus erythematosus. *Semin. Arthritis Rheum. 8*:33–51, 1978.
43. Isaacson, D, Elgart, M, Turner, ML: Antimalarials in dermatology. *Int. J. Dermatol. 21*:379–395, 1982.
44. Bernstein, HN, Svaifler, NI, Rubin, M, Mausour, AM: The ocular deposition of chloroquine. *Invest. Ophthalmol. Vis. Sci. 2*:384–392, 1963.
45. Olansky, AJ: Antimalarials and ophthalmologic safety. *J. Am. Acad. Dermatol. 6*: 19–23, 1982.
46. Good, MI, Shader, RI: Lethality and behavioral side effects of chloroquine. *J. Clin. Psychopharmacol. 2*:40–47, 1982.
47. Bell, GH, Sumner, JW, Patchen, LC, Brown, WJ: Antibody response to preexposure human diploid-cell rabies vaccine given concurrently with chloroquine. *N. Engl. J. Med. 314*:280–284, 1986.

III. QUININE AND THE CINCHONA ALKALOIDS

Quinine is the main alkaloid of the several obtained from cinchona bark. The cinchona tree is indigenous to certain regions of South America. The use of cinchona was described by an Augustinian monk named Calancha, from Lima, Peru, and appeared in a religious book published in Spain in 1639: "A tree grows which they call *the fever tree* in the country of Loxa, whose bark, the color of cinnamon, is made into powder amounting to the weight of two small silver coins and given as a beverage, cures the fevers and tertians; it has produced miraculous results in Lima." According to a popular version, the bark was used successfully in 1638 to treat the wife of the viceroy of Peru, Countess Ana del Chinchon. The following year the drug was introduced in Spain, and by 1640 it was employed for fevers in Europe. The Belgian Herman van der Heyden was the first to mention it in the medical literature, in 1643. Linnaeus termed cinchona the species of plant from which the drug is obtained. The word is likely to have been derived from the name of Countess Ana del Chinchon; others think it a derivative of the Incan word *kinia*, which means bark. The exact circumstances leading to the introduction of quinine to European medicine are not known (1). The Jesuits were the principal importers and distributors of cinchona in Europe, for which reason the drug came to be called Jesuits' bark. It was also known as Cardinal's bark because of its sponsoring in Rome by the Cardinal de Lugo. The conservative medical groups disregarded the new antipyretic because it did not conform to the teachings of Galen. Besides, that it was used by the Jesuits arose suspicion. It remained for many years a secret remedy dispensed mostly by charlatans. In 1677, cinchona was included for the first in the *London Pharmacopeia* as *Cortex Peruanus*. For almost two centuries the bark was employed in medicine as powder, extract, or infusion. Opinions differed widely as to the optimum therapeutic regimens, frequency of doses, and routes of administration (2). Quinine and cinchonine were isolated from cinchona in 1820 by Pelletier and Caventou. The use of these alkaloids as such spread rapidly.

A. Chemistry

Quinine and related alkaloids are still obtained entirely from natural sources, their synthesis having proved impractical owing to its complexity and high cost.

Cinchona contains a mixture of more than 20 alkaloids. Of these, the most important is quinine, which is also the most potent of the crystallizable alkaloids (quinine, quinidine, cinchonine, and cinchonidine).

Quinine and quinidine are optical isomers with qualitatively identical pharmacological actions. The most specific effect of quinine is on malaria parasites, whereas quinidine is most effective on the cardiac muscle. Cinchonine and cinchonidine are also optical isomers.

Quinine, 6-methoxy-α-(5-vinyl-2-quinuclidinyl)-4-quino-linemethanol, has the following structural formula:

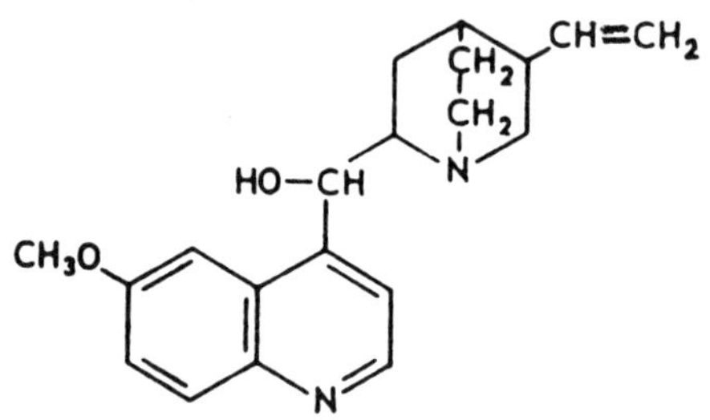

Quinine contains a quinoline group attached through a secondary alcohol linkage to a quinuclidine ring. A methoxy side chain is attached to the quinoline ring and a vinyl to the quinuclidine.

Quinidine has the same structure as quinine except in the steric configuration of the secondary alcohol group. The other natural alkaloids related to quinine differ mainly in substitution on the side chain. Each alteration in the chemical structure of quinine correlates with quantitative and qualitative changes in the pharmacological actions of the resulting compounds.

Antimalarial potency and other pharmacological actions have been studied in relation to chemical alterations in the quinine molecule. None of the derivatives has shown more antimalarial effectiveness than quinine (3). The methoxy and the vinyl radicals are not involved in antimalarial activity. The secondary alcohol group, on the other hand, is absolutely essential. Its reduction increases toxicity and abolishes antiplasmodial potency. Stereoisomerism is relatively unimportant, for which reason the antimalarial activity of quinidine is similar to that of quinine. Important data drawn from the study of these interactions have contributed to the development of more effective and less toxic antimalarials, such as mefloquine.

B. Mechanisms of Action

Quinine has spectra of activity similar to those of chloroquine. It is believed that their mechanisms of action may be related. A number of studies have been conducted in order to elucidate the mechanism of action specific to quinine; however, this remains largely unknown. The selective activity of quinine on blood schizonts most likely corresponds to the ability of parasitized erythrocytes to concentrate the drug (4). Quinine concentration in invaded red cells is much higher than in parasite-free red cells. Quinine, unlike chloroquine, does not cause pigment clumping; on the other hand, it can inhibit competitively the clumping effect that the 4-aminoquinolines induce (5).

Quinine, like chloroquine, also inhibits macromolecular synthesis in malaria parasites. Its effect on DNA (6) is greater than its effect on RNA and protein synthesis. For a description of the binding interactions of these drugs with DNA, the reader is referred to the section on chloroquine.

C. Clinical Pharmacology

Quinine is rapidly and almost completely absorbed from the intestine. Absorption takes place mainly from the upper small intestine, even in patients with diarrhea. Peak plasma concentration in healthy adults has been found to be 5.1 ± 1.3 μg/ml (7). In patients with malaria, however, there is increased quinine concentration in plasma (8–10). According to a study by White and co-workers (11), quinine plasma concentrations are higher during acute malaria than in convalescence. This is due to a decrease in clearance and volume of distribution values. The route of administration also affects plasma concentration. Following oral administration, plasma concentrations of quinine were 10–20% lower than with intravenous infusion (7). The same difference has been observed in children (12). Red blood cell concentrations of quinine were found to be similar to plasma concentration before infection (10), whereas during malaria plasma concentrations became considerably higher than those in erythrocytes. Using the extraction fluorescence technique, White and co-workers (13) reported erythrocyte-plasma concentration ratios to vary considerably between individuals with acute malaria, although exceeding unity in only 1 of 23 cases. Quinine elimination from red cells was more rapid than from plasma elimination, half-lives being half those derived from corresponding plasma values. The difference in concentration is proportional to parasitemia and to the stage of parasite development (13).

After absorption, quinine is distributed throughout most of the body fluids, the distribution phase in healthy adults being 1.89 ± 0.54 min (7). The total apparent volume of distribution has been estimated as 1.8 ± 0.37 liter/kg with a distribution of the central compartment of 0.56 ± 0.32 liter/kg, representing approximately one-third of the total volume of distribution (7).

A significant fraction, approximately 70%, of plasma quinine in healthy individuals is bound to proteins (7). In uncomplicated malaria and convalescence, protein binding increases (89.9 ± 5.8% and 89.0 ± 5.5%, respectively) and is even higher in cerebral malaria (92.8 ± 3.5%) (14). In patients with cerebral malaria, the CSF-plasma concentration ratio was 0.07 ± 0.03 and was inversely correlated with the total plasma concentration (11). In another study (14), the CSF-free quinine ratio was 0.55 ± 0.33.

Clearance of quinine occurs predominantly by hepatic metabolism. Metabolites have lower antimalarial activity than the parent compound (15). Quinine is excreted partly unchanged but mainly in the form of the hydroxylated metabolite. The drug and its metabolite appear in the urine within 1 hr of administration; very small quantities remain in the body after 48 hr (11,16). Total clearance in healthy adults has been reported to be 1.92 ± 0.45 ml/min kg^{-1}, with an elimination half-life of 11.1 ± 2.1 hr (7). Garnham et al. (17) estimated similar half-lives following oral administration of quinine in adults.

Urinary clearance represents only 20% of the total clearance. Renal excretion has been found to be twice as rapid when the urine is acidic as when it is alkaline (18).

Pharmacokinetic parameters of quinine in children differ from those in adults. In healthy children, lower values have been observed for elimination half-life and volume of distribution, but rates of total clearance are similar to those of adults. In a series of 22 children aged 2–12 years, Sabcharoen and co-workers (12) reported volumes of distribution of 1.1 and 1.4 liter/kg, elimination half-lives of 6.1 and 3.2 hr, and total clearance rates of 2.6 and 5.0 ml/min kg^{-1} after intravenous and oral administration, respectively.

Pharmacokinetic differences have also been noted between children with acute falciparum malaria and convalescent children.

In a study conducted by Shann and co-workers (19), a dose of 300 mg/m^2 of quinine dihydrochloride was given by three different routes of administration. In the group receiving intravenous infusion over 4 hr, the peak serum concentration of 9.7 ± 3.7 μg/ml was recorded at the end of infusion (at hour 4); the volume of distribution was 1.5 ± 0.4 liter/kg and the elimination half-life 12.5 ± 4.0 hr. The second group received the drug by deep intramuscular injection. Absorption was rapid, the highest serum concentration of 10.6 ± 4.4 μg/ml being measured 1 hr after injection; the volume of distribution was 1.3 ± 0.3 liter/kg and the elimination half-life 8.4 ± 2.8 hr. In six children belonging to this group, quinine dihydrochloride was given intramuscularly every 12 hr and serum concentrations measured again on day 5. Mean peak serum concentration was 11.3 ± 4.0 μg/ml 1 hr after the injection and 6.5 ± 4.6 μg/ml at 12 hr; elimination half-life was 9.8 ± 1.9 hr. In the third group the drug was administered by nasogastric tube. The highest serum concentration of 10.3 ± 5.7 μg/ml was reached at 3 hr; the elimination half-life was 13.1 ± 6.5 hr and volume of distribution 1.4 ± 0.5 liter/kg. In four children with cerebral malaria, the elimination half-life was 8.48 ± 2.56 hr and volume of distribution 1.44 ± 0.01 liter/kg.

It is generally held that quinine serum concentrations should not exceed 10 μg/ml to avoid the risk of toxicity. However, the minimum inhibitory concentration (MIC) of quinine in Thailand approaches 20 μg/ml (20). Therefore, quinine therapy is bound to fail unless serum concentrations of the drug are maintained above the MIC for 7 days. No serious cardiotoxicity has been reported (11) at quinine concentration between 10 and 20 μg/ml. Hence Shann and co-workers suggest that if 10-μg/ml serum concentrations of quinine are required, children be given a loading dose of 20 mg/kg quinine dihydrochloride by intravenous infusion over 4 hr followed by 7.5 mg/kg infused over 2 hr every 8 hr. Once the child begins to recover, 10 mg/kg of quinine sulfate may be given orally; this higher dose is suggested because the half-life of quinine usually falls during the recovery period (11).

Pharmacokinetic differences have also been observed in women with falciparum malaria in the third trimester of pregnancy when compared with other adults (21). These differences more or less parallel those found in children. Elimination half-lives are shorter (11.3 ± 4.3 hr), volume of distribution is smaller (0.96 ± 0.27 liter/kg), and total clearance is reduced (1.22 ± 0.77 ml/min kg^{-1}). Cord plasma concentration has been estimated to be approximately one-third that in maternal plasma (15).

In the presence of acute renal failure, quinine plasma and serum concentrations were reported to increase considerably (22,23). However, as nonspecific assay methods were used, the metabolite contribution to the overall quinine concentration could not be estimated. Clearance in the peritoneal dialysate was low (<8 ml/min). Although no toxic effects were observed, it was concluded that the dose of quinine in renal failure should be reduced by one-half or two-thirds (i.e., 600 mg in 24 hr in normal adults). White and co-workers (11) found no differences in the pharmacokinetics of quinine in cerebral malaria patients with serum creatinine concentrations above 3 mg/dl, compared with similar patients with creatinine concentrations below 3 mg/dl. As urinary clearance of quinine accounts for only 20% of the total clearance in healthy subjects and in nonoliguric malaria patients, it was suggested that the high quinine plasma concentration in acute renal failure relates more to the severity of the malarial infection and to associated pharmacokinetic changes than to decreased glomerular filtration.

D. Preparation, Dosage, Regimens, and Routes of Administration

In the United States, the pure alkaloids are employed rather than the galenic preparations (Quinimax 3394 RP). Many preparations of cinchona alkaloids are available in tropical communities where malaria is endemic and inexpensive medication is essential.

Quinine sulfate is the salt most commonly used. It is supplied as 3-grain (186-mg) or 6-grain (372-mg) capsules or tablets. Quinine dihydrochloride comes in 2-ml ampuls containing 300 mg/ml.

The usual dose of quinine sulfate in adults for treatment in areas where the 4-aminoquinolines and antifolate-sulfonamide combinations are considered ineffective is 600 mg three times daily (total 1800 mg) for 3 days. Administration may continue for 10–14 days in areas of Southeast Asia where diminished sensitivity to quinine has been noted (24). The pediatric dose of quinine sulfate is 25 mg/kg day^{-1}, divided in three doses for 3 days.

Quinine dihydrochloride is used for parenteral treatment of patients unable to tolerate oral medication, in the presence of vomiting, severe diarrhea, comatous state, or high parasite count (100,000 mm^{-3}) (24). Therapy with quinine dihydrochloride must be administered to either children or adults in a slow intravenous drip (over 2–4 hr), repeated if necessary after 8 hr until oral medication is tolerated. In children, quinine dihydrochloride is infused as follows: 10 mg/kg salt diluted in normal saline solution, 1 mg/ml, and administered 1 ml/min every 8 hr (maximum, 600 mg every 8 hr) until oral medication is tolerated. For example, for a child weighing 20 kg, 200 mg quinine dihydrochloride = 200 ml; time of infusion is around 3 hr.

As a general rule, quinine dihydrochloride, 10 mg/kg body weight in physiological saline solution (10 ml/kg body weight) is administered by intravenous infusion over 2–4 hr every 8–12 hr until the patient is able to take oral medication. Some authors suggest that quinine dihydrochloride be diluted at 0.5 mg/ml and administered at a rate of 1 ml/min (25).

In *adults*, the dose is 60 mg quinine dihydrochloride in 300 ml normal saline given by slow intravenous drip (over 2–4 hr) every 8–12 hr, up to a maximum of 1800 mg/day.

Blood glucose monitoring is desirable during drug administration in the event of intravenous infusion and/or high parasitemia, since in both cases there may be associated hypoglycemia. Subcutaneous and intramuscular injection should be avoided because local tissue damage may ensue.

When it is known for certain that the patient has not taken prior medication, a loading dose of quinine may be given, i.e., 20 mg/kg as above (24).

E. Drug Assays

The protein-precipitation fluorescence assay technique developed by Brodie and Udenfriend (26) is regarded as relatively nonspecific, although it represented a considerable advance with respect to earlier fluorescence methods that quantitated equally quinine, quinidine, and some more polar metabolites. Quinine is usually measured by the extraction fluorescence (EF) method devised by Spinks and Tottey (27) and later modified by Cramer and Isaksson (28). The more sensitive method of high-performance liquid chromatography has been recently introduced (29,30). Quinine values obtained by EP are generally considerably higher than those recorded by HPLC (29). This difference might be accounted for by EF quantitation of metabolites, although this has not been confirmed by comparative studies of quinidine assay methods, which resulted in similar values for EF and more sensitive techniques (31). It is expected that HPLC will be consistently used in the future to obtain more precise discrimination and quantitiation of quinine and its metabolites.

F. Therapeutic Indications

Quinine acts primarily as a schizontocide; it has little effect on sporozoites or pre-erythrocytic forms of malarial parasites. The alkaloid is also gametocidal for *P. vivax* and *P. malariae*, but not for *P. falciparum*. As both a suppressive and a therapeutic agent, quinine is more toxic and less effective than chloroquine. However, it is especially valuable for the treatment of severe illness due to chloroquine and multidrug-resistant strains of *P. falciparum*. The drug should not be used alone because it is less effective and more toxic than the synthetic antimalarial compounds. It is given concurrently with primaquine to achieve a radical cure of relapsing vivax malaria. It is also administered with pyrimethamine and a sulfonamide or with tetracycline for the suppressive cure of patients with multidrug-resistant malaria (31,32).

G. Toxicity

Toxicity may arise from overdosage or from hypersensitivity. An oral dose of 8 g quinine is fatal to adults. When quinine is repeatedly administered in full doses, typical symptoms occur, termed cinchonism. In mild cases, symptoms include ringing in the ears, nausea, headache, and disturbed vision. If medication is continued, more severe gastrointestinal, cardiovascular, and dermal symptoms may appear.

Vision and hearing are affected. Functional impairment of the eighth nerve results in vertigo, tinnitus, and decreased auditory acuity. Visual signs consist of photophobia, blurred vision, altered color perception, diplopia, night blindness, mydriasis, constricted visual fields, and scotomata. It is not known whether the visual and the auditory effects are of neural origin or secondary to vascular changes. Retinal vessels are constricted and retinal ischemia occurs. The disks are pale and retinal edema may ensue. Severe optic atrophy may occur. Spiral ganglion cells similar to those noted in the ganglion cells of the retina support the notion that cellular injury from quinine is direct. Both vascular and neural components of injury are probably involved.

Gastrointestinal symptoms are present in cinchonism. The local irritant action of quinine results in abdominal pain, nausea, and vomiting, although the latter may also have a central nervous origin.

Central nervous system symptoms include headache, fever, vomiting, excitement, confusion, and syncope. As poisoning progresses, body temperature and blood pressure diminish, respiratory distress follows initial stimulation, cyanosis appears, and the pulse weakens. The patient becomes comatose and may die in a few hours from respiratory arrest. In case of recovery, symptoms generally subside. In some patients, however, the visual and auditory sequelae of varied severity may persist.

Anuria and uremia may ensue from renal injury by quinine. An infrequent complication of quinine therapy is massive hemolysis, hemoglobinemia, and hemoglobinuria, seen mainly in pregnant women. Hypoprothrombinemia may be observed sometimes, but vitamin K administration neutralizes the prolongation of prothrombin time. Agranulocytosis or purpura is rare and may appear in hypersensitive individuals.

If toxic signs occur after the administration of small doses of quinine or related alkaloids, the patient is usually hypersensitive to these agents. Cutaneous flushing, pruritus, gastric distress, and ringing in the ears are common manifestations of hypersensitivity. Hemoglobinuria and asthma are rare types of idiosyncrasy.

H. Contraindications

The drug should not be used in patients with optic neuritis or tinnitus. In adult patients with atrial fibrillations, quinine administration necessitates the same precautions as quinidine, owing to the risk of embolism following conversion of atrial fibrillation to sinus rhythm. Fibrillating atria do not contract, and thrombi often develop in the left atrium. After sinus rhythm resumes, atrial contraction may dislodge thrombi and embolization occurs.

I. Drug Interactions

Quinine antagonizes with anticholinesterase agents, such as physostigmine. It is therefore contraindicated in myasthenia gravis.

Quinine increases the concentration of digoxin in plasma. Appropriate adjustment of digoxin dosage is necessary to avoid toxicity.

References

1. Haggis, AW: Fundamental errors in the early history of cinchona. *Bull. Hist. Med. 10*:568–592, 1941.
2. Wesselhoeft, C: The early history of malaria, the discovery of cinchona, the introduction and early use of cinchona bark. *New Orleans Med. Surg. J. 68*:693–727, 1916.
3. Wiselogle, FY (ed.): *A Survey of Antimalarial Drugs, 1941–1945*, J. W. Edwards, Publishers, Ann Arbor, Michigan, 1946.
4. Peters, W: Chemotherapy of malaria. In: *Malaria*, Vol. 1 (JP Kreier, ed.), Academic Press, New York, 1980, pp. 145–283.
5. Chou, AC, Chevli, R, Fitch, CD: Ferriprotoporphyrin IX fulfills the criteria for identification as the chloroquine receptor of malaria parasites. *Biochemistry 19*: 1543–1549, 1980.
6. Davidson, MW, Griggs, BG, Jr., Boykin, DW, Wilson, WD: Molecular structural effects involved in the interaction of quinolinemethanolamines with DNA. Implications for antimalarial action. *J. Med. Chem. 20*:1117–1122, 1977.
7. White, NJ, Chanthavanich, P, Krishna, S, Bunch, C, Silamut, K: Quinine disposition kinetics. *Br. J. Clin. Parmacol. 16*:399–403, 1983.
8. Brooks, MH, Malloy, JP, Bartelloni, PJ, Sheehy, TW, Barry, KG: Quinine, pyrimethamine and sulphuorthodimethoxine: Clinical response, plasma levels and urinary excretion during the initial attack of naturally acquired falciparum malaria. *Clin. Pharmacol. Ther. 10*:85–91, 1969.
9. Hall, AP, Hanchalay, S, Doberstyn, E, Bumntphund, S: Quinine dosage and serum levels in falciparum malaria. In: *Annual Report, SEATO Medical Research Laboratories*, 1975, pp. 241–250.
10. Trenholme, GM, Williams, RL, Rieckmann, KH, Frischer, H, Carson, PE: Quinine disposition during malaria and during induced fever. *Clin. Pharmacol. Ther. 19*: 459–467, 1976.
11. White, NJ, Looareesuwan, S, Warrell, DA, Warrell, MJ, Bunnag, D, Harinasuta, T: Quinine pharmacokinetics and toxicity in cerebral and uncomplicated falciparum malaria. *Am. J. Med. 73*:564–571, 1982.

12. Sabcharoen, A, Chongsuphajaisiddhi, T, Attanath, P: Serum quinine concentrations following the initial dose in children with falciparum malaria. *Southeast Asian J. Trop. Med. Public Health 13*:556–562, 1982.
13. White, NJ, Looareesuwan, S, Silamut, K: Red cell quinine concentrations in falciparum malaria. *Am. J. Trop. Med. Hyg. 32*:456–460, 1983.
14. Silamut, K, White, NJ, Looareesuwan, S, Warrell, DA: Binding of quinine to plasma proteins in falciparum malaria. *Am. J. Trop. Med. Hyg.* (in press, 1985).
15. White, NJ: Clinical pharmacokinetics of antimalarial drugs. *Clin. Pharmacokinet. 10*: 187–215, 1985.
16. Hall, AP, Czerwinski, AW, Madonia, EC, Evensen, KL: Human plasma and urine quinine levels following tablets and intravenous infusion. *Clin. Pharmacol. Ther. 14*: 580–585, 1973.
17. Garnham, JC, Raymond, K, Shotton, E, Turner, P: The bioavailability of quinine. *J. Trop. Med. Hyg. 70*:264–169, 1976.
18. Haag, HB, Larson, PS, Schwartz, JJ: The effect of urinary pH on the elimination of quinine in man. *J. Pharmacol. Exp. Ther. 79*:136–139, 1943.
19. Shann, F, Stace, J, Edstein, M: Pharmacokinetics of quinine in children. *J. Pediatr. 106*:506–510, 1985.
20. Chongsuphajaisiddhi, T, Sabcharoen, A, Attanath, P: Treatment of quinine-resistant falciparum malaria in Thai children. *Southeast Asian J. Trop. Med. Public Health 14*: 357–362, 1983.
21. Looareesuwan, S, Karbwang, J, White, NJ, Phillips, RE, Warrell, DA, Kietinun, S: Effect of quinine on uterine function and the fetus in women suffering from severe falciparum malaria in the final trimester of pregnancy (abstract). *International Congress Tropical Medicine and Malaria*, Calgary, 1984, p. 87.
22. Donadio, JV, Whelton, A, Kazyak, L: Quinine therapy and peritoneal dialysis in acute renal failure complicating malarial haemoglobinuria. *Lancet 1*:375–379, 1968.
23. Canfield, CJ, Miller, LH, Bartelloni, PJ, Eichler, P, Barry, KG: Acute renal failure in *Plasmodium falciparum* malaria. *Arch. Intern. Med. 122*:199–203, 1968.
24. World Health Organization: Use of antimalarial drugs. In: *Advances in Malaria Chemotherapy*, Technical Report Series 711, World Health Organization, Geneva, 1984, pp. 60–90.
25. Randall, G, Seidel, JS: Malaria. *Pediatr. Clin. North Am. 32*:893–916, 1985.
26. Brodie, BB, Udenfriend, S: The estimation of quinine in human plasma with a note on the estimation of quinindine. *J. Pharmacol. Exp. Ther. 78*:154–158, 1943.
27. Spinks, A, Tottey, MM: Studies on synthetic antimalarial drugs. XVI. The absorption, distribution and excretion of 2-*p*-chlorophenylguanidino-4-8-diehtylaminoethylamino-6-methylpyrimidine (3349) in experimental animals. *Ann. Trop. Med. Parasitol. 40*:145–152, 1948.
28. Cramer, G, Isaksson, B: Quantitative determination of quinidine in plasma. *Scand. J. Clin. Lab. Invest. 15*:553–556, 1963.
29. Edstein, M, Stace, J, Shann, F: Quantification of quinine in human serum by high performance liquid chromatography. *J. Chromatogr. 278*:445–451, 1983.
30. Furner, RL, Brown, GB, Scott, J: A method for differentiation and analysis of quinine and quinidine by gas chromatography/mass spectrometry. *J. Anal. Toxicol. 5*:275–278, 1981.
31. Ochs, HR, Greenblatt, DJ, Woo, E: Clinical pharmacokinetics of quinindine. *Clin. Pharmacokin. 5*:150–168, 1980.
32. Reacher, M, Campbell, CC, Freeman, J, Doberstyn, EB, Brandling-Bennett, AD: Drug therapy for *Plasmodium falciparum* malaria resistant to pyrimethamine-sulfadoxine (FANSIDAR). A study of alternate regimens in Eastern Thailand. *Lancet 2*:1066–1069, 1980.

IV. QUINIDINE

Quinidine is the dextrostereoisomer of quinine. Van Heyningen, in 1848, was the first to describe this compound, which was prepared and given its present name by Pasteur in 1853. It shares the antimalarial effects of quinine. Quinidine is more active on the cardiac muscle than quinine. The earliest recorded reference to the use of cinchona in atrial fibrillations is that of the French physician Jean Baptiste de Sénoc of Paris, in 1749 (1).

Over 100 years ago, quinidine was found to be effective against *P. falciparum* malaria in India (2). A later study in Malaya (2) revealed that quinidine was as active an antimalarial as quinine. This was confirmed by Sanders (3) and Taggart and colleagues (4), who assumed quinidine to be superior to quinine. The interest in the cinchona alkaloids and their antimalarial potency subsequently declined, dimmed by the success of new synthetic drugs, such as chloroquine.

However, a number of circumstances prompted resumed interest in the antimalarial therapeutic potential of quinidine. *Plasmodium falciparum* in Southeast Asia is becoming resistant to all available agents, including quinine. No other drug can be administered parenterally for the treatment of severe chloroquine-resistant infections. Furthermore, White and colleagues (5) and Oduola and colleagues (6) have reported in vitro findings suggesting that African and Asian strains of *P. falciparum* are more sensitive to quinidine. Moreover, resurgence of malaria has been noted together with the increasing prevalence of drug-resistant infections on all continents (7–9). Because quinine, the only drug still effective against most strains of falciparum infections, is not manufactured in the United States and not readily available in Europe, Latin America, and Japan, the recovery of patients may be seriously compromised by the delay in obtaining it from special centers, e.g., the Centers for Disease Control (CDC) in the United States. Cases are known of patients who died before the drug could be obtained (10). Parenteral quinidine, on the other hand, is widely distributed for use in cardiac arrhythmias and at present is recommended and used for malaria in the United States (11) and in the United Kingdom (12,13). White and colleagues (5) showed that oral quinidine cured the uncomplicated attack of chloroquine-resistant falciparum malaria, and in a double-blind trial (14), quinidine proved to be more effective than quinine.

A. Chemistry

Quinidine has the same structure as quinine except for the steric configuration of the secondary alcohol group. As a dextrostereoisomer, quinidine shares the antimalarial activity of quinine (See Section III).

1. Quinidine Sulfate

When used as an antimalarial, quinidine sulfate is given by the oral route. It is a white, odorless fine powder or acidular crystals, with an intensely bitter taste, darkening on exposure to light. The base equivalence is 217 mg quinidine sulfate approximately equivalent to 200 mg quinidine base.

2. Quinidine Gluconate

Quinidine gluconate is used in intravenous solution for the treatment of severe falciparum malaria. It is also a white, odorless powder with a very bitter taste, containing no more than 20% dihydroquinidine gluconate. It is freely soluble in water and slightly soluble in alcohol. A solution in water is dextrorotatory. It should be protected from light. Base equivalence: 289 mg quinidine gluconate is equivalent to 200 mg quinidine base.

The U.S.P. describes quinidine as an alkaloid that may be derived from various species of cinchona and their hybrids, from *Remijia pedunculata*, or prepared from quinine.

B. Mechanism of Action and Antimalarial Activity

Quinidine is at least as potent as, and possibly more potent than quinine as an antimalarial (5,15,16). Like quinine, it is a blood schizontocide and its mechanism of action is similar to that described for quinine and chloroquine.

During World War II, quinidine proved more effective against *P. falciparum* and *P. vivax* than equimolar doses of quinine (4,17). Later work with *Plasmodium gallinaceum* showed that a quinine-resistant strain remained fully sensitive to quinidine (18). The appearance of malaria resistant to quinine after centuries of use has been blamed on the substitution for cinchona bark extracts of more highly purified quinine salts that lack synergistic amounts of minor alkaloids, including quinidine (19).

C. Clinical Pharmacology

1. Pharmacokinetic Properties in Patients Without Malaria

An extensive literature is available on the pharmacokinetics of quinidine in healthy volunteers and in patients with cardiovascular disease (20), but there have been no studies comparing the diastereomers in humans.

Quinidine clearance rates in the dog were 56% lower and elimination half-lives 54% shorter than those of quinine, but steady-state volumes of distribution were similar (21). A comparison of quinidine pharmacokinetic data in healthy volunteers (20) with those of quinine indicates a difference in the opposite direction: volume of distribution estimates were larger (2.0–3.5 liter/kg), total clearance rates slightly larger (2.5–5.0 ml/min kg^{-1}), and terminal elimination half-lives generally shorter (5–12 hr). Similar values were derived from patients with falciparum malaria.

As with quinine, the clearance of quinidine occurs predominantly by hepatic metabolism, which accounts for 60–85% of the total clearance, and renal clearance represents 15–40%. Kinetic data on quinidine in children and pregnancy are limited to an early report by Brodie and Udenfriend (22), in which measurements were done by the protein-precipitation fluorescence technique, and a case report on a woman who had received quinidine sulfate during pregnancy and at delivery. Concentrations in the neonate were 82%, and breast milk concentrations 70% of the serum values in the mother (23).

Quinidine is moderately well absorbed after oral administration; mean bioavailability was estimated in 70% (24). Congestive heart failure delays absorption (25). About 90% of plasma quinidine is bound to α_1-acid glycoprotein and albumin. Following intramuscular administration, the absorption of quinidine is erratic (26). Bioavailability by this route was 85–90%. Rectal absorption is incomplete, with bioavailability about 30% (27,28). Swerdlow and colleagues (29) showed that the intravenous administration of quinidine is safe even in the presence of intraventricular conduction delays and heart failure, provided that the drug is infused slowly, i.e., over 2–4 hr, in malaria patients.

2. Pharmacokinetics in Malaria Patients

Taggart and colleagues (4), in 1948, were the first to measure plasma concentrations of quinidine in malaria patients. The drug was found to be well absorbed, with less than 5%

of the administered dose excreted unchanged in the feces. With daily doses from 0.1 to 1.5 g, mean plasma concentrations ranged between 0.2 and 5.0 mg/liter. Mean concentrations above 1.0 mg/liter for 6 days were considered effective in the treatment of volunteers infected with the McClendon strain of falciparum malaria. Comparing these data with earlier results obtained with quinine, the authors concluded that quinidine was twice as potent as quinine.

White and coworkers (5), in 1981, re-evaluated quinidine in a clinical trial performed in Thailand, where falciparum malaria is highly resistant to chloroquine and is becoming increasingly resistant to quinine. Quinidine sulfate was given orally to 14 patients with uncomplicated falciparum malaria at a dose of 11 mg/kg salt (9.1 mg/kg base) three times daily for 1 week. Treatment was successful, and no cardiotoxicity was noted. QT_c prolongation in the ECG was observed, which was four times greater than with equivalent quinine plasma concentrations (30). Peak plasma concentrations after the first dose, measured by a double-extraction fluorescence technique, were reached within 3 hr (mean, 1.1 hr). Elimination half-lives varied between 6.4 and 16.5 hr (mean, 10.0 hr), with volume of distribution estimates between 0.93 and 1.77 liter/kg (mean, 1.33 liter/kg). Total clearance ranged between 0.78 and 2.38 ml/min kg^{-1} (mean, 1.68 ml/min kg^{-1}). Peak plasma concentrations were recorded on the second and third days of treatment (range, 4.4–13.6 mg/liter), then declined toward the end of treatment. Urinary clearance was not measured.

3. Pharmacokinetics of Intravenous Quinidine Gluconate in Severe Malaria

Phillips and colleagues (2) studied the pharmacokinetics of quinidine gluconate given intravenously to 14 patients admitted with severe falciparum malaria to a hospital in eastern Thailand.

Quinidine gluconate (80 mg salt = 50 mg base per milliliter) in a loading dose of 15 mg base per kilogram body weight, was dissolved in 250 ml normal saline and infused over 4 hr. Conscious patients were asked twice a day about side effects; pulse rate and blood pressure were monitored, and ECG was displayed continuously. Subsequent doses of 7.5 mg base per kilogram were given every 8 hr for 7 days in 4-hr infusions. Patients who were able to swallow were given quinidine sulfate capsules (300 mg salt = 248 mg base) orally, at a dose as near as possible to that given intravenously.

Mean plasma concentration was 9.4 mg/liter, compared with a mean quinine concentration of 12.8 mg/liter in an earlier study. In 10 patients, plasma concentrations were consistently above 6 mg/liter during the first 72 hr of treatment. CSF concentrations of quinidine in three patients with cerebral malaria were 6.8, 10.0, and 16.7% of the plasma values. Mean values were: terminal elimination half-life, 12.8 ± 5.3 hr; volume of distribution, 1.68 ± 0.54 liter/kg; total clearance, 1.75 ± 0.88 ml/min kg^{-1}; and renal clearance, 0.62 ± 0.18 ml/min kg^{-1}, representing a mean of 32% of total clearance.

D. Preparation, Dosage, Regimens, and Routes of Administration

Quinidine sulfate (Cin-Quin, Quinora; also distributed by Schein and Geneva Laboratories) is available in tablets (100–300 mg), capsules (200–300 mg), sustained-release tablets (300 mg), and ampuls (200 mg/ml). Base equivalence: quinidine sulfate 217 mg is approximately equivalent to 200 mg quinidine base.

Quinidine gluconate (Geneva, Schein) is presented in 324-mg tablets (206 mg quinidine base) and 330-mg sustained-release tablets (206 mg quinidine base) (Duraquin

Parke Davis).It is also available from Eli Lilly in ampuls containing 80 mg salt per milliliter (50 mg base per milliliter) (2).

1. Treatment of Uncomplicated Falciparum Malaria

The oral adult dose of quinidine is 11 mg/kg salt (equivalent to 9.1 mg/kg base) three times daily for 1 week.

Children should be given a test dose of 2 mg base per kilogram to exclude idiosyncrasy, followed by 10 mg base per kilogram dose every 8 hr for 1 week (31).

2. Quinidine Gluconate Dosage for Treatment of Severe Falciparum Malaria or Cerebral Malaria

Adults should receive a loading dose of 15-mg base per kilogram body weight, dissolved in 250 ml normal saline, by intravenous infusion over 4 hr (1 ml/min). Subsequent doses of 7.5 mg base per kilogram are given every 8 hr for 7 days by 4-hr intravenous infusions. When patients are well enough to swallow, quinidine sulfate capsules (300 mg salt, 248 base) can be administered orally in a dose as near as possible to that given intravenously.

Children should be given a test dose of 2 mg base per kilogram orally or intravenously to exclude idiosyncrasy, followed by 7.5 mg base per kilogram dissolved in normal saline (2 mg/ml), infused over 4 hr, every 8 hr for 7 days. If the child is able to swallow, it can be switched to oral quinidine sulfate at a dose of 7.5–10 mg/kg body weight every 8 hr.

E. Drug Assays

Early measurements were done with nonspecific assay techniques, e.g., the protein precipitation method, which quantitated equally quinine, quinidine, and various more polar metabolites (22). The double-extraction fluorescence technique is now widely used (5, 32). Although this method still quantitates a series of metabolites (24), it has been found to compare well with more specific assay techniques, such as gas chromatography, gas chromatography-mass spectrometry, and high-performance liquid chromatography (20).

F. Therapeutic Indications

The long-established existence of highly chloroquine-resistant strains in Southeast Asia (33,34), together with the appearance of quinine-resistant strains, have created a crisis in the chemotherapy of falciparum malaria. A recent re-evaluation of quinidine (4) as an antimalarial has shown it to be effective in severe malaria, producing a prompt and sustained fall in parasite counts in all patients and, in the survivors, providing defervescence and parasite clearance times comparable to those obtained with quinine.

Pharmacokinetic data for malaria suggest that dosage recommendations and adjustments for quinidine should be approximately the same as for quinine (35).

Quinidine appears as a valuable alternative drug for the treatment of severe cases of malaria in areas of multidrug-resistant *P. falciparum*. If quinine-resistant strains remain sensitive to quinidine in vivo, this advantage may come to be of the utmost importance.

G. Toxicity and Side Effects

1. Cardiovascular Side Effects and Toxicity

Quinidine is a potentially dangerous drug, chiefly because of its action on the cardiovascular system. Both quinine and quinidine have antiarrhythmic properties, but quinidine is judged superior in this regard, long-term suppression of supraventricular arrhythmia and ventricular premature beats being the main contemporary usage of the drug.

Quinidine therapy prolongs the refractory period of the myocardial action potential, and the lengthening of the QT interval is an approximate but useful guide to plasma quinidine levels in patients with malaria (26,30). This effect is greater than that of equimolar concentrations of quinine (30). As quinidine concentration in plasma rises above 2 μg/ml, the QRS complex and the QT_c interval will widen progressively (36). If the duration of the QRS complex increases by 50% or more, a reduction in dosage should be considered. At high plasma concentrations of quinidine, cardiac toxicity may become severe; S-A block or arrest, high-grade A-V block, ventricular tachyarrhythmias, or asystole may occur. Conduction is slowed in all parts of the heart. Depolarization of Purkinje fibers has been observed, with ensuing abnormal automaticity. Severe poisoning with quinidine may induce bizarre arrhythmias. Polymorphic ventricular tachycardia caused by quinidine toxicity must be treated with the utmost caution. Sodium lactate, catecholamines, glucagon, and magnesium sulfate may be useful in counteracting ventricular tachyarrhythmias caused by this drug (37,38). Quinidine and its hydroxy metabolite can be recovered by dialysis (39).

The rapid administration of quinidine or quinine may produce serious hypotension (40), attributable to a peripheral α-adrenergic blocking effect (41). Hemodynamic studies indicate that hypotension due to quinidine is caused by vasodilatation without a significant decrease in cardiac output. Therapeutic levels of quinidine have no significant adverse effects on myocardial performance. Very high concentrations may adversely affect myocardial contractility (42).

Intravenous quinidine appears to be well tolerated, provided it is given slowly (20,43).

The most dreaded toxic effect of quinidine is syncope with refractory myocardial failure (44). This phenomenon was described as early as 1925 (15). Parasite sequestration within the myocardial microvasculature might predispose patients to this effect (45). Hypotension may occur during the loading dose. Decreased myocardial contractility may cause blood pressure to fall, but dehydration, which is often seen in severe malaria, makes the patient more vulnerable to the peripheral vasodilatory action of quinidine (44), as indicated by the beneficial effect of saline infusions.

ECG monitoring is necessary in severely ill malaria patients and may help to predict quinidine toxicity. However, early and precise correction of circulatory volume deficits, careful timing of infusions, and close observation of the patient are crucial.

Lower doses of quinidine are used to treat multidrug-resistant falciparum malaria (46). If these doses prove adequate, there will be a greater margin of safety when the drug has to be given intravenously. Recrudescence might be prevented by adding a pyrimethamine-sulfonamide combination or tetracycline, depending on the local patterns of sensitivity.

2. Other Side Effects

Like other cinchona alkaloids, quinidine can cause cinchonism, which is described in the context of quinine (see Section III). Fever, anaphylactic reactions, and thrombocytopenia may develop. The latter is uncommon but life threatening and occurs mainly during prolonged treatment. Asthmalike respiratory difficulty may result from hypersensitivity.

H. Contraindications

Quinidine sulfate is contraindicated in patients with complete heart block or intraventricular conduction defects. It should not be given in the presence of untreated cardiac insufficiency. It is also contraindicated in digitalis overdosage. It should be avoided in patients with myasthenia gravis.

I. Drug Interactions

Drugs, such as phenobarbital and phenytoin, which induce drug-metabolizing enzymes in the liver, may significantly shorten the duration of action of quinidine by increasing its rate of elimination (47). Concomitant administration of quinidine and digoxin results in markedly increased plasma concentrations of digoxin, owing to a decrease in its clearance (48). Prothrombin time will rise in patients receiving oral anticoagulants when quinidine administration begins (49). The mechanism underlying this reaction is not clear.

As an α-adrenergic blocking agent, quinidine interacts additively with drugs that induce vasodilation or decreased blood volume. Nitroglycerin can cause severe postural hypotension in patients receiving quinidine.

If a high concentration of potassium is present in plasma, any given concentration of quinidine will have a greater effect on the heart.

An initial test dose of quinidine should always be given to detect hypersensitivity.

References

1. Willius, FA, Keis, TE: Cardiac clinics. XCIV. A remarkably early reference to the use of cinchona in cardiac arrythrmia. *Proc. Staff Meet. Mayo Clin. 17*:294–296, 1942.
2. Phillips, RE, Warrell, DA, White, NJ, Looareesuwan, S, Karbwang, J: Intravenous quinidine for the treatment of severe falciparum malaria. Clinical and pharaceutical studies. *N. Engl. J. Med. 312*:1273–1278, 1985.
3. Sanders, JP: Treatment of malaria with a short course of quinidine. *Am. J. Trop. Med. 15*:651–660, 1935.
4. Taggart, JV, Earle, DP, Jr., Berliner, RW, Zubrod, CG, Welch, WJ, Bowman-Wise, N, Schroeder, EF, London, IM, Shannon, JA: Studies on the chemotherapy of human malarias. III. The physiological disposition and antimalarial activity of the cinchona alkaloids. *J. Clin. Invest. 27*:80–86, 1948.
5. White, NJ, Looareesuwan, S, Warrell, DA, Chonogsuphajaisiddhi, T, Bunnag, D, Harinasuta, T: Quinidine in falciparum malaria. *Lancet 2*:1069–1071, 1981.
6. Oduola, AM, Rogers, MD, Weatherly, NF, Bowdre, JH, Desjardins, RE: Relative antiplasmodial activities of quinine and quinidine in vitro. *Proc Annual Meet Am Soc Trop Med Hyg*, Cleveland, Ohio, November 7–11, 1982.
7. Bruce-Chwatt, LJ: Imported malaria: An uninvited guest. *Br. Med. Bull. 38*:179–185, 1982.
8. Wyler, DJ: Malaria resurgence, resistance and research (two parts). *N. Engl. J. Med. 308*:875–878, 934–940, 1983.
9. Centers for Disease Control: Imported malaria among travellers. *MMWR 33*:388–399, 1984.
10. Kapila, M, Lee, SH, Gray, W, Robson, A: Fatal falciparum malaria and the availability of parenteral antimalarial drugs in hospitals. *Br. Med. J. 284*:1547–1548, 1982.
11. Markell, EK, Voge, M: *Medical Parasitology*, 5th ed., W. B. Saunders, Philadelphia, 1981.
12. Ellis, CJ, Chiodini, PL: The treatment of falciparum malaria. *J. Antimicrob. Chemother. 13*:311–314, 1984.

13. Gilles, HM, Harinasuta, T, Bunnag, D: Malaria. In: *Recent Advances in Tropical Medicine* (HM Gilles, ed.), Churchill Livingstone, Edinburgh, 1984, pp. 1–22.
14. Suntharasamai, P, Vanijanond, S, Harinasuta, T, Bunnag, D: A double-blind randomised trial of quinine vs quinidine in chloroquine-resistant falciparum malaria. *XI Internat Congr Trop Med Malaria*, Calgary, September 16–22, 1984.
15. Medical Research Council: Clinical comparison of quinine and quinidine. In: *Special Report Series 96*, Medical Research Council, London, 1925, pp. 1–27.
16. Sanders, JP, Dawson, WT: Efficacy of quinidine in malaria. *JAMA 99*:1773–1777, 1932.
17. Wiselogle, FY: *A Survey of Antimalarial Drugs, 1941–1945*, J. W. Edwards Publishers, Ann Arbor, Michigan, 1946.
18. Knoppers, AT: Twofold quinine resistance of *Plasmodium falciparum*, induced by regular administration of the drug. *Doc. Nederl. Indon. Morb. Trop. 1*:55–66, 1949.
19. Smit, EHD: The rediscovery of cinchona alkaloids as antimalarial drugs. *XI Internat Congr Trop Med Malaria*, Calgary, September 16–22, 1984.
20. Ochs, HR, Greenblatt, DJ, Woo, E: Clinical pharmacokinetics of quinidine. *Clin. Pharmacokinet. 5*:150–168, 1980.
21. Clohisy, DR, Gibson, TP: Comparison of pharmacokinetic parameters of intravenous quinidine and quinine in dogs. *J. Cardiovasc. Pharmacol. 4*:107–110, 1982.
22. Brodie, BB, Udenfriend, S: The estimation of quinine in human plasma with a note on the estimation of quinidine. *J. Pharmacol. Exp. Ther. 78*:154–158, 1943.
23. Hill, LM, Malkasian, GD: The use of quinidine sulfate throughout pregnancy. *Obstet. Gynecol. 54*:366–368, 1979.
24. Guentert, TW, Upton, RA, Holford, NHG, Riegelman, S: Divergence of pharmacokinetic parameters of quinidine obtained by specific and nonspecific assay methods. *J. Pharmacokinet. Biopharm. 7*:303–311, 1979.
25. Crouthamel, WG: The effect of congestive heart failure on quinidine pharmacokinetics. *Am. Heart J. 90*:335–339, 1975.
26. Greenblatt, DJ, Pfiefer, HJ, Ochs, HR, Franke, K, MacLaughlin, DS, Smith, TW, Kochweser, J: Pharmacokinetics of quinidine in humans after intravenous, intramuscular and oral administration. *J. Pharmacol. Exp. Ther. 202*:365–378, 1977.
27. Kalmasohn, RW, Sampson, JJ: Studies of plasma quinidine content. I. Relation to single dose administration by three routes. *Circulation 1*:564–568, 1950.
28. Ditlefsen, EML: Concentration of quinidine in blood following oral, parenteral and rectal administration. *Acta Med. Scand. 146*:81–92, 1953.
29. Swerdlow, CD, Yu, JO, Jacobson, E, Mann, S, Winkle, RA, Griffin, JC, Ross, DL, Mason, JW: Safety and efficacy of intravenous quinidine. *Am. J. Med. 75*:36–42, 1983.
30. White, NJ, Looareesuwan, S, Warrell, DA: Quinine and quinidine: An EKG comparison in the treatment of falciparum malaria. *J. Cardiovasc. Pharmacol. 5*:173–175, 1983.
31. Nelson, JD: Antiparasitic therapy. In: *1985 Pocketbook of Pediatric Antimicrobial Therapy*, 6th ed., Williams and Wilkins, Baltimore, 1985, pp. 56–62.
32. Cramer, G, Isaksson, B: Quantitative determination of quinidine in plasma. *Scand. J. Clin. Lab. Invest. 15*:553–556, 1963.
33. Hall, AP, Segal, HE, Pearlman, EJ, Phintuyothin, P, Kosakal, S: Amodiaquine-resistant falciparum malaria in Thailand. *Am. J. Trop. Med. Hyg. 24*:575–580, 1975.
34. Phillips, RE, Looareesuwam, S, Karbwang, J, et al.: Failure of chloroquine-erythromycin and chloroquine-tetracycline combinations in the treatment of chloroquine-resistant falciparum malaria in eastern Thailand. *Lancet 1*:300–302, 1984.

35. White, NJ: Clinical pharmacokinetics of antimalarial drugs. *Clin. Pharmacokinet. 10*: 187–215, 1985.
36. Heissenbuttel, RH, Bigger, JT, Jr.: The effect of oral quinidine on intraventricular conduction in man. Correlation of plasma quinidine with changes in intraventricular conduction time. *Am. Heart J. 80*:453–462, 1970.
37. Bellet, S, Hamdan, G, Somlyo, A, Lara, R: The reversal of cardiotoxic effects of quinidine by molar sodium lactate: An experimental study. *Am. J. Med. Sci. 237*: 165–176, 1959.
38. Wasserman, F, Brodsky, L, Kathe, JH, Rodensky, PL, Dick, MM, Denton, PS: The effect of molar sodium lactate in quinidine intoxication. *Am. J. Cardio. 3*:294–299, 1959.
39. Conrad, KA, Molk, BL, Chidsey, CA: Pharmacokinetic studies of quinidine in patients with arrhythmias. *Circulation 55*:1–7, 1977.
40. Strahan, JH: Quinine by continuous intravenous drip in the treatment of acute falciparum malaria. *Trans. R. Soc. Trop. Med. Hyg. 41*:669–676, 1948.
41. Ferrer, MI, Harvey, RM, Werko, L, Dresdale, DT, Cournand, A, Richards, DW: Some effects of quinidine sulfate on the heart and circulation in man. *Am. Heart J. 36*: 816–837, 1948.
42. Bigger, JY, Jr., Hoffman, BF: Antiarrhythmic drugs. In: *The Pharmacological Basis of Therapeutics*, 7th ed., (A Goodman, LS Goodman, TW Rall, and F Murad, eds.), Macmillan, New York, 1985, pp. 748–783.
43. Markiewicz, W, Winkle, R, Binetti, G, Kernoff, R, Harrison, DC: Normal myocardial contractile state in the presence of quinidine. *Circulation 53*:101–106, 1976.
44. Bigger, JT, Jr.: Management of arrhythmias. In: *Heart Disease. Textbook of Cardiovascular Medicine*, Vol. I (E Braunwald, ed.), W. B. Saunders, Philadelphia, 1980, pp. 691–743.
45. Garnham, PCC: Malarial immunity in Africans: Effects in infancy and early childhood. *Ann. Trop. Med. Parasitol. 43*:47–61, 1949.
46. Ris, HB, Stahel, E, Pittet, JF, Friedemann, M: Das antiarrhythmikun Chinidin als Alternative in der Behandlung der schweren Falciparum-Malaria. *Schweiz. Med. Wochenschr. 113*:254–258, 1983.
47. Data, JL, Wilkinson, GR, Nies, AS: Interaction of quinidine with anticonvulsant drugs. *N. Engl. J. Med. 294*:699–702, 1976.
48. Bigger, JT, Jr.: The quinidine-digoxin interaction. *Mod. Concepts Cardiovasc. Dis. 51*:73–78, 1982.
49. Koch-Weser, J: Quinidine-induced hypoprothrombinemic hemorrhage in patients on chronic warfarin therapy. *Ann. Intern. Med. 68*:511–517, 1968.

V. PRIMAQUINE

By the end of the nineteenth century, a few years after Ehrlich's discovery of a moderate plasmocidal effect by methylene blue, 8-aminoquinolines were found to have a weak schizontocidal activity in infected canaries. It was also shown that by substituting a dialkylaminoalkyl group for one of the N-methyl groups of methylene blue, the moderate plasmodicidal effect of the dye could be enhanced. As in quinine, the quinoline ring with a methoxy group was thought to be important for antimalarial activity. Hence, investigators began to synthesize quinoline derivatives featuring the methoxy and substituted 8-amino groups. Mühlens (1), in 1926, introduced pamaquine for the treatment of malaria. It was the first 8-aminoquinoline to be synthesized. During World War II, several hundred derivatives of 8-aminoquinolines were investigated in an effort to find other compounds more active and less toxic than pamaquine (2,3). Only three agents were selected for further study: pentaquine, isopentaquine, and primaquine.

Nowadays only primaquine is widely used, after extensive field trials with U.S. forces in Korea. This drug remains the nearest approach to a reasonably tolerated, all-purpose antimalarial agent. Quinocide, a substance very similar in structure to primaquine, is employed in some parts of the world.

A. Chemistry

Primaquine, 6-methoxy-8-(4′-amino-1′-methylbutylamino)quinoline, has the following structural formula:

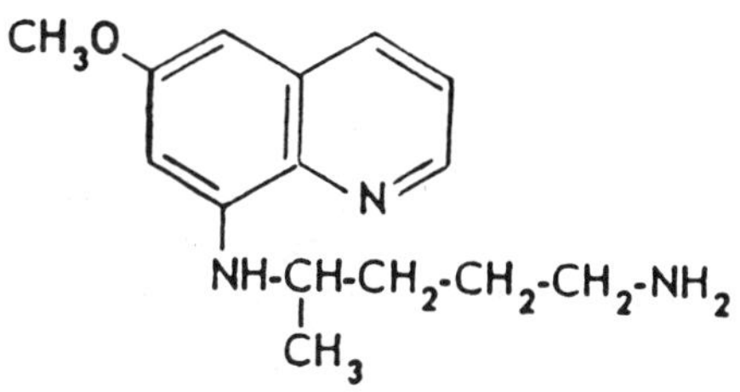

It is available as a diphosphate salt that forms stable solutions in water. However, some decomposition may occur when exposed to light and air.

A low therapeutic index was the main handicap that limited the use of a former derivative, pamaquine. This caused it to be substituted for by primaquine, that has equivalent antimalarial potency but lower toxicity. The degree of toxicity relates to the degree of substitution of the terminal amino group. Both pamaquine and primaquine are 6-methoxy-8-aminoquinoline compounds differing only in the terminal substituents of the alkylamino-alkylamino side chain. Pamaquine has a tertiary terminal amine, as shown below, but primaquine has a primary terminal amine:

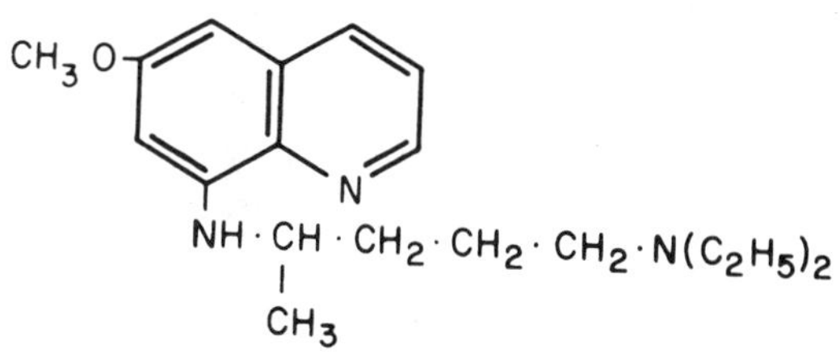

Intermediate between these two drugs lies isopentaquine, isomeric with pamaquine but with a secondary terminal amine (4). Although the 6-methoxy substituent is not essential for the activity of these drugs, it is present in all the congeners that have proved clinically effective.

B. Mechanism of Action

The mechanism of action of primaquine and the other 8-aminoquinolines has not been established. Reactivity with plasmodial mitochondria indicates interference with energy metabolism. There is evidence of a blocking action by primaquine and other 8-aminoquinolines on the mitochondria of pre-erythrocytic schizonts, but this effect has been obtained so far only in rodent malaria (5,6). A similar action of primaquine has been noted on the mitochondria of intraerythrocytic forms (7). However, the initial disruptive effect of primaquine on parasite mitochondria appears to be rapidly compensated for by an increase in the synthesis of these organelles (7).

Studies on isolated nucleic acids show that 8-aminoquinolines bind to DNA and other nucleic acids. The degree of binding is comparable to that with chloroquine, but these associations are not intercalative. Primaquine and its derivatives, however, are far less effective than chloroquine on macromolecular synthesis in nonhuman malaria parasites. The inhibitory effects of primaquine on DNA and RNA function were observed in studies on mammalian tissue systems, which may have little or no relevance to its antiparasitic action.

Primaquine itself appears to account for antimalarial activity, whereas metabolites of primaquine may be more active than the parent compound in causing hemolysis (8).

C. Antimalarial Activity and Resistance

Primaquine acts as a primary tissue schizontocide (causal prophylaxis drug) affecting preerythrocytic (PE) schizonts, and as a hypnozoitocide affecting the latent forms (hypnozoites), now believed to be responsible for true relapses in *P. vivax* infections and possibly also in *P. ovale* infections. The 8-aminoquinolines, of which only primaquine is currently employed, are the only clinically useful drugs with definite hypnozoitocidal activity. It has been postulated, although not yet demonstrated, that it is a metabolite of primaquine, not the parent compound, that is active against PE schizonts and hypnozoites.

Primaquine is used to achieve radical cure of vivax malaria and as a supplement to suppression with chloroquine in the uncommon cases in whom chloroquine therapy has proven unsuccessful. Primaquine is also effective against the primary exoerythrocytic forms of *P. falciparum*; this activity, however, is of limited practical value. It is completely ineffective against the asexual blood forms of *P. falciparum*, for which reason it is almost always used in association with a blood schizontocide.

The drug exerts a strong gametocytocidal effect on all four plasmodium species that infect humans, especially *P. falciparum*. This gametocytocidal activity could be an invaluable tool in reducing human reservoirs. Its effectiveness against gametocytes of *P. falciparum* strains persists irrespective of whether parasites have become resistant to chloroquine or other blood schizontocides. A single dose of 45 mg can eliminate gametocytes in adult patients after clinical cure has been achieved. The use of primaquine as a gametocytocide for falciparum infection is important in areas where reservoirs of the parasite have been considerably reduced but receptivity remains. A small, safe single dose is highly effective in killing fully or almost mature gametocytes. In some areas, a daily dose is given for up to 5 days, thus increasing the probability of eliminating all gametocytes.

The acute initial clinical attack in both vivax and ovale malaria is effectively suppressed by blood schizontocides, but the latent tissue forms may need to be eradicated by primaquine in patients no longer residing in malarious areas. Radical cure is of no real value if the threat of reinfection persists.

Resistance to 8-aminoquinoline compounds can be developed in experimental animal models. Resistance of *P. vivax* to primaquine is not yet a major clinical problem. However, some strains of *P. vivax* have shown reduced susceptibilities to the action of primaquine in humans. It is therefore of the utmost importance to avoid misuse of the drug and to develop new drugs of similar characteristics (8).

D. Clinical Pharmacology

After oral administration, primaquine is rapidly absorbed from the intestine. Following a single dose of 45 mg primaquine base, a peak plasma level of 153.3 ± 23 μg/ml is reached within 3 ± 1 hr (9). Bioavailability has been estimated in 74% (9). The drug is distributed throughout the body fluid, with an apparent volume of distribution of 205 ± 37 liters/kg (9). Only a very small amount is fixed in the tissues.

It is rapidly eliminated from the body. The elimination phase of the plasma concentration-time curve is monoexponential, with a half-life of 7.1 ± 1.6 hr. It is almost completely eliminated from the body within 24 hr of administration. The rate of systemic clearance is 21.1 ± 7.1 liter/hr. The plasma clearance is likely to be predominantly due to metabolic degradation, since only 1.3 ± 0.9% of the administered dose (9) is recovered in the urine as unchanged primaquine in 24 hr. The three oxidative metabolites of primaquine identified to date are 8-(3-carboxyl-1-methylpropylamino)-6-methoxyquinoline, 5-hydroxyprimaquine, and 5-hydroxy-6-desmethylprimaquine (10). The major metabolite of primaquine found in the plasma of rodents and humans has been identified as the carboxylic acid derivative (9,14). The antimalarial potency of the metabolites is considerably lower than that of primaquine. In contrast, their hemolytic activity is greater than that of the parent compound, as assessed by the in vitro formation of methemoglobin (8). According to the primaquine degradation scheme devised by Tarlov and co-workers (12), the 6-methoxy group is converted to hydroxy, a second hydroxy group is added in position 5, and the resultant compound is converted to quinonimine via the 5,6-quinone derivative of the parent compound. Quinonimine is or may be transformed into a resonating compound capable of acting as an oxidation-reduction mediator. This agent may accelerate the oxidation of essential substances in sensitive erythrocytes by acting as an electron acceptor, thereby promoting hemolysis. This redox activity might also contribute to antimalarial activity by interfering with parasite electron transfer pathways or by generating active oxygen species, such as superoxide free radical.

Greaves and co-workers (13) did not find any significant differences between primaquine kinetics in British and Thai subjects, and neither were kinetics altered in subjects deficient in glucose-6-phosphate dehydrogenase.

E. Preparation, Dosage, Regimens, and Routes of Administration

Primaquine (diphosphate; proprietary name and synonyms: Neo-Quipenyl, 4516 R.P., diphosphate; SN 13,272; WR 2,975) is supplied in tablets containing 26.3 mg of the salt, equivalent to 15 mg base. The dosage is usually expressed in terms of the base, and 17.6 mg diphosphate corresponds to 10 mg base.

Primaquine is always administered by the oral route. It is used mainly for the treatment of infections caused by sensitive strains of *P. vivax* and *P. ovale*. It is given in association with chloroquine according to the following schedule. After full doses of chloroquine base on days 1 (900 mg), 2 (300 mg), and 3 (300 mg), primaquine is administered on days 4–17 at a daily dosage of 15 mg base. The pediatric dose is 0.3 mg/kg day^{-1} up to a maximum of 15 mg base per day, also for 14 days. This regimen is recommended if radical cure is desirable, e.g., in malaria-free areas or in those with low endemicity. Patients infected by resistant strains of *P. vivax* (Southwest Pacific) may require three times the daily dosage of primaquine stated above. In these cases, the recommended regimen for adults is 600 mg chloroquine base, followed 6 hr later by 300 mg chloroquine base combined with 45 mg primaquine base in one dose. Thereafter, 300 mg chloroquine base jointly with 45 mg primaquine base should be given as a single dose on the same day of each week for 7 additional weeks (14). The pediatric dose should be increased accordingly, i.e., 0.9 mg/kg day^{-1} up to a maximum of 45 mg base per day. When glucose-6-phosphate dehydrogenase deficiency is known or suspected to be present, an alternative regimen of 45 mg primaquine base weekly for 8 weeks may be considered.

F. Drug Assays

The pharmacokinetics of primaquine have been analyzed by high-performance liquid chromatography (10,15) and gas chromatography-mass spectrometry techniques (16). Mihaly and co-workers (9) also applied HPLC to study the kinetics of both primaquine and its main plasma metabolite, the carboxylic acid derivative.

G. Therapeutic Indications

This drug is used mainly for the radical cure of vivax and other relapsing malarias. Radical cure can be achieved by administering primaquine during the long-term latent period of the infection. Its use during an acute clinical attack prevents subsequent recrudescence. Primaquine should always be given in conjunction with full doses of a schizontocide (chloroquine) in order to diminish the possibility of resistance development. Sometimes the combination of primaquine and a 4-aminoquinoline may be used for prophylaxis or interruption of transmission, especially of *P. falciparum.*

H. Toxicity

Primaquine administration in the usual therapeutic doses is largely free of side effects in white subjects. Abdominal cramps and epigastric distress may occur with higher doses. Cyanosis (methemoglobinemia), anemia, and leukocytosis are other occasional side effects.

Higher doses (60–240 mg primaquine base daily for adults) accentuate the abdominal symptoms and cause methemoglobinemia and cyanosis in most subjects, and leukopenia may be noted in some patients. Abdominal distress is milder if the drug is taken at mealtime. Subjects congenitally deficient in nicotinamide adenine dinucleotide (NADH) methemoglobin reductase may exhibit severe methemoglobinemia (17). Overdosage may also induce granulocytopenia and agranulocytosis. Hepatic function is usually normal during primaquine therapy.

Glucose-6-phosphate dehydrogenase deficiency affects a certain proportion of black individuals (10% of black males in the United States). These patients may suffer from anemia due to intravascular hemolysis if given primaquine base at a daily dose of 15 mg or higher. Some other, darker skinned individuals, such as Sephardic Jews, Greeks, Sardinians, and Iranians, may exhibit a higher degree of erythrocyte sensitivity to primaquine than black subjects.

A simple test for detecting primaquine sensitivity was devised by Brewer and coworkers in 1960 (18). The authors observed that the rate of methemoglobin reduction by erythrocytes from these patients is much slower than normal in the presence of methylene blue. The tests correlate very well with the severity of hemolysis. Hemolysis is often of intermediate severity in females. Primaquine sensitivity is inherited by a gene carried on the X chromosome; hence, heterozygous females are less affected. Because of "variable penetrance," females present primaquine sensitivity less frequently than would be predicted.

The severity of hemolysis is dose dependent. If the initial dose is not too large, hemolysis is self-limited even when the same dose is maintained. This self-limitation is due to the fact that, after destruction of older erythrocytes, which are most susceptible, there remain younger cells and newly produced reticulocytes that are relatively resistant to hemolysis. However, the severity of hemolysis can be enhanced or mitigated by a variety of factors and may often be unpredictable. Primaquine should be immediately discontinued if marked darkening of the urine or a sudden decrease in hemoglobin occurs (19). Pretreatment determination of GGPD deficiency should be mandatory.

I. Contraindications

Primaquine is contraindicated in acutely ill patients suffering from systemic disease characterized by a tendency to granulocytopenia, such as very active cases of rheumatoid arthritis and lupus erythematosus. It should not be given simultaneously with agents capable of depressing the myeloid elements of the bone marrow.

J. Drug Interactions

Primaquine should not be administered at the same time as quinine or within 3 weeks of terminating a course of this drug, because quinine increases toxicity (20).

References

1. Mühlens, P: Die Behandlung der natürlichen menschlichen Malaria-Infektion mit Plasmochin. *Naturwissenschaften 14*:1162–116, 1926.
2. Elderfield, RC, et al.: Alkylaminoalkyl derivatives of 8-aminoquinoline. *J. Am. Chem. Soc. 68*:1524–1529, 1946.
3. Wiselogle, FY (ed.): *A survey of Antimalarial Drugs, 1941–1945* (two volumes), J. W. Edwards Publishers, Ann Arbor, Michigan, 1946.
4. Hill, J: Chemotherapy of malaria. Part 2. The antimalarial drugs. In: *Experimental Chemotherapy*, Vol. 1 (RJ Schnitzer and F Hawking, eds.), Academic Press, New York, 1963, pp. 513–601.
5. Boulard, Y, et al.: The chemotherapy of rodent malaria. XXXIV. Casual prophylaxis. Part III. Ultrastructural changes induced in exo-erythrocytic schizpnts of *Plasmodium yoelii* by primaquine. *Ann. Trop. Med. Parasitol. 77*:555–568, 1983.
6. Peters, W, et al.: The chemotherapy of rodent malaria. XXXVI. Causal prophylaxis. Part IV. The activity of a new 8-aminoquinoline, WR 225,448 against exo-erythrocytic schizonts of *P. yoelii yoelii. Ann. Trop. Med. Parasitol. 78*:467–478, 1984.
7. Howells, RE, et al.: The chemotherapy of rodent malaria. XIII. Fine structural changes observed in the erythrocytic stages of *Plasmodium berghei berghei* following exposure to primaquine and menoctone. *Ann. Trop. Med. Parasitol. 64*:203–207, 1970.
8. World Health Organization: *Report of the Steering Committee of the Scientific Working Groups on Malaria*, World Health Organization, Geneva, 1984.
9. Mihaly, GW, Ward, SA, Edwards, G, Orme, ML'E, Breckenridge, AM: Pharmacokinetics of primaquine in man: Identification of the carboxylic acid derivative as a major plasma metabolite. *Br. J. Clin. Pharmacol. 17*:441–446, 1984.
10. Baker, JK, McChesney, JD, Hufford, CD, Clark, AM: High-performance liquid chromatographic analysis of the metabolism of primaquine and the identification of a new mammalian metabolite. *J. Chromatogr. 230*:69–77, 1982.
11. World Health Organization: Recent progress in chemotherapeutic research. In: *Advances in Malaria Chemotherapy*, Technical Report Series 711, World Health Organization, Geneva, 1984, pp. 91–156.
12. Tarlov, AR, Brewer, GJ, Carson, PE, Alving, AS: Primaquine sensitivity. *Arch. Intern. Med. 109*:209–234, 1962.
13. Greaves, J, Evans, DAP, Gilles, HM, Fletcher, KA, Bernnag, D, Harinasuta, T: Plasma kinetics and urinary excretion of primaquine in man. *Br. J. Clin. Pharmacol. 10*: 399–405, 1980.

14. Webster, LT, Jr.: Drugs used in the chemotherapy of protozoal infections. Malaria. In: *The Pharmacological Basis of Therapeutics*, 7th ed., (A Goodman, LS Gilman, TW Rall, and F Murad, eds.), Macmillan, New York
15. Ward, SA, Edwards, G, Orme, ML'E, Breckenridge, AM: Determination of primaquine in biological fluids by reversed phased high-performance liquid chromatography. *J. Chromatogr. 305*:239–243, 1983.
16. Greaves, J, Evans, DAP, Gilles, HM, Baty, JD: A selected ion monitoring assay for primaquine in plasma and urine. *Biomed. Mass Spectrom. 6*:109–112, 1979.
17. Cohen, RJ, Sachs, JR, Wicker, DJ, Conrad, ME: Methemoglobinemia provoked by malarial chemoprophylasix in Vietnam. *N. Engl. J. Med. 279*:1127–1131, 1968.
18. Brewer, GJ, Tarlov, AR, Alving, AS: Methemoglobin reduction test: A new simple, in vitro test for identifying primaquine sensitivity. *Bull. WHO 22*:633–640, 1960.
19. Kellermeyer, RW, Tarlov, AR, Brewer, GJ, Carson, PE, Alving, AS: Hemolytic effect of therapeutic drugs; clinical considerations of the primaquine-type hemolysis. *JAMA 180*:388–394, 1962.
20. Markell, EK, Voge, M: *Medical Parasitology*, 5th ed., W. B. Saunders, Philadelphia, 1981.

VI. MEFLOQUINE

Mefloquine is a most promising investigational antimalarial compound. It was developed and tested initially by the U.S. Army; since 1976 it has been developed by the World Health Organization in collaboration with the Walter Reed Army Institute of Research and Hoffman LaRoche. Clinical trials showed it to be a readily tolerated antimalarial agent, highly active against both the usual and the multidrug-resistant strains of *P. falciparum* (1,2).

Promising alternatives to mefloquine have been identified—among others halofantrine—but extensive clinical evaluations are yet to be done (3).

A. Chemistry

Mefloquine is structurally related to quinine (racemic α-(2-piperydil)-2,8-bis-(trifluoromethyl)-4-quinolinemethanol). It has the following formula:

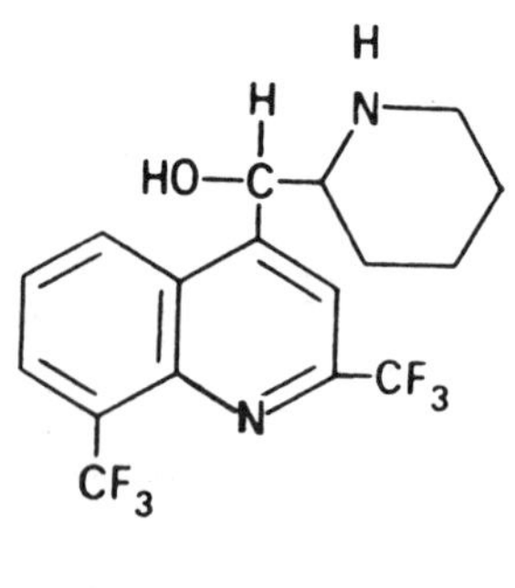

The hydrochloride is a white, odorless, bitter powder.

B. Mechanisms of Action

In some respects mefloquine behaves like quinine; however, its precise mechanism of action is not known. Mefloquine does not compound by intercalation with guanine-containing double-stranded DNA (4,5). However, failure to demonstrate intercalation does not rule out other interactions of mefloquine with DNA.

Mefloquine and quinine produce similar morphological changes in early ring stages of *P. falciparum* and *P. vivax* (1). Mefloquine alters the membranes of malaria parasites (6). Like quinine, it interferes with the pigment clumping induced by chloroquine and related 4-aminoquinolines (7,8). Mefloquine competes with chloroquine for accumulation in infected erythrocytes, owing to its high-affinity binding to red blood cell membranes (8,9). However, although changes in chloroquine-resistant strains may result in the exclusion of chloroquine, the avidity for mefloquine appears to be retained.

C. Resistance

Data on resistance are limited to date to those collected from studies on induced resistance and from extensive field trials.

Type II mefloquine resistance has been observed in Thailand (10). In that area, mefloquine was available only for limited clinical trial use, but it is possible that resistance to quinine already existed. Mefloquine resistance also occurred in an isolate of *P. falciparum* in Tanzania (11). Another clinical trial in Gabon (12) revealed that in some instances there was reduced sensitivity to mefloquine in strains highly resistant to chloroquine. Reduced sensitivity was also found among *P. falciparum* isolates in the Philippines (11).

Resistance to mefloquine may be easily induced in experimental models, but mefloquine-resistant strains of *P. berghei* appear to be more susceptible than expected to mefloquine-pyrimethamine-sulfadoxine combination. This suggests a potentiating effect rather than the additive effect observed with *P. berghei* strains that are normally sensitive to mefloquine (13). Resistant strains of *P. falciparum* were present in some areas even before mefloquine was deployed (10,11).

D. Clinical Pharmacology

Mefloquine is well absorbed after oral administration. The bioavailability of preparations used at present is above 85%. The drug is known to have great affinity to the red blood cell membranes and therefore concentrates more in red cells than in plasma. Erythrocytic concentration in healthy volunteers (14) was found to double that in plasma, whereas in vitro concentrations in red blood cells may be up to 60 times higher than those in the extracellular medium (15). As a result, pharmacokinetic parameters may differ widely, depending on whether they are derived from whole blood or plasma measurements. Desjardins and co-workers (16) studied the kinetics of mefloquine in healthy volunteers receiving single oral doses ranging from 250 to 1000 mg, on the basis of whole blood concentrations. Absorption was more rapid and more complete from aqueous suspension than from tablets, mean absorption half-lives being 1.1 and 3.8 hr, respectively, and the area under the concentration-time curves 35% greater with the suspension than with tablets. Peak plasma concentrations of 250–1220 μg/liter were reached in 11–48 hr. In most cases the whole blood concentration data fit a triexponential decline. The volume of distribution ranged between 9.4 and 19.2 liter/kg; mean, 13.3 liter/kg. Considerable variations in the terminal elimination half-lives were recorded: from 6.5 to 22.7 days; mean, 13.9 days. These data suggest slow clearance and a very small first-pass effect.

Schwartz and co-workers (14) measured both blood and plasma concentrations of mefloquine in a pharmacokinetic study performed in healthy volunteers. The drug was rapidly absorbed after single doses of 250–1000 mg. Absorption half-lives varied from 22 to 120 min. Plasma terminal elimination half-lives ranged between 15.6 and 33 days, and volume of distribution values between 13.5 and 29.1 liter/kg. Mean total clearance was calculated in approximately 0.4 ml/min kg^{-1}, from values ranging from 18 to 40 ml/min. Urinary excretion accounted for 1.5–8.7% of the unchanged mefloquine.

Despite differences in volume of distribution and elimination half-live values, the studies by Desjardins and colleagues and Schwartz and colleagues confirm the extensive tissue distribution and slow clearance of mefloquine.

Plasma mefloquine is largely bound to proteins. In both healthy volunteers and malaria patients, approximately 2% of the administered drug is in the free form (17).

Several metabolites are formed; two have been identified as 2,8-bis-trifluoromethyl-quinoline-4,4-methanol and 2,8-trifluoromethylquinoline-4-carboxylic acid. The drug is eliminated mainly by biotransformation within 4 hr of oral intake; measurable amounts of the carboxylic acid metabolite can be detected in the plasma. After a few days the concentrations of this metabolite exceed those of mefloquine, and the area under the plasma concentration-time curve is about 3.4 times greater than that of the active unchanged drug (17). The metabolite has a smaller volume of distribution (in the dog it is 30 times smaller than that of the parent compound); it does not diffuse into tissue compartments or into erythrocytes (18). These metabolites do not affect the toxicity of mefloquine.

Plasma concentrations gradually increase as weekly doses are repeated, reaching a steady level after only a few months. A tolerance trial was performed by administering to volunteers weekly doses of 250 mg mefloquine base; mean mefloquine steady-state plasma concentrations of 0.56–1.25 mg/liter were found. Mean plasma concentrations of the metabolites, measured at the same time, were 3.5–8.6 times higher. After 6 months of weekly doses, the elimination half-life of mefloquine from plasma was assessed (multiple-dose kinetics) and found to range from 17 to 35 days, which indicates that no enzyme induction inhibition is to be expected after prolonged therapy.

Data on mefloquine kinetics in malaria patients are scarce, despite extensive field trials. A comparative study (17) was conducted in five Thai patients with uncomplicated falciparum malaria and a group of healthy volunteers receiving either a deuterium-labeled suspension or unlabeled tablets. Peak concentrations following a 250-mg dose in Thai patients were 706–1439 μg/liter, approximately tripling those of the white volunteers. Plasma protein binding was similar in both groups (98%), whereas other parameters differed: the volume of distribution was smaller (6.0 ± 1.0 liter/kg), terminal elimination half-life shorter (10.3 ± 2.5 days), and total clearance slower (0.29 ± 0.07 ml/min kg^{-1}). These kinetic differences may be partly explained by the ethnic differences but are also likely to reflect malaria-induced changes (15). The absorption of mefloquine in comatose patients with cerebral malaria is remarkably rapid. In most cases of the studied series it was less than 4 hr. Steady-state concentrations were found to vary between 300 and 105 μg/liter (15). The drug was not detected in CSF or in the peritoneal dialysate of patients in acute renal failure.

The kinetics of a combination of mefloquine (250 mg), sulfadoxine (500 mg), and pyrimethamine (25 mg) was studied in children following a single dose (15). The values recorded for mefloquine were: volume of distribution, 8.4 to 18.4 liter/kg; elimination half-life, 223 hr; and total clearance, 0.60 ml/min kg^{-1}. The clearance of all three drugs was higher than in adults.

No data have been reported on the pharmacokinetics of mefloquine in pregnancy or in the presence of hepatic dysfunction or renal insufficiency.

E. Preparation, Dosage, Regimens, and Routes of Administration

Mefloquine (Lariam, WR 142,490) is an investigational drug that is still undergoing extensive clinical evaluation. The Walter Reed Army Institute of Research supplies tables of 250 mg.

Based on the results of clinical trials (13) the following dosages can be recommended for effective cure of *P. falciparum* infections:

Adults, 18-20 mg/kg body weight (750-1250 mg) in a single dose. When the calculated dose amount exceeds 750 mg, 750 mg should be administered first, followed 8 hr later by 250-500 mg.
Children, 25 mg/kg body weight in a single dose.

Half this dose is sufficient to eliminate *P. vivax* from the blood; however, hypnozoites will persist unless primaquine is given. If in acute falciparum malaria parenteral therapy is required, quinine dihydrochloride should be administered initially (see quinine for dosage and mode of infusion), followed by mefloquine 8-12 hr after the last infusion (when the patient is able to take oral medication).

For suppressive treatment, 250 mg mefloquine base is the standard dose for adults, given at weekly intervals. Half this dose might suffice in the steady state (i.e., after about 2 months). In children, suppressive treatment requires 4-6 mg of mefloquine base per kilogram body weight.

Dosage recommendations for suppressive treatment with tablets containing 250 mg mefloquine base are as follows:

Adults and children above 45 kg body weight; 1 tablet weekly
Children* 15-19 kg, 1/4 tablet weekly; 20-30 kg, 1/2 tablet weekly; 31-45 kg, 3/4 tablet weekly

If mefloquine is used in combination with sulfadoxine and pyrimethamine, there are, for research purposes only, tablets containing 250 mg mefloquine, 500 mg sulfadoxine, and 25 mg pyrimethamine (ratio 10:20:1). This combination is administered at a mefloquine dosage of 12.5-15 mg/kg body weight in a single dose. It is used for the treatment of resistant falciparum malaria, and as a rule, patients receive two or three tablets as a single dose.

In a Thai field trial a simplified dosage table of combined mefloquine, sulfadoxine, and pyrimethamine was used in children as single-dose treatment (19).

6-10 kg, 1/2 tablet
10-15 kg, 3/4 tablet
16-19 kg, 1 tablet
20-30 kg, 1 1/2 tablets
31-45 kg, 2 tablets

*No clinical experience is available with mefloquine in infants (19).

F. Drug Assays

The pharmacokinetics of mefloquine have been studied using three assay techniques. These are thin-layer chromatography (18), with a lower limit of detection of 50 μg/liter, high-performance liquid chromatography (16,20), apt for concentrations below 10 μg/liter, and gas chromatography-mass spectrometry (21), with a lower limit of detection of 1 μg/liter.

G. Therapeutic Indications

Mefloquine is used mainly for the prevention and treatment of chloroquine-resistant falciparum malaria. It is currently the only agent that, when used alone, is capable of ensuring suppression and cure of infections caused by multidrug-resistant strains of *P. falciparum*. It is recommended that the drug be used only for the treatment and prevention of infections by such strains, because its misuse can result in the development and rapid spread of mefloquine-resistant *P. falciparum*.

On the basis of potential resistance, many investigators emphasize that it would be unwise to make widespread the use of mefloquine alone and that rational combinations with other antimalarials should be developed with a view to delaying the emergence of mefloquine resistance. Early studies by Peters (22) demonstrated that specific combinations of antimalarials succeeded in delaying the development of resistance in experimental models. The pharmacokinetics of the different component drugs have to be well matched, so that two or three active drugs remain together and in contact with the parasites in the erythrocytes for a sufficient length of time. In suppressive therapy, effective concentrations of all the drugs administered should be maintained in the blood during the dosage intervals (23). The combination of mefloquine with sulfadoxine pyrimethamine fulfills these requirements.

Experiments based on the *P. berghei* model for inducing resistance to mefloquine demonstrated that if the sulfadoxine-pyrimethamine combination is given together with mefloquine, the induced level of resistance to these drugs and also the rate of induction are lower in comparison with the rapid development and the high degree of resistance induced by mefloquine alone (24-26). Following evaluation of these findings, the activity, toxicology, and pharmacokinetics of this triple combination were studied in animal models.

The additive antimalarial activity of these three substances in the absence of increased toxicity allowed clinical trials to be initiated using tablets containing 250 mg mefloquine, 500 mg of sulfadoxine, and 25 mg pyrimethamine (24,27,28). Clinical trials were performed in Thailand (21) comparing the triple combination to mefloquine. A total of 47 patients received a single dose of mefloquine alone (750 mg), and 49 patients received a single dose of the triple combination (mefloquine, 750 mg; sulfadoxine, 1500 mg; and pyrimethamine, 75 mg). Follow-up was for 42 days. Among patients treated with mefloquine alone, recrudescence with low parasitemia occurred in one case on day 14. In a second case, parasites reappeared on day 42. In the group treated with the triple combination there was a single recrudescence; however, because of vomiting shortly after treatment, the amount of drug absorbed might have been insufficient.

In Ndola (Zambia) and in Belem (Brazil), studies were carried out on three groups of 50 patients each. One group received one tablet containing 250 mg mefloquine, 500 mg sulfadoxine, and 25 mg pyrimethamine; the second group, two tablets, and the third group, three tablets, in all cases as single doses. The Zambian study showed good tolerance and no recrudescence in any of the groups after a 63-day follow-up. The remarkable success of this trial was probably because no resistance to sulfadoxine-pyrimethamine existed in the area.

In Belem (State of Para, Brazil), where resistance to sulfadoxine-pyrimethamine is common, recrudescences occurred in 6 of 35 patients treated with one tablet only, whereas there was complete cure in the groups treated with two or three tablets (19).

Another study was performed in the Kuchinarai District in Thailand with outpatients (male adults). Three tablets as a single dose (750 mg mefloquine, 1500 mg sulfadoxine, and 75 mg pyrimethamine) were administered to 49 patients; 47 patients received a 750-mg single dose of mefloquine alone. The follow-up extended for 42 days. In the mefloquine group one patient became positive on day 42, suggesting that reinfection might have occurred. In the triple-drug combination group, recrudescence occurred on day 21 in a patient who had vomited 70 min after receiving medication. In both groups there was good tolerance; parasite clearance and clinical response were similar (19).

In June 1983, a large field trial of the triple-drug combination was launched in Thailand for the curative treatment of malaria in several "hard core" areas of *P. falciparum* multidrug-resistant strains, mainly near the Kampuchean border. Patients with *P. falciparum* infections diagnosed by blood smears were treated with either a single dose of the triple combination of mefloquine, 250 mg, sulfadoxine, 500 mg, and pyrimethamine, 25 mg per tablet, or, in the case of the control group, with quinine-tetracycline (quinine, 10 mg/kg per dose three times per day for 3 days; tetracycline, 5 mg/kg per dose four times per day for 7 days).

In the first group, all individuals infected with *P. falciparum, except* pregnant women and children below 1 year, received the triple drug combination at a dosage of mefloquine of 12.5-15 mg/kg body weight per day. Pregnant women and infants received quinine (10 mg/kg per dose three times a day) for 7 days.

All patients were followed for 12 weeks. Tolerance of both regimens was excellent (100 patients were admitted to each group). Two failures were reported in the group treated with the combination, one recrudescence (or reinfection) on day 28 and one RII-type persistence of parasitemia. The results are encouraging, and further trials in progress will clarify the value of the drug combination (19).

Administration of one or more doses of quinine, together with mefloquine, avoids the delay with the time needed for the latter drug to achieve a therapeutic concentration in blood. This association is suggested for serious *P. falciparum* infections, although it still requires confirmation. Also, the possibility of enhanced toxicity needs to be investigated (19). This association should optimize the therapeutic action of mefloquine.

A single dose of 45 mg primaquine (adult dose) may be given with a therapeutic dose of mefloquine in order to sterilize any existing *P. falciparum* gametocytes. This combination should minimize or interrupt the transmission of parasites in areas where vectors are present.

H. Toxicity

Mefloquine given orally in single doses up to 1500 mg or in 500-mg doses each week is well tolerated in humans. The patterns of adverse reactions seen in healthy volunteers were similar to those seen in malarious patients.

The main adverse reactions reported, all of them mild to moderate, were nausea, dizziness, vomiting, abdominal pain, and diarrhea. Itching or skin rashes occurred in a few cases. Asymptomatic sinus bradycardia was observed in some patients of the Ndole (Zambia) and Bangkok (Thailand) studies. It usually occurred 5-7 days after mefloquine administration and reverted to normal after 7-14 days.

The overall incidence of reactions was nausea, 17.7%; vomiting, 13.3%; diarrhea, 14.9%; dizziness, 14.7%; abdominal pain, 8.3%; sinus bradycardia, 8.9%; skin itching or rash, 1.4%; and neuropsychiatric changes, 0.9%. Most of these symptoms required no treatment and were reversible. In some areas (Ndole and Belem), the incidence of abdominal pain was higher, probably because concomitant multiple helmintic infections were present in 90-100% of the patients. Neuropsychiatric changes characterized by behavior disorders, paranoid ideas, and hallucinations were seen in Bangkok and Ndole. All of these patients received symptomatic treatment and remained well.

Mefloquine induces no adverse hematologic or biochemical reactions. Studies on mutagenicity, carcinogenicity, and teratogenicity have been negative to date (19).

I. Contraindications

Because of lack of information, the use of mefloquine in women in childbearing age, pregnant women, and infants is not yet recommended.

This new compound is highly effective in the management of multiple drug-resistant falciparum malaria. It is also effective for the prophylaxis and treatment of human infections due to all species of malaria parasites. The risk that *P. falciparum* might develop resistance to this valuable compound is always present; hence certain precautions aimed at avoiding misuse should be taken when deploying the drug:

1. Strict drug control through exacting government regulations concerning importation and distribution.
2. Limitation of use. The World Health Organization, national governments and manufacturers should see that supplies of mefloquine are made available only to those countries in which there is a clear indication for its use.
3. Time limit for the use of mefloquine. It is dangerous to depend on mefloquine or any other antimalarial to control the disease indefinitely, in the absence of other control measures. A time limit should therefore be set for its use in community protection.
4. Sensitivity monitoring. It is advisable to determine the baseline sensitivity of local strains of *P. falciparum* to this drug, using the in vitro microtest (29,30), and again whenever a change in clinical response to the drug is suspected.
5. Integrated control. Mefloquine should be used only as one of the tools in an integrated attack on malaria, as part of a long-term control program or for the emergency handling of an epidemic. Reliance only on antimalarials is not enough and may lead to the emergence of drug resistance.

J. Drug Interactions

As mefloquine has been combined with sulfadoxine and pyrimethamine in preparations available so far only for research purposes, eventual interactions with these two drugs would be important from a therapeutic point of view. However, studies on single-drug and multiple-drug kinetics of the individual drugs have revealed no significant interactions (15). Concurrent administration with quinine appears to lower mefloquine concentrations in plasma (15).

References

1. Schmidt, LH, Crosby, R, Rasco, J, Vaughan, D: Antimalarial activities of various 4-quinolinemethanols with special attention to WR-142, 490 (mefloquine). *Antimicrob. Agents Chemother. 13*:1011–1030, 1978.
2. World Health Organization: Development of mefloquine as an antimalarial drug. *Bull. WHO 61*:169–178, 1983.
3. Canfield, CJ: Antimalarial aminoalcohol alternatives to mefloquine. *Acta Trop. (Basel) 37*:232–237, 1980.
4. Davidson, MW, Griggs, BG, Jr., Boykin, DW, Wilson, WD: Mefloquine, a clinically useful quinolinemethanol antimalarial which does not significantly bind to DNA. *Nature 254*:632–634, 1975.
5. Davidson, MW, Griggs, BG, Jr., Boykin, DW, Wilson, WD: Molecular structural effects involved in the interaction of quinolinemethanolamines with DNA. Implications for antimalarial action. *J. Med. Chem. 20*:1117–1122, 1977.
6. Brown, RE, Stancatto, FA, Wolfe, AD: The effects of mefloquine on *Escherichia coli. Life Sci. 25*:1857–1864, 1979.
7. Warhurst, DC, Thomas, SC: The chemotherapy of rodent malaria. XXXI. The effect of some metabolic inhibitors upon chloroquine-induced pigment clumping (CIMPC) in *Plasmodium berghei. Ann. Trop. Med. Parasitol. 72*:203–211, 1978.
8. Fitch, CD, Cham, RL, Chevli, R: Chloroquine resistance in malaria: Accessibility of drug receptors to mefloquine. *Antimicrob. Agents Chemother. 15*:258–262, 1979.
9. San George, RC, Nagel, RL, Fabry, ME: On the mechanism for the cell accumulation of mefloquine, an antimalarial drug. *Biochim. Biophys. Acta 803*:174–181, 1984.
10. Boudreau, EF, et al.: Type II mefloquine resistance in Thailand. *Lancet 2*:1335, 1982.
11. Bygbjerg, IC, et al.: Mefloquine resistance of falciparum malaria from Tanzania enhanced by treatment. *Lancet 1*:774–775, 1983.
12. Burchard, GD: Untersuchungen zur Chloroquin-Empfindlichkeit von *P. falciparum* im Gabun. *Meeting German Speaking Soc Trop Med*, Garmisch-Partenkirchen, Federal Republic of Germany, 1983.
13. Leimer, R, Wedekamm, E: Pharmacokinetics, efficacy and tolerance of the combination mefloquine plus Fansidar (sulfadoxine pyrimethamine). *XIIIth International Congress of Chemotherapy*, Vienna, August–September 1983, Abstracts SY42, part 21, pp. 32–36.
14. Schwartz, DE, Eckert, G, Hartmann, D, Weber, E, Richard-Lenoble, D, Ekue, JMK, Gentilini, M: Single dose kinetics of mefloquine in man. *Chemotherapy 28*:70–84, 1982.
15. White, NJ: Clinical pharmacokinetics of antimalarial drugs. *Clin. Pharmacokinet. 10*: 187–215, 1985.
16. Desjardins, RE, Pamplin, CL, Von Bredow, J, Barry, KG, Canfield, CJ: Kinetics of a new antimalarial, mefloquine. *Clin. Pharmacol. Ther. 26*:372–379, 1979.
17. Schwartz, DE, Warrell, DA, Dubach, VC, Ranalder, VB, White, NJ, Looareesuwan, S: Pharmacokinetic parameters of mefloquine in adult male Thai patients and Swiss volunteers (abstract). *Proc II Internat Congr Trop Med Malaria*, Calgary, 1984, p. 136.
18. Schwartz, DE, Weber, W, Richard-Lenoble, D, Gentilini, M: Kinetic studies of mefloquine and one of its metabolites in the dog and in man. *Acta Trop. (Basel) 37*:238–242, 1980.
19. World Health Organization: Recent progress in chemotherapeutic research. In: *Advances in Malaria Chemotherapy*, Technical Report Series 711, World Health Organization, Geneva, 1984, pp. 91–156.

20. Kapetanovic, IM, Di Giovanni, JD, Bartosevich, J, Meledez, V, Von Bredow, J, Hieffer, M: Analysis of the antimalarial mefloquine in blood and plasma using high performance liquid chromatography. *J. Chromatogr. 277*:209–215, 1983.
21. Schwartz, DE, Ranalder, WB: Highly sensitive and specific determination of mefloquine in biological fluids using GC-MS with selected ion monitoring. *Biomed. Mass Spectrom. 8*:589–592, 1981.
22. Peters, W: *Chemotherapy and Drug Resistance in Malaria*, Academic Press, London, 1970.
23. Fernex, M: Drug combination in malaria. In: *Advances in Pharmacology and Therapeutics. Proceedings of the VIIth International Congress of Pharmacology, Paris, 1978*, Vol 10 (JR Boissier et al., eds.), Pergamon Press, Oxford, 1979, pp. 91–98.
24. Merkli, B, Richle, RW: Studies on the resistance to single and combined antimalarials in the *Plasmodium berghei* mouse model. *Acta Trop. (Basel) 37*:228–231, 1980.
25. Peters, W, Robinson, BL: The chemotherapy of rodent malaria. XXXIV. Further studies on the retardation of drug resistance by the use of a triple combination of mefloquine, pyrimethamine and sulfadoxine in mice infected with *Plasmodium berghei* and *P. berghei* NS. *Ann. Trop. Med. Parasitol. 78*:459–466, 1984.
26. Peters, W, et al.: The chemotherapy of rodent malaria. XXVIII. The development of resistance to mefloquine (WR 142,490). *Ann. Trop. Med. Parasitol. 71*:419–427, 1977.
27. Richle, R, Merkli, B: Chemotherapeutische Wirksamkeit von Malaria-Mitteln bei der experimentellen Mäusemalaria. *Meeting German Speaking Soc Trop Med, Garmisch-Partenkirchen*, Federal Republic of Germany, 1983.
28. Weidekamm, E, Schwartz, DE: Pharmakokinetik und Dosierung der neuen Antimalariakombination Fansidar/Mefloquine (Ro 13-5112). *Meeting German Speaking Soc Trop Med*, Garmisch-Partenkirchen, Federal Republic of Germany, 1983.
29. Rieckmann, KH: Susceptibility of cultured parasites of *Plasmodium falciparum* to antimalarial drugs. In: *The In Vitro Cultivation of the Pathogens of Tropical Diseases*, Tropical Diseases Research Series 3, UNDP/World Bank/WHO Special Programme for Research Training in Tropical Diseases, 1980, pp. 35–50.
30. Yinsunsri, L, Rieckmann, K: In vitro microtechnique for determining the drug susceptibility of cultured parasites of *Plasmodium falciparum. Trans. R. Soc. Trop. Med. Hyg. 74*:809–810, 1980.

VII. PYRIMETHAMINE AND RELATED COMBINATIONS

Many 2,4-diaminopyrimidines have been synthesized and tested for antimicrobial activity. Two of them are widely used. The first, pyrimethamine, was developed and employed as an antimalarial agent. The second, trimethoprim, originally created as an antibacterial agent, was later found to have antimalarial properties. Some of the earlier 2,4-diaminopyrimidines were found to competitively antagonize folic and folinic acids in the growth of *Lactobacillus casei*. Investigators predicted that *L. casei* would not be unique in its sensitivity to these compounds and that useful chemotherapeutic agents would be developed from this group. Shortly afterward, research demonstrated that these new compounds had high antimalarial activity. The most active, pyrimethamine, was later found to be very effective against plasmodia that infect humans (1,2). Nowadays it is widely used for malaria prophylaxis and suppression.

A. Chemistry

Pyrimethamine, 2-4-diamino-5-chlorophenyl-6-ethylpyrimidine (Daraprim), has the following structural formula:

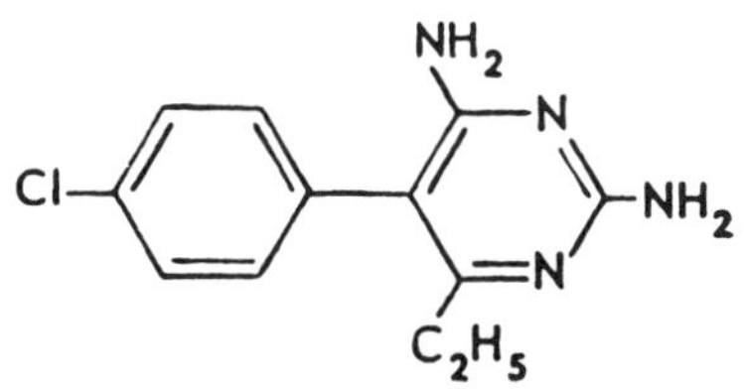

It is a white, crystalline, odorless and tasteless powder insoluble in water, with a melting point of 238–242°C. It is soluble in alcohol (1:200), in chloroform (1:125), and in warm dilute mineral acids and slightly soluble in acetone. It must be stored in airtight containers and protected from light.

B. Mechanisms of Action

Diaminopyrimidines act by inhibiting dihydrofolate reductase of plasmodia at concentrations far below those required to produce comparable inhibitions of the mammalian enzyme (3). Dihydrofolate reductase (DHFR) catalyzes the reduction of dihydrofolate to tetrahydrofolate, which in turn is needed for the biosynthesis of purines, pyrimidines, and nucleic acids.

Malaria parasites utilize the same folate cofactor mechanism as bacteria for macromolecular synthesis. As in host mammalian cells, the essential substance is tetrahydrofolate (FA_4), which is formed from dihydrofolic acid (FA_2) by enzymic reduction through dihydrofolate reductase. Microbial cells cannot utilize the available preformed folic acid (FA) as a source of FA_2 as do host cells and therefore have to synthesize it from para-aminobenzoic acid (PABA) (see Figure 3).

In malarial parasites, two sites along the synthetic pathway of folate cofactors are susceptible to drug effects (see Figure 4).

African children infected with *P. falciparum* and *P. malariae* were treated in 1959 with the combination of sulfadiazine and pyrimethamine. Clinical cure was obtained with the combination of less than 1/10 of the curative dose of pyrimethamine plus less than 1/4 of the curative dose of sulfadiazine (3). This enhanced effectiveness allows dosage to be reduced while maintaining the level of efficacy and diminishing or delaying the possibility of resistance to either or both drugs. Moreover, sulfonamides and sulfones have a negligible effect on host tissue; also pyrimethamine, proguanil, and trimethoprim have very low affinity to host DHFR.

C. Antimalarial Activity and Resistance

Resistance develops rapidly after the use of pyrimethamine alone for mass treatment or as a medicated salt. Such use is therefore contraindicated (4).

There may be cross-resistance to chloroproguanil, cycloguanil, proguanil, and trimethoprim (5).

D. Clinical Pharmacology

Pyrimethamine absorption from the intestine is relatively rapid. Peak plasma concentrations are reached in 2–6 hr after administration of an oral dose (6,7). In one study in healthy volunteers the peak plasma concentration was 234 ± 21 μg/liter (8). Clearance is slow (24.8 ± 3.8 ml/min kg^{-1}) (8), and bioavailability is presumably high; it was approximately 100% in monkeys (9). The concentrations achieved in plasma are suppressive for

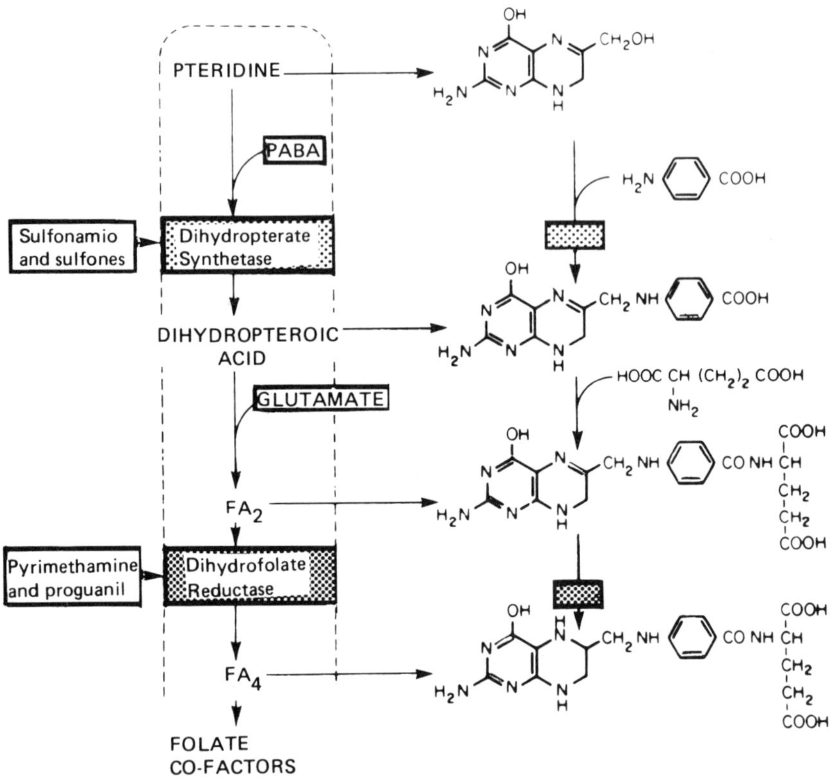

Figure 3 The processes of folate cofactor synthesis in both parasitic and host cells. (Authorized reproduction from James DM and Gilles HM: *Human Antiparasitic Drugs. Pharmacology and Usage*. Copyright 1985 by John Wiley and Sons Ltd., Chichester, New York, Brisbane, Toronto, Singapore.)

drug-sensitive strains (10,11). The amount of drug bound to plasma protein was found to be 87 ± 1% (8). Salivary concentration was about 20% that in plasma, reflecting the unbound drug concentration in the plasma (8). Pyrimethamine is distributed throughout the body fluids, the apparent volume of distribution being estimated as 2.93 ± 0.52 liter/kg. Plasma concentrations decline slowly with an elimination half-life of 83 ± 14 hr (8,12). Urinary clearance has been found to be 0.41 ± 0.6 ml/min kg^{-1} (6,8). Pyrimethamine is also excreted in the milk of nursing mothers. Several metabolites appear in the urine; however, their structure and antimalarial activity are still largely unknown. No kinetic changes were detected in pyrimethamine when administered with dapsone.

Brooks and colleagues (13) studied the pharmacokinetics of pyrimethamine in 15 patients with uncomplicated falciparum malaria receiving a 50-mg oral dose of pyrimethamine in addition of 1 g sulfadoxine and 650 mg quinine, the latter at 8-hr intervals. Mean plasma concentrations ranged from 300 to 600 μg/liter throughout the duration of the study (14 days). Urinary excretion declined from 4.2 mg on day 1 to 2.2 mg on day 7.

No data have been reported so far on pyrimethamine disposition in children, pregnant women, or patients with severe malaria, renal failure, or hepatic dysfunction. The drug has been shown to rapidly enter the brain of animals. However, CSF concentrations in humans are not known to date (14).

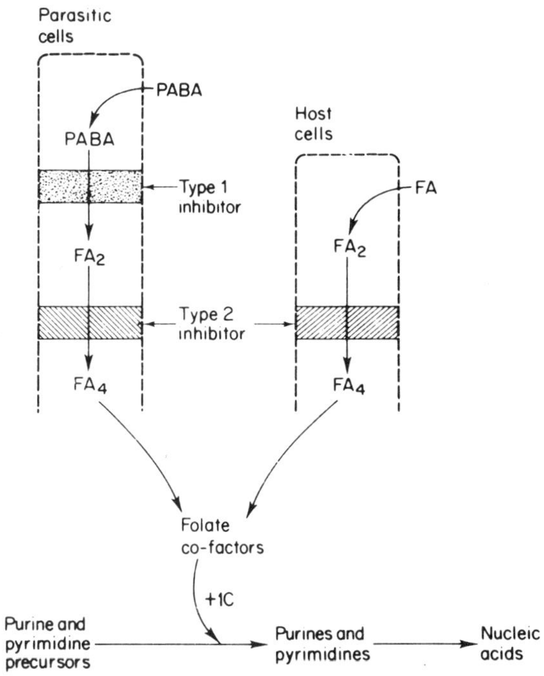

Figure 4 The site and mechanism of action of both groups of antifolate antimalarials. (Authorized reproduction from James DM and Gilles HM: *Human Antiparasitic Drugs. Pharmacology and Usage*. Copyright 1985 by John Wiley and Sons Ltd., Chichester, New York, Brisbane, Toronto, Singapore.)

E. Preparation, Dosage, Regimens, and Routes of Administration

Pyrimethamine is marketed in tablets containing 25 mg. For antimalarial therapy, however, the drug is practically always used together with a sulfonamide or a sulfone.

Pyrimethamine (25 mg) is available in a fixed combination tablet with sulfadoxine (500 mg). Sulfadoxine is a sulfonamide with a particularly long half-life (7-9 days). Pyrimethamine (12.5 mg) is also available in combination with dapsone (100 mg). These preparations are given weekly for prophylaxis and suppressive therapy.

Oral adult dose: pyrimethamine, 25 mg once weekly during and for 6 weeks after exposure in a malarious area
Oral pediatric dose: pyrimethamine, 0.5 mg/kg once weekly up to the maximum adult dose during and for 6 weeks after exposure in a malarious area
Oral adult dose: pyrimethamine, 25 mg, plus sulfadoxine, 500 mg (Fansidar, 1 tablet), once weekly during and for 6 weeks after exposure in a malarious area
Oral pediatric dose: pyrimethamine, 0.5 mg/kg, plus sulfadoxine, 10 mg/kg, once weekly up to the maximum adult dose for the same duration

Dosage guide (pyrimethamine, 25 mg, + sulfadoxine, 500 mg [Fansidar]):

4–10 kg, 3.12 mg + 62.5 mg = 1/8 tablet weekly
10–15 kg, 6.25 mg + 125 mg = 1/4 tablet weekly

15-30 kg, 12.5 mg + 250 mg = 1/2 tablet weekly
30-50 kg, 18.75 mg + 375 mg = 3/4 tablet weekly
>50 kg, 25 mg + 500 mg = 1 tablet weekly

Oral adult dose: pyrimethamine, 12.5 mg, plus dapsone, 100 mg (Maloprim, 1 tablet), once weekly during and for 6 weeks after leaving a malarious area
Oral pediatric dose: pyrimethamine and dapsone combination not recommended for children
Oral adult dose: pyrimethamine, 25 mg, plus sulfalene, 500 mg (Metakelfin, 1 tablet), once weekly during and for 6 weeks after exposure in a malarious area
Oral pediatric dose: pyrimethamine, 0.5 mg/kg, plus sulfalene, 10 mg/kg, once weekly up to the maximum adult dose for the same duration.

Dosage guide (pyrimethamine, 25 mg, + sulfalene, 500 mg, Metakelfin): as for Fansidar.

Maloprim and Metakelfin are not available in the United States. Pyrimethamine may also be used for the treatment of active chloroquine-resistant *P. falciparum* malaria (uncomplicated attack).

Oral adult regimen: pyrimethamine, 25 mg twice a day for 3 days, plus quinine sulfate, 650 mg three times a day for 3 days, plus sulfadiazine, 500 mg four times a day for 5 days
Oral pediatric regimen: pyrimethamine, 0.5 mg/kg per dose twice a day for 3 days up to a maximum of 25 mg twice a day, plus quinine sulfate, 8 mg/kg per dose three times a day for 3 days, plus sulfadiazine, 100-200 mg/kg day^{-1} in four doses for 5 days up to a maximum of 2 g/day

The pyrimethamine-sulfadoxine combination is used for treatment in areas where strains sensitive to the antifolate sulfonamide association are present, but where 4-aminoquinolines are considered ineffective. The oral adult dose for treatment is pyrimethamine, 75 mg, plus sulfadoxine, 1500 mg, in a single dose. The oral pediatric dose for treatment is pyrimethamine, 1 mg/kg body weight, plus sulfadoxine, 20 mg/kg body weight, in a single dose. This medication is associated with quinine sulfate, 650 mg (adult dose) or 8 mg/kg per dose (pediatric dose), three times a day for 3 days (15).

The same single dose of the pyrimethamine-sulfadoxine combination is used for the acute attack of vivax malaria, followed by primaquine, 15 mg per base daily for adults or 0.3 mg/kg per base daily for children, for 2 weeks.

In areas of highly chloroquine-resistant, sulfadoxine- and pyrimethamine-resistant *P. falciparum* with *P. vivax* also present (Asia east of India, Australia, Oceania, America south of the Panama Canal, except Argentina and Paraguay), the combination of pyrimethamine, 25 mg, plus sulfadoxine, 500 mg, *plus* chloroquine or amodiaquine (300 mg base), or mefloquine (250 mg base), can be given to adults at weekly intervals for malaria suppression. The regimen for children is as follows (16):

	Sulfadoxine, 500 mg Pyrimethamine, 25 mg	Plus	Chloroquine or Amodiaquine	Or	Mefloquine
9–12 years	3/4 tablet	plus	200–300 mg base	or	125 mg base
5–8 years	1/2 tablet	plus	150–200 mg base	or	125 mg base
1–4 years	1/4 tablet	plus	50–100 mg base	or	63 mg base
<1 year	–	–	37.5–50 mg base	or	30 mg base

Pyrimethamine has been used for research purposes in combination with mefloquine and sulfadoxine in tablets containing 250 mg mefloquine, 500 mg sulfadoxine, and 25 mg pyrimethamine (ratio 10:20:1). This combination is administered at a dosage of mefloqune of 12.5–15 mg/kg body weight in a single dose (see Section VI).

F. Drug Assays

Several methods have been used to study the pharmacokinetics of pyrimethamine: thin-layer chromatography (8,17), gas chromatography (12,18), high-performance liquid chromatography (12,19), and microbiological assay. HPLC techniques have been recently devised (16,20) for the simultaneous quantitation of pyrimethamine and sulfadoxine (Fansidar), including the major metabolite of the latter, N_4-acetylsulfadoxine, and pyrimethamine and dapsone (Maloprim).

G. Therapeutic Indications

Pyrimethamine is used at present almost exclusively in combination with sulfonamides and sulfones. The combination of pyrimethamine with a sulfonamide (sulfadoxine) has been widely employed for prophylaxis and suppression and has proven effective against chloroquine-resistant strains of *P. falciparum* when given once weekly. However, even this combination is becoming less effective owing to the increasing prevalence of multidrug-resistant strains of *P. falciparum*. The same combination does not provide radical cure of vivax malaria, owing to the widespread resistance of *P. vivax* to pyrimethamine. However, suppressive cure of certain strains can be attained if suppression therapy continues for 10 weeks after leaving a malarious area.

Pyrimethamine is of limited value in treating the acute primary attack of malaria. It clears parasitemia very slowly but prevents the development of the fertilized gamete.

In combination with a short-acting sulfonamide (sulfadiazine), pyrimethamine is useful for the treatment of acute attacks of uncomplicated chloroquine-resistant falciparum malaria. Quinine should be included in this regimen to assure a prompt schizontocidal effect. This combination should never be used as a first-line agent for malaria control in areas where parasites are sensitive to 4-aminoquinolines. It should be available and reserved as a second-line drug.

H. Toxicity, Precautions, and Contraindications

At the recommended doses, pyrimethamine alone causes no significant clinical toxicity, except occasional skin rashes and depression of hematopoiesis due to the interference with folic acid metabolism by the drug. With larger doses, allergic reactions, megaloblastic anemia, leukopenia, thrombocytopenia, pancytopenia, exfoliative dermatitis, and athrophic glossitis are more likely to occur. Overdosage may cause severe vomiting, convulsions, respiratory failure, and death in children (21).

Megaloblastic anemia resembles that of folic acid deficiency; it reverses readily if treatment is discontinued or folic acid is administered.

Doses of pyrimethamine should not be increased over those recommended for suppression, except when used in combination with other agents for the treatment of strains resistant to multiple drugs. Bone marrow suppression may result from higher doses of sulfadoxine-pyrimethamine combination. Even aplastic anemias have been reported. In areas where chloroquine-resistant *P. falciparum* is highly prevalent, the pyrimethamine-sulfadoxine combination (Fansidar) is widely used as a suppressive agent. It has been reported to be well tolerated for as long as 2 years of continued prophylaxis, although users should have a leukocyte differential count every 3-6 months (15). In the last few years, however, a number of severe cutaneous reactions to Fansidar have been documented, e.g., erythema multiforme, toxic epidermic necrolysis, Lyell's syndrome, and Stevens-Johnson syndrome (22,23). Hornstein and Ruprecht (22) reported a case of Fansidar-induced Stevens-Johnson syndrome in an adult white patient, presenting with severe febrile malaise, generalized bullous skin rash, and pluriorificial mucous membrane involvement, 2 days after returning from a 3-week trip to the Sahara. The patient had taken one tablet weekly shortly before and during the trip. Major complications ensued that required a 3-month hospitalization. It is worthwhile noting that in this case pyrimethamine was specifically identified as the causative agent by a lymphocyte-transformation test done 2 months after discharge. The same test performed at an earlier date, i.e., during the recovery phase, had resulted in minimal increase of blast transformation by pyrimethamine and Fansidar, respectively. These observations have led to revise the general recommendations for Fansidar for chemoprophylaxis in combination with chloroquine (23), stressing the need for individual prescription and limiting the geographic areas in which it is specifically indicated, i.e., east and central Africa with chloroquine-resistant *P. falciparum*. Travelers to chloroquine-resistant *P. falciparum* regions in Asia and South America should take Fansidar in addition to chloroquine only if they plan to stay overnight in rural areas.

Young children receiving Fansidar should be given supplementary calcium folinate-cyanocomplex. When this combination was first introduced in 1970, the manufacturers indicated in the accompanying literature that it should not be used during pregnancy because of the known teratogenicity of pyrimethamine (preventable by supplementary folate administration) and the fear that sulfadoxine might cause kernicterus in the neonate if given in late pregnancy. Experience to date has not corroborated these warnings (24). Pyrimethamine, either alone or in combination with a sulfonamide, has been given to a large number of pregnant women during the past 30 years for malaria prophylaxis, and no teratogenic effects have been reported (25). It has been found to protect the infants and their mothers from the effects of malaria attacks, such as severe placental infections, infarcts, and inadequate fetal nutrition (26). The drug combination is unlikely to cause kernicterus at the doses used for malaria treatment and prophylaxis (27). However, since the teratogenic potential of pyrimethamine in humans has not yet been definitely resolved, other authors (28) suggest that the use of other drugs for malaria prophylaxis by pregnant women or their avoidance of travel may be more acceptable alternatives. Folinic acid supplement should be given during the first trimester of pregnancy to women receiving the pyrimethamine-sulfadoxine combination (15).

References

1. Falco, EA, Goodwin, LG, Hitchings, GH, Rollow, IM, Russel, PB: 2,4-Diaminopyrimidines, a new series of antimalarials. *Br. J. Pharmacol. Chemother. 6*:185–200, 1951.
2. Symposium on Daraprim (various authors): *Trans. R. Soc. Trop. Med. Hyg. 46*:467–508, 1952.
3. Hurly, MGD: Potentiation of pyrimethamine by sulphadiazine in human malaria. *Trans. R. Soc. Trop. Med. Hyg. 53*:412–413, 1959.
4. James, DM, Gilles, HM: Malaria. In: *Human Antiparasitic Drugs* (DM James and HM Gilles, eds.), John Wiley, Chichester, 1985, pp. 120–164.

5. World Health Organization: *Chemotherapy of Malaria and Resistance to Antimalarials*, Technical Report Series 529, World Health Organization, Geneva, 1973.
6. Cavallito, JC, Nichol, CA, Brenckman, WD, et al.: Lipid soluble inhibitors of dihydrofolate reductase. I. Kinetics, tissue distribution and extent of metabolism of pyrimethamine, methopurine and etoprine in the rat, dog, and man. *Drug Metab. Dispos.* *6*:329–337, 1978.
7. Weidekamm, E, Plozza-Notebrock, H, Forgo, I. Dubach, UC: Plasma concentrations of pyrimethamine and sulfadoxine and evaluation of pharmacokinetic data by computerized curve fitting. *Bull. WHO* *60*:115–122, 1982.
8. Ahmad, RA, Rogers, HJ: Pharmacokinetics and protein binding interactions of dapsone and pyrimethamine. *Br. J. Clin. Pharmacol.* *10*:519–524, 1980.
9. Smith, CC, Schmidt, LH: Observations on the absorption of pyrimethamine from the gastrointestinal tract. *Exp. Parasitol.* *13*:178–185, 1963.
10. Stickney, DR, Simmons, WS, De Angelis, RL, Rundles, RW, Nichol, CA: Pharmacokinetics of pyrimethamine (PRM) and 2,4-diamino-5-(3′,4′-dichlorophenyl)-6-methyl pyrimidine (DMP) relevant to meningeal leukemia. *Proc. Am. Assoc. Cancer Res.* *14*:52, 1973.
11. Brodie, BB, Barr, JE, Craig, LC: Metabolic products of the cinchona alkaloids in human urine. *J. Biol. Chem.* *188*:567–581, 1951.
12. Jones, CR, Ovenell, SM: Determination of plasma concentrations of dapsone, aminoacetyl dapsone and pyrimethamine in human subjects dosed with Maloprim. *J. Chromatogr.* *163*:179–185, 1979.
13. Brooks, MH, Malloy, JP, Bartelloni, PJ, Sheehy, TW, Barry, KG: Quinine, pyrimethamine and sulphorthodimethoxine: Clinical response, plasma levels and urinary excretion during the initial attack of naturally acquired falciparum malaria. *Clin. Pharmacokinet.* *10*:187–215, 1985.
14. White, NJ: Clinical pharmacokinetics of antimalarial drugs. *Clin. Pharmacokinet.* *10*:187–215, 1985.
15. World Health Organization: Use of antimalarial drugs. In: *Advances in Malaria Chemotherapy*, Technical Report Series 711, World Health Organization, Geneva, 1984, pp. 60–90.
16. Edstein, M: Quantification of antimalarial drugs. I. Simultaneous measurement of sulphadoxine. N_4-acetylsulphadoxine and pyrimethamine in human plasma. *J. Chromatogr.* *305*:502–507, 1984.
17. De Angelis, RL, Simmons, WS, Nichol, CA: Quantitative thin layer chromatography of pyrimethamine and related diaminopyrimidines in body fluids and tissues. *J. Chromatogr.* *106*:41–49, 1975.
18. Cala, PC, Trenner, NR, Buhs, RP, Dowing, GV, Smith, JL, Van Den Heuvel, WJ: Gas chromatographic determination of pyrimethamine in tissue. *J. Agr. Food Chem.* *20*:337–340, 1972.
19. Timm, U, Weidekamm, E: Determination of pyrimethamine in human plasma after administration of Fansidar or Fansidar-mefloquine by means of high-performance liquid chromatography with fluorescence detection. *J. Chromatogr.* *230*:107–114, 1982.
20. Edstein, M: Quantification of antimalarial drugs. II. Simultaneous measurement of dapsone, monoacetyldapsone and pyrimethamine in human plasma. *J. Chromatogr.* *307*:426–431, 1984.
21. Reynolds, JEF, Prasad, AB (eds.): Chloroquine and other antimalarials. In: *Martindale. The Extra Pharmacopeia*, 28th ed., The Pharmaceutical Press, London, 1982, pp. 394–407.
22. Hornstein, OP, Ruprecht, KW: Fansidar-induced Stevens-Johnson syndrome. *N. Engl. J. Med.* *307*:1529–1530, 1982.

23. Centers for Disease Control: Revised recommendation for preventing malaria in travelers to areas with chloroquine-resistant *Plasmodium falciparum*. *MMWR 34*: 185–195, 1985.
24. Anonymous: Pyrimethamine combinations in pregnancy. *Lancet 2*:1005–1007, 1983.
25. Hengst, P: Untersuchungen zur Teratogenität des Daraprim (Pyrimethamin) beim Menschen. *Zentralbl. Gynaekol. 94*:551–555, 1972.
26. McGregor, IA, et al.: Malaria infection of the placenta in The Gambia, West Africa: Its incidence and relationship to stillbirth, birthweight and placental weight. *Trans. R. Soc. Trop. Med. Hyg. 77*:232–244, 1983.
27. Scholer, HJ: Assessment of the safety of Fansidar to pregnancy. Animal and human data, 1983. Unpublished World Health Organization Document MSP/SGCM/INF/83.6.
28. Schwartz, IK, Campbell, CC: Indications for the use of Fansidar in malaria. *N. Engl. J. Med. 307*:194, 1982.

33
Anthelmintic Drugs

JOSE ANTONIO JESUS BODINO and EDUARDO L. LOPEZ
Children's Hospital of Buenos Aires, Buenos Aires, Argentina

Helminthiasis is the most common disease in the world. More than 2 billion people are hosts to various types of worms; this number is increasing, and infection with more than one type of helminth is common in many developing countries, particularly in tropical regions.

Human parasitic helminths are endoparasitic like the protozoa, but their highly developed functional systems and morphology are distinctive and their infections are by transmission of infective eggs or larvae. Helminths vary with respect to bodily structure, physiology, habitat, and susceptibility to the different anthelmintic drugs.

The majority of helminths do not multiply in the definitive human host. They have been defined as guerrillas repeatedly infiltrating host defense as individuals or in small groups and gradually building up into larger forces; warfare is usually by attrition and tends to be prolonged (1). Important exceptions are *Strongyloides stercoralis*, whose larvae may become infectious while in the dog, and *Echinococcus granulosus*, whose larval multiplication forms the hydatid cyst.

Substantial progress in the discovery and development of antiparasitic drugs, especially in veterinary medicine, has provided the physician with effective agents that are very useful tools in the treatment of intestinal infections. However, new drugs are needed to treat several types of systemic helminthiasis, such as echinococcosis, filariasis, and trichinoses.

The anthelmintics not only act locally, expelling worms from the gastrointestinal tract, but several drugs also have activity against several types of systemic worms that penetrate in tissues. Therefore, the term "anthelmintics" will be referred to in a wide sense: drugs used to treat local and systemic infections.

I. THIABENDAZOLE

This was the first broad-spectrum anthelmintic to be developed for use in human medicine. It was the product of investigation of several substitute benzimidazole compounds; therefore it belongs to the benzimidazole group, such as mebendazole, albendazole, flubendazole, and ciclobendazole (2).

A. Chemistry

Thiabendazole has the following chemical structural formula:

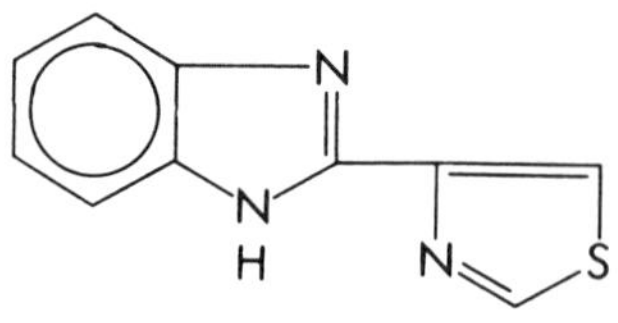

It is a stable, white crystalline compound, almost insoluble in water but soluble in dilute alkali or acid.

B. Mechanism of Action and Anthelmintic Action (Table 1)

As do other benzimidazoles, thiabendazole has high activity against a group of nematodes, and it has a complete larvicidal activity in vitro at 10 μg/ml (3). It is effective against adult worms and the larvae stage. Its ovicidal activity can be achieved in vitro at very low concentrations, and Egerton showed that a concentration 1 ppm prevents the embryonic development of *Ascaris lumbricoides* eggs in vitro (4).

Although its mechanism of action is unknown, thiabendazole has been shown to inhibit the fumarase reductase system in the sheep nematode, *Haemonchus contortus*. The mitochondrial fumarase reductase system is essential for anaerobic metabolism, the energy source for the intestinal helminths. Watts et al. showed that thiabendazole suppresses assembly of the microtubules of *Strongyloides*, leading to inhibition of secretion of parasite acetylcholinesterase and dislodgment of the *Strongyloides* (5).

Thiabendazole has no effect on filariasis.

C. Clinical Pharmacology

After oral administration, thiabendazole is rapidly and almost completely absorbed. The peak concentration in plasma occurs around 1 hr after ingestion and is approximately 15 μg/ml.

More than 40% of the drug and its metabolites (5-hydroxythiabendazole, glucoronide of thiabendazole, and sulfate ester of thiabendazole) are excreted within the first 4 hr and 80% within the first 24 hr after oral administration (6). Thiabendazole is almost completely metabolized to the 5-hydroxy form, which appears in the urine, largely as glucoronide or sulfate conjugates (7). Of the unchanged drug, 5% is found in the feces.

D. Preparation, Dosage, and Route of Administration

Thiabendazole is available as a flavored suspension containing 125, 250, or 500 mg per 5 ml. Pediatric drops containing 100 mg/ml and thiabendazole are also available as chewable tablets of 500 mg. The drug is preferably given after meals.

The standard dose for treating all roundworms is 25 mg/kg twice a day. The duration of treatment is 1 day for pinworms and 2 successive days for all other infections.

The treatment of cutaneous larva migrans (*Ancylostoma caninum*) must be continued for 5 days, and for trichinosis 5–7 days are necessary.

Table 1 Anthelmintic Activity[a]

Drug	*A. lumbricoides*	*T. trichuria*	*E. vermicularis*	*N. americans*	*A. duodenalis*	*S. stercolaris*
Mebendazole	++++	+++	++++	+++	++	++
Thiabendazole	+++	–	++	++	++	++++
Pyrantel	++++	++	+++	++	++	–
Piperazine	+++	–	+++	–	–	–
TCE	–	–	–	++	++++	–
Bephenium	+++	–	–	+++	+++	–
Levamisole	+++	–	–	++	++	–

[a]Anthelmintic activity: ++++ very high, +++ high, ++ moderate, – nil or low.

E. Drug Assay

There are two analytic procedures for the detection of thiabendazole in biologic fluids and tissues: radiometric and chemical assay methods. The radiometric method employs three forms of thiabendazole: [^{14}C] thiabendazole, tritiated thiabendazole, and [^{35}S]-thiabendazole. In the chemical assay procedure, thiabendazole and its metabolite 5-hydroxythiabendazole are determined by fluorescence after previous extraction into ethyl acetate (8).

F. Therapeutic Indications

Thiabendazole is a major drug in the treatment of *S. stercoralis* infections and of cutaneous larva migrans. There is some evidence that the drug may be useful in the treatment of visceral larva migrans. Although thiabendazole kills larvae in the muscle of pigs experimentally infected with *Trichinella spiralis*, its efficacy in established infections is questionable. However, several early cases of human trichinosis have shown marked clinical improvement (9). Other authors showed actively motile larvae in muscle biopsies after 7 days of treatment (10).

Thiabendazole produces a cure rate of 90% in pinworm. It has inconsistent efficacy in infections caused by *A. lumbricoides*, hookworm, and whipworm.

G. Toxicity (11)

Adverse effects tend to occur 3–4 hr after ingestion and they include nausea, vomiting, epigastric distress, and vertigo. Other adverse effects that occur less frequently include pruritus, skin rashes, diarrhea, headache, drowsiness, giddiness, and sensory changes. Bone marrow suppression and dermatologic changes are seen very infrequently.

Fever, chills, facial flush, and lymphadenopathy have been reported, and they may represent hypersensitivity to the drug or an allergic response to the parasite. Crystalluria, which promptly subsided on discontinuation of treatment, has also been reported. Metabolites excreted in urine and sweat may cause a foul odor. Approximately 30% of patients receiving the recommended dose experience some adverse reaction; thiabendazole is probably the least well tolerated of the currently used intestinal antinematode drugs.

H. Precautions and Contraindications

Thiabendazole is contraindicated in patients with a history of hypersensitivity and should be discontinued at the first sign of hypersensitivity. The drug is best avoided if there is renal or hepatic dysfunction.

Since central nervous system (CNS) adverse effects occur frequently, thiabendazole must not be given to patients who must operate vehicles or machinery where loss of attention could cause accidents.

References

1. Warren, KS: The guerilla worm. *N. Engl. J. Med. 282*:810–815, 1970.
2. Van Den Bossche, H, Rochette, F, Harig, C: Mebendazole and related anthelmintics. *Adv. Pharmacol. Chemother. 19*:67–128, 1982.
3. Brown, HD, Matzuk, AR, Ilves, IR, Peterson, LH, Harris, SA, Sarret, LH, Egerton, JR, Yakstis, JJ, Campbell, WC, Cuckler, AC: Antiparasitic drugs. IV. 2-(4-Thiazolyl)benzimidazole, a new anthelmintic. *J. Am. Chem. Soc. 83*:1764–1765, 1961.

4. Egerton, JR: The effect of thiabendazole upon *Ascaris* and *Stephanurus* infections. *J. Parasitol. 47*(2):37, 1961.
5. Watts, SD, Rapson, EB, Atkins, AM, Lee, DL: Inhibition of acetylcholinesterase from *Nippostrongylus brasiliensis* by benzimidazole anthelmintics. *Biochem. Pharmacol. 3*:3035–3040, 1982.
6. Tocco, DJ, Rosemblum, C, Martin, CM, Robinson, HJ: Absorption, metabolism and excretion of thiabendazole in man and laboratory animals. *Toxicol. Appl. Pharmacol. 9*:31–39, 1966.
7. Robinson, HJ, Silber, RH, Glaessle, OE: Thiabendazole: Toxicological, pharmacological and antifungal properties. *Texas Rep. Biol. 27*(Suppl. 2):537–560, 1969.
8. Tocco, DJ, Egerton, JR, Bowers, W, Christensen, VW, Rosenblum, C: Absorption, metabolism and elimination of thiabendazole in farm animals and a method for its estimation in biological materials. *J. Pharmacol. Exp. Ther. 149*:263–271, 1965.
9. Campbell, WC, Cuckler, AC: Effect of thiabendazole with treatment and control of parasitic infections in man. *Texas Rep. Biol. Med. 27*(Suppl. 2):665–684, 1965.
10. Kean, BH, Hoskins, DW: Treatment of trichinosis with thiabendazole. *JAMA 190*: 852–853, 1964.
11. Council on Drugs: Evaluation of a broad-spectrum anthelmintic thiabendazole (Mintezol). *JAMA 205*:172–173, 1968.

II. MEBENDAZOLE

Mebendazole (MBZ) is a broad-spectrum anthelmintic. It was introduced for the treatment of roundworm infection after the successful research undertaken by Brugmans and collaborators in 1971. It was approved by the Food and Drug Administration (FDA) for the treatment of infections caused by *Ascaris lumbricoides, Enterobius vermicularis*, hookworm species, and *Trichuris trichiura* in 1974.

Mebendazole and its congeners form a group of benzimidazole anthelmintics with a different spectrum from that of thiabendazole.

A. Chemistry

Mebendazole has the following structural formula:

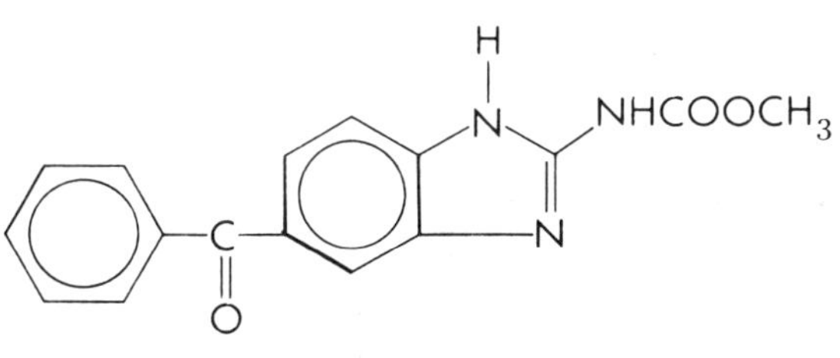

Its empirical formula is $C_{16}H_{13}N_3D_3$. It is a methyl-5-benzoylbenzimidazole-2-carbamate. Structurally, the 2-carbamomethoxy group replaces the thiazole ring substituent in thiabendazole.

Its specifications are as follows:

1. Appearance: an off-white to slightly yellow powder
2. Melting point: melts with descomposition above 280°C

3. Practically insoluble in water, ether, alcohol, and dilute mineral acids, freely soluble (50%) in formic acid

Its most important derivatives are flubendazole, cyclobendazole, and albendazole.

B. Mechanism of Action

Mebendazole selectively and irreversibly blocks glucose uptake by adult intestinal-dwelling helmintics (nematodes and cestodes) and their tissue-dwelling larvae (2,3). This leads to increased utilization of parasite glycogen, depriving parasites of their main energy source. The lack of glycogen results in decreased formation of the adenosine triphosphate required for survival and reproduction of the helminth.

Since its introduction, new information has accumulated showing the effects of glycogen depletion on the ultrastructure of the helminth. After the administration of mebendazole, the primary change is the degeneration of cytoplasmic microtubules in the teguments and intestinal cells of affected worms (4). This microtubular deterioration results in a blockage of transport secretory granules from within the Golgi apparatus of the cytoplasm. As a result of great amounts of these granules, the cytoplasm cells are lysed and death of the helminth occurs. Mebendazole also binds to host tubulin but it is more selective for the parasitic tubulin (4,5).

C. Anthelmintic Activities

Mebendazole is highly active and effective against intestinal helminths, especially *A. lumbricoides*, *Enterobius*, *T. trichiura*, and hookworms (*Ancylostoma* and *Necator*) (Table 1). It is also used in the treatment of capillariasis, and it is possibly effective against tapeworms (taeniasis). Its activity is inconsistent against *S. stercoralis.*

There is some evidence that mebendazole may be a useful alternative to diethylcarbamazine in onchocerciasis (6).

Mebendazole is a rather slow acting drug. Death of the parasites is slow, and their clearance from the gastrointestinal tract occurs more than 3 days after treatment (7).

The antiparasitic activity of mebendazole occurs at different stages of parasite development. In roundworm, hookworm, whipworm, and pinworm, it is very effective against both helminth adults and larvae. In addition, it has been found to be ovicidal, with egg failing to develop to the larval stage (8,9).

D. Clinical Pharmacology

Published data about the pharmacokinetics of mebendazole in humans is quite limited, especially in children. Absorption from the intestine is poor in experimental animals, and 80% of the given dose appears in the stools while 5% appears in the urine.

In humans receiving 200 mg/day, the plasma concentrations do not exceed 30 μg/ml. Brugmans and colleagues reported only minimal absorption after a single 0.1-mg/kg body weight oral dose of ^{14}C-labeled mebendazole in three healthy adult volunteers. Only 5–10% of the oral dose was absorbed, as judged by the total amount of radioactivity in the urine. The reason for this is the very low solubility of the compound. The remaining radioactivity was apparently excreted unchanged in the feces. Peak plasma concentrations of the drug and its metabolites represent no more than 0.5% of the total radioactivity. The peak concentration was reached within 2–4 hr (10).

Wilson and colleagues treated two patients with a high dose of oral mebendazole (40 mg/kg body weight daily) for hydatid cysts. Peak concentrations of about 0.080 μg/ml were detected at 1/2-2 hr after oral administration. Although concentrations ranged from 0.012 to 0.040 μg/ml after a 1-g dose of the drug (11), plasma concentrations did not exceed 0.030 μg/ml of unchanged mebendazole (12) in four children after ingestion of a 100-mg dose.

Recently, Dawson and colleagues, using a tracer oral dose of [^{3}H] mebendazole in five adult volunteers, showed that the average elimination half-life was 0.93 hs, the apparent clearance rate was 0.846 liter/min, and the average time to peak plasma concentration was 0.42 hs (13). The absorbed fraction was mostly metabolized in the liver, and the major metabolite detected in the urine was the 2-amino-5(6)α-benzoylbenzimidazole. It has been recently postulated that 2-amino-5(6)α-hydroxybenzoylbenzimidazole is the most important metabolite excreted in urine (14). The metabolites are excreted in 24-48 hr and represent 5-10% of the single dose.

E. Preparation, Dosage, and Route of Administration

Mebendazole is available as a suspension containing 100 mg in each 5 ml and as scored chewable tablets of 100 mg. It is also available with the same trademark in Canada, Germany, Belgium, South Africa, Australia, Italy, and The Netherlands. Other trademarks are Mebutar in Argentina and Mebendacin in Spain.

Mebendazole is given orally, and the dosage schedule is the same for adults and children. Fasting or purging is not required.

Table 2 Mebendazole: Schedule of Treatment

Infection	Dosage	Days	Follow-up
Ancylostoma duodenale	100 mg twice a day	3	Fecal examination 3-4 weeks after treatment; if eggs are present repeat therapy
Ascaris lumbricoides	100 mg twice a day	3	Fecal examination: 2-4 weeks
Capillaria philippinensis	200 mg twice a day	10-25	Multiple fecal examinations are needed over several months
Echinococcus granulo (hydatid cyst); see clinical indication	400-600 mg three times a day	30	Ultrasonography, computed tomography, and/or radionucleotide
Enterobius vermicularis	100 mg, single dose	1	Scotch tape of perianal area if symptoms persist
Necator americanus	100 mg twice a day	3	Same as *Ancylostoma*
Trichinella spiralis	300-400 mg three times a day, then 400-500 mg three times a day	3 10	Clinical muscle biopsy is necessary in severe cases
Trichuris trichiura	100 mg twice a day	3	Same as *Ascaris lumbricoides*

Table 2 shows the dosages of mebendazole and days of treatment for the different helminths.

F. Drug Assay

Two assays are available. One uses mebendazole labeled with tritium (^3H) and the other is a high-pressure liquid chromatography method. For more details, see References 10, 13, and 14.

G. Therapeutic Indications

Mebendazole is the drug of choice for the most common parasites in pediatric patients. The poor intestinal absorption of mebendazole is a therapeutic advantage in the treatment of intestinal helminths. It is extremely effective in the treatment against *T. trichiura*, *A. lumbricoides*, *E. vermicularis*, and hookworms.

Before the introduction of mebendazole, the cure rate of trichuriasis with thiabendazole was less than 35%, whereas with the use of mebendazole the mean cure rate is approximately 75% (15,20).

Mebendazole is very effective against *Ascaris lumbricoides*. One study showed a cure rate of 98.8%, with egg reduction of 99.5% after 3 days of treatment (15). Souza and colleagues showed a success rate of 100% against roundworm in 85 children (21).

The cure rates using mebendazole for pinworms range from 91% to 100% (10,12,16), and most of the studies showed that mebendazole was as efficacious as piperazine citrates, pyrantel pamoate, and pyrvinium pamoate (10,12).

Mebendazole is also indicated against both species of hookworms (*Necator* and *Ancylostoma*). In one study, 97.5% of the patients were cured of their hookworm with a 3-day course of treatment (21).

Mebendazole is also effective in the treatment of taeniasis (solium and saginata). Pena Chavarria and colleagues cured 100% of their patients, treating them with 300 mg twice a day for 3 days; however, other authors indicate cure rates of 73–90% using mebendazole for 4 days (23,24).

Finally, mebendazole is effective against *Capillaria philippinensis*. Singson and colleagues reported a 100% cure rate after a 20-day course of treatment with mebendazole (25).

H. Toxicity and Side Effects

Mebendazole is relatively free of side effects or toxic reactions (10,18). This high degree of safety probably results from its poor absorption. Mild and transient diarrhea and colicky abdominal phase occurred in children with severe ascaridiasis (7). In another report, 2 of over 100 patients treated with mebendazole complained of slight headache and dizziness (17). Rare patients treated with high doses have manifest allergic reactions, alopecia, and reversible neutropenia (26).

Mebendazole is embryotoxic and teratogenic in rats.

I. Precautions and Contraindications

Mebendazole should not be given to pregnant women, and it should not be used in patients who have experienced allergic reactions to the drug.

References

1. Van Den Bossche, H, Rochette, F, Horig, C: Mebendazole and related anthelmintics. *Adv. Pharmacol. Chemother. 19*:67–128, 1982.
2. Van Den Bossche, H: Biochemical effects of the anthelmintic drug Mebendazole. In: *Comparative Biochemistry of Parasites*, Academic Press, New York, 1972, pp. 139–157.
3. Van Den Bossche, H: The molecular basics of anthelmintic action. In: *Biochemistry of Parasites and Host-Parasite Relationships*, Elsevier-North Holland, New York, 1976, pp. 553–572.
4. Van Den Bossche, H: A look at the mode of action of some old and new antifilarial compounds. *Ann. Soc. Belg. Med. Trop. 61*:287–296, 1981.
5. Verheyen, A, Borger, SM, Vanparis, SO, Thienpont, D: The effects of mebendazole on the ultrastructure of cestodes. In: *Biochemistry of Parasites and Host-Parasite Relationships*, Elsevier-North Holland, New York, 1976, pp. 605–618.
6. Rivas Alcala, AR, Greene, BM, Taylor, HR, Dominguez Vazquez, A, Rivalcaba Macias, AM, Lugo Pfeiffer, C, Mackenzie, CD, Beltran, HF: Chemotherapy of onchocerciasis: A controlled comparison of mebendazole, levanisole and diethylcarbamazine. *Lancet 2*:485–490, 1981.
7. Pena Chavarria, A, Swartzwelder, JC, Villarejos, VM, Zeledon, R: Mebendazole, an effective broad spectrum anthelmintic. *Am. J. Trop. Med. Hyg. 22*:592–595, 1975.
8. Wagner, ED, Pena Chavarria, A: In vivo effects of a new anthelmintic, mebendazole (R 17.635) on the eggs of *Trichuria* and hookworm. *Am. J. Trop. Med. Hyg. 23*: 151–153, 1974.
9. Wagner, ED, Reyinger, DD: In vivo effects of mebendazole and levanisole in the treatment of trichuriasis and enterobiasis. *Am. J. Trop. Med. Hyg. 27*:203–205, 1979.
10. Brugmans, JP, Thienpon, DC, Van Wisngaarden, I, Vanpariss, OF, Schvermans, VL, Lavwers, HL: Mebendazole in enterobiasis: Radiochemical and pilot clinical study in 1278 subjects. *JAMA 217*:313–316, 1971.
11. Wilson, JF, Davidson, M, Rausch, RL: A clinical trial of mebendazole in the treatment of alveolar hydatid disease. *Am. Rev. Respir. Dis. 118*:747–757, 1978.
12. Committee on Drugs: Commentary on anthelmintics. *J. Pediatr. 62*:251–252, 1978.
13. Dawson, M, Braithwhite, PA, Roberts, MS, Watson, TR: The pharmacokinetics and bioavailability of a tracer dose of (^{3}H)-Mebendazole in man. *Br. J. Clin. Pharmacol. 19*:79–86, 1985.
14. Dawson, M, Watson, TR: The effect of dose form on the bioavailability of mebendazole in man. *Br. J. Clin. Pharmacol. 19*:87–90, 1985.
15. Wolfe, MS, Wershing, JM: Mebendazole: Treatment of trichuriasis and ascariasis in Bahamian children. *JAMA 230*:1408–1411, 1974.
16. Miller, MS, Krupp, JM, Little, MD, Santos, C: Mebendazole: An effective anthelmintic for trichuriasis and enterobiasis. *JAMA 230*:1412–1414, 1974.
17. Seah, SK: Mebendazole in the treatment of helminthiasis. *Can. Med. Assoc. J. 115*: 777–779, 1976.
18. Blechman, MG: Clinical effectiveness of mebendazole in the treatment of trichinosis. *Curr. Ther. Res. Clin. Exp. 18*:800–803, 1975.
19. Scragg, JN, Proctor, EM: Mebendazole in the treatment of severe symptomatic trichuriasis in children. *Am. J. Trop. Med. Hyg. 26*:198–203, 1977.
20. Scragg, JN, Proctor, EM: Further experience with mebendazole in the treatment of symptomatic trichuriasis in children. *Am. J. Trop. Med. Hyg. 27*:255–257, 1978.
21. Souza, DWC, De Souza, MS, De Neves: The therapeutic action of mebendazole in patients with multiple parasite infection. *Rev. Inst. Med. Trop. Sao Paulo 15*:30–33, 1973.

22. Pena Chavarria, A, Villarejos, VM, Zeledon, R: Mebendazole in the treatment of *Taeniasis solium* and *Taeniasis saginata*. *Am. J. Trop. Med. Hyg. 26*:118–120, 1977.
23. de Oliveira Gomes, MC: The treatment of taeniasis with mebendazole. *Folha Med. 68*:87–95, 1973.
24. Katz, N, Zicker, F: Clinical trial with mebendazole in patients with taeniasis. *Rev. Soc. Bras. Med. Trop. 7*:225–229, 1973.
25. Singson, CN, Banzon, TC, Cross, JH: Mebendazole in the treatment of intestinal cappillariasis. *Am. J. Trop. Med. Hyg. 24*:932–934, 1975.
26. Schantz, PM, Van Den Bossche, H, Eckert, J: Chemotherapy for larval echinococcosis in animals and humans: Report of a workshop. *Z. Parasitenkd. 67*:5–26.

III. PIPERAZINE

Piperazine was initially used for the treatment of gout. It was ineffective for this indication, but its anthelminthic activity has proved to be of clinical value.

Piperazine induces a flaccid muscle paralysis in the worms, which results in their expulsion with peristaltic activity.

A. Chemistry

Piperazine has the following structural formula:

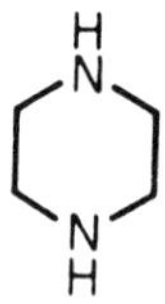

It is available as hydrate and various salts: citrate, phosphate, or as chelate compound with calcium edetate.

Hydrate piperazine is a colorless, glassy crystalline compound with a faint characteristic odor and a saline taste. Citrate piperazine is a white, odorless crystalline or granular powder with an acid taste. Phosphate piperazine is also a white, odorless crystalline powder with a slight taste. The citrate, phosphate, and calcium edetate salts are soluble in water.

The dosage of the salts of piperazine is expressed in terms of piperazine hydrate, such that 100 mg piperazine hydrate is equivalent to 120 mg piperazine adipate, 214 mg piperazine calcium edetate, 125 mg piperazine citrate, and 104 mg piperazine phosphate.

B. Mechanism of Action

The action of piperazine has been studied on isolated *Ascaris* preparations. It reversibly antagonizes the stimulating effect of acetylcholine on the *Ascaris*. It is assumed, therefore, that the drug produces a neuromuscular blockade by preventing the despolarizating effect of acetylcholine on neuromuscular function. The suggested basis of this mechanism of action is that piperazine alters the permeability of the cell membrane of ions responsible for maintaining the resting potential. This action is reversible since affected worms recover their activities if incubated in drug-free medium (1).

After paralysis is established in the worms, they are easily dislodged from the intestinal mucusa by peristalsis and are then expelled in the stools.

Piperazine affects all stages of the parasite in the gut, but it appears to have no effect on tissue larvae.

C. Anthelmintic Activity

Piperazine exerts its activity on *Ascaris lumbricoides* and *Enterobius vermicularis*. It has little activity against hookworms, tapeworms, or whipworms.

D. Clinical Pharmacology

Only sparse information exists on the disposition of piperazine. Piperazine hexahydrate and all derivatives behave in a pharmacologically similar manner. All of them are administered orally (2).

They are well absorbed from the intestine and excreted in urine mainly in unchanged form. Part of the absorbed drug is metabolized.

E. Preparation, Dosage, and Route of Administration

Piperazine is available in different forms.

Piperazine citrate is available as tablets of 250 and 550 mg and as syrups containing 550 mg per 5 ml (equivalent to 250, 550, and 500 mg hexahydrate).

Piperazine phosphate is available in other countries as tablets, each containing 500 mg piperazine hexahydrate.

The dosage is:

1. For *Ascaris* (common roundworm), adult patients: 75 mg/kg (maximum 3.5 g) as a single daily dose for 2 consecutive days. For children, give 75 mg/kg as a single daily dose for 2 consecutive days. In severe infection, the treatment course may be repeated after a 1-week interval.
2. For *Enterobius* (common pinworm), adults and children, a single daily dose of 65 mg/kg is given with a maximum daily dose of 2.5 g for 7 consecutive days.

Piperazine preparations are always given orally. The use of laxatives or enemas and dietary restriction is not necessary.

F. Therapeutic Indications

Piperazine is indicated in the treatment of ascariasis and oxyuriasis.

In circumstances in which it is desired to apply mass therapy of ascariasis as a public health measure and repeated therapy is not practical, a single dose of 70 mg/pound may be used (3,4). This procedure is successful in removing the worms in the great majority of cases.

The major practical difficulty in using piperazine to treat pinworm infection is that therapy must be continued for 7 days, and owing to reinfections a second course of treatment is necessary.

G. Toxicity

Piperazine has been used widely in humans, and it is very well tolerated; serious adverse effects are rare. Nausea, vomiting, diarrhea, abdominal pain, headache, and urticaria occasionally occur and usually disappear rapidly when the therapy is stopped. Severe neurotoxicity has been reported, and cataract formation and hypersensitivity have been reported rarely. Piperazine has been used in pregnancy without adverse reactions.

H. Precautions and Drug Interaction

The drug is contraindicated in patients with epilepsy or severe neurological disease and liver disease. Piperazine in high serum concentrations may enhance the effect of chlorpromazine.

References

1. Saz, HJ, Bueding, E: Relationships between anthelmintic effects and biochemical and physiological mechanisms. *Pharmacol. Res. 18*:871–894, 1966.
2. Rogers, EW: Excretion of piperazine salts in urine. *Br. Med. J. 1*:136–137, 1958.
3. Schwartzwelder, C, Miller, JH, Sappenfield, RW: Treatment of ascariasis in children with a single dose of piperazine citrate. *Pediatrics 16*(1):115–118, 1955.
4. Goodwin, LG, Standen, OD: Treatment of ascariasis with various salts of piperazine. *Br. Med. J. 1*:131–133, 1958.

IV. PYRANTEL PAMOATE

Pyrantel was first introduced as a broad-spectrum anthelmintic for veterinary use against roundworms, hookworms, and pinworms (1). Its effectiveness and lack of toxicity led to its use in humans (2). Successful clinical studies have resulted in its acceptance for the treatment of several nematode infections.

A. Chemistry

Pyrantel belongs to the tetrahydropirimidine group, and it is employed as the pamoate salt. Its structural formula is as follows:

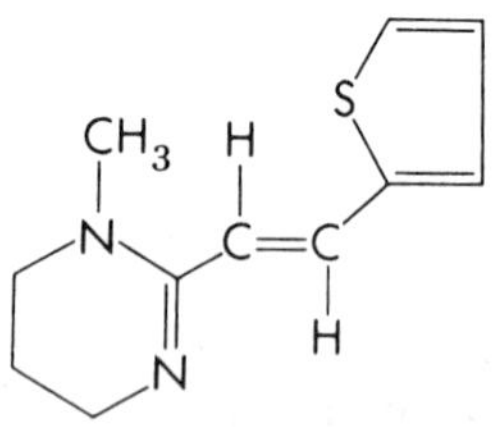

Chemically, pyrantel pamoate is 1,4,5,6-tetrahydro-1-methyl-2-[(CE)-2-(2-thienyl)-vinyl)] pyrimidine-4,4′-methylene-bis-(3-hydroxy-2-naphthoate), and its molecular weight is 594.7. The pamoate is a yellow to tan colored, odorless, tasteless crystalline powder. Pyrantel pamoate, 2.9 g, is equivalent to 1 g of pyrantel. It is practically insoluble in water, alcohol, and methylalcohol and is soluble in dimethylsulfoxide; it must be protected from light.

Two other derivatives ar oxantel pamoate, which is an m-oxyphenol analog of pyrante, and morantel.

B. Mechanism of Action

Pyrantel and its analogs owe their anthelmintic activity to their action on the worm neuromuscular system. They are depolarizing neuromuscular blocking agents. Pyrantel has a spastic effect on the worm that resembles more closely that of ganglionic stimulation in automatically innervated mammalian systems. Pyrantel's spastic effect on the worm is similar to that of nicotine and is abolished by specific ganglionic blocking agents, such as pempidine (3). In single muscle cells of *Ascaris*, pyrantel produces depolarization accompanied by increase in tension of the muscle cell. In contrast, piperazine causes hyperpolarization and relaxation in single muscle cells; thus pyrantel and piperazine are mutal antagonists (4,5).

C. Anthelmintic Action

Pyrantel pamoate has anthelmintic action against roundworm (*Ascaris*), pinworm (*Enterobius*), and hookworm. It is possibly less active against *Necator*. Pyrantel pamoate is not effective against *T. trichiura*, unlike its analog oxantel.

D. Clinical Pharmacology

Less than 10% of pyrantel pamoate is absorbed from the gastrointestinal tract. After a standard oral dose (1 g), the plasma concentrations of unchanged drug are low; peak concentrations of 0.05-0.13 μg/ml are reached in 1-3 hr. More than 50% of the dose is excreted in the feces as the unchanged form. Less than 15% is excreted in urine as parent drug and metabolites. The drug is given orally at any time without regard to ingestion of food or beverages.

E. Preparation, Dosage Regimen, and Route of Administration

Pyrantel pamoate is supplied as a pleasant-tasting caramel-flavored suspension that contains the equivalent of 50 mg pyrantel base per milligram. The bottles must be protected from light.

The dosage and administration are as follows for children and adults: a single dose of 11 mg pyrantel base per kilogram of body weight, maximum total dose 1 g. Purging is not necessary prior to, during, or after therapy. It may be taken with milk or fruit juices.

F. Therapeutic Indications

Pyrantel pamoate is effective against infections caused by *Ascaris* and *Enterobius*. It is less effective against hookworm infections.

Cure rates of 92.6% against roundworm (*Ascaris*) infections and 85.7% against hookworms have been reported (6). A group of 69 children with pinworm infections were treated with pyrantel pamoate with a cure rate of 95% (2).

Oxantel is effective against whipworm (*T. trichiura*): in mild to moderate infections a single dose of 10-20 mg/kg body weight is enough. It may be repeated after 10-14 days.

G. Toxicity

The most frequently encountered adverse reactions are related to the gastrointestinal system: anorexia, nausea, vomiting, epigastic pain, abdominal cramps, diarrhea, and tenesmus. Occasionally it may cause elevation of serum glutamic-oxaloacetic transaminase (SGOT) values, drowsiness, and insomnia.

It should be used with caution in patients with impaired liver function.

H. Drug Interactions

Because pyrantel pamoate and piperazine appear to be mutally antagonistic, it would be unwise to use them together.

References

1. Austin, WC, Courtney, W, Danilewicz, JC, Morgan, DH, Conover, LH, Howes, HL, Lynch, JE, McFarland, JW, Cornwald, RL, Theodorives, VA: Pyrantel tartrate, a new anthelmintic effective against infections of domestic animals. *Nature 212*:1273–1274, 1966.
2. Bumbalo, TS, Fugazzoto, D, Wyczalek, JV: Treatment of enterobiasis with pyrantel pamoate. *Am. J. Trop. Med. Hyg. 18*:50–52, 1969.
3. Janes, DH, Gilles, HM: Introduction of parasitic helminths. In: *Human Antiparasitic Drugs: Pharmacology and Usage*, John Wiley and Sons, Chichester, 1985, pp. 210–211.
4. Aubry, ML, Cowell, P, Davey, MJ, Shevde, S: Aspects of the pharmacology of a new anthelmintic: Pyrantel. *Br. J. Pharmacol. 38*:332–344, 1970.
5. Eyre, P: Some pharmacodynamic effects of the nematicides: Methyridine, tetramisole and pyrantel. *J. Pharm. Pharmacol. 22*:26–36, 1970.
6. Iscam, N, Chowdhury, NA: Efficacy of pyrantel pamoate in mixed parasitic infections. *Asian J. Trop. Med. Public Health 7*:81–84, 1977.

V. NICLOSAMIDE

Niclosamide was developed originally as a molluscicide (1). It has been found to be the most successful drug in treating a variety of tapeworm infections in humans and animals. It was introduced as an anthelmintic drug in 1960 (2).

A. Chemistry

Niclosamide is a chlorinated salicylanilide of relatively simple structure.

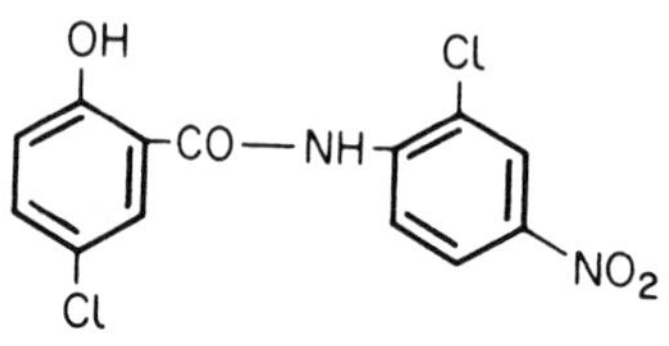

Its chemical name is 2′,5-dichloro-4′-nitrosalicylanilide. It is a cream-colored, almost odorless tasteless powder. Niclosamide is practically insoluble in water and is soluble in 1 in 150 of alcohol and 1 in 350 of ether. It is soluble in acetone, and it is necessary to protect it from light.

A large number of structural analogs of niclosamide have been synthesized to improve the biologic profile of the drug. The sodium and piperazine salts of niclosamide have been found to possess activity against a number of tapeworms. Introduction of the groups of different electronic nature in both the benzene rings of niclosamide has yielded a large variety of potent antitapeworm drugs: Terenol, oxyelzamide, and rafoxanide are particularly important.

B. Mechanisms of Action

Niclosamide exerts its anthelmintic action against a wide range of cestodes. It has a lethal effect on mature adult worms that induces the scoleces to detach and the worms to disintegrate before they are eliminated in the stools.

There is considerable evidence that niclosamide interferes with the energy metabolism of helminths. The principal action of the drug may be to inhibit anaerobic phosphorylation of adenosine diphosphate (ADP) by the mitochondria of the parasite (3,4). It is noteworthy that only parasite mitochondria are affected at therapeutic concentrations.

The other properties of niclosamide are (1) the inhibition of glucose uptake, which it shares with other anthelmintics, and (2) induction of complete muscular paralysis in the *Dipylidium caninum* (4).

C. Clinical Pharmacology

Niclosamide is not significantly absorbed from the gastrointestinal tract, and no systemic pharmacological effects have been published.

D. Preparation, Dosage, and Regimen

Niclosamide is available in 500-mg chewable tablets. These must be chewed thoroughly before swallowing and washed down with a small amount of water. For infections caused by *Taenia saginata, Taenia solium* and/or *Diphyllobothrium latum*, the patient should abstain from solid food from the evening before treatment (5).

Children weighing more than 35 kg should receive a single dose of 1.5 g. Children weighing less than 35 kg should receive 1 g. A brisk purgative is recommended to expel the killed worms 2 hr after a dose. This is to minimize the possibility of migration of *T. solium* eggs released by the disintegration of segments into the stomach with the consequent risk of cysticercosis.

The recommended dose in the treatment of infections caused by dwarfworm (*Hymenolepes nana*) should be given once daily for 7 days. A second treatment after 3 weeks is also recommended (6).

E. Therapeutic Indications

Niclosamide is the drug of choice for infections with *D. latum, Diphylidium caninum, H. nana, T. saginata*, and *T. solium* (7,8). The use of niclosamide against *T. solium* is dangerous because of the risk of provoking cysticercosis following its administration. Quinacrine is preferred by some clinicians because it causes the expulsion of *T. solium* intact.

Usually, the cure rate is around 95% with a single dose. In the case of *H. nana*, a similar cure rate is achieved if treatment is continued for up to 7 days. This duration is necessary since the parasite is embedded more deeply in the intestinal tract.

F. Toxicity

Occasional gastrointestinal upsets may occur: nausea, gastrointestinal pain, or discomfort. Moreover, the drug has no direct irritant effect. There are no alterations in hepatic or renal function or in blood counts in treated patients (9).

G. Precautions and Contraindications

No contraindications exist for the use of niclosamide as a taeniacide. No drug interactions have been described.

References

1. Agrawal, VK, Sharma, S: Salicylanilides in the treatment of helminth diseases. *Pharmazie 39*:373–378, 1983.
2. Gonnert, R, Schraufstatter, E: Experimentelle Untersuchugen Mit *N*-(2-chlor-4-Nitrophenil)-5-Chlorsalicylamid, Einen Neven Brandwurmmitel. I. Mitterlung. Chemotherapeutische Versuche. *Arzneimittel forsch. 10*:881–884, 1960.
3. Scheibel, LW, Saz, HJ: The pathway for anaerobic carbohydrate dissimilation in *Hymenolepis diminuta. Comp. Biochem. Physiol. 18*:151–162, 1968.
4. Scheibel, LW, SAZ, HJ, Bueding, E: The anaerobic incorporation of ^{32}P into adenosine triphosphate by *Hymenolepis diminuta. J. Biol. Chem. 243*:2229–2235, 1968.
5. Niclosamide. In: *Martindale. The Extra Pharmacopeia*, 28th ed. (J Reynolds, ed.), The Pharmaceutical Press, London, 1982, p. 100.
6. WHO Scientific Group: Intestinal protozoan and helmintic infections. *666*:114–115, 1985.
7. Brown, HW: Anthelmintics, new and old. *Clin. Pharmacol. Ther. 10*:5–21, 1968.
8. Jones, W: Niclosamide as a Treatment for *Hymenolepis diminuta* and *Dipylidium caninum* infection in man. *Am. J. Trop. Med. Hyg. 28*:300–302, 1979.
9. Abdallah, A, Saif, M: The efficacy of *N*-2-chloro-4-nitrophenil 5-chlorosalicylamide in the treatment of taeniasis. *J. Egypt Med. Assoc. 44*:379–381, 1961.

34
Antifilarials

JOSE ANTONIO JESUS BODINO and EDUARDO L. LOPEZ
Children's Hospital of Buenos Aires, Buenos Aires, Argentina

I. DIETHYLCARBAMAZINE

The occurrence of more than 15,000 cases of filariasis among American military personnel assigned to the Western Pacific area during World War II stimulated the search for effective filaricides. Diethylcarbamazine, a piperazine derivative, emerged as the most promising antifilarial compound (1-3). It has a broad spectrum of activity against the Filarioidea in vivo, including the microfilariae of the species *Wuchereria bancrofti, Brugia malayi, Brugia timori, Loa loa,* and *Onchocerca volvulus*, and all adult worms except *O. volvulus.*

A. Chemistry

The chemical name of diethylcarbamazine is 1-diethylcarbamyl-4-methylpiperazine. It is a derivative of piperazine, and although piperazine itself has no antifilarial activity, the piperazine ring in its structure is an essential prerequisite.

Diethylcarbamazine has the following structural formula:

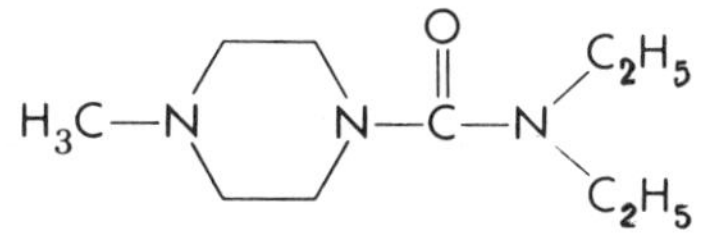

Diethylcarbamazine (DEC) was first used as the chloride but is now produced as the dihydrogen citrate, which contains only half its weight of base. For convenience and because the chloride is no longer in use, the abbreviation DEC refers in most modern textbooks to diethylcarbamazine citrate as well as to the base. In reporting doses, it is important to indicate whether the doses refer to a specific salt or to the base. *Unless otherwise indicated, it is to be assumed that the dose refers to the citrate.*

The drug is marketed as the dicitrate salt, a colorless crystalline solid, freely soluble in water, with an unpleasant sweetish taste. It is stable under all ordinary laboratory conditions, including autoclaving and cooking, when used as the medicated salt.

B. Mechanism of Action and Antiparasitic Activity

1. Microfilaricidal Effects

DEC causes the microfilariae to leave the circulation for the liver, where they become trapped and are subject to phagocytosis. However, it has been demonstrated in vitro that therapeutic concentrations of DEC have no significant effect on the microfilariae of any species. It has also been shown that the microfilaricidal action depends on the proper function of the humoral and cellular immune mechanisms of the host. Reticuloendothelial cells of the liver destroy most microfilariae, but some may remain unaffected even after repeated courses of DEC (4). The microfilariae of *W. bancrofti* in hydrocele fluid are not affected by DEC despite penetration in the fluid (4).

The drug has two types of action on susceptible microfilariae. The initial factor in their destruction is a decrease in the muscular activity of the organisms and eventually their immobilization; this may result from a hyperpolarizing effect of the piperazine moiety, causing dislocation from their normal habitat in the host (5). This is followed by changes on the surface membranes of microfilariae, increasing their susceptibility to the host defense system (2,3). The morphological changes that DEC is known to induce on the surface coat of some microfilariae may expose the parasitic antigens. The antigens, in the presence of specific antibodies, form antigen-antibody complexes that facilitate phagocytosis. This theory conforms with the finding that phagocytic destruction of microfilariae occurs only after immunity has been established (6).

The drug causes microfilariae of *O. volvulus* to disappear from the skin but does not kill microfilariae in nodules that contain adult female worms.

DEC may not achieve a complete clearing of microfilariae in all individuals. Surviving microfilariae may develop in the insect host after exposure to repeated course of DEC (4).

DEC has no effect on third-stage larvae of *W. bancrofti* in vitro, but it has a prophylactic action on *B. malayi* in cats and *Presbytis* monkeys. DEC given orally at 5 mg/kg body weight to *Prebytis* 2 days before and up to 7 days after infection was lethal to the infective larvae. With the same dosage given 29-35 days after infection, fourth-stage larvae were killed and the monkeys were protected from developing a patent infection. The possible chemotherapeutic action of DEC against *W. bancrofti* and *B. malayi* in humans is currently under investigation (4).

2. Action on Adult Worms

DEC has a considerable macrofilaricidal action against lymphatic filarial parasites in humans. Dying or dead adult worms surrounded by degenerated cells are observed in lymphatic nodular reactions after treatment with DEC. DEC has been shown to kill adult worms of *L. loa*, and there is presumptive evidence that it kills most *W. bancrofti* and *B. malayi* and *B. timori*. However, it has little action against adult *O. volvulus*. The mechanism by which DEC kills adult worms is not clear (2).

3. Action on the Recurrence of Acute Clinical Manifestations

DEC has proven effective in diminishing the frequency of attacks of funiculitis, epididymitis, orchitis, and adenolymphangitis. Longitudinal studies have demonstrated that DEC therapy also reduces the possibility of developing chronic obstructive lesions.

4. Action on Chronic Clinical Manifestations

Patients with transient lymphedema, small developing hydrocele, or chyluria usually respond well to treatment with DEC. Sometimes repeated courses are necessary to eliminate all the adult worms. Treatment of microfilariae carriers with DEC reduces the incidence of chronic diseases. DEC therapy is also beneficial to patients with early elephantiasis and pitting edema. However, patients with a large hydrocele and/or elephantiasis with deformities do not show any improvement after DEC treatment.

5. Action on Occult Filariasis

DEC is the drug of choice for tropical pulmonary eosinophilia (7). Marked clinical and hematologic improvement is achieved within a few days, but relapses may occur in as many as 20% of patients.

C. Resistance

No experimental or clinical evidence of resistance to DEC has yet been reported for any filarial parasite. Persistent microfilaremia after treatment with DEC is probably not due to resistance to the drug. Instead, it is likely to result from malabsorption of the drug or from some deficiency of the host immune system. Additional courses of DEC usually eliminate the residual microfilaremia (4).

D. Clinical Pharmacology

DEC is readily absorbed after oral (as well as cutaneous or ocular) administration, with a peak blood concentration of about 100 ng/ml, 1-2 hr after an oral dose of 50 mg. Higher doses (800 mg) generally result in peak blood concentrations of 4-5 μg/ml (4,8). DEC rapidly equilibrates with all tissues (including hydrocele and presumably other body fluids).

Metabolism of DEC is both rapid and extensive (9). Excretion is nearly all urinary, with the blood half-life depending on the urine pH. In acid urine, the blood half-life is only 2-3 hr, but in alkaline urine it is about 10-12 hr. In acid urine, 60-80% of DEC is excreted unchanged in the urine within 48 hr, with 10% appearing as DEC-*N*-oxide; 4-5% of the DEC dose is excreted in the feces (4).

E. Preparations, Dosages, Regimens, and Routes of Administration

Diethylcarbamazine citrate (Hetrazan) is available in tablets containing 50 mg.

The product is stable even under conditions of high temperature and humidity. The dosage of DEC used to treat filarial disease may be adjusted effectively according to local experience.

For *W. bancrofti, B. malayi, L. loa*, and *Dipetalonema perstans*, DEC is used at a dose of 6 mg/kg body weight per day orally, divided in three doses of 2 mg/kg per dose after meals for 7 days. This schedule aims at reducing microfilaremia to subinfective levels for mosquitoes.

DEC is used for treatment toward possible cure (10,11) as follows:

Adult dose: day 1, 50 mg; day 2, 50 mg three times daily; day 3, 100 mg three times daily; days 4-21, 2 mg/kg three times daily (6 mg/kg day^{-1})

Pediatric dose: day 1, 25-50 mg (daily dose); day 2, 25-50 mg (daily dose); day 3, 50-100 mg (daily dose); days 4-21, 2 mg/kg per dose three times daily (6 mg/kg day^{-1})

For tropical eosinophilia:

Adult dose: DEC, 2 mg/kg per dose three times daily for 7-10 days
Pediatric dose: DEC, 2 mg/kg per dose three times daily for 7-10 days

For *O. volvulus* (11):

Adult dose: days 1-3, 25 mg daily (3 days); days 4-8, 50 mg daily (5 days); days 9-11, 100 mg daily (3 days); days 12-23, 150 mg daily (12 days)
Pediatric dose: days 1-3, 0.5 mg/kg three times daily (maximum 25 mg daily); days 4-6, 1.0 mg/kg three times daily (maximum 50 mg daily); days 7-9, 1.5 mg/kg three times daily (maximum 100 mg daily); days 10-24, 2.0 mg/kg three times daily (maximum 150 mg daily)

This treatment is followed by administration of suramin IV.

Adult dose: 100-200 mg (test dose) IV, followed by 1 g IV at weekly intervals for 5 weeks (11)
Pediatric dose: 10-20 mg (test dose) IV, followed by 20 mg/kg IV at weekly intervals for 5 weeks

Seidel (12) indicates the following *pediatric* dosage for Suramin: 50 mg (test dose) IV, followed by 10-15 mg/kg IV weekly for 5 weeks (maximum 1 g weekly). Some authors use suramin only if microfilariae persist after DEC therapy and nodulectomy.

In DEC regimens for large-scale campaigns (4), repeated courses of DEC tablet administration for *W. bancrofti* filariasis, 6 mg/kg body weight for 12 days, may be necessary to lower microfilariae prevalence and density to the desired level. DEC has also been given weekly, monthly, or even yearly with successful results (13).

For *B. Malayi-B. timori* filariasis, the regimen employed varies from country to country and from time to time within a country. The range is 3-6 mg DEC per kilogram body weight per day, with a total dose of 18-72 mg/kg body weight. Repeated courses may be necessary.

The use of DEC in a mixture with salt is a special form of mass therapy using very low doses of the drug over a long period.

Common salt medicated with 1-4 g DEC per kilogram is used for filariasis control in some endemic areas of *W. bancrofti* and *B. malayi*, particularly after an initial reduction in prevalence has been achieved by mass or selective treatment of microfilaria carriers. This form of treatment is feasible only if people accept medicated salt and when health authorities exert an adequate control of the salt supply. Treatment should be continued for at least 6-9 months. In China, DEC-medicated salt has been distributed to more than 18 million people with no observed side effects and with satisfactory results.

In India, 300 million people live in zones where lymphatic filariasis is endemic. There are estimated to be at least 6 million attacks of acute filarial disease per year, and at least 15 million persons currently have one or more chronic filarial lesions. It was found that the total dose of DEC, not the size or spacing of individual doses, is more important in terms of reducing microfilaria rates and densities.

DEC was successfully used in Indonesia for filariasis control. A low-dose scheme was developed in 1977 in West Flores, an island highly endemic for *B. timori*. Health education and community participation were essential (knowledge of the parasite as a causative agent, role of mosquitoes as transmitters, recognition of the acute and chronic manifestations of filariasis, and DEC efficacy and side effects). Weekly doses were 25 mg for children below 10 years and 50 mg for adults and children aged 10 years and above. Treatment was continued for 18 months; the total dosage of DEC for an adult was thus about 4.0 g. After mass treatment with DEC was stopped, all acute cases of clinical filariasis that occurred subsequently in the community were immediately treated with 100 mg DEC three times daily for 10 days for adults and children aged 10 or more, and 50 mg DEC three times daily for 10 days for children below 10 years. With this regimen, microfilaria rates decreased dramatically to very low levels (confirmed by Nucleopore filtration) and have remained low for 3-4 years. A considerable proportion of people with lymphedema and long-standing elephantiasis have also gradually become normal again.

It is now widely recognized that it is essential to incorporate the control of lymphatic filariasis into the primary health care system. For further information on regimens of DEC administration for large-scale campaigns, the reader is referred to the Fourth Report of the WHO Expert Committee on Filariasis (14).

F. Drug Assays

Estimations of DEC concentrations in blood, body fluids, and urine can usually be made by a simple colorimetric method in the field. More accurate estimations can be obtained in the laboratory using gas-liquid chromatography (4).

G. Therapeutic Indications

DEC can be used effectively to treat infections caused by *W. bancrofti, B. malayi, B. timori, L. loa*, and *O. volvulus*. In the first four parasites, radical cure can be achieved by either single or multiple courses of treatment. For the treatment of infections caused by *O. volvulus*, radical cure is unlikely because of the drug's inability to eliminate the adult worms. Control can be achieved with short periodic courses of treatment. DEC is also effective in treating filariasis due to *D. (Acanthocheilonema) perstans*, and *Dipetalonema streptocerca* (15). It seems ineffective against *Mansonella ozzardi* (16), filaria found in Yucatan (Mexico), Panama, Venezuela, Columbia, Guyana, and the upper Amazon region of Brazil, and Argentina. *M. ozzardi* and *D. perstans* are considered nonpathogenic (10).

In patients with eosinophilic lung (tropical eosinophilia), treatment with DEC brings about a rapid disappearance of the symptoms.

H. Toxicity

Two types of reaction may occur during DEC treatment of lymphatic filariasis. The first is a pharmacological dose-dependent response to the chemical properties of the drug itself, which is equally frequent in infected and noninfected recipients. The second type of reaction is a response of the infected host to the destruction and death of the parasites, which, within limits, is independent of dose but directly related to the parasite burden.

Untoward reactions to DEC, although fairly frequent, are not severe and usually disappear within a few days despite continuation of the therapy. Drug side effects in persons without filarial infection are dose dependent and include headache, general malaise, weakness, dizziness, joint pains, anorexia, nausea, vomiting, lethargy, and hypotension. These symptoms begin within 1-2 hr of taking the drug and persist for a few hours.

There is no accumulation of the drug following prolonged administration, and chronic toxicity does not occur. No abortifacient or teratogenic effects have been reported.

Almost all patients receiving therapy exhibit leukocytosis, first evident on the second day, reaching its peak on the fourth or fifth day, and gradually subsiding over a period of a few weeks. Reversible proteinuria may occur. The eosinophilia frequently seen in patients with filariasis can be intensified by drug therapy. Ocular complications include limbitis, punctate keratitis, uveitis, atrophy of the retinal pigment epithelium, and optical neuritis (17,18). DEC may induce severe encephalitis in *L. loa* infections.

In patients infected with *O. volvulus* or *B. malayi* and to a lesser extent in those infected with *W. bancrofti* and *L. loa*, the initial systemic and/or local reactions provoked by the massive destruction of microfilariae, macrofilariae, or both during treatment may be severe. In such cases the dosage should be lowered or the drug stopped temporarily. Relief of the symptoms in heavily infected patients may be afforded by pretreatment with dexamethasone (2-4 mg per dose twice daily) or antihistaminics (19). Once the initial reactions have subsided, continued treatment should not provoke a further series of reactions. These are thought to be immunologic responses to the disintegrating microfilariae and dead adult worms. Fever may or may not be present.

Systemic reactions include headache, aches in other parts of the body, joint pains, dizziness, anorexia, malaise, urticaria, vomiting, and sometimes attacks of asthma in asthmatic patients. These side effects are observed more or less in decreasing frequency in the order given above and in varying combinations. They occur a few hours after the first dose of DEC and generally do not last more than 3 days. Fever and systemic reactions are positively associated with microfilaremia and with the density of microfilariae in the blood. By spacing doses, systemic reactions become less frequent and less intense after the second dose of DEC and rarely appear after subsequent doses. A similar reduction in reactions can be achieved by giving repeated small doses, the ultimate example being the use of DEC-medicated salt (1-4 g of DEC per kilogram of common salt). These reactions eventually cease spontaneously, and an interruption of treatment is rarely necessary. Symptomatic treatment with antipyretics or analgesics may be helpful.

Local reactions include lymphadenitis, lymphangitis, abscess, ulceration, and transient lymphedema, in decreasing frequency in the order given above and in varying combinations. In *W. bancrofti* infections, local reactions also include funiculitis, epididymitis, and orchitis. These reactions tend to occur later in the course of treatment, beginning 3-5 days up to 3-4 weeks after the first oral dose. These usually disappear spontaneously, and interruption of treatment is not necessary. Lymphedema may persist for several months after treatment, but development of elephantiasis has not been observed in well-documented follow-up studies (4).

There are no contraindications to the use of DEC. However, it is advisable to use low doses for the initial therapy, especially in onchocerciasis and loasis, with a view to minimizing adverse reactions to the destruction of parasites. Pretreatment with corticosteroids may be helpful (19). Side effects may be specially severe in patients with mixed infections due to *O. volvulus* and *L. loa*. In patients with onchocerciasis, there is usually a typical reaction within 16 hr after the first oral dose. The clinical complaint consists of intense itching and skin rashes, enlargement and tenderness of the inguinal lymph nodes, hyperpyrexia, tachycardia, and headache. These symptoms persist for 3-7 days and then subside, after which high doses can be tolerated.

References

1. Hewitt, RI, White, DE, Kushner, S, Wallace, WS, Stuart, MW, Subba Row, Y: Parasitology of piperazines in the treatment of filariasis. *Ann. N.Y. Acad. Sci. 50*: 128–140, 1948.
2. Hawking, F: Diethylcarbamazine and new compounds for the treatment of filariasis. *Adv. Pharmacol. Chemother. 16*:129–194, 1979.
3. Van Den Bossche, H: A look at the mode of action of some old and new antifilarial compounds. *Ann. Soc. Belg. Med. Trop. 61*:287–296, 1981.
4. World Health Organization: Chemotherapy. In: *Lymphatic Filariasis*, Fourth Report of the WHO Expert Committee on Filariasis, Technical Report Series 702, World Health Organization, Geneva, 1984, pp. 48–66.
5. Langham, ME, Kramer, TR: The in vitro effect to diethylcarbamazine on the motility and survival of *Onchocerca volvulus* microfilariae. *Tropenmed. Parasitol. 31*: 59–66, 1980.
6. Piessens, FW, et al.: Effect of treatment with diethylcarbamazine on immune responses to filarial antigens in patients infected with *Brugia malayi. Acta Trop. (Basel) 38*:227–234, 1981.
7. Neva, FA, Ottensen, EA: Current concepts in parasitology. Tropical (filarial) eosinophilia. *N. Engl. J. Med. 298*:1129–1131, 1978.
8. Ree, GH, Hall, AP, Hutchison, DBA, Weatherley, BC: Plasma levels of diethylcarbamazine in man. *Trans. R. Soc. Trop. Med. Hyg. 71*:542–543, 1978.
9. Faulker, JK, Smith, KH: Dealkylation and N-oxidation in the metabolism of 1-diethyl-4-methylpiperazine in the rat. *Xenobiotica 2*:59–68, 1972.
10. Markell, EK, Voge, M: The blood and tissue-dwelling nematodes. In: *Medical Parasitology*, 5th ed., W. B. Saunders, Philadelphia, 1981, pp. 232–270.
11. Anonymous: Drugs for parasitic infections. *Med. Lett. Drug Ther. 26*:27–34, 1984.
12. Seidel, JS: Treatment of parasitic infections. *Pediatr. Clin. North Am. 32*:1077–1095, 1985.
13. Partono, F, Purnomo, OS, Oemijati, S, Soewarta, A: The long term effects of repeated diethylcarbamazine administration with special reference to microfilaremia and elephantiasis. *Acta Trop. (Basel) 38*:217–225, 1981.
14. World Health Organization: *Lymphatic Filariasis*, Fourth Report of the WHO Expert Committee on Filariasis, Technical Report Series 702, World Health Organization, Geneva, 1984.
15. Ottensen, EA: Filariases and tropical eosinophilia. In: *Tropical and Geographical Medicina* (KS Warren and AA Mahmoud, eds.), McGraw-Hill, New York, 1984, pp. 390–412.
16. Bartholomew, CF, Nathan, MB, Tikasingh, ES: The failure of diethylcarbamazine in the treatment of *Manzonella ozzardi* infections. *Trans. R. Soc. Trop. Med. Hyg. 72*:423–424, 1978.
17. Rivas Alcala, AR, Greene, BM, Taylor, HR, Dominguez Vazquez, A, Ruvalcaba Macias, AM, Lugo Pfeiffer, C, Mackenzie, CD, Beltran, HF: Chemotherapy of onchocerciasis: A controlled comparison of mebendazole, levamisole and diethylcarbamazine. *Lancet 2*:485–490, 1981.
18. Dominguez Vazquex, A, Taylor, HR, Greene, BM, Ruvalcaba Macias, AM, Rivas Alcala, AR, Murphy, RP, Beltran Hernandez, F: Comparison of flubendazole and diethylcarbamazine in treatment of onchocerciasis. *Lancet 1*:137–143, 1983.
19. Greene, BM: Onchocerciasis. In: *Tropical and Geographical Medicine* (KS Warren and AAF Mahmoud, eds.), McGraw-Hill, New York, 1984, pp. 413–422.

II. IVERMECTIN

Ivermectin, a semisynthetic macrocytic lactone, is highly effective against a broad range of helmintic parasites and arthropods. It is widely used in veterinary medicine (1,2). The drug is undergoing initial clinical trials in persons infected with *O. volvulus* (3,4). Ivermectin has shown to have microfilaricidal action and minimal toxic effects. Follow-up studies suggest a sustained reduction in microfilarial counts (4,5).

Ivermectin appears to be a clearly superior agent in comparison with diethylcarbamazine. In a clinical trial performed on 30 employees (aged 19–45 years) of the Liberian Agricultural Company (6) (Grand Basse County), ivermectin was as effective for infections caused by *O. volvulus* as DEC although it was administered in a single oral dose whereas DEC was given for 8 days. Ivermectin was given in a single total dose of 12 mg (200 μg/kg) and DEC in a single dose of 50 mg/daily for 2 days, followed by 100 mg twice a day to complete an 8-day course. Treatment with ivermectin was associated with less severe and fewer systemic and ocular reactions than treatment with DEC. Ivermectin did not cause significant changes in the posterior segment of the eye (6). The efficacy of ivermectin, judging from its ability to eliminate microfilariae from the skin and ocular tissues, was at least as good as that of DEC and, as a result of its more sustained effect, probably better.

Thus, ivermectin might have the advantage of being given in a single dose and less frequently than DEC (6).

It has been assumed that the severe side effects observed with DEC therapy result from the massive death of microfilariae. However, the disparity between the microfilaricidal activity of ivermectin and the relative lack of adverse reactions noted with its use suggests that, in addition to microfilarial killing, other factors may play a part in the reactions to DEC.

The precise mechanism of action of ivermectin against helminths is not yet known. Its behavior as an agonist of γ-antibutyric acid is thought to explain its activity against nematodes (1,7).

The trials being currently performed support a predominantly microfilaricidal effect, but additional studies are obviously necessary to establish the optimal dose, the precise mechanism of action against *O. volvulus*, and the degree of safety, mainly in patients with advanced ocular damage.

The suggested pediatric dose is 0.05 mg/kg orally as a single dose (8).

References

1. Campbell, WC, Fischer, MH, Stapley, EO, Albers-Schonberg, G, Jacob, TA: Ivermectin, a potent new antiparasitic agent. *Science 221*:823–828, 1983.
2. Campbell, WC, Benz, GW: Ivermectin, a review of efficacy and safety. *J. Vet. Pharmacol. Ther. 7*:1–16, 1984.
3. Aziz, MA, Diallo, S, Lariviere, M, Porta, M: Efficacy and tolerance of ivermectin in human onchocerciasis. *Lancet 2*:171–173, 1982.
4. Awadzi, K, Dadzie, KY, Schulz-Key, H, Haddock, DRW, Gilles, HM, Aziz, MA: The chemotherapy of onchocerciasis. X. An assessment of four single-dose treatment regimens of MK-933 (IVERMECTIN) in human onchocerciasis. *Ann. Trop. Med. Parasitol. 79*:63–78, 1985.
5. Aziz, MA, Diallo, S, Lariviere, M, Diop, IM, Porta, M, Gaxotte, JP: Ivermectin in onchocerciasis. *Lancet 2*:1456–1457, 1982.

6. Greene, BM, Taylor, HR, Cupp, EW, Murphy, RP, White, AT, Aziz, MA, Schulz-Key, H, D'Anna, SA, Newland, HS, Goldschmidt, LP, Aver, CH, Hanson, AP, Freeman, SV, Reber, EW, Williams, PN: Comparison of ivermectin and diethylcarbamazine in the treatment of onchocerciasis. *N. Engl. J. Med. 313*:133–138, 1985.
7. Terada, M, Ishii, AI, Kino, H, Sand, M: *Angiostrongylus cantonensis* paralysis due to avermectin B_1a and ivermectin. *Exp. Parasitol. 57*:149–157, 1984.
8. Nelson, JD; Antiparasitic therapy. In: *1985 Pocketbook of Pediatric Antimicrobial Therapy*, 6th ed., Williams and Wilkins, Baltimore, 1985, pp. 56–62.

35
Schistosomiasis Drugs

JOSE ANTONIO JESUS BODINO and EDUARDO L. LOPEZ
Children's Hospital of Buenos Aires, Buenos Aires, Argentina

Three species of schistosomes or blood flukes cause the disease in humans, i.e., *Schistosoma mansoni, Schistosoma haematobium*, and *Schistosoma japonicum*. The exact prevalence of schistosomiasis is uncertain, but there are probably no fewer than 200 million infected persons worldwide and at least half a billion at risk. The disease is widely distributed in Africa, the Middle and Far East, and areas of South America. It is considered the second major cause of morbidity and mortality in the tropics. *S. mansoni* infections are most widespread and occur in Africa, parts of South America, the Caribbean, and the Middle East. *S. haematobium* prevails in North Africa, the Middle East, and large areas of sub-Saharan Africa. *S. japonicum* infections are restricted to China, Japan, and Southeast Asia. Marked regional variations are seen in the distribution of the disease.

The existence of the disease is determined by the presence of susceptible snail species that act as intermediate hosts and their aquatic environment. Rural development involving irrigation projects and the construction of lakes and canals may result in increased infection prevalence.

This group of trematodes, belonging to the schistosomatidial family, is unique in its morphology and many aspects of its biology.

I. METRIFONATE

Metrifonate was introduced as an organophosphorus compound with irreversible anticholinesterase properties; it was first used as an insecticide and afterward as an anthelmintic. Its first activity as anthelmintic was demonstrated in vitro against *Ascaris lumbricoides*; later it was seen that it is active against other parasites, but its schistosomicidal activity is almost exclusively against *S. haematobium.*

A. Chemical Structure

Metrifonate has the following structural formula:

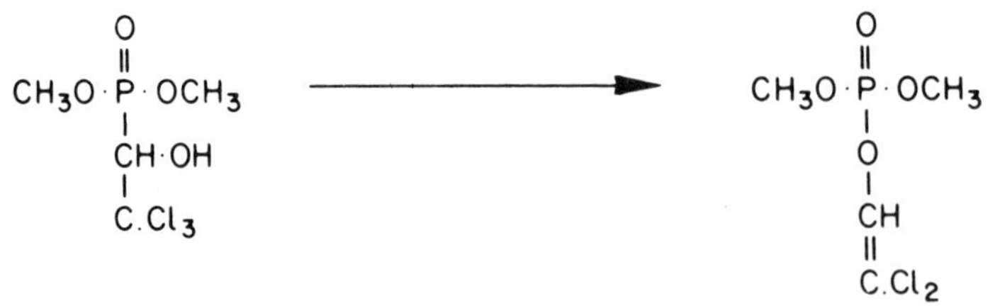

Metrifonate Dichlorovos

It is dimethyl 2,2,2-trichloro-1-hydroxyethylphosphonate. It is a white or pale yellow crystalline powder with a characteristic musty odor. It is soluble in 1 in 7 of water and soluble in alcohol and in hydrocarbons, such as xylenes and methylnaphthalenes. Solutions should be prepared immediately before use.

B. Mechanisms of Action

Metrifonate is rapidly and spontaneously transformed at physiological pH to dichlorovos (2,2-dichlorovinyl dimethyl phosphate) in vivo, and this metabolite is the active agent.

The neurotoxicity of anticholinesterases is common to insects, helminths, and mammals. In all three, cholinesterases have the same function, that is, to convert the active transmitter, acethylcholine, to the inactive base, choline. Metrifonate is an anticholinesterase with more specificity for helminth cholinesterase than mammalian cholinesterases (1,2).

Although in vitro both *S. haematobium* and *S. mansoni* cholinesterases are inhibited, *S. mansoni* infections do not respond well to the drug despite its high anticholinesterase effect in vitro. The location of *S. haematobium* in the plexus of the bladder rather than in the mesenteric venous plexus may be an important factor in the clinical effectiveness of metrifonate (3,4). The most prominent finding after the treatment of *S. haematobium* infections in humans is the reduction in the number of eggs passed in the urine, probably owing to a physical effect causing worm displacement from the vesicular veins to other sites.

C. Clinical Pharmacology

Oral administration results in peak serum concentrations of metrifonate (30 μg/ml) and of its active metabolite, dichlorvos (0.3 μg/ml), within 2 hr after a metrifonate single oral dose of 10 mg/kg. The concentrations can be detected for at least 8 hr. The half-life of both compounds in plasma is about 1.5 hr (5). Once formed, dichlorvos is rapidly metabolized in the plasma by several enzymatic degradative processes as well as by schistosomal arylesterases (6).

D. Preparation, Dosage, and Regimen

In the United States, metrifonate is available only from the Parasitic Disease Drug Service of the Centers for Disease Control (CDC).

The recommended dosage is 10 mg/kg given orally every other week in three doses.

Although it also has limited prophylactic application, it was used in highly endemic areas with good results. The prophylactic dosage is 7.5 mg/kg given once every 4 weeks (7).

E. Therapeutic Indications

Its use is practically confined to *S. haematobium* infections. The cure rate for *S. haematobium* infections is approxiamtely 50–80% (7).

F. Toxicity

The toxicity and side effects of metrifonate are related to its anticholinesterase activity. When it is indicated at the usual dosage, the plasma cholinesterase activity is rapidly reduced to a negligible level and returns to normal when therapy is stopped. However, despite these changes, the drug is well tolerated.

Other side effects include diarrhea, vomiting, abdominal pain, and vertigo; however, these adverse reactions are mild and transient.

References

1. Reiner, E, Krauthacker, B, Simeon, V, Skrinjaric-Spoljar, M: Mechanism of inhibition in vitro of mammalian acetylcholinesterase and cholinesterase in solutions of $0_1 0_1$-dimethyl $2_1 2_1 2_1$-trichloro-1-hydroxyethyl phosphonate (Trichlorophon). *Biochem. Pharmacol. 24*:717–722, 1975.
2. Symposium (various authors): Metrifonate and dichlorvos: Theoretical and practical aspects. *Acta Pharmacol. Toxicol. (Copenh.) 49*(Suppl. V):7–113, 1981.
3. Omer, AHS, Teesdale, CH: Metrifonate trial in the treatment of various presentations of *S. haematobium* and *S. mansoni* infections in the Sudan. *Am. Trop. Med. Parantol. 72*:145–150, 1978.
4. Feldmeier, H, Doehring, E, Daffala, AA, Omer, AHS, Dietrich: Efficacy of metrifonate in urinary schistosomiasis: Comparison of reduction of *S. haematobium* and *S. mansoni* eggs. *Am. J. Trop. Med. Hyg. 31*:1188–1194, 1982.
5. Nordgren, I, Bengtsson, E, Homstedt, B, Petterson, BM: Levels of metrifonate and bichlorvos in plasma and erythrocytes during treatment of schistosomiasis with bilarcil. *Acta Pharmacol. Toxicol. (Cophenh.) 49*(Suppl. V):79–86, 1981.
6. Reiner, E, Simeon, V, Skrinjaric-Spoljar, M: Hydrolysis of $0_1 0_x$-dimethyl-2-2-dichlorovinyl phosphate (DDUP) by esterases in parasitic helminths, and in vertebrate plasma and erythrocytes. *Comp. Biochem. Physiol. (C) 66C*:149–152, 1980.
7. Jewsbury, JM, Cooke, MJ, Weber, MC: Field trial of Metrifonate in the treatment and prevention of schistosomiasis infection in man. *Scand. Trop. Med. Parasitol. 71*:67–83, 1977.

II. OXAMNIQUINE

A. Chemistry

It has the following structural formula:

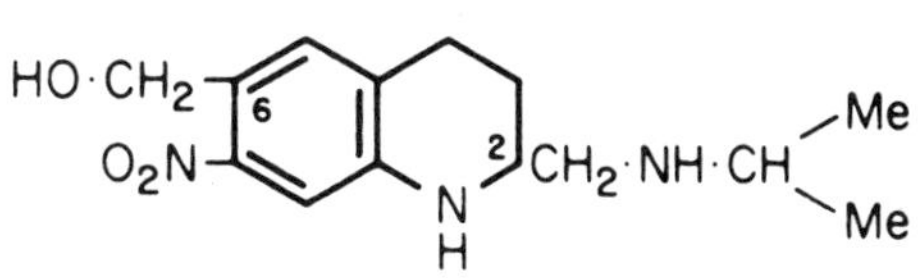

It is 1,2,3,4-tetrahydro-2-isopropylaminomethyl-7-nitro-6-quinolylmethanol. It is a light organge crystalline powder, soluble as about 1 in 3300 of water at 27°C. It is also soluble in acetone and methyl alcohol.

B. Mechanism of Action

Oxamniquine exerts its lethal effect on juvenile and adult worms. Male worms are more susceptible than female worms. Although the primary mechanism of action is unknown, the drug exhibits anticholinergic activities. The latter are evidenced by stimulation of motor activity in *S. mansoni* and inhibition of carbachol-induced paralysis. Acetylcholinesterase is not affected (1,2).

In experimental animals, a single dose of the drug causes male worms to be retained in the liver. Oxamniquine is concentrated and retained in the worms for several days, mainly as metabolites. The nature and significance of these metabolites need further investigation and could assist to clarify the exact mechanism of action.

C. Anthelmintic Activity

Oxamniquine is an effective agent in experimental and human infections due to *S. mansoni*. It has no value in the treatment of infections caused by *S. haematobium* or *S. japonium.*

D. Clinical Pharmacology

Oxamniquine is rapidly absorbed by the oral route. Peak serum concentrations are attained within 1-3 hr. Following an oral dose of 15 mg/kg, peak concentrations of 0.3–2.5 μg/ml occur, although there may be wide variation in concentrations. No detectable concentrations are measured 12 hr after an oral dose. The presence of meals delays absorption; hence the concentrations achieved in the plasma during the first hours after ingestion are low (2,3).

When the drug is administered by the intramuscular route (7.5 mg/kg), plasma concentrations rarely exceed 0.15 μg/ml. These low concentrations persist longer than after an equivalent oral dose. Most of administered dose is excreted as metabolites in the urine. Less than 2% of the dose is excreted unchanged. The main metabolite is 6-carboxyl derivative, accounting for about 70% of the excreted drug. This and the other metabolites are biologically inactive. They are excreted in urine in the first 12 hr after administration (2,3). The major metabolite is found in the gut wall during absorption. Its plasma concentrations exceed by 10-fold those of oxamniquine (4).

E. Preparation, Dosage, and Route of Administration

Oxamniquine (Vansil) is available as capsules containing 250 mg of the drug. The oral route is preferred to the intramuscular because of the severe local pain following intramuscular injection. The dosage is usually 12–15 mg/kg in a single dose. Children weighing less than 30 kg should be given 20 mg/kg in a single dose or two doses of 10 mg/kg each with an interval of 6–8 hr. The drug is better tolerated after food.

It is noteworthy that some African strains of *S. mansoni* are more resistant and require a total dosage ranging between 15 and 60 mg/kg given over 3–4 days. Thus the most appropriate regimen of administration must be conditioned by the geographic area and the characteristics of the strain.

F. Therapeutic Indications

Oxamniquine is useful only in the treatment of infections caused by *S. mansoni*. Cure rates ranging from 70 to 95% have been published (5-9). Katz et al. reported a cure rate of 73.7% achieved in 19 children with *S. mansoni* infections given a single oral dose of 20 mg/kg (7).

It is also effective in all stages of infection and in patients with toxemic and hepatosplenic involvement. Finally, oxamniquine has been used successfully in combination with metrifonate to treat mixed *S. mansoni* and *S. haematobium* infections.

G. Toxicity

The drug is usually well tolerated, but abdominal pain, dizziness, headache, vomiting, and nausea may occur. Only very rarely have other side effects been described. These include diarrhea, skin eruptions, small increases in SGOT and SGPT, excitement, and hallucinations. Convulsions have occurred very rarely in patients with a history of epilepsy. Mild eosinophilia may occur after treatment, probably due to the host reaction to dead worms.

A reddish discoloration of urine has been reported, probably due to a metabolite.

There is no experimental evidence to show that the drug exhibits mutagenicity, carcinogenicity, or teratogenicity. No drug interactions have been described.

References

1. Foster, L: The preclinical development of Oxamniquine. *Rev. Inst. Med. Trop. Sao Paulo 15*:1–9, 1973.
2. Kaye, B: Oxamniquine: metabolism, pharmacokinetics and mode of action. WHO Scientific Working Group on the Biochemistry and Chemotherapy of Schistosomiasis. WHO, Geneva 1–19, 1984.
3. Kaye, B, Woolhouse, NM: The metabolism of Oxamniquine, a new schistosomicide. *Ann. Trop. Med. Parasitol. 70*:323–328, 1976.
4. Kaye, B, Roberts, DW: The metabolism of oxamniquine in gut wall. *Xarobiotica 10*: 97–101, 1980.
5. Bassily, S, Farid, G, Higashi, I, Watten, RH: Treatment of complicated *Schistosomiasis mansoni* with oxamniquine. *Am. J. Trop. Med. Hyg. 27*:1284–1286, 1978.
6. Katz, N: Chemotherapy of *Schistosomiasis mansoni. Adv. Pharmacol. Chemother. 14*: 1–70, 1977.
7. Katz, N, Zicker, F, Pereira, SP: Field trials with oxamniquine in a schistosomiasis mansoni endemic area. *Am. J. Trop. Med. Hyg. 26*:234–237, 1977.
8. Omer, AHS: Oxamniquine for treating *Schistosoma mansoni* infection in Sudan. *Br. Med. J. 2*:163–165, 1978.
9. Abdel-Wahab, MF, Oldfield, EC, Strickland, ET, El-Shaly, A: Oxamniquine therapy of schistosomiasis in an Egyptian village. *Current Chemotherapy and Infectious Disease, Proc. XI Int. Cong. of Chemother. II*:1108–1109, 1980.

III. PRAZIQUANTEL

Praziquantel is a pyrazinoisoquinoline derivative synthesized by Seubert et al. in 1977 (1).

A. Chemistry

Praziquantel has the following structural formula:

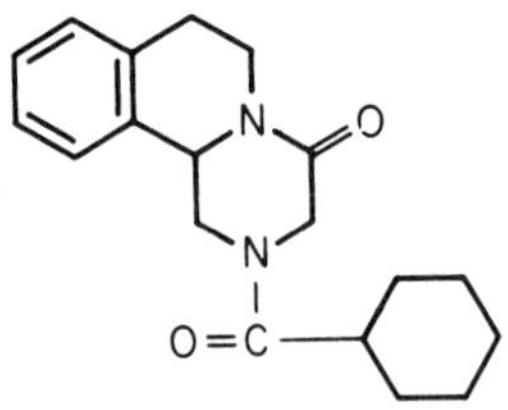

It is 2-(cyclohexylcarbanyl)-1,2,3,6,7,11b-hexahydro-2H-pyrazino-[2,1α]-isoquinolin-4-one. It is a crystalline and almost colorless powder with a distinctly bitter taste.

B. Mechanism of Action

Praziquantel exerts a rapid cestocidicidal effect in vivo, causing the worms to detach from the intestinal wall and disintegrate. Concentrations as low as 1 μg/ml cause motility changes in adult worms, such as *Taenia* and *Hymenolepis nana*. Praziquantel also has a rapid effect on *Schistosoma* (2). Animal experiments have shown that when praziquantel is administered to infested animals, it is rapidly taken up by the parasites, which fail to transform it metabolically. It causes a rapid muscular contraction in the parasites, probably by altering the permeability of cell membranes to mono- and divalent cations (2). This action probably causes the worms to lose their attachment to host tissue. It also appears to result in a reduction of endogenous glycogen and an increase in lactate release (3). Moreover, at higher concentrations, praziquantel causes vacuolization and disintegration of the teguments of worms (3). This tegumental effect is important as it is well correlated with the clinical efficacy of praziquantel (4).

C. Anthelmintic Activity

The cestodes and trematodes are most susceptible to the praziquantel action. They are paralyzed at concentrations of 0.3 μg/ml. The schistosomicidal activity of praziquantel has been confirmed in experimental studies, in which adult *S. japonicum*, the most difficult of all three important *Schistosoma* species, proved to be highly sensitive to praziquantel in mice, rabbits, and dogs (5).

Praziquantel is the only drug currently available that has activity against liver flukes (*Clonorchis sinensis, Opisthorchis viverrini, Opisthorchis filivens*, and *Fasciola hepatica*).

Praziquantel is active against Cestodiasis: *Taenia saginata* and *Taenia solium* and *H. nana*. Another important activity is against larval cestode infestations, especially cysticercosis (see Section F).

D. Clinical Pharmacology

Approximately 80% of an oral praziquantel is rapidly and readily absorbed after oral administration, with extent of absorption of 80%. Maximal serum concentrations are achieved in about 1-2 hr after a dose of 15–45 mg/kg. Despite good absorption, only a small fraction of the drug (5%) enters the systemic circulation owing to a very pronounced first-pass metabolism in the liver (5).

The recommended single dose of 20–40 mg/kg results in plasma concentrations of unchanged drug in excess of 0.3 μg/ml, which is adequate to induce paralysis of the cestodes. More than 10% of the parenterally administered drug and its metabolites are secreted into the gastrointestinal lumen (6).

Unmetabolized praziquantel is eliminated with a half-life of 1-1.5 hr; the metabolites (hydroxylation products containing one or more hydroxyl groups) have a half-life of approximately 4 hr. About 80% of a dose of praziquantel is recovered as metabolites in the urine after 4 days, and 90% of this amount is excreted within 24 hr. Praziquantel appears in breast milk in a concentration of about one-quarter that in maternal blood.

E. Preparation, Dosage, and Route of Administration

Praziquantel is provided in 600-mg tablets with three scores. To date, it is approved in the United States only for the treatment of schistosomiasis. The dosage recommended for this disease is

A single oral dose of 40 mg/kg: *S. mansoni* and *S. haematobium* (7,8)
Two to three oral doses of 30 mg/kg 4-6 hr apart: *S. japonicum*

It is recommended that the tablets be washed down with some liquid during meals.

F. Therapeutic Indications

The indications of praziqunatel are presented in Table 1.

1. Schistosomiasis

Praziquantel is the best broad-spectrum schistosomicidal drug. Several trials using a single dose of 30-40 mg/kg praziquantel against *S. haematobium* have observed success rates of 75-95% (7,9).

With respect to *S. mansoni*, a single dose of 30 mg/kg resulted in cures of 36.5-50% in children and 45-75% in adults (10). Cure rates of approximately 93% (11) have been noted in clinical trials carried out in Venezuela.

With respect to *S. japonicum*, publications from the People's Republic of China showed an almost 100% cure rate (6).

2. Other Indications

Praziquantel is also effective for the therapy of infections caused by *C. sinensis, O. viverini*, and *H. nana*.

Clinical trials were recently carried out with praziquantel for the treatment of cysticercosis in different countries (12). The drug was given at a dosage of 5-10 mg/kg to 75 mg/kg body weight daily during 7-14 days, and the results were generally encouraging; however, it is necessary to perform more double-blind clinical trials before the drug is accepted as the therapy of choice for central nervous system cysticercosis (13).

G. Toxicity

Abdominal pain and discomfort, headache, and dizziness may occur. These adverse reactions are transient and dose related.

No carcinogenciity, teratogenicity, or mutagenciity was encountered. When used in higher doses, as in the treatment of neurocysticercosis, reactions may occur that have been attributed to the death of the larvae. These reactions may include seizures, fever, headache, hypotension, and shock. Anaphylaxis has also been reported; therefore, patients who are treated with praziquantel for neurocysticercosis must be hospitalized during treatment.

Table 1 Praziquantel: Indications and Dosage

Infection	Dosage	Follow-up and comments
Schistosoma haematobium	40 mg/kg single dose	Urine examination for eggs 1 month after treatment; eventually: bladder or rectal biopsy
Schistosoma mansoni	40 mg/kg single dose	Stool examination for eggs: 1 month after treatment; eventually rectal biopsy
	30 mg/kg every 4–6 hr, two or three doses	Stool examination for eggs: 1 month after treatment or rectal biopsy
Heterophyes (intestinal fluke)	25 mg/kg every 4–6 hr, two or three doses	Stool examination for eggs: 1 month after treatment
Fasciola hepatica (liver fluke) or *Fasciolopsis buski* (intestinal fluke)	25 mg/kg every 4–6 hr, two or three doses	Stool examination for eggs: 1 month after therapy; efficacy is controversial
Metagonimus yoka gawai (intestinal fluke)	25–30 mg/kg every 4–6 hr, three doses on the same day	Stool examination for eggs: 2–4 weeks after treatment
Clonorchis sinensis (Chinese liver fluke)	Same as above	Stool examination for eggs: 1–3 months after therapy
Paragonimus westermani (lung fluke)	Same as above	Sputum and stool examination: 1–2 months after therapy
Cysticercus cellulosae (*Taenia solium*)	15–20 mg/kg twice a day, 14 days (50–60 mg/kg day^{-1} in three divided doses)	Clinical course and CAT scans

H. Precautions and Contraindications

It is contraindicated in patients with hypersensitivity to the drug. Since parasite destruction within the eye may cause severe and irreparable lesions, ocular cysticercosis should not be treated with praziquantel.

References

1. Seubert, K, Pohlke, R, Loebish, F: Synthesis and properties of praziquantel, a novel broad spectrum anthelmintic with excellent activity against schistosomal infections. *Experientia 33*:1036–1037, 1977.
2. Pax, RA, Bennet, JL, Fetterer, R: A benzodiazepine derivative and praziquantel: Effects on musculature of *Schistosoma mansoni* and *Schistosoma japonicum. Naunyn Schmeidebergs Arch. Pharmacol. 304*:309–315, 1978.
3. Andrews, P: A summary of the efficacy of praziquantel against schistosomes in animal experiments and notes on its mode of action. *Arzneimittelforsch. 31*:538–541, 1981.
4. Xiao, S, Catto, BA, Webster, LT, Jr.: Effects of praziquantel on different stages of *Schistosoma mansoni* in vitro and in vivo. *J. Infect. Dis. 151*:1130–1137, 1985.
5. Leopold, G, Ungenthum, W, Growll, E, Diekmann, HW, Nowak, H, Wegner, DHE: Clinical pharmacology in normal volunteers of praziquantel, a new drug against schistosomes and cestodes. *Eur. J. Clin. Pharmacol. 14*:281–291, 1978.
6. Pearson, RD, Guerrant, RL: Praziquantel: A major advance in anthelmithic therapy. *Ann. Intern. Med. 99*:195–198, 1983.
7. McMahon, JF, Kalstrup, N: Praziquantel: A new schistosomicide against *Schistosoma haematobium. Br. Med. J. 2*:1396–1399, 1979.
8. Katz, N, Rocha, RS, Chavez, A: Preliminary trials of praziquantel in human infections due to *Schistosoma mansoni. Bull. WHO 57*:781–785, 1979.
9. Oyediran, A, Kofie, B, Bammeke, AD, Bambboye, A: Clinical experience with praziquantel in the treatment of Nigerian patients infected with *Schistosoma haematobium. Arzneimittelforsch. 31*:581–584, 1981.
10. Prata, A, Coutinho, A, Berti, JJ, Paez de Molina, B, Coura, JR, Argento, CA, Santos, ML, Dias, LC, Katz, N, Rocha, RS, Pedro, RJ: Experience with praziquantel. *Presentations at 3rd. Workshop on praziquantel.* Rio de Janeiro 1978.
11. Webbe, G: Schistosomiasis: Some advances. *Br. Med. J. 283*:1104–1106, 1981.
12. Groll, EW: Chemotherapy of human cysticercosis with praziquantel. In: *Cysticercosis: Present State of Knowledge and Perspectives* (A Flisser, ed.), Academic Press, New York, 1982.
13. Lawner, PM: Medical management of neurocysticercosis with praziquantel. *Bull. Clin. Neurosci. 487*:102–105, 1983.

IV. NIRIDAZOLE

Niridazole was selected as the most active member of a group of 5-nitrothiazoles developed for a special drug program. It is active by oral administration against the three species of schistosomiasis.

A. Chemistry

Niridazole has the following structural formula:

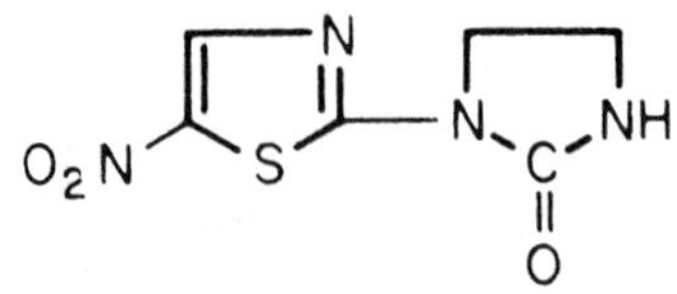

The clinical formula is 1-(5-nitrothiazol-2-yl)imidazolidin-2-one. It is a yellow, odorless, tasteless crystalline powder, practically insoluble in water and most organic solvents.

B. Mechanism of Action

Niridazole is selectively concentrated in worms and exerts its effect directly on the reproductive system. The drug acts in both sexes, but female worms are more susceptible to niridazole. The pathological effects are first noted in the gonads of both sexes: changes in the vitelline gland lead to abnormal egg formation and eventual disruption; spermatogenesis is also affected, with the formation of defective spermatozoids. The gonadal lesions are followed by the death of the worms. Enzymatic reduction of the nitro group of the niridazole by the schistosoma is required for antiparasitic activity (1).

In addition, niridazole reduces the inflammatory response to infection with *Dracunculus medinensis* and to *S. mansoni* eggs deposited in the tissues. This action is probably due to 1-thiocarbamoyl-2-imidazolidinone, a niridazole metabolite that suppresses cell-mediated immunity (2–4).

C. Anthelmintic Activity

Niridazole is very active against *D. medinensis*, and it is an alternative to praziquantel for the treatment of *S. japonicum* infections. However, in the case of dracunculiasis, some authors believe that the efficacy of niridazole has to be attributed to its anti-inflammatory properties, not to a direct effect on the adult female worm.

D. Clinical Pharmacology

Following oral administration, the drug is relatively well absorbed over a period of several hours to achieve maximum plasma concentrations in about 6 hr. The drug is rapidly metabolized during the first pass through the liver to an inactive metabolite. Because of its slow absorption and rapid metabolism, the plasma peak concentrations are low, around 0.3–0.6 μg/ml, but its different metabolites achieve higher concentrations in serum and may persist a long time because the metabolites have a high binding affinity for plasma protein (5,6).

The drug is found to concentrate in the germinal cell of the parasites, and niridazole is almost entirely eliminated as metabolic product in the urine and stools. Urine becomes dark and has an unpleasant odor.

E. Preparation, Route of Administration, and Dosage

Niridazole is not available in the market in the United States, although it is used in the United Kingdom where it is supplied in scored tables of 100 and 500 mg. Niridazole is taken orally in a dose of 25 mg/kg up to a maximum of 1.5 g in two divided doses. The duration of treatment is usually 7–10 days (see below).

F. Therapeutic Indications

Niridazole is a schistosomicide; it accumulates in eggs and gut cells of the adult worms, and it is particularly active against *S. haematobium* owing to the high concentration achieved in the portal blood; the duration of treatment for this infection is usually 7 days. It has been the drug of choice for this infection in children; however, it is being replaced by newer and safer drugs, such as praziquantel. Patients with hepatosplenic schistosomiasis should be treated in the hospital.

It is also used in the treatment of guinea worm (*D. medinenisis*). The dosage is 25 mg/kg day^{-1} in two divided doses. The duration is usually 7-10 days, although it is controversial whether it has a direct effect on the worms (7).

G. Toxicity

Niridazole is associated with numerous side effects, and there is some degree of intolerance, especially in adults. The drug may produce changes in the electroencephalograph (EEG) and cause convulsions, confusion, insomnia, and hallucinations. Central nervous system (CNS) toxicity is more frequent in patients with hepatic disease. Niridazole may produce hemolysis in patients with glucose-6-phosphate dehydrogenase deficiency (8). Depression of spermatogenesis and testicular damage have been induced in experimental animals, but in humans there is no conclusive evidence that spermatogenesis is affected to any significant degree.

The commonest side effects involve the gastrointestinal tract, with anorexia, nausea, vomiting, abdominal spasm, and headache occurring frequently. Skin reactions are uncommon. The incidence and severity of these side effects are considerably less common in children. Niridazole is carcinogenic in mice and hamsters (9,10).

H. Precautions and Contraindications

Impairment of hepatic function demands close attention to patients who receive niridazole; reduction of drug dosage may be necessary. Niridazole may also be contraindicated in patients with epilepsy, psychotic or severe neurotic behavior, or marked debilitation. Because of its possible carcinogenciity, niridazole should not be used indiscriminately.

References

1. Tracy, JW, Catto, BA, Webster, LT, Jr.: Metabolism of niridazole by adult *Schistosoma mansoni*: Correlation to covalent drug binding to parasite macromolecules. *Mol. Pharmacol. 24*:291–299, 1983.
2. Mahmoud, AAF, Mandel, MA, Warren, KS, Webster, LT, Jr.: Niridazole: A potent long-acting suppressant of cellular hypersensitivity. *J. Immunol. 114*:279–283, 1975.
3. Tracy, JW, Kazura, JW, Webster, LT, Jr.: The formation of 1-thiocarbamoyl-2-imidazolidinone. *Immunopharmacology 4*:187–200, 1982.
4. Gautam, SC, Sissors, DL, Webster, LT, Jr.: Further observations on the effect of 1-thiocarbamoyl-2-imidazolidinone in cell-mediated immunity. *Immunopharmacology 4*:201–212, 1982.
5. Valencia, CI, Catto, BA, Fairchild, EM, Wilson, SB, Maramba, NC, Webster, LT, Jr.: The concentration-time course of niridazole and six metabolites in the serum of four Filipinos with *Schistosoma japonicum* infection given niridazole. *J. Pharmacol. Exp. Ther. 230*:133–140, 1984.

6. Symposium (various authors): The pharmacological and chemotherapeutical properties of niridazole and other schistosomal compounds. *Ann. N.Y. Acad. Sci. 160*: 426–946, 1969.
7. Kothari, ML, Pardnani, DS, Anand, MP: Niridazole in dracunculiasis. *Am. J. Trop. Med. Hyg. 17*:864–866, 1968.
8. Doyen, A, Leonard, J, Mbendi, S, Sonnet, J: Influence des doses therapeutique du CIBA 32644-Ba sur l'hematopoiese des patients atteints de bilharziose et d'amibiase. *Acta Trop. (Basel) 24*:59–77, 1967.
9. Bulay, O, Urman, H, Clayson, DB, Shubik, P: Carcinogenic effects of niridazole on rodents infected with *Schistosoma mansoni. JNCI 59*:1625–1629, 1977.
10. Webster, LT, Jr., Tracy, JW, Blumer, JL, Catto, BA, Sissors, DL: Relationships of niridazole metabolism to antiparasitic efficacy and host toxicity. In: *Proceedings of IUPHAR 9th. International Congress*, Macmillan Press, London, 1984, pp. 363–367.

36
Drugs Used in the Chemotherapy of Other Protozoal Infections

JOSE ANTONIO JESUS BODINO and EDUARDO L. LOPEZ
Children's Hospital of Buenos Aires, Buenos Aires, Argentina

I. THE LEISHMANIASES: THE ANTIMONIALS: SODIUM STIBOGLUCONATE

Early in the sixteenth century, Paracelsus introduced antimony into medical treatment. Antimony gained much popularity because of its emetic effect. Although it became a popular medication during the sixteenth century, it was later abandoned because of its toxicity and lack of specific medicinal properties. Early in this century, antimonial emetic was reintroduced as a therapeutic agent, mainly because of the discovery of specific antiparasitic properties. It was first used against trypanosomiasis. Following Vianne's work on leishmaniasis in 1912, the toxic antimony compound potassium antimonyl tartrate ("tartar emetic") was used in cases of mucocutaneous leishmaniasis (Figure 1, Table 1). This subsequently led to its use against visceral leishmaniasis. The drug was employed successfully in clinical cases, as well as in controlling extensive epidemics in Assam in 1915. However, as toxicity was still a major problem, the search for better tolerated derivatives became a priority.

Trivalent antimonial compounds, notably antimony sodium tartrate, stibophen, and anthiolimine, were found to be as effective and less toxic than tartar emetic.

Later, the successful syntheses of pentavalent antimonial derivatives of phenylstibonic acid were followed by the introduction of a variety of drugs that were also effective and far less toxic than the former, thus permitting the use of larger doses and a reduction in the period of treatment.

An early member of the pentavalent antimony compound group was sodium stibogluconate. This drug has gained wide acceptance, together with meglumine antimonate, a similar compound used in French-speaking countries for the treatment of leishmaniasis (1,2).

A. Chemistry

Sodium stibogluconate has the following structural formula:

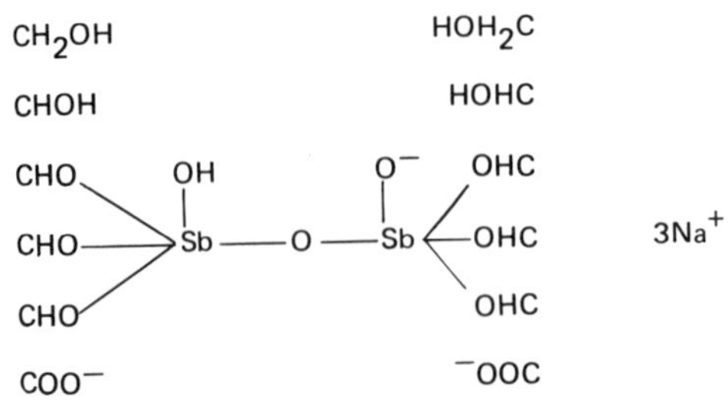

It is a colorless, amorphous powder, readily soluble in water, and contains 30–34% pentavalent antimony. It belongs to the newer pentavalent compounds that have been synthesized as substitutes for tartar emetic, which fall into two groups: (1) *p*-aminophenyl stibonic acid derivatives, in which antimony is directly linked to carbon; these compounds were probably structurally analogous to atoxyl, and the following structure was proposed:

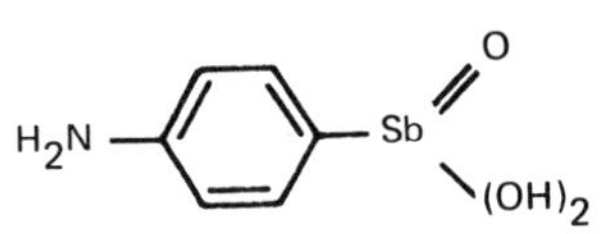

and (2) antimony acid derivatives, in which antimony is attached via an oxygen to one

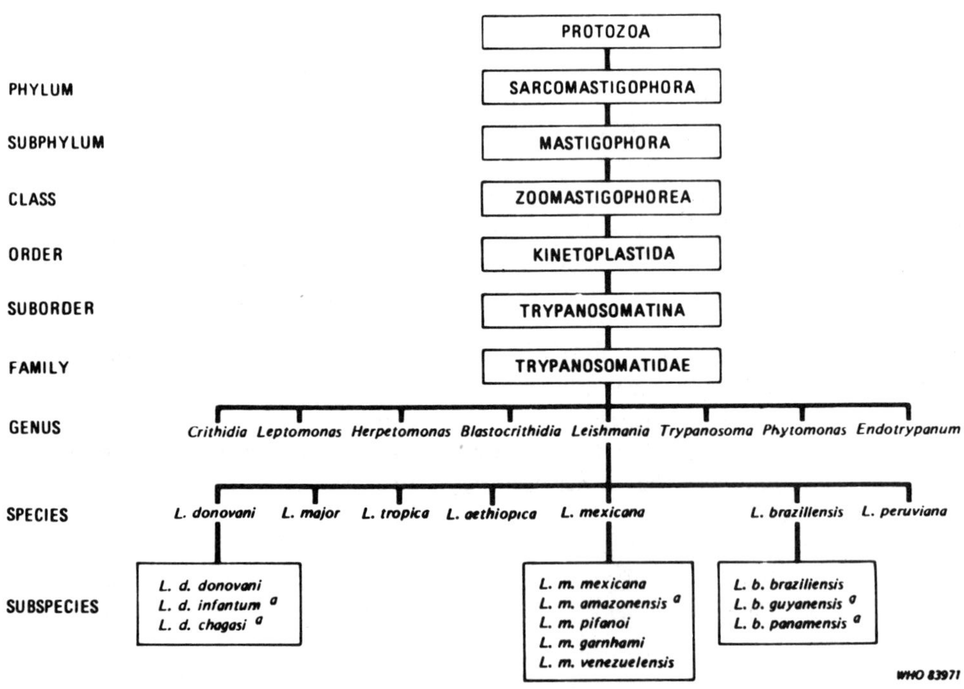

Figure 1 The taxonomy of the named species of *Leishmania* that are known to infect humans. (Reproduction authorized by the World Health Organization.)

Table 1

Species or complex	Subspecies	Geographic distribution	Type of lesion
Leishmania mexicana	*mexicana*	Mexico, Guatemala, Honduras, United States (Texas)	Cutaneous, mild "chiclero's ear ulcer"
	amazonensis	Amazon basin	Cutaneous, mild, single, diffuse
	pifarwi	Venezuela	Cutaneous, rarely seen, diffuse
	garnhanis	Venezuela	Rare, single or multiple
Leishmania braziliensis	*braziliensis*	Brazil, eastern Andes, northern Argentina, Colombia, Bolivia, Peru, Costa Rica, Paraguay	Cutaneous and mucocutaneous, extensive
	guyanensis	French Guyana, Brazil, Venezuela, Suriname	Cutaneous, multiple
	panamensis	Panama, Colombia	Cutaneous, single, multiple
	peruviana	Peru	Cutaneous, "uta," single or scarce
Leishmania tropica	*minor*	Asia, Mediterranean coast	Cutaneous, mild, self-healing
	major	Asia, North Africa	Cutaneous, acute and severe
	aethiopica	Ethiopia, Kenya	Cutaneous, mild
Leishmania donovani	*donovani*	China, India, Central and East Africa	Visceral, diffuse, severe, high fatality
	infantins	Mediterranean coast, southern USSR	Visceral, same as *L. d. donovani*
	chagasi	Brazil, Colombia, El Salvador, Honduras, Martinique, Mexico, Venezuela	Visceral, same as *L. d. donovani*

carbon, in a chain bearing a number of hydroxyl groups, such as aliphatic hydroxy acids or sugar derivatives.

Stibonic acid derivatives are structurally more complex than indicated by the structure proposed. They are unpredictable in their composition and stability and have variable biologic effects, this being probably due to certain properties, such as hydration, polymerization, and the weakness of the –C–Sb– bond. The production of these compounds is difficult because stability of the standardized product cannot be ensured.

Despite these shortcomings, stibonic acid derivatives have played an important role in the development of leishmanicidal drugs. Pentavalent antimonials have proven effective and relatively safe agents. Few derivatives are still available for use in certain areas; these include urea stibamine and ethylstibamine.

The *p*-aminophenyl stibonic acid derivatives are now mostly displaced by the antimonic acid derivatives.

Sodium stibogluconate is one of the two antimonic acid derivatives now in common use and is the drug of choice in all cases of leishmaniasis that respond to antimonials. Meglumine antimonate is preferred in French-speaking countries. Both produce similar therapeutic responses: there are few side effects, and the choice is determined by availability.

B. Mechanisms of Action and Antiprotozoal Activity

Sodium stibogluconate has little effect on leptomonads growing in tissue culture. This difference between in vitro and in vivo effectiveness suggests that activity depends on antimony reduction to the trivalent form. However, it might also be explained by a difference in sensitivity between the free flagellated forms and the intracellular forms, which cannot be readily cultured. The known pentavalent antimonials exert a high degree of leishmanicidal activity, but their active form as well as the mechanism responsible for their activity is not known.

The concentration of the pentavalent antimonials in the macrophage is likely to be greatly facilitated by their aggregative and polymeric properties. Once an effective concentration has been reached, the parent compound or a metabolite may facilitate lysosomal activity by the enveloping macrophage (3,4). Sodium stibogluconate has recently been shown to be effective in the in vitro macrophage model at concentrations attained in vivo, indicating that its activity is exclusive to its target site. The newly introduced in vitro macrophage model, which reflects the antileishmanial activity of known drugs, is an invaluable addition to the available screening methods. The finding that lysosomes can greatly enhance the delivery of the standard drugs in experimental models in vivo is based on the location of the parasite within the reticuloendothelial system and on the lysosome affinity of the carrier. It is anticipated that this will lead to improved methods of drug delivery in humans.

C. Clinical Pharmacology

Sodium stibogluconate is not bound by erythrocytes and attains much higher concentrations in plasma than the trivalent compounds.

After an injection of either sodium stibogluconate or meglumine antimonate, Sb^{5+} is excreted in the urine so that blood antimony concentrations fall to less than 10% of the peak concentrations about 8 hr after injection. Peak concentrations of antimony of about mg/liter occur 1-2 hr after intramuscular injection, and concentrations of up to 100 mg/liter occur immediately after intravenous injection of a dose of Sb^{5+} of 10 mg/kg body weight.

The slight accumulation of the drug in the body is reflected by a small increase in blood concentrations some 24 hr after injection, compared with the preinjection concentration. There is no further incremental accumulation after about 10 days. For example, a Sb concentration of 0.05 mg/liter 24 hr after the first dose may rise to 0.1-0.3 mg/liter before injection on day 10 of treatment (5). After intramuscular injection, over 80% of the administered dose appears in the urine within 6 hr. After intravenous injection, 95% of the dose appears in the urine within the same time, indicating that sodium stibogluconate is not metabolized appreciably. The drug is rapidly cleared by the kidney, with minimal tissue binding, mainly in the liver and spleen. Daily injections are adequate to maintain therapy.

D. Preparation

Sodium stibogluconate is available through the Parasitic Disease Drug Service, Centers for Disease Control, Atlanta, Georgia, as a 33% solution containing 330 mg of the drug per milliliter, equivalent to 100 mg pentavalent antimony (Sb^{5+}).

E. Administration

The drug may be given intramuscularly or by careful intravenous injection. The latter should be made slowly in no less than 5 min through a fine needle (23-25 gauge; 0.6-0.5 mm) to minimize the risk of thrombosis.

F. Dosage

On a weight-for-weight basis, children require more Sb^{5+} than adults and tolerate it better. No toxic signs were observed following a dose of 20 mg/kg body weight once daily. In both adults and children, tolerance is adversely affected by impaired renal function. The results of a study carried out in Kenya showed that a dose of 10 mg/kg body weight given every 8 hr for 10 days was not toxic and resulted in a significantly more rapid clearance of parasites from splenic aspirates than did the same dose given daily. Single pentavalent antimony doses of 30 mg/kg, on the other hand, are associated with increased toxicity (5).

First-line therapy is intended to provide an adequate daily dosage of Sb^{5+} for long enough to achieve parasitological cure without relapse. The regimen should be simple but must allow for the greater requirements of Sb^{5+} in children. As the drug is only slightly accumulated in the body and rapidly excreted by the kidney, there is no risk of cumulative toxicity and no need to interrupt treatment with rest periods.

G. Treatment Regimen

The initial treatment of *visceral leishmaniasis* (or kala-azar), caused by *Leishmania donovani*, should be based on a daily injection of 20 mg Sb^{5+} per kilogram body weight to a maximum of 850 mg (5). This implies a maximum daily dose of 8.5 mg sodium stibogluconate (or 10 ml meglumine antimonate). The injections should be given for a minimum of 20 days. The duration of treatment varies from one endemic area to another, but therapy should be continued in any case for 2 weeks after parasitological cure. Pentamidine is used for relapsed and irresponsive patients.

For *Leishmania braziliensis* (American mucocutaneous leishmaniasis), and *Leishmania mexicana* (American cutaneous leishmaniasis):

Adult dose: 10 mg/kg daily (maximum 600 mg daily) IM or IV for 10 days (may be repeated)

Pediatric dose: 10 mg/kg daily (maximum 600 mg daily) IM or IV for 10 days

An alternative is amphotericin B. For *Leishmania tropica* (oriental sore, cutaneous leishmaniasis):

Adult dose: 10 mg/kg daily (maximum 600 mg daily) IM or IV for 10 days (may be repeated)
Pediatric dose: 10 mg/kg daily (maximum 600 mg daily) IM or IV for 10 days

H. Therapeutic Indications

Treatment objectives are to cure the patient (who is often malnourished and immunosuppressed) of an intracellular parasite infection, to prevent relapse and the development of unresponsiveness, and to minimize hospitalization. To achieve these goals an appropriate drug must be given at an adequate dose level and frequency for a suitable period of time.

Sodium stibogluconate is the drug of choice for leishmaniasis, given either intravenously or by the intramuscular route, in courses of 10 days or more depending on the clinical form or on the endemic area.

Infants tolerate rather larger doses in proportion to body weight than do adults. In very debilitated patients who appear to react unfavorably to the initial dose, it may be advisable to administer the drug on alternate days or at longer intervals.

In the treatment of oriental sore (*L. tropica*), rapid disappearance of parasites has been reported following infiltration of the solution around the edges of the lesions. The total volume used should not exceed 2 ml at any one time. Otherwise, a single course of 10 days should prove effective in almost all cases.

Sodium stibogluconate may not be effective in some cases of mucocutaneous leishmaniasis (*L. braziliensis*). Cuatious treatment with amphotericin B may be successful in this condition (6).

I. Toxicity

Pentavalent antimony compounds are less toxic than the trivalent derivatives. This low toxicity is attributable to their rapid clearance.

Tolerance is generally good, except when dosage is increased to compensate for a poor response to therapy or in patients with renal insufficiency.

Common side effects include headache, lethargy, anorexia, vomiting, nausea, severe coughing, itching, and malaise. Myalgia, arthralgia, bradycardia, pneumonitis, and mild rashes may occur. Electrocardiographic changes are dose dependent, the most common being T-wave inversion, prolonged Q-T interval, and fusion of the S-T segment and T wave. Renal damage is rarely reported. Less common complications are hepatocellular damage, hemolysis, anemia, thrombocytopenia, and anaphylaxis associated with urticaria, laryngeal edema, and visceral collagen.

The patient should be assessed before treatment for nutritional status. Baseline measurements should include serum albumin, hemoglobin and leukocyte count, coagulation function, liver enzymes, urea, and creatinine. The electrocardiogram (ECG) should be taken if the doses of pentavalent antimonial compounds are higher than recommended.

Hypersensitivity reactions are rare and occur only after multiple courses of treatment.

J. Contraindications

Sodium stibogluconate is given in life-threatening situations, but myocarditis, hepatitis, liver disease, and concurrent bacterial and viral infections contraindicate its use. An ECG should be obtained if concurrent heart disease is suspected. Treatment with sodium stibogluconate should be discontinued if there is progressive proteinuria, severe arthralgia, or rash. Hemorrhagic complications, especially epistaxis, hemoptysis, or intestinal bleeding, may occur. These are probably due to either hypoprothrombinemia or thrombocytopenia and may be precipitated by the intake of salicylates (aspirin).

II. MEGLUMINE ANTIMONATE

The drug is also known as *N*-methylglutamine antimonate. The combination of antimonic acid with organic amines was known to result in a product that could be stabilized by adding a carbohydrate. A stable preparation was thus obtained by combining antimonic acid with *N*-methylglutamine, an aminosugar and product of glucose and methylamine. Although the chemical structure of meglumine antimonate has not been established, it is likely to be complex as with all derivatives of the polymeric antimonic acid.

Its mechanisms of action, antiprotozoal (leishmanicidal) activity, pharmacokinetics, therapeutic indications, toxicity, and contraindications are similar to those of sodium stibogluconate. It is widely used in French-speaking countries.

Meglumine antimonate solution contains about 8.5% Sb^{5+} (85 mg/ml), whereas sodium stibogluconate solution contains about 10% Sb^{5+} (100 mg/ml). The same doses are used as for sodium stibogluconate.

Drug equivalence: 10 ml meglumine antimonate contains 850 mg Sb^{5+}; 8.5 ml sodium stibogluconate contains 850 mg Sb^{5+}.

References

1. Findlay, GM: *Recent Advances in Chemotherapy*, Vol. 1, Churchill, London, 1950.
2. Beveridge, E: Chemotherapy of leishmaniasis. In: *Experimental Chemotherapy*, Vol. 1 (RJ Schnitzer and F Hawking, eds.), Academic Press, New York, 1963, pp. 257–287.
3. Steck, EA: The chemotherapy of protozoal infections: Whither? *J. Protozool. 28*:30–35, 1981.
4. Chang, KP: Cellular and molecular mechanisms of intracellular symbiosis in leishmaniasis. *Int. Rev. Cytol. 14* (Suppl.):267–305, 1983.
5. World Health Organization: Control methods. In: *The Leishmaniases*, Technical Report Series 701, World Health Organization, Geneva, 1984, pp. 99–115.
6. Sampaio, SA, Godoy, JT, Paiva, L, Dillon, NL, Lacas, C da S: The treatment of American (mucocutaneous) leishmaniasis with amphotericin B. *Arch. Dermatol. 82*:627–635, 1960.

III. THE TRYPANOSOMIASES: PENTAMIDINE

Pentamidine is a member of the diamidine group of drugs. Diamidines are derivatives of synthalin (decamethylenguanidine), a hypoglycemic drug with a high degree of hepatotoxicity. Several derivative compounds were developed on the premise that hypoglycemia in the host might effectively induce a trypanocidal effect by interfering with trypanosome glycolysis. This activity, however, was soon found to be unrelated to trypanosomal glycolysis interference but likely to have some bearing on the drug's ability to bind with DNA. The discovery of the chemotherapeutic activity of the diamidines was quite fortituous (1,2). The three compounds that were found to possess outstanding activity in African trypanosomiasis and visceral leishmaniasis are 4,4′-diamidinostilbene (stilbamidine), 4,4′-diamidinophenoxypentane (pentamidine), and 4,4′-diamidinophenoxypropane (propamidine). Pentamidine has proved to be the most useful, being most stable, least toxic, and easy to administer. Hydroxystilbamidine isethionate (2-hydroxy-4,4′-diamidinostilbene diisethionate) have proven useful in the treatment of North American blastomycosis and visceral leishmaniasis.

A. Chemistry

Pentamidine, 4,4′-diaminodiphenoxypentane di-(β-hydroxyethane sulfonate), has the following structural formula:

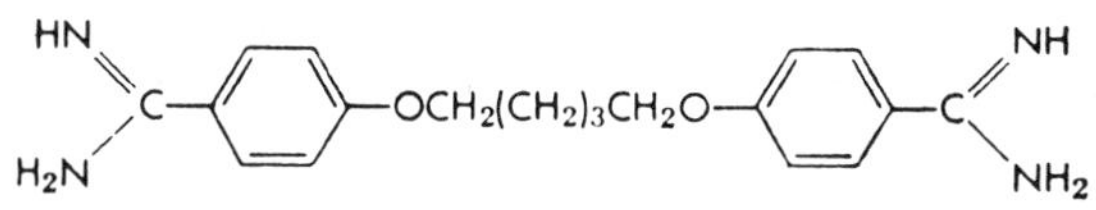

Pentamidine isethionate, the preparation currently available, is a white powder soluble in water to the extent of 10%. It is presented as a dry powder in vials containing 300 mg of the drug (Pentam 300). Solutions must be used shortly after preparation and protected from light to prevent the formation of hepatotoxic substances.

B. Mechanism of Action

The biologic activity of the aromatic diamidines is dependent on two intact terminal amidine groups and their separation by phenyl as well as by methylene and/or O and N linkages, which form a bridge.

The trypanocidal action of pentamidine and other diamidines is attributed to the two amidine groupings in the molecule. Their spatial positioning with respect to each other, which depends on the length of the bridge that separates them and on the conformation the molecule assumes, appears to be a determining factor for activity in related compounds of pentamidine and diminazene. Both compounds concentrate in the parasites. In the case of pentamidine, concentration is a carrier-mediated process.

The mechanism of action of the diamidines has not yet been precisely established. Their trypanocidal activity may emanate from interactions of these compounds with DNA or nucleotides and their derivatives. There is a binding affinity for DNA that is non-intercalative, with high affinity for kinetoplast DNA (kDNA) causing suppression of kinetoplast replication and function. This preferential binding results from permeability factors rather than from molecular differences in the macromolecules, since DNA from all sources can bind effectively to these drugs in vitro. The binding to kDNA results in structural kinetoplast changes and the production of dyskinetoplastic trypanosomes, which, although unable to infect the insect vector, are still capable of dividing in the mammal. This effect, therefore, cannot alone account for the trypabocidal activity of the diamidines. Other mechanisms may act independently or may be inhibited as a consequence of the drug's selective effect on the kinetoplast.

The fine structural changes that diamidines induce in trypanosomes resemble those induced by known inhibitors of DNA synthesis. Thus function may be a vulnerable target in trypanosomes, owing to their inability to synthesize purine de novo.

It has also been suggested that these drugs interfere with the uptake or function of polyamines (3–5). Further studies are needed for the correct understanding and interpretation of these and other structural and biochemical changes in parasites exposed to diamidine drugs.

C. Antiprotozoal Activity

A number of protozoa are vulnerable to diamidines, but the action of these agents has been shown to be quite selective. Pentamidine is curative in *Trypanosoma rhodesiense* and *Trypanosoma congolense* infections in experimental animals but ineffective against *Trypanosoma cruzi*-infected mice. It cures *Babesia canis* infections in puppies and *L. donovani* infections in hamsters. The treatment of human leishmaniasis and trypanosomiasis with diamidines is based on these experimental findings.

Pentamidine may be useful in the treatment of pneumonia caused by *Pneumocystis carinii* (6–9).

Diamidines are also fungicidal. This activity has been demonstrated in vitro against *Blastomyces dermatitidis*. These drugs have proven effective in curing systemic blastomycosis. Although amphotericin B is preferred to the diamidines for the initial treatment of this disease, hydroxystilbamidine is a good alternative in the absence of an adequate response to the antibiotic.

D. Clinical Pharmacology

The pharmacokinetics of pentamidine have not been extensively studied but are inferred from data on other diamidines, particularly stilbamidine. Pentamidine isethionate is thought to be incompletely absorbed when given by the oral route. This assumption is derived from studies done with stilbamidine and diminazene, the latter a diamidine used in animal trypanosomiasis. Pentamidine isethionate is fairly well absorbed from parenteral sites of administration. After being injected, it is detectable in the blood for only a brief period and then excreted slowly in the urine in the unchanged form. Peak blood concentrations after daily doses of 4 mg/kg body weight are generally less than 1 mg/liter, but concentrations of 0.2–0.4 mg/liter persist for at least 24 hr and urinary excretion extends for several weeks. Experimental studies by Waalkes and co-workers (10) showed that the drug was stored for months in the liver and kidney of laboratory animals.

The value of pentamidine for trypanosomiasis prophylaxis seems to reside in its tissue-binding properties. However, the drug is ineffective in the later stages of African trypanosomiasis, owing to its poor penetrability into the central nervous system (CNS).

E. Preparation, Dosages, Regimens, and Routes of Administration

Pentamidine isethionate is supplied in single-dose ampuls containing 200 mg. In the United States, the drug is available from the Parasitic Disease Division, Centers for Infectious Diseases, Atlanta, Georgia.

In adults the drug should be dissolved in no more than 3 ml sterile distilled water. Children should be given a 100 mg/ml solution. The drug must be kept refrigerated.

Pentamidine is preferably given by intramuscular injection in individual doses of 2–4 mg base per kilogram body weight, daily or every other day. Intravenous administration causes severe adverse reactions. A course of 10 injections is given in the early (hemolymphatic) stage of *Trypanosoma gambiense* infections. The drug is ineffective once the CNS is involved. As neurological involvement may be expected to occur very early in *T. rhodesiense* infections (especially in non-Africans), pentamidine is not used because it does not penetrate the blood-brain barrier. It is used for treatment of *L. donovani* infections (visceral leishmaniasis) and in some cases of *P. carinii* pneumonia.

For early African trypanosomiasis (*T. gambiense*),

Therapeutic doses (children and adults): 4 mg/kg daily IM, course of 10 injections
Prophylactic doses (children and adults): 3–5 mg/kg in a single dose IM, given at intervals not longer than 6 months

For *L. dovonani* infection (visceral leishmaniasis or kala-azar), for children and adults give 2–4 mg/kg daily IM, course of 15 doses. A second course, given after a 2-week interval, may be necessary in areas where response to treatment is known to be poorer.

For *P. carinii* infections in children and adults, give 4 mg/kg daily IM, course of 12–14 doses.

F. Therapeutic Indications

Pentamidine is indicated as a alternative treatment in the early (hemolymphatic) stages of *T. gambiense* infections. The drug is far less effective in *T. rhodesiense* than in *T. gambiense* infections because of the early invasion of the CNS by *T. rhodesiense* (11,12).

Pentamidine has been used successfully as an alternative agent in the treatment of visceral leishmaniasis. A second course, given after an interval of 1 or 2 weeks, is administered in some endemic areas where the infection is known to be less responsive to treatment. Pentamidine is particularly useful in cases who have failed to respond to antimonials. For example, many Chinese patients are hypersensitive to antimonial compounds, and in the Sudan high doses of antimonials are needed to treat visceral leishmaniasis. For patients who are unresponsive to pentavalent antimonials, treatment with pentamidine or amphotericin B is recommended. Some success in the treatment of cutaneous leishmaniasis (*L. tropica* infection or Oriental sore) has been reported (13).

Treatment of *P. carinii* infections involves courses of pentamidine of 12–14 days. If treatment succeeds, clinical improvement will be observed 4–6 days after the first injection. Improvement also depends on supportive therapy and on the elimination of predisposing conditions. Debilitated patients with altered immunity or concomitant neoplastic disease have a poorer prognosis (7). Trimethoprim-sulfamethoxasole combination is preferred for these infections.

G. Toxicity

Intravenous injection of pentamidine and other diamidines very often brings about dangerous reactions, such as breathlessness, tachycardia, vomiting, dizziness, or loss of consciousness. These reactions are likely to result from the abrupt fall of blood pressure, which may be partly due to the release of histamine or to a too rapid intravenous administration. It is advisable that resuscitation equipment always be available in the setting where drug therapy is administered, for prompt use in cases of hypotension or profound shock. Although sterile abscesses may occur at sites of injection, the intramuscular route is better tolerated. Intramuscular injection may also be followed by hypotension, tachycardia, nausea, vomiting, and metallic taste.

Acute renal failure has been reported in the course of therapy. Hypoglycemia may occur on days 5-7 of therapy and may be life threatening if not recognized (14,15). However, it is usually reversible in patients with normal renal function prior to treatment (16).

Mild anemia, leukopenia, and elevation of the liver transaminases also may occur.

References

1. King, H, Lourie, EM, Yorke, W: Studies in chemotherapy. XIX. Further report on new trypanocidal substances. *Ann. Trop. Med. Parasitol. 32*:177–192, 1938.
2. Lourie, EM, Yorke, W: Studies in chemotherapy. The trypanocidal action of certain aromatic diamidines. *Ann. Trop. Med. Parasitol. 33*:289–304, 1939.
3. Damper, D, Patten, CL: Pentamidine transport and sensitivity in *bruceu*-group trypanosomes. *J. Protozool. 23*:349–346, 1976.
4. Bacchi, CJ: Content, synthesis and function of polyamines in trypanosomatids: Relationship to chemotherapy. *J. Protozool. 28*:20–27, 1981.
5. Meshnick, SR: The chemotherapy of African trypanosomiasis. In: *Parasitic Diseases*, Vol. 2 (JM Mansfield, ed.), Marcel Dekker, New York, 1984, pp. 165–199.
6. Ivady, G, Paldy, L, Koltay, M, Toth, G, Kovaks, Z: *Pneumocystis carinii* pneumonia. *Lancet 1*:616–617, 1967.
7. Walzer, PD, Perl, DP, Krogstad, DJ, Rawson, PG, Schultz, MG: *Pneumocystis carinii* pneumonia in the United States. *Ann. Intern. Med. 80*:83–93, 1974.
8. Hughes, WE, Feldman, S, Chaudhary, SC, Ossi, MJ, Cox, F, Sanyal, SK: Comparison of pentamidine isethionate and trimethoprim-sulfamethoxazole in treatment of *Pneumocystis carinii* pneumonia. *J. Pediatr. 92*:285–291, 1978.
9. Hughes, WE, Kuhn, S, Chaudhary, S, Feldman, S, Verzosa, M, Aur Jar, Pratt, C, George, SL: Successful chemoprophylaxis for *Pneumocystis carinii* pneumonitis. *N. Engl. J. Med. 297*:1419–1426, 1977.
10. Waalkes, TP, Denham, C, De Vita, VT: Pentamidine: Clinical pharmacological correlations in man and mice. *Clin. Pharmacol. Ther. 11*:505–512, 1970.
11. Apted, FIC: Present status of chemotherapy and chemoprophylaxis of human trypanosomiasis in the Eastern Hemisphere. *Pharmacol. Ther. 11*:391–413, 1980.
12. Brener, Z: Present status of chemotherapy and chemoprophylaxis of human trypanosomiasis in the Western Hemisphere. *Pharmacol. Ther. 7*:71–90, 1979.
13. Beveridge, E: Chemotherapy of leishmaniasis. In: *Experimental Chemotherapy*, Vol. 1 (RJ Schnitzer and F Hawking, eds.), Academic Press, New York, 1963, pp. 257–287.
14. Wang, JJ, Freeman, AI, Gaeta, JF, Sinks, LF: Unusual complications of pentamidine in the treatment of *Pneumocystis carinii* pneumonia. *J. Pediatr. 77*:311–314, 1970.
15. Sharpe, SM: Pentamidine and hypoglycemia. *Ann. Intern. Med. 99*:128, 1983.
16. De Vita, VT, Emmer, M, Levine, A, Jacobs, B, Berard, C: *Pneumocystis carinii* pneumonia. *N. Engl. J. Med. 280*:287–291, 1969.

IV. MELARSOPROL

Malarsoprol is an arsenical compound. Arsenical compounds were the first trypanocidal drugs to be introduced early in this century. The intial clinical trials carried out in Africa in 1907 were encouraging enough for Ehrlich to decide to focus on this group of chemicals. He studied a variety of arsenical compounds in order to find one with the most favorable chemotherapeutic index.

A. Chemistry

Melarsoprol has the following structural formula:

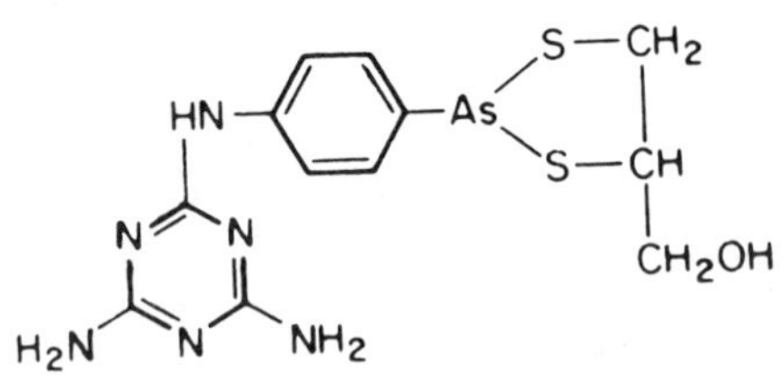

It is derived from Melarsen, and its phenylarsenoxide with the melaminyl moiety in the p-position. Investigators introduced arsenic and antimony compounds containing this group on the premise that nitrogen-containing groups conferred antitrypanosome activity. The melaminyl structure with its six symmetrically arranged nitrogen atoms was an interesting choice. Melarsen, the pentavalent form, was no more toxic than Atoxyl, but was more active than both Atoxyl and tryparsamide. The trivalent Melarsen arsenoxide was highly trypanocidal and had a good therapeutic index; however, problems arose during the clinical trials owing to its toxicity and side effects. Finally, melarsoprol, its dimercaprol derivative, proved to be successful in increasing the safety of arsenic treatment (1,2).

It is available in the United States only from the Parasitic Disease Division, Centers for Disease Control, Atlanta, Georgia.

Melarsoprol is provided as a 3.6% (w/v) sterile solution in propylene glycol.

B. Mechanisms of Action and Antiprotozoal Effects

The mechanism of action of the arsenoxide structure is based on its attachment to the trypanosome by covalent bonding. Ehrlich suggested that the attachment involves essential sulfydryl (–SH) groupings, and this is substantiated by the protective action that exogenous sulfydryl compounds induce against arsenoxide activity and toxicity. Such compounds mask the arsenoxide grouping and prevent its combination with endogenous –SH, which probably forms part of the arsenoxide receptor in parasite and host tissue.

Although the endogenous reaction is slowly reversible, such a combination involving essential parasitic –SH groups can readily exert its lethal effect by blocking these biologically active groups. Host tissue is also susceptible to arsenoxide effects, but to a lesser degree. It is now generally accepted that these vital groups in the parasite are attached to enzymes. They are distributed very abundantly on the parasite surface and account for the rapid concentration of arsenicals on parasites following drug exposure. An enzyme with a high affinity for arsenoxide may form part of the parasite's unique glycolytic process. Phosphopyruvate kinase is highly sensitive (3). Flynn and Bowman (3) demonstrated that arsenical drugs act differently upon this terminal glycolytic enzyme, phosphopyruvate kinase, depending on whether the source of the enzyme is trypanosomal or mammalian. Mammalian tissues oxidize the drug to nontoxic and readily excreted pentavalent compounds more rapidly than does the protozoan. Besides, melarsoprol may be able to enter the parasite more readily than mammalian tissue cells.

Some arsenic-resistant parasites may resemble host cells in that they have become less permeable to organic arsenicals (4).

C. Clinical Pharmacology

The drug is relatively insoluble in water and is available as a solution in propylene glycol for intravenous administration. Despite the many dangers involved, this is the preferred route because it ensures that the desired blood concentration is rapidly achieved. Blood concentrations of 0.3-0.5 μg/ml are obtained, which decrease gradually over a period of several days. A small but therapeutically significant amount of the drug enters the cerebrospinal fluid and has a lethal effect on trypanosomes affecting the CNS. Low concentrations may be detected by biologic methods (less than 0.01 μg/ml), the arsenic content being equivalent to that in blood. Concentrations were measured chemically. These determinations confirm penetrability into the CNS (5,6).

The drug is excreted quickly. However, more pharmacokinetic data are needed at both experimental and clinical levels (5,6).

D. Preparation, Dosage, Regimes, and Routes of Administration

Melarsoprol is available through the Parasitic Disease Service, Centers for Disease Control, as a 3.6% solution in propylene glycol in 6-ml ampuls. The drug must be kept refrigerated.

It is administered by slow intravenous injection through a fine needle, avoiding extravasation into surrounding tissues because it is intensely irritating. All syringes and needles used must be sterilized dry.

For pediatric patients (7,8), a total dose of 18-25 mg/kg should be given over 1 month. The initial dose is 0.36 mg/kg IV, increasing gradually to a maximum of 3.6 mg/kg at intervals of 1-5 days for a total of 9-10 doses.

According to other authors (6), maximal single doses in children should not exceed 1.8 mg/kg.

For adult patients (8), give 2-3.6 mg/kg daily IV for 3 consecutive days; after 1 week, 3.6 mg/kg daily IV for 3 consecutive days; repeat again after 10-21 days, 3.6 mg/kg daily IV for 3 consecutive days.

Smaller doses should be given to debilitated patients. Particularly in late *T. rhodesiense* infections, the initial dose may be 1.8 mg/kg, the full dosage being given at the end of the first course.

Following such regimens, about 80-90% of patients are cured. Some may relapse, and some of the relapsing cases will be refractory to further treatment with melarsoprol.

E. Therapeutic Indications

Melarsoprol is indicated for the treatment of the meningoencephalitic stage (late stage) of African trypanosomiasis. It is extremely effective in all advanced cases of both Gambian and Rhodesian varieties of disease. Its therapeutic action is invaluable in the more acute Rhodesian infections, which so far have proven refractory to all other available drugs. It is not effective against *T. cruzi*.

Melarsoprol is very active against both the early and late stages of trypanosomiasis; it is effective against tryparsamide-resistant strains and does not produce ocular toxicity. For these reasons it has largely superseded tryparsamide. The drug is also effective in the treatment of the early hemolymphatic stage of the disease. However, because of its toxicity, it is used only for treatment of cases with CNS involvement. For the same reasons, it has no place in prophylaxis. Its use requires considerable care; hospitalization is essential, and patients need to be assessed before being subjected to therapy.

F. Toxicity

Toxicity correlates with blood concentrations of arsenic above 3 μg per 100 ml. Fatalities occur at concentrations between 100 and 1500 μg per 100 ml.

Side effects are common during treatment with melarsoprol (9). A febrile reaction may occur soon after drug injection, mainly if parasitemia is high. The greatest danger is the reaction the drug may induce by its rapid lethal effect on the trypanosomes within the CNS. This is referred to as the Javisch-Hercheimer type of reactive encephalopathy and occurs between days 4 and 12 after the first dose of melarsoprol. It usually subsides, and additional treatment does not produce further deterioration. It is estimated that around 2-10% of the cases treated react to melarsoprol in this manner. The condition is fatal in approximately 1-5%. However, deaths have become less frequent due to better knowledge of the use of the drug. Patients with pronounced cerebrospinal fluid changes are prone to this complication. Hemorrhagic encephalopathy during treatment, although uncommon, may be fatal. Hypersensitivity reactions may develop later after successive courses of treatment. After recovery, a small dose provokes a lesser reaction, and desensitization may be attained by starting with smaller doses and increasing these slightly, allowing time for recovery, until it is possible to give a final 3 to 4-day course in full dosage. Corticosteroids are sometimes indicated in these cases. Agranulocytosis is very seldom observed.

Treatment must be modified if casts are detected in the urine or if there is evidence of hepatic disturbance.

Other toxic effects observed are those involving the cardiovascular system, peripheral nervous system, and skin. Vomiting and abdominal colic may be present but their occurrence can be reduced by injecting the drug slowly in the supine, fasting patient. The patient should remain in bed, not erect, for several hours after the drug is injected.

Immediate reactions to drug administration are common; some are due to the solvent (propylene glycol), which is highly irritant to tissues. A brown swelling may appear at the site of injection, which will take quite a long time to be absorbed.

G. Contraindications

The use of the drug is contraindicated during epidemics of influenza. Patients with glucose-6-phosphate dehydrogenase deficiency treated with melarsoprol may present severe hemolytic reactions. Administration of the drug to leprous patients may precipitate erythema nodosum.

Melarsoprol should be given only to hospitalized patients, and the initial dosage should be based upon clinical assessment of the general condition of the patient rather than on body weight.

References

1. Friedheim, EAH: L'acide triazine-arsinique dans le traitement de la maladie du sommeil. *Ann. Inst. Pasteur (Paris) 65*:108–118, 1940.
2. Vanhoof, LMJJ: Observations on trypanosomiasis in Belgian Congo. *Trans. R. Soc. Trop. Med. Hyg. 40*:728–761, 1947.
3. Flynn, IW, Bowman, IBR: Further studies on the mode of action of arsenicals on trypanosome pyruvate kinase. *Trans. R. Soc. Trop. Med. Hyg. 63*:121, 1969.

4. Eagle, H, Doak, GO: The biological activity of arsenosobenzenes in relation to their structure. *Pharmacol. Rev. 3*:107–143, 1951.
5. James, D, Gilles, HM: The trypanosomiasis. In: *Human Antiparasitic Drugs. Pharmacology and Usage* (D James and HM Gilles, eds.), John Wiley, Chichester, 1985, pp. 72–91.
6. Hawking, F: Chemotherapy of trypanosomiasis. In: *Experimental Chemotherapy*, Vol. 1 (RJ Schnitzer and F Hawking, eds.), Academic Press, New York, 1963, pp. 129–256.
7. Committee on Infectious Diseases (American Academy of Pediatrics): *Report of the Committee on Infectious Diseases (Red Book)*, 19th ed., American Academy of Pediatrics, Evanston, Illinois, 1982, pp. 193–197.
8. Anonymous: Drugs for parasitic infections. *Med. Lett. Drug Ther. 26*:27–34, 1984.
9. Robertson, DHH: Chemotherapy of African trypanosomiasis. *Practitioner 188*:80–83, 1962.

V. SURAMIN

Suramin evolved from the dye substances in which Ehrlich first established antitrypanosoma activity. Such dyestuffs as trypan red, trypan blue, and afridol violet showed trypanocidal activity, and after several years of research in Germany, suramin was introduced into therapy in 1920. It is a nonmetabolic, symmetrical derivative of urea similar to the dyes but devoid of their staining properties. It is used primarily for treatment of early cases of both Gambian and Rhodesian trypanosomiasis without CNS involvement, and for onchocerciasis.

A. Chemistry

Suramin sodium has the following structural formula:

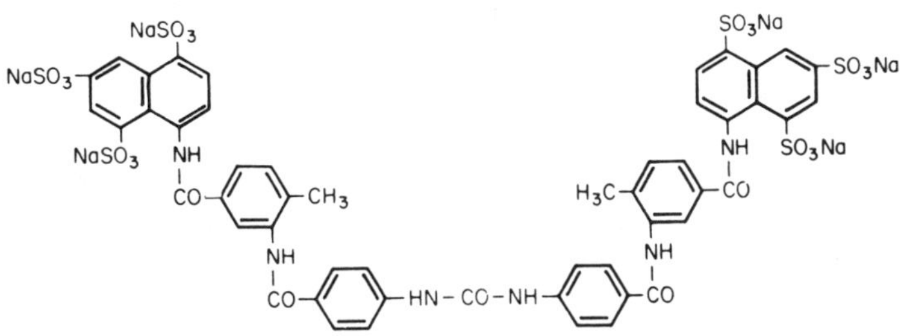

It is a white, microcrystalline powder, readily soluble in water to yield a neutral solution. Only freshly prepared solutions should be employed. Suramin is not marketed in the United States but is available from the Parasitic Disease Division, Centers for Disease Control, Atlanta, Georgia.

B. Mechanism of Action and Antiprotozoal Effects

Investigators are still unable to explain the mode of trypanocidal action of suramin, particularly because the drug inhibits so many trypanosomal enzymes (1). Inhibition is achieved at very low concentrations, thus making it difficult to study such system in isolation for investigating the specific antiparasitic action. Inhibition of glycerol phosphate oxidase, a parasite enzyme involved in energy metabolism, correlates with the antitrypanosomal activity of several derivatives of suramin (2). Furthermore, the energy metabolism of trypanosomes obtained from suramin-treated animals is reduced; the delayed onset of drug activity may be due to slow endocytic uptake by the parasite of a suramin-plasma protein complex. Besides its affinity for proteins, with which it combines, forming complexes, suramin readily combines with other large molecules, including some cationic drugs.

Its prompt effect in vivo suggests that the drug is effective in its unchanged form. Perceptible changes in the parasite, however, are slow to develop. The parasite loses infectivity (its ability to divide in a fresh host), and in the infected host it divides more slowly. This altered replicative process might be related to the drug's known inhibitory effect on RNA polymerase. As mentioned before, the effect on glycolytic enzymes (glycerol phosphate oxidase) is almost certain.

C. Clinical Pharmacology

Absorption of suramin from the intestine is poor, and the intravenous route is therefore employed. Intramuscular and subcutaneous administration are avoided because they cause intense local irritation. The plasma concentration of the drug following intravenous administration falls fairly rapidly for a few hours, then more slowly for a few days, and then achieves a low concentration, which is maintained for as long as 3 months. This persistence is mainly due to its firm binding to plasma protein, but the slow excretion of unbound drug is also contributory. There is no evidence of metabolism, and the large, polar compound apparently lacks appreciable penetration into red blood cells.

Tissue concentrations are uniformly lower than those in the plasma. The drug is present in the form of accumulated intracellular granules found within the cells of the reticuloendothelial system and the kidney tubules. Kidneys of experimental animals have been found to contain considerably more suramin than other organs. This retention in the kidney may account for the fairly frequent occurrence of albuminuria following injection of suramin in humans. The drug does not penetrate into the cerebrospinal fluid in appreciable amounts.

D. Preparation, Dosage, Regimens, and Routes of Administration

Suramin sodium is available through the Parasitic Disease Drug Service, Centers for Disease Control, Atlanta, Georgia, as capsules containing 1.0 g powder. Solutions must be prepared just before use by adding 10 ml sterile, distilled water. It should not be used if it has been in solution more than 30 min.

It is usually given by slow intravenous injection in 10% aqueous solution. It is the drug of choice for the acute hemolymphatic stage of African trypanosomiasis of African sleeping sickness (*T. gambiense* and *T. rhodesiense*) before CNS involvement. Treatment of active African trypanosomiasis should not be started until 24 hr after diagnostic lumbar puncture is performed.

In case of CNS involvement, melarsoprol should be used.

Suramin is used in children at the dose of 20 mg/kg day^{-1} IV on days 1, 3, 7, 14, and 21, after a test dose of 2 mg/kg. The daily dose should not exceed 1 g.

The adult dose is 100–200 mg (test dose) IV, then 1 g IV on days 1, 3, 7, 14, and 21.

In onchocerciasis, suramin is used after treatment with diethylcarbamazine. The pediatric dosage (3,4) is 10–20 mg IV (test dose), followed by 15–20 mg/kg IV at weekly intervals for 5 weeks. The adult dosage is 100–200 mg IV (test dose), followed by 1 g IV at weekly intervals for 5 weeks.

E. Therapeutic Indications

Suramin is used to treat African trypanosomiasis caused by *T. gambiense* and *T. rhodesiense*. It is not effective against *T. cruzi* or South American trypanosomiasis.

The drug is effective only in the early stage or hemolymphatic stage of the disease (with no CNS involvement), producing a high rate of cure of both Gambian and Rhodesian forms.

In later stages of the disease with definite CNS involvement, suramin is commonly used before or in conjunction with a course of arsenical therapy, because of the low concentrations of suramin achieved in cerebrospinal fluid.

Suramin may be used in the prophylaxis of Rhodesian and Gambian trypanosomiasis, but pentamidine is preferable for this purpose.

Chemoprophylaxis is not recommended to travelers on occasional brief visits to endemic areas, since the risk of serious drug toxicity outweighs that of acquiring the disease.

Suramin is the most effective drug for clearing the adult filariae in onchocerciasis. A single dose of 20 mg/kg IV weekly for 5-6 weeks is used in children. A test dose of 10 mg is given before initiating the treatment.

F. Toxicity

A variety of untoward reactions may follow the administration of suramin. Immediate toxic reactions are especially likely to occur in the weak and malnourished patient. These include nausea, vomiting, shock, and loss of consciousness. The incidence can be minimized to 0.1-0.3% by reducing the initial dose (test dose) and by slowing the rate of injection. Colic and acute urticaria are other immediate reactions. Later reactions within the first 24 hr include fever, papular reactions, paresthesia, lacrimation, photophobia, edema, and hyperesthesia of the palms of the hands and the soles of the feet.

The most serious and common effect of suramin is nephrotoxicity, which becomes manifest several days after treatment. It is caused by the irritant effect resulting from drug accumulation in the epithelial cells of the proximal convoluted tubules. These cells undergo degenerative changes as the amount of deposition increases. The appearance of toxicity may be detected by testing for albuminuria, hematuria, and cylindruria. This is a routine procedure that should be applied regularly before and throughout the period of treatment. The drug must be discontinued at the first indication of renal damage. Moderate albuminuria occurs often during the acute phase, but persisting, heavy albuminuria calls for caution; the schedule and dosage of treatment should be modified. Suramin should be discontinued if casts are present in the urine. Palmar and plantar hypersthesia may be the first symptom of peripheral neuritis.

Other delayed toxic effects are jaundice and exfoliative dermatitis. Agranulocytosis and hemolytic anemia occur rarely.

G. Contraindications

The drug should not be administered to pregnant women or to children under 6 years of age. Therapy should be discontinued in patients who show intolerance to the initial doses. In renal insufficiency, the drug should be employed cautiously.

References

1. Meshnick, SR: The chemotherapy of African trypanosomiasis. In: *Parasitic Diseases*, Vol. 2 (ED Mansfield, ed.), Marcel Dekker, New York, 1984, pp. 165–199.

2. Fairlamb, AH, Bowman, IBR: *Trypanosoma brucei*: Suramin and other trypanocidal compounds: Effects on *sn*-glycerol-3-phosphate oxidase. *Exp. Parasitol. 43*: 353–361, 1977.
3. Seidel, JS: Treatment of parasitic infections. *Pediatr. Clin. North Am. 32*:1077–1095, 1985.
4. Anonymous: Drugs for parasitic infections. *Med. Lett. Drug Ther. 26*:27–34, 1984.

VI. BENZNIDAZOLE

A number of compounds of the nitroimidazole group were synthesized and tested following the discovery of azomycin (2-nitroimidazole) by Nakamura in 1955 and the demonstration of its trichomonacidal activity by Horie shortly afterwards. The most widely known is metronidazole (1959), 1-(β-hydroethyl)-2-methyl-5-nitroimidazole, highly active against *Trypanosoma vaginalis, Entamoeba histolytica*, and *Giardia lamblia*. Other clinically effective 5-nitroimidazoles closely related in structure and activity to metronidazole are currently available in some parts of the world, but not in the United States. These include tinidazole (Fasigyne), nimorazole (Naxogin), and ornidazole (Tiberal).

Benznidazole, a 2-nitroimidazole derivative, has the uncommon property of being effective against the acute Chagas-Mazza's infection. It was synthesized in 1968 by Wineholt and Liebman.

A. Chemistry

Benznidazole has the following structural formula:

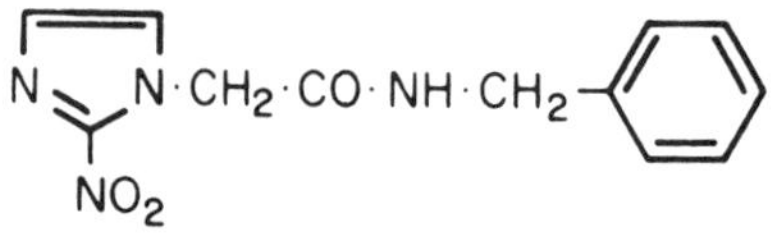

Its generic name is N-benzil-2-nitro-1 imidazole acetamide. Benznidazole is an unchanged molecule, devoid of the acid-base functional groups in the pH range of physiological interest. It is rather poorly soluble in water (approximately 40 mg per 100 mg at 37°C). The partition coefficients of the drug between organic solvents and water, however, are high (7.0 in 1-octanol-buffer, pH 7.4, and 5.1 in chloroform buffer, pH 7.4, at RT).

B. Mechanisms of Action and Antimicrobial Activity

Benznidazole does not immediately manifest its lethal effect in *T. cruzi*. Microscopic observation reveals that the inhibitory effect increases with the period of drug contact, and the pattern of cell death is similar to that of aging cultures. First the movement becomes slower, then the cells change their shape and form rosettes, and finally lysis takes place.

Benznidazole affects protein and RNA synthesis in growing cultures of *T. cruzi*. As the nitrofuran derivatives also induce these effects and the neurological reactions, one wonders whether the nitroaryl radical is responsible. Onset and degree of inhibition correlate with drug concentration. This correlation manifests itself particularly in the inhibitory effect on protein synthesis. Total inhibition with 100 μg/ml benznidazole occurs in

1 hr, whereas with 50 μg/ml total inhibition is achieved in 4 hr. With lower concentrations, total inhibition was not achieved during the observed period. Partial inhibition is induced with 25 μg/ml after 2 hr and with 12.5 μg/ml after 3 hr. DNA synthesis is far less susceptible to the inhibitory effect of the drug than are RNA and protein synthesis.

Since the decrease in oxygen consumption and carbon dioxide production by the parasite takes place even after a longer period of time, these are considered a result of the increasing cellular immobility and lysis, rather than primary drug effects. The anaerobic respiration of *T. cruzi* being minimal, no measurable inhibition by the drug was observed. Thus, inhibition of respiration by benznidazole was not demonstrated, whereas the 5-nitroimidazoles, i.e., metronidazole and ornidazole, were shown to suppress immediately the anaerobic respiration of *T. vaginalis* and *Clostridia*, as reflected by an immediate nonmobility (1).

Benzidazole did not show any antibacterial activity in the anaerobic species tested. Its lethal effect on protozoa (and probably that of the 2-nitroimidazole derivatives generally) is presumably brought about by the inhibition of protein and RNA synthesis (2).

C. Clinical Pharmacology

a. Single-dose kinetics. After a single oral dose of 100 mg benznidazole, absorption was fairly rapid (3). Peak plasma concentrations of 2.2–2.8 μg/ml were reached after 3–4 hr, and average bioavailability is high (92%). The mean fraction of protein-bound benznidazole was 44.1%. The physicochemical properties of benznidazole suggest that the drug readily penetrates the blood-brain barrier. The value of distribution was approximately 0.55 liter/kg. The average elimination half-life was 12 hr.

b. Multiple-dose kinetics. When patients were given 7 mg/kg day^{-1} in two divided doses, the average calculated steady-state peak concentration was 12.3 μg/ml among eight patients. The average value for each patient in the four samples ranged from 9.15 to 14.6 μg/ml.

The average calculated steady-state trough concentration was 8.05 μg/ml among eight patients, ranging from 5.92 to 10.70 μg/ml.

The elimination half-life of benznidazole ranged between 11.7 and 15.5 hr. The relatively small interindividual variations in this parameter found in the previous study in healthy volunteers (3) also held true for the patients in this study. The highest individual maximum measured concentration was 16.4 μg/ml, and the lowest minimum concentration was 5.4 μg/ml. This demonstrates that, in all the patients during the full-dose period of treatment, i.e., days 10–30, the drug concentration was permanently above the minimal trypanosomicidal concentration of 3–6 μg/ml, as found effective in tissue cultures (5). Also, the drug concentration never exceeded the limit of 20 μg/ml at which toxic effects are more likely to occur.

D. Preparation, Dosage, Regimens, and Routes of Administration

Benznidazole is available in South America in scored tablets of 100 mg.

The benznidazole adult dose for acute Chagas' disease is 5 mg/kg orally per day in two divided doses, for 30 days.

The pediatric dose for acute or congenital Chagas' disease is 5 mg/kg day^{-1} orally in two divided doses, for 30 days.

It is advisable to begin with 2 mg/kg day^{-1} administered in two doses, increasing the dose progressively to reach the full dose of 5 mg/kg day^{-1} on day 5 or 6 of treatment, then continuing for 4 weeks.

E. Drug Assays

Benznidazole, as the other nitroimidazoles in biologic fluids, can be conveniently determined by differential pulse polarography (reduction of the nitro group in the range of -0.50 to -0.60 V versus saturated calomel electrode) (3).

F. Therapeutic Indications

Benznidazole is an effective antiprotozoal drug. It is very active against *T. cruzi* and is effective in concentrations ranging from 3 to 6 μg/ml (5). It is also useful in the treatment of *T. vaginalis* and *E. histolytica* infections, although to a lesser degree than are other nitroimidazoles (ornidazole).

Experimental studies showed it to be moderately effective against *T. rhodesiense, T. congolense, L. donovani*, and *L. mexicana* (6).

The drug is effective in the acute stage of the disease, inducing a rapid remission of fever, hepato- and splenomegaly, adenopathy, and involution of the initial lesion or "chagoma" (7-10 days), with negativization of parasitemia in 80-90% of cases (7). It is also effective in cases of congenital disease. In the chronic phase, a decrease in parasitemia may be obtained with the use of benznidazole, but the drug does not provide complete parasitological cure.

G. Toxicity

During the first or second week of treatment, skin rashes may appear, sometimes subsiding spontaneously. More severe cutaneous reactions may be observed, with fever, purpura, or generalized polymorphic nonbullous erythema. Eruptions may be macular, morbiliform, or urticariform. These reactions, which usually appear on day 8 or 9 of treatment, may be avoided by starting therapy with lower doses (2 mg/kg day^{-1}), to reach the therapeutic dose of 5 mg/kg day^{-1} by the end of the first week. Other adverse effects are vomiting, gastrointestinal distress, diarrhea, and anorexia. Granulocytopenia and thrombocytopenia have been reported.

Higher doses (8-10 mg/kg day^{-1}) may induce a peripheral polyneuropathy of unpredictable severity, mainly in adult patients. In these cases, the drug must be discontinued.

The relationship linking side effects and dosage is illustrated by a clinical study, in which patients were divided in three groups, each receiving less than 5 mg/kg day^{-1} of benznidazole, 5-6 mg, and more than 7 mg, respectively. Side effects occurred in 24.2% of cases in the low-dose group, in 33.3% of those in the medium-dose group, and in 77.8% of the high-dose group (8). The most common adverse effect was cutaneous eruption (17.4%), followed in a decreasing order of prevalence by anorexia (5%), intestinal cramps (3%), nausea and/or vomiting (3%), and dizziness and other neurological signs (1-2%).

H. Precautions and Contraindications

Unless absolutely necessary, pregnant women should not be treated with benznidazole. The drug is relatively contraindicated in patients with renal, hepatic, hematologic, and neurological pathology.

I. Drug Interactions

Alcohol should be avoided during treatment with benznidazole. Current ingestion of alcohol may induce a disulfiramlike reaction, including abdominal distress, vomiting, flushing, and headache.

References

1. Edwards, DI, Mathison, GE: The mode of action of metronidazole against *Trichomonas vaginalis*. *J. Gen. Microbiol. 63*:297–302, 1970.
2. Polak, A, Richle, R: Mode of action of the 2-nitroimidazole derivative benznidazole. *Ann. Trop. Med. Parasitol. 72*:45–53, 1978.
3. Raaflaub, J, Ziegler, WH: Single-dose pharmacokinetics of the trypanosomicide benznidazole in man. *Arzneimittelforsch. 29*:1601–1617, 1979.
4. Wagner, JG: *Biopharmaceutics and Relevant Pharmacokinetics*, 1st ed., Hamilton Press, Hamilton, Illinois, 1971.
5. Richle, W, Raaflaub, J: Difference of effective anti-trypanosomal dosages of benznidazole in mice and man. Chemotherapeutic and pharmacokinetic results. *Acta Trop. (Basel) 37*:257–261, 1980.
6. Richle, R: Antiparasitic activity of Ro 7-1051 against *Trypanosoma cruzi*, in vitro, in experimental Chagas' disease and other experimental protozoal infections, Investigation Dept., Hoffman-La Roche, Basel, 1976.
7. Barclay, CA, Cerisola, JA, Lugones, H, Ledesma, O: Status of the clinical and seroparasitological evaluation of benznidazole in the treatment of acute Chagas' disease. X Internat Cong Chemother, Zurich, September 18–23, 1977.
8. Barclay, CA: Internal Report (on file) 96/78, Research Division, Productos Roche, Buenos Aires, Argentina.

VII. AMEBIASIS, GIARDIASIS, AND TRICHOMONIASIS: DILOXANIDE

Of the haloacetamide derivatives prepared for a development program for potential amebicides, diloxanide was the most promising. It is a dichloroacetamide derivative introduced by Bristow et al. in 1956 (1). It proved to be more effective than emetine in vitro and considerably potent against chronic intestinal amebiasis. However, it had little effect on acute amebic dysentery and none on extraintestinal amebiasis when administered alone. It was also effective in the treatment of cyst-passing patients. Among the many diloxanide derivatives prepared, the furoate ester was shown to be much more effective than the parent compound in experimentally infected rats (2). In clinical trials, it also proved effective against the noninvasive parasites (3,4).

A. Chemistry

Diloxanide furoate has the following structural formula:

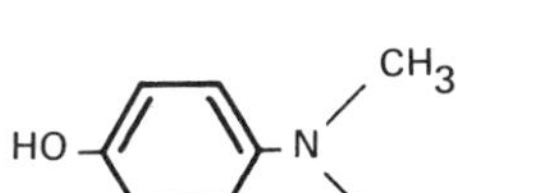

After oral ingestion, the ester is hydrolyzed to diloxanide and furoic acid.

Teclozan and etofamide are other dichloroacetamide compounds that have proven effective as intraluminal amebicides (5).

B. Mechanism of Action

Both diloxanide and its furoate are directly amebicidal when tested in vitro and are more active than emetine. The furoate ester is effective within a concentration range of

0.01-0.1 μg/ml. Its activity appears to be directed at the lumen-dwelling trophozoites, and this probably takes place well before the encystment process begins.

Little is known of its mechanism of action. It has been suggested, on the basis of structural similarities, that its action may be related to that of chloramphenicol on bacterial cells. However, this comparison seems unlikely because the inhibitory effect of chloramphenicol on bacterial protein synthesis depends on its ability to bind to the type of ribosome subunit found only in bacterial cells. Moreover, chloramphenicol lacks direct therapeutic effectiveness in both experimental and clinical amebiasis.

C. Clinical Pharmacology

A large proportion of an oral dose of diloxanide furonate is rapidly absorbed from the gastrointestinal tract, with most of the ester hydrolyzed to diloxanide before absorption. Thus, only diloxanide appears in the systemic circulation (6). Peak concentrations are reached in the blood within 1 hr, but fall to a fraction of this within 6 hr.

The drug is eliminated mainly via the kidney. Urinary excretion accounts for 60-90% of the administered dose, much of it in the form of glucuronide, within 48 hr. About half of this appears in the urine within 6 hr. Less than 10% is excreted in the feces. This probably represents the biologically active fraction derived from the unabsorbed residue or from extraintestinal sites by excretory processes.

D. Preparation, Dosage, Regimens, and Routes of Administration

Diloxanide furoate is available in the United States from the Parasitic Diseases Division, Centers for Disease Control, Atlanta, Georgia.

The adult dose is 500 mg orally three times daily for 10 days. If necessary, a second course may be given immediately following the first.

The pediatric dose is 20 mg/kg day^{-1} in three divided doses for 10 days.

E. Therapeutic Indications

Diloxanide is the drug of choice in the treatment of asymptomatic passers of cysts and also in the treatment of invasive and extraintestinal amebiasis (4,7). In the former case it is administered alone, whereas in the latter it is given in combination with an appropriate systemic or mixed amebicide. If given alone, it is ineffective against extraintestinal amebiasis. It may be useful as a prophylactic in areas with a high risk of infection. There is no agreement on its efficacy when used alone in the treatment of acute amebiasis with frank dysentery. Satisfactory results have been reported from some areas, but in others the drug has proven less effective (8,9).

Low cost is an important advantage of diloxanide, particularly in underdeveloped countries.

F. Toxicity

The drug is generally well tolerated. Only minor and transient side effects have been observed in humans, mainly affecting the gastrointestinal tract. Flatulence is most commonly reported; vomiting, pruritus, and urticaria occur occasionally (10). It is a remarkably safe drug with no other known pharmacological effects.

References

1. Bristow, NW, Oxley, P, Williams, GAH, Woolfe, G: Entamide, a new amoebicide; preliminary note. *Trans. R. Soc. Trop. Med. Hyg. 50*:182, 1956.

2. Main, PT, Bristow, NW, Oxley, P, Watkins, TI, Williams, GAH, Wilmshurst, EC, Woolfe, G: Entamide. *Ann. Biochem. Exp. Med. 20*:441–448, 1960.
3. Shaldon, S: Entamide furoate in the treatment of acute amoebic dysentery. *Trans. R. Soc. Trop. Med. Hyg. 54*:469–470, 1960.
4. Woodruff, AW, Bell, S: Clinical trials with entamide furoate and related compounds. 1. In a non-tropical environment. *Trans. R. Soc. Trop. Med. Hyg. 54*:389–395, 1960.
5. Neal, RA: Experimental amoebiasis and the development of anti-amoebic compounds. *Parasitology 8*:175–191, 1983.
6. Wilmshurst, EC, Cliffe, EE: Absorption and distribution of amoebicides. In: *Absorption and Distribution of Drugs* (TB Binns, ed.), Livingstone, Edinburgh, 1964, pp. 191–198.
7. Krogstad, DJ, Spencer, HC, Jr., Healy, GR: Amebiasis. *N. Engl. J. Med. 298*:262–265, 1978.
8. Suchak, NG, Satoskar, RS, Sheth, UK: Entamide furoate in the treatment of intestinal amoebiasis. *Am. J. Trop. Med. Hyg. 11*:330–332, 1962.
9. Wilmot, AJ, Powell, SJ, McLeod, I, Elsdon-Dew, R: Some newer amoebicides in acute amoebic dysentery. *Trans. R. Soc. Trop. Med. Hyg. 56*:85–86, 1962.
10. Wolfe, MS: Nondysenteric intestinal amebiasis. Treatment with diloxanide furoate. *JAMA 224*:1601–1604, 1973.

VIII. EMETINE AND DEHYDROEMETINE

Emetine was the first effective drug for the treatment of amebiasis. It is an alkaloid obtained from ipecac, the ground root of the Brazilian shrub, *Uragoga ipecacuanha*. It is also prepared semisynthetically by methylation of cephaeline, another ipecacuanha alkaloid. Preparations of the powdered root were used for centuries for treating dysentery before its highly specific activity against isolated amebic trophozoites was demonstrated by Vedder in 1912. Emetine has since been used widely in the treatment of invasive intestinal amebiasis, amebic hepatitis, and amebic abscesses.

Dehydroemetine is a close structural analog of emetine but less toxic. However, amebicides of the nitroimidazole group are gradually replacing both emetine and dehydroemetine since they have proven equally effective and far less toxic.

A. Chemistry

Emetine has the following structural formula:

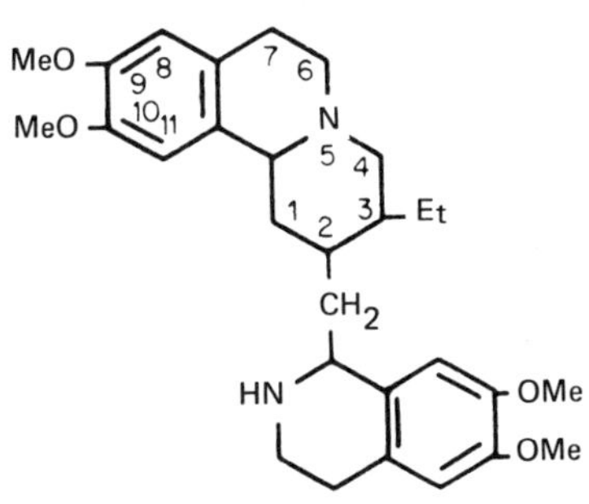

The natural alkaloid is biologically the most active of the many possible stereoisomers of the accepted configuration for emetine. Of the many congeners tested, only one, 2,3-dihydroemetine, has shown to be promising enough to undergo clinical evaluation.

Emetine derived from natural sources is levorotatory; (−)-emetine is obtained from synthetic sources and is available as the hydrated hydrochloride.

Both emetine and dihydroemetine are administered intramuscularly because their highly irritant and cardiotoxic properties contraindicate other routes of administration.

Emetine bismuth iodide, an insoluble preparation, may be safely administered by the oral route of release the active form in the small intestine. This compound is given to supplement the effect of the parenterally injected drug and has limited uses.

Dihydroemetine appears to be identical to emetine in all aspects other than the pharmacokinetic. Its elimination rate is about twice that of emetine, but the route is not yet clear. Because it is less cumulative, it is less toxic.

B. Mechanisms of Action

Emetine exerts a lethal effect on trophozoites of *E. histolytica* in vitro at concentrations equal to those obtained in the blood following therapy. Cysts and parasites present in the intestinal lumen are less susceptible to the drug's lethal action than are the active forms, which invade the tissues. Emetine induces degenerative changes in the trophozoites by interfering with their division.

The drug can irreversibly inhibit protein synthesis in these parasitic protozoa as well as in mammalian cells. This finding was the result of a comparative study of emetine and cycloheximide, based on their close configurational and conformational similarities. Both substances inhibited protein synthesis in mammalian cells by what appeared to be an identical mechanism, acting specifically at the elongation stage to inhibit part of the translocation process, that involving the movement of mRNA along the ribosome. The two drugs inhibit the same molecular mechanism, but the inhibitory effect of cycloheximide is reversible. Furthermore, this drug can also inhibit the initial and terminal phases of protein synthesis.

The effect of emetine is therefore more selective. In addition, this may not be the only mechanism implicated in its amebicidal activity. This does not depend on active protein synthesis, and that some drugs are amebicidal at concentrations that do not affect protein synthesis indicates this mechanism is probably only part of the whole process or that alternative mechanisms may operate.

Thus, the complete mechanism of action of emetine is not known, but whatever it is, it is likely also to be implicated in drug toxicity. The inhibitory effect of emetine on protein synthesis was studied on isolated cells. It was found to correlate quantitatively with amebicidal activity as well as with toxicity in mammalian cells.

Differential distribution of the drug and other kinetic factors may be responsible for the limited selectivity toward the parasite in vivo.

C. Clinical Pharmacology

All the available data are derived from studies in experimental animals. Studies in small mammals indicate complete absorption after parenteral administration of radiolabeled emetine hydrochloride. Only 20% is absorbed when given by the oral route. The half-life is about 5 days, and there is selective tissue binding.

The drug concentrates mainly in the liver, spleen, lung, and kidney. Amebicidal concentrations were detected in the liver even 4 weeks after the administration of a single parenteral dose. Smaller amounts can be found in the heart; those in the brain are insignificant.

Data on metabolism and excretion are incomplete. It is thought that the drug is mainly excreted in the urine; however, none could be recovered by a chemical method from the urine of patients medicated with full doses of emetine, or from dogs receiving intraperitoneally to guinea pigs. Only 5% radioactivity was detected in the urine, but over 80% appeared in the feces. Much of the drug is probably excreted unchanged in the feces (1,2).

D. Preparation, Dosage, Regimens, and Routes of Administration

Emetine hydrochloride is available as an injection containing 65 mg/ml. Dihydroemetine is supplied by the Parasitic Diseases Division, Centers for Disease Control, Atlanta, Georgia.

Doses for invasive intestinal and extraintestinal amebiasis are as follows.

Adult dose. Emetine: 1 mg/kg day^{-1} (maximum 60 mg/day) IM for up to 5 days; dihydroemetine: 1-1.5 mg/kg day^{-1} (maximum 90 mg/day) IM for up to 5 days

Pediatric dose. Emetine: 1 mg/kg day^{-1} in two doses (maximum 60 mg/day) IM for up to 5 days; dihydroemetine: 1-1.5 mg/kg day^{-1} in two doses (maximum 90 mg/day) IM for up to 5 days

Treatment should preferably not be repeated; if necessary, the second course should be given before 14 days of the first.

E. Therapeutic Indications

Emetine and dihydroemetine are indicated for the treatment of invasive forms of intestinal or extraintestinal amebiasis. Both drugs belong to the group of the systemic amebicides. They are rarely used nowadays, having been replaced by mixed amebicides of the nitroimidazole class. Thus, emetine and dihydroemetine should be used only if the nitroimidazoles are ineffective or contraindicated. Although emetine and dihydroemetine may be lifesaving owing to their potent amebicidal activity, neither can be used alone for curative purposes.

F. Toxicity

Emetine is a very toxic drug. Its adverse effects, at therapeutic doses, primarily involve the cardiovascular system, the neuromuscular system, the centeral nervous system, and the gastrointestinal tract.

Gastrointestinal symptoms, such as nausea, vomiting, diarrhea, and abdominal cramps, may follow parenteral administration. Neuromuscular symptoms include generalized weakness, muscular fatigue, pain, and stiffness. The effects precede the more serious cardiovascular effects and persist until the drug is withdrawn. These side effects may be related to a neuromuscular blocking effect or to the drug-induced inhibition of protein synthesis. These effects are generalized and distinct from the local effects that occur at injection sites.

Cardiotoxicity is the most serious effect induced by both emetine and dihydroemetine. It develops during treatment, producing ECG changes, tachycardia, and precordial pain (2).

Because of the toxic effects on the heart, patients receiving emetine should have ECG monitoring and should remain sedentary during therapy.

G. Precautions and Contraindications

The use of emetine or dihydroemetine is contraindicated in pregnancy and in patients with cardiac, renal, or neuromuscular disease.

References

1. Harries, J: Amebiasis: A review. *J. R. Soc. Med. 75*:190–197, 1982.
2. Yang, WCT, Dubick, M: Mechanism of emetine cardiotoxicity. *Pharmacol. Ther. 10*: 15–26, 1980.

IX. IODOQUINOL AND THE HALOGENATED 8-HYDROXYQUINOLINES

Quinoline derivatives were tested for amebicidal activity because of the isoquinoline moiety in the emetine structure. The first isoquinoline compounds tested were found to have limited efficacy. However, some 8-hydroxyquinolines proved promising, and this led eventually to the halogenated derivatives. Of these, di-iodohydroxyquin, i.e., iodoquinol, is the most widely used.

A. Chemistry

Iodoquinol is a dihalogenated derivative of the 8-hydroxyquinolines (8-quinolinol). It has the following structural formula:

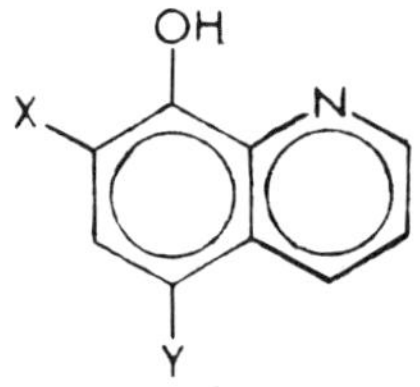

Iodoquinol (X = Y = I)

Clioquinol (X = I; Y = Cl)

Iodoquinol is of a light yellowish to tan color, almost odorless, and stable in air. It is practically insoluble in water and sparingly soluble in most other solvents. It contains 64% organically bound iodine.

Clioquinol (iodochlorhydroxyquin) is another well-known derivative of this class of compounds.

B. Mechanism of Action

The 8-hydroxyquinolines are effective amebicides, active against both trophozoites and cystic forms. The mechanism through which iodoquinol exerts its amebicidal activity remains unknown.

C. Clinical Pharmacology

The drug is fairly well absorbed following oral administration. In humans, 25% of the administered dose of clioquinol may be found in the urine as a glucuronide; either sulfate is also formed. Iodoquinol is the least absorbed derivative, three times less than clioquinol. It is not known whether the effectiveness of these compounds in intestinal amebiases is due to their action in the intestinal lumen or to drug accumulation in the blood.

After an oral dose of 250 mg clinoquinol, plasma concentrations reach an average of 5 μg/ml after 4–8 hr. Half-life ranges from 11 to 14 hr.

D. Preparation, Dosage, Regimens, and Routes of Administration

Iodoquinol is available in tablets containing 210 or 650 mg drug.

Clioquinol is no longer marketed in tablets for oral use in the United States. It is available only as 3% ointment or cream in 1-ounce tubes for dermatologic use (eczema, athlete's foot, and other fungal infections).

The iodoquinol dosage to treat asymptomatic carriers of intestinal amebiasis is as follows.

Oral adult dose: 650 mg three times daily for 20 days
Oral pediatric dose: 30–40 mg/kg daily divided in three doses for 20 days (maximum dose, 2 g)

The drug can be given with meals. It may be taken as a suspension containing 200-400 mg in 5 ml by mixing a pulverized tablet with cherry syrup.

Iodoquinol may be associated with metronidazole to treat mild, moderate, or severe intestinal disease. It is also combined with emetine.

E. Therapeutic Indications

Iodoquinol is used for the treatment of asymptomatic intestinal amebiasis. It is also used in combination with metronidazole or emetine to treat mild, moderate, and severe forms of intestinal amebiasis. In combination with these drugs, it has also been used to treat hepatic abscesses.

F. Toxicity

These compounds were once considered to have very low toxicity. Thus, they were widely used to treat traveler's diarrhea and nonspecific diarrhea in children. Unfortunately, these drugs were later found to be associated with substantial risk, particularly with prolonged administration at high doses. The most important toxic reaction, primarily attributed to clioquinol, is subacute myelo-optic neuropathy. This is a myelitislike illness, first described in epidemic form in Japan, where thousands of patients were affected. Only sporadic cases have been reported elsewhere, and the actual prevalence of this condition is unknown. The disease was studied in Japan by a special research committee, which ascribed the toxic effect to clioquinol. As a result, the use of this drug was prohibited in Japan in 1970 and later in other countries as well, including the United States. The controlled use of clioquinol in Japan brought about an immediate and dramatic decrease in the prevalence of the disease, thus confirming the role played by clioquinol as the causative agent (1,2). The early symptoms were abdominal pain and persistent diarrhea, followed by bilateral sensory disorders, such as paresthesia predominantly affecting the distal portion of the lower limbs, signs of pyramidalism, and slight involvement of the upper limbs. Less common were blurred vision and blindness, disturbances in the autonomic nervous system, psychological alterations, and a greenish coloration of the tongue. Although the disease was endemic only in Japan and it appeared to be caused by clioquinol, similar toxic effects have been noted elsewhere with relation to other 8-hydroxyquinolines (2).

The administration of high doses of iodoquinol to children with chronic diarrhea has been associated with optic atrophy and permanent loss of vision.

Other toxic reactions are furunculosis, generalized dermatitis, urticaria, and pruritus. Adverse effects related to the gastrointestinal tract include nausea, abdominal pain, diarrhea, vomiting, and pruritus ani. Chills, fever, headache, vertigo, and enlargement of the thyroid have also been reported.

G. Precautions and Contraindications

Iodoquinol should be used with caution in patients with thyroid disease. Protein-bound serum iodine levels may increase during treatment with the drug and therefore interfere with certain thyroid function tests. These effects may persist for as long as 6 months after discontinuation of therapy. This is unrelated to thyroid function.

The safety of the drug in pregnancy or during lactation has not been established.

The drug is contraindicated in patients with known hypersensitivity to iodine and 8-hydroxyquinolines and in those with hepatic damage.

References

1. Cavanagh, JB: Peripheral neuropathy caused by chemical agents. *CRC Crit. Rev. Toxicol. 2*:365–417, 1973.
2. Oakley, GP, Jr.: The neurotoxicity of the halogenated hydroxyquinolines. *JAMA 225*:395–397, 1973.

X. QUINACRINE

Quinacrine, a derivative of acridine, was used as an antimalarial drug during World War II. However, it was soon abandoned for this usage, because of its toxicity and inability to cure vivax malaria or act as a causal prophylactic.

Nowadays, the major indication of quinacrine is for the treatment of *G. lamblia* infections (1).

A. Chemistry

Quinacrine has the following structural formula:

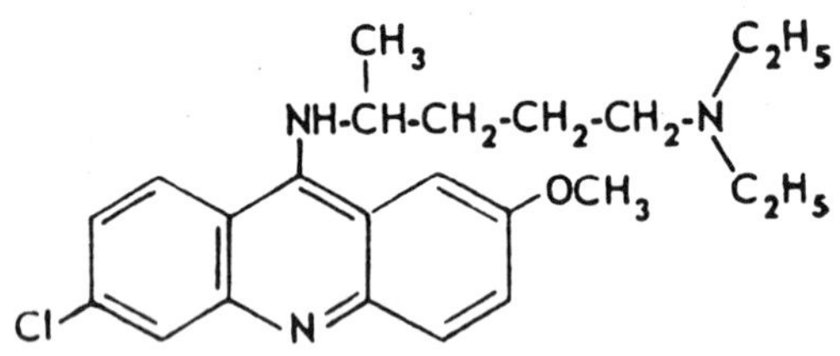

B. Mechanism of Action

It is not known whether quinacrine is effective per se or after metabolic transformation. The parent drug is likely to be the active substance, if one considers its ready intercalation with DNA. Its selective toxicity is a function of relative distribution rather than specificity of action (2).

C. Clinical Pharmacology

Quinacrine is well absorbed from the gastrointestinal tract and appears in the blood within 2 hr. It concentrates in the liver, spleen, pancreas, and lung. Higher concentrations are found in erythrocytes and leukocytes than in the plasma. The drug is also detected in all body fluids, and it crosses the placental barrier. Its half-life has been estimated to be 5 days. It is very slowly excreted in the urine and feces. Significant amounts can be detected in the urine for at least 2 months after discontinuation of the drug. It accumulates progressively when administered for long periods of time. Quinacrine hydrochloride has been found to bind to serum proteins in vitro.

D. Preparation, Dosages, Regimens, and Routes of Administration

Quinacrine is available as the dihydrochloride designated quinacrine hydrochloride. It is supplied as tablets containing 100 mg of the dihydrochloride equivalent to 80% quinacrine base.

The adult dose for giardiasis is 100 mg three times daily for 5-7 days. A second course of treatment may be necessary 1 or 2 weeks later.

The pediatric dose is 2 mg/kg body weight three times daily (up to a maximum of 300 mg daily) for 5-7 days.

The drug is extremely bitter; so, if pulverized, it needs to be sweetened.

Stools must be followed for 2 weeks to 1 month after treatment. Enterotest should be performed if stools are negative and the patient is still symptomatic.

E. Therapeutic Indications

Quinacrine is currently used mainly for the treatment of giardiasis.

F. Toxicity and Side Effects

The toxic effects of quinacrine have been well documented (3). These are common and most frequently involve the gastrointestinal tract, e.g., abdominal pain, nausea, and vomiting. Dizziness and headache may occur. Blood dyscrasias, urticaria, and exfoliative dermatitis have also been described.

A yellow-orange discoloration of the skin may follow prolonged therapy or inappropriate dosage, due to deposition of the drug. Blue or black pigmentation of the nails may also occur.

Ocular toxicity, similar to that induced by chloroquine, is rare. Lichenoid skin eruptions have been reported in infrequent instances, as have acute hepatic necrosis and convulsions.

G. Precautions and Contraindications

Quinacrine is contraindicated in pregnancy because it readily passes the placental barrier and reaches the fetus.

Great caution should be exercised in prescribing this drug to patients with psoriasis. Pronounced exacerbations may occur, and exfoliative lesions sometimes develop.

H. Drug Interactions

Concomitant administration of quinacrine and primaquine results in markedly elevated concentrations of the latter, thus enhancing its toxicity.

References

1. Wolfe, MS: Giardiasis. *JAMA 233*:1362–1365, 1975.
2. Albert, A: *Selective Toxicity: The Physico-Chemical Basis of Therapy*, 6th ed., Chapman & Hall, London, 1979.
3. Findlay, GM: *Recent Advances in Chemotherapy*, Vol. II, J & A. Churchill, London, 1951.

37
Nitroimidazoles

EDWARD D. RALPH*
The University of Western Ontario, London, Ontario, Canada

Metronidazole was the first and is the best known of the clinically applicable nitroimidazole group of drugs. It was developed through intensive research for an effective drug against *Trichomonas vaginalis* by Rhone-Poulenc in France (1). In 1956, a 2-nitroimidazole compound known as azomycin from a *Streptomyces* species (previously isolated and described by Japanese investigators in 1953) (2) was found to possess good activity against *T. vaginalis*. Systematic chemical manipulation of this compound determined that the nitro group at position 5 of the imidazole gave compounds with the best antimicrobial activity and least toxicity (3). Additional side-chain substitutions ultimately resulted in the synthesis in 1957 of metronidazole. Subsequently, other 5-nitroimidazoles were developed which have clinical application including tinidazole (1969) (4) and ornidazole (1974) (Figure 1) (5).

Structure-activity studies determined that a side chain at position 1 containing fewer than five alkyl groups (CH_2) and the absence of, or a short chain at, position 2 produced the best antimicrobial activity (1). The substitutions at position 1, which vary among the nitroimidazoles, result in different pharmacokinetic properties.

I. MECHANISM OF ACTION

The mechanism of action of the nitroimidazoles has been studied most extensively using metronidazole in various protozoal, whole bacterial, or cell extract systems. However, the exact mechanism has yet to be firmly elucidated. The activity appears to be dependent upon or associated with the electrochemical reduction of the nitro group at position 5 of metronidazole to produce an active but labile "intermediate," which then exerts a lethal or inhibitory effect on DNA (6). Fragmentation of the imidazole ring ultimately occurs with the formation of acetamide (7).

**Present affiliation*: University Hospital, London, Ontario, Canada

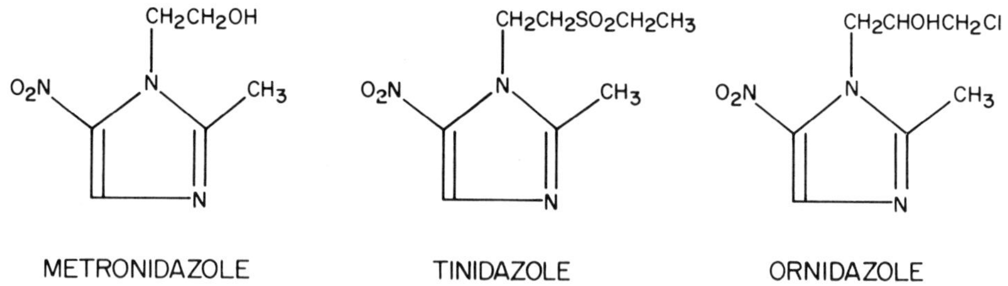

Figure 1 Three 5-nitroimidazoles.

In metabolic studies in various anaerobes, metronidazole has been shown to be a powerful "electron syphon" during its reduction. It avidly accepts electrons from reduced ferrodoxin, for example, and can thereby inhibit other metabolic pathways (for example, the phosphoroclastic reaction present in *Clostridium pasteurianum*) (8). In this system, therefore, it exerts an antimicrobial effect in the process of being reduced in addition to its effect on DNA. Because of their unique mechanism of action, the spectrum of activity of nitroimidazoles is primarily restricted to obligate anaerobic organisms that possess the intracellular electrochemical conditions necessary for the reduction of the drug. Moreover, oxygen inhibits the effect of nitroimidazoles through interference with the nitro group reduction (6). Development of resistance is very rare. In one resistant *Bacteroides fragilis* strain, it was noted that there was decreased uptake of metronidazole by the organism associated with reduced reduction to its active form (9).

II. ANTIMICROBIAL ACTIVITY AND RESISTANCE

The nitroimidazoles are primarily active against obligate anaerobic protozoa and bacteria, and their activity is essentially similar. A large amount of susceptibility data is available, especially for metronidazole against anaerobic bacteria, and for some organisms, susceptibility data for tinidazole and ornidazole must be inferred. Sensitivity testing of protozoal organisms is unstandardized, and there are few data for *Entamoeba histolytica* and *Giardia lamblia*. Table 1 summarizes the average minimum inhibitory concentrations of nitroimidazoles for various organisms.

Gram-negative anaerobic rods (*Bacteroides* and *Fusobacterium*) and spore-forming gram-positive rods (*Clostridium* species) are very susceptible and resistance is very unusual. However, gram-positive cocci (especially *Peptostreptococcus* species), non-spore-forming rods (*Bifidobacterium* species), and gram-negative cocci (*Veillonella*) are less susceptible. *Propionibacterium* and *Actinomyces* species are usually very resistant. The nitroimidazoles demonstrate a consistently bactericidal effect against exponential and stationary-phase organisms.

In studies with metronidazole, no antagonism with other antibiotics active against *B. fragilis* was seen. Metronidazole usually demonstrates an additive or partially synergistic effect with other antibiotics (15).

The metabolites of metronidazole and tinidazole, especially the hydroxy compounds, demonstrate bioactivity. This is less than the parent drugs against obligate anaerobes but greater against some facultative anaerobes, including *Gardnerella vaginalis* (16,17).

Table 1 Representative MIC of Nitroimidazoles (Metronidazole, Tinidazole, and Ornidazole) for Various Protozoa and Anaerobic Bacteria

Organism	MIC (μg/ml)	Reference
Protozoa		
Entamoeba histolytica	0.17[a]	10
Giardia lamblia	0.5	11
Trichomonas vaginalis	1.5	12
Bacteria		
Bacteroides fragilis (and related species)	1.6	13, 14
Bacteroides melaninogenicus	0.8	
Fusobacterium spp.	0.4	
Clostridium perfringens	0.8	
Peptostreptococcus spp.	12.5	
Peptococcus spp.	1.6	
Veillonella spp.	6.25	
Bifidobacterium	6.25	

[a] ED_{50}.

III. CLINICAL PHARMACOLOGY

A. Absorption and Bioavailability

Table 2 summarizes serum concentrations of metronidazole, tinidazole, and ornidazole after oral and intravenous administration from representative studies in both pediatric and adult patients. It should be noted that there are few studies providing data in pediatric patients, and these have involved the use of metronidazole only. Therefore, data from adult patients have been provided for tinidazole and ornidazole. Where possible, studies in which specific assays (e.g., high-pressure liquid chromatography; HPLC) have been used to measure unmetabolized drug have been quoted.

As noted in the table, peak serum concentrations after single doses of metronidazole (on a miligram per kilogram basis) are approximately in the same range for pediatric and adult patients. Moreover, from comparative data in adults, these concentrations are also similar after dosing with tinidazole and ornidazole. In contrast, serum concentrations at 8 and 12 hr (which are commonly used dosage intervals) differ among the three drugs, reflecting the longer half-lives of tinidazole and ornidazole compared with that of metronidazole. This is also noted with metronidazole in infants of different gestational ages: higher concentrations are present at 8 and 12 hr in younger patients.

When the rates of absorption of oral doses are examined in various studies, there is a wide range in the time to peak concentration (T_{max}) for all drugs from as short as 15 min to as long as 4 hr. In one infant of 6 weeks, the T_{max} of metronidazole was 4 hr. In general, from comparative studies, metronidazole appears to be the most rapidly absorbed, with an average T_{max} of 1-2 hr, followed by tinidazole and ornidazole with a T_{max} of 2–4 hr. In one study in adults, food significantly delayed the rate of absorption of metronidazole compared with the fasting state (139 vs. 71 min for T_{max}) (25).

Table 2 Serum Level Data After Single Oral and Intravenous Doses of Metronidazole, Tinidazole, and Ornidazole in Pediatric and Adult Patients

Drug	Age group, mean weight (g)	Dose	Route of administration	T_{max} (hr)	Serum level concentrations (μg/ml)			Assay	Reference
					Peak	8 hr	12 hr		
Metronidazole	< 21 weeks' gestation (1020)	7.5 mg/kg	IV	-	8[a]	–	6.5[a]	HPLC[b]	18
		15 mg/kg	IV	–	30[a]	–	28[a]	HPLC	18
	32–35 weeks' gestation (1860)	7.5 mg/kg	IV	–	18[a]	–	14[a]	HPLC	18
	6 weeks (2830)	22.1 mg/kg	PO	4	22.2	14[a]	12[a]	Polar[c]	19
	9–13 years (30–50 kg)	11.8 mg/kg	PO	3	12[a]	9[a]	7[a]	Polar	19
	10–14 years (>50 kg)	8.5 mg/kg	PO	3	10[a]	6[a]	5[a]	Polar	19
	Adults	500 mg	IV	–	18	7[a]	–	HPLC	20
		500 mg	PO	0.33–3	13.1	7	–	HPLC	20
		500 mg	IV	–	9.4	4.5[a]	–	HPLC	21
		500 mg	PO	2	9.0	5[a]	–	HPLC	21
		750 mg	PO	0.5–1	12.3	7[a]	5[a]	TLC[d]	22
Tinidazole	Adults	500 mg	IV	–	7.5[a]	6[a]	–	HPLC	21
		500 mg	PO	3	10.1[a]	7[a]	–	HPLC	21
Ornidazole	Adults	750 mg	PO	2–4	10.9	8	7	HPLC	22
		500 mg	IV	–	13	–	–	BA[e]	23
		1500 mg	PO	1–2	33.2	–	14.5	TLC	24

[a]Data extrapolated from graphs.
[b]High-pressure liquid chromatography.
[c]Polarography.
[d]Thin-layer chromatography.
[e]Bioassay.

Bioavailability studies for metronidazole, tinidazole, and ornidazole, in which the area under the time-concentration curves after oral and intravenous administration have been compared, demonstrate bioavailability for all three compounds of approximately 90–100% (26).

In a comparative study in adults, metronidazole and tinidazole given rectally produced peak concentrations approximately 50% those of oral doses and absorption was delayed with a T_{max} of about 4 hr (21). Bioavailability was also decreased (39% tinidazole vs. 53% metronidazole). Other studies with metronidazole given rectally have shown a bioavailability of 70% or greater (27).

Intravaginal metronidazole and tinidazole produce serum concentrations that are quite low (15–20% of oral dose levels) and bioavailability of 25% for metronidazole and only 10% for tinidazole (21).

Multiple doses of nitroimidazoles, because of their long half-lives, show some drug accumulation over the first few days of dosing. In one study in adults, after oral doses of 500 mg every 6 hr of metronidazole, minimum serum concentrations averaged 17.7 μg/ml on day 3 with no evidence of further accumulation by day 7 (28). In an intravenous study of multiple doses of 500 mg metronidazole every 8 hr, between days 2 and 6, maximum serum concentrations ranged between 14 and 60 μg/ml and minimum concentrations were 5.6–21 μg/ml (29).

B. Protein Binding

Metronidazole, tinidazole, and ornidazole have a low degree of protein binding. With an equilibrium dialysis technique, ornidazole at concentrations of 1 and 10 μg/ml had a mean protein binding of 12.2% and metronidazole 9.7% (22). In other studies, the protein binding of metronidazole ranged from 0 to 20% (27). Tinidazole, with an ultrafiltration technique, was found to be 12% bound (30).

C. Distribution

All three drugs appear to be well distributed in tissues throughout the body, although most data available apply to metronidazole and tinidazole. Pharmacokinetic data relating to distribution are shown in Table 3. The large apparent volumes of distribution are predictive of high tissue concentrations. The half-life of distribution of metronidazole was determined to be 0.30 and 1.24 hr in two studies using two-compartment open models in adults (31,32).

In examining the volumes of distribution in both pediatric and adult age groups with metronidazole, there appears to be no significant difference. Moreover, in adult patients the volumes of distribution of tinidazole and ornidazole appear to be fairly similar to that of metronidazole.

Maximum tissue concentrations generally lag behind peak serum concentrations by a factor of several hours. Table 4 shows representative tissue levels as a percentage of serum concentrations for metronidazole and tinidazole. Although these data are from adult studies, it would be expected that similar ratios would exist for pediatric patients.

D. Elimination

1. Metabolism

The nitroimidazoles are metabolized, primarily in the liver, to various oxidative metabolites that have been detected in the urine and serum. Metronidazole and ornidazole

Table 3 Volumes of Distribution for Metronidazole, Tinidazole, and Ornidazole in Pediatric and Adult Patients

Drug	Age group, mean weight (g)	Volume of distribution (V_d) % Body weight	Liters/kg	Liters	Reference
Metronidazole	<32 weeks' gestation (1020)		0.65		18
	>32–35 weeks' gestation (1860)		0.71		18
	35 weeks' gestation (3150)		0.69		18
	6 weeks (2830)		0.87		19
	9–14 years (30–>50 kg)		0.64		19
	Adults		0.76		19
	Adults			53.2	21
	Adults	83.0			22
	Adults		0.85		31
	Adults		1.02		32
Tinidazole	Adults		0.81		33
	Adults			57.0	21
Ornidazole	Adults	86.7			22
	Adults		1.12		23

Table 4 Representative Tissue Levels as % Serum Levels in Humans for Metronidazole and Tinidazole

Drug	Tissue or fluid	% Concentration of serum level	Reference
Metronidazole	CSF	60–100	27
	Synovial fluid	100	34
	Bile	100	35
	Breast milk	100	36
	Saliva	100	19
	Bone	75	37
	Uterus, fallopian tube	95	38
	Aqueous humor	38	39
Tinidazole	CSF	100	40
	Gallbladder bile	121	33
	Breast milk	162	33
	Liver	31	33
	Intestine	60–118	33
	Muscle	119	33
	Skin	81	33
	Aqueous humor	47	39

undergo proportionately greater metabolic transformation than tinidazole (26), and the metabolites of the latter drug have been detected in only a few studies. The major metabolites of metronidazole are [1-(2-hydroxyethyl)-2-hydroxymethyl-5-nitroimidazole), the hydroxy metabolite, and (1-acetic acid-2-methyl-5-nitroimidazole) the acid metabolite. Following single doses in adults, the hydroxy metabolite is detected in the serum at concentrations approximately 10–20% of unchanged drug with peak concentrations occurring approximately 8 hr after peak concentrations of the parent compound, with the acid metabolite usually undetectable in serum (41). With multiple doses, the hydroxy metabolite may be detected at concentrations up to 30% of those of unchanged drug and the acid metabolite at only 3% (41).

The hydroxy metabolite has been detected in the serum and urine of a 19-day-old term infant, as well as in the serum of infants greater than 35 weeks' gestation. It is undetectable in infants less than 35 weeks' gestation unless previously exposed to betamethasone (through the maternal circulation) (18). Therefore, oxidative metabolic pathways in term infants are present to metabolize metronidazole but are not yet developed in preterm infants (less than 35 weeks' gestation). Betamethasone, however, stimulated the hepatic mono-oxygenase in preterm infants, resulting in hydroxylation (18).

The degree of metabolism of tinidazole as reported in studies is variable. Most studies have detected no metabolites, but one found traces of the hydroxy metabolite [1-(2-ethylsulfonyl-ethyl)-2-hydroxymethyl-5-nitroimidazole] in the serum and it represented 2% of the total administered dose excreted in the urine after a large single dose of 1600 mg (33). The major metabolites of ornidazole are 1-(3-chloro-2-hydroxypropyl)-2-hydroxymethyl-5-nitroimidazole, the hydroxy metabolite, and 3-(2-methyl-5-nitroimidazole 1-yl) 1,2-propane diol. These two compounds represent approximately 70% of the metabolites of ornidazole in the urine (42).

2. Excretion

The nitroimidazoles and their metabolites are excreted through the kidney primarily by glomerular filtration with little or no tubular reabsorption. Table 5 summarizes the urinary excretion of these drugs and is dependent upon the type of assay used. In ^{14}C tracer studies with metronidazole and ornidazole, approximately 60% of the total dose was excreted in the urine over 48 hr. By bioassay, however, only 17% of the total dose of metronidazole was detected as bioactivity. When HPLC methods are used, only 8% of metronidazole and 19% of tinidazole are excreted within 24 hr as unchanged drug. For ornidazole, 4% of the administered dose is excreted as unchanged drug over 48 hr. The hydroxy and acid metabolites of metronidazole in the urine account for approximately 16% of the administered dose over 24 hr.

Glucuronide and sulfated conjugates of metronidazole and its metabolites have been also detected in the urine (44).

Another route of elimination is through fecal excretion, although the percentage of dose excreted is much less compared with the urinary route. For metronidazole and ornidazole, 14 and 22% of the administered dose, respectively, are excreted in feces as unchanged drugs and metabolites in adults as determined by ^{14}C tracer studies (22).

The elimination and clearance rates (total body and renal) for the nitroimidazoles derived from various studies are summarized in Table 6. The average half-life for metronidazole in infants and older patients is shorter (approximately 8 hr) than for ornidazole (12 hr) and tinidazole (13 hr). For preterm infants, however, the half-life of metronidazole is much longer, presumably due to the decreased metabolism of the drug. In one

Table 5 Urinary Excretion of Nitroimidazoles in Pediatric and Adult Patients

Drug	Dose	Time interval	% Total dose (unchanged drug + metabolites)	% Total dose as unchanged drug	% Total dose as metabolites	Average urine concentration (time interval)	Assay	Reference
Metronidazole								
4–14 years	10 mg/kg	0–24	30–38			235 (6–9 hr)	Polar	19
Adults	750 mg	0–48	70	7.7			^{14}C tracer	22
	500 mg	0–48	17	–		98 (4–8 hr)	BA	27
	500 mg	0–24	27	9	I[a] 12		HPLC	20
					II[b] 6			
	500–2000 mg	0–24	20	4	I 11		HPLC	32
					II 5			
Tinidazole								
Adults	5 mg/kg	0–24	19				HPLC	43
	1600 mg	0–72	37	25.1	I 2	131 (4–8 hr)	HPLC	33
Ornidazole								
Adults	750 mg	0–48	54	4			^{14}C tracer	22

[a]Hydroxy metabolite.
[b]Acid metabolite.

Table 6 Elimination and Clearance Rates for Metronidazole, Tinidazole, and Ornidazole in Pediatric Patients and Adults

				Clearance				
				Total body				
Dose	Age group, mean weight (g)	Dose	$T_{1/2\beta}$ (hr)	ml/kg min^{-1}	ml/min	Renal (ml/min)	Assay	Reference
Metronidazole	<32 weeks' gestation (1020)		75.3	0.12			HPLC	18
	32–35 weeks' gestation (1860)		35.4	0.27			HPLC	18
	36–40 weeks' gestation (3150)		24.8	0.31			HPLC	18
	Infant, 6 weeks	22 mg/kg PO	10.66	0.94			Polar	19
	9–14 years	10.2 mg/kg PO	8.98	0.94			Polar	19
	Adults		8.31	1.07			Polar	19
	Adults	500 mg IV	7.9	1.04	80.1		HPLC	21
	Adults	750 mg PO	8.4				TLC	22
	Adults	500 mg PO	8.7			10.2	BA	27
	Adults	500 mg IV	8.3		81.3		HPLC	45
	Adults	500–2000 mg IV	9.8		107		HPLC	32
	Adults	500 mg IV	6.57		103		HPLC	31
Tinidazole	Adults	500 mg IV	14.0		47.6		HPLC	21
	Adults	150 mg PO	12.7				TLC	30
	Adults	1600 mg IV	13.3	0.71		12.6	HPLC	33
	Adults	500 mg IV	13.1		46.0		HPLC	45
Ornidazole	Adults	750 mg PO	14.4				TLC	22
	Adults	500 mg IV	10.8		76		BA	23
	Adults	1500 mg PO	13.8				TLC	24

study, the mean half-lives varied between 75 hr for infants of less than 32 weeks' gestation to 24 hr for infants 36–40 weeks' gestational age with proportionately low total body clearance (18). In one infant at 6 weeks, the half-life was 10.7 hr, only slightly longer than for children and adults. No specific data are available for ornidazole or tinidazole in this very young age group.

As a result of the decreased clearance, the dosing interval for preterm and term infants has been recommended to be every 48 and every 24 hr, respectively, after an initial loading dose of 15 mg/kg (18).

3. Elimination in Organ Failure

a. Renal Failure. Data are not available for the disposition of the nitroimidazoles in pediatric patients with renal failure. In adult subjects, renal failure does not change significantly the serum half-lives of metronidazole (31), tinidazole (46), or ornidazole (47) after single intravenous or oral doses. However, for metronidazole, with single as well as multiple doses, there was an accumulation of both the hydroxy and acid metabolites that increased up to two to three times those concentrations seen in normal subjects after a single intravenous dose (31). Also, there is a disproportionate increase in the concentration of the acid metabolite, which in renal failure was estimated to have a half-life of approximately 138 hr compared with the hydroxy metabolite, which had a half-life of 34 hr (48). The volumes of distribution for metronidazole were similar in normal and renal failure patients (31). For tinidazole, there was no accumulation of the major metabolite (hydroxy metabolite) and there appeared to be no clinically important pharmacokinetic changes in patients with renal failure (46). For ornidazole, the half-life is similar but the total plasma clearance of 46.3 ml/min was approximately one-half that of 90 ml/min found in normal patients (47).

With hemodialysis, the half-life of unchanged metronidazole was reduced approximately 50% to 3 hr (31,49), and for tinidazole the half-life was reduced from 15 to 4.25 hr (50). Hemodialysis also reduces the half-life of ornidazole, but in one study the reduction was not possible to calculate accurately (47). Hemodialysis is an important mechanism to eliminate the accumulated metabolites of metronidazole and reduces the half-life of the hydroxy metabolite to 8 hr (from 34 hr) and the acid metabolite from 138 to 7.9 hr (49). Because of the increased clearance of the nitroimidazoles during hemodialysis, full dosage regimens may be followed as in patients without renal failure but the doses should be given after hemodialysis rather than before to ensure adequate postdialysis doses.

Peritoneal dialysis had very little effect on the elimination of metronidazole (or its major metabolites) (51) and ornidazole (47). Although no specific data are available, it is unlikely that the pharmacokinetics of tinidazole are affected by peritoneal dialysis. In summary, in patients with severe renal failure, either on no dialysis or on peritoneal dialysis, the dose of metronidazole and possibly ornidazole should be reduced approximately 30% to avoid the potential accumulation of metabolites. This dosage reduction is likely unnecessary in patients receiving tinidazole.

b. Liver Failure. No data are available regarding the disposition of metronidazole or other nitroimidazoles in pediatric patients with liver failure. In adults with cirrhosis and hepatic fibrosis secondary to schistosomiasis, the half-life of metronidazole was slightly longer in cirrhotic patients and the concentrations of the hydroxy metabolite were lower in patients with schistosomal liver disease (52). It is possible in these patients that oxidative enzyme activity is decreased with reduced clearance of metronidazole.

Also, in one case of hepatic amyloid infiltration and renal failure, the half-life of metronidazole was prolonged to 20.6 hr compared with an average of 6.5 hr in other patients with renal failure alone (31). Reducing the dose of metronidazole by 30% in patients with severe liver impairment may be a reasonable dose adjustment. Additional pharmacokinetic data are necessary before specific dosage adjustments can be made relative to liver dysfunction.

E. Preparations, Dosages, Regimens, and Routes of Administration

The nitroimidazoles are available as oral, intravenous, vaginal, rectal, and topical cream preparations; however, not all forms or drugs are available universally.

Oral capsules and tablets range in potency from 200 to 500 mg, whereas vaginal and rectal suppositories usually contain 500–1000 mg of the drug. A topical cream preparation contains 10% metronidazole.

The intravenous preparations of metronidazole, tinidazole, and ornidazole usually contain 500–800 mg of the drug.

The long half-lives of all the nitroimidazoles enable single-dose regimens for some infections, as well as only twice or thrice daily doses to maintain high therapeutic concentrations. For example, dosage regimens for metronidazole include a single high dose of 50 mg/kg (to a maximum of 2 g) for trichomoniasis to daily doses of 25–50 mg/kg given in divided doses every 8 or 12 hr. For tinidazole or ornidazole, dosing intervals are usually every 12 or 24 hr. For serious infections, the intravenous form of the nitroimidazoles is initially used, but because of excellent bioavailability of the oral and rectal preparations and their low cost, these are preferred as the patient's condition improves.

The nitroimidazoles have a very bitter taste that must be masked in suspensions for palatability in young children. A tasteless compound of metronidazole, metronidazole benzoate, has been used, although its bioavailability appears to be about 30% lower than pure metronidazole (53).

IV. DRUG ASSAYS

The assay of nitroimidazoles in serum or plasma and other tissues has evolved over the past 20 years from polarographic and microbiologic techniques to various chromatographic methods. The least specific polarographic assay detects all compounds possessing a nitroimidazole structure (parent compound and metabolites) without regard to bioactivity (54). Bioassays that use various rapidly growing anaerobic organisms (e.g., *Clostridium* species) are clinically very useful in that they measure total bioactivity present (55). For example, the hydroxy metabolite of metronidazole has approximately 30–50% the activity of metronidazole against anaerobic organisms and therefore would contribute to the level of bioactivity determined. However, for this reason, the bioassay does not enable accurate pharmacokinetic studies of individual parent compounds and their metabolites. Also, other antibiotics effective against the test organism in the bioassay would cross-react with the nitroimidazoles, producing a spuriously high value. High-pressure (performance) liquid chromatography appears to have superseded other chromatographic techniques, including thin-layer and gas-liquid chromatography, because of its precision and simplicity (41,42,56). Very small quantities of plasma are required for HPLC, as low as 100 μl, with quantities of approximately 500 μl required for bioassay. Both types of assay can usually measure levels as low as 0.5 μg/ml).

V. THERAPEUTIC INDICATIONS

All three nitroimidazoles appear to be equally effective against a wide range of anaerobic organisms. These encompass protozoal infections, including vaginal trichomoniasis, intestinal giardiasis, and intestinal and hepatic amebiasis, and anaerobic bacterial infections caused by clinically important pathogens, including *Bacteroides, Fusobacterium, Clostridium, Peptococcus*, and *Peptostreptococcus* species. Because of their excellent bactericidal action and penetration of most body tissues, they are effective in infections of the central nervous system (meningitis and cerebral abscess), upper (chronic otitis media and sinusitis), and lower respiratory tract (aspiration pneumonia, lung abscess, and empyema), cardiovascular (endocarditis), musculoskeletal (septic arthritis and osteomyelitis), and intra-abdominal and intrapelvic sepsis. Because many of the above infections are polymicrobial with aerobic organisms, antibiotics effective against aerobes are also included in treatment regimens.

The nitroimidazoles have been used successfully as chemoprophylactic agents in various intra-abdominal and pelvic surgical procedures where anaerobes are important pathogens.

Metronidazole has also been shown to be effective in the treatment of *Clostridium difficile* associated colitis (57) and bacterial vaginosis (nonspecific vaginitis) caused by *G. vaginalis* in association with various anaerobic organisms (58).

VI. TOXICITY

The nitroimidazoles are generally well tolerated by pediatric patients (59). However, various toxic effects, especially with high doses, have been reported for all three drugs, although these have been best documented with metronidazole.

Studies with metronidazole demonstrated a variable tumorigenic effect in certain laboratory animals and a mutagenic effect in particular bacterial strains (the Ames test); however, the significance of these effects in humans and the teratogenic potential have been questioned and never clearly demonstrated despite over 20 years of use (60–62).

Toxic effects that are likely dose dependent that have been demonstrated in patients on metronidazole include a disulfuramlike intolerance when given with alcohol (63) and a neutropenia that is reversible with discontinuation of the drug (64). Central nervous system effects (headache, dizziness, psychosis, and seizures) are usually seen after large single or daily doses (65,66). In a 12-year-old patient with intra-abdominal sepsis given intravenous metronidazole at a dose of 250 mg every 6 hr (total, 4 g), generalized seizures occurred followed by a prolonged organic brain syndrome (67). In one report with tinidazole, an acute toxic reaction characterized by a vasovagal attack, hypotension, and nausea occurred in an adult after 1600 mg were infused over 80 min (68). Sensory peripheral neuropathy (asymptomatic and symptomatic) was found in 11 of 13 patients with Crohn's disease aged 12–22 years who had been treated for 4–11 months with metronidazole at doses from 10 to 33 mg/kg day^{-1}. Discontinuation of metronidazole in 9 patients resulted in resolution or improvement in all but one patient (69). It is postulated that prolonged metronidazole administration (total dose greater than 30 g) causes axonal degeneration because of inhibition of neuronal RNA (70,71). Antibiotic-associated colitis has also been reported after metronidazole (72).

Hypersensitivity reactions including rashes have also been reported. Less serious side effects include nausea, vomiting, a metallic taste, and a brown discoloration of the urine (produced by an azo metabolite of metronidazole).

Whether pediatric patients are more or less susceptible to toxicity to the nitroimidazoles is unknown, but no extraordinary effects have been reported when the drug has been used in these patients.

VII. CONTRAINDICATIONS

No absolute contraindications exist for the use of the nitroimidazoles, except in patients who have experienced a serious hypersensitivity reaction, which is rare. Because of the disulfuramlike reaction noted with the simultaneous ingestion of ethanol, pharmaceutical preparations containing alcohol should not be given with the nitroimidazoles or for 48 hr following their discontinuation. Patients with severe renal disease should be carefully watched to avoid the accumulation and potential toxic effects of metronidazole and possibly ornidazole and their metabolites. Also, patients with severe hepatic disease because of the slower metabolism of the nitroimidazoles may also have unexpected side effects on usual dosage regimens. Patients with a history of seizures should be carefully observed while receiving metronidazole, and in patients with pre-existing neutropenia, an alternate drug should be considered, if appropriate.

VIII. DRUG INTERACTIONS

Metronidazole increases the serum concentration of warfarin owing to an interaction with racemic and *S*(−)-warfarin. The interaction is stereoselective, and therefore the use of *S*(+)-warfarin would obviate this problem (73). Pretreatment with metronidazole for 6 days in adults did not affect the pharmacokinetics of diazepam, antipyrine, or phenytoin, whose disposition is dependent upon oxidative drug metabolism (cytochrome P_{450} system) (74). Also, metronidazole did not modify the disposition of intravenous theophylline (75), but in contrast, cimetidine administration (probably as a result of inhibition of the microsomal P_{450} mono-oxygenases in the liver) decreased the plasma clearance and prolonged the half-life of metronidazole (76).

REFERENCES

1. Jolles, GE: Origin and anti-infective activities of metronidazole. In: *Metronidazole*, Proceedings of the International Metronidazole Conference, Montreal, Quebec, Canada, May 26–28, 1976 (SM Finegold, ed.; JA McFadzean and FJC Roe, assoc. eds.), Excerpta Medica, Princeton, 1977, pp. 3–11.
2. Maeda, K, Osata, T, Umezawa, H: A new antibiotic azomycin. *J. Antibiot. 6A*:182, 1953.
3. Cosar, C, Crisan, C, Horclois, R, Jacob, R, Robert, J, Tchelitcheff, S, Vaupre, R: Nitro-imidazoles. Preparation et activite chimiotherapeutique. *Arzneimittelforsch. 16*:23–29, 1966.
4. Miller, MW, Howes, LT, English, AR: Tinidazole, a potent new antiprotozoal agent. *Antimicrob. Agents Chemother. 9*:257–260, 1969.
5. Hoffer, M, Grunberg, E: Synthesis and antiprotozoal activity of 1-(3-chloro-2-hydroxypropyl) substituted nitroimidazoles. *J. Med. Chem. 17*:1019–1020, 1974.
6. Muller, M: Action of clinically utilized 5-nitroimidazoles on microorganisms. *Scand. J. Infect. Dis. (Suppl.) 26*:31–41, 1981.
7. Yeung, T-C, Beaulieu, BB, Jr., McLafferty, MA, Goldman, P: Interaction of metronidazole with DNA repair mutants of *Escherichia coli*. *Antimicrob. Agents Chemother. 25*:65–70, 1984.

8. Lockerby, DL, Rabin, HR, Laishley, EJ: Role of the phosphoroclastic reaction of *Clostridium pasteurianum* in the reduction of metronidazole. *Antimicrob. Agents Chemother. 27*:863–867, 1985.
9. Tally, FP, Malamy, MH: Mechanism of antimicrobial resistance and resistance transfer in anaerobic bacteria. *Scand. J. Infect. Dis. (Suppl.) 35*:37–44, 1982.
10. Cederno, JR, Krogstad, DT: Susceptibility testing of *Entamoeba histolytica. J. Infect. Dis. 148*:1090–1095, 1983.
11. Jokipii, L, Jokipii, AMM: In vitro susceptibility of *Giardia lamblia* trophozoites to metronidazole and tinidazole. *J. Infect. Dis. 1412*:317–325, 1980.
12. Ralph, ED, Darwish, R, Austin, TW, Smith, EA, Pattison, FLM: Susceptibility of *Trichomonas vaginalis* strains to metronidazole: Response to treatment. *Sex. Transm. Dis. 10*:119–122, 1983.
13. Wust, J: Susceptibility of anaerobic bacteria to metronidazole, ornidazole, and tinidazole and routine susceptibility testing by standardized methods. *Antimicrob. Agents Chemother. 11*:631–637, 1977.
14. Chow, AW, Bednorz, D, Guze, LB: Susceptibility of obligate anaerobes to metronidazole: An extended study of 1054 clinical isolates. In: *Metronidazole*, Proceedings of the International Metronidazole Conference, Montreal, Quebec, Canada, May 26–28, 1976 (SM Finegold, ed.; JA MacFadzean and FJC Roe, assoc. eds.), Excerpta Medica, Princeton, 1977, pp. 286–292.
15. Ralph, ED, Amatnieks, Y: Potentially synergistic antimicrobial combinations with metronidazole against *Bacteroides fragilis. Antimicrob. Agents Chemother. 17*:379–382, 1980.
16. Ralph, ED, Austin, TW, Pattison, FLM, Schieven, B: Inhibition of *Haemophilus vaginalis (Corynebacterium vaginale)* by metronidazole, tetracycline, and ampicillin. *Sex. Transm. Dis. 6*:199–202, 1979.
17. Shanker, S, Monro, R: Sensitivity of *Gardnerella vaginalis* to metabolites of metronidazole and tinidazole. *Lancet 1*:167, 1982.
18. Jager-Roman, E, Doyle, PE, Baird-Lambert, J, Cvejic, M, Buchanan, N: Pharmacokinetics and tissue distribution of metronidazole in the newborn infant. *J. Pediatr. 100*:651–654, 1982.
19. Amon, I, Amon, K, Scharp, H, Franke, G, Nagel, F: Disposition kinetics of metronidazole in children. *Eur. J. Clin. Pharmacol. 24*:113–119, 1983.
20. Houghton, GW, Thorne, PS, Smith, J, Templeton, R, Colier, J: Comparison of the pharmacokinetics of metronidazole in healthy female volunteers following either a single oral or intravenous dose. *Br. J. Clin. Pharmacol. 8*:337–381, 1979.
21. Mattila, J, Mannisto, PT, Mantyla, R, Nykanen, S, Lamminsivu, U: Comparative pharmacokinetics of metronidazole and tinidazole as influenced by administration route. *Antimicrob. Agents Chemother. 23*:721–725, 1983.
22. Schwartz, DE, Jeunet, F: Comparative pharmacokinetic studies of ornidazole and metronidazole in man. *Chemotherapy 22*:19–29, 1976.
23. Luthy, R, Weber, F, Siegenthaler, W: In vitro and in vivo properties of ornidazole. Abstract 454, 16th Interscience Conference on Antimicrobial Agents and Chemotherapy, October 27–29, 1976, Chicago, American Society for Microbiology.
24. Matheson, I, Hernborg Johannesen, K, Bjorkvoll, B: Plasma levels after a single oral dose of 1.5 g ornidazole. *Br. J. Vener. Dis. 53*:236–239, 1977.
25. Mecander, A, Kahlmeter, G, Kamme, C, Ursing, B: Bioavailability of metronidazole in fasting and non-fasting healthy subjects and in patients with Crohn's disease. *Eur. J. Clin. Pharmacol. 12*:69–72, 1977.
26. Anderson, KE: Pharmacokinetics of nitroimidazoles. Spectrum of adverse reactions. *Scand. J. Infect. Dis. (Suppl.) 26*:60–67, 1981.

27. Ralph, ED: Clinical pharmacokinetics of metronidazole. *Clin. Pharmacokinet. 8*: 43–62, 1983.
28. Ralph, ED, Clarke, JT, Libke, RD, Luthy, RP, Kirby, WMM: Pharmacokinetics of metronidazole as determined by bioassay. *Antimicrob. Agents Chemother. 6*:691–696, 1974.
29. Houghton, GW, Thorne, PS, Smith, J, Templeton, R, Collier, J, Moesgaard, F, Lykkegaard-Nielsen, M: The pharmacokinetics of intravenous metronidazole (single and multiple dosing). In: *Metronidazole*, Proceedings of the Second International Symposium on Anaerobic Infections, Geneva, April 25–27 (I Phillips and J Collier, eds.), The Royal Society of Medicine, London Academic Press, London; Grune and Stratton, New York, 1979, pp. 35–40.
30. Taylor, JA, Jr., Migliardi, JR, Von Wittenau, MS: Tinidazole and metronidazole pharmacokinetics in man and mouse. *Antimicrob. Agents Chemother.* 267–270, 1969.
31. Kreeft, JH, Olgivie, RI, Dufresne, LR: Metronidazole kinetics in dialysis patients. *Surgery 93*(Part 2):149–153, 1983.
32. Rabin, HR, Urtusun, RC, Partington, J, Koziol, D, Sharon, M, Walker, K: High dose metronidazole: Pharmacokinetics and bioavailability using an iv preparation and application of its use as a radiosensitizer. *Cancer Treat. Rep. 64*:1087–1095, 1980.
33. Wood, BA, Faulkner, JK, Munro, AM: The pharmacokinetics, metabolism and tissue distribution of tinidazole. *J. Antimicrob. Chemother. (Suppl. A) 10*:43–57, 1982.
34. Sattar, MA, Sankey, MG, Cawley, MID, Kaye, CM, Holt, JE: The penetration of metronidazole into the synovial fluid. *Postgrad. Med. J. 58*:20–24, 1982.
35. Nielsen, ML, Justeben, T: Excretion of metronidazole in human bile. Investigations of hepatic bile, common duct bile, and gall bladder bile. *Scand. J. Gastroenterol. 12*:1003–1008, 1977.
36. Erickson, SH, Oppenheim, GL, Smith, GH: Metronidazole in breast milk. *Obstet. Gynecol. 57*:48–50, 1981.
37. Rood, JP, Collier, J: Metronidazole levels in alveolar bone. In: *Metronidazole*, Proceedings of the Second International Symposium on Anaerobic Infections, Geneva, April 25–27 (I Phillips and J Collier, eds.), The Royal Society of Medicine, London Academic Press, London; Grune and Stratton, New York, 1979, pp. 45–47.
38. Elder, MG, Kane, JL: The pelvic tissue levels achieved by metronidazole after single or multiple dosing—oral or rectal. In: *Metronidazole*, Proceedings of the Second International Symposium on Anaerobic Infections, Geneva, April 25–27 (I Phillips and J Collier, eds.), The Royal Society of Medicine, London Academic Press, London; Grune and Stratton, New York, 1979, pp. 55–58.
39. Mattila, J, Nerdrum, K, Rouhianen, H, Mannisto, P, Tuovinen, E, Lamminsivu, U: Penetration of metronidazole and tinidazole into the aqueous humor in man. *Chemotherapy 29*:188–191, 1983.
40. Jokipii, AMM, Myllyla, VV, Hokkanen, E, Jokipii, L: Penetration of the blood brain barrier by metronidazole and tinidazole. *J. Antimicrob. Chemother. 3*:239–245, 1977.
41. Wheeler, LA, DeMeo, M, Halula, M, George, L, Hesseltine, P: Use of high pressure liquid chromatography to determine plasma levels of metronidazole and metabolites after intravenous administration. *Antimicrob. Agents Chemother. 13*:205–209, 1978.
42. Merdjan, H, Bonnat, C, Singlas, E, Diquet, B: Measurement of ornidazole by high-performance liquid chromatography. *J. Chromatogr. 273*:475–480, 1983.
43. Vinge, E, Andersson, K-E, Ando, G, Lunell, E: Biological availability and pharmacokinetics of tinidazole after single and repeated doses. *Scand. J. Infect. Dis. 15*: 391–397, 1983.

44. Stambaugh, JE, Feo, LG, Manthei, RW: The isolation and identification of the urinary oxidative metabolites of metronidazole in man. *J. Pharmacol. Exp. Ther.* *161*:373–381, 1968.
45. Mattie, A, Dijkmans, BAC, Van Gulpen, C: The pharmacokinetics of metronidazole and tinidazole in patients with mixed aerobic-anaerobic infections. *J. Antimicrob. Chemother. (Suppl. A) 10*:59–64, 1982.
46. Robson, RA, Bailey, RR, Sharman, JR: Tinidazole pharmacokinetics in severe renal failure. *Clin. Pharmacokinet. 9*:88–94, 1984.
47. Merdjan, H, Baumelou, A, Duquet, B, Chick, O, Singlas, E: Pharmacokinetics of ornidazole in patients with renal insufficiency; influence of haemodialysis and peritoneal dialysis. *Br. J. Clin. Pharmacol. 19*:211–217, 1985.
48. Gabriel, R, Page, CM, Weller, IVD, Collier, J, Houghton, GW, Templeton, R, Thorne, PS: The pharmacokinetics of metronidazole in patients with chronic renal failure. In: *Metronidazole*, Proceedings of the Second International Symposium on Anaerobic Infections, Geneva, April 25–27 (I Phillips and J. Collier, eds.), The Royal Society of Medicine, London Academic Press, London; Grune and Stratton, New York, 1979, pp. 50–54.
49. Roux, AF, Moirot, E, Delhotal, B, Leroy, JA, Bonmarhand, GP, Humbert, G, Flouvat, B: Metronidazole kinetics in patients with acute renal failure on dialysis: A cumulative study. *Clin. Pharmacol. Ther. 36*:363–368, 1984.
50. Flouvat, BL, Imbert, C, Dubois, DM, Temperville, BP, Roux, AF, Chevalier, GC, Humbert, G: Pharmacokinetics of tinidazole in chronic renal failure and patients on hemodialysis. *Br. J. Clin. Pharmacol. 15*:735–741, 1983.
51. Guay, DR, Meatherall, RC, Baxter, H, Jacyk, WR, Penner, B: Pharmacokinetics of metronidazole in patients undergoing continuous ambulatory peritoneal dialysis. *Antimicrob. Agents Chemother. 25*:306–310, 1984.
52. Daneshmend, TK, Homeida, M, Kaye, CM, Elamin, AA, Roberts, CJC: Disposition of oral metronidazole in hepatic cirrhosis and in hepatosplenic schistosomiasis. *Gut 23*:807–813, 1982.
53. Alestig, K, Freij, L, Arnold, E: Absorption and excretion of metronidazole after administration of metronidazole benzoate mixture. *Scand. J. Infect. Dis. 12*:149–152, 1980.
54. Kane, PO, McFadzean, JA, Squires, S: Absorption and excretion of metronidazole. Serum concentration and urinary excretion after oral administration. *Br. J. Vener. Dis. 37*:273–275, 1961.
55. Ralph, ED, Kirby, WMM: Bioassay of metronidazole with either anaerobic or aerobic incubation. *J. Infect. Dis. 132*:587–591, 1975.
56. Nilsson-Ehle, I, Ursing, B, Nilsson-Ehle, P: Liquid chromotographic assay for metronidazole and tinidazole: Pharmacokinetic and metabolic studies in human subjects. *Antimicrob. Agents Chemother. 19*:754–760, 1981.
57. Pashby, NL, Bolton, RP, Sherriff, RJ: Oral metronidazole in *Clostridium difficile* colitis. *Br. Med. J. 1*:1605–1606, 1979.
58. Pheifer, TA, Forsyth, PS, Durfee, MA, Pollock, HM, Holmes, KK: Nonspecific vaginitis. Role of *Haemophilus vaginalis* and treatment with metronidazole. *N. Engl. J. Med. 298*:1429–1434, 1978.
59. Brook, I: Treatment of anaerobic infections in children with metronidazole. *Dev. Pharmacol. Ther. 6*:187–198, 1983.
60. Roe, FJC: A critical appraisal of the toxicology of metronidazole. In: *Metronidazole*, Proceedings of the Second International Symposium on Anaerobic Infections, Geneva, April 25–27 (I Phillips and J Collier eds.), The Royal Society of Medicine, London Academic Press, London; Grune and Stratton, New York, 1979, pp. 215–222.

61. Beard, C, Noller, KL, O'Fallon, M, Karland, LT, Dockerty, MB: Lack of evidence for cancer due to use of metronidazole. *N. Engl. J. Med. 301*:519–522, 1979.
62. Friedman, GD: Cancer after metronidazole. *N. Engl. J. Med. 302*:519, 1980.
63. Semer, JM, Friedland, P, Vaisberg, M, Greenberg, M. The use of metronidazole in the treatment of alcoholism. *Am. J. Psychiatr. 123*:722–724, 1966.
64. Smith, JA: Neutropenia associated with metronidazole therapy. *Can. Med. Assoc. J. 123*:202, 1980.
65. Frytak, S, Moertel, CG, Childs, DS, Albers, JW: Neurologic toxicity associated with high dose metronidazole. *Ann. Intern. Med. 88*:361–362, 1978.
66. Thomas, GM, Rauth, AM, Bush, RS, Black, BE, Cummings, BJ: A toxicity study of daily dose metronidazole with pelvic irradiation. *Cancer Clin. Trials 3*:223–230, 1980.
67. Bailes, J, Willis, J, Priebe, C, Strub, R: Encephalopathy with metronidazole in a child. *Am. J. Dis. Child. 137*:290–291, 1983.
68. Aase, S, Olsen, AK, Roland, M, Fagerhol, MK, Liavag, I, Bergan, T, Leinb, O: Severe toxic reaction to tinidazole. *Eur. J. Clin. Pharmacol. 24*:425–427, 1983.
69. Duffy, LF, Daum, F, Fisher, SE, Selman, J, Vishnubhakat, SM, Aiges, HW, Markowitz, JF, Silverberg, M: Peripheral neuropathy in Crohn's disease patients treated with metronidazole. *Gastroenterology 8*:681–684, 1985.
70. Bradley, WG, Karlson, IJ, Rassol, CG: Metronidazole neuropathy. *Br. Med. J. 3*: 610–611, 1977.
71. Karlsson, IJ, Hamlyn, AN: Metronidazole neuropathy. *Br. Med. J. 3*:832, 1977.
72. Thomson, G, Clark, AH, Hare, K, Spilg, WG: Pseudomembranous colitis after treatment with metronidazole. *Br. Med. J. 282*:864–865, 1981.
73. O'Reilly, RA: The stereoselective interaction of warfarin and metronidazole in man. *N. Engl. J. Med. 295*:354–357, 1976.
74. Jensen, JC, Gugler, R: Interaction between metronidazole and drugs eliminated by oxidative metabolism. *Clin. Pharmacol. Ther. 37*:407–410, 1985.
75. Reitberg, DP, Klarnet, JP, Carlson, JK, Schentag, JJ: Effect of metronidazole on theophylline pharmacokinetics. *Clin. Pharm. 2*:441–444, 1983.
76. Gugler, R, Jensen, JC: Interaction between cimetidine and metronidazole. *N. Engl. J. Med. 309*:1518–1519, 1983.

Part VII
Summary

38
Drugs of Choice

CHARLES G. PROBER
Stanford University School of Medicine, Stanford, California

The three principal factors to be considered in selecting an antimicrobial agent for a specific clinical situation are

1. The proven or presumed identity of the pathogen(s)
2. The measured or presumed antimicrobial susceptibility of the infecting pathogen(s)
3. A variety of host factors

Therefore, a brief discussion of each of these factors is relevant before presenting in tabular form specific "drugs of choice."

I. IDENTIFICATION OF PATHOGENS

Whenever possible, the antimicrobial agent should be chosen on the basis of isolation of a pathogen. However, most patients present with an acute problem mandating immediate empirical therapy. In such cases, the antimicrobial agent is selected upon knowledge of pathogens likely to cause infection at a specific site in that specific patient. Results of rapid diagnostic tests may be helpful in the initial antimicrobial selection. For example, in cases of suspected bacterial meningitis, Gram stain and latex particle agglutination of the cerebrospinal fluid may suggest a specific pathogen. If neither rapid techniques nor cultures identify an etiologic agent(s), therapy is continued on the basis of the original "best guess." If, on the other hand, a pathogen is isolated, specific antimicrobial therapy can be substituted for the original empirical therapy.

II. SUSCEPTIBILITY OF PATHOGENS

In the selection of empirical therapy, both pathogen identity and antimicrobial susceptibility must be presumed. If a pathogen is never isolated, this presumed susceptibility and response to treatment will determine the entire course of therapy.

If a specific pathogen is isolated, in vitro antimicrobial susceptibility testing allows the determination of the most suitable antimicrobial agent. Susceptibility testing of viruses, parasites, and fungi is not routinely available. The techniques of bacterial susceptibility testing are discussed in Chapter 1. The usual spectrum of activity of specific antimicrobial agents is outlined in the chapter dealing with each agent. It must be emphasized that these general susceptibility data do not apply to all geographic areas. The susceptibility patterns of bacterial pathogens are under constant evolution influenced by local antibiotic-prescribing patterns. In view of these geographic variations, local susceptibility data should be considered when developing specific empirical treatment regimens. In some cases, the susceptibility of certain pathogens need not be confirmed as they have demonstrated stable susceptibility over time. For example, all meningococci remain sensitive to penicillin. However, the number of bacteria for which susceptibility testing is not routinely indicated is ever diminishing.

III. HOST FACTORS

Host age and the clinical setting determine the most probable etiologic agent(s) and therefore the most suitable empirically selected antibiotic(s), (see Tables 1-14). Other host factors influence the pharmacokinetics and toxicities of selected antimicrobials.

The single most important factor that determines the choice, dose, and route of administration of antimicrobial agents is the site of infection. The distribution characteristics of the antimicrobials under consideration will determine which agents are most likely to penetrate to the site of infection in therapeutically adequate concentrations. The distribution characteristics of each antimicrobial agent are discussed in the chapter concerning the specific agent. In addition, there may be factors at the site of infection that influence antimicrobial activity. These factors include local pH and ionic content, as well as the local presence of pus, blood, or β-lactamase producing bacteria.

For example, reduced local pH increases the biologic activity of certain antibiotics (e.g., methenamine, nitrofurantoin, and chlorotetracycline), whereas an elevated local pH increases the biologic activity of others (e.g., erythromycin, clindamycin, and aminoglycosides) (1-3). The local concentrations of calcium and magnesium have a substantial influence on the minimum inhibitory concentrations (MIC) of aminoglycosides against *Pseudomonas aeruginosa*; higher ionic concentrations resulting in higher MIC (4). The presence of pus results in reduced activity of aminoglycosides (5) whereas the presence of blood results in reduced activity of penicillins and tetracyclines (6). Hemoglobin may bind and hence inactivate these antibiotics. The presence of β-lactamase producing organisms can inactivate any of the β-lactam antibiotics.

Host factors that can influence both the pharmacokinetics and toxicity of certain antibiotics include age, genetic characteristics, pregnancy, and renal and hepatic function. Drug disposition in neonates differs markedly from disposition in older children and adults. The reduced renal and hepatic function present in the early weeks of life result in substantial alterations in the kinetics of drugs excreted by the kidneys or liver or metabolized by the liver. Chapter 4 discusses the factors to be considered when prescribing antimicrobial agents to neonates. Another effect of age on pharmacokinetics results from the increased gastric pH of most children less than 3 years of age and some adults more than 60 years of age. The oral absorption of a variety of antimicrobial agents is altered by the alkaline gastric pH evident at these age extremes.

Table 1 Empirical Antibiotic Selection for Bacterial Infections of the Abdomen

Diagnosis	Host factors	Etiologies	Suggested antibiotic(s)	
			First choice	Alternative
Peritonitis	Primary (e.g., with nephrotic syndrome)	Pneumococci, *E. coli*	Ampicillin + tobramycin	Erythromycin + tobramycin
Peritonitis	Secondary to bowel perforation	*Bacteroides* sp., Enterobacteriaceae, enterococci	Clindamycin + tobramycin	Cefoxitin
Peritonitis	Secondary to continuous ambulatory peritoneal dialysis	Staphylococci, Enterobacteriaceae	Vancomycin + cefotaxime	Vancomycin + tobramycin
Necrotizing enterocolitis	In neonates	Enterobacteriaceae, *Bacteroides* sp.	Clindamycin + tobramycin	Cefoxitin

Table 2 Empirical Antibiotic Selection for Bacterial Infections of the Blood stream

Diagnosis	Host factors	Etiologies	Suggested antibiotic(s)	
			First choice	Alternative
Sepsis	Neonate	Streptococci, Enterobacteriaceae, staphylococci, *Listeria*	Ampicillin + tobramycin	Vancomycin + cefotaxime
Sepsis	Child	Pneumococci, *Hemophilus influenzae*, meningococci	Cefotaxime	Ampicillin + chloramphenicol
Sepsis	Adolescent	Staphylococci, meningococci	Nafcillin + cefotaxime	Vancomycin + chloramphenicol
Sepsis	Nosocomial	Staphylococci, Enterobacteriaceae	Vancomycin + cefotaxime	Nafcillin + tobramycin
Sepsis	Central intravenous catheter related	Staphylococci, Enterobacteriaceae	Vancomycin + cefotaxime	Nafcillin + tobramycin

Table 3 Empirical Antibiotic Selection for Bacterial Infection of the Bone

Diagnosis	Host factors	Etiologies	Suggested antibiotic(s)	
			First choice	Alternative
Osteomyelitis	Neonates	Staphylococci, streptococci, Enterobacteriaceae	Nafcillin + tobramycin	Vancomycin + tobramycin
Osteomyelitis	Acute hematogenous or chronic	Staphylococci	Nafcillin	Clindamycin
Osteomyelitis	Associated with hemoglobino-pathy	Staphylococci, *Salmonella*	Nafcillin + ampicillin	Vancomycin + chloramphenicol
Osteomyelitis	Postoperative	Staphylococci, Enterobacteriaceae	Nafcillin + tobramycin	Vancomycin + tobramycin
Osteomyelitis	Foot, after puncture wound	*Pseudomonas* sp.	Ticarcillin + tobramycin	Ceftazidime

Table 4 Empirical Antibiotic Selection for Bacterial Infections of the Central Nervous System

Diagnosis	Host factors	Etiologies	Suggested antibiotic(s)	
			First choice	Alternative
Abscess	Not associated with trauma	Streptococci, anaerobic species	Penicillin + chloramphenicol	Metronidazole
Abscess	Associated with chronic ear disease	*Pseudomonas*	Ceftazidine + chloramphenicol	Ceftazidine + metronidazole
Abscess	Associated with trauma or surgery	Staphylococci, streptococci, anaerobic species	Nafcillin + chloramphenicol	Vancomycin + metronidazole
Meningitis	Neonate	Enterobacteriaceae, group B streptococci, *Listeria*	Ampicillin + tobramycin	Cefotaxime + ampicillin
Meningitis	Infant and child	*Hemophilus influenzae*, pneumococci, meningococci	Ampicillin + chloramphenicol	Cefotaxime
Shunt infection	Ventriculoperitoneal shunt in place	Staphylococci, Enterobacteriaceae	Nafcillin + tobramycin	Vancomycin + cefotaxime

Table 5 Empirical Antibiotic Selection for Bacterial Infections of the Ear and Sinuses

Diagnosis	Host factors	Etiologies	Suggested antibiotic(s)	
			First choice	Alternative
Otitis externa, "malignant"	Diabetes mellitis	*Pseudomonas* sp.	Ticarcillin + tobramycin	Ceftaxidime
Acute otitis media	Infant and child	Pneumococci, *Hemophilus influenzae*, *Neisseria catarrhalis*	Amoxicillin	TMP-SMZ
Sinusitis	—	Pneumococci, *Hemophilus*, streptococci	Amoxicillin	TMP-SMZ

Table 6 Empirical Antibiotic Selection for Bacterial Infections of the Eye

Diagnosis	Host factors	Etiologies	Suggested antibiotic(s)	
			First choice	Alternative
Preseptal cellulitis	Without trauma	*Hemophilus influenzae*	Cefuroxime	Ampicillin + chloramphenicol
Preseptal cellulitis	With trauma	Staphylococci, streptococci, *H. influenzae*	Nafcillin + chloramphenicol	Vancomycin + cefuroxime
Orbital cellulitis	–	Staphylococci, pneumococci	Nafcillin + chloramphenicol	Vancomycin + cefuroxime
Ophthalmia neonatorum	Onset 2–5 days of age	Gonococci	Penicillin	–
Ophthalmia neonatorum	Onset after 5 days of age	*Chlamydia*	Erythromycin	Sulfonamide

Table 7 Empirical Antibiotic Selection for Bacterial Infections of the Genital Tract

Diagnosis	Host factors	Etiologies	Suggested antibiotic(s)	
			First choice	Alternative
Epididymoorchitis	No urinary tract infection	Gonococci, *Chlamydia*	Erythromycin	Tetracycline
Epididymoorchitis	With urinary tract infection	Enterobacteriaceae	TMP-SMZ	Amoxicillin
Purulent cervicitis	–	Gonococci, *Chlamydia*	Erythromycin	Tetracycline
Urethritis	Gram-negative diplococci seen on gram stain	Gonococci	Penicillin	Spectinomycin
Urethritis	Bacterial cultures negative	*Chlamydia*, *Ureaplasma*	Erythromycin	Tetracycline
Pelvic inflammatory disease	–	Gonococci, *Chlamydia*, *Bacteroides* sp., Enterobacteriaceae, *Mycoplasma*	Cefoxitin + tetracycline	Metronidazole + tetracycline
Nonspecific vaginitis	Malodorous discharge	*Gardnerella vaginalis*, *Bacteroides* sp.	Metronidazole	Ampicillin

Table 8 Empirical Antibiotic Selection for Bacterial Infections of the Heart

Diagnosis	Host factors	Etiologies	Suggested antibiotic(s)	
			First choice	Alternative
Endocarditis	Congenital heart disease	Staphylococci, enterococci, *Streptococcus viridans*	Nafcillin + gentamicin	Vancomycin + gentamicin
Endocarditis	Prosthetic valves	Staphylococci, Enterobacteriaceae	Vancomycin + gentamicin	Nafcillin + gentamicin
Endocarditis	Normal valves	Staphylococci	Nafcillin + gentamicin	Vancomycin + gentamicin
Pericarditis	–	Staphylococci, *Hemophilus influenzae*	Nafcillin + chloramphenicol	Nafcillin + cefuroxime

Table 9 Empirical Antibiotic Selection for Bacterial Infections of the Joint

			Suggested antibiotic(s)	
Diagnosis	Host factors	Etiologies	First choice	Alternative
Septic arthritis	Neonates	Staphylococci, streptococci, Enterobacteriaceae	Nafcillin + tobramycin	Vancomycin + tobramycin
Septic arthritis	Infants and children	Staphylococci, *Hemophilus influenzae*, streptococci	Nafcillin + chloramphenicol	Cefuroxime
Septic arthritis	Sexually active adolescent	Staphylococci, streptococci, gonococci	Nafcillin + penicillin	Vancomycin + cefoxitin
Septic arthritis	Postoperative	Staphylococci, Enterobacteriaceae	Nafcillin + tobramycin	Vancomycin + tobramycin

Table 10 Empirical Antibiotic Selection for Bacterial Infections of the Kidney

Diagnosis	Etiologies	Suggested antibiotic(s)	
		First choice	Alternative
Pyelonephritis	Enterobacteriaceae	Ampicillin + gentamicin	Cefotaxime
Cystitis	Enterobacteriaceae	Sulfonamide	Amoxicillin
Asymptomatic bacteriuria	Enterobacteriaceae	Sulfonamide	Amoxicillin
Perinephric abscess	Staphylococci, Enterobacteriaceae	Nafcillin + cefotaxime	Nafcillin + tobramycin

Table 11 Empirical Antibiotic Selection for Bacterial Infections of the Lungs

Diagnosis	Host factors	Etiologies	Suggested antibiotic(s)	
			First choice	Alternative
Pneumonia	Neonate	Streptococci, Enterobacteriaceae, staphylococci	Ampicillin + cefotaxime	Ampicillin + tobramycin
Pneumonia	<2 years of age	Pneumococci, *Hemophilus influenzae*, staphylococci	Nafcillin + cefuroxime	Nafcillin + chloramphenicol
Pneumonia	>2 years of age	Pneumococci, *H. influenzae*	Cefuroxime	Ampicillin + chloramphenicol
Pneumonia	Aspiration	Oral anaerobic species, Enterobacteriaceae	Clindamycin + tobramycin	Chloramphenicol + tobramycin
Pneumonia	Cystic fibrosis	*Pseudomonas* sp.	Piperacillin + tobramycin	Ceftazidime
Pneumonia	Nosocomial	Enterobacteriaceae, staphylococci	Vancomycin + cefotaxime	Nafcillin + tobramycin

Table 12 Empirical Antibiotic Selection for Bacterial Infections of the Mouth

Diagnosis	Host factors	Etiologies	Suggested antibiotic(s): First choice	Suggested antibiotic(s): Alternative
Vincent's angina	–	Fusospirochetal	Penicillin	Erythromycin
Orofacial infection	Odontogenic origin	Anaerobic species	Penicillin	Erythromycin
Dental root abscess	–	Anaerobic species	Penicillin	Erythromycin
Buccal cellulitis	Young child	*Hemophilus influenzae*	Cefuroxime	Ampicillin + chloramphenicol

Table 13 Empirical Antibiotic Selection for Bacterial Infections of the Skin and Soft Tissues

Diagnosis	Host factors	Etiologies	Suggested antibiotic(s)	
			First choice	Alternative
Burn	Local or systemic infection evident	*Pseudomonas* sp., staphylococci, streptococci, Enterobacteriaceae	Piperacillin + tobramycin	Ceftazidime + tobramycin
Cellulitis	Trauma related	Staphylococci, streptococci	Nafcillin	Clindamycin
Cellulitis	Intravenous catheter related	Staphylococci, Enterobacteriaceae	Vancomycin + cefotaxime	Nafcillin + tobramycin
Cellulitis	Facial	*Hemophilus influenzae*	Cefuroxime	Ampicillin + chloramphenicol
Impetigo	–	Group A streptococci	Penicillin	Erythromycin
Fasciitis	Trauma or varicella related	Group A streptococci	Penicillin	Clindamycin
Myositis	–	Staphylococci	Nafcillin	Vancomycin
"Gas gangrene"	Contaminated wound	*Clostridia perfringens*	Penicillin	Metronidazole

Table 14 Empirical Antibiotic Selection for Bacterial Infections of the Upper Airway

Diagnosis	Etiologies	Suggested antibiotic(s) First choice	Alternative
Exudative pharyngitis	Group A streptococci	Penicillin	Erythromycin
Membranous pharyngitis	*Corynebacterium diphtheriae*	Erythromycin	Penicillin
Epiglottitis	*Hemophilus influenzae*	Cefuroxime	Ampicillin + chloramphenicol

Age is also related to the frequency of certain toxic reactions. Hypersensitivity reactions and nephrotoxicity are in general more commonly observed among older patients. The incidence of isoniazid hepatotoxicity increases with increasing age. Sulfonamides, which can displace bilirubin from albumin, increase the risk of kernicterus among neonates. The capacity of tetracycline to bind to dental enamel is responsible for the age-related dental toxicity of this antibiotic.

Several genetic characteristics may affect disposition and response to antimicrobial agents. For example, ethnic groups who have more rapid acetylators (e.g., the Chinese) tend to metabolize isoniazid more rapidly than those who have more slow acetylators (e.g., whites). On the other hand, this acetylation status may also influence the frequency of isoniazid-related neurotoxicity. Slow acetylators appear to have an increased incidence of isoniazed related polyneuritis. Glucose-6-phosphate dehydrogenase (G6PD) deficiency is a genetic abnormality that influences antimicrobial toxicity. This condition predisposes to hemolysis when patients are exposed to oxidizing agents, such as sulfonamides and nitrofurans.

Pregnancy may also modify the disposition and toxicity of antimicrobial agents. Whenever a drug is administered to a pregnant woman, effects on the fetus must also be considered. Certain agents may be potentially teratogenic, whereas others may adversely affect certain developing organs (e.g., aminoglycosides and the ear). Chapter 7 discusses aspects of antimicrobial therapy in pregnancy. The status of both renal and hepatic function can influence the pharmacokinetics and toxicity of a wide variety of antimicrobial agents. Chapter 5 outlines the effects of renal and hepatic dysfunction on antimicrobial chemotherapy.

IV. DRUGS OF CHOICE

Considering all the factors outlined above that may influence the selection of an antimicrobial agent, it should be evident that recommending a drug of choice for every possible clinical situation is not possible. The tables in this chapter are meant to provide guidelines for the most common and least complicated situations. Unfortunately, clinical reality frequently deals with less common and more complicated situations than outlined.

Three sets of tables are presented in this chapter. The first (Tables 1-15) deals with empirical antibiotic selection. The second (Tables 16-24) deals with antimicrobial agents of choice for specific pathogens. The third set (Tables 25-30) deals with specific dosage guidelines. The duration of therapy for specific infectious conditions is dependent upon

Table 15 Empirical Antibiotic Selection for Bacterial Infections in the Febrile Neutropenic Immunosuppressed Host

Diagnosis	Etiologies	Suggested antibiotic(s): First choice	Suggested antibiotic(s): Alternative
Sepsis	Enterobacteriaceae, *Pseudomonas* sp., staphylococci	Piperacillin + tobramycin	Ceftazidime + tobramycin
		Add amphotericin B if fever and neutropenia persist >7 days on antibiotics	
Pneumonia	*Pneumocystis carinii*, Enterobacteriaceae, *Pseudomonas* sp., staphylococci	TMP-SMZ + tobramycin	TMP-SMZ + ceftazidime
		Add amphotericin B if pneumonia has developed during antibiotic therapy	
Typhilitis or perirectal abscess	*Bacteroides* sp., *Pseudomonas* sp., Enterobacteriaceae, enterococci	Piperacillin + tobramycin	Clindamycin + ceftazidime

Table 16 Preferred Therapy for Infections Caused by Gram-Positive Cocci

Bacteria	Types of infection	Antibiotic of first choice	Alternative
Staphylococci			
Penicillin sensitive	All	Penicillin	Vancomycin
Penicillin resistant	All	Nafcillin	Vancomycin
Methicillin resistant	All	Vancomycin	TMP-SMZ + rifampin
Streptococci			
Group A	All	Penicillin	Erythromycin
Group B	Sepsis, meningitis	Penicillin + gentamicin	Cefotaxime
Enterococci	Endocarditis	Penicillin + gentamicin	Vancomycin + gentamicin
	Others	Penicillin	Vancomycin
Pneumococci	Meningitis	Penicillin	Chloramphenicol
	Others	Penicillin	Cefazolin
Anaerobic species	All	Penicillin	Chloramphenicol

Table 17 Preferred Therapy for Infections Caused by Gram-Positive Bacilli

Bacteria	Types of infection	Antibiotic of first choice	Alternative
Bacillus anthracis	All	Penicillin	Erythromycin
Clostridium perfringens	All	Penicillin	Chloramphenicol
C. tetani	All	Penicillin	Erythromycin
Corynebacterium diphtheriae	All	Erythromycin	Penicillin
Diphtheroids	All	Erythromycin	Penicillin
Listeria	All	Ampicillin + tobramycin	TMP-SMZ

Table 18 Preferred Therapy for Infections Caused by Gram-Negative Cocci

Bacteria	Types of infection	Antibiotic of first choice	Alternative
Gonococci			
Penicillin sensitive	Genital	Penicillin	Spectinomycin
	Pharyngeal	Penicillin	TMP-SMZ
	Disseminated	Penicillin	Cefoxitin
	Neonatal	Penicillin	Cefotaxime
	Genital	Spectinomycin	Cefoxitin
	Pharyngeal	TMP-SMZ	—
	Disseminated	Cefoxitin	Cefotaxime
	Neonatal	Cefotaxime	Tobramycin
Meningococci	All	Penicillin	Chloramphenicol

Table 19 Preferred Therapy for Infections Caused by Gram-Negative Bacilli[a]

Bacteria	Types of infection	Antibiotic of first choice	Alternative
Bacteroides sp.	All	Clindamycin	Metronidazole
Brucella	All	Chloramphenicol	TMP-SMZ
Campylobacter fetus	All	Chloramphenicol	Tobramycin
C. jejuni	All	Erythromycin	Chloramphenicol
Escherichia coli	All	Tobramycin	Cefotaxime
Enterobacter aerogenes	All	Tobramycin	Cefotaxime
Francisella tularensis	All	Streptomycin	Chloramphenicol
Fusobacterium nucleatum	All	Penicillin	Clindamycin
Hemophilus influenzae	Otitis, sinusitis	Amoxicillin	Erythromycin - sulfisoxazole
	Serious	Cefotaxime	Ampicillin + chloramphenicol
Klebsiella pneumoniae	All	Tobramycin	Cefotaxime
Legionella sp.	All	Erythromycin + rifampin	–
Pasteurella multocida	All	Penicillin	Cefazolin
Proteus sp.	All	Tobramycin	Cefotaxime
Pseudomonas sp.	All	Ticarcillin + tobramycin*	Ceftazidime*
Salmonella	Gastroenteritis	None	–
	All others	Chloramphenicol	TMP-SMZ
Serratia	All	Gentamicin*	Cefotaxime
Shigella	All	TMP-SMZ	Ampicillin
Vibrio cholerae	All	Tetracycline	TMP-SMZ
Yersinia sp.	Gastroenteritis	TMP-SMZ	–
	All others	Chloramphenicol	Tobramycin

[a]The asterisk signifies bacteria for which the recommended antibiotic is consistently more active in vitro than other members of the same antibiotic class.

Table 20 Preferred Therapy for Infections Caused by Acid-Fast Bacilli

Bacteria	Types of infection	Antibiotic of first choice	Alternative
Mycobacterium tuberculosis	Pulmonary	Isoniazid + rifampin	Isoniazid + ethambutol
	Extrapulmonary	Isoniazid + rifampin + streptomycin	Isoniazid + rifampin + ethambutol
M. leprae	Leprosy	Dapsone + rifampin	Clofazimine

Table 21 Preferred Therapy for Infections Caused by Spirochetes

Spirochete	Types of infection	Antibiotic of first choice	Alternative
Treponema pallidum	Syphilis	Penicillin	Erythromycin
Borrelia recurrentis	Relapsing fever	Penicillin	Tetracycline
Leptospira	Leptospirosis	Penicillin	Tetracycline
Borrelia burgdorferi	Lyme disease	Penicillin	Tetracycline

Table 22 Preferred Therapy for Infections Caused by Miscellaneous Agents

Agent	Types of infection	Antibiotic of first choice	Alternative
Actinomyces israelii	All	Penicillin	Tetracycline
Chlamydia psittaci	All	Chloramphenicol	Tetracycline
C. trachomatis	Conjunctivitis, pneumonia	Erythromycin	Sulfisoxazole
	Urethritis	Erythromycin	Tetracycline
Mycoplasma pneumoniae	All	Erythromycin	Tetracycline
Nocardia	All	TMP-SMZ	Amikacin
Rickettsia	All	Chloramphenicol	Tetracycline
Ureaplasma urealyticum	All	Erythromycin	Tetracycline

Table 23 Preferred Therapy for Infections Caused by Fungi

Fungus	Types of infection	Antifungal of first choice	Alternative
Aspergillus	All	Amphotericin B	–
Blastomyces dermatitidis	All	Amphotericin B	Ketoconazole
Candida sp.	Skin and mucosal	Nystatin	Ketoconazole
	Urinary tract	Flucytosine	Amphotericin B
	Disseminated	Amphotericin B	–
Coccidioides immitis	Lung	Ketoconazole	Amphotericin B
	Bone, Joint	Amphotericin B	Ketoconazole
	Meningeal	Amphotericin B	
Cryptococcus neoformans	All	Amphotericin B + flucytosine	–
Histoplasma capsulatum	Lung	Ketoconazole	Amphotericin B
	Disseminated	Amphotericin B	Ketoconazole
Mucor	All	Amphotericin B	–
Sporothrix schenckii	All	Iodides	Amphotericin B

Table 24 Viral Infections for Which Antiviral Therapy Should Be Considered

Diagnosis	Host factors	Virus	Suggested antiviral	
			First choice	Alternative
Herpes labialis	Immunosuppressed	HSV	Acyclovir (topical, oral, or IV)	–
Herpes genitalis	First episode, primary	HSV	Acyclovir (topical, oral, or IV)	–
	Recurrent	HSV	Acyclovir (oral)	–
Herpes encephalitis	–	HSV	Acyclovir (IV)	Vidarabine
Neonatal herpes	–	HSV	Acyclovir (IV)	Vidarabine
Keratoconjunctivitis	–	HSV	Vidarabine	Idoxuridine (topical)
Varicella	Immunosuppressed	VZV	Acyclovir (IV)	Vidarabine
Zoster	Immunosuppressed	VZV	Acyclovir (IV)	Vidarabine
Pneumonia	–	Influenza A	Amantadine (oral)	Ribavirin (aerosol)
Pneumonia	–	Influenza B	Ribavirin (aerosol)	–
Pneumonia	Immunosuppressed	CMV	DHPG[a] (IV)	–
Retinitis	Immunosuppressed	CMV	DHPG[a] (IV)	–
Bronchiolitis	–	RSV	Ribavirin (aerosol)	–

[a]9-(1,3-Dihydroxy-2-propoxymethyl)guanine.

Table 25 Dosage Guidelines for Parenteral Antibacterial Agents

Antibiotic	Unit dose (mg/kg)	Dosing interval (hr)	Daily dose (mg/kg)	Maximum daily dose (g)
Amikacin	7.5	8	22	1
Ampicillin	25–50	4–6	100–200	10
Azlocillin	50–75	4–6	200–300	24
Carbenicillin	100–150	4–6	400–600	40
Cefazolin	17–33	8	50–100	6
Cefoperazone	50–75	8–12	100–150	12
Cefotaxime	25–50	4–6	100–200	12
Cefoxitin	20–40	4–6	80–160	12
Ceftazidime	50–75	8	200–300	6
Ceftriaxone	25–50	12–24	100	2
Ceftizoxime	25–50	4–6	100–200	12
Cefuroxime	25–75	8	75–225	6
Cephalothin	20–30	4–6	75–125	10
Chloramphenicol	12.5–25	6	50–100	4
Clindamycin	6.5–10	6	25–40	4
Cloxacillin	25–50	6	100–200	8
Erythromycin	5–12.5	6	20–50	4
Fusidic acid	7.0	8	20	1.5
Gentamicin	2.5	8	7.5	0.3
Kanamycin	10	8	30	1.0
Lincomycin	7–10	8–12	10–20	2.0
Methicillin	25–50	6	100–200	10
Metronidazole	7.5	6	30	4

Table 25 (Continued)

Antibiotic	Unit dose (mg/kg)	Dosing interval (hr)	Daily dose (mg/kg)	Maximum daily dose (g)
Mezlocillin	50–75	4–6	200–300	24
Minocycline	2	12	4	0.2
Moxalactam	50–70	6–8	150–200	10
Nafcillin	37.5	6	150	10
Netilmicin	2.5	8	7.5	0.3
Nitrofurantoin	1.5–2	6	5–7	0.4
Oxacillin	25–50	6	100–200	10
Oxytetracycline	7.5–12.5	8–12	15–25	2
Penicillin				
G-benzathine	50,000 U	Once	50,000 U	2.4 million U
G-potassium or sodium	25,000–60,000 U	4	100,000–250,000 U	20 million U
G-procaine	12,500–50,000 U	12–24	25,000–50,000 U	4.8 million U
Piperacillin	50–75	4–6	200–300	24
Spectinomycin	30–40	Once	30–40	2
Streptomycin	10–15	12	20–30	2
Sulfadiazine	25–33	6–8	100	6
Sulfisoxazole	25–33	6–8	100	6
Tetracycline	5–15	8–12	15–30	2
Ticarcillin	50–75	4–6	200–300	24
Tobramycin	2.5	8	7.5	0.3
TMP-SMZ	2.5–10 (of TMP)	6–12	5–20 (of TMP)	1.2 (of TMP)
Vancomycin	10	6	40	4

Table 26 Dosage Guidelines for Oral Antibacterial Agents

Antibiotic	Unit dose (mg/kg)	Dosing interval (hr)	Daily dose (mg/kg)	Maximum daily dose (g)
Amoxicillin	10–15	8	30–45	3
Ampicillin	12.5–25	6	50–100	3
Bacampicillin	12.5–25	12	25–50	2
Cefaclor	13	8	40	2
Cefadroxil	15	12	30	2
Cephalexin	6.5–12.5	6	25–50	3
Cephradine	6.5–12.5	6	25–50	2
Chloramphenicol	12.5–25	6	50–100	3
Clindamycin	2.5–6.5	6	10–25	2
Cloxacillin	12.5–50	6	50–200	4
Cyclacillin	17–33	8	50–100	3
Demeclocyline	2–6	6–12	8–12	0.6
Dicloxacillin	6.5–25	6	25–100	2
Doxycycline	2.5–5	12–24	5	0.2
Erythromycin	5–20	6–12	20–40	2
Flucloxacillin	6.5–25	6	25–100	2
Fusidic acid	7–13	8	20–40	1.5
Lincomycin	10–20	8	30–60	3
Methacycline	2.5–5	6–12	10	0.6
Methenamine				
Bippurate	12.5–25	12	25–50	2
Mandelate	12.5–20	6	50–75	4

Table 26 (Continued)

Antibiotic	Unit dose (mg/kg)	Dosing interval (hr)	Daily dose (mg/kg)	Maximum daily dose (g)
Metronidazole	5–10	8	15–30	2
Minocycline	2	12	4	0.2
Nalidixic acid	12.5	6	50	4
Nafcillin	12.5–25	6	50–100	3
Neomycin	20–30	6–8	50–100	12
Nitrofurantoin	1.5–2	6	5–7	0.4
Oxacillin	12.5–25	6	50–100	3.0
Oxytetracycline	6.5–12.5	6	25–50	0.6
Penicillin				
G	8–17	6–8	25–50	3
V	8–17	6–8	25–50	3
Rifampin	10–20	12–24	20	1.2
Sulfadiazine	30–37.5	4–6	120–150	6
Sulfamethizole	7.5–11	6	30–45	4
Sulfamethoxazole	25–30	12	50–60	3
Sulfasalazine	10–20	4–8	30–60	6
Sulfisoxazole	30–37.5	4–6	120–150	6
Tetracycline	6.5–12.5	6	25–50	3
Trimethoprim	2	12	4	1
TMP-SMZ	2.5–10 (of TMP)	6–12	5–20 (of TMP)	0.32 (of TMP)
Vancomycin	12.5	6	50	4

Table 27 Dosage Guidelines for Antimycobacterial Agents

Agent	Unit dose (mg/kg)	Dosing interval (hr)	Daily dose (mg/kg)	Maximum daily dose
Cycloserine	3.5–5	12	7–10	1 g
Ethambutol	15	24	15	15 mg/kg day^{-1}
Ethionamide	5–10	12	10–20	1 g
Isoniazid	10–20	12–24	10–20	0.6 g
Para-aminosalicyclic acid	66.6–75	6–8	200–300	12 g
Pyrazinamide	5–15	6–12	20–30	3 g
Rifampin	10–20	12–24	20	1.2 g
Streptomycin	10–15	12	20–30	2 g

Table 28 Dosage Guidelines for Antifungal Agents

Agent	Unit dose (mg/kg)	Dosing interval (hr)	Daily dose (mg/kg)	Maximum daily dose
Amphotericin B	0.25–1.0	24–48	0.25–1.0	1 mg/kg
Flucytosine	12.5–37.5	6	50–150	150 mg/kg
Griseofulvin	3–11	1–4	11	2 g
Ketoconazole	5–10	24	5–10	1 g
Miconazole	6.6–13.3	8	20–40	3.6 g
Nystatin	250,000–500,000 U	6	1–2 million U	4 million U

Table 29 Dosage Guidelines for Antiviral Agents

Antiviral	Unit dose (mg/kg)	Dosing interval (hr)	Daily dose (mg/kg)	Maximum daily dose
Acyclovir	5–10	8	15–30	30 mg/kg
Amantadine	2.2–4.4	12	4.4–8.8	150–200 mg
Ribavirin	0.82 hr^{-1}	Aerosol	1.9	1.9 mg/kg
Vidarabine	15–30	24	15–30	15 mg/kg

Table 30 Dosage Guidelines for Parenteral Antibacterial Therapy of Neonates During the First Week of Life

Antibiotic	Unit dose (mg/kg)	Dosing interval (hr) ⩽2000 g	Dosing interval (hr) >2000 g
Amikacin	7.5	12	12
Ampicillin	25–50[a]	12	12
Carbenicillin	100	12	12
Cefazolin	20	12	12
Cefotaxime	50	12	12
Cephalothin	20	12	12
Chloramphenicol	12.5–25	24	24
Gentamicin	2.5	12	12
Kanamycin	7.5–10	12	12
Methicillin	25–50	12	8
Metronidazole	7.5	12	12
Mezlocillin	75	12	8
Moxalactam	50	12	12
Nafcillin	20	12	12
Netilmicin	2.5	12	12
Oxacillin	25–50	12	8
Sodium penicillin G	25,000–50,000 U[a]	12	12
Benzathine penicillin G	50,000 U	Once	Once
Procaine penicillin G	50,000 U	24	24
Ticarcillin	75	12	8
Tobramycin	2	12	12
Vancomycin	15	24–36	24

[a]Higher dose for meningitis.

the severity of the infection and the clinical response to treatment. There are few controlled trials defining the optimal duration of treatment for specific infections.

V. EMPIRICAL ANTIBIOTIC SELECTION

Tables 1–14 present recommendations for the empirical therapy of a variety of infections. These infections are grouped according to the principal organ involved. Each of these 14 tables presents a specific diagnosis by organ site, major relevant host factors to consider, and most likely etiologies. Therapeutic options for the initiation of therapy are outlined. Although they are labeled "first choice" and "alternative," this is not meant to represent a rigid order of preference. Only two therapeutic options are presented for the sake of simplicity. This is not meant to imply that other therapeutic regimens are not acceptable. In general, if one of the recommended therapeutic regimens includes a β-lactam antibiotic, the optional regimen does not. Therefore, a therapeutic option for a patient with an allergy to β-lactams is available. When a combination of antimicrobials is recommended, care has been taken, whenever possible, to avoid agents toxic to the same organ. For example, rather than recommend an aminoglycoside and vancomycin combination (both nephrotoxic), a third-generation cephalosporin and vancomycin combination is more often recommended. I have elected to recommend a specific antibiotic rather than simply a class of antibiotics, e.g., recommending "an aminoglycoside." Therefore, the substitution of one member of an antibiotic group for another is generally acceptable. This substitution will often be determined in a specific locale by patterns of bacterial resistance, relative costs, and personal preferences.

Table 15 relates to the empirical treatment of infections in a specific subpopulation; the febrile, neutropenic host. Only the four most common sites of infection observed in this population of patients are presented.

Tables 16-24 outline the antimicrobial agents indicated for specific pathogens. Tables 16-23 outline the pathogen and type of infection, and two therapeutic options (where available) are provided.

Table 24 outlines the diagnosis and host factors important in the choice of antiviral therapy. These antiviral agents have proven efficacy in the specified clinical situation.

Tables 25-30 specify dosage guidelines. The larger doses and/or more frequent dosing intervals are recommended for the most serious infections. The dosage recommendations provided are guidelines, based upon available pharmacokinetic, pathogen susceptibility, and in vivo efficacy data. Although some clinicians tend to use doses in excess of those recommended here, there are no data to support the therapeutic advantage of this "megadose" approach. Table 30 provides dosing guidelines for neonates in the first week of life, according to two birth weight categories. Beyond the first week of life, the dosing recommendations found in Tables 24-29 apply.

The recommendations presented in this chapter represent only guidelines. Thoughtful patient management requires individualization of therapy in which all pertinent antimicrobial, pharmacokinetic, and host factors are considered.

REFERENCES

1. Moellering, RC, Principles of anti-infective therapy. In: *Anti-infective Therapy* (GL Mandell, RG Douglas, and JE Bennett, eds.), Wiley Interscience, New York, 1985, pp. 1-29.
2. Zinner, SH, Sabath, LD, Casey, JI, Finland, M: Erythromycin and alkalinisation of the urine in the treatment of urinary tract infections due to gram-negative bacilli. *Lancet 1*:1267-1268, 1971.
3. Sabath, LD, Gerstein, DA, Leaf, CD, Finland, M: Increasing the usefulness of antibiotics: Treatment of infections caused by gram-negative bacilli. *Clin. Pharmacol. Ther. 11*:161-167, 1970.
4. Pollock, HM, Minshew, BH, Kenny, MA, Schoenknecht, FD: Effect of different lots of Mueller-Hinton agar on the interpretation of the gentamicin susceptibility of *Pseudomonas aeruginosa. Antimicrob. Agents Chemother. 14*:360-367, 1978.
5. Bryant, RE, Hammond, D: Interaction of purulent material with antibiotics used to treat *Pseudomonas* infections. *Antimicrob. Agents Chemother. 6*:702-707, 1974.
6. Craig, WA, Kunin, CM: Significance of serum protein and tissue binding of antimicrobial agents. *Annu. Rev. Med. 27*:287-300, 1976.

39

Guidelines for Intravenous Administration of Antimicrobial Drugs

L. LEE DUPUIS and SUSAN STANSFIELD
The Hospital for Sick Children, Toronto, Ontario, Canada

Appropriate drug administration technique ensures delivery of the total dose in its active form and seeks to prevent adverse effects. These goals may be difficult to accomplish when drugs are administered intravenously. Complications may arise due to drug-equipment, drug-solution, or drug-drug incompatibilities. Administration of the drug with inappropriate equipment or technique, in an inappropriate concentration, or at an inappropriate rate may result in adverse effects or suboptimal therapy.

The information provided in this chapter will assist the reader in providing safe and effective intravenous antibiotic therapy. Various intravenous administration techniques will be discussed, and specific guidelines for the intravenous administration of antibiotics will be provided.

I. DRUG DELIVERY CONSIDERATIONS

Pediatric drug dosing frequently involves small doses to be given in small volumes. An understanding of the specific methods used to administer these doses is needed to adapt theoretical data on drug utilization to the clinical setting. The mechanics and limitations of the drug delivery system will influence a drug's pharmacokinetic profile in each patient and can help to explain unexpected results in therapeutic drug monitoring or efficacy.

The following information highlights characteristics of some methods and equipment that can affect drug delivery. Some problems typical of infusion to the small infant are discussed in Chapter 8.

A. Slow Infusion Rates

These can result in lengthy times to onset and completion of drug delivery. Microbore tubing with diameters of 0.06–0.14 cm can minimize this effect.

B. Drug Specific Gravity

In a slow-moving intravenous fluid, the specific gravity can cause the drug to settle or float and pool in a bend of the intravenous tubing. The drug can fail to be administered on schedule. Shortening and streamlining the tubing may obviate this problem.

C. In-Line Filters

These can also allow drug separation by specific gravity and/or result in some loss of drug by adsorption to the filter membrane. Newly designed filters and chambers attempt to overcome this shortcoming.

D. Intermittent Administration

A great many methods of intermittent intravenous administration are possible, each with its own limitations. They all allow the rate to be controlled by mechanical infusion devices.

1. Volume Control Set (Buretrol or Burette)

In the mixing chamber a drug can be diluted to any specific volume appropriate for the dose, but it may then have to flow through up to 20 ml of standard tubing to arrive at the patient. Small-volume doses given at slow rates will have delayed delivery. Sets with microbore tubing and a method whereby the drug is administered closer to the patient are preferable.

2. Minibags (or Bottles)

The dose is diluted in a prefilled intravenous bag, which may be 25, 50, or 100 ml in size. This may involve more fluid than an infant can tolerate, and the fixed dilutions that result can give an inappropriate concentration of the drug. There may also be inaccuracy in the dose delivered. For example: a 25-ml minibag is slightly overfilled by the manufacturer. A bag may contain approximately 27-33 ml, a 24% variation. This bag must then be completely administered to deliver an entire drug dose that has been added. The dose is given through a set that could retain perhaps 7 ml, approximately 23% of the dose. This may be flushed into the patient, administering additional fluid, discarded with a set change, or left to be administered at the start of the next dose after possible degradation. This set may also be attached to a primary infusion line far from the patient, causing the additional delay in dosing described in Section I.D.1.

3. Syringes

a. Manual Injections. Very small volumes can be injected into the tubing at a site near the patient and the administration rate controlled by the rate of the intravenous solution flow. Injections may be toward the patient (antegrade) if the dose volume is less than the volume of the tubing between the injection site and the patient or away from the patient (retrograde) if somewhat larger. The time for drug delivery then depends upon the drug volume and the flow rate. Microbore tubing can decrease the delay in delivery. The amount of drug delivered can depend upon the amount of drug sequestered in the dead space of the injection site, which can be $\geqslant$0.05 ml. This can be a significant proportion of small-volume doses, and injection ports with the smallest dead spaces should be selected to minimize this effect and decrease the need to flush small doses through.

b. Syringe Pumps. Syringes can be prepared with desired drug dilutions and can be administered through microbore tubing connected close to the patient. Doses can be administered at a rate independent of the primary solution. The tubing will retain a portion of the dose, however, and tubing with the smallest priming volume should be used or it may require flushing.

E. Summary

These comments on particular aspects of drug delivery illustrate a few of the potential problems to be encountered in pediatric intravenous therapy. Detailed information on the subject may be found in more extensive reviews of the subject (1).

II. COMPATIBILITY

Combinations of a drug solution and a diluent or two drug solutions are chemically compatible if the potency of all components is retained for a specified time period. Combinations that are physically compatible do not change in color or transparency or form a precipitate within a specified time period. A combination that is physically compatible may not be chemically compatible. Chemical compatibility data are obviously preferable to physical compatibility data but are often unavailable.

Many different factors, including pH, solubility, chemical reaction potential, and concentration, may determine physical or chemical compatibility. Drug manufacturers are required to provide information regarding the chemical and physical compatibility of their product in primary intravenous solutions. This information is more often than not geared toward administration to adults, and it may be inappropriate to apply this information to children. For example, the suggested volume of administration may exceed the child's fluid requirements. This problem can be avoided by administering some drugs by direct intravenous injection, but others (e.g., fusidic acid) must be diluted as directed to avoid complications. Drug administration in a diluent or concentration other than recommended by the manufacturer is not advised unless compatibility and stability information exist to support the alternative method.

Systems in which two or more drugs are administered together in the same primary intravenous solution or that mix in the same intravenous tubing distal to the patient are more complicated. Although the bank of drug-drug compatibility information is increasing, it is often difficult, if not impossible, to extrapolate from published information to the situation at hand. For example, amikacin, 5 g/l in Normsol R, is physically and chemically compatible with erythromycin gluceptate, 1 g/l in Normsol R. However, it cannot be assumed that amikacin and erythromycin gluceptate mixtures are always compatible. When these drugs are mixed together in the same concentrations in dextrose 5% in water, there is significant degradation of erythromycin within 4 hr. Diluents and drug concentrations must be considered when assessing compatibility.

Mixing two or more drugs together in the same primary intravenous solution is not recommended. If the drugs are known to be compatible, they can be administered together via the same intravenous tubing ("piggybacked"). If compatibility is unknown or if incompatibility is suspected, the drugs should be administered separately and the intravenous tubing flushed after the administration of each drug.

Table 1 provides general guidelines for the intravenous administration of specific antibiotics to children. Diluents are recommended for administration of each antibiotic

Table 1 IV Antibiotic Administration Guidelines

Drug	Direct IV injection	IV additive	Compatibility	Comments
Acyclovir	Not recommended	Dilute solution to a concentration of 7 mg/ml or less; infuse over 60 min	Solutions: compatible with commonly used IV fluids[a]; drugs: no information	Monitor infusion site for signs of phlebitis and irritation; avoid extravasation; do not use paraben-preserved water for injection for reconstitution
Amikacin	Neonates: dilute solution to 50 mg/ml; administer using retrograde technique; not recommended for infants or older children	Dilute solution to a concentration of 2 mg/ml or less; infuse over 30–60 min	Solutions: compatible with commonly used IV fluids[a]; drugs: incompatible with amphotericin B, cephalosporins, penicillins	
Amphotericin B	Not recommended	Dilute reconstituted solution to a concentration of 0.1 mg/ml or less; infuse over 2–6 hr	Solutions: compatible with D5W with pH $\geqslant$ 4.2; incompatible with amikacin, carbenicillin, gentamicin, kanamycin, penicillin G K/Na, tetracycline	Monitor infusion site for phlebitis and irritation; too rapid administration may cause hypotension, arrhythmias, cardiac arrest; do not filter
Ampicillin	Neonates: administer reconstituted solutions (250 mg/ml or less) undiluted over 3–5 min using retrograde technique; other: dilute reconstituted solution to a concentration of 100 mg/ml or less; administer over 3–5 min at a rate not to exceed 100 mg/min	Dilute reconstituted solution to a concentration of 100 mg/ml or less; infuse over 20–30 min at a rate not to exceed 100 mg/min	Solutions: compatible with NS, D5W; drugs: incompatible with erythromycin, gentamicin, kanamycin, tetracycline	

Azlocillin	Administer reconstituted solution (200 mg/ml) over 5 min; use retrograde technique for neonates	Dilute reconstituted solution to a concentration of 60 mg/ml or less; infuse over 30 min	Solutions: compatible with commonly used IV fluids[a]; drugs: incompatible with aminoglycosides	Monitor injection site for signs of phlebitis and irritation
Carbenicillin	Administer reconstituted solution (100 mg/ml) at a rate not to exceed 200 mg/min; use retrograde technique for neonates	Dilute reconstituted solution to a concentration of 140 mg/ml or less; infuse over at least 15 min at a rate not to exceed 200 mg/min	Solutions: compatible with commonly used IV fluids[a]; drugs: incompatible with aminoglycosides, amphotericin B	Monitor injection site for signs of phlebitis and irritation
Cefamandole	Dilute reconstituted solution to a concentration of 50–100 mg/ml; administer over 3–5 min; use retrograde technique for neonates	Dilute reconstituted solution to a concentration of 20 mg/ml; infuse over 15–60 min	Solutions: compatible with commonly used IV fluids[a]; drugs: incompatible with aminoglycosides	Monitor infusion site for signs of phlebitis and irritation
Cefazolin	Dilute reconstituted solution to a concentration of 50–100 mg/ml; administer over 3–5 min; use retrograde technique for neonates	Dilute reconstituted solution to a concentration of 20 mg/ml or less; infuse over 30–60 min	Solutions: compatible with commonly used IV fluids[a]; drugs: incompatible with erythromycin gluceptate, kanamycin, tetracycline	Monitor infusion site for signs of phlebitis and irritation
Cefonicid	Administer reconstituted solution (220 or 325 mg/ml) over 3–5 min; use retrograde technique for neonates	Dilute reconstituted solution to a concentration of 40 mg/ml or less; infuse over 20–30 min	Solutions: compatible with commonly used IV fluids[a]; drugs: incompatible with aminoglycosides	
Cefoperazone	Administer reconstituted solution (100 mg/ml) over 3–5 min; use retrograde technique for neonates	Dilute reconstituted solution to a concentration of 20–100 mg/ml; infuse over 15–60 min	Solutions: compatible with commonly used IV fluids[a]; drugs: incompatible with aminoglycosides	Monitor injection site for signs of phlebitis and irritation
Cefotaxime	Administer reconstituted solution (95 mg/ml or less) over 3–5 min; use retrograde technique for neonates	Dilute reconstituted solution to a concentration of 20 mg/ml or less; infuse over 30–60 min	Solutions: compatible with commonly used IV fluids[a]; drugs: no information	Monitor injection site for signs of phlebitis and irritation

Table 1 (Continued)

Drug	Direct IV injection	IV additive	Compatibility	Comments
Cefoxitin	Administer reconstituted solution (180 mg/ml or less) over 3–5 min; use retrograde technique for neonates	Dilute reconstituted solution to a concentration of 20 mg/ml or less; infuse over 30–60 min	Solutions: compatible with commonly used IV fluids[a]; drugs: incompatible with aminoglycosides	Monitor injection site for signs of phlebitis and irritation
Cefsulodin	Administer reconstituted solution (100 mg/ml) over 5 min; use retrograde technique for neonates	Dilute reconstituted solution to a concentration of 20 mg/ml or less; infuse over 20–30 min	Solutions: compatible with NS, D5W; drugs: incompatible with aminoglycosides	Monitor injection site for signs of phlebitis and irritation
Ceftazidime	Administer reconstituted solution (180 mg/ml or less) over 3–5 min; use retrograde technique for neonates	Dilute reconstituted solution to a concentration of 180 mg/ml or less; infuse over 15–30 min	Solutions: compatible with commonly used IV fluids[a]; drugs: incompatible with aminoglycosides	Monitor injection site for signs of phlebitis and irritation
Ceftizoxime	Administer reconstituted solution (95 mg/ml) over 3–5 min; use retrograde technique for neonates	Dilute reconstituted solution to a concentration of 40 mg/ml or less; infuse over 15–30 min	Solutions: compatible with commonly used IV fluids[a]; drugs: incompatible with aminoglycosides	Monitor injection site for signs of phlebitis and irritation
Ceftriaxone	Administer reconstituted solution (100 mg/ml) over 3–5 min; use retrograde technique for neonates	Dilute reconstituted solution to a concentration of 40 mg/ml or less; infuse over 10–30 min	Solutions: compatible with commonly used IV fluids[a]; D5W with KCl 10 mmol/l, D5W and NaCl 0.2% with KCl 20 mmol/l; drugs: incompatible with aminoglycosides	Monitor injection site for signs of phlebitis and irritation
Cefuroxime	Administer reconstituted solution (100 mg/ml or less) over 3–5 min; use retrograde technique for neonates	Dilute reconstituted solution to a concentration of 30 mg/ml or less; infuse over 30 min	Solutions: compatible with commonly used IV fluids[a]; drugs: incompatible with aminoglycosides	Monitor injection site for signs of phlebitis and irritation

Cephalothin	Administer reconstituted solution (100 mg/ml) over 3–5 min; use retrograde technique for neonates	Dilute reconstituted solution to 20 mg/ml or less; infuse over 30–60 min	Solutions: compatible with commonly used IV fluids[a]; incompatible with solutions of pH < 4 or > 8.5; drugs: incompatible with aminoglycosides, erythromycin, penicillin G, sulfisoxazole, tetracycline	Monitor injection site for signs of phlebitis and irritation
Chloramphenicol	Administer reconstituted solution (neonates; 25 mg/ml; others, 100 mg/ml) over 3–5 min; use retrograde technique for neonates	Dilute reconstituted solution to a concentration of 20 mg/ml or less; infuse over 30–60 min	Solutions: compatible with commonly used IV fluids[a]; drugs: incompatible with tetracycline, vancomycin	
Clindamycin	Neonates: dilute solution to 30 mg/ml; administer using retrograde technique; not recommended for infants or children	Dilute solution to 6 mg/ml or less; infuse over 15–30 min at a rate not to exceed 30 mg/min	Solutions: compatible in commonly used IV fluids[a]; drugs: incompatible with ampicillin	
Cloxacillin	Dilute reconstituted solution to 50 mg/ml or less (neonates, 125 mg/ml or less); administer over 2–5 min; use retrograde technique for neonates	Dilute reconstituted solution to a concentration of 100 mg/ml or less; dilute doses of 1 g or more in 100 ml IV fluid if possible; infuse over 30–40 min	Solutions: compatible with commonly used IV fluids[a]; drugs: no information	Monitor injection site for signs of phlebitis and irritation
Cotrimoxazole	Neonates: administer using retrograde technique; not recommended for infants or older children	Dilute 1 ml solution in 25 ml diluent; infuse over 60–90 min; fluid restriction: dilute 1 ml solution in 10–24 ml diluent; extreme fluid restriction: dilute 1 ml solution in 4 ml diluent	Solutions: compatible with D5W, stable for 4 hr; drugs: no information	

Table 1 (Continued)

Drug	Direct IV injection	IV additive	Compatibility	Comments
Doxycycline	Not recommended	Dilute to a concentration of 0.1–1 mg/ml; infuse over 1–4 hr	Solutions: compatible with NS, D5W, Ringer's solution, lactated Ringer's solution; drugs: incompatible with acid-sensitive drugs	
Erythromycin gluceptate	Neonates: administer using retrograde technique; not recommended for infants or older children	Dilute reconstituted solution to a concentration of 1 mg/ml; administer as a continuous infusion *or* dilute reconstituted solution to a concentration of 2–5 mg/ml; infuse over 20–60 min	Solutions: compatible in commonly used IV fluids[a]; NS is preferred diluent; drugs: incompatible with amikacin, tetracycline	Monitor injection site for signs of phlebitis and irritation
Flucytosine	Not recommended	Administer 10 mg/ml solution over 20 min to 6 hr	Solutions: compatible with NS, D5W; drugs: no information	A commercially manufactured injection is unavailable in Canada; injection may be prepared extemporaneously
Metronidazole	Not recommended	Infuse solution (5 mg/ml) at a rate not to exceed 25 mg/min	Solutions: compatible with commonly used IV fluids[a]; drugs: no information	
Mezlocillin	Administer reconstituted solution (100 mg/ml) over 3–5 min; use retrograde technique for neonates	Dilute reconstituted solution to a concentration of 80 mg/ml or less; infuse over 30 min	Solutions: compatible with commonly used IV fluids[a]; drugs: incompatible with aminoglycosides	Monitor injection site for signs of phlebitis and irritation
Miconazole	Not recommended	Dilute 10 mg/ml solution to a concentration of 6 mg/ml or less; infuse over 30–60 min	Solutions: compatible with NS, D5W; drugs: no information	Parenteral miconazole has investigational/emergency release status in Canada
Moxalactam	Administer reconstituted solution (100 mg/ml) over	Dilute reconstituted solution to a concentration of 20 mg/ml or	Solutions: compatible with commonly used IV fluids[a];	Monitor injection site for signs of phlebitis

	3–5 min; use retrograde technique for neonates	less; infuse over 30–60 min	drugs: incompatible with aminoglycosides	and irritation
Nafcillin	Dilute reconstituted solution (250 mg/ml) to 33 mg/ml or less; administer over 5–10 min at a rate not to exceed 200 mg/min; use retrograde technique for neonates	Dilute reconstituted solution to a concentration of 20 mg/ml or less; infuse over 10–20 min at a rate not to exceed 200 mg/min	Solutions: compatible with commonly used IV fluids[a]; drugs: no information	Monitor injection site for signs of phlebitis and irritation; avoid extravasation
Netilmicin	Neonates: administer using retrograde technique; not recommended for infants or older children	Dilute solution to a concentration of 1 mg/ml; doses > 50 mg may be diluted in 50 ml; infuse over 15–60 min	Solutions: compatible with commonly used IV fluids[a]; drugs: incompatible with amphotericin B, cephalosporins, penicillins	
Oxacillin	Administer reconstituted solution (100 mg/ml or less) over 10 min at a rate not to exceed 100 mg/min; use retrograde technique for neonates	Dilute reconstituted solution to a concentration of 100 mg/ml or less; infuse over 10–20 min at a rate not to exceed 100 mg/min	Solutions: compatible with commonly used IV fluids[a]; drugs: incompatible with tetracycline	
Penicillin G potassium	Dilute reconstituted solution to a concentration of 100,000 IU/ml or less; administer over 5 min; use retrograde technique for neonates	Dilute reconstituted solution to a concentration of 10,000–50,000 IU/ml; infuse over 20–60 min	Solutions: compatible with commonly used IV fluids[a]; drugs: incompatible with amphotericin B, tetracycline	Monitor injection site for signs of phlebitis or irritation
Penicillin G sodium	Dilute reconstituted solution to a concentration of 100,000 IU/ml or less; administer over 5 min; use retrograde technique for neonates	Dilute reconstituted solution to a concentration of 10,000–50,000 IU/ml; infuse over 20–60 min	Solutions: compatible with commonly used IV fluids[a]; drugs: incompatible with amphotericin B, cephalothin	Monitor injection site for signs of phlebitis or irritation

Table 1 (Continued)

Drug	Direct IV injection	IV additive	Compatibility	Comments
Pentamidine	Not recommended	Dilute solution in 50–100 ml; infuse over at least 60 min	Solutions: compatible with D5W; drugs: no information	Monitor injection site for signs of phlebitis or irritation; too rapid IV infusion may result in abrupt hypotension
Piperacillin	Administer reconstituted solution (400 mg/ml) over 3–5 min; use retrograde technique for neonates	Dilute reconstituted solution to a concentration of 67 mg/ml or less; infuse over 20–30 min	Solutions: compatible with commonly used IV fluids[a]; drugs: incompatible with aminoglycosides	Monitor injection site for signs of phlebitis or irritation
Rifampin	Not recommended	Dilute to a concentration of 1.2 mg/ml; infuse over 3 hr	Solutions: compatible with NS, D5W, D10W, lactated Ringer's solution, and Ringer's solution; drugs: incompatible with cefamandole, tetracycline, rolitetracycline, doxycycline	Monitor injection site for signs of phlebitis or irritation; parenteral rifampin has investigational/emergency release status in Canada
Tetracycline	Not recommended	Dilute to a concentration of 10 mg/ml or less; infuse over 40 min to 2 hr	Solutions: compatible with commonly used IV fluids[a]; drugs: incompatible with cephalothin, cefazolin, erythromycin, methicillin, oxacillin, penicillin G, and acid-sensitive drugs	Monitor injection site for signs of phlebitis or irritation; avoid extravasation

Tobramycin	Neonates: administer using retrograde technique; not recommended for infants or older children	Dilute solution to a concentration of 1 mg/ml; doses > 50 mg may be diluted in 50 ml; infuse over 15–60 min	Solutions: compatible with commonly used IV fluids[a]; drugs: incompatible with amphotericin B, cephalosporins, penicillins	
Ticarcillin	Dilute reconstituted solution (200 mg/ml) to a concentration of 100 mg/ml; administer over 5 min; use retrograde technique for neonates	Dilute reconstituted solution to a concentration of 50 mg/ml or less; infuse over 30–120 min	Solutions: compatible with commonly used IV fluids[a]; drugs: incompatible with aminoglycosides, vancomycin	Monitor injection site for signs of phlebitis and irritation
Vancomycin	Not recommended	Dilute reconstituted solution (50 mg/ml) to a concentration of 2.5–5 mg/ml; infuse over 1 hr	Solutions: compatible with commonly used IV fluids[a]; drugs: incompatible with chloramphenicol, methicillin, penicillin G, sulfisoxazole, ticarcillin	Monitor injection site for signs of phlebitis and irritation; avoid extravasation; too rapid administration may result in "red man" syndrome
Vidarabine	Not recommended	Dilute suspension (200 mg/ml) to a concentration of 0.33–0.45 mg/ml; infuse over 12–24 hr	Solutions: compatible with commonly used IV fluids[a]; drugs: no information	Monitor injection site for signs of phlebitis and irritation; final filtration with an in-line 0.45-μm filter is recommended

[a]Commonly used IV fluids: D5W, NS, common dextrose-saline solutions (e.g., 2/3–1/3, D5NS), Ringer's solution, lactated Ringer's solution; D5W: dextrose 5 % in water; NS: normal saline.

as an intravenous additive. Drugs that are incompatible with the antibiotic under discussion are also listed. For more complete compatibility information, the reader is advised to consult specific texts (2,3) on this subject or a pharmacist.

REFERENCES

1. Leff, RD, Roberts, RJ: *Practical Aspects of Intravenous Drug Therapy Techniques*, American Society of Hospital Pharmacists, Bethesda, Maryland, 1985.
2. Trissel, LA: *Handbook on Injectable Drugs*, American Society of Hospital Pharmacists, Bethesda, Maryland, 1986.
3. King, JC: *Guide to Parenteral Admixtures*, Cutter Laboratories, St. Louis, 1985.

40

Approaching Adverse Reactions to Antimicrobial Therapy in Children

NEIL H. SHEAR
The Hospital for Sick Children, Toronto, Ontario, Canada

Of all children exposed to antimicrobials, 5-10% will develop a reaction that is believed to be secondary to the drug (1,2). The toxicity section of each chapter illustrates the huge variety of adverse reactions and the associated difficulty in making a definitive diagnosis. Since no physician would want to knowingly re-expose a patient to a potentially harmful medication, adverse reactions tend to be overdiagnosed. This approach (i.e., to call adverse reactions all adverse events that occur during therapy) is both simple and safe. However, there are several caveats.

Many drugs are part of a large, clinically important group of antimicrobials, and a reaction to one drug may exclude the future use of many compounds. For example, does a putative reaction to amoxicillin mean that the patient can never receive any penicillin (or cephalosporin) for therapy? Clearly, the label of "penicillin allergy" may have far-reaching effects, and such a conclusion could make both the physician and patient ill at ease.

If an adverse event develops in a patient during multiple drug exposures, the conclusion that an adverse reaction occurred will have tremendous impact. Antibiotic exposure often occurs in a sequential fashion. A common clinical history is that of a child with otitis media who is put on amoxicillin and develops a "rash" after two doses. The pediatrician changes therapy to sulfamethoxazole-trimethoprim, and the patient develops "hives." Subsequent therapy with erythromycin results in severe gastrointestinal upset, and the parents believe their child is allergic to everything.

Physicians feel more comfortable in diagnosing well-defined dose-dependent toxicity. Predisposing factors often exist that make these reactions predictable (i.e., renal or hepatic insufficiency secondary to disease or immaturity). An elevated serum concentration of the drug is also reassurance of the cause-and-effect relationship in this circumstance. Reactions that appear to be dose-independent or hypersensitivity reactions create the majority of diagnostic problems. These reactions involve only a small percentage of patients exposed to the drug, have the potential to be severe or life-threatening, and appear to have no predictive factors.

Table 1 Hypersensitivity Reactions

Reaction	Clinical features	Known mechanisms	References
Urticaria	Transient, pruritic, erythematous papules and plaques	IgE-mediated	3, 4
Anaphylaxis	Urticaria, hypotension, bronchospasm	IgE-mediated	5
Hypersensitivity syndromes (mononucleosis-like reaction, toxic erythema, etc.)	Sequential occurrence of some or all of the following Fever Skin rash (exanthem-like, erythema multiforme, vasculitis, toxic epidermal necrolysis) Atypical lymphocytosis Toxicity to liver, kidneys, bone marrow, heart, brain, etc. Blood eosinophilia Note: This is a multisystemic disease	Pharmacogenetic defect in the ability to detoxify oxidative metabolites of the parent drug (e.g., sulfonamides); other antimicrobials can cause a similar syndrome and the mechanisms are unknown	6, 7

Table 2 Steps in the Approach to a Suspected Adverse Reaction

1. Clinical diagnosis
2. Analysis of drug exposure
3. Differential diagnosis
4. Literature search
5. Confirmation
6. Advice to the patient
7. Reporting
8. Learning to cope

The Hospital for Sick Children in Toronto has started an adverse reaction clinic to help answer some of the dilemmas posed to physicians and the families under their care. This has been a collaborative effort of the divisions of clinical pharmacology, allergy, and dermatology. Several patterns of hypersensitivity reactions have emerged to help the clinician with the diagnostic process. These are outlined in Table 1. The approach and techniques that have been developed are summarized in Table 2, and each step is illustrated below with examples.

I. APPROACH TO A SUSPECTED ADVERSE REACTION

Step 1. Clinical Diagnosis of an Adverse Event

An accurate diagnosis is critical. Help from laboratory tests and consultations is often important and necessary. The definition of some reactions may be relatively straightforward (e.g., leukopenia). In contrast, the diagnosis of erythema multiforme can be difficult and the combined efforts of clinical and laboratory specialists are needed (8). Urticaria is not difficult to diagnose, but the diagnosis may be based purely on a description of the reaction by the patient. A misdiagnosis at this early stage can have far-reaching effects. It has been shown that 24% of skin eruptions designated as adverse reactions by generalists (general practitioners, pediatricians, and internists) were subsequently diagnosed as other non-drug-related conditions (e.g., scabies or psoriasis) by a dermatologist (9).

Examples of adverse events	Basis of diagnosis
Leukopenia	Blood count
Erythema multiforme	1. Clinical diagnosis–generalist
	2. Clinical diagnosis–dermatologist
	3. Pathological diagnosis–generalist
	4. Pathological diagnosis–specialist
Urticaria	1. Clinical description–witness
	2. Clinical diagnosis–physician
	3. Pathological diagnosis–pathologist

The following data (which are extraneous to the diagnosis) must be compiled to enable recognition of adverse reaction syndromes (see Table 1).

Other necessary information	Examples
Timing of reaction	Exact dates relative to drug exposure
Other clinical features	Fever
Other target organ damage	Bone marrow, blood cells, skin, liver, kidney, etc.

Step 2. Analysis of Drug Exposure

The drugs suspected of causing the reaction should be known in detail. A complete history of drug exposure is needed, as well as any past history of drug exposure. It is extremely helpful to know which drugs the patient has or has not tolerated in the past.

Complete list of all drug exposure, including	Example
Trade name	Amoxil
Formulation	Suspension
Concentration	50 mg/ml
Dosage	40 mg/kg day^{-1}
Known excipients (10)	Color, flavor, preservatives, suspending agent
Timing of dosing	Every 8 hr; reaction occurred 2 hr after dose 5
Serum concentrations	Not available

Consider drugs that may provide alternative choices for therapy. This is a good point to begin to consider alternative therapies (as described in Chapter 38). Many of the following steps can be used to find appropriate alternatives for the specific circumstances of the adverse reaction.

Step 3. Differential Diagnosis

There are several aspects to consider in differential diagnosis. First, as in Step 1, all possible clinical diagnoses should be considered (e.g., are the red plaques on the skin erythema multiforme or urticaria?). The other aspects to investigate are the cause of the clinical problem, nondrug etiologies, and predisposing factors.

Examples of adverse events	Alternative etiology	Confirm diagnosis by
Leukopenia	Viral infection	Serology
Erythema multiforme	Herpes simplex	Serology
Urticaria	Wheat	History, skin test

How well documented is the association between the adverse event and the drug?

Examples of adverse events	Drug	Association
Leukopenia	Ampicillin	Known (but may be transient) (11)
Erythema multiforme	Ampicillin	Well known
Urticaria	Ampicillin	Well known

Consider predisposing factors.

Example of adverse event	Drug	Predisposition	Importance
Exanthematous rash	Ampicillin	Concurrent Epstein-Barr (EB) virus infection	Ampicillin (and other penicillins) should be safe to use in the future when the patient is not infected with EB virus

Step 4. Literature Search

For expected associations do a literature search. The extent of the search will depend on the degree to which the association is known.

Stage of search	References	Possible sources
Start	Office textbooks	*AMA Drug Evaluations* (12)
	Product monograph	Pharmaceutical company
	Standard (library) textbooks	*Meyler's Side Effects of Drugs* (13)
		Textbook of Adverse Drug Reactions (14)
	Journals and periodicals	Specialty journal: Reactions (15)
		Information letters: *FDA Drug Bulletin* (16)
		Review articles: Adverse reactions to anti-infective agents (17)
	Consultations	Specialist (in disease of the target organ)
		Clinical pharmacologist
		Hospital pharmacist
More help	Self-directed search (18)	*Index Medicus*
		Computer services (19)
	Assisted search	
	Hospital librarian	
	Drug information officer	Hospital pharmacy
	Regulatory agency	FDA
	Pharmaceutical company	Manufacturer of the drug

If no association is found or the documentation is poor,

1. Reconsider the clinical diagnosis.
2. Review the history.
3. Consider additives (fillers, excipients, and solvents) (10).
4. Continue with the following steps (the reaction may be new and unreported).

Step 5. Confirmation

If a drug reaction is suspected it is critical that the physician try to prove causality (20). Even though the association may be strong in the literature (i.e., the definitive studies have been done), this does not mean that the patient has had a true adverse reaction. The three most commonly used methods involve algorithms and in vivo and in vitro testing. These methods have changed over the years (21), and the most current methods (which we use in our clinic) are described below. The utility of these methods will depend on how well they stand up under scrutiny and general availability.

Method used	Examples	Advantages	Limitations
Algorithm	Flowsheets that assign a numerical score for the likelihood of a reaction having been drug related (22–24)	Quantitative, no risk to the patient, can be standardized	Ultimate result qualitative; variability among users high (25)
In vivo testing	Rechallenge (26)	Can demonstrate that drug use will be safe; patient acts as own model; cheaper than in vitro investigations	Potentially very dangerous for patients who have had hypersensitivity reactions
	Penicillin skin testing (27,28)	Simple, safe; negative test result allows safe oral challenge; positive result may help confirm weak clinical history	Best done by experienced team; reagents may be difficult to obtain and can be unreliable if rarely used; test results cannot be easily extrapolated to all penicillins
In vitro testing	Lymphocyte toxicity assay for sulfonamide hypersensitivity reactions (6)	Allows confirmation of sensitivity; may be of use to identify family members at risk of reaction	Not widely available; expensive; is still a research tool

Step 6. Advice to the Patient

Even if it has been possible to confirm the diagnosis of an adverse reaction and to identify the drug that caused the reaction, many questions remain.

Issue	Patient's question	Answer
The drug in question	How certain are you that the drug caused the reaction?	The answer is based on the preceeding steps, particularly confirmatory testing.
	Could it happen again?	The answer depends on whether there is a predisposition (permanent or temporary).
	What if I need the drug in the future?	Desensitization has been successful with some antimicrobials (29,30).
Other drugs	What alternative drugs are available?	Alternative therapy can be decided upon.
	Will other drugs cross-react?	This information may be available from the literature search or the confirmation testing. The answer is dependent on understanding the mechanism of the reaction and experience published about related antimicrobials.
Relatives of the patient	Will my siblings or children be at increased risk with respect to the general population?	The predisposition to hypersensitivity reactions may be inherited, and close relatives may be at an increased risk; for example, idiosyncratic reactions to sulfonamides (6).
Notification	How can I ensure that I will not be needlessly exposed to the drug again?	Register with Medic Alert. Notify all physicians involved in patient's care.

Step 7. Reporting the Reaction

It is the duty of the physician to report adverse drug reactions. Spontaneous reporting is an important method of identifying adverse reactions to drugs that have been recently released for widespread use (31,32). Many new local and national organizations now take part in the collation and analysis of adverse reaction data.

Report the reaction to	This involves
Manufacturer of the drug	Telephone call
Hospital pharmacy	Telephone call
ADRRS (adverse drug reaction reporting system of the American Academy of Dermatology)	Telephone call (33)
State medical association	Filling out a form
FDA adverse reaction report	Filling out a form (16)
Medical journal	Writing a letter (34,35)

Step 8. Aftermath, or Learning to Cope

Adverse events are common. Reidenberg and Lowenthal (36) asked healthy people taking no medication if they had experienced the usually reported minor side effects of drugs (including headache, skin rash, nausea, diarrhea) during the previous 3 days. These "adverse non-drug reactions" were present in 81% of these people. True adverse reactions are also common. Up to 10% of people exposed to a drug will have what is believed to be an adverse reaction. Severe reactions are rare. The usually quoted rate of hypersensitivity reactions to sulfonamides is 1 per 10,000 exposures. These rare events, however, have a tremendous impact on the way we react to adverse events and make the prescribing physician wary.

Examples of adverse reactions	Concern that the reaction may evolve into
Leukopenia	Aplastic anemia
Erythema multiforme	Toxic epidermal necrolysis
Urticaria	Anaphylaxis

Every time an antibiotic is prescribed, the physician is faced with the balance of necessity versus safety. Generally, antibiotics have an impressive safety profile and can cure life-threatening diseases. It is a difficult task for the prescriber to be aware of all adverse reactions and to be able to convey available information in a meaningful manner to the patient. Many attempts at monitoring drug therapy (serum concentrations, repeat blood counts, and liver enzymes) are not helpful in allaying concerns.

Once an adverse reaction has occurred, it is often difficult for the prescribing physician to deal with the guilt of having made the choice of treatment. Patients can appear distrustful when clear-cut answers are not forthcoming. This can result in a breakdown of the doctor-patient relationship.

It is important for physicians to understand the possible consequences of adverse reactions on medical practice. Open discussion of these issues, it is hoped, will help both doctor and patient feel less isolated. It may be productive to consider reactions as a "disease" so that proper diagnosis and treatment may ensue.

II. CASE HISTORY

This stepwise analysis is concluded with a recent referral to our adverse reaction clinic, highlighting some of the points made in this chapter.

A 16-month-old boy was admitted to the hospital with pneumonia and otitis media. He was initially treated with Zinacef (cefuroxime) but developed a skin rash and therapy was changed to intravenous cloxacillin. Oral therapy began after 2 days, and 2 days later he developed generalized urticaria (2 hr after a dose of cloxacillin). The reaction responded to antihistamine treatment, and he was discharged from the hospital on Pediazole (erythromycin-sulfisoxazole). The patient had no known atopy, but there was a family history of atopic dermatitis and allergic rhinitis. The patient had not been exposed to penicillins prior to this admission.

We were asked to assess him for penicillin sensitivity.

A. Diagnosis

As I stated at the outset, the easiest approach is to say that this patient is allergic to penicillin (and likely cephalosporins) and should avoid these antibiotics.

If we take the stepwise approach, however, we find

1. Clinical diagnosis: generalized urticaria (by history).
2. Assessment of drug exposure related to the diagnosis: (1) cloxacillin and (2) cefuroxime (much less likely because of timing).
3. Differential diagnosis: For this we have to take a probing history. An astute physician in our division found that the patient had eaten a peanut-containing chocolate bar immediately prior to developing urticaria.
4. Literature search: Peanuts, chocolate, and cloxacillin are well-established causes of urticaria.
5. Confirmation: Skin testing for peanut was strongly positive but was negative to penicillin and its components. A RAST (radioallergosorbent test for allergen-specific IgE antibodies) for peanut was also positive.
6. Advice to the patient: The parents were told that penicillins should be safe to use in the future and that peanuts (and related allergens) must be avoided.

B. Summary

The role of peanuts in the reaction was a surprise. This type of information can easily be overlooked if adverse reactions are not approached in an organized fashion. The ultimate goal is to give accurate, meaningful information to the patient. I believe that this approach will help improve our ability to deal with adverse reactions and to use antimicrobials more wisely.

ACKNOWLEDGMENTS

I would like to thank the members of the Adverse Reaction Clinics in Toronto (Drs. Stephen Spielberg, Barry Zimmerman, Elizabeth Weber, Sasi Lavi, Jack Uetrecht, and Allan Knight) and Dr. Michael Rieder, an astute physician.

This work was supported in part by a Career Scientist Award of the Ontario Ministry of Health, the Medical Research Council of Canada (grant MA-9716), and a grant-in-aid from the Canadian Dermatology Foundation.

REFERENCES

1. Goldstein, RA, Patterson, MD: Drug allergy: Prevention, diagnosis, and treatment. *Ann. Intern. Med. 100*:302–303, 1984.
2. Kramer, MS, Hutchinson, TA, Flegel, KM, Naimark, L, Contardi, R, Leduc, DG: Adverse drug reaction in general pediatric out patients. *J. Pediatr. 106*:305–310, 1985.
3. Keahey, TM: The pathogenesis of urticaria. *Dermatol. Clin. 3*:13–28, 1985.
4. Synkowski, D, Dore, N, Provost, TT: Urticaria and urticaria-like lesions. *Clin. Rheum. Dis. 8*:383–395, 1982.
5. Boston Collaborative Drug Surveillance Program: Drug-induced anaphylaxis. *JAMA 224*:613–615, 1973.
6. Shear, NH, Spielberg, SP, Grant, DM, Tang, BK, Kalow, W: Differences in metabolism of sulfonamides predisposing to idiosynciatic toxicity. *Ann. Intern. Med. 105*: 179–184, 1986.
7. Deswarte, RD: Drug allergy—problems and strategies. *J. Allergy. Clin. Immunol. 74*:209–221, 1984.
8. Howland, WW, Golitz, LE, Weston, WL, Huff, JC: Erythema multiforme: Clinical, histopathologic, and immunologic study. *J. Am. Acad. Dermatol. 10*:438–446, 1984.
9. Lloyd, M: A drug reaction survey. *Trans. St. John's Hosp. Dermatol. Soc. 55*:64–68, 1986.
10. Simon, RA: Adverse reactions to drug additives. *J. Allergy Clin. Immunol. 74*: 623–630, 1984.
11. Feldman, S, Doolittle, M, Lott, L, Roberson, P, Hughes, WT: Similar hematologic changes in children receiving trimethoprim-sulfamethoxasole or amoxicillin for otitis media. *J. Pediatr. 106*:995–1000, 1985.
12. AMA Department of Drugs, *AMA Drug Evaluation*, John Wiley & Sons, New York, 5th ed., 1983.
13. Dukes, MNG, ed.: *Meyler's Side Effects of Drugs*, Excerpta Medica, Amsterdam, 10th ed., 1984.
14. Davies, DM, ed.: *Textbook of Adverse Drug Reactions*, Oxford University Press, New York, 2nd ed., 1981.
15. Heel, RC, ed.: *Reactions*, ADIS Press, Aukland, New Zealand.
16. FDA Drug Bulletin, Circulation Dept., HFI-43, 5600 Fishers Lane, Rockville, MD 20857.
17. Rahal, JJ, Simberkoff, MS: Adverse reactions to anti-infective agents. *Disease-a-month 25*:1–67, 1978.
18. Haynes, RB, McKibbon, KA, Fitzgerald, D, Guyatt, GH, Walker, CJ, Sackett, DL: How to keep up with the medical literature. IV. Using the literature to solve clinical problems. *Ann. Intern. Med. 105*:636–640, 1986.
19. Haynes, RB, McKibbon, A, Walker, CJ, et al.: Computer searching of the medical literature: An evaluation of MEDLINE searching systems. *Ann. Intern. Med. 103*: 812–816, 1985.
20. Deciding whether your treatment has done harm. In: *Clinical Epidemiology* (DL Sackett, RB Haynes, and PR Tugwell, eds.), Little, Brown, Boston, 1985, pp. 223–241.
21. Assem, ESK: Tests for detecting drug allergy. In: *Textbook of Adverse Drug Reactions* (DM Davies, ed.), Oxford University Press, New York, 1981, pp. 554–568.
22. Naranjo, CA, Busto, U, Sellers, EM, et al.: A method for estimating the probability of adverse drug reactions. *Clin. Pharmacol. Ther. 30*:239–245, 1981.
23. Lane, D, Naranjo, CA, Jones, J, Hutchinson, T: A Bayesian method for improving the assessment of drug safety. *Clin. Pharmacol. Ther. 39*:205, 1986.

24. Kramer, MS, Leventhal, JM, Hutchinson, TA, Feinstein, AR: An algorithm for the operational assessment of adverse drug reactions. I. Background, description, and instructions for use. *JAMA 242*:623–638, 1979.
25. Louik, C, Lacouture, PG, Mitchell, AA, et al.: A study of adverse reaction algorithms in a drug surveillance program. *Clin. Pharmacol. Ther. 38*:183–187, 1985.
26. Kauppinen, K: Rational performance of drug challenge in cutaneous hypersensitivity. *Semin. Dermatol. 2*:227–230, 1983.
27. Sussman, GL, Davis, K, Kohler, PF: Penicillin allergy: A practical approach to management. *Can. Med. Assoc. J. 134*:1353–1356, 1986.
28. Mendelson, LM, Ressler, C, Rosen, JP, Selcow, JE: Routine elective penicillin allergy skin testing in children and adolescents: Study of sensitization. *J. Allergy Clin. Immunol. 73*:76–81, 1984.
29. Sullivan, TJ, Yecies, LD, Shatz, GS, Parker, CW, Wedner, HJ: Desensitization of patients allergic to penicillin using orally administered β-lactam antibiotics. *J. Allergy Clin. Immunol. 69*:275–282, 1982.
30. Purdy, BH, Philips, DM, Summer, S: Desensitization of sulfasalazine skin rash. *Ann. Intern. Med. 100*:512–514, 1984.
31. Faich, GA: Adverse-drug-reaction monitoring. *N. Engl. J. Med. 314*:1589–1592, 1986.
32. Lortie, FM: Postmarketing surveillances of adverse drug reactions: Problems and solutions. *Can. Med. Assoc. J. 136*:27–32, 1986.
33. ADRRS (adverse drug reaction reporting system) telephone (toll free) number: (800) 323–1473.
34. Jones, JJ: Criteria for journal reports of suspected adverse drug reactions. *Clin. Pharm. 1*:554–555, 1982.
35. Berneker, GC, Ciucci, AG, Joyce, J: Standards for reporting adverse drug reactions. *Br. Med. J. 287*:1720, 1983.
36. Reidenberg, MM, Lowenthal, DD: Adverse nondrug reactions. *N. Engl. J. Med. 279*: 678–679, 1968.

Index

Q

V

W

Z

About the Editors

GIDEON KOREN is a staff member of the Divisions of Clinical Pharmacology and Hematology-Oncology in the Department of Pediatrics at The Hospital for Sick Children's Research Institute in Toronto, Canada. He also serves as a Career Scientist for the Ontario Ministry of Health, Assistant Professor of Pediatrics and Pharmacology at the University of Toronto, and Director of the Motherisk Program of Antenatal Counseling for Drug/Chemical Exposure. His chief areas of research include pediatric pharmacology, renal handling of drugs, and perinatal toxicology. The author or coauthor of over 220 articles, book chapters, abstracts, and other publications, Dr. Koren has made numerous presentations at professional society meetings in the United States, Canada, and Israel. He is an editorial board member of the *Journal of Toxicology--Clinical Toxicology* (Marcel Dekker, Inc.) and a member of the Israeli Society of Clinical Pediatrics, Canadian Society of Clinical Pharmacology, American Board of Medical Toxicology, and American Society of Clinical Pharmacology and Therapeutics. Dr. Koren received the M.D. degree (1974) from the Sackler School of Medicine, Tel-Aviv University, Israel.

CHARLES G. PROBER is Associate Professor of Pediatrics at Stanford University School of Medicine in Stanford, California, where he is also Co-Director of the Pediatric Infectious Disease Division. Previously he was Associate Professor of Pediatrics, Microbiology, and Pharmacology at the University of Toronto and served in the Infectious Disease Division at The Hospital for Sick Children in Toronto, Canada. Dr. Prober has published over 50 articles in the field of pediatric infectious diseases. He is a member of the Infectious Disease Society of America, Canadian Infectious Disease Society, Society for Pediatric Research, and Canadian Society for Clinical Investigation. Dr. Prober received the M.D. degree (1973) from the University of Manitoba in Winnipeg, Manitoba, Canada.

RONALD GOLD is Chief of the Division of Infectious Diseases and Senior Staff Physician at The Hospital for Sick Children in Toronto, Canada. He is also Professor of Pediatrics and Microbiology in the Faculty of Medicine at the University of Toronto. The author or coauthor of more than 80 articles, book chapters, abstracts, and other publications, Dr. Gold is the coeditor of the *Third Edition* of the text *Epidemiology and Public Health.* He is a Fellow of the Royal College of Physicians and Surgeons (Canada), American Academy of Pediatrics, and Infectious Diseases Society of America, and a member of the Canadian Infectious Disease Society, and American Association for the Advancement of Science. Dr. Gold received the M.D. degree (1962) from Harvard Medical School and M.P.H. degree (1967) from the Harvard School of Public Health in Boston, Massachusetts.